STOLLER'S

ATLAS OF

Orthopaedics and Sports Medicine

David W. Stoller, MD, FACR

Director, MRI and Musculoskeletal Imaging
California Pacific Medical Center
San Francisco, California

Director, National Orthopaedic Imaging Associates
San Francisco, California

Illustrated by **Salvador Beltran**

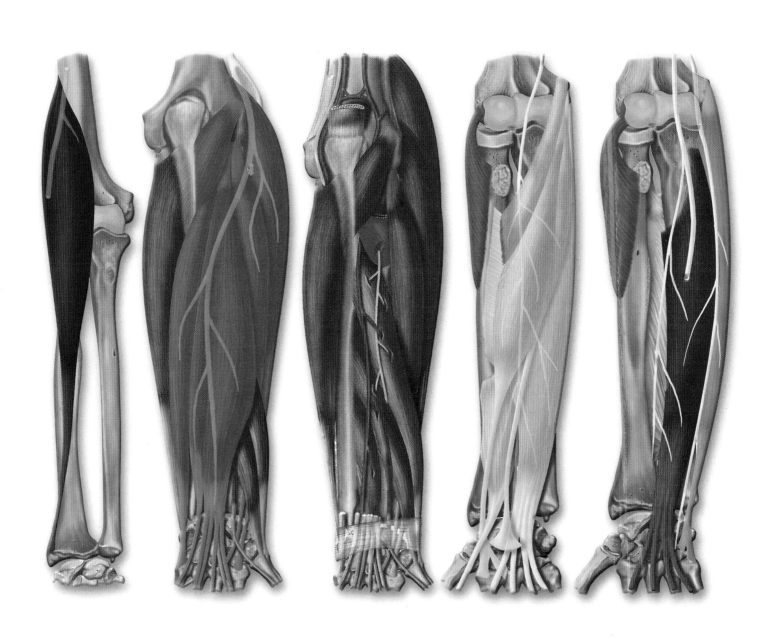

STOLLER'S
ATLAS OF
Orthopaedics and Sports Medicine

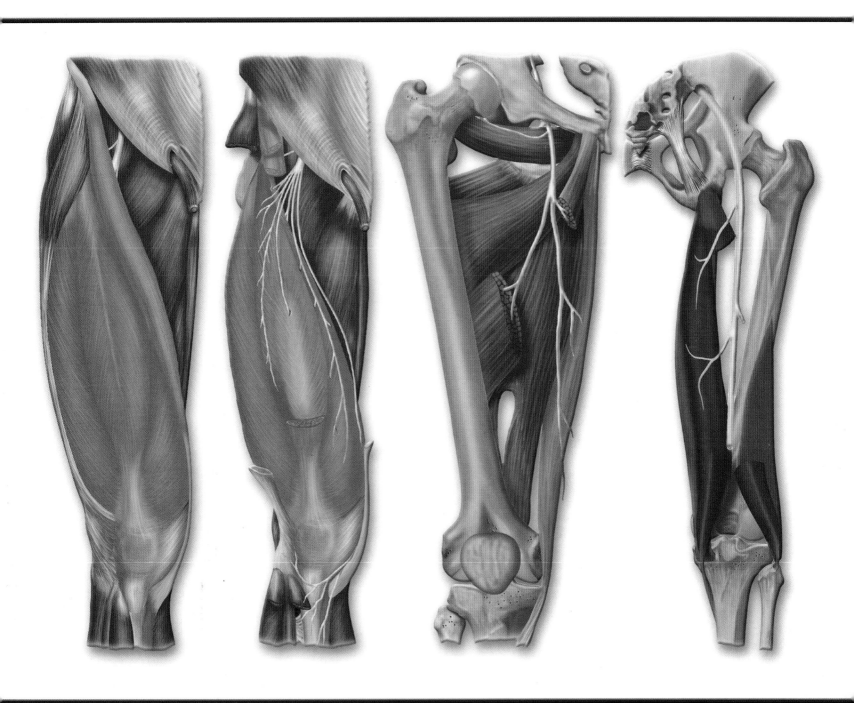

Wolters Kluwer | Lippincott Williams & Wilkins
Health

Philadelphia · Baltimore · New York · London
Buenos Aires · Hong Kong · Sydney · Tokyo

Acquisitions Editor: Lisa McAllister
Managing Editor: Kerry Barrett
Marketing Manager: Angela Panetta
Production Editor: Bridget H. Meyer
Senior Production Manager: Caren Erlichman
Creative Director: Doug Smock
Designer: Wanda Espana
Compositor: Maryland Composition

351 West Camden Street   530 Walnut Street
Baltimore, MD 21201   Philadelphia, PA 19106

Printed in China

9 8 7 6 5 4 3 2 1

Library of Congress Cataloging-in-Publication Data

Stoller's atlas of orthopaedics and sports medicine / [edited by] David W. Stoller.
    p. ; cm.
  Includes bibliographical references and index.
  ISBN-13: 978-0-7817-8389-7 (alk. paper)
  ISBN-10: 0-7817-8389-5 (alk. paper)
1. Musculoskeletal system—Magnetic resonance imaging—Atlases.   2. Orthopedics—Atlases.   3. Sports medicine—Atlases.
I. Stoller, David W.   II. Title: Atlas of orthopaedics and sports medicine.
  [DNLM: 1. Musculoskeletal System—anatomy & histology—Atlases. 2. Magnetic Resonance Imaging—Atlases.
  3. Musculoskeletal Diseases—pathology—Atlases. 4. Musculoskeletal System—pathology—Atlases. WE 17 S8749 2008]

QM100.S76 2008

616.7'07458—dc22

DISCLAIMER
Care has been taken to confirm the accuracy of the information present and to describe generally accepted practices. However, the authors, editors, and publisher are not responsible for errors or omissions or for any consequences from application of the information in this book and make no warranty, expressed or implied, with respect to the currency, completeness, or accuracy of the contents of the publication. Application of this information in a particular situation remains the professional responsibility of the practitioner; the clinical treatments described and recommended may not be considered absolute and universal recommendations.

The authors, editors, and publisher have exerted every effort to ensure that drug selection and dosage set forth in this text are in accordance with the current recommendations and practice at the time of publication. However, in view of ongoing research, changes in government regulations, and the constant flow of information relating to drug therapy and drug reactions, the reader is urged to check the package insert for each drug for any change in indications and dosage and for added warnings and precautions. This is particularly important when the recommended agent is a new or infrequently employed drug.

Some drugs and medical devices presented in this publication have Food and Drug Administration (FDA) clearance for limited use in restricted research settings. It is the responsibility of the health care provider to ascertain the FDA status of each drug or device planned for use in their clinical practice.

To purchase additional copies of this book, call our customer service department at **(800) 638-3030** or fax orders to **(301) 223-2320**. International customers should call **(301) 223-2300**.

Visit Lippincott Williams & Wilkins on the Internet: *http://www.lww.com*. Lippincott Williams & Wilkins customer service representatives are available from 8:30 am to 6:00 pm, EST.

Dedication

To my cherished son Griffin, and my lovely wife Marcia, for their extraordinary love, support, and understanding, and for accommodating the sacrifices of personal time.

To my parents Adele and the late Nat Stoller, for their inspiration, love, and encouragement.

Contributors

Jenny T. Bencardino, M.D.
Musculoskeletal Radiologist
Melville, New York

Simon Blease, M.D.
Honorary Senior Clinical Lecturer
University of Bristol
United Kingdom

Miriam A. Bredella, M.D.
Assistant Professor in Radiology
Harvard Medical School
Massachusetts General Hospital
Boston, Massachusetts

Jean-Luc Drapé, M.D.
Department of Radiology B
Hospital Cochin
University Paris-France
Paris, France

Richard D. Ferkel, M.D.
Assistant Clinical Professor of Orthopaedic Surgery
University of California
Los Angeles, California
Director of Sports Medicine Fellowship and Attending Surgeon
Southern California Orthopaedic Institute
Van Nuys, California

Arthur E. Li, M.D.
California Advanced Imaging Associates
San Mateo, California

David M. Lichtman, M.D.
Chairman, Department of Orthopaedic Surgery
University of North Texas College of Medicine
Adjunct Professor of Orthopaedics
Baylor College of Medicine and Uniformed Services
University of Health Sciences
Houston, Texas
Clinical Professor of Orthopaedic Surgery
U.T. Southwestern Medical Center
Dallas, Texas

Hollis G. Potter, M.D.
Professor of Radiology
Weill Medical College of Cornell University
New York, New York
Chief, Magnetic Resonance Imaging
Hospital for Special Surgery
New York, New York

Zehava S. Rosenberg, M.D.
Professor of Radiology
New York School of Medicine
Hospital for Joint Diseases
New York, New York

Marc R. Safran, M.D.
Professor of Orthopaedic Surgery
Stanford University
Palo Alto, California

Thomas G. Sampson, M.D.
Associate Professor of Orthopaedic Surgery
University of California
San Francisco, California
Director, Hip Arthroscopy
Post Street Surgery Center
Medical Director, Total Joint Center
Saint Francis Memorial Hospital
San Francisco, California

David W. Stoller, M.D., FACR
Director, MRI and Musculoskeletal Imaging
California Pacific Medical Center
San Francisco, California
Director, National Orthopaedic Imaging Associates
San Francisco, California

Eugene M. Wolf, M.D.
Department of Orthopaedic Surgery
St. Mary's Medical Center
San Francisco, California

Preface

Stoller's Atlas of Orthopaedics and Sports Medicine represents a unique and comprehensive undertaking for both myself and Lippincott Williams & Wilkins. *Stoller's Atlas* was conceived and produced to allow access to the entire Stoller-Beltran collection of color illustrations in a dedicated single volume format using an oversized 9½″ x 12″ book.

I have collaborated with Salvador Beltran to enhance our orthopaedic anatomy and pathology collection by approximately 250 new color plates. Novel 3D color illustrations of muscle innervations accompany each of the joint chapters to improve the interpretation of muscle trauma and denervation patterns.

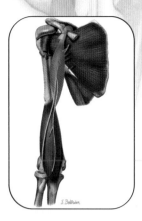

High resolution MR images are displayed two per page and 5 inches in height. Normal muscle color plates are displayed one per page and up to 10 inches in height for easy reference. *Pearls and Pitfalls* are grouped together for an improved overview in one location using color thumbnail icons. MR anatomy pathology and plates are displayed from 5 inches to 10 inches in height to reinforce concepts and further advance our understanding of the spectrum of orthopaedic pathology. Cross reference features are included within the *Pearls and Pitfalls* section as well as between all color illustrations and the corresponding pages of the 3rd Edition of *Magnetic Resonance Imaging in Orthopaedics and Sports Medicine*.

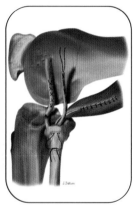

Salvador Beltran and I have attempted to incorporate developments afforded by the advent of arthroscopic experience in orthopaedics and sports medicine. I am hopeful that our efforts to produce an oversized single volume atlas will make the navigation of orthopaedic and sports medicine less intimidating.

David W. Stoller, M.D., FACR
Director, MRI and Musculoskeletal Imaging
California Pacific Medical Center
San Francisco, California
Director, National Orthopaedic Imaging Associates
San Francisco, California

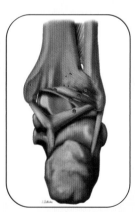

Acknowledgments

Undertaking the writing of this atlas has provided a unique opportunity to contribute to the emerging field or orthopaedic magnetic resonance imaging. Orthopaedic MRI has earned respect and a distinct subspecialty and has become a primary modality in the diagnosis of internal derangement of the joints.

I would like to acknowledge the contribution of the following individuals:

Arthur E. Li, M.D. for his assistance in the normal MR section.

I would like to acknowledge the contributors of the 3rd Edition of *Magnetic Resonance Imaging in Orthopaedics and Sports Medicine* whose efforts assisted in the preparation of the *Pearls and Pitfalls* section. These authors include Jenny T. Bencardino, M.D., Simon Blease, M.D., Miriam A. Bredella, M.D., Jean-Luc Drapé, M.D., Hollis G. Potter, M.D., and Zehava S. Rosenberg, M.D.

The orthopaedic surgeons who contributed their arthroscopic expertise in the 3rd edition of *Magnetic Resonance Imaging Orthopaedics and Sports Medicine*. These contributors include: Lesley J. Anderson, M.D., Gordon A. Brody, M.D., W. Dilworth Cannon, M.D., Richard D. Ferkel, M.D., James O. Johnston, M.D., David M. Lichtman, M.D., Roger A. Mann, M.D., Wesley M. Nottage, M.D., Marc R. Safran, M.D., Thomas G. Sampson, M.D., and Eugene M. Wolf, M.D.

John C. Loh, M.D., and Neil Kennedy, M.D. for medical text editing. National orthopaedic imaging associates 2007—2008 fellows John C. Loh, M.D., Neil Kennedy, M.D., Meghan Blake, M.D., Jean-Pierre Phancao, M.D., and Rajiv Chopra, M.D., for manuscript review.

Kim Dick, RT, for organizing thousands of images. Her accomplishments deserve special mention.

The expert staff at Lippincott Williams & Wilkins, for their efforts and appreciation of the necessary quality required to bring this text to fruition, including Lisa McAllister, Executive Editor, Caren Erlichman, Senior Production Manager, Kerry Barrett, Senior Managing Editor, Doug Smock, Creative Director, and Bridget Meyer, Production Editor.

A number of books and articles were particularly helpful as references for both the manuscript and illustrations. I offer the following list both in acknowledgment for their usefulness and as a recommended reading/reference resource list.

Byrd JWT. Operative hip arthroscopy, 2nd ed. New York: Springer, 2005.

Canale ST. Campbell's Operative Orthopaedics, 10th ed. St. Louis: Mosby, 2002.

Craig EJ. Master techniques in orthopaedic surgery: the shoulder, 2nd ed. Philadelphia: Lippincott Williams & Wilkins, 2004.

DeLee JC, Drez D Jr, Miller MD. Delee & Drez's orthopaedic sports medicine: principles and practice, 2nd ed. Philadelphia: W.B. Saunders, 2002.

De Palma AF. Surgery of the shoulder. Philadelphia: Lippincott Williams & Wilkins, 1983.

Lichtman DM, Alexander AH. The wrist and its disorders, 2nd ed. Philadelphia: WB Saunders, 1997.

Miller MD, Howard RF, Plancher KD. Surgical atlas of sports medicine. Philadelphia: W.B. Saunders, 2003.

Netter FH. Atlas of human anatomy, 4th ed. Philadelphia: W.B. Saunders, 2006.

Rockwood CA Jr, Matson FA III, Wirth MA, et al. The shoulder, 3rd ed. Philadelphia: W.B. Saunders, 2004.

Rosenberg Z. MR imaging of the hip. Magnetic resonance imaging clinics of North America. Philadelphia: W.B. Saunders, 2005.

Schmidt H-M, Lanz U. Surgical anatomy of the hand. New York: Thieme Medical Publishers, 2004.

Schünke M, Schulte E, Schumacher U. Thieme Atlas of Anatomy. New York: Thieme Medical Publishers, 2005.

Snyder SJ. Shoulder arthroscopy. Philadelphia: Lippincott Williams & Wilkins, 2003.

Spinner R. Peroneal intraneural ganglia; the importance of the articular branch. J Neurosurg 2003; 99: 319-329.

Standring S. Gray's anatomy, the anatomical basis of clinical practice, 39th ed. Philadelphia: Elsevier Churchill Livingstone, 2005.

Table of Contents

Chapter

1

MR Normal Anatomy: *Lower Extremity*

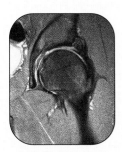

The Hip

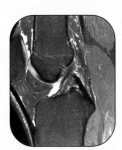

The Knee

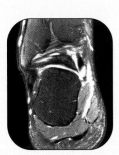

The Ankle and Foot

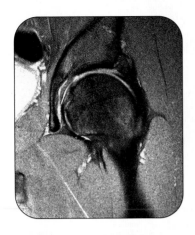

The Hip
MR Normal Anatomy

Coronal

Figures 1.1A to 1.1N
Pages 4–10

Axial

Figures 1.2A to 1.2L
Pages 11–16

Sagittal

Figures 1.3A to 1.3L
Pages 17–22

Hip - Coronal

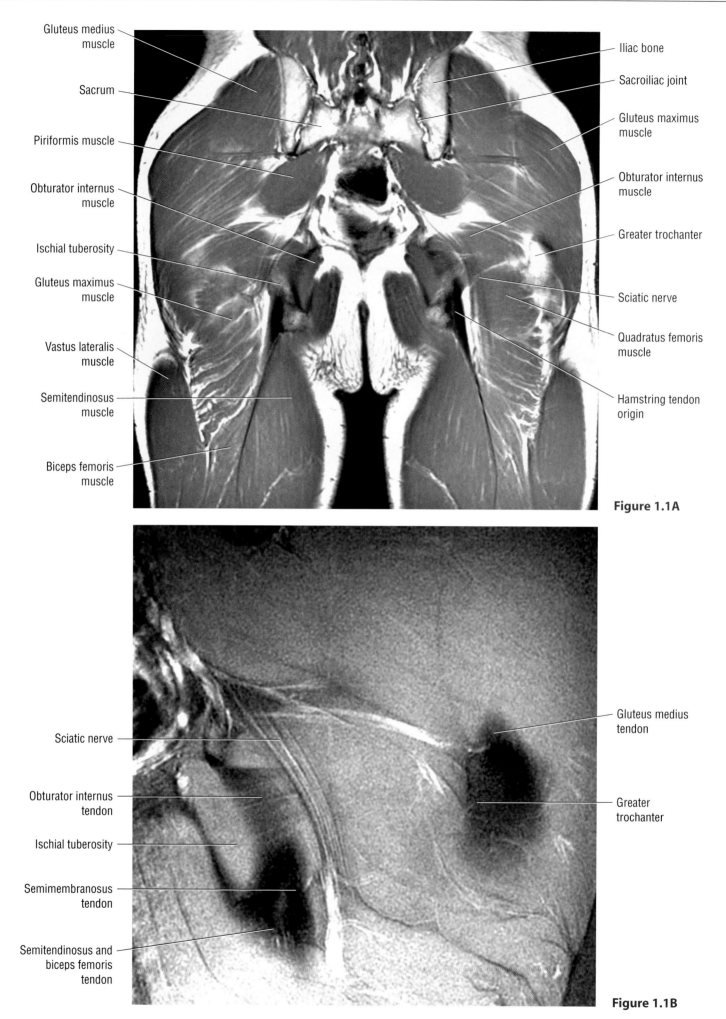

Gluteus medius muscle

Sacrum

Piriformis muscle

Obturator internus muscle

Ischial tuberosity

Gluteus maximus muscle

Vastus lateralis muscle

Semitendinosus muscle

Biceps femoris muscle

Iliac bone

Sacroiliac joint

Gluteus maximus muscle

Obturator internus muscle

Greater trochanter

Sciatic nerve

Quadratus femoris muscle

Hamstring tendon origin

Figure 1.1A

Sciatic nerve

Obturator internus tendon

Ischial tuberosity

Semimembranosus tendon

Semitendinosus and biceps femoris tendon

Gluteus medius tendon

Greater trochanter

Figure 1.1B

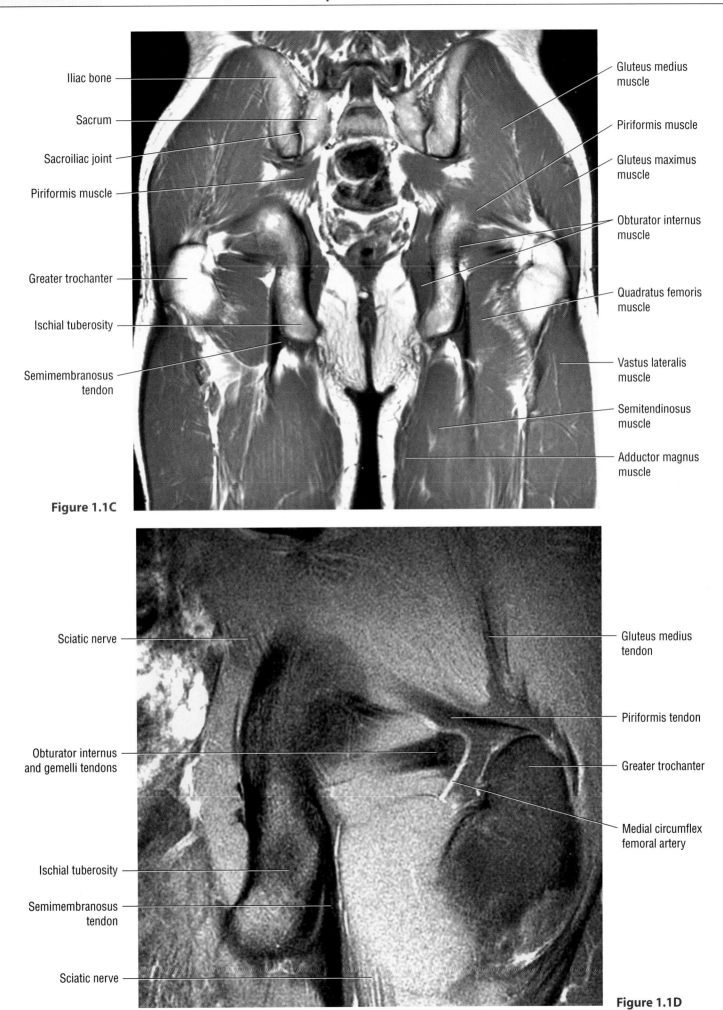

Iliac bone

Sacrum

Sacroiliac joint

Piriformis muscle

Greater trochanter

Ischial tuberosity

Semimembranosus tendon

Gluteus medius muscle

Piriformis muscle

Gluteus maximus muscle

Obturator internus muscle

Quadratus femoris muscle

Vastus lateralis muscle

Semitendinosus muscle

Adductor magnus muscle

Figure 1.1C

Sciatic nerve

Obturator internus and gemelli tendons

Ischial tuberosity

Semimembranosus tendon

Sciatic nerve

Gluteus medius tendon

Piriformis tendon

Greater trochanter

Medial circumflex femoral artery

Figure 1.1D

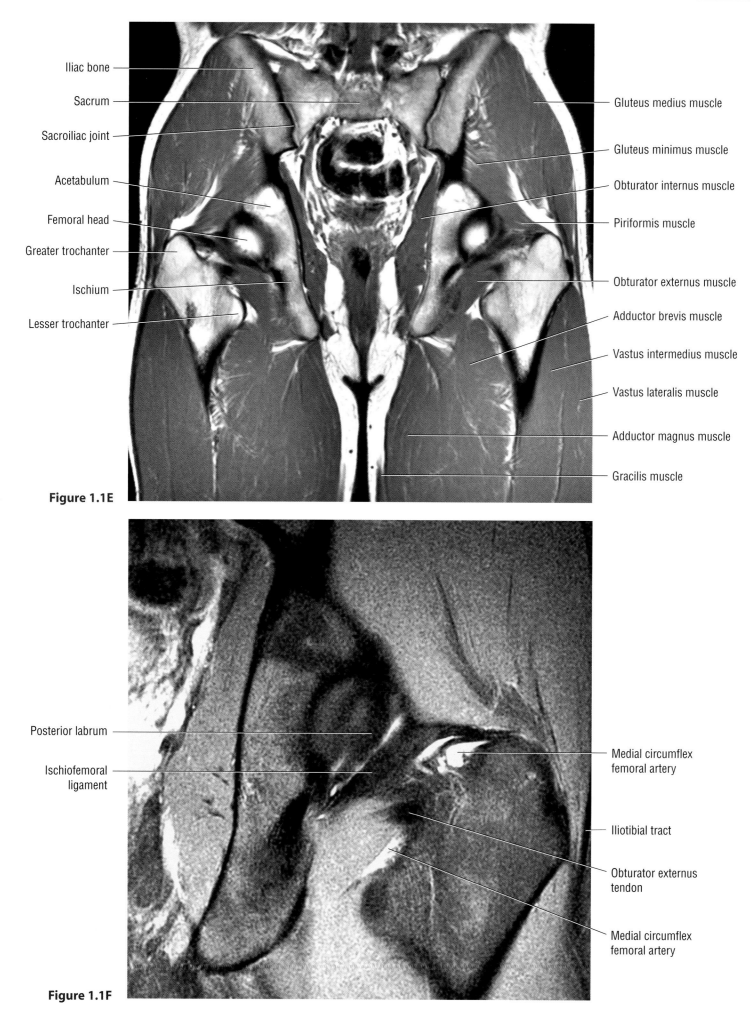

Iliac bone

Sacrum

Sacroiliac joint

Acetabulum

Femoral head

Greater trochanter

Ischium

Lesser trochanter

Gluteus medius muscle

Gluteus minimus muscle

Obturator internus muscle

Piriformis muscle

Obturator externus muscle

Adductor brevis muscle

Vastus intermedius muscle

Vastus lateralis muscle

Adductor magnus muscle

Gracilis muscle

Figure 1.1E

Posterior labrum

Ischiofemoral ligament

Medial circumflex femoral artery

Iliotibial tract

Obturator externus tendon

Medial circumflex femoral artery

Figure 1.1F

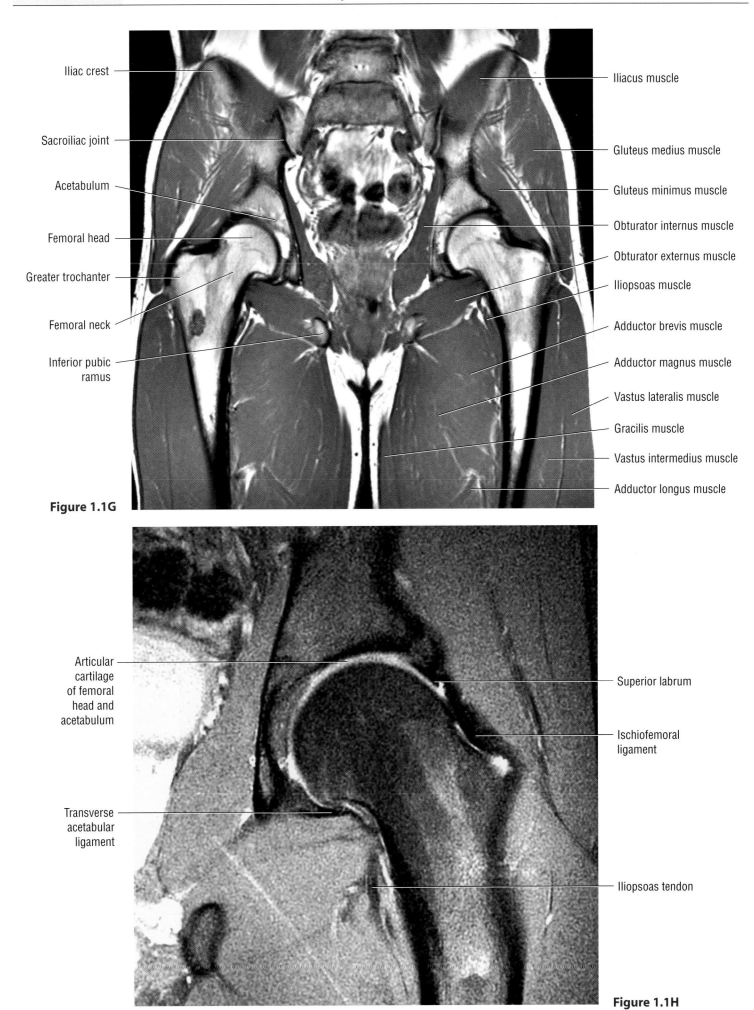

Iliac crest

Sacroiliac joint

Acetabulum

Femoral head

Greater trochanter

Femoral neck

Inferior pubic ramus

Iliacus muscle

Gluteus medius muscle

Gluteus minimus muscle

Obturator internus muscle

Obturator externus muscle

Iliopsoas muscle

Adductor brevis muscle

Adductor magnus muscle

Vastus lateralis muscle

Gracilis muscle

Vastus intermedius muscle

Adductor longus muscle

Figure 1.1G

Articular cartilage of femoral head and acetabulum

Transverse acetabular ligament

Superior labrum

Ischiofemoral ligament

Iliopsoas tendon

Figure 1.1H

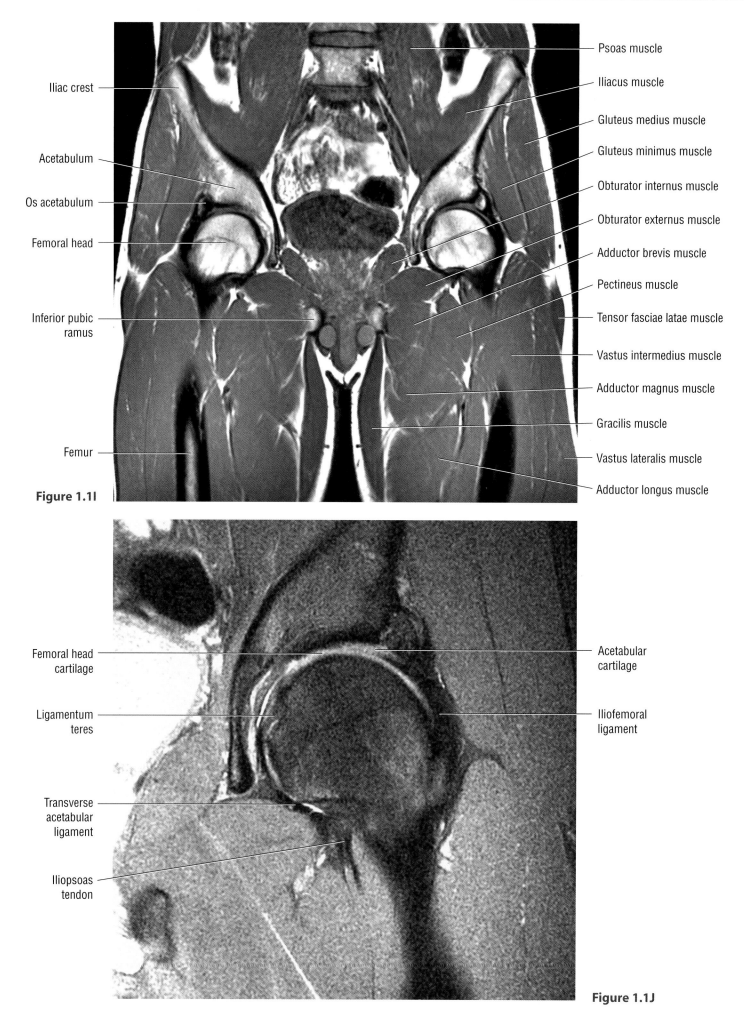

Iliac crest

Acetabulum

Os acetabulum

Femoral head

Inferior pubic
ramus

Femur

Figure 1.1I

Psoas muscle

Iliacus muscle

Gluteus medius muscle

Gluteus minimus muscle

Obturator internus muscle

Obturator externus muscle

Adductor brevis muscle

Pectineus muscle

Tensor fasciae latae muscle

Vastus intermedius muscle

Adductor magnus muscle

Gracilis muscle

Vastus lateralis muscle

Adductor longus muscle

Femoral head
cartilage

Ligamentum
teres

Transverse
acetabular
ligament

Iliopsoas
tendon

Acetabular
cartilage

Iliofemoral
ligament

Figure 1.1J

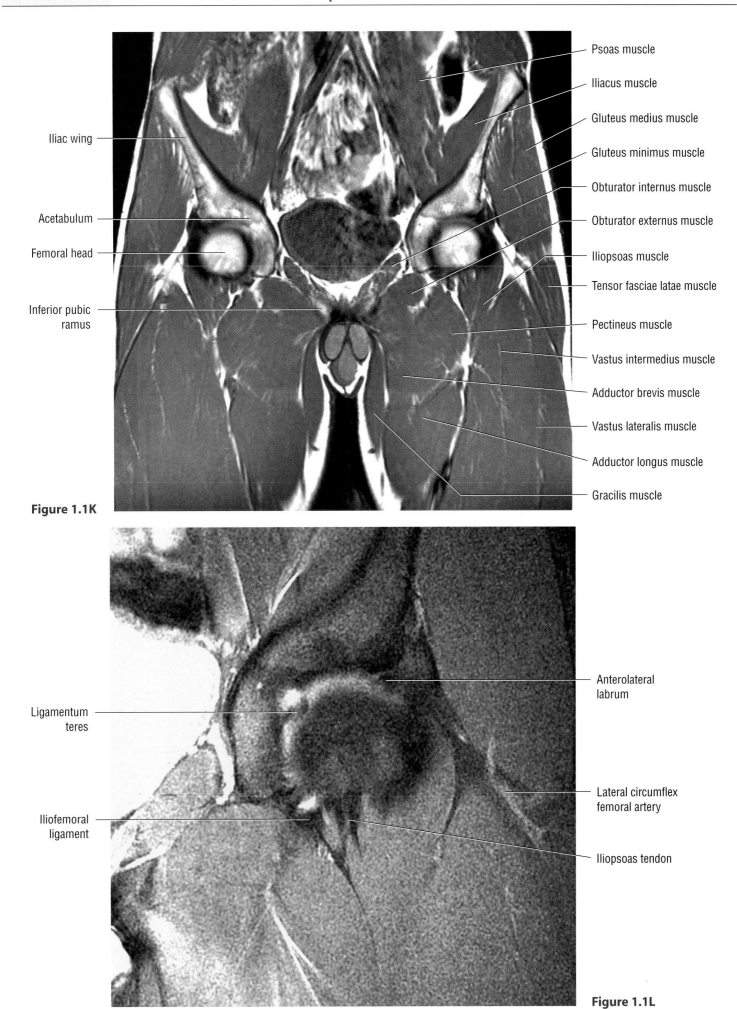

Iliac wing

Acetabulum

Femoral head

Inferior pubic
ramus

Psoas muscle

Iliacus muscle

Gluteus medius muscle

Gluteus minimus muscle

Obturator internus muscle

Obturator externus muscle

Iliopsoas muscle

Tensor fasciae latae muscle

Pectineus muscle

Vastus intermedius muscle

Adductor brevis muscle

Vastus lateralis muscle

Adductor longus muscle

Gracilis muscle

Figure 1.1K

Ligamentum
teres

Iliofemoral
ligament

Anterolateral
labrum

Lateral circumflex
femoral artery

Iliopsoas tendon

Figure 1.1L

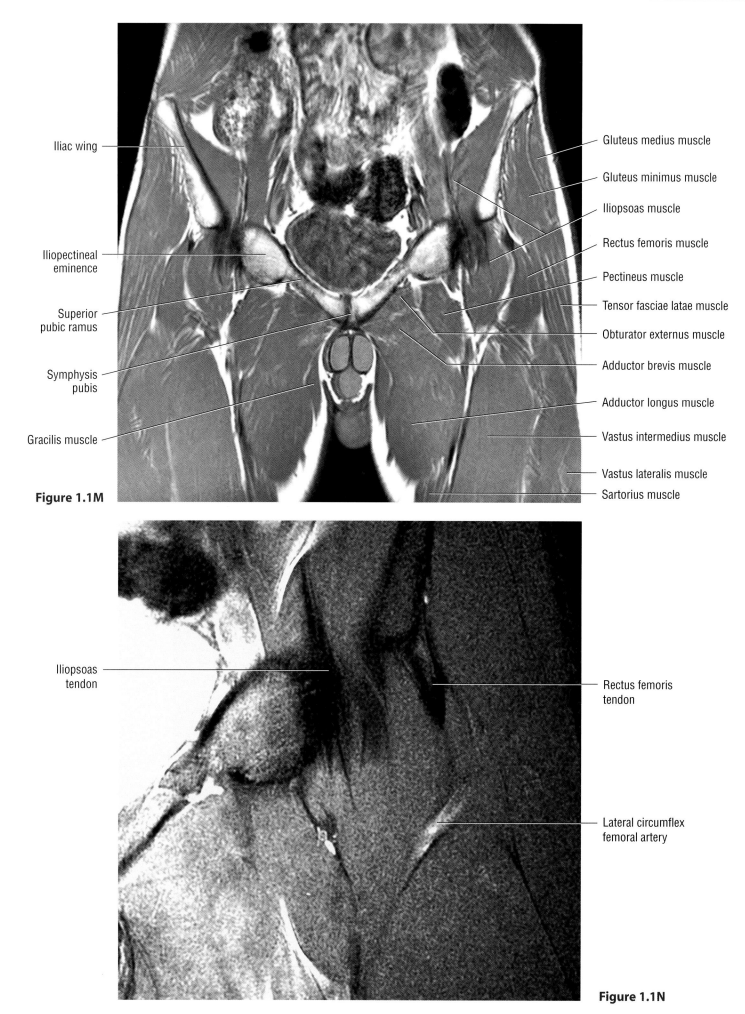

Iliac wing

Iliopectineal eminence

Superior pubic ramus

Symphysis pubis

Gracilis muscle

Gluteus medius muscle

Gluteus minimus muscle

Iliopsoas muscle

Rectus femoris muscle

Pectineus muscle

Tensor fasciae latae muscle

Obturator externus muscle

Adductor brevis muscle

Adductor longus muscle

Vastus intermedius muscle

Vastus lateralis muscle

Sartorius muscle

Figure 1.1M

Iliopsoas tendon

Rectus femoris tendon

Lateral circumflex femoral artery

Figure 1.1N

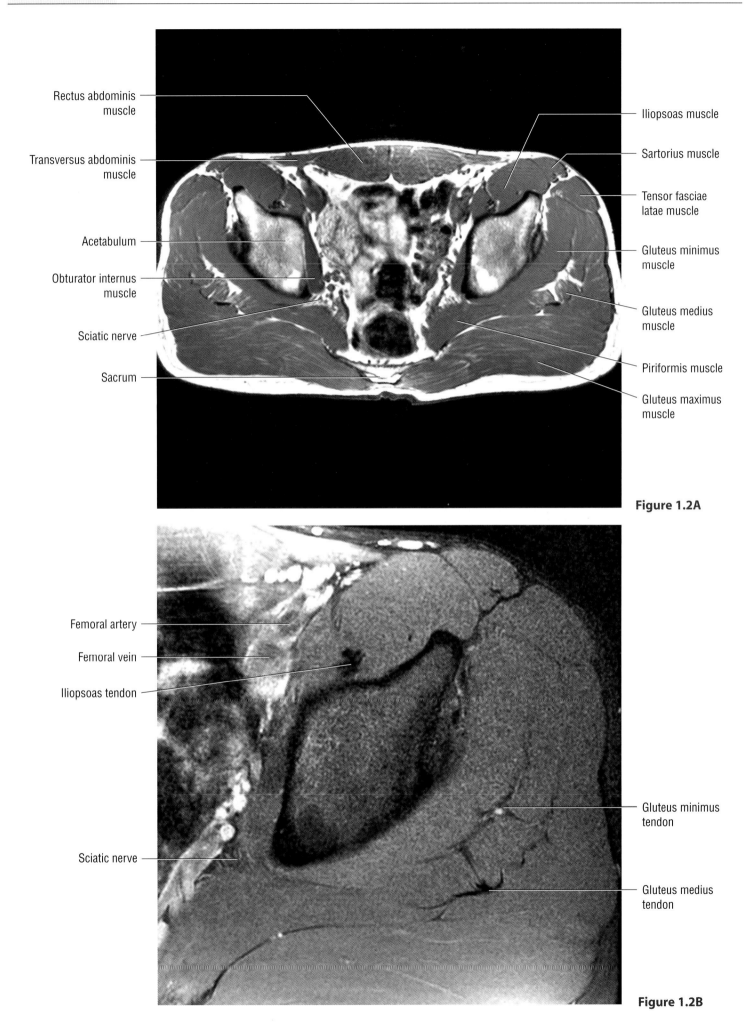

Rectus abdominis muscle

Transversus abdominis muscle

Acetabulum

Obturator internus muscle

Sciatic nerve

Sacrum

Iliopsoas muscle

Sartorius muscle

Tensor fasciae latae muscle

Gluteus minimus muscle

Gluteus medius muscle

Piriformis muscle

Gluteus maximus muscle

Figure 1.2A

Femoral artery

Femoral vein

Iliopsoas tendon

Sciatic nerve

Gluteus minimus tendon

Gluteus medius tendon

Figure 1.2B

Hip - Axial

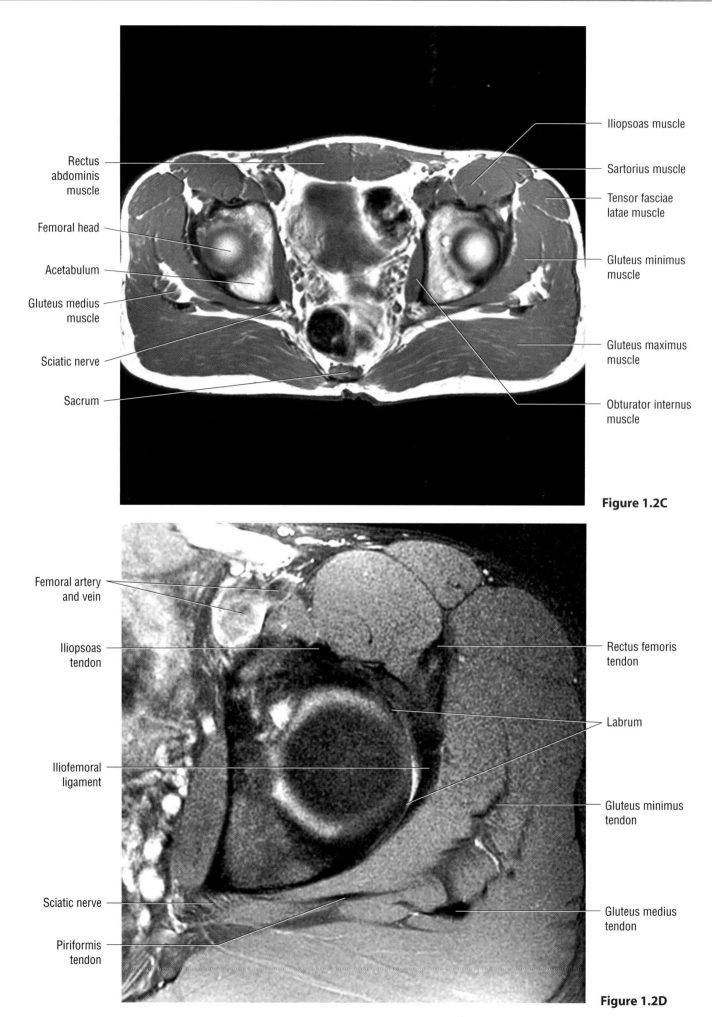

Rectus abdominis muscle

Femoral head

Acetabulum

Gluteus medius muscle

Sciatic nerve

Sacrum

Iliopsoas muscle

Sartorius muscle

Tensor fasciae latae muscle

Gluteus minimus muscle

Gluteus maximus muscle

Obturator internus muscle

Figure 1.2C

Femoral artery and vein

Iliopsoas tendon

Iliofemoral ligament

Sciatic nerve

Piriformis tendon

Rectus femoris tendon

Labrum

Gluteus minimus tendon

Gluteus medius tendon

Figure 1.2D

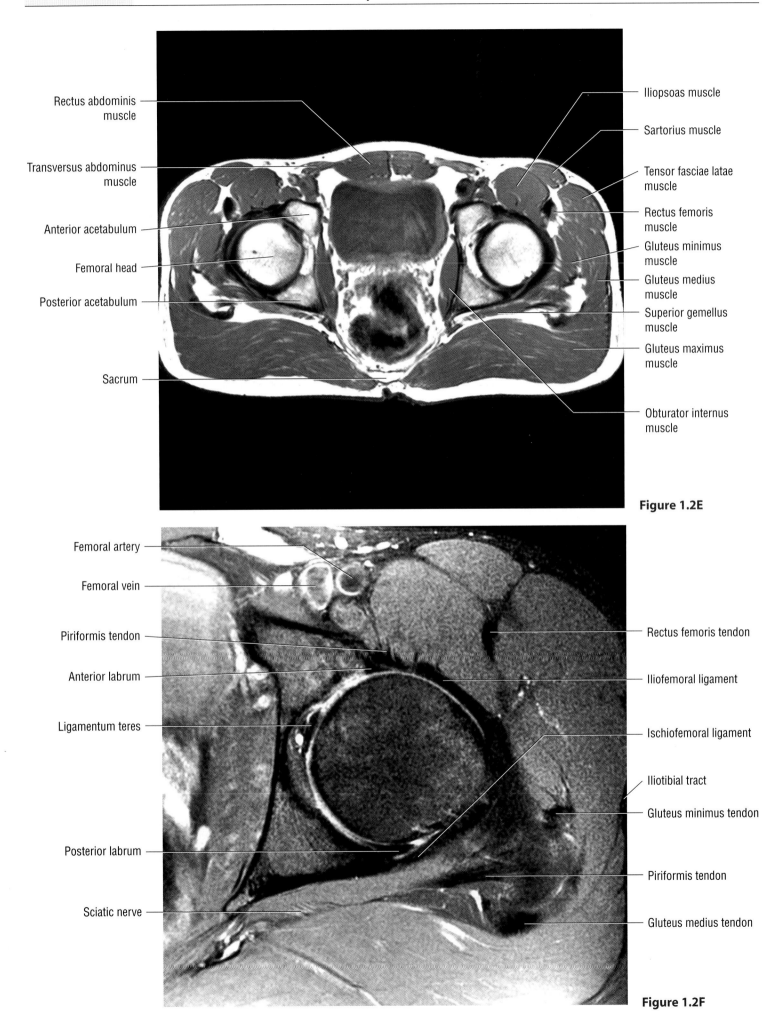

Rectus abdominis muscle

Transversus abdominus muscle

Anterior acetabulum

Femoral head

Posterior acetabulum

Sacrum

Iliopsoas muscle

Sartorius muscle

Tensor fasciae latae muscle

Rectus femoris muscle

Gluteus minimus muscle

Gluteus medius muscle

Superior gemellus muscle

Gluteus maximus muscle

Obturator internus muscle

Figure 1.2E

Femoral artery

Femoral vein

Piriformis tendon

Anterior labrum

Ligamentum teres

Posterior labrum

Sciatic nerve

Rectus femoris tendon

Iliofemoral ligament

Ischiofemoral ligament

Iliotibial tract

Gluteus minimus tendon

Piriformis tendon

Gluteus medius tendon

Figure 1.2F

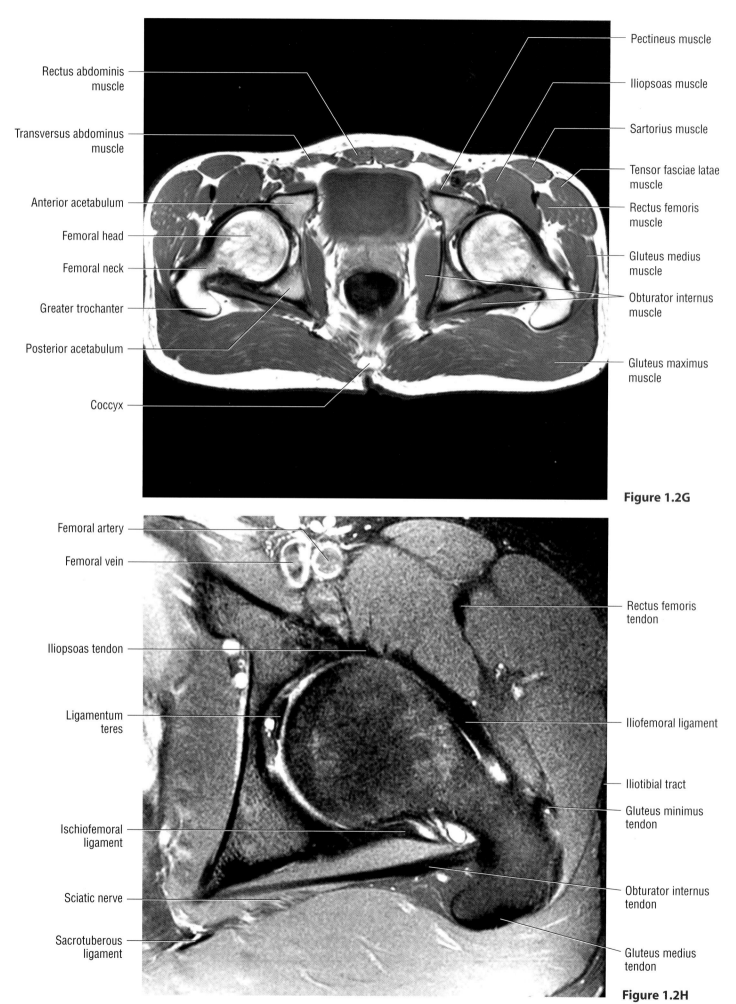

Rectus abdominis muscle

Transversus abdominus muscle

Anterior acetabulum

Femoral head

Femoral neck

Greater trochanter

Posterior acetabulum

Coccyx

Pectineus muscle

Iliopsoas muscle

Sartorius muscle

Tensor fasciae latae muscle

Rectus femoris muscle

Gluteus medius muscle

Obturator internus muscle

Gluteus maximus muscle

Figure 1.2G

Femoral artery

Femoral vein

Iliopsoas tendon

Ligamentum teres

Ischiofemoral ligament

Sciatic nerve

Sacrotuberous ligament

Rectus femoris tendon

Iliofemoral ligament

Iliotibial tract

Gluteus minimus tendon

Obturator internus tendon

Gluteus medius tendon

Figure 1.2H

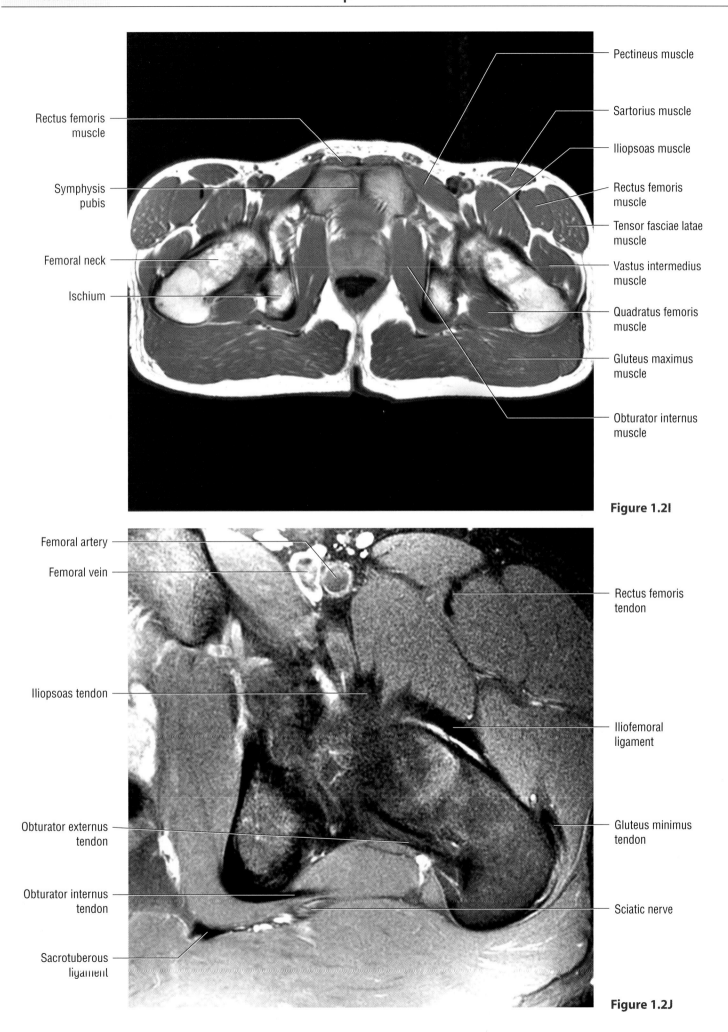

Pectineus muscle

Sartorius muscle

Iliopsoas muscle

Rectus femoris muscle

Tensor fasciae latae muscle

Vastus intermedius muscle

Quadratus femoris muscle

Gluteus maximus muscle

Obturator internus muscle

Rectus femoris muscle

Symphysis pubis

Femoral neck

Ischium

Figure 1.2I

Femoral artery

Femoral vein

Rectus femoris tendon

Iliopsoas tendon

Iliofemoral ligament

Obturator externus tendon

Gluteus minimus tendon

Obturator internus tendon

Sciatic nerve

Sacrotuberous ligament

Figure 1.2J

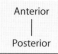
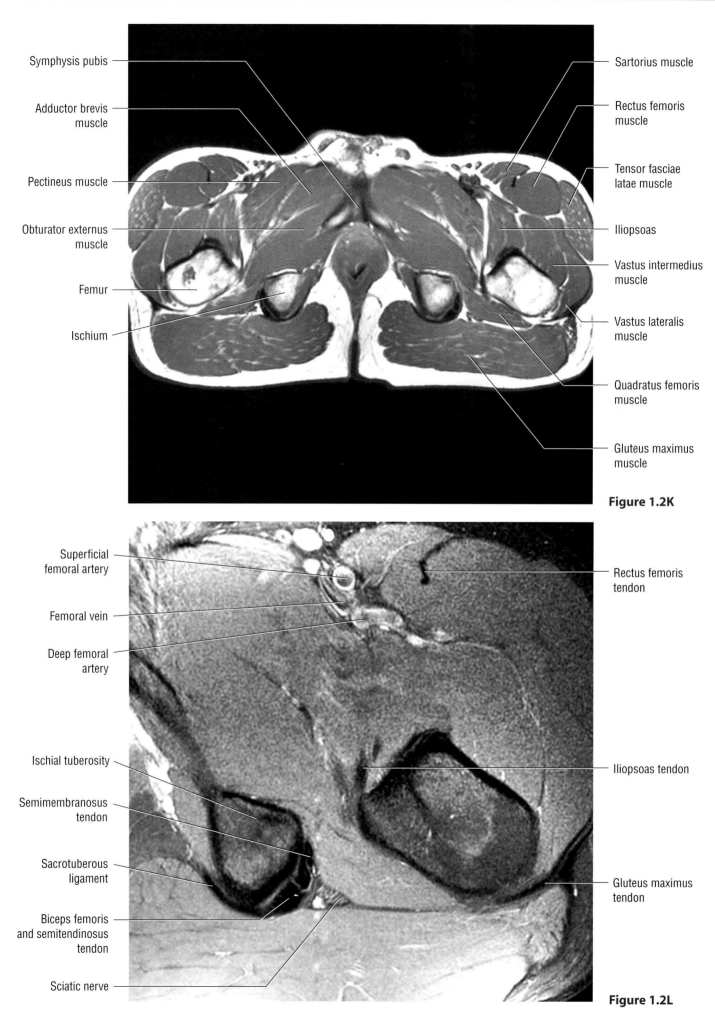

Symphysis pubis

Adductor brevis
muscle

Pectineus muscle

Obturator externus
muscle

Femur

Ischium

Sartorius muscle

Rectus femoris
muscle

Tensor fasciae
latae muscle

Iliopsoas

Vastus intermedius
muscle

Vastus lateralis
muscle

Quadratus femoris
muscle

Gluteus maximus
muscle

Figure 1.2K

Superficial
femoral artery

Femoral vein

Deep femoral
artery

Ischial tuberosity

Semimembranosus
tendon

Sacrotuberous
ligament

Biceps femoris
and semitendinosus
tendon

Sciatic nerve

Rectus femoris
tendon

Iliopsoas tendon

Gluteus maximus
tendon

Figure 1.2L

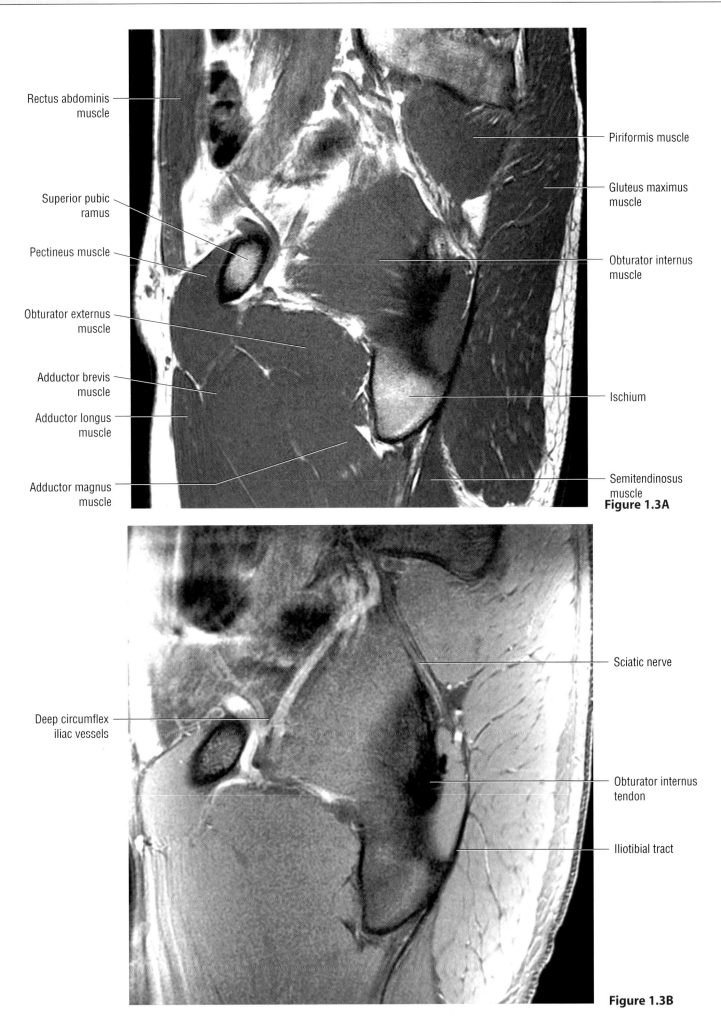

Rectus abdominis muscle

Superior pubic ramus

Pectineus muscle

Obturator externus muscle

Adductor brevis muscle

Adductor longus muscle

Adductor magnus muscle

Piriformis muscle

Gluteus maximus muscle

Obturator internus muscle

Ischium

Semitendinosus muscle

Figure 1.3A

Deep circumflex iliac vessels

Sciatic nerve

Obturator internus tendon

Iliotibial tract

Figure 1.3B

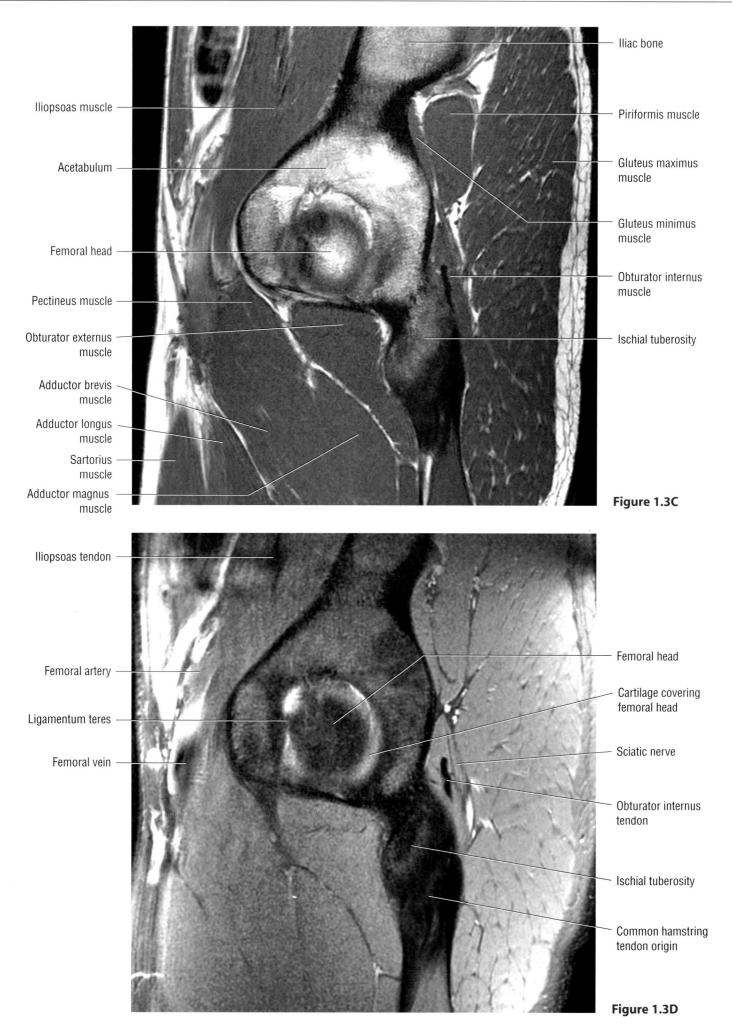

Iliopsoas muscle

Acetabulum

Femoral head

Pectineus muscle

Obturator externus
muscle

Adductor brevis
muscle

Adductor longus
muscle

Sartorius
muscle

Adductor magnus
muscle

Iliac bone

Piriformis muscle

Gluteus maximus
muscle

Gluteus minimus
muscle

Obturator internus
muscle

Ischial tuberosity

Figure 1.3C

Iliopsoas tendon

Femoral artery

Ligamentum teres

Femoral vein

Femoral head

Cartilage covering
femoral head

Sciatic nerve

Obturator internus
tendon

Ischial tuberosity

Common hamstring
tendon origin

Figure 1.3D

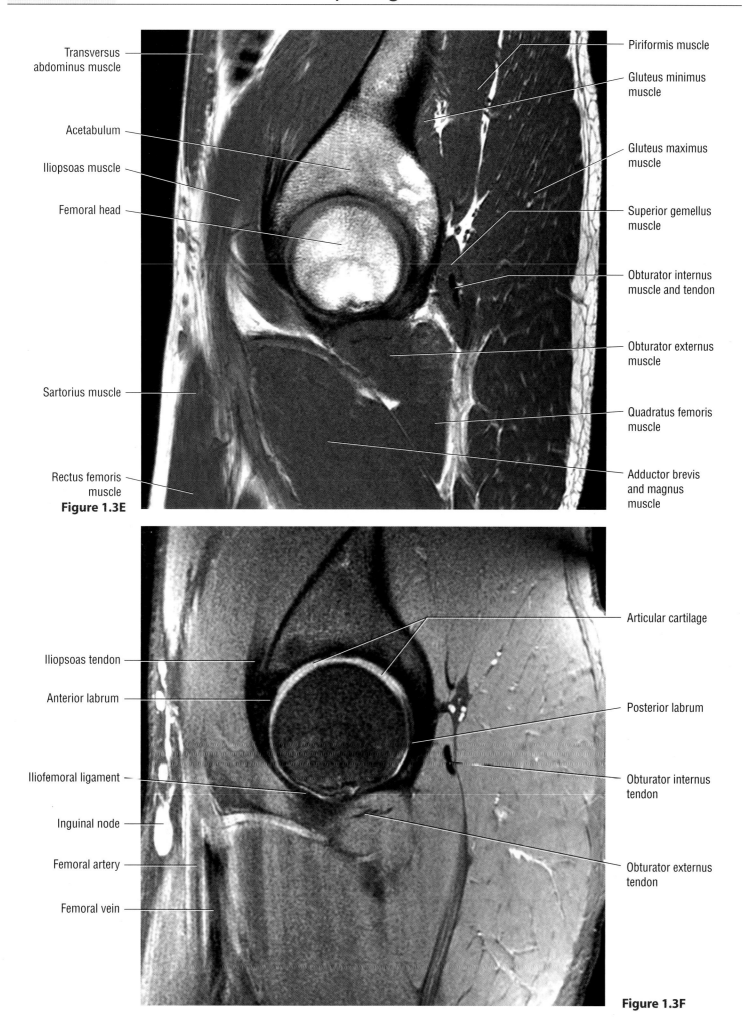

Transversus abdominus muscle

Piriformis muscle

Gluteus minimus muscle

Acetabulum

Gluteus maximus muscle

Iliopsoas muscle

Femoral head

Superior gemellus muscle

Obturator internus muscle and tendon

Obturator externus muscle

Sartorius muscle

Quadratus femoris muscle

Rectus femoris muscle

Adductor brevis and magnus muscle

Figure 1.3E

Articular cartilage

Iliopsoas tendon

Anterior labrum

Posterior labrum

Iliofemoral ligament

Obturator internus tendon

Inguinal node

Femoral artery

Obturator externus tendon

Femoral vein

Figure 1.3F

Hip - Sagittal

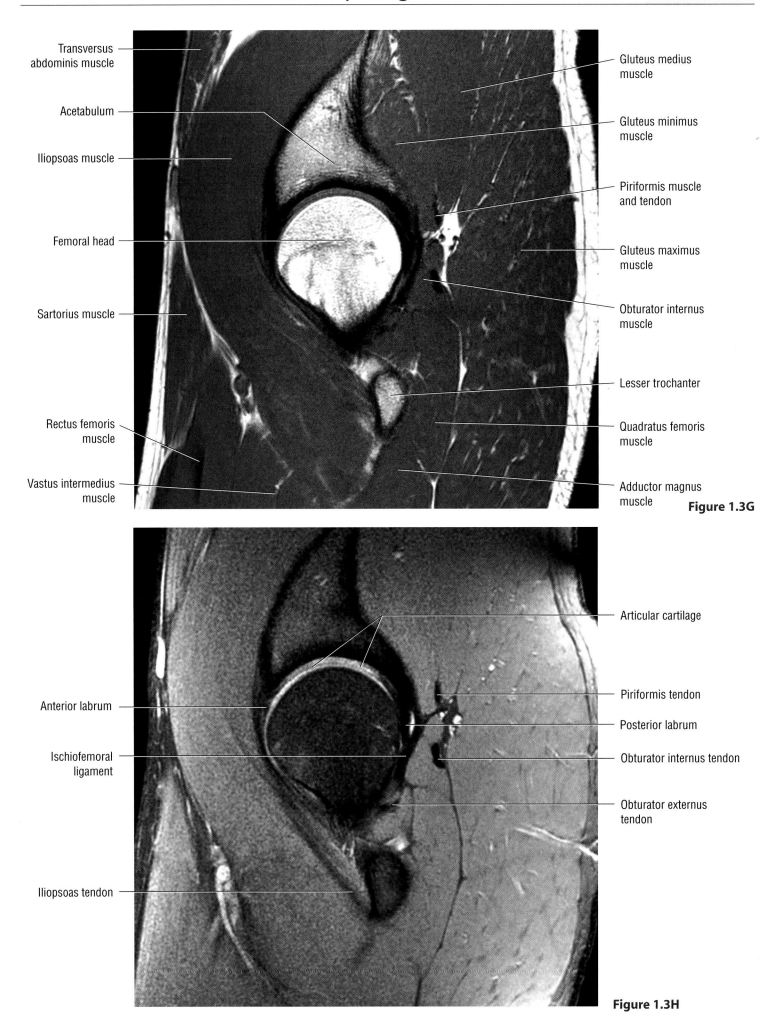

Transversus abdominis muscle

Acetabulum

Iliopsoas muscle

Femoral head

Sartorius muscle

Rectus femoris muscle

Vastus intermedius muscle

Gluteus medius muscle

Gluteus minimus muscle

Piriformis muscle and tendon

Gluteus maximus muscle

Obturator internus muscle

Lesser trochanter

Quadratus femoris muscle

Adductor magnus muscle

Figure 1.3G

Anterior labrum

Ischiofemoral ligament

Iliopsoas tendon

Articular cartilage

Piriformis tendon

Posterior labrum

Obturator internus tendon

Obturator externus tendon

Figure 1.3H

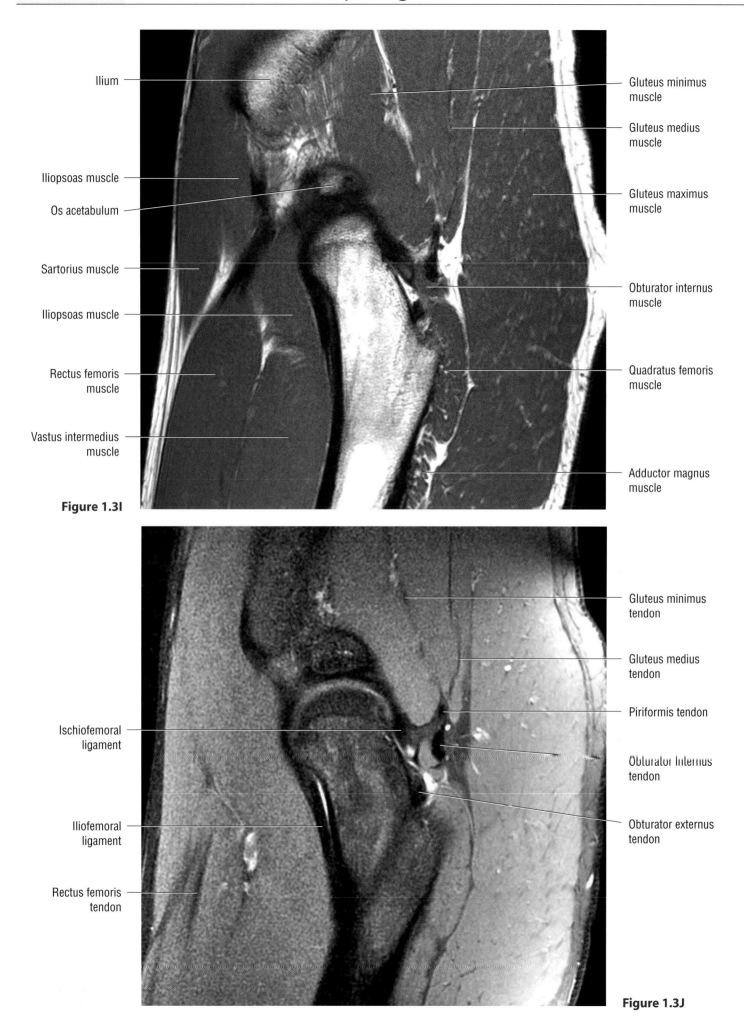

Ilium

Iliopsoas muscle

Os acetabulum

Sartorius muscle

Iliopsoas muscle

Rectus femoris muscle

Vastus intermedius muscle

Gluteus minimus muscle

Gluteus medius muscle

Gluteus maximus muscle

Obturator internus muscle

Quadratus femoris muscle

Adductor magnus muscle

Figure 1.3I

Ischiofemoral ligament

Iliofemoral ligament

Rectus femoris tendon

Gluteus minimus tendon

Gluteus medius tendon

Piriformis tendon

Obturator Internus tendon

Obturator externus tendon

Figure 1.3J

Hip - Sagittal

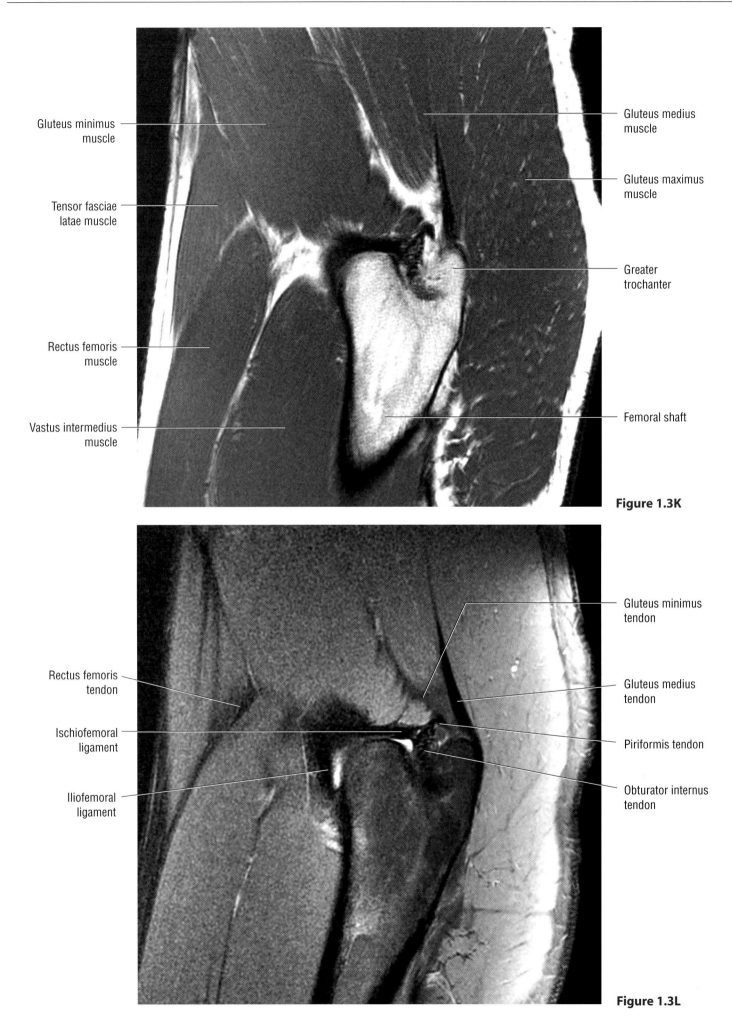

Gluteus minimus muscle

Tensor fasciae latae muscle

Rectus femoris muscle

Vastus intermedius muscle

Gluteus medius muscle

Gluteus maximus muscle

Greater trochanter

Femoral shaft

Figure 1.3K

Rectus femoris tendon

Ischiofemoral ligament

Iliofemoral ligament

Gluteus minimus tendon

Gluteus medius tendon

Piriformis tendon

Obturator internus tendon

Figure 1.3L

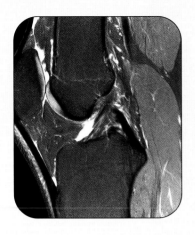

The Knee

MR Normal Anatomy

Axial

Sagittal

Coronal

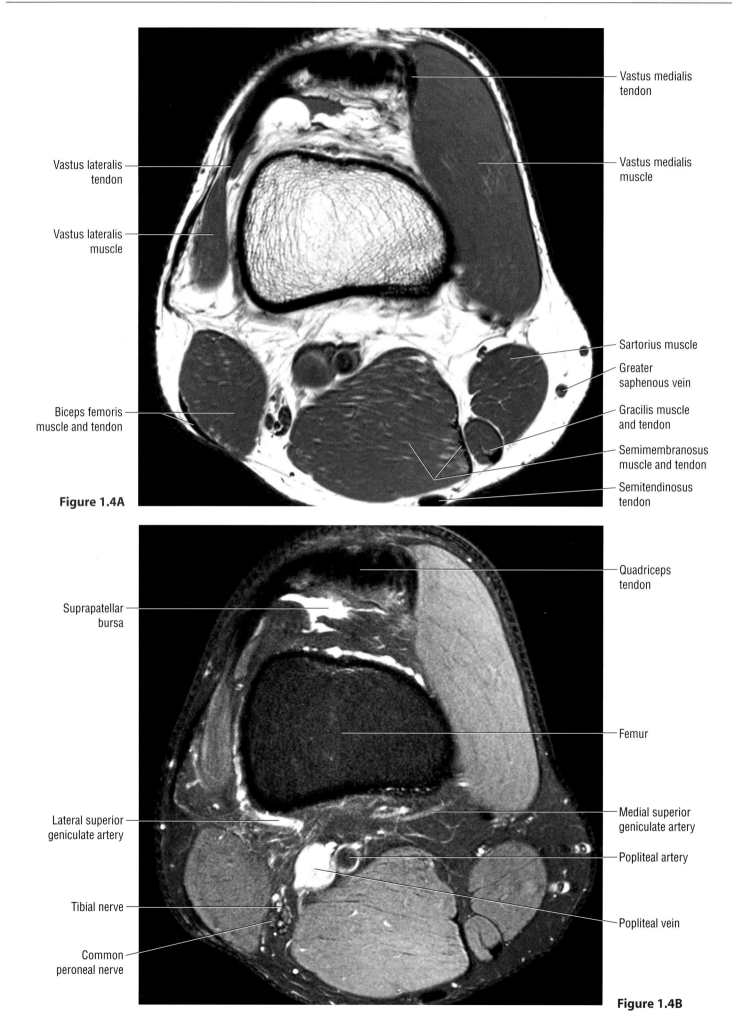

Figure 1.4A

Vastus medialis tendon

Vastus medialis muscle

Vastus lateralis tendon

Vastus lateralis muscle

Sartorius muscle

Greater saphenous vein

Gracilis muscle and tendon

Biceps femoris muscle and tendon

Semimembranosus muscle and tendon

Semitendinosus tendon

Figure 1.4B

Quadriceps tendon

Suprapatellar bursa

Femur

Lateral superior geniculate artery

Medial superior geniculate artery

Popliteal artery

Tibial nerve

Common peroneal nerve

Popliteal vein

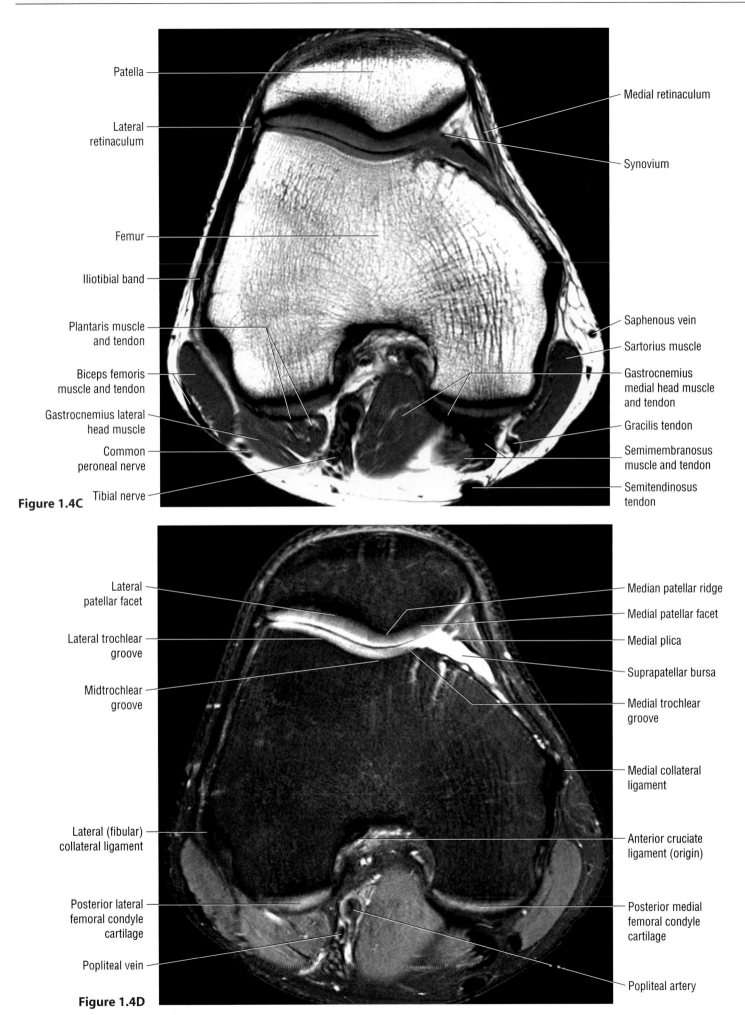

Patella
Lateral retinaculum
Femur
Iliotibial band
Plantaris muscle and tendon
Biceps femoris muscle and tendon
Gastrocnemius lateral head muscle
Common peroneal nerve
Tibial nerve

Medial retinaculum
Synovium
Saphenous vein
Sartorius muscle
Gastrocnemius medial head muscle and tendon
Gracilis tendon
Semimembranosus muscle and tendon
Semitendinosus tendon

Figure 1.4C

Lateral patellar facet
Lateral trochlear groove
Midtrochlear groove
Lateral (fibular) collateral ligament
Posterior lateral femoral condyle cartilage
Popliteal vein

Median patellar ridge
Medial patellar facet
Medial plica
Suprapatellar bursa
Medial trochlear groove
Medial collateral ligament
Anterior cruciate ligament (origin)
Posterior medial femoral condyle cartilage
Popliteal artery

Figure 1.4D

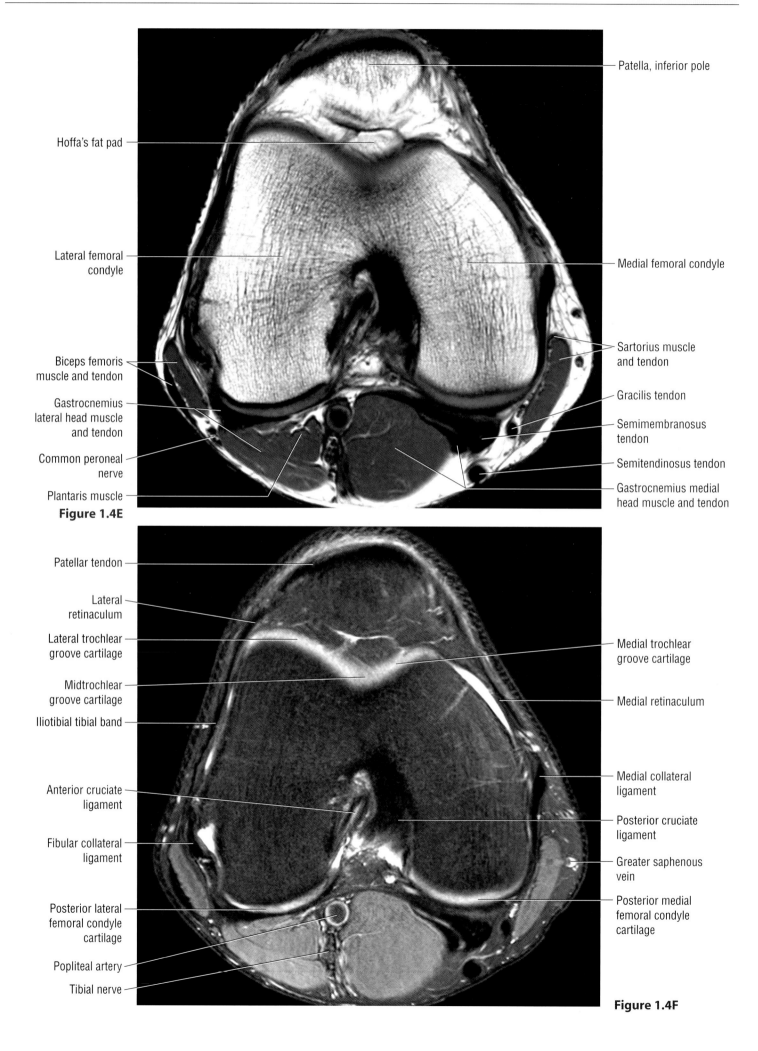

Figure 1.4E

- Hoffa's fat pad
- Lateral femoral condyle
- Biceps femoris muscle and tendon
- Gastrocnemius lateral head muscle and tendon
- Common peroneal nerve
- Plantaris muscle
- Patella, inferior pole
- Medial femoral condyle
- Sartorius muscle and tendon
- Gracilis tendon
- Semimembranosus tendon
- Semitendinosus tendon
- Gastrocnemius medial head muscle and tendon

Figure 1.4F

- Patellar tendon
- Lateral retinaculum
- Lateral trochlear groove cartilage
- Midtrochlear groove cartilage
- Iliotibial tibial band
- Anterior cruciate ligament
- Fibular collateral ligament
- Posterior lateral femoral condyle cartilage
- Popliteal artery
- Tibial nerve
- Medial trochlear groove cartilage
- Medial retinaculum
- Medial collateral ligament
- Posterior cruciate ligament
- Greater saphenous vein
- Posterior medial femoral condyle cartilage

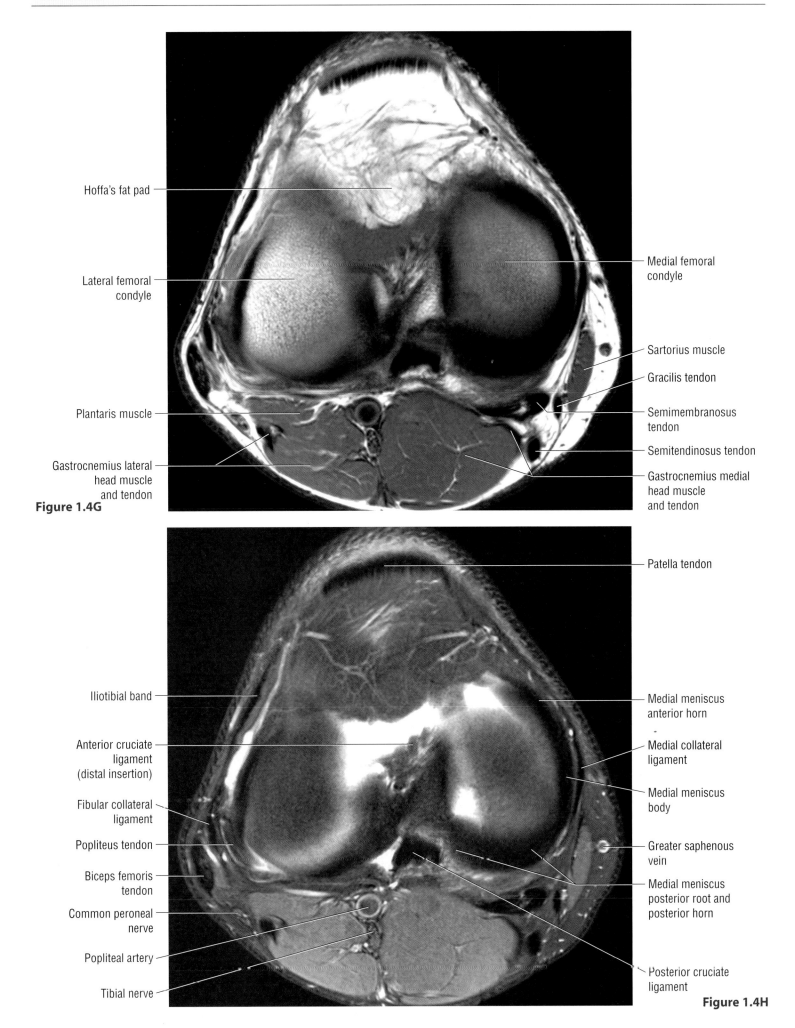

Hoffa's fat pad

Lateral femoral condyle

Plantaris muscle

Gastrocnemius lateral head muscle and tendon

Medial femoral condyle

Sartorius muscle

Gracilis tendon

Semimembranosus tendon

Semitendinosus tendon

Gastrocnemius medial head muscle and tendon

Figure 1.4G

Iliotibial band

Anterior cruciate ligament (distal insertion)

Fibular collateral ligament

Popliteus tendon

Biceps femoris tendon

Common peroneal nerve

Popliteal artery

Tibial nerve

Patella tendon

Medial meniscus anterior horn

Medial collateral ligament

Medial meniscus body

Greater saphenous vein

Medial meniscus posterior root and posterior horn

Posterior cruciate ligament

Figure 1.4H

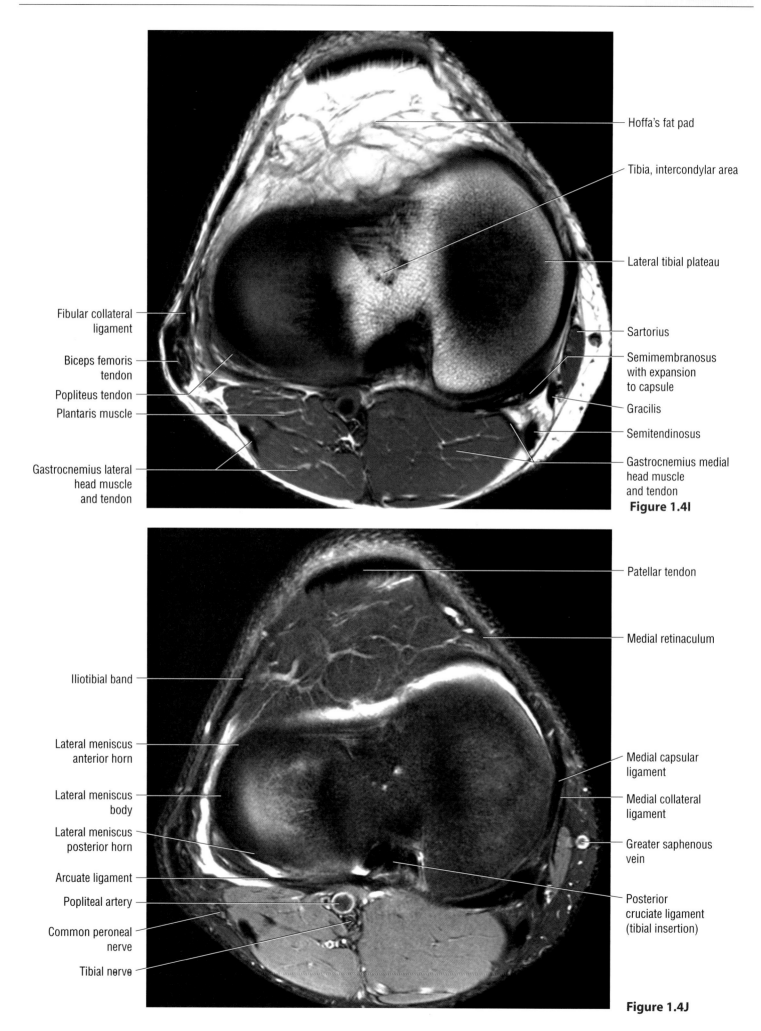

Hoffa's fat pad

Tibia, intercondylar area

Lateral tibial plateau

Sartorius

Semimembranosus with expansion to capsule

Gracilis

Semitendinosus

Gastrocnemius medial head muscle and tendon

Fibular collateral ligament

Biceps femoris tendon

Popliteus tendon

Plantaris muscle

Gastrocnemius lateral head muscle and tendon

Figure 1.4I

Patellar tendon

Medial retinaculum

Medial capsular ligament

Medial collateral ligament

Greater saphenous vein

Posterior cruciate ligament (tibial insertion)

Iliotibial band

Lateral meniscus anterior horn

Lateral meniscus body

Lateral meniscus posterior horn

Arcuate ligament

Popliteal artery

Common peroneal nerve

Tibial nerve

Figure 1.4J

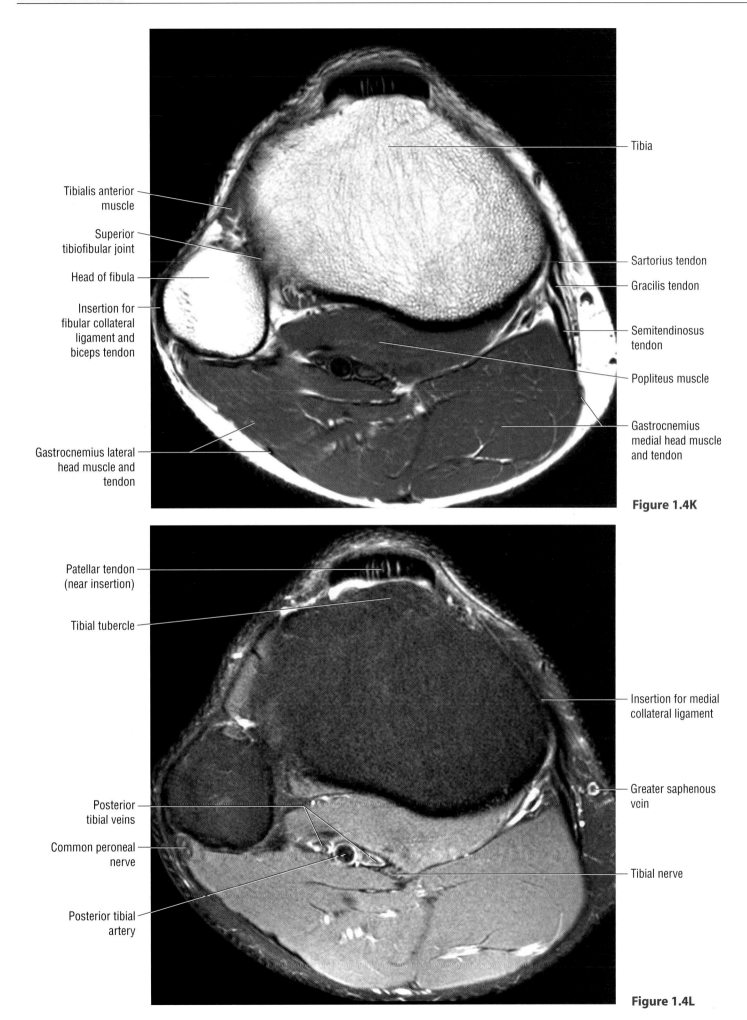

Tibialis anterior muscle

Superior tibiofibular joint

Head of fibula

Insertion for fibular collateral ligament and biceps tendon

Gastrocnemius lateral head muscle and tendon

Tibia

Sartorius tendon

Gracilis tendon

Semitendinosus tendon

Popliteus muscle

Gastrocnemius medial head muscle and tendon

Figure 1.4K

Patellar tendon (near insertion)

Tibial tubercle

Posterior tibial veins

Common peroneal nerve

Posterior tibial artery

Insertion for medial collateral ligament

Greater saphenous vein

Tibial nerve

Figure 1.4L

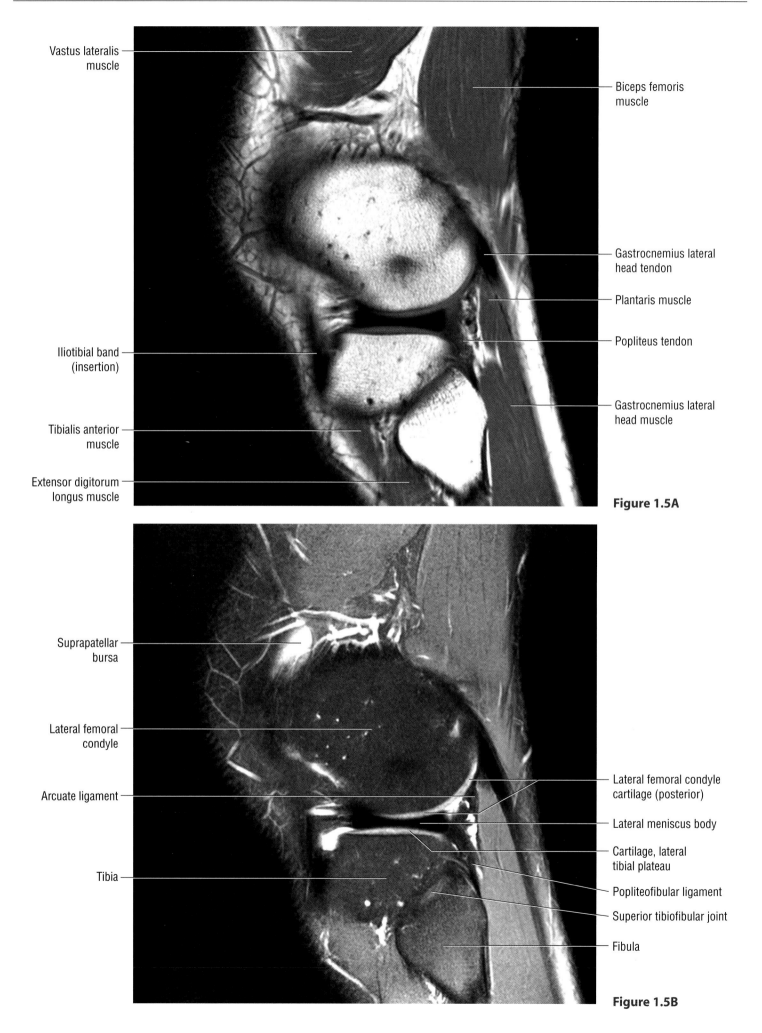

Vastus lateralis muscle

Biceps femoris muscle

Gastrocnemius lateral head tendon

Plantaris muscle

Popliteus tendon

Iliotibial band (insertion)

Gastrocnemius lateral head muscle

Tibialis anterior muscle

Extensor digitorum longus muscle

Figure 1.5A

Suprapatellar bursa

Lateral femoral condyle

Arcuate ligament

Lateral femoral condyle cartilage (posterior)

Lateral meniscus body

Cartilage, lateral tibial plateau

Tibia

Popliteofibular ligament

Superior tibiofibular joint

Fibula

Figure 1.5B

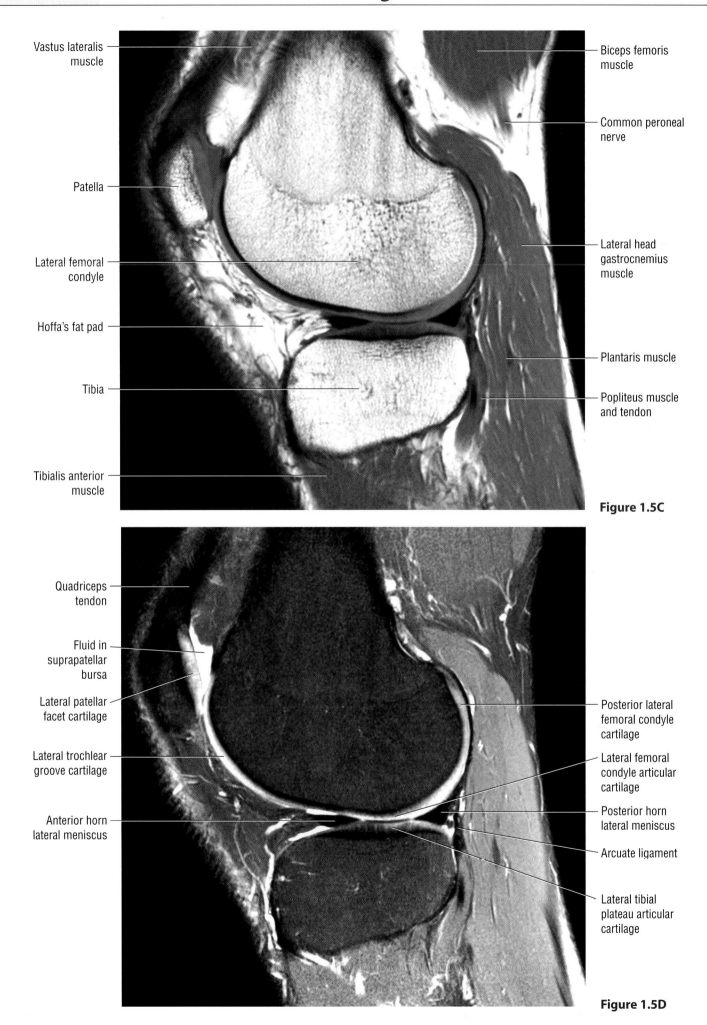

Vastus lateralis muscle

Patella

Lateral femoral condyle

Hoffa's fat pad

Tibia

Tibialis anterior muscle

Biceps femoris muscle

Common peroneal nerve

Lateral head gastrocnemius muscle

Plantaris muscle

Popliteus muscle and tendon

Figure 1.5C

Quadriceps tendon

Fluid in suprapatellar bursa

Lateral patellar facet cartilage

Lateral trochlear groove cartilage

Anterior horn lateral meniscus

Posterior lateral femoral condyle cartilage

Lateral femoral condyle articular cartilage

Posterior horn lateral meniscus

Arcuate ligament

Lateral tibial plateau articular cartilage

Figure 1.5D

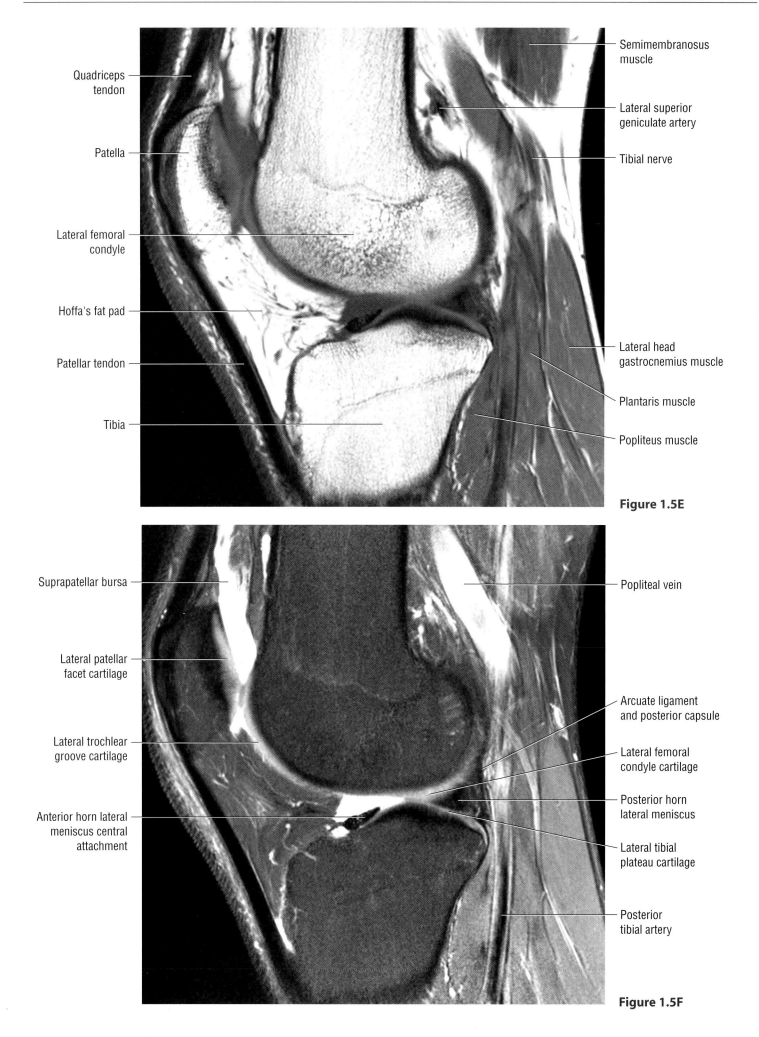

Quadriceps tendon

Patella

Lateral femoral condyle

Hoffa's fat pad

Patellar tendon

Tibia

Semimembranosus muscle

Lateral superior geniculate artery

Tibial nerve

Lateral head gastrocnemius muscle

Plantaris muscle

Popliteus muscle

Figure 1.5E

Suprapatellar bursa

Lateral patellar facet cartilage

Lateral trochlear groove cartilage

Anterior horn lateral meniscus central attachment

Popliteal vein

Arcuate ligament and posterior capsule

Lateral femoral condyle cartilage

Posterior horn lateral meniscus

Lateral tibial plateau cartilage

Posterior tibial artery

Figure 1.5F

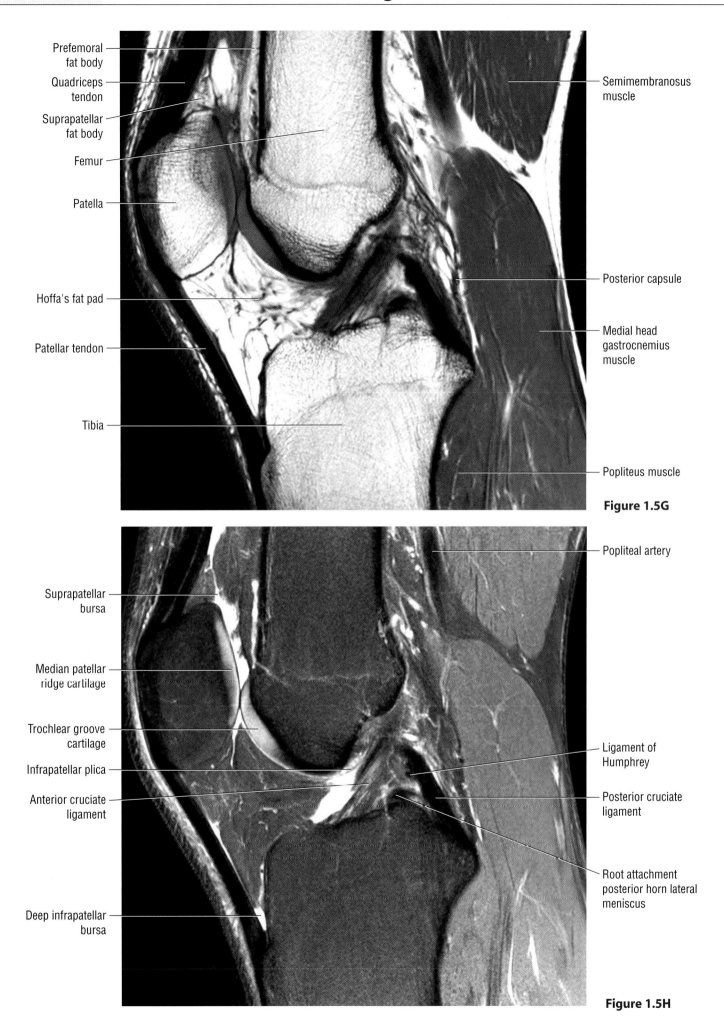

Prefemoral fat body

Quadriceps tendon

Suprapatellar fat body

Femur

Patella

Hoffa's fat pad

Patellar tendon

Tibia

Semimembranosus muscle

Posterior capsule

Medial head gastrocnemius muscle

Popliteus muscle

Figure 1.5G

Suprapatellar bursa

Median patellar ridge cartilage

Trochlear groove cartilage

Infrapatellar plica

Anterior cruciate ligament

Deep infrapatellar bursa

Popliteal artery

Ligament of Humphrey

Posterior cruciate ligament

Root attachment posterior horn lateral meniscus

Figure 1.5H

Knee - Sagittal

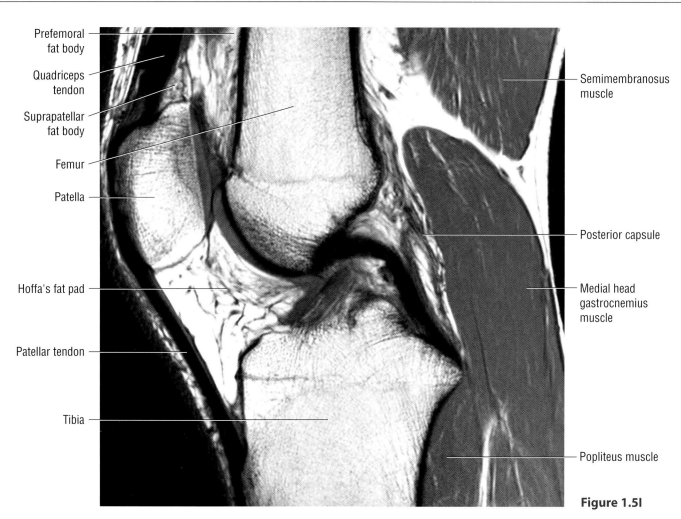

Prefemoral fat body

Quadriceps tendon

Suprapatellar fat body

Femur

Patella

Hoffa's fat pad

Patellar tendon

Tibia

Semimembranosus muscle

Posterior capsule

Medial head gastrocnemius muscle

Popliteus muscle

Figure 1.5I

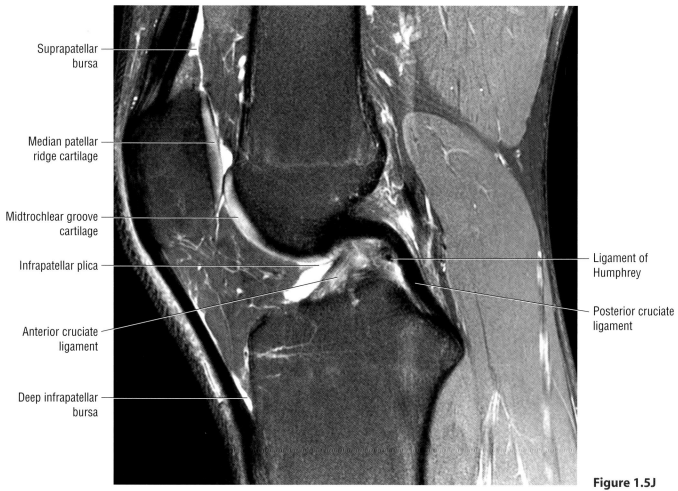

Suprapatellar bursa

Median patellar ridge cartilage

Midtrochlear groove cartilage

Infrapatellar plica

Anterior cruciate ligament

Deep infrapatellar bursa

Ligament of Humphrey

Posterior cruciate ligament

Figure 1.5J

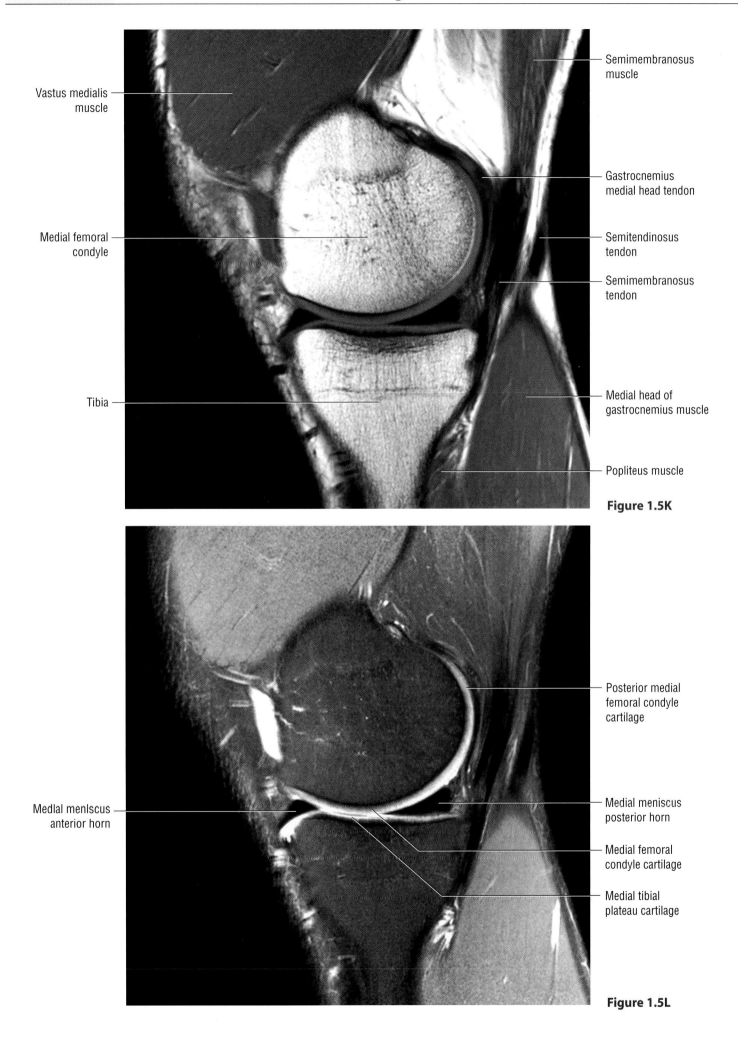

Vastus medialis muscle

Medial femoral condyle

Tibia

Semimembranosus muscle

Gastrocnemius medial head tendon

Semitendinosus tendon

Semimembranosus tendon

Medial head of gastrocnemius muscle

Popliteus muscle

Figure 1.5K

Medial meniscus anterior horn

Posterior medial femoral condyle cartilage

Medial meniscus posterior horn

Medial femoral condyle cartilage

Medial tibial plateau cartilage

Figure 1.5L

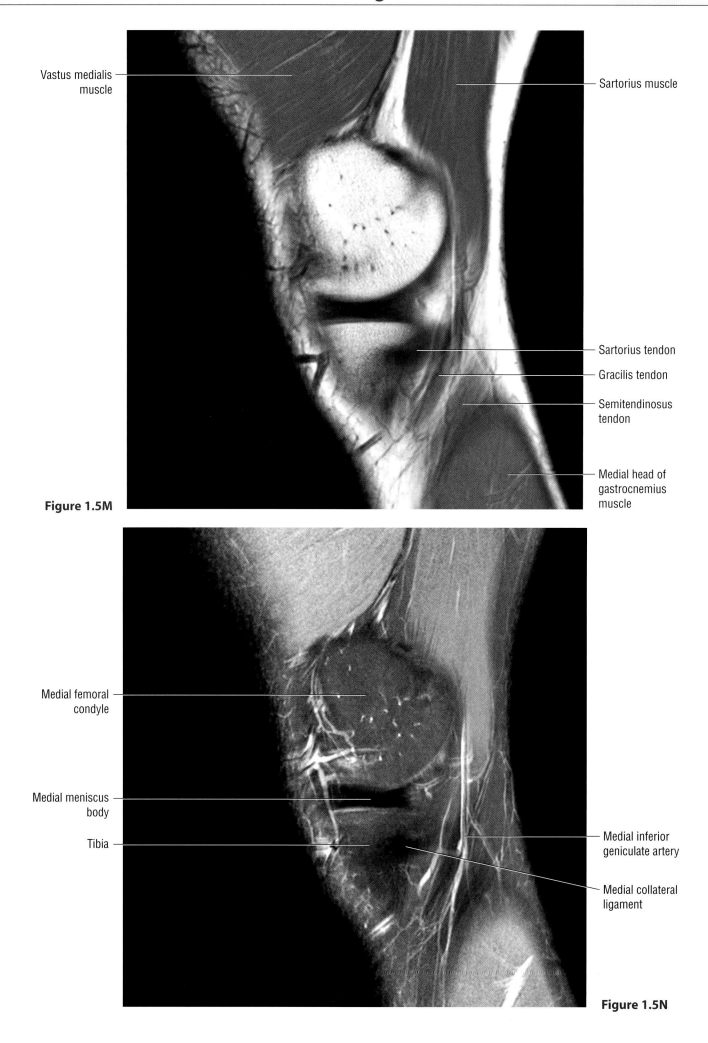

Vastus medialis
muscle

Sartorius muscle

Sartorius tendon

Gracilis tendon

Semitendinosus
tendon

Medial head of
gastrocnemius
muscle

Figure 1.5M

Medial femoral
condyle

Medial meniscus
body

Tibia

Medial inferior
geniculate artery

Medial collateral
ligament

Figure 1.5N

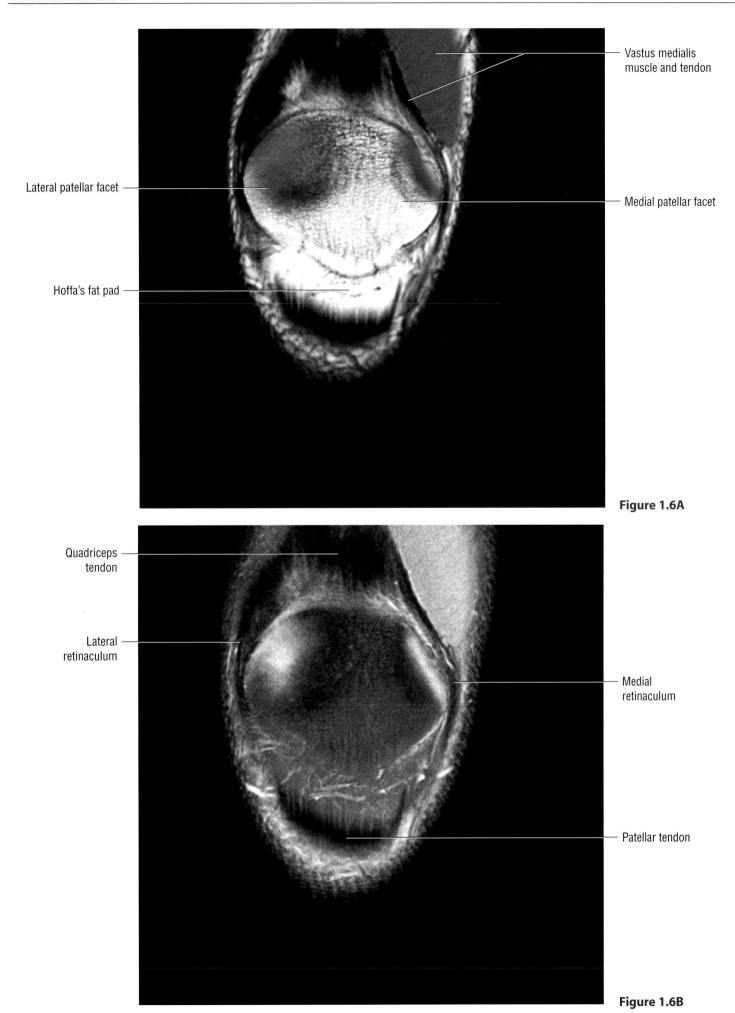

Lateral patellar facet

Hoffa's fat pad

Vastus medialis muscle and tendon

Medial patellar facet

Figure 1.6A

Quadriceps tendon

Lateral retinaculum

Medial retinaculum

Patellar tendon

Figure 1.6B

Knee - Coronal

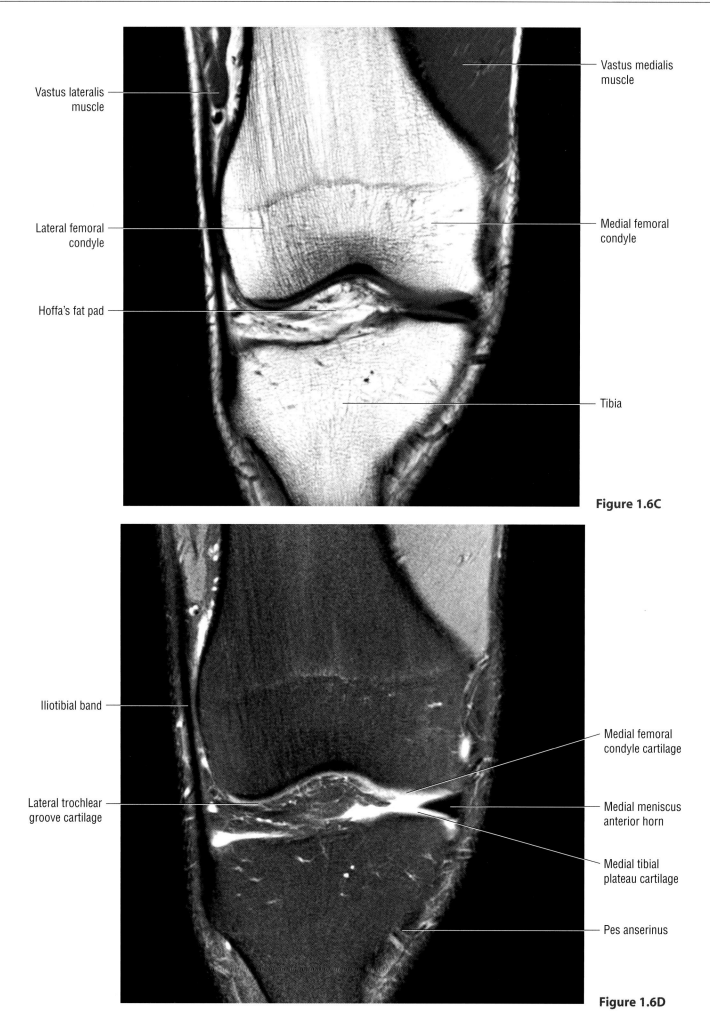

Vastus lateralis muscle

Vastus medialis muscle

Lateral femoral condyle

Medial femoral condyle

Hoffa's fat pad

Tibia

Figure 1.6C

Iliotibial band

Medial femoral condyle cartilage

Lateral trochlear groove cartilage

Medial meniscus anterior horn

Medial tibial plateau cartilage

Pes anserinus

Figure 1.6D

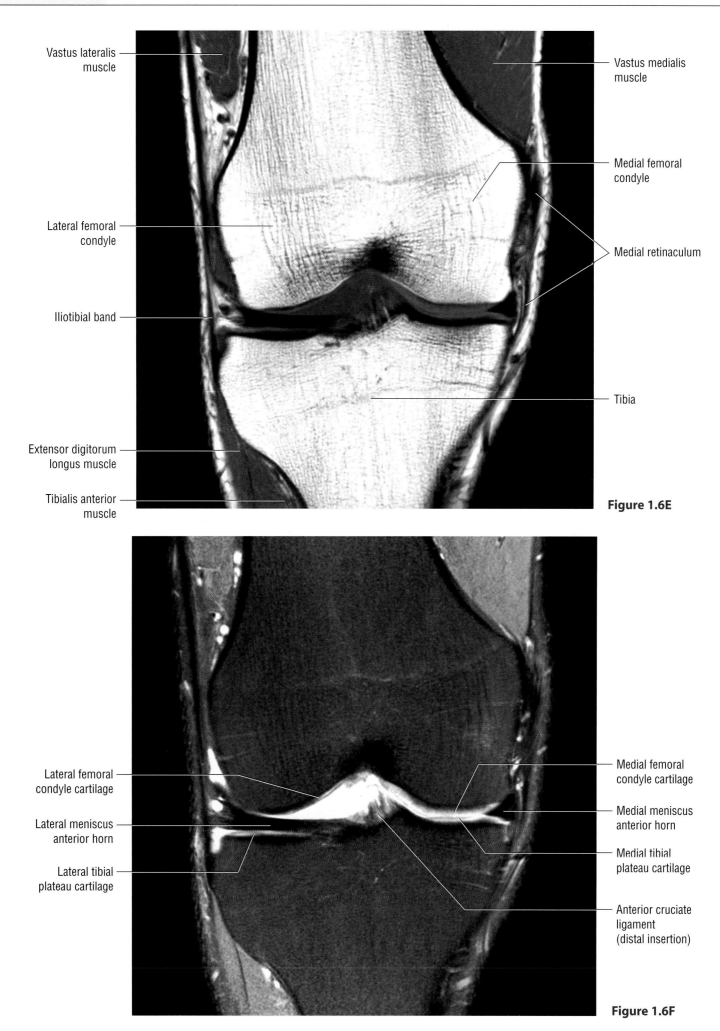

Vastus lateralis muscle

Vastus medialis muscle

Medial femoral condyle

Lateral femoral condyle

Medial retinaculum

Iliotibial band

Tibia

Extensor digitorum longus muscle

Tibialis anterior muscle

Figure 1.6E

Lateral femoral condyle cartilage

Medial femoral condyle cartilage

Lateral meniscus anterior horn

Medial meniscus anterior horn

Lateral tibial plateau cartilage

Medial tibial plateau cartilage

Anterior cruciate ligament (distal insertion)

Figure 1.6F

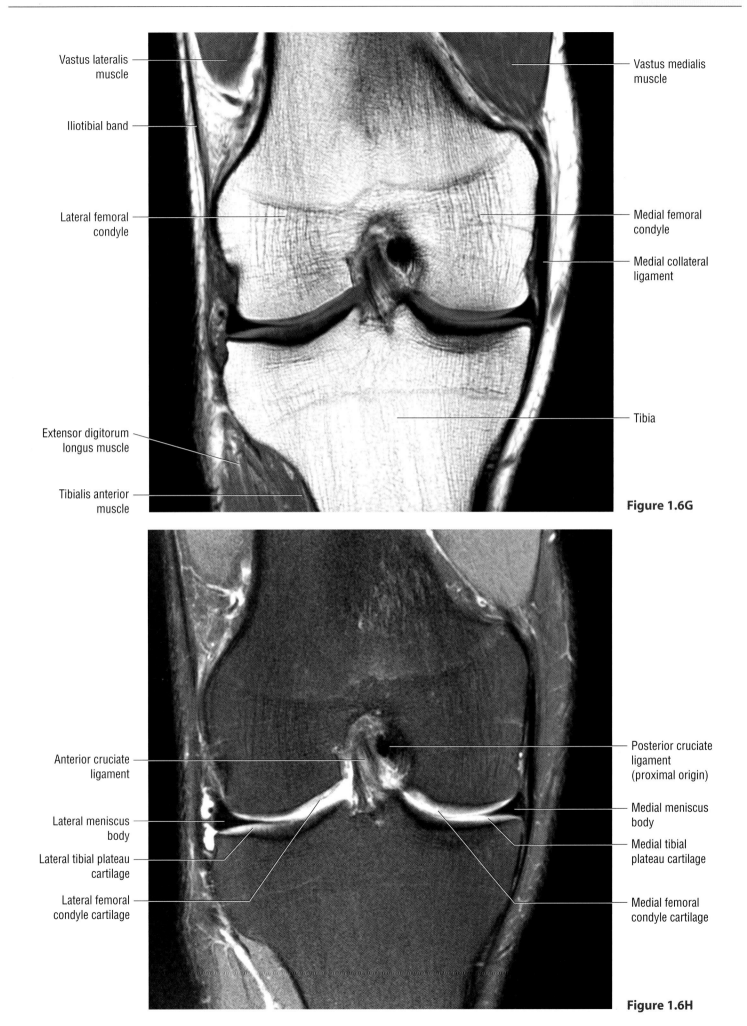

Vastus lateralis muscle

Iliotibial band

Lateral femoral condyle

Extensor digitorum longus muscle

Tibialis anterior muscle

Vastus medialis muscle

Medial femoral condyle

Medial collateral ligament

Tibia

Figure 1.6G

Anterior cruciate ligament

Lateral meniscus body

Lateral tibial plateau cartilage

Lateral femoral condyle cartilage

Posterior cruciate ligament (proximal origin)

Medial meniscus body

Medial tibial plateau cartilage

Medial femoral condyle cartilage

Figure 1.6H

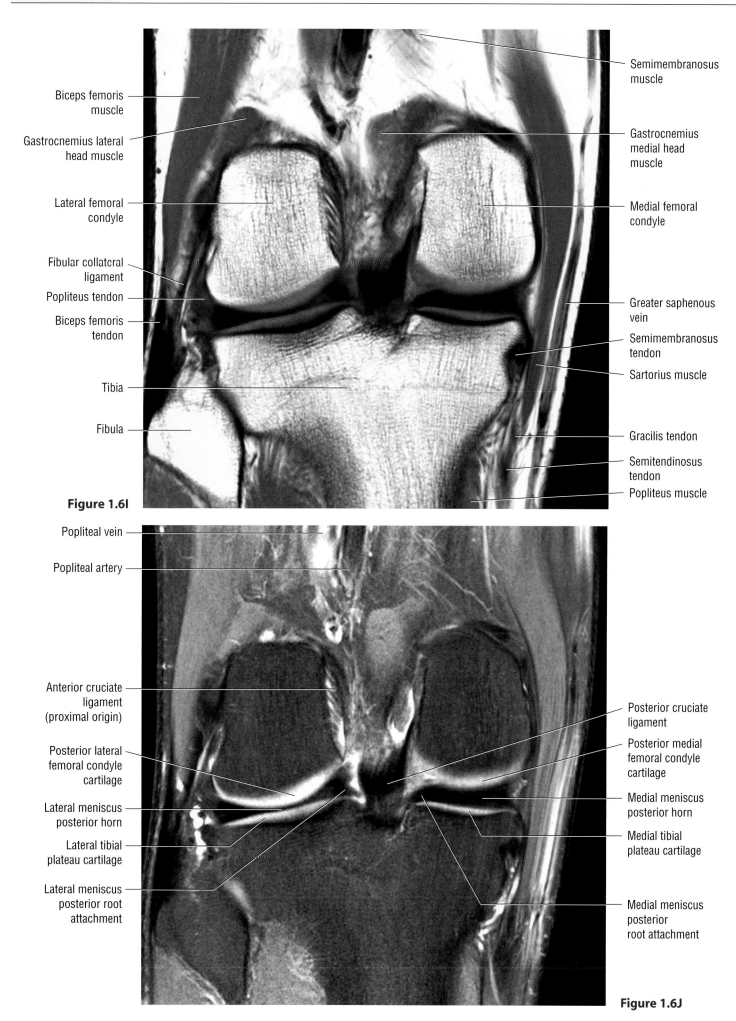

Superior
Lateral ─┼─ Medial
Inferior

Biceps femoris muscle

Gastrocnemius lateral head muscle

Lateral femoral condyle

Fibular collateral ligament

Popliteus tendon

Biceps femoris tendon

Tibia

Fibula

Figure 1.6I

Semimembranosus muscle

Gastrocnemius medial head muscle

Medial femoral condyle

Greater saphenous vein

Semimembranosus tendon

Sartorius muscle

Gracilis tendon

Semitendinosus tendon

Popliteus muscle

Popliteal vein

Popliteal artery

Anterior cruciate ligament (proximal origin)

Posterior lateral femoral condyle cartilage

Lateral meniscus posterior horn

Lateral tibial plateau cartilage

Lateral meniscus posterior root attachment

Posterior cruciate ligament

Posterior medial femoral condyle cartilage

Medial meniscus posterior horn

Medial tibial plateau cartilage

Medial meniscus posterior root attachment

Figure 1.6J

Knee - Coronal

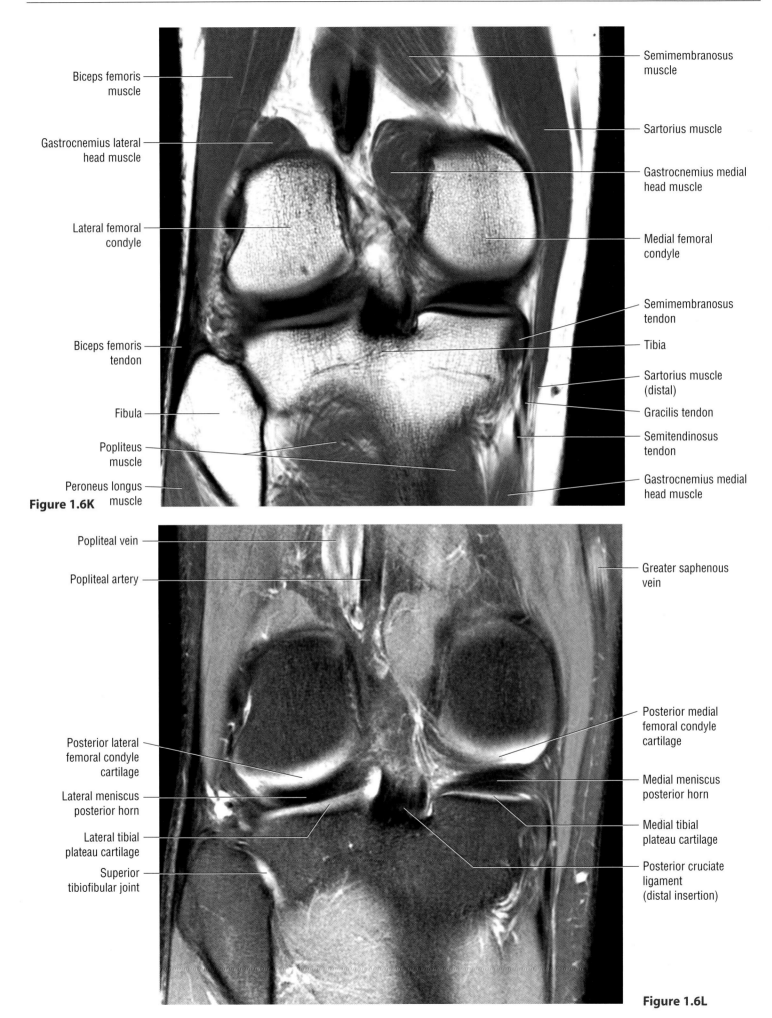

Biceps femoris muscle

Gastrocnemius lateral head muscle

Lateral femoral condyle

Biceps femoris tendon

Fibula

Popliteus muscle

Peroneus longus muscle

Semimembranosus muscle

Sartorius muscle

Gastrocnemius medial head muscle

Medial femoral condyle

Semimembranosus tendon

Tibia

Sartorius muscle (distal)

Gracilis tendon

Semitendinosus tendon

Gastrocnemius medial head muscle

Figure 1.6K

Popliteal vein

Popliteal artery

Posterior lateral femoral condyle cartilage

Lateral meniscus posterior horn

Lateral tibial plateau cartilage

Superior tibiofibular joint

Greater saphenous vein

Posterior medial femoral condyle cartilage

Medial meniscus posterior horn

Medial tibial plateau cartilage

Posterior cruciate ligament (distal insertion)

Figure 1.6L

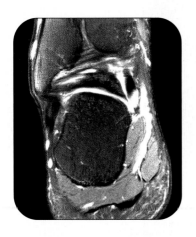

The Ankle and Foot
MR Normal Anatomy

Sagittal

Coronal

Axial

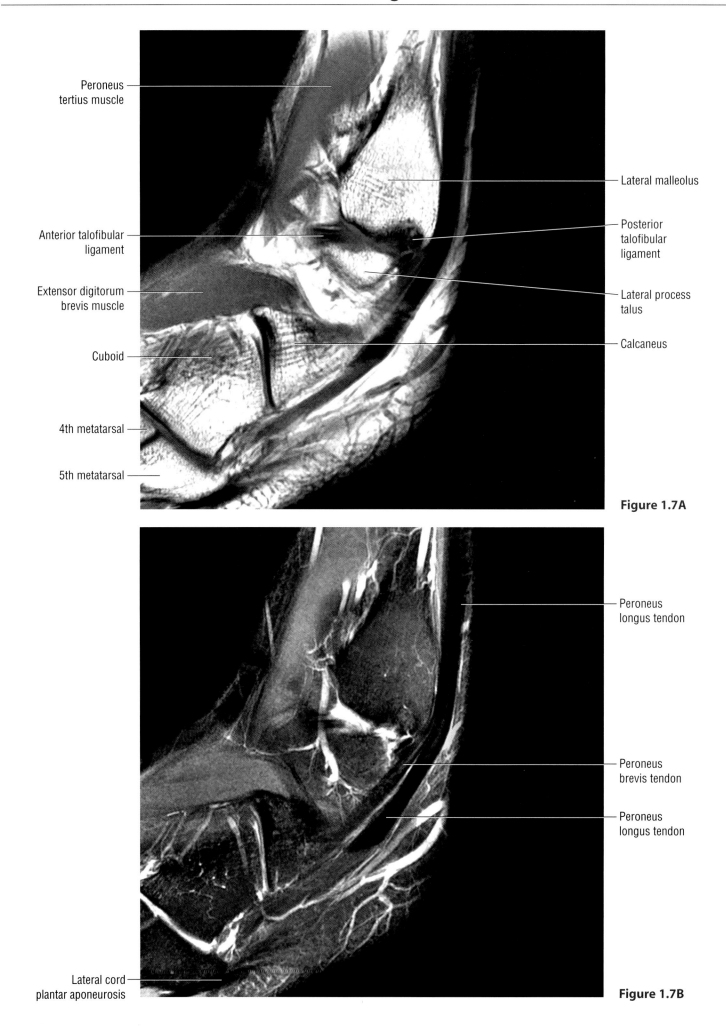

Peroneus tertius muscle

Lateral malleolus

Anterior talofibular ligament

Posterior talofibular ligament

Extensor digitorum brevis muscle

Lateral process talus

Cuboid

Calcaneus

4th metatarsal

5th metatarsal

Figure 1.7A

Peroneus longus tendon

Peroneus brevis tendon

Peroneus longus tendon

Lateral cord plantar aponeurosis

Figure 1.7B

Superior
Anterior — Posterior
Inferior

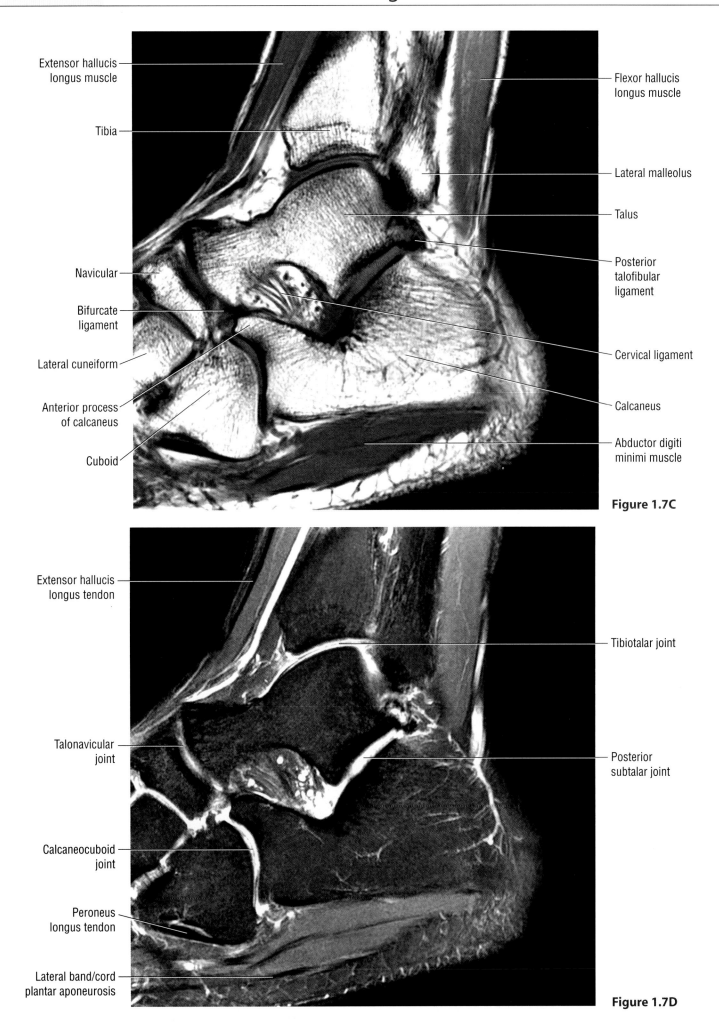

Extensor hallucis
longus muscle

Tibia

Navicular

Bifurcate
ligament

Lateral cuneiform

Anterior process
of calcaneus

Cuboid

Flexor hallucis
longus muscle

Lateral malleolus

Talus

Posterior
talofibular
ligament

Cervical ligament

Calcaneus

Abductor digiti
minimi muscle

Figure 1.7C

Extensor hallucis
longus tendon

Talonavicular
joint

Calcaneocuboid
joint

Peroneus
longus tendon

Lateral band/cord
plantar aponeurosis

Tibiotalar joint

Posterior
subtalar joint

Figure 1.7D

Ankle - Sagittal

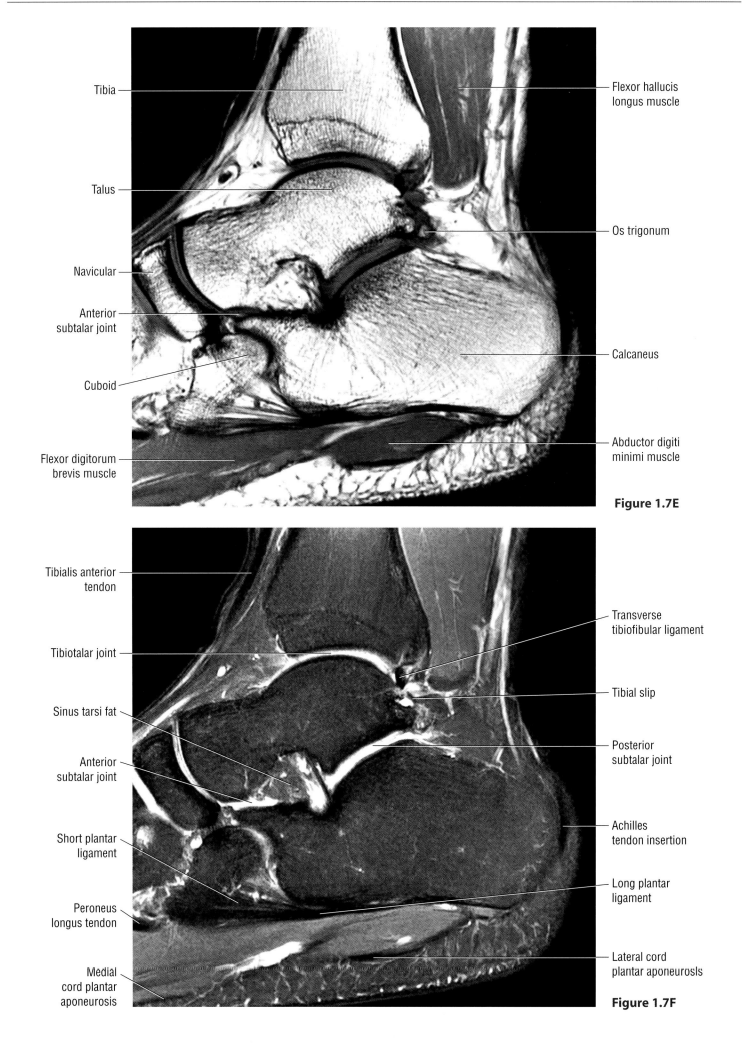

Tibia

Talus

Navicular

Anterior subtalar joint

Cuboid

Flexor digitorum brevis muscle

Flexor hallucis longus muscle

Os trigonum

Calcaneus

Abductor digiti minimi muscle

Figure 1.7E

Tibialis anterior tendon

Tibiotalar joint

Sinus tarsi fat

Anterior subtalar joint

Short plantar ligament

Peroneus longus tendon

Medial cord plantar aponeurosis

Transverse tibiofibular ligament

Tibial slip

Posterior subtalar joint

Achilles tendon insertion

Long plantar ligament

Lateral cord plantar aponeurosis

Figure 1.7F

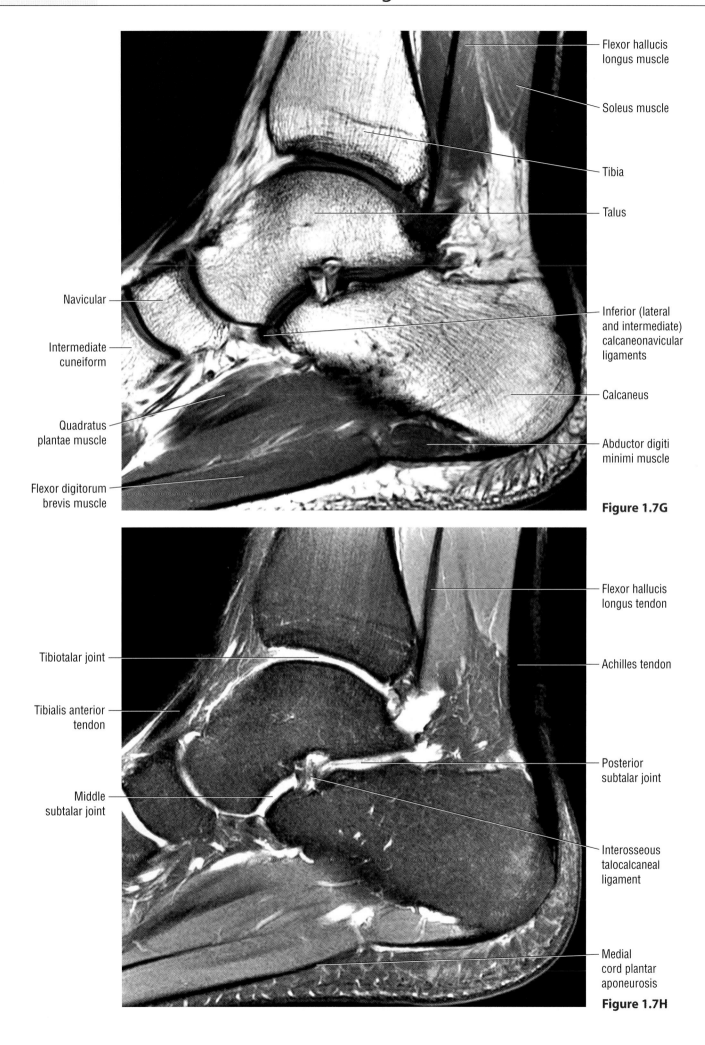

Flexor hallucis longus muscle

Soleus muscle

Tibia

Talus

Navicular

Inferior (lateral and intermediate) calcaneonavicular ligaments

Intermediate cuneiform

Calcaneus

Quadratus plantae muscle

Abductor digiti minimi muscle

Flexor digitorum brevis muscle

Figure 1.7G

Flexor hallucis longus tendon

Tibiotalar joint

Achilles tendon

Tibialis anterior tendon

Posterior subtalar joint

Middle subtalar joint

Interosseous talocalcaneal ligament

Medial cord plantar aponeurosis

Figure 1.7H

Ankle - Sagittal

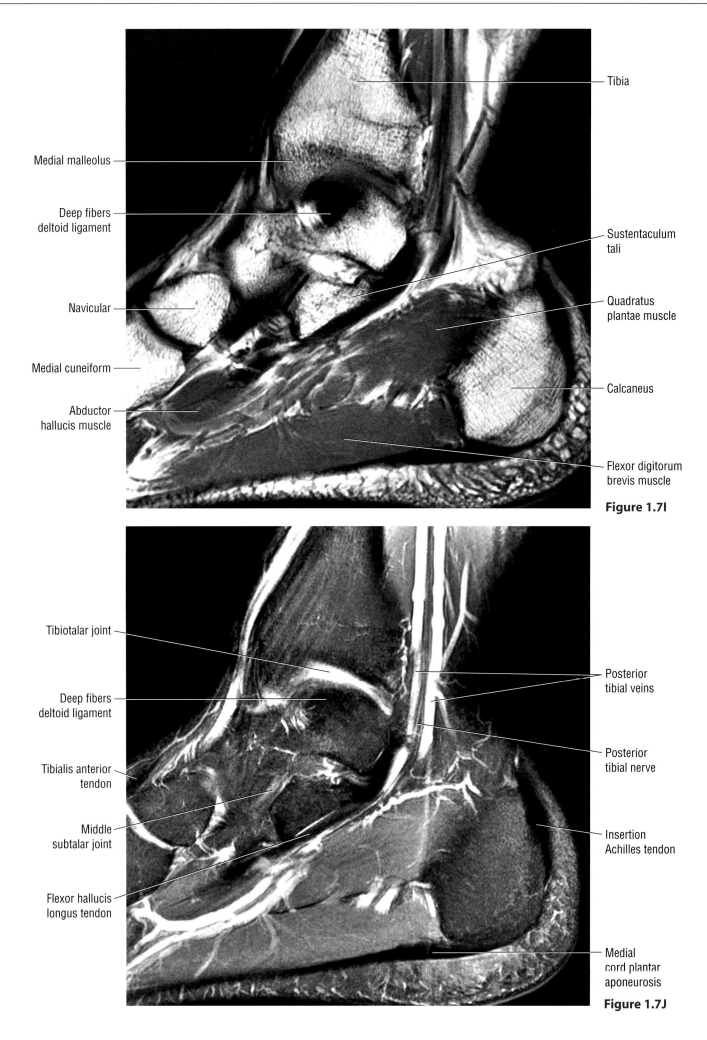

Tibia

Medial malleolus

Deep fibers
deltoid ligament

Sustentaculum
tali

Navicular

Quadratus
plantae muscle

Medial cuneiform

Abductor
hallucis muscle

Calcaneus

Flexor digitorum
brevis muscle

Figure 1.7I

Tibiotalar joint

Posterior
tibial veins

Deep fibers
deltoid ligament

Tibialis anterior
tendon

Posterior
tibial nerve

Middle
subtalar joint

Insertion
Achilles tendon

Flexor hallucis
longus tendon

Medial
cord plantar
aponeurosis

Figure 1.7J

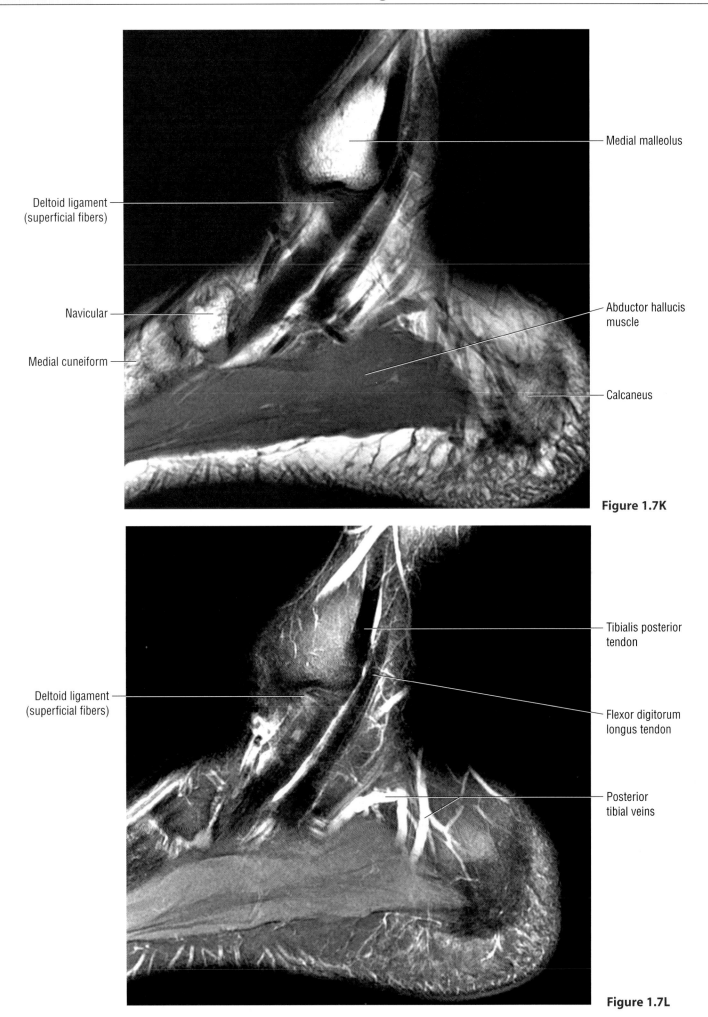

Medial malleolus

Deltoid ligament
(superficial fibers)

Navicular

Medial cuneiform

Abductor hallucis
muscle

Calcaneus

Figure 1.7K

Tibialis posterior
tendon

Deltoid ligament
(superficial fibers)

Flexor digitorum
longus tendon

Posterior
tibial veins

Figure 1.7L

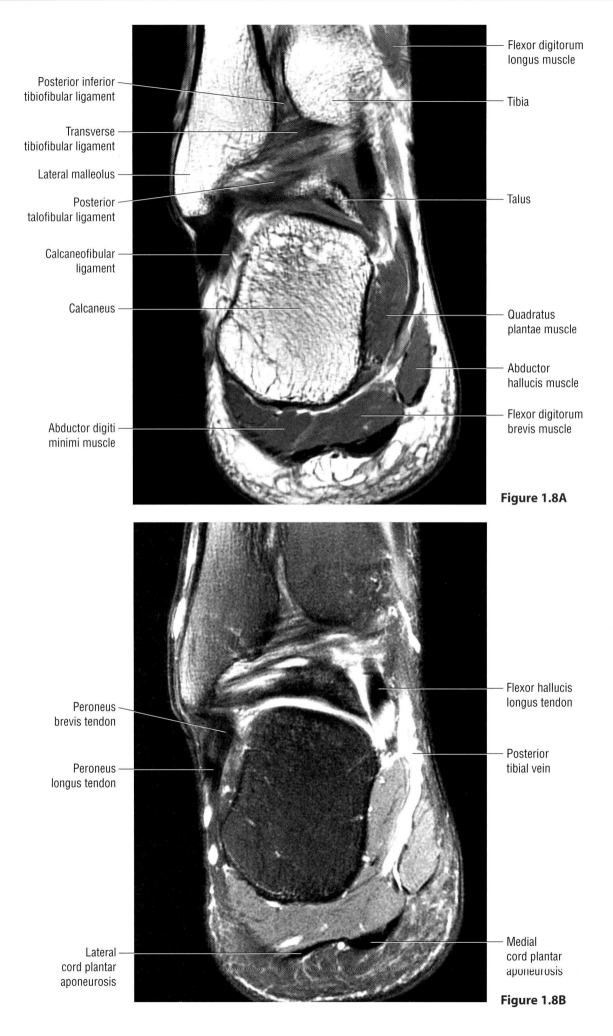

Posterior inferior tibiofibular ligament

Transverse tibiofibular ligament

Lateral malleolus

Posterior talofibular ligament

Calcaneofibular ligament

Calcaneus

Abductor digiti minimi muscle

Flexor digitorum longus muscle

Tibia

Talus

Quadratus plantae muscle

Abductor hallucis muscle

Flexor digitorum brevis muscle

Figure 1.8A

Peroneus brevis tendon

Peroneus longus tendon

Lateral cord plantar aponeurosis

Flexor hallucis longus tendon

Posterior tibial vein

Medial cord plantar aponeurosis

Figure 1.8B

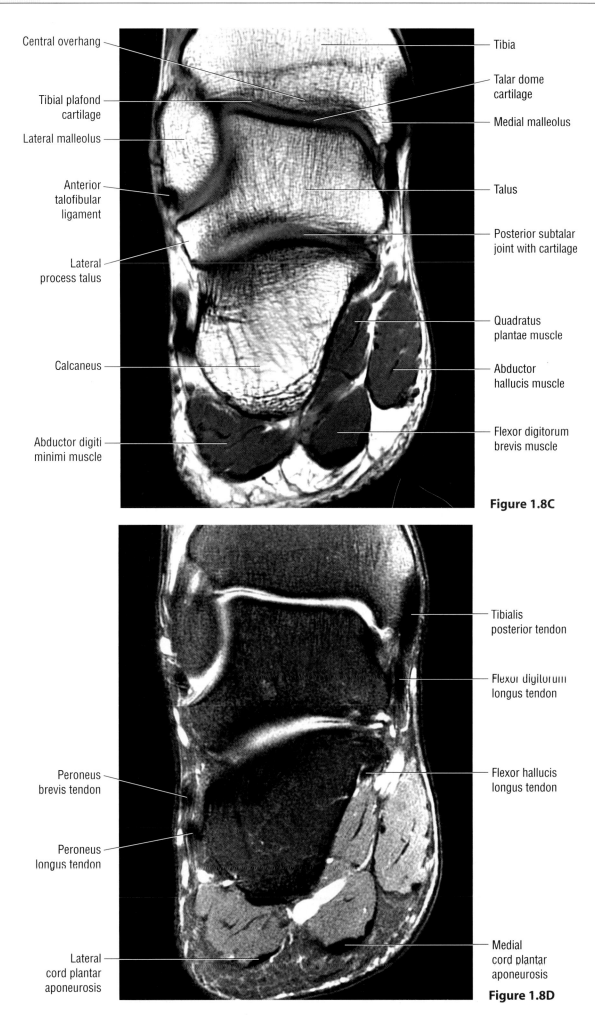

Central overhang

Tibial plafond cartilage

Lateral malleolus

Anterior talofibular ligament

Lateral process talus

Calcaneus

Abductor digiti minimi muscle

Tibia

Talar dome cartilage

Medial malleolus

Talus

Posterior subtalar joint with cartilage

Quadratus plantae muscle

Abductor hallucis muscle

Flexor digitorum brevis muscle

Figure 1.8C

Peroneus brevis tendon

Peroneus longus tendon

Lateral cord plantar aponeurosis

Tibialis posterior tendon

Flexor digitorum longus tendon

Flexor hallucis longus tendon

Medial cord plantar aponeurosis

Figure 1.8D

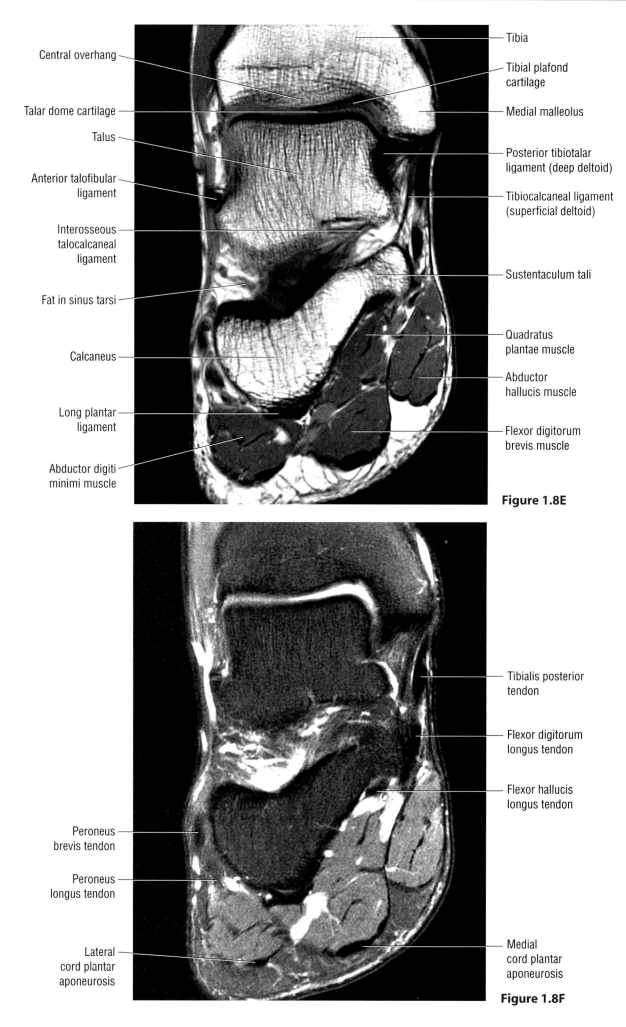

Central overhang

Talar dome cartilage

Talus

Anterior talofibular
ligament

Interosseous
talocalcaneal
ligament

Fat in sinus tarsi

Calcaneus

Long plantar
ligament

Abductor digiti
minimi muscle

Tibia

Tibial plafond
cartilage

Medial malleolus

Posterior tibiotalar
ligament (deep deltoid)

Tibiocalcaneal ligament
(superficial deltoid)

Sustentaculum tali

Quadratus
plantae muscle

Abductor
hallucis muscle

Flexor digitorum
brevis muscle

Figure 1.8E

Peroneus
brevis tendon

Peroneus
longus tendon

Lateral
cord plantar
aponeurosis

Tibialis posterior
tendon

Flexor digitorum
longus tendon

Flexor hallucis
longus tendon

Medial
cord plantar
aponeurosis

Figure 1.8F

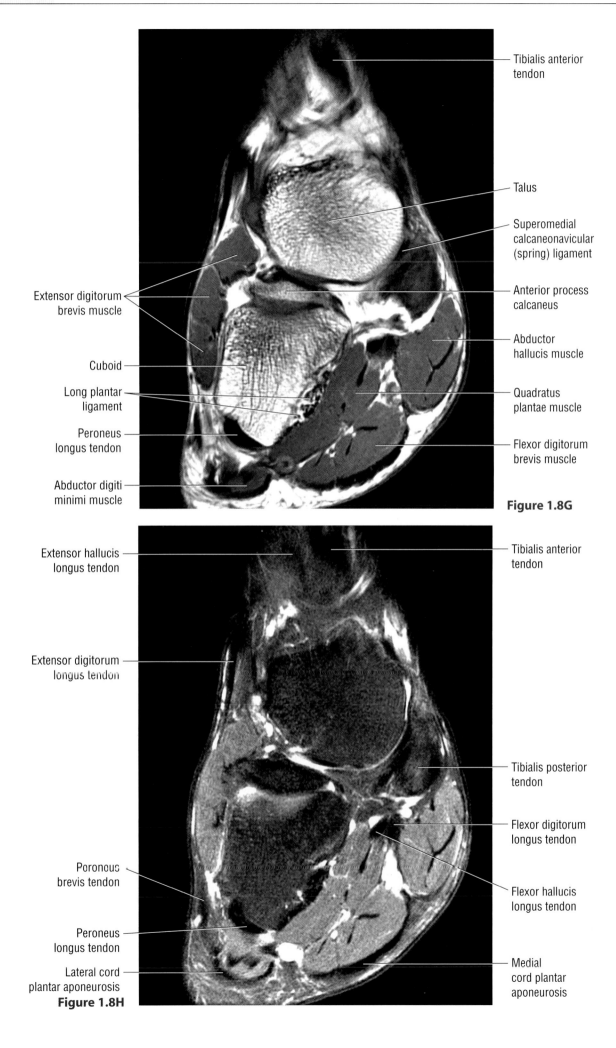

Tibialis anterior tendon

Talus

Superomedial calcaneonavicular (spring) ligament

Anterior process calcaneus

Abductor hallucis muscle

Quadratus plantae muscle

Flexor digitorum brevis muscle

Extensor digitorum brevis muscle

Cuboid

Long plantar ligament

Peroneus longus tendon

Abductor digiti minimi muscle

Figure 1.8G

Extensor hallucis longus tendon

Tibialis anterior tendon

Extensor digitorum longus tendon

Tibialis posterior tendon

Flexor digitorum longus tendon

Peroneus brevis tendon

Flexor hallucis longus tendon

Peroneus longus tendon

Lateral cord plantar aponeurosis

Medial cord plantar aponeurosis

Figure 1.8H

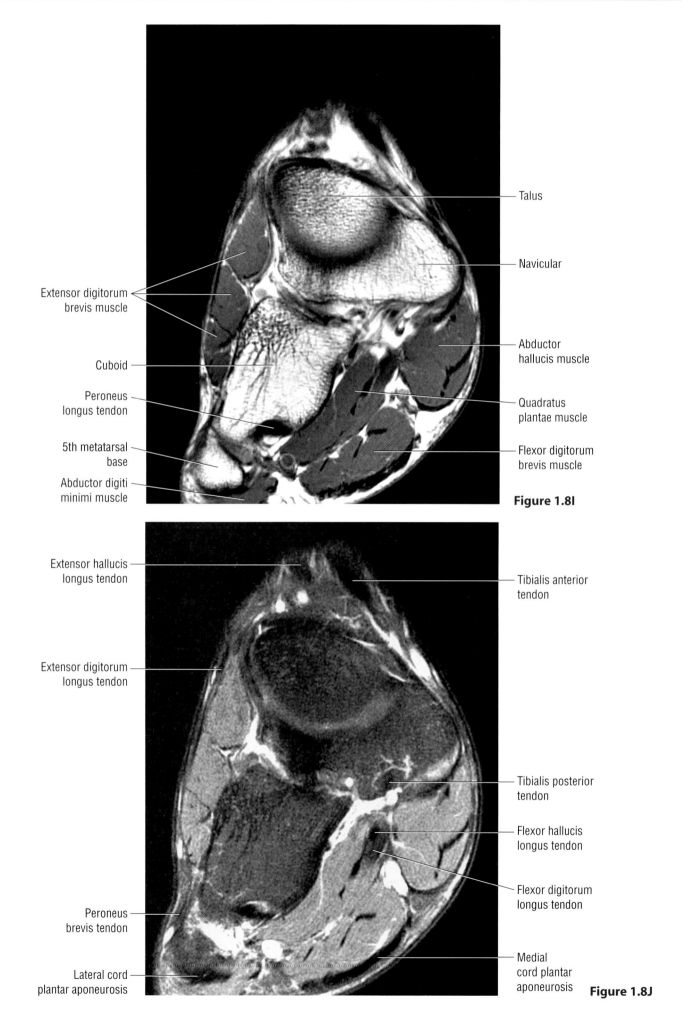

Talus

Navicular

Extensor digitorum
brevis muscle

Abductor
hallucis muscle

Cuboid

Peroneus
longus tendon

Quadratus
plantae muscle

5th metatarsal
base

Flexor digitorum
brevis muscle

Abductor digiti
minimi muscle

Figure 1.8I

Extensor hallucis
longus tendon

Tibialis anterior
tendon

Extensor digitorum
longus tendon

Tibialis posterior
tendon

Flexor hallucis
longus tendon

Flexor digitorum
longus tendon

Peroneus
brevis tendon

Lateral cord
plantar aponeurosis

Medial
cord plantar
aponeurosis

Figure 1.8J

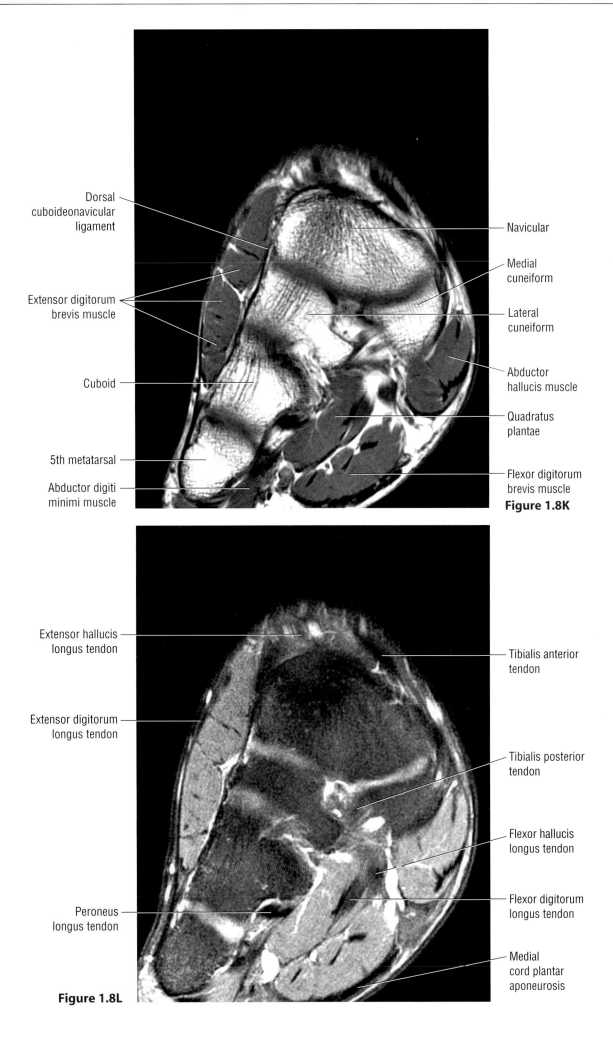

Dorsal cuboideonavicular ligament

Extensor digitorum brevis muscle

Cuboid

5th metatarsal

Abductor digiti minimi muscle

Navicular

Medial cuneiform

Lateral cuneiform

Abductor hallucis muscle

Quadratus plantae

Flexor digitorum brevis muscle

Figure 1.8K

Extensor hallucis longus tendon

Extensor digitorum longus tendon

Peroneus longus tendon

Tibialis anterior tendon

Tibialis posterior tendon

Flexor hallucis longus tendon

Flexor digitorum longus tendon

Medial cord plantar aponeurosis

Figure 1.8L

Ankle - Axial

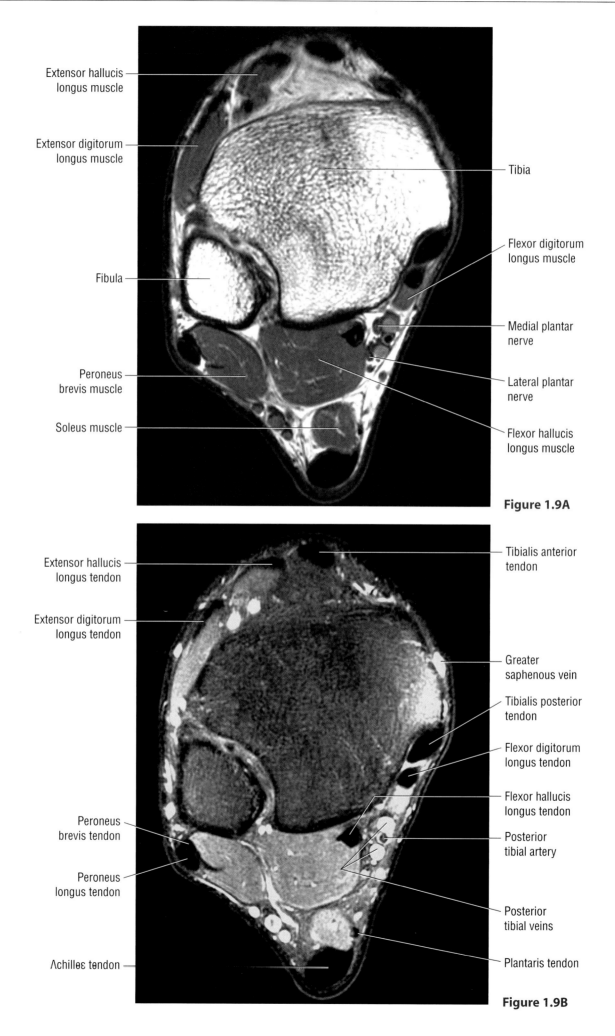

Extensor hallucis longus muscle

Extensor digitorum longus muscle

Fibula

Peroneus brevis muscle

Soleus muscle

Tibia

Flexor digitorum longus muscle

Medial plantar nerve

Lateral plantar nerve

Flexor hallucis longus muscle

Figure 1.9A

Extensor hallucis longus tendon

Extensor digitorum longus tendon

Peroneus brevis tendon

Peroneus longus tendon

Achilles tendon

Tibialis anterior tendon

Greater saphenous vein

Tibialis posterior tendon

Flexor digitorum longus tendon

Flexor hallucis longus tendon

Posterior tibial artery

Posterior tibial veins

Plantaris tendon

Figure 1.9B

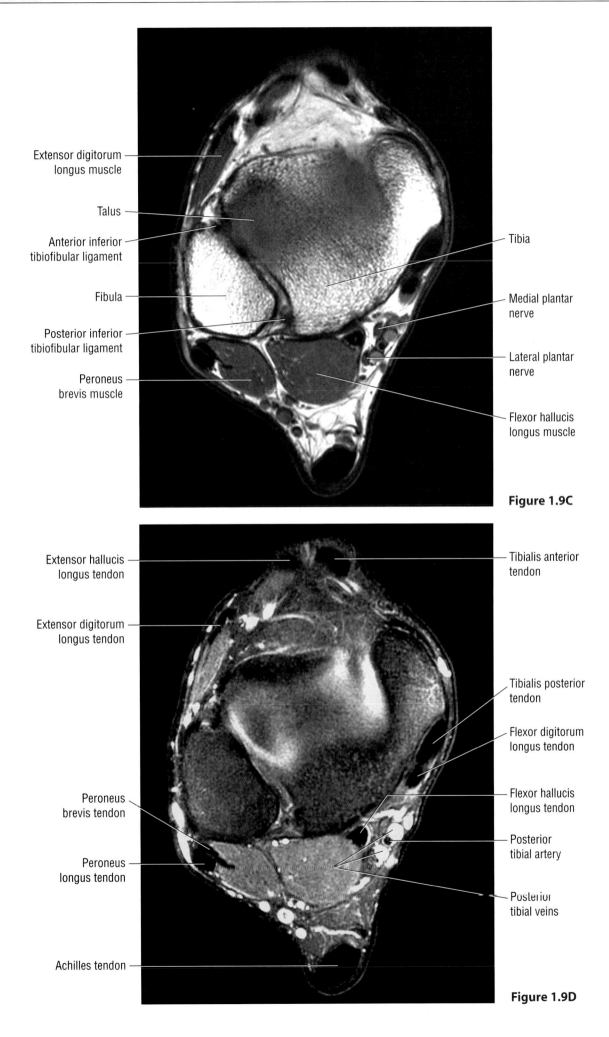

Extensor digitorum longus muscle

Talus

Anterior inferior tibiofibular ligament

Fibula

Posterior inferior tibiofibular ligament

Peroneus brevis muscle

Tibia

Medial plantar nerve

Lateral plantar nerve

Flexor hallucis longus muscle

Figure 1.9C

Extensor hallucis longus tendon

Extensor digitorum longus tendon

Peroneus brevis tendon

Peroneus longus tendon

Achilles tendon

Tibialis anterior tendon

Tibialis posterior tendon

Flexor digitorum longus tendon

Flexor hallucis longus tendon

Posterior tibial artery

Posterior tibial veins

Figure 1.9D

Anterior
Lateral ─┼─ Medial
Posterior

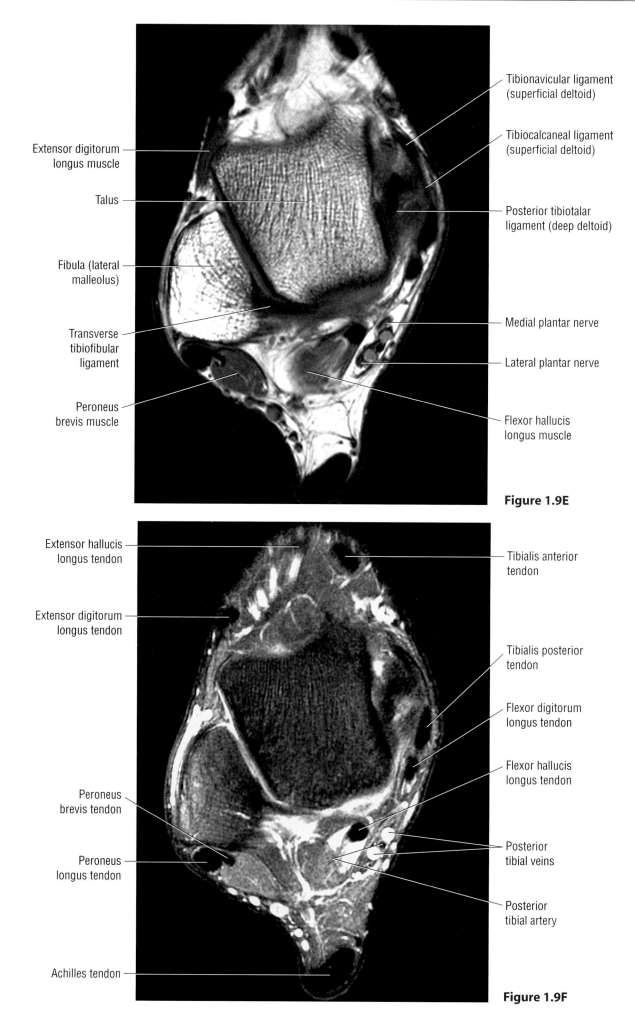

Extensor digitorum longus muscle

Talus

Fibula (lateral malleolus)

Transverse tibiofibular ligament

Peroneus brevis muscle

Tibionavicular ligament (superficial deltoid)

Tibiocalcaneal ligament (superficial deltoid)

Posterior tibiotalar ligament (deep deltoid)

Medial plantar nerve

Lateral plantar nerve

Flexor hallucis longus muscle

Figure 1.9E

Extensor hallucis longus tendon

Extensor digitorum longus tendon

Peroneus brevis tendon

Peroneus longus tendon

Achilles tendon

Tibialis anterior tendon

Tibialis posterior tendon

Flexor digitorum longus tendon

Flexor hallucis longus tendon

Posterior tibial veins

Posterior tibial artery

Figure 1.9F

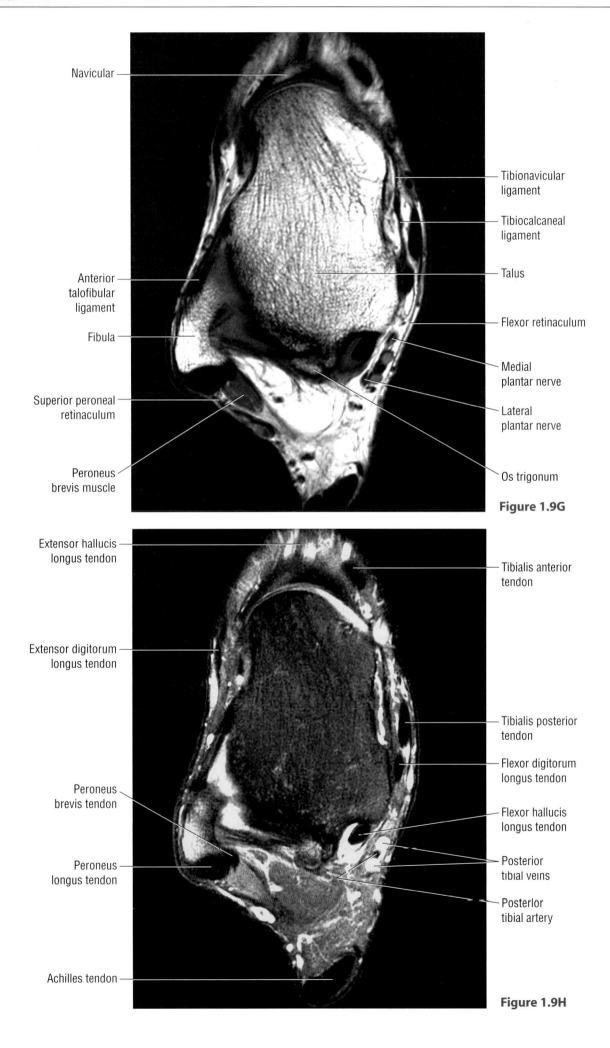

Navicular

Tibionavicular ligament

Tibiocalcaneal ligament

Anterior talofibular ligament

Talus

Flexor retinaculum

Fibula

Medial plantar nerve

Superior peroneal retinaculum

Lateral plantar nerve

Peroneus brevis muscle

Os trigonum

Figure 1.9G

Extensor hallucis longus tendon

Tibialis anterior tendon

Extensor digitorum longus tendon

Tibialis posterior tendon

Flexor digitorum longus tendon

Peroneus brevis tendon

Flexor hallucis longus tendon

Peroneus longus tendon

Posterior tibial veins

Posterior tibial artery

Achilles tendon

Figure 1.9H

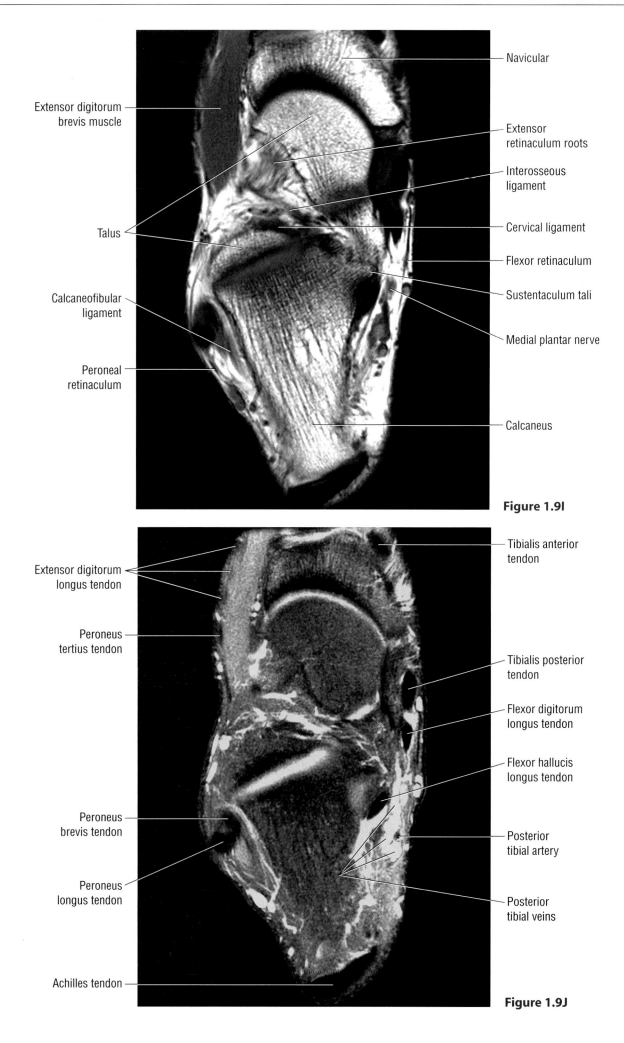

Navicular

Extensor digitorum brevis muscle

Extensor retinaculum roots

Interosseous ligament

Talus

Cervical ligament

Flexor retinaculum

Calcaneofibular ligament

Sustentaculum tali

Medial plantar nerve

Peroneal retinaculum

Calcaneus

Figure 1.9I

Tibialis anterior tendon

Extensor digitorum longus tendon

Peroneus tertius tendon

Tibialis posterior tendon

Flexor digitorum longus tendon

Flexor hallucis longus tendon

Peroneus brevis tendon

Posterior tibial artery

Peroneus longus tendon

Posterior tibial veins

Achilles tendon

Figure 1.9J

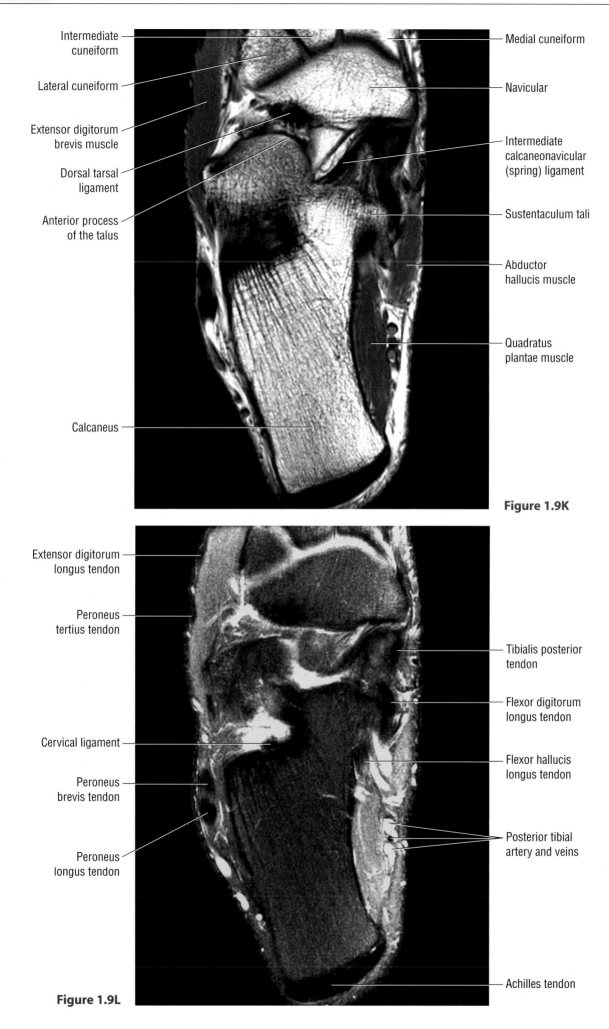

Intermediate cuneiform

Lateral cuneiform

Extensor digitorum brevis muscle

Dorsal tarsal ligament

Anterior process of the talus

Calcaneus

Medial cuneiform

Navicular

Intermediate calcaneonavicular (spring) ligament

Sustentaculum tali

Abductor hallucis muscle

Quadratus plantae muscle

Figure 1.9K

Extensor digitorum longus tendon

Peroneus tertius tendon

Cervical ligament

Peroneus brevis tendon

Peroneus longus tendon

Tibialis posterior tendon

Flexor digitorum longus tendon

Flexor hallucis longus tendon

Posterior tibial artery and veins

Achilles tendon

Figure 1.9L

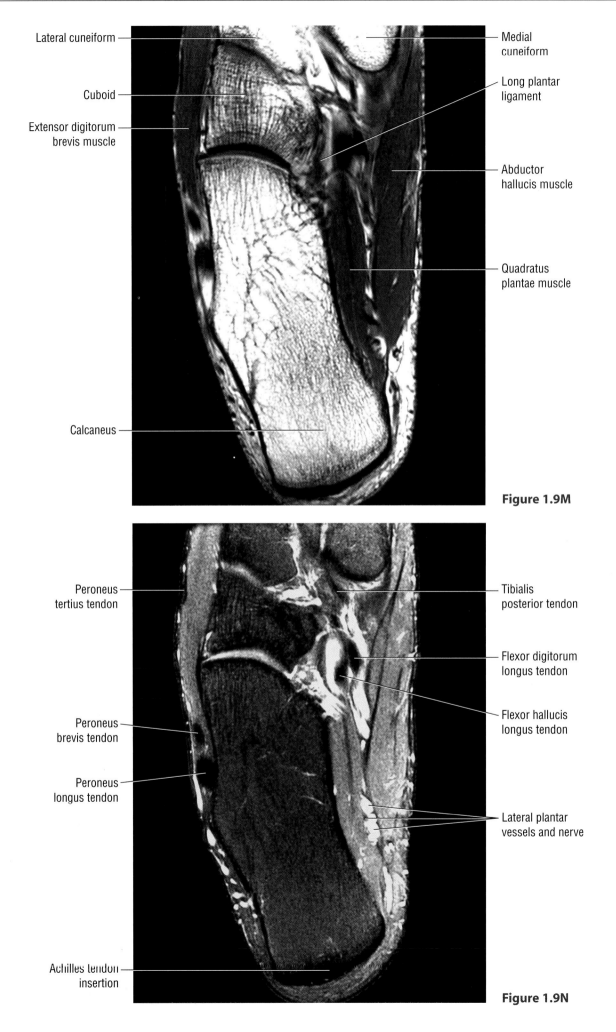

Lateral cuneiform

Cuboid

Extensor digitorum
brevis muscle

Calcaneus

Medial
cuneiform

Long plantar
ligament

Abductor
hallucis muscle

Quadratus
plantae muscle

Figure 1.9M

Peroneus
tertius tendon

Peroneus
brevis tendon

Peroneus
longus tendon

Achilles tendon
insertion

Tibialis
posterior tendon

Flexor digitorum
longus tendon

Flexor hallucis
longus tendon

Lateral plantar
vessels and nerve

Figure 1.9N

Chapter

2

MR Normal Anatomy: *Upper Extremity*

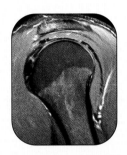

The Shoulder

Figures 2.1 to 2.3
Pages 65–84

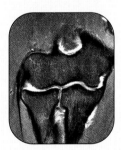

The Elbow

Figures 2.4 to 2.6
Pages 85–104

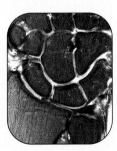

The Wrist

Figures 2.7 to 2.9
Pages 105-124

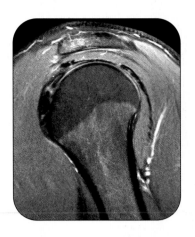

The Shoulder
MR Normal Anatomy

Coronal

Axial

Sagittal

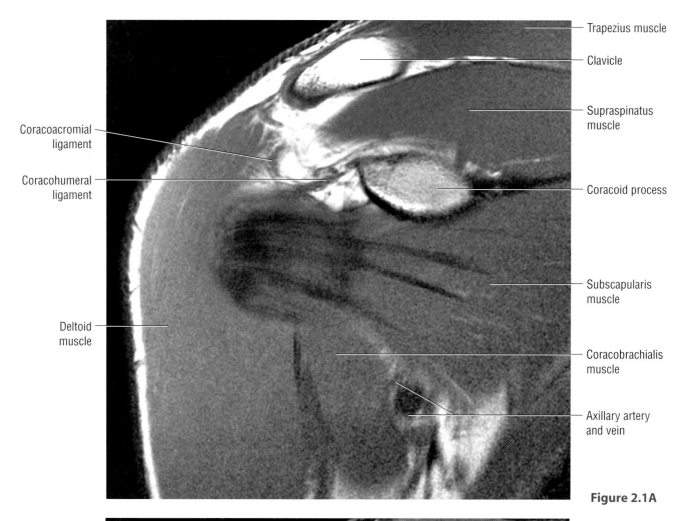

Trapezius muscle

Clavicle

Supraspinatus
muscle

Coracoacromial
ligament

Coracohumeral
ligament

Coracoid process

Subscapularis
muscle

Deltoid
muscle

Coracobrachialis
muscle

Axillary artery
and vein

Figure 2.1A

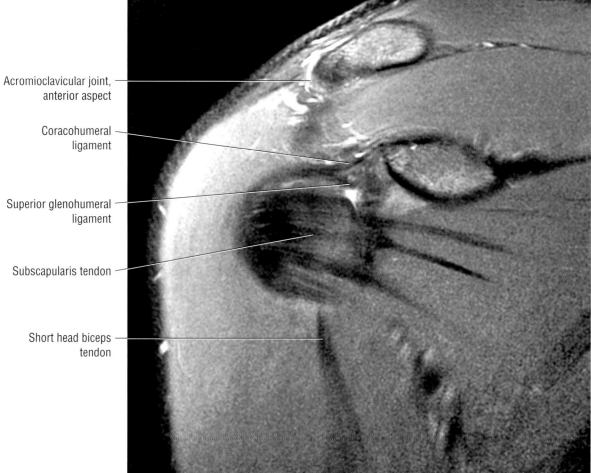

Acromioclavicular joint,
anterior aspect

Coracohumeral
ligament

Superior glenohumeral
ligament

Subscapularis tendon

Short head biceps
tendon

Figure 2.1B

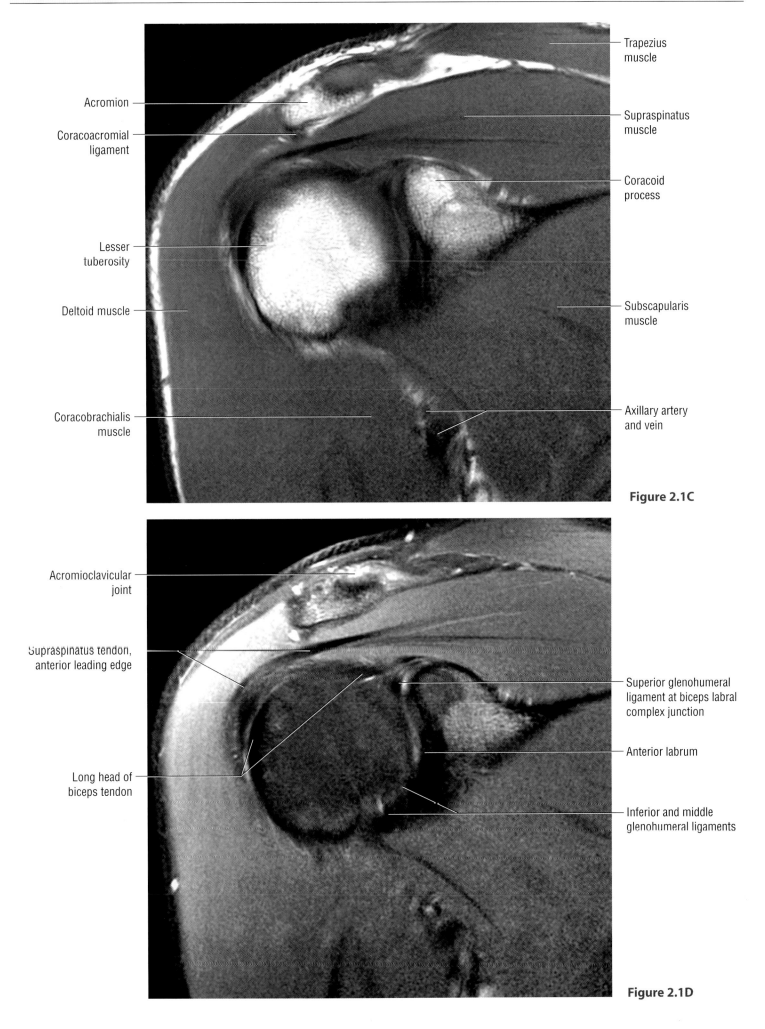

Trapezius
muscle

Acromion

Supraspinatus
muscle

Coracoacromial
ligament

Coracoid
process

Lesser
tuberosity

Deltoid muscle

Subscapularis
muscle

Coracobrachialis
muscle

Axillary artery
and vein

Figure 2.1C

Acromioclavicular
joint

Supraspinatus tendon,
anterior leading edge

Superior glenohumeral
ligament at biceps labral
complex junction

Anterior labrum

Long head of
biceps tendon

Inferior and middle
glenohumeral ligaments

Figure 2.1D

Shoulder - Coronal

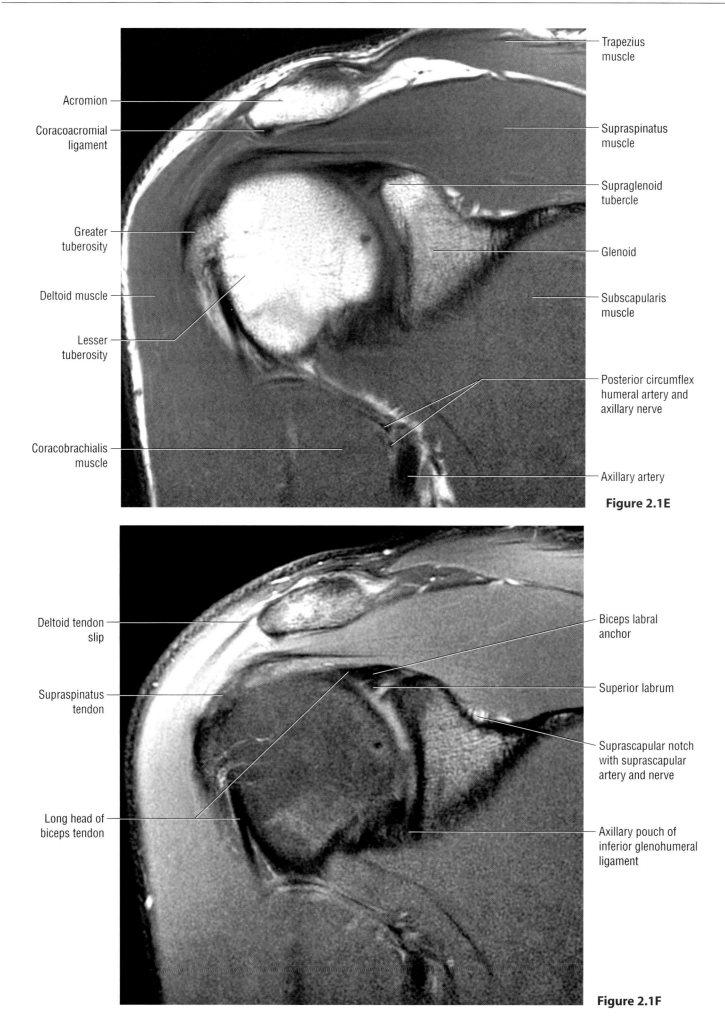

Trapezius
muscle

Acromion

Coracoacromial
ligament

Supraspinatus
muscle

Supraglenoid
tubercle

Greater
tuberosity

Glenoid

Deltoid muscle

Subscapularis
muscle

Lesser
tuberosity

Posterior circumflex
humeral artery and
axillary nerve

Coracobrachialis
muscle

Axillary artery

Figure 2.1E

Deltoid tendon
slip

Biceps labral
anchor

Supraspinatus
tendon

Superior labrum

Suprascapular notch
with suprascapular
artery and nerve

Long head of
biceps tendon

Axillary pouch of
inferior glenohumeral
ligament

Figure 2.1F

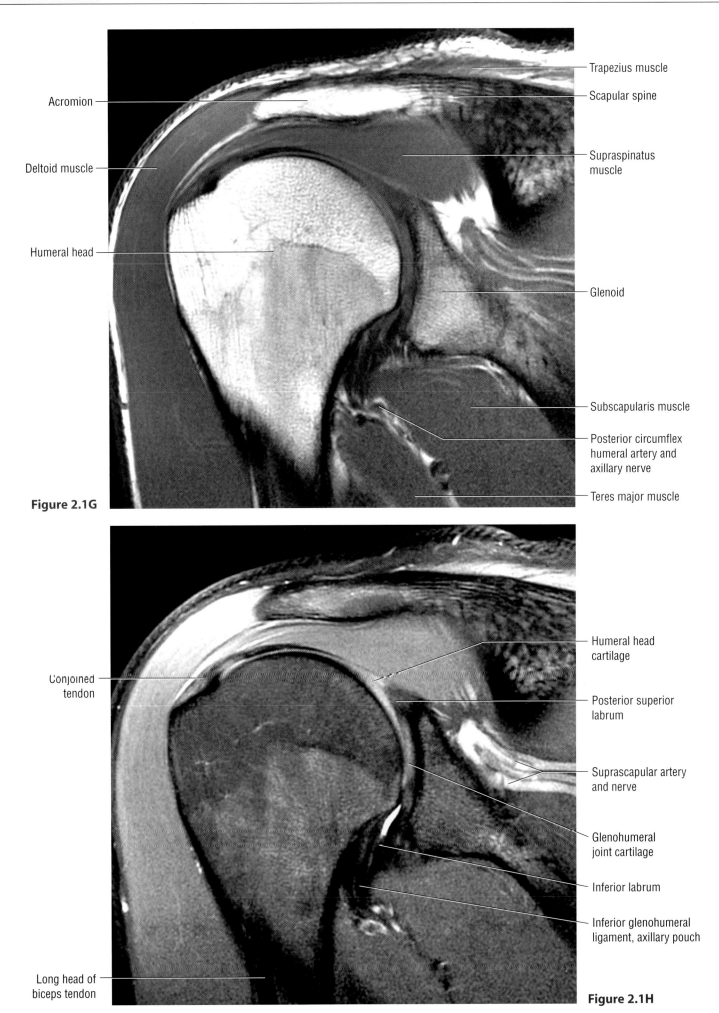

Acromion

Deltoid muscle

Humeral head

Trapezius muscle

Scapular spine

Supraspinatus muscle

Glenoid

Subscapularis muscle

Posterior circumflex humeral artery and axillary nerve

Teres major muscle

Figure 2.1G

Conjoined tendon

Long head of biceps tendon

Humeral head cartilage

Posterior superior labrum

Suprascapular artery and nerve

Glenohumeral joint cartilage

Inferior labrum

Inferior glenohumeral ligament, axillary pouch

Figure 2.1H

Shoulder - Coronal

Superior
Lateral ✛ Medial
Inferior

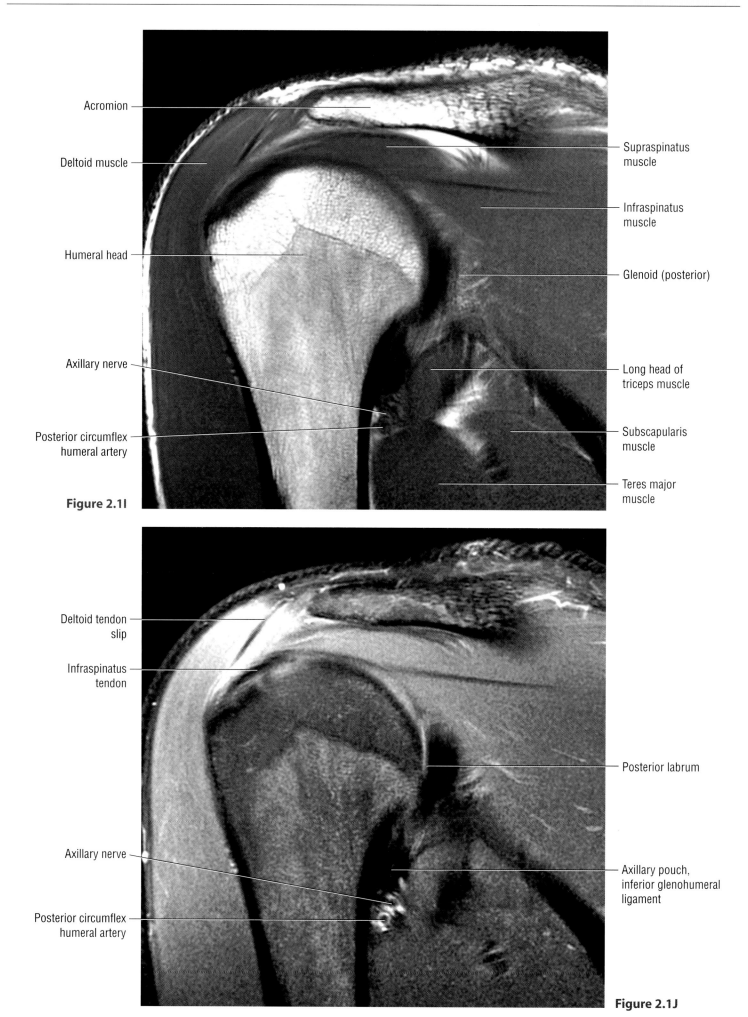

Acromion

Deltoid muscle

Humeral head

Axillary nerve

Posterior circumflex
humeral artery

Supraspinatus
muscle

Infraspinatus
muscle

Glenoid (posterior)

Long head of
triceps muscle

Subscapularis
muscle

Teres major
muscle

Figure 2.1I

Deltoid tendon
slip

Infraspinatus
tendon

Axillary nerve

Posterior circumflex
humeral artery

Posterior labrum

Axillary pouch,
inferior glenohumeral
ligament

Figure 2.1J

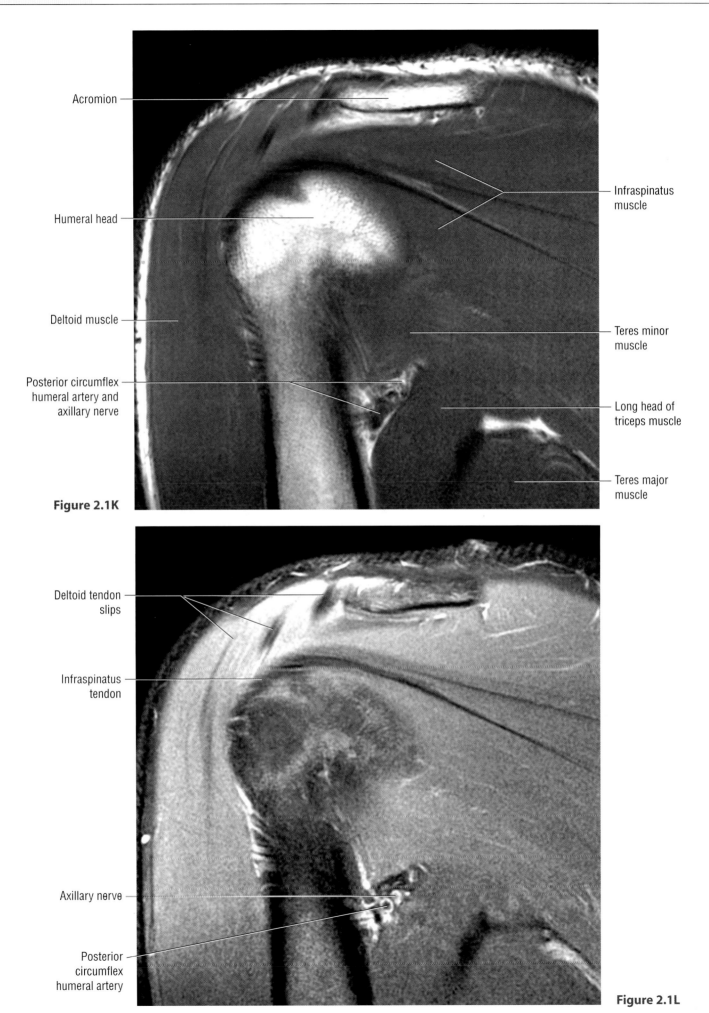

Acromion

Humeral head

Deltoid muscle

Posterior circumflex
humeral artery and
axillary nerve

Infraspinatus
muscle

Teres minor
muscle

Long head of
triceps muscle

Teres major
muscle

Figure 2.1K

Deltoid tendon
slips

Infraspinatus
tendon

Axillary nerve

Posterior
circumflex
humeral artery

Figure 2.1L

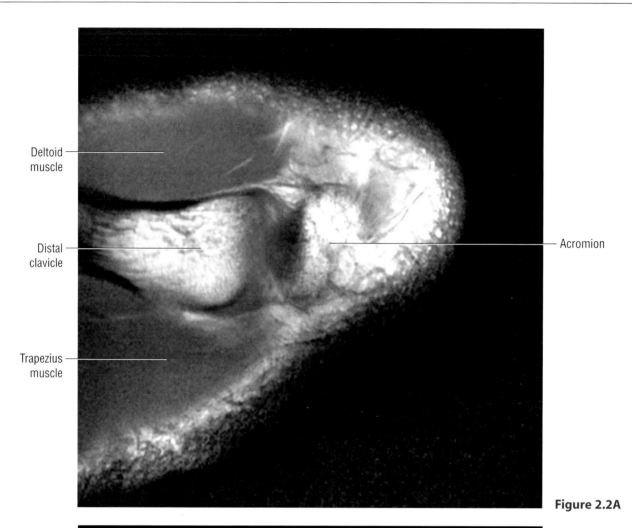

Deltoid muscle

Distal clavicle

Trapezius muscle

Acromion

Figure 2.2A

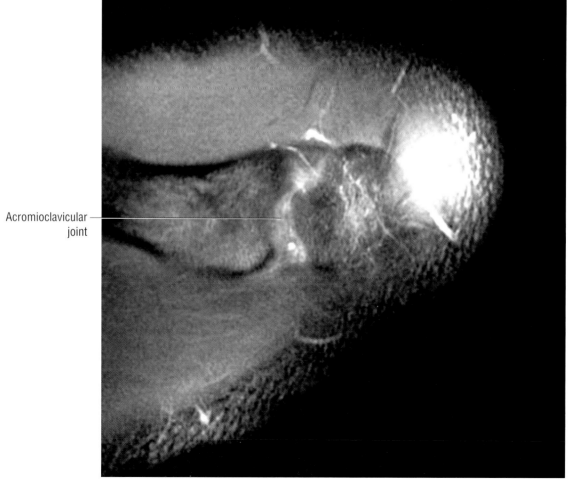

Acromioclavicular joint

Figure 2.2B

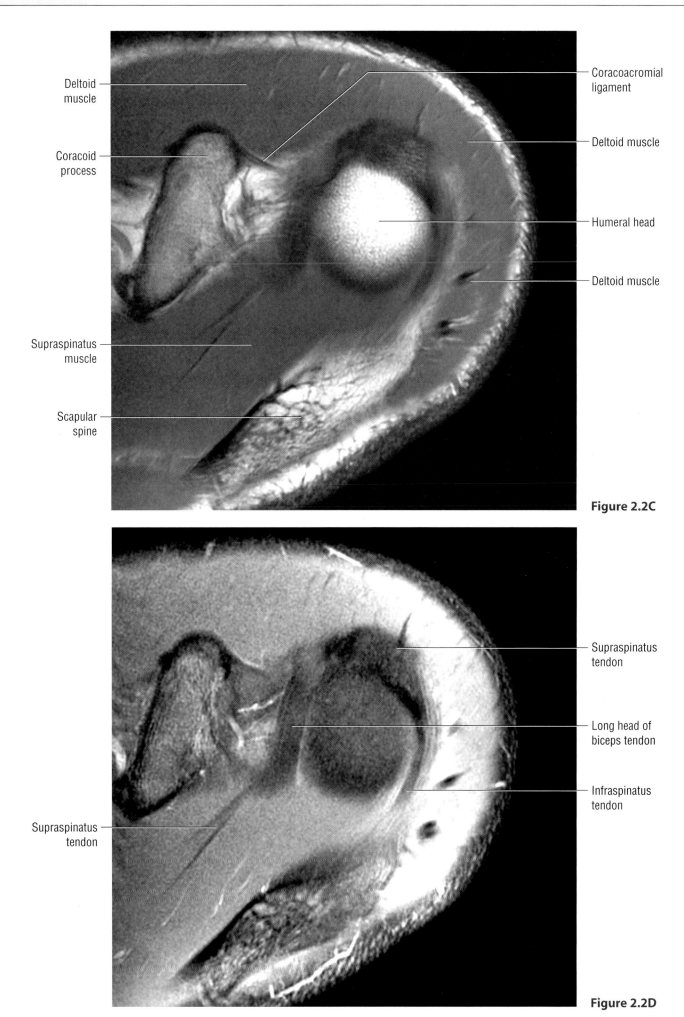

Deltoid muscle

Coracoid process

Supraspinatus muscle

Scapular spine

Coracoacromial ligament

Deltoid muscle

Humeral head

Deltoid muscle

Figure 2.2C

Supraspinatus tendon

Long head of biceps tendon

Infraspinatus tendon

Supraspinatus tendon

Figure 2.2D

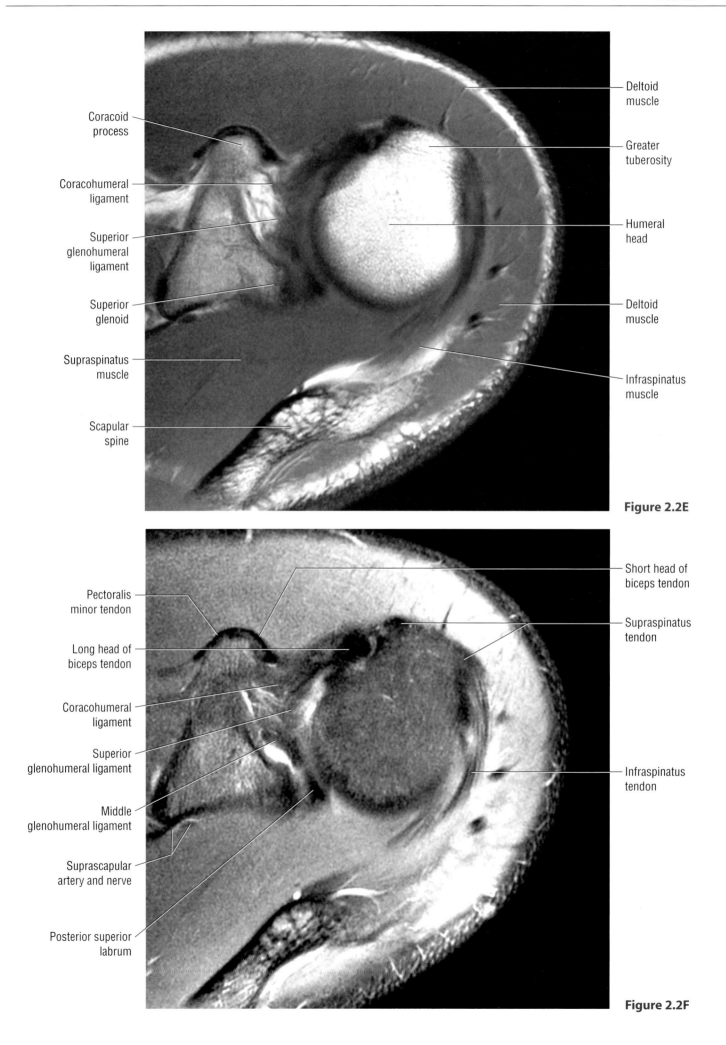

Coracoid process

Coracohumeral ligament

Superior glenohumeral ligament

Superior glenoid

Supraspinatus muscle

Scapular spine

Deltoid muscle

Greater tuberosity

Humeral head

Deltoid muscle

Infraspinatus muscle

Figure 2.2E

Pectoralis minor tendon

Long head of biceps tendon

Coracohumeral ligament

Superior glenohumeral ligament

Middle glenohumeral ligament

Suprascapular artery and nerve

Posterior superior labrum

Short head of biceps tendon

Supraspinatus tendon

Infraspinatus tendon

Figure 2.2F

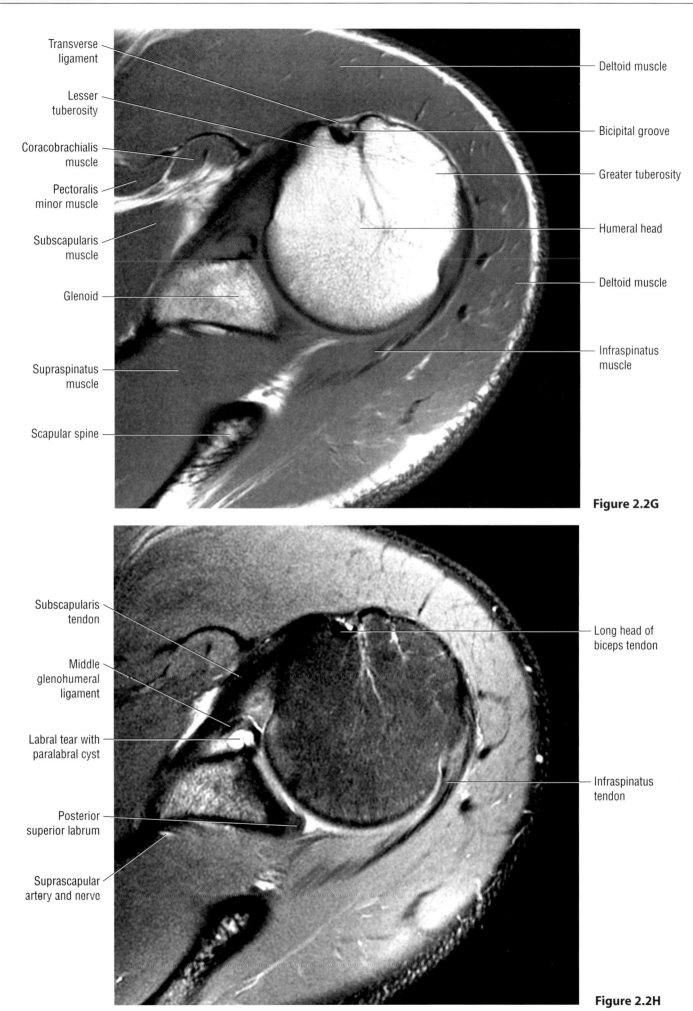

Transverse ligament

Lesser tuberosity

Coracobrachialis muscle

Pectoralis minor muscle

Subscapularis muscle

Glenoid

Supraspinatus muscle

Scapular spine

Deltoid muscle

Bicipital groove

Greater tuberosity

Humeral head

Deltoid muscle

Infraspinatus muscle

Figure 2.2G

Subscapularis tendon

Middle glenohumeral ligament

Labral tear with paralabral cyst

Posterior superior labrum

Suprascapular artery and nerve

Long head of biceps tendon

Infraspinatus tendon

Figure 2.2H

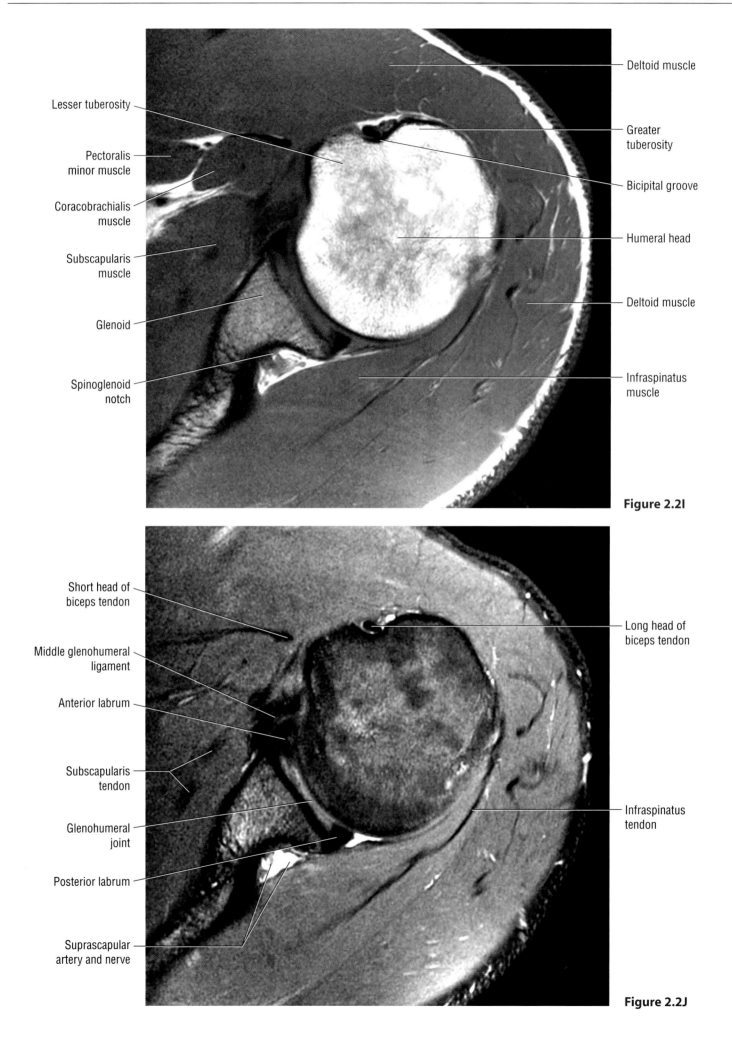

Lesser tuberosity

Pectoralis minor muscle

Coracobrachialis muscle

Subscapularis muscle

Glenoid

Spinoglenoid notch

Deltoid muscle

Greater tuberosity

Bicipital groove

Humeral head

Deltoid muscle

Infraspinatus muscle

Figure 2.2I

Short head of biceps tendon

Middle glenohumeral ligament

Anterior labrum

Subscapularis tendon

Glenohumeral joint

Posterior labrum

Suprascapular artery and nerve

Long head of biceps tendon

Infraspinatus tendon

Figure 2.2J

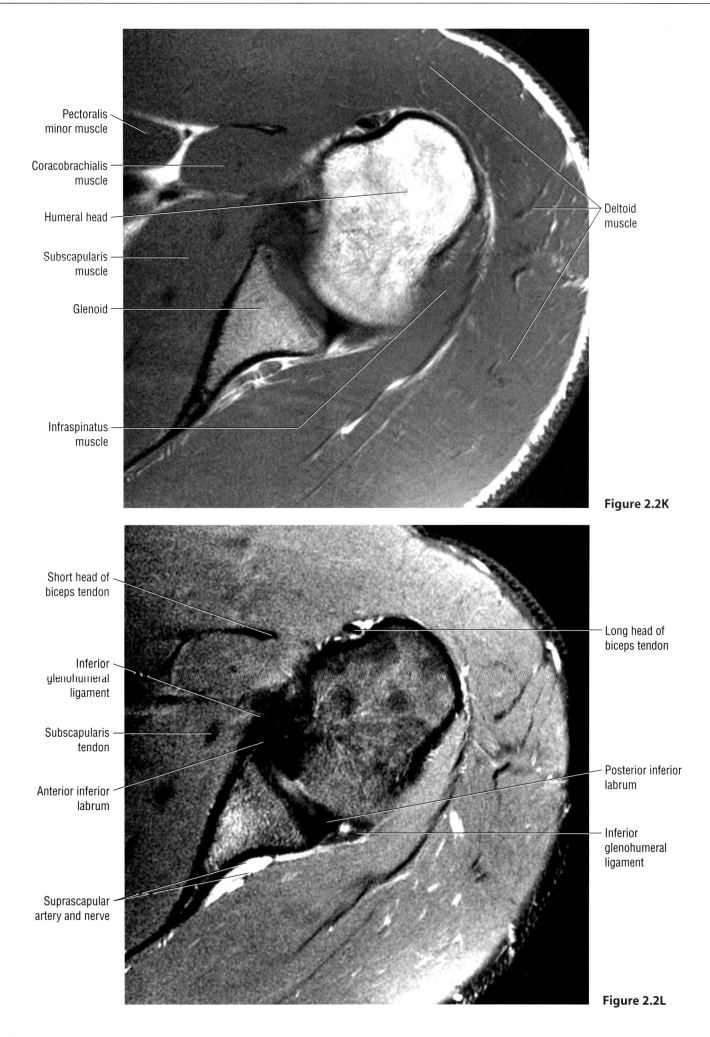

Pectoralis minor muscle

Coracobrachialis muscle

Humeral head

Subscapularis muscle

Glenoid

Infraspinatus muscle

Deltoid muscle

Figure 2.2K

Short head of biceps tendon

Inferior glenohumeral ligament

Subscapularis tendon

Anterior inferior labrum

Suprascapular artery and nerve

Long head of biceps tendon

Posterior inferior labrum

Inferior glenohumeral ligament

Figure 2.2L

Shoulder - Sagittal

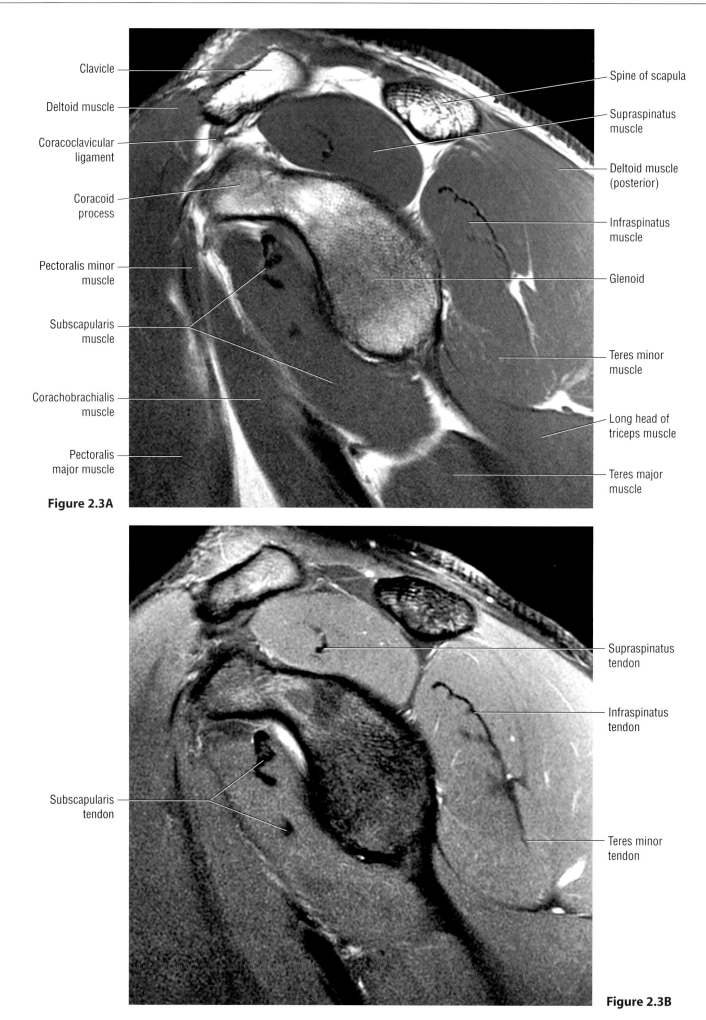

Clavicle

Deltoid muscle

Coracoclavicular ligament

Coracoid process

Pectoralis minor muscle

Subscapularis muscle

Corachobrachialis muscle

Pectoralis major muscle

Spine of scapula

Supraspinatus muscle

Deltoid muscle (posterior)

Infraspinatus muscle

Glenoid

Teres minor muscle

Long head of triceps muscle

Teres major muscle

Figure 2.3A

Subscapularis tendon

Supraspinatus tendon

Infraspinatus tendon

Teres minor tendon

Figure 2.3B

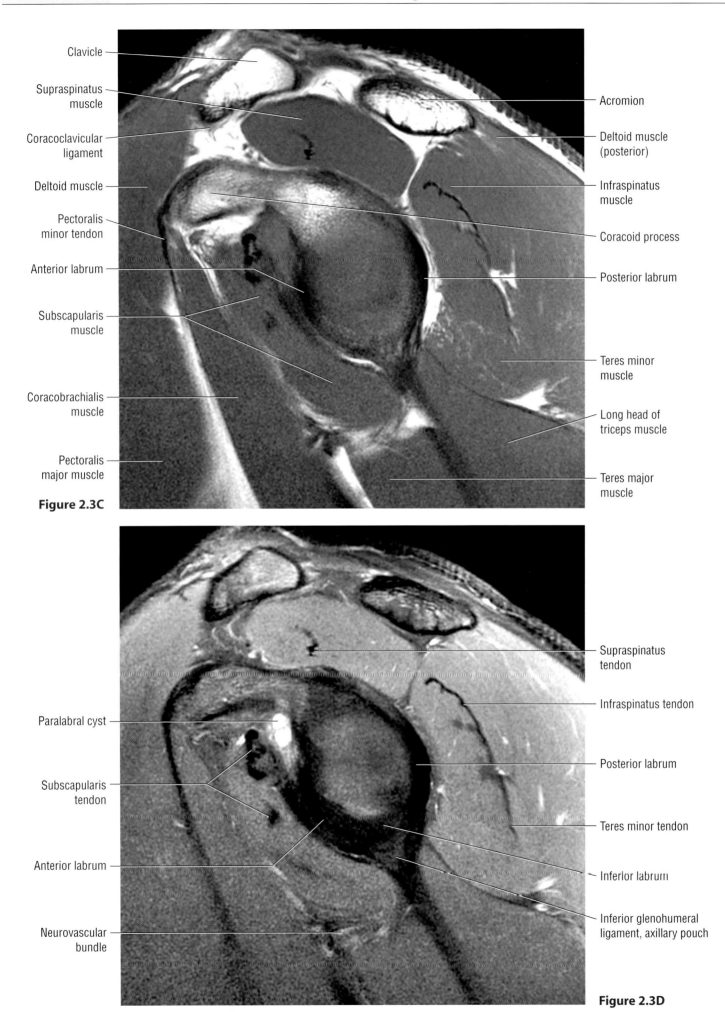

Clavicle

Supraspinatus
muscle

Coracoclavicular
ligament

Deltoid muscle

Pectoralis
minor tendon

Anterior labrum

Subscapularis
muscle

Coracobrachialis
muscle

Pectoralis
major muscle

Acromion

Deltoid muscle
(posterior)

Infraspinatus
muscle

Coracoid process

Posterior labrum

Teres minor
muscle

Long head of
triceps muscle

Teres major
muscle

Figure 2.3C

Paralabral cyst

Subscapularis
tendon

Anterior labrum

Neurovascular
bundle

Supraspinatus
tendon

Infraspinatus tendon

Posterior labrum

Teres minor tendon

Inferior labrum

Inferior glenohumeral
ligament, axillary pouch

Figure 2.3D

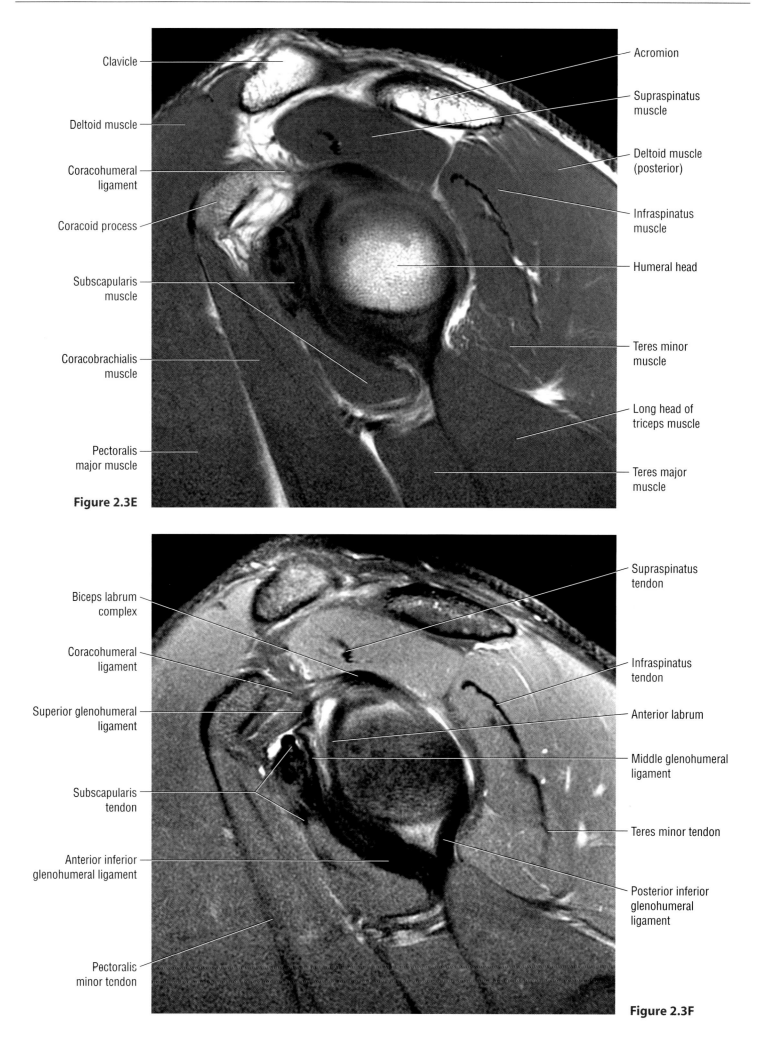

Clavicle

Deltoid muscle

Coracohumeral
ligament

Coracoid process

Subscapularis
muscle

Coracobrachialis
muscle

Pectoralis
major muscle

Acromion

Supraspinatus
muscle

Deltoid muscle
(posterior)

Infraspinatus
muscle

Humeral head

Teres minor
muscle

Long head of
triceps muscle

Teres major
muscle

Figure 2.3E

Biceps labrum
complex

Coracohumeral
ligament

Superior glenohumeral
ligament

Subscapularis
tendon

Anterior inferior
glenohumeral ligament

Pectoralis
minor tendon

Supraspinatus
tendon

Infraspinatus
tendon

Anterior labrum

Middle glenohumeral
ligament

Teres minor tendon

Posterior inferior
glenohumeral
ligament

Figure 2.3F

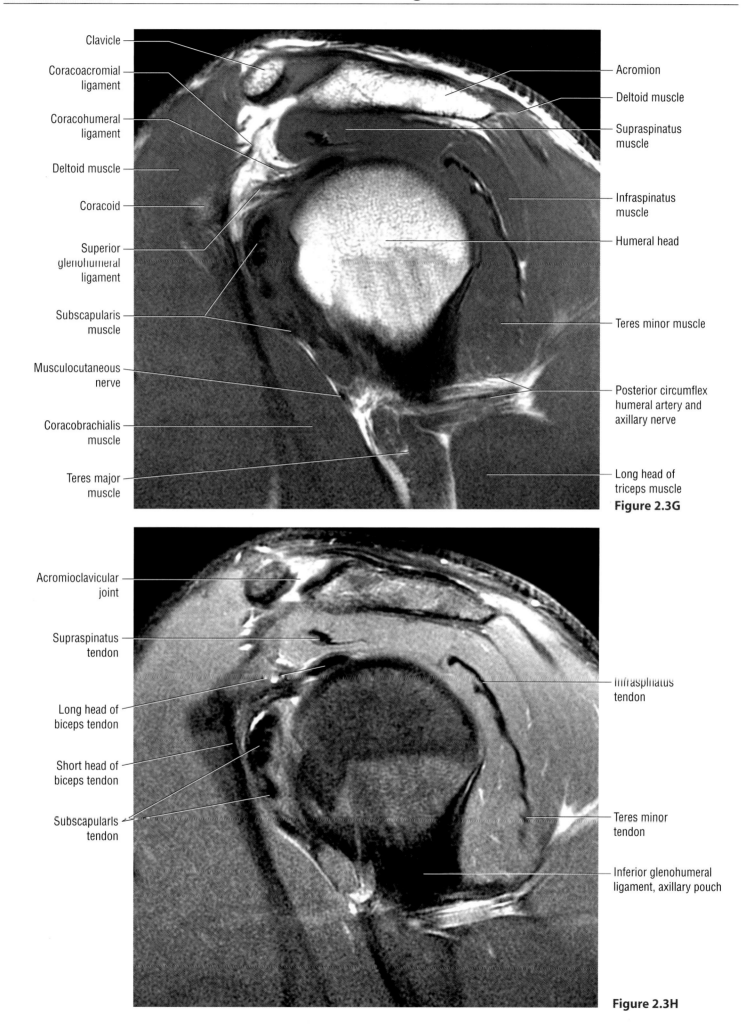

Clavicle

Coracoacromial
ligament

Coracohumeral
ligament

Deltoid muscle

Coracoid

Superior
glenohumeral
ligament

Subscapularis
muscle

Musculocutaneous
nerve

Coracobrachialis
muscle

Teres major
muscle

Acromion

Deltoid muscle

Supraspinatus
muscle

Infraspinatus
muscle

Humeral head

Teres minor muscle

Posterior circumflex
humeral artery and
axillary nerve

Long head of
triceps muscle

Figure 2.3G

Acromioclavicular
joint

Supraspinatus
tendon

Long head of
biceps tendon

Short head of
biceps tendon

Subscapularis
tendon

Infraspinatus
tendon

Teres minor
tendon

Inferior glenohumeral
ligament, axillary pouch

Figure 2.3H

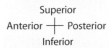

Superior
Anterior ─┼─ Posterior
Inferior

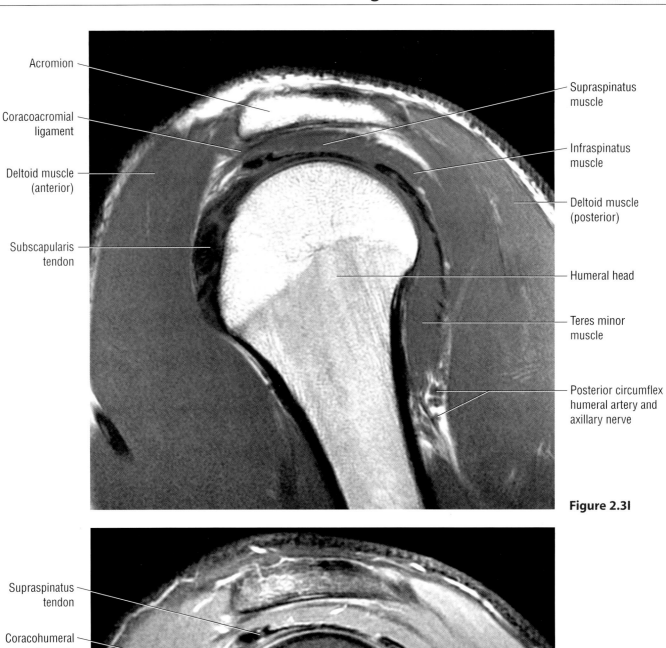

Acromion

Coracoacromial
ligament

Deltoid muscle
(anterior)

Subscapularis
tendon

Supraspinatus
muscle

Infraspinatus
muscle

Deltoid muscle
(posterior)

Humeral head

Teres minor
muscle

Posterior circumflex
humeral artery and
axillary nerve

Figure 2.3I

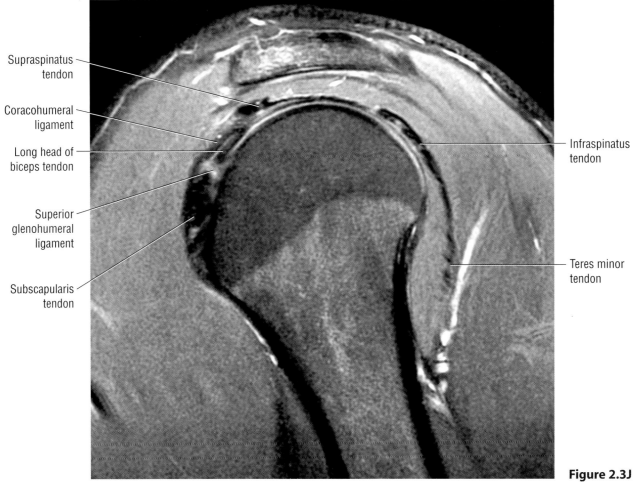

Supraspinatus
tendon

Coracohumeral
ligament

Long head of
biceps tendon

Superior
glenohumeral
ligament

Subscapularis
tendon

Infraspinatus
tendon

Teres minor
tendon

Figure 2.3J

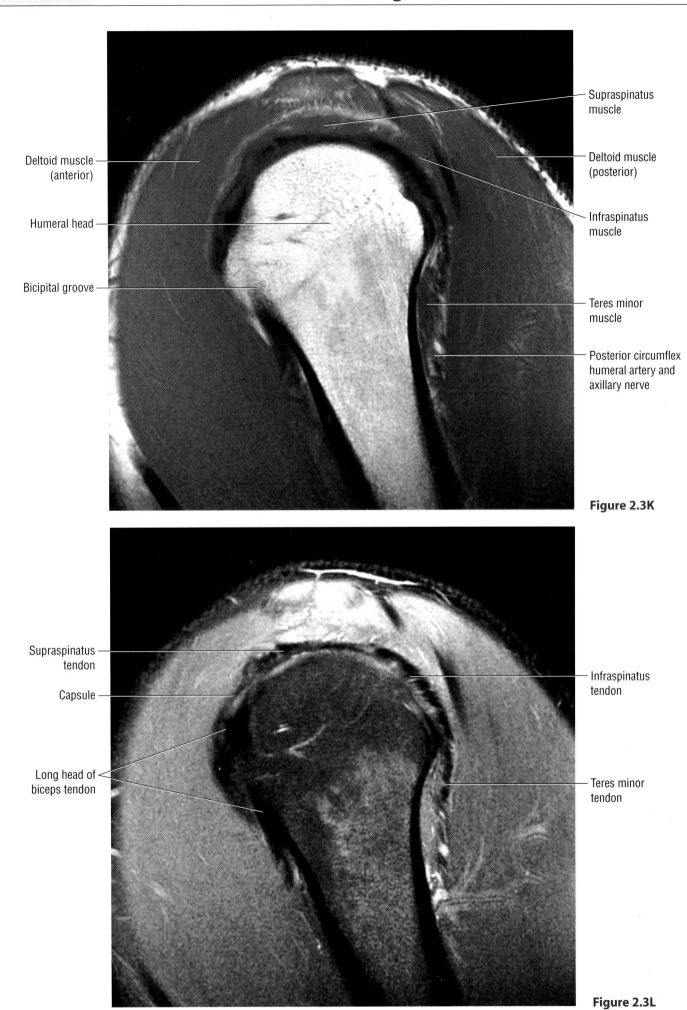

Deltoid muscle
(anterior)

Humeral head

Bicipital groove

Supraspinatus
muscle

Deltoid muscle
(posterior)

Infraspinatus
muscle

Teres minor
muscle

Posterior circumflex
humeral artery and
axillary nerve

Figure 2.3K

Supraspinatus
tendon

Capsule

Long head of
biceps tendon

Infraspinatus
tendon

Teres minor
tendon

Figure 2.3L

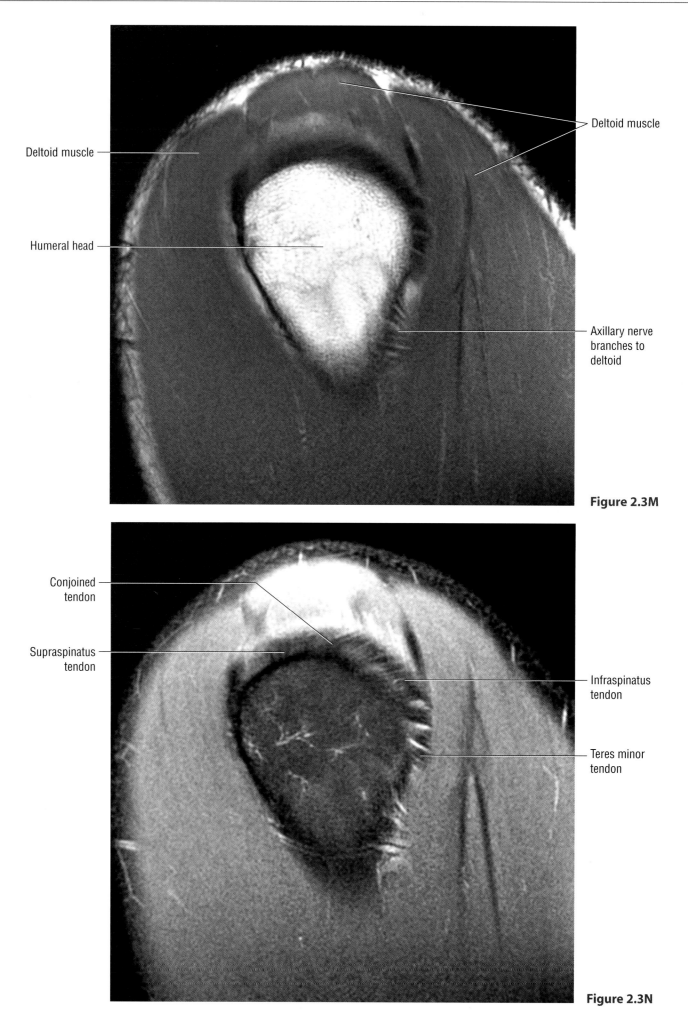

Deltoid muscle

Deltoid muscle

Humeral head

Axillary nerve branches to deltoid

Figure 2.3M

Conjoined tendon

Supraspinatus tendon

Infraspinatus tendon

Teres minor tendon

Figure 2.3N

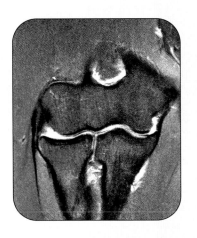

The Elbow
MR Normal Anatomy

Coronal

Figures 2.4A to 2.4L
Pages 86–91

Axial

Figures 2.5A to 2.5L
Pages 92-97

Sagittal

Figures 2.6A to 2.6N
Pages 98-104

Elbow - Coronal

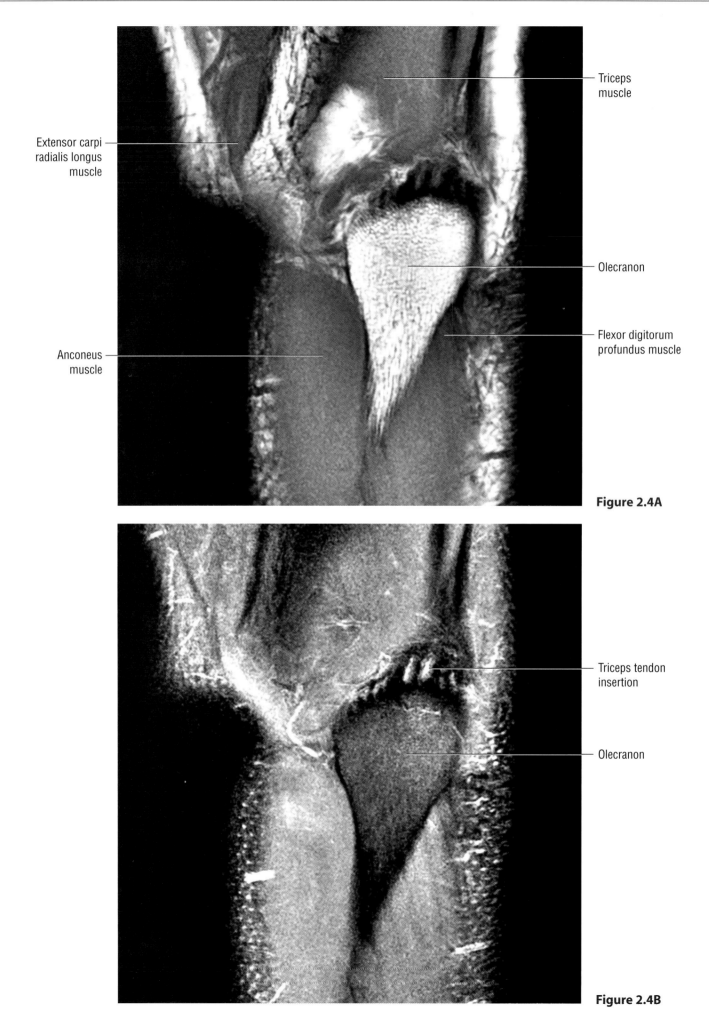

Triceps muscle

Extensor carpi radialis longus muscle

Olecranon

Flexor digitorum profundus muscle

Anconeus muscle

Figure 2.4A

Triceps tendon insertion

Olecranon

Figure 2.4B

Proximal
Lateral ┼ Medial
Distal

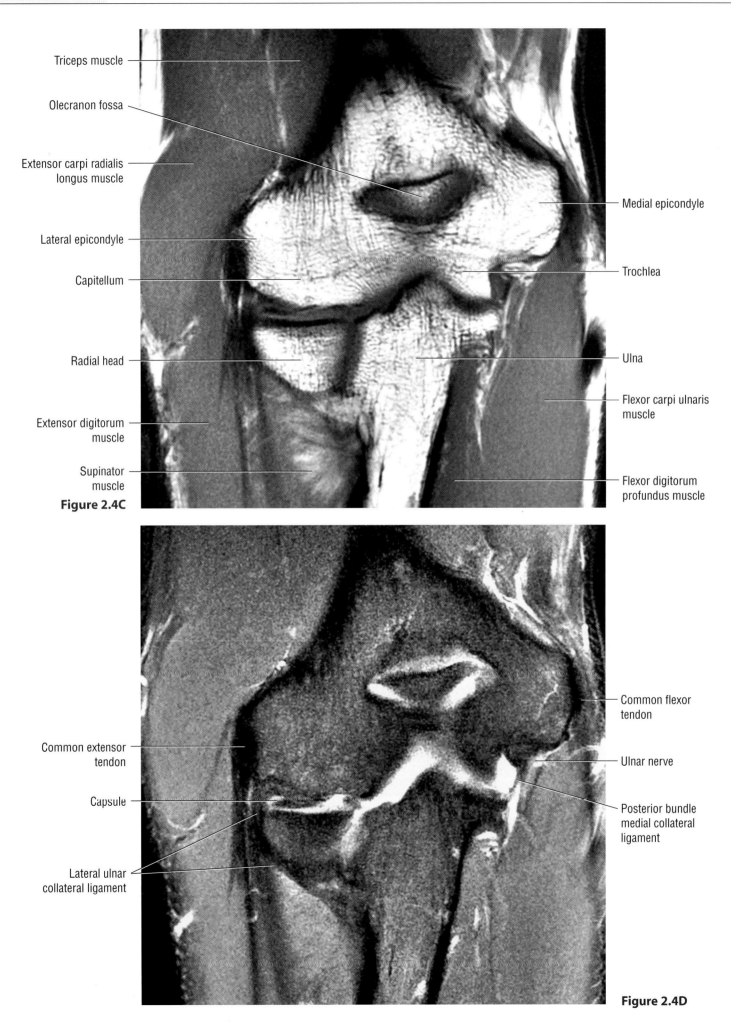

Triceps muscle

Olecranon fossa

Extensor carpi radialis
longus muscle

Medial epicondyle

Lateral epicondyle

Capitellum

Trochlea

Radial head

Ulna

Flexor carpi ulnaris
muscle

Extensor digitorum
muscle

Supinator
muscle

Flexor digitorum
profundus muscle

Figure 2.4C

Common extensor
tendon

Common flexor
tendon

Ulnar nerve

Capsule

Posterior bundle
medial collateral
ligament

Lateral ulnar
collateral ligament

Figure 2.4D

Elbow - Coronal

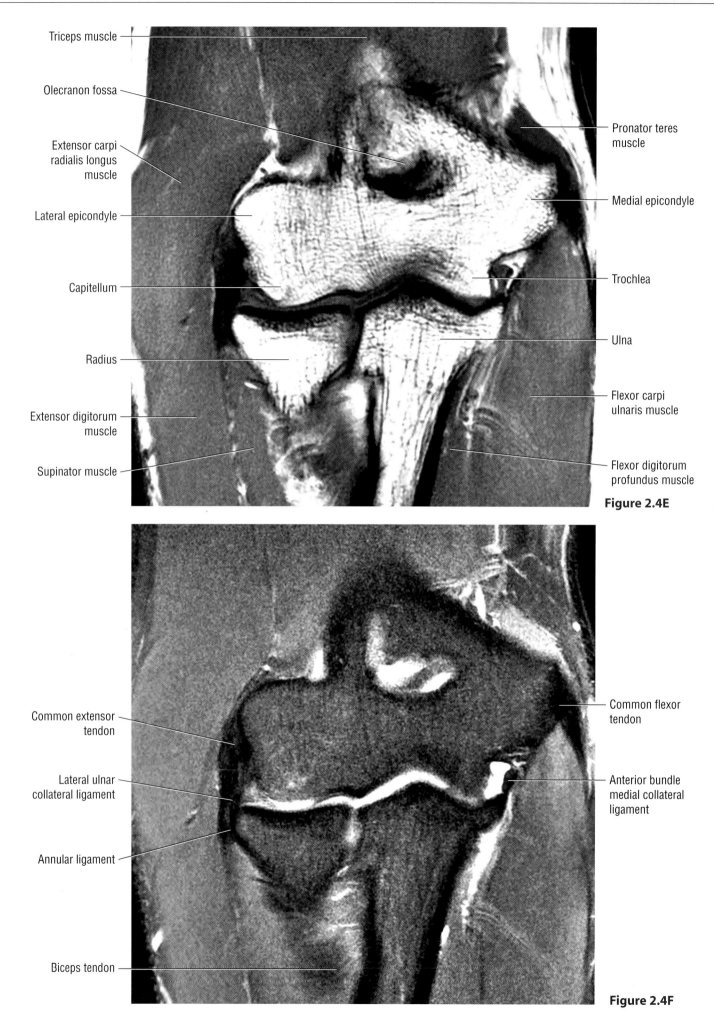

Triceps muscle

Olecranon fossa

Extensor carpi radialis longus muscle

Lateral epicondyle

Capitellum

Radius

Extensor digitorum muscle

Supinator muscle

Pronator teres muscle

Medial epicondyle

Trochlea

Ulna

Flexor carpi ulnaris muscle

Flexor digitorum profundus muscle

Figure 2.4E

Common extensor tendon

Lateral ulnar collateral ligament

Annular ligament

Biceps tendon

Common flexor tendon

Anterior bundle medial collateral ligament

Figure 2.4F

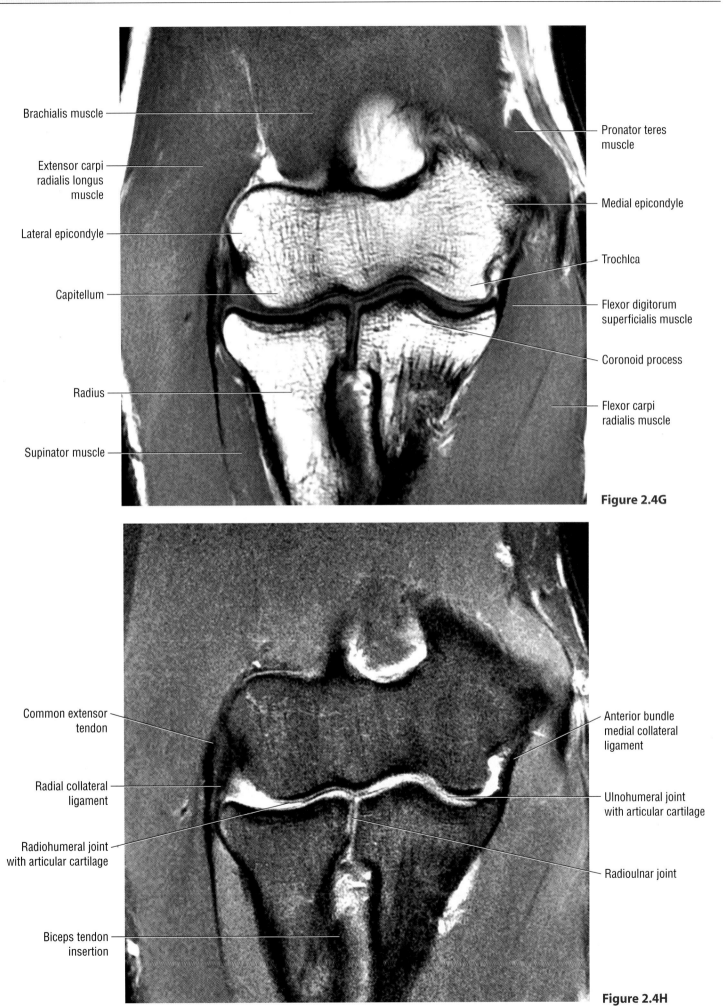

Brachialis muscle

Extensor carpi radialis longus muscle

Lateral epicondyle

Capitellum

Radius

Supinator muscle

Pronator teres muscle

Medial epicondyle

Trochlca

Flexor digitorum superficialis muscle

Coronoid process

Flexor carpi radialis muscle

Figure 2.4G

Common extensor tendon

Radial collateral ligament

Radiohumeral joint with articular cartilage

Biceps tendon insertion

Anterior bundle medial collateral ligament

Ulnohumeral joint with articular cartilage

Radioulnar joint

Figure 2.4H

Elbow - Coronal

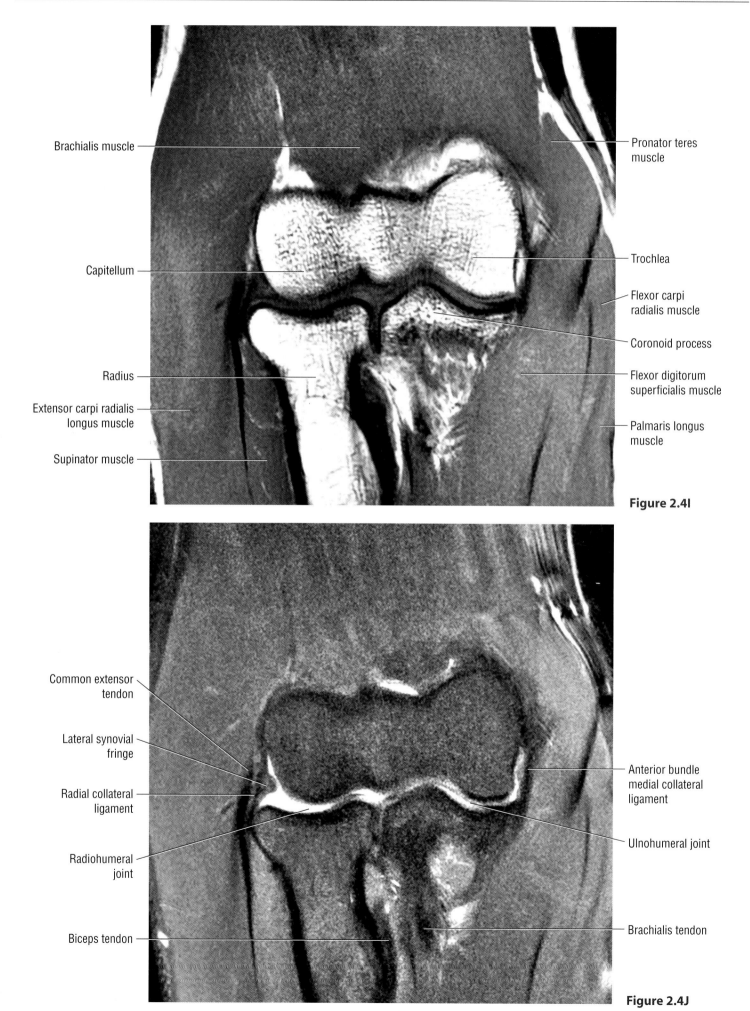

Brachialis muscle

Capitellum

Radius

Extensor carpi radialis longus muscle

Supinator muscle

Pronator teres muscle

Trochlea

Flexor carpi radialis muscle

Coronoid process

Flexor digitorum superficialis muscle

Palmaris longus muscle

Figure 2.4I

Common extensor tendon

Lateral synovial fringe

Radial collateral ligament

Radiohumeral joint

Biceps tendon

Anterior bundle medial collateral ligament

Ulnohumeral joint

Brachialis tendon

Figure 2.4J

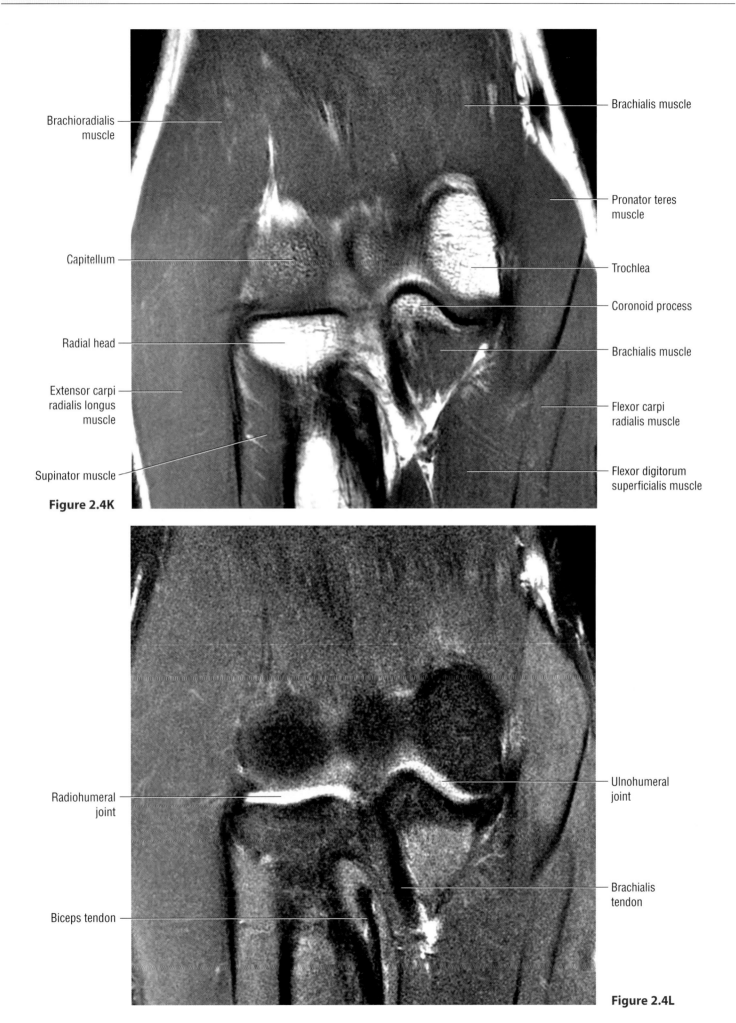

Brachioradialis muscle

Brachialis muscle

Capitellum

Pronator teres muscle

Radial head

Trochlea

Extensor carpi radialis longus muscle

Coronoid process

Brachialis muscle

Supinator muscle

Flexor carpi radialis muscle

Flexor digitorum superficialis muscle

Figure 2.4K

Radiohumeral joint

Ulnohumeral joint

Biceps tendon

Brachialis tendon

Figure 2.4L

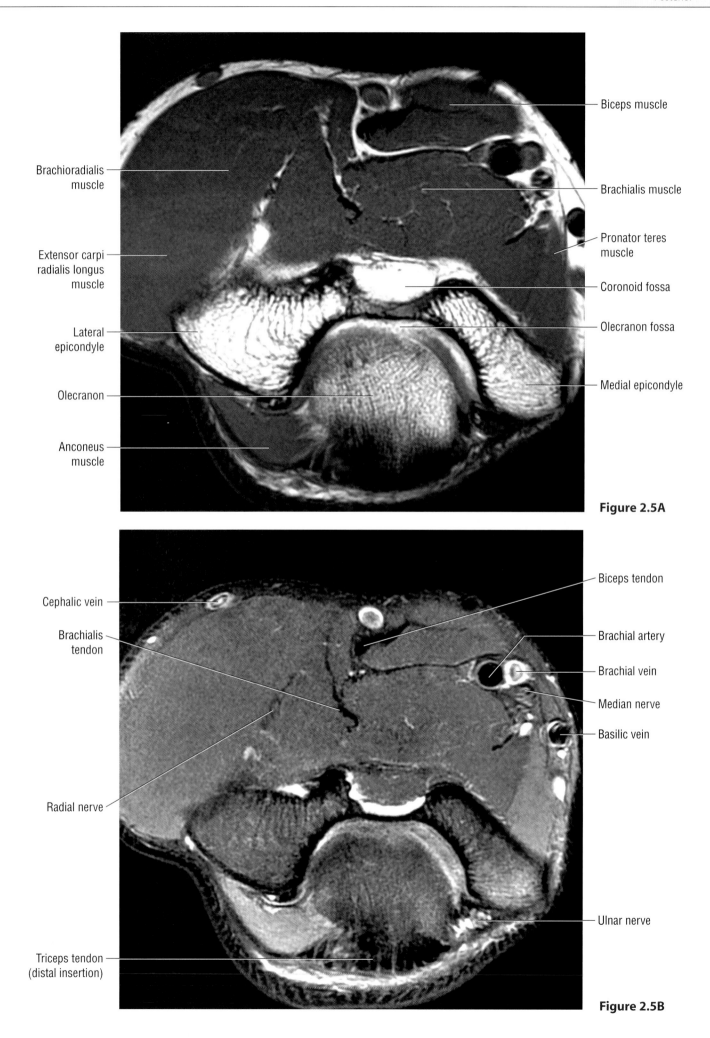

Biceps muscle

Brachioradialis muscle

Brachialis muscle

Pronator teres muscle

Extensor carpi radialis longus muscle

Coronoid fossa

Olecranon fossa

Lateral epicondyle

Olecranon

Medial epicondyle

Anconeus muscle

Figure 2.5A

Cephalic vein

Biceps tendon

Brachialis tendon

Brachial artery

Brachial vein

Median nerve

Basilic vein

Radial nerve

Ulnar nerve

Triceps tendon (distal insertion)

Figure 2.5B

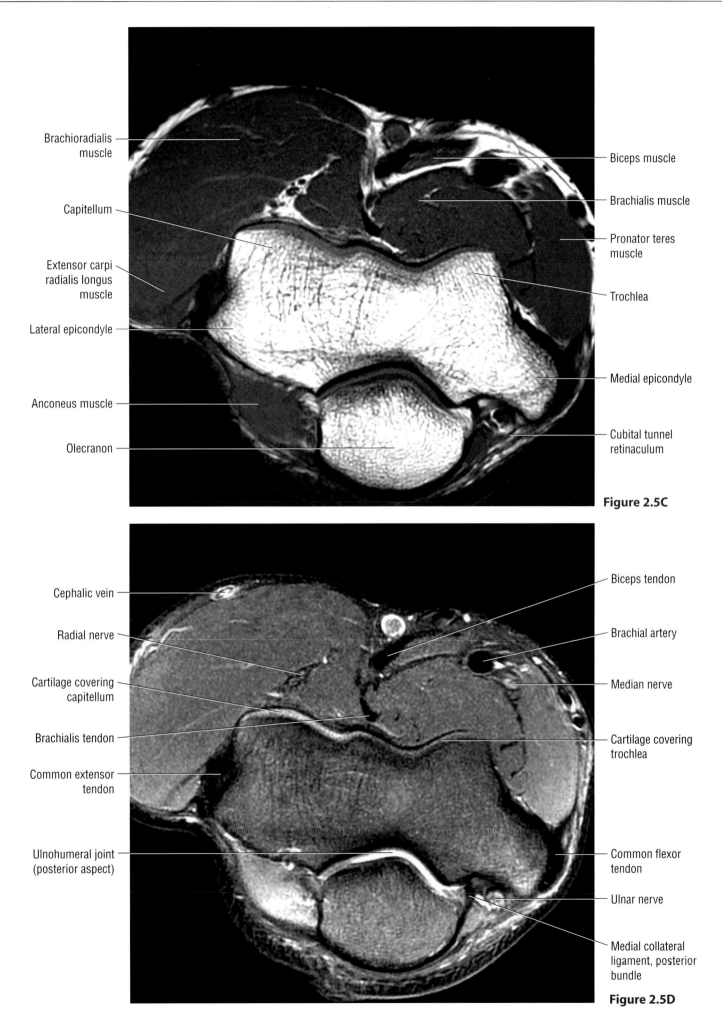

Brachioradialis muscle

Biceps muscle

Capitellum

Brachialis muscle

Extensor carpi radialis longus muscle

Pronator teres muscle

Lateral epicondyle

Trochlea

Anconeus muscle

Medial epicondyle

Olecranon

Cubital tunnel retinaculum

Figure 2.5C

Cephalic vein

Biceps tendon

Radial nerve

Brachial artery

Cartilage covering capitellum

Median nerve

Brachialis tendon

Cartilage covering trochlea

Common extensor tendon

Ulnohumeral joint (posterior aspect)

Common flexor tendon

Ulnar nerve

Medial collateral ligament, posterior bundle

Figure 2.5D

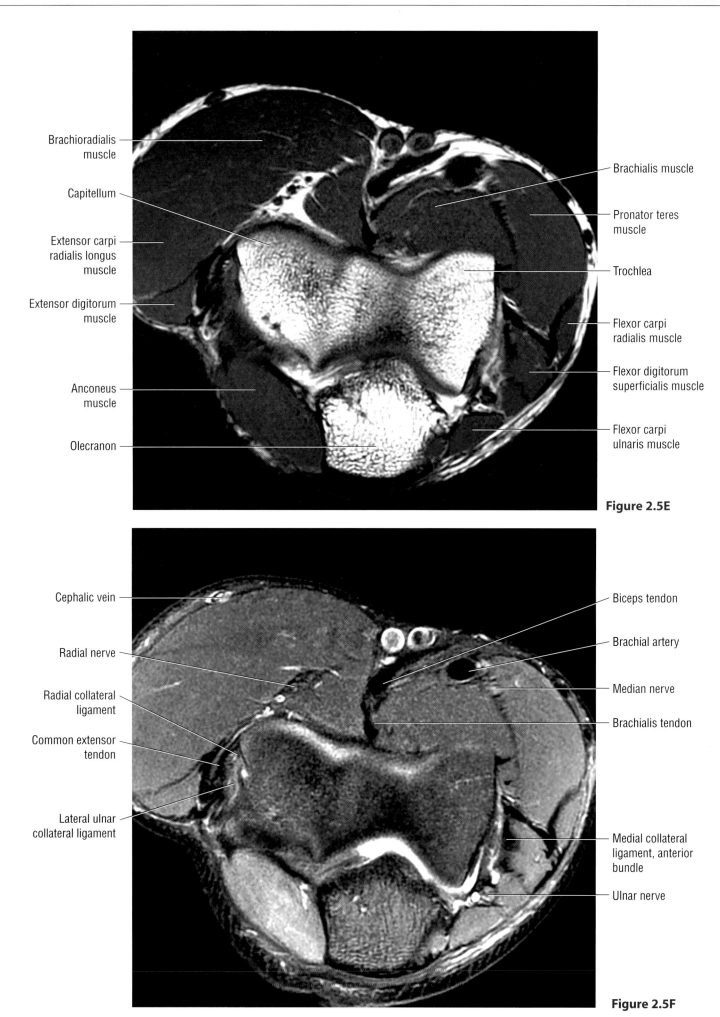

Brachioradialis muscle

Capitellum

Extensor carpi radialis longus muscle

Extensor digitorum muscle

Anconeus muscle

Olecranon

Brachialis muscle

Pronator teres muscle

Trochlea

Flexor carpi radialis muscle

Flexor digitorum superficialis muscle

Flexor carpi ulnaris muscle

Figure 2.5E

Cephalic vein

Radial nerve

Radial collateral ligament

Common extensor tendon

Lateral ulnar collateral ligament

Biceps tendon

Brachial artery

Median nerve

Brachialis tendon

Medial collateral ligament, anterior bundle

Ulnar nerve

Figure 2.5F

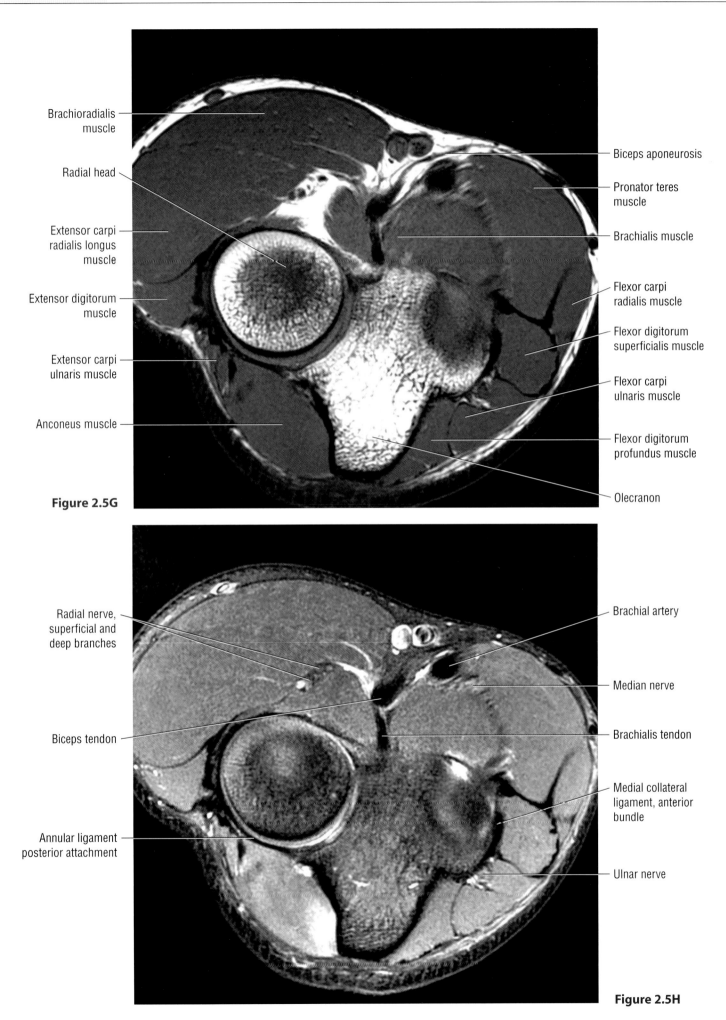

Brachioradialis muscle

Radial head

Extensor carpi radialis longus muscle

Extensor digitorum muscle

Extensor carpi ulnaris muscle

Anconeus muscle

Biceps aponeurosis

Pronator teres muscle

Brachialis muscle

Flexor carpi radialis muscle

Flexor digitorum superficialis muscle

Flexor carpi ulnaris muscle

Flexor digitorum profundus muscle

Olecranon

Figure 2.5G

Radial nerve, superficial and deep branches

Biceps tendon

Annular ligament posterior attachment

Brachial artery

Median nerve

Brachialis tendon

Medial collateral ligament, anterior bundle

Ulnar nerve

Figure 2.5H

Elbow - Axial

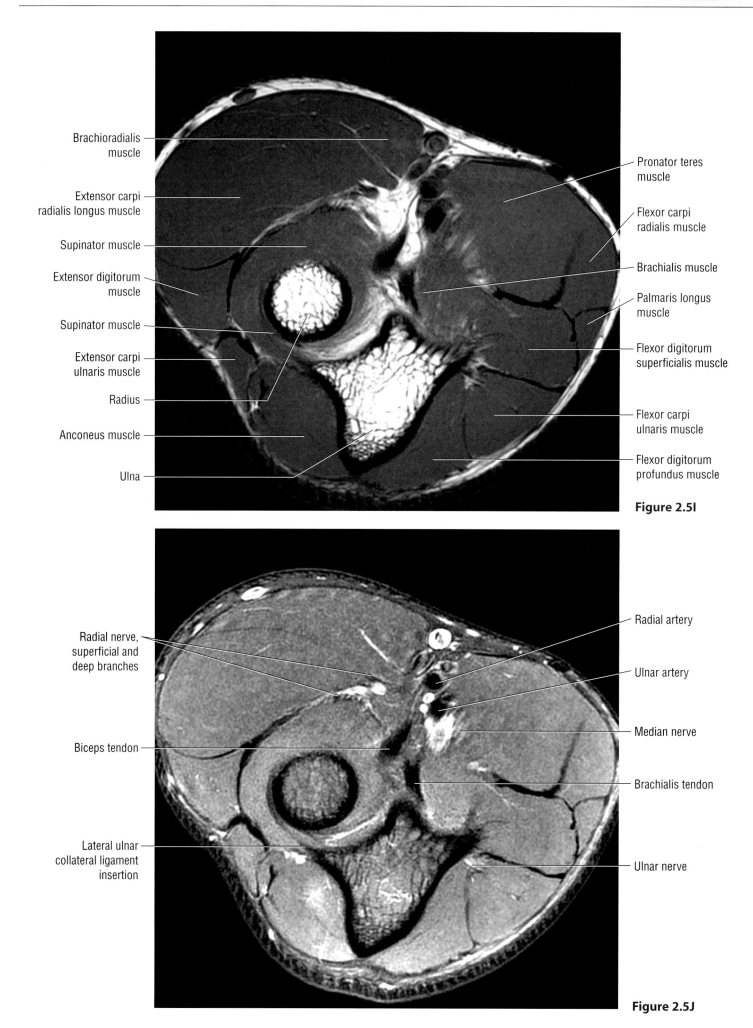

Brachioradialis muscle

Extensor carpi radialis longus muscle

Supinator muscle

Extensor digitorum muscle

Supinator muscle

Extensor carpi ulnaris muscle

Radius

Anconeus muscle

Ulna

Pronator teres muscle

Flexor carpi radialis muscle

Brachialis muscle

Palmaris longus muscle

Flexor digitorum superficialis muscle

Flexor carpi ulnaris muscle

Flexor digitorum profundus muscle

Figure 2.5I

Radial nerve, superficial and deep branches

Biceps tendon

Lateral ulnar collateral ligament insertion

Radial artery

Ulnar artery

Median nerve

Brachialis tendon

Ulnar nerve

Figure 2.5J

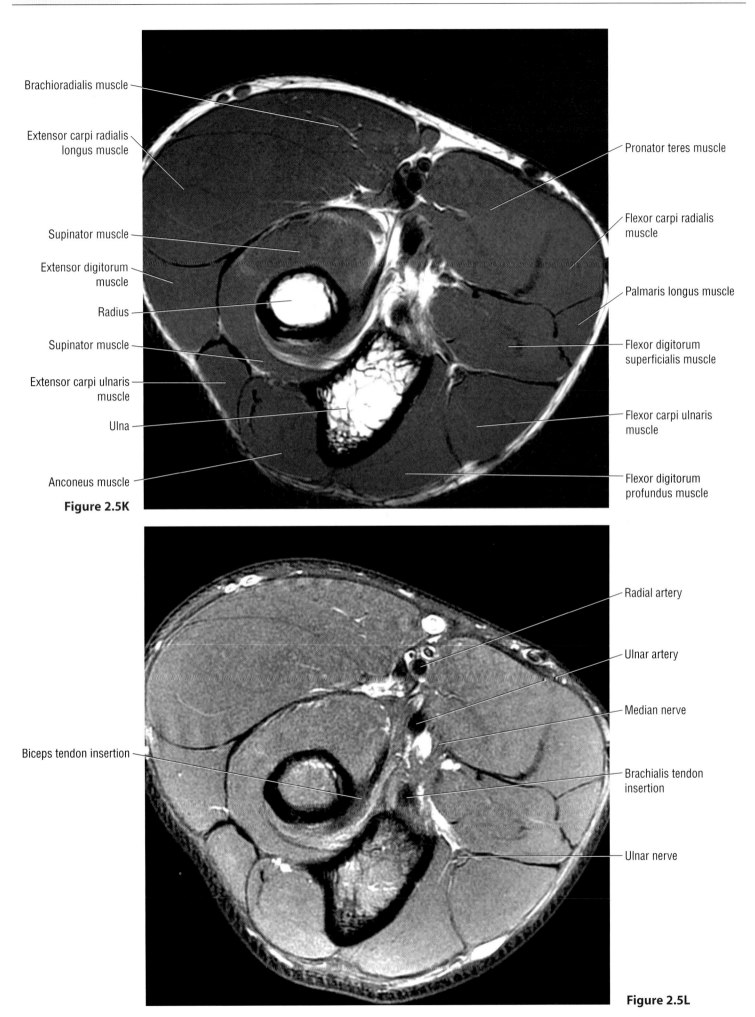

Brachioradialis muscle

Extensor carpi radialis longus muscle

Supinator muscle

Extensor digitorum muscle

Radius

Supinator muscle

Extensor carpi ulnaris muscle

Ulna

Anconeus muscle

Pronator teres muscle

Flexor carpi radialis muscle

Palmaris longus muscle

Flexor digitorum superficialis muscle

Flexor carpi ulnaris muscle

Flexor digitorum profundus muscle

Figure 2.5K

Biceps tendon insertion

Radial artery

Ulnar artery

Median nerve

Brachialis tendon insertion

Ulnar nerve

Figure 2.5L

Proximal
Anterior ─┼─ Posterior
Distal

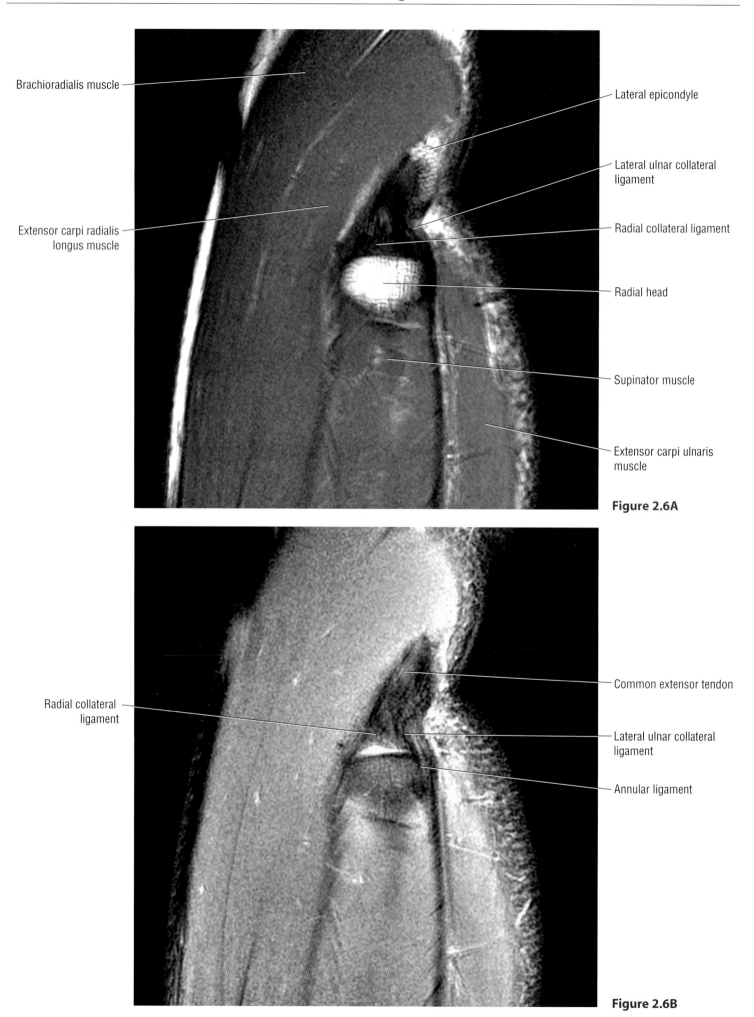

Brachioradialis muscle

Lateral epicondyle

Lateral ulnar collateral ligament

Extensor carpi radialis longus muscle

Radial collateral ligament

Radial head

Supinator muscle

Extensor carpi ulnaris muscle

Figure 2.6A

Radial collateral ligament

Common extensor tendon

Lateral ulnar collateral ligament

Annular ligament

Figure 2.6B

Proximal
Anterior ─┼─ Posterior
Distal

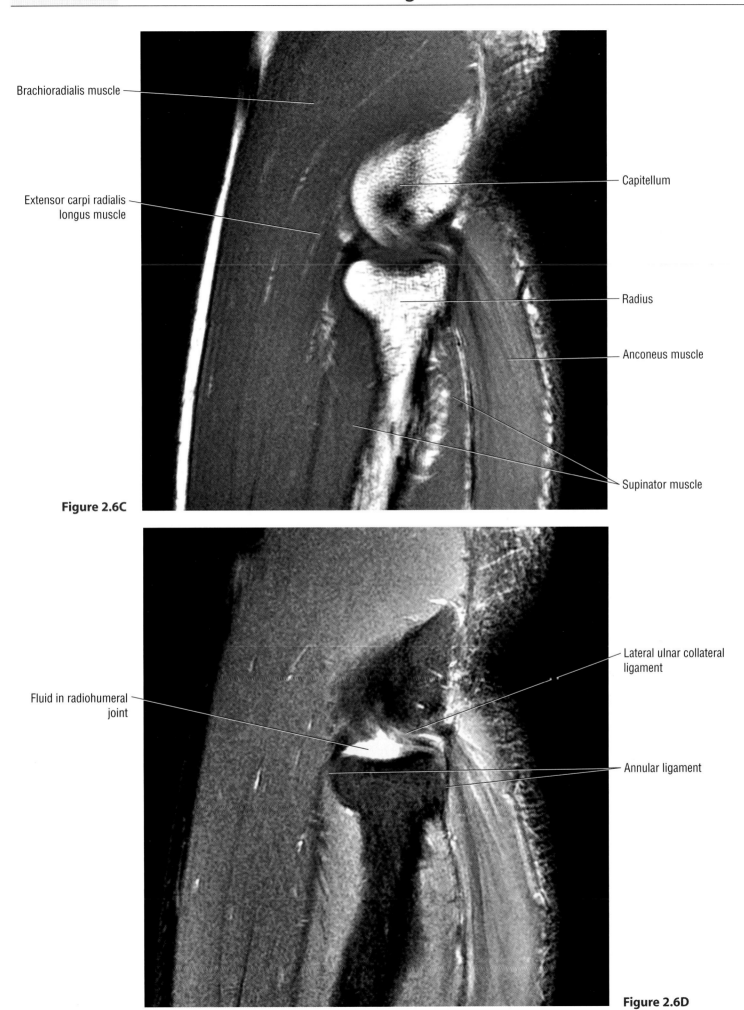

Brachioradialis muscle

Extensor carpi radialis longus muscle

Capitellum

Radius

Anconeus muscle

Supinator muscle

Figure 2.6C

Fluid in radiohumeral joint

Lateral ulnar collateral ligament

Annular ligament

Figure 2.6D

Elbow - Sagittal

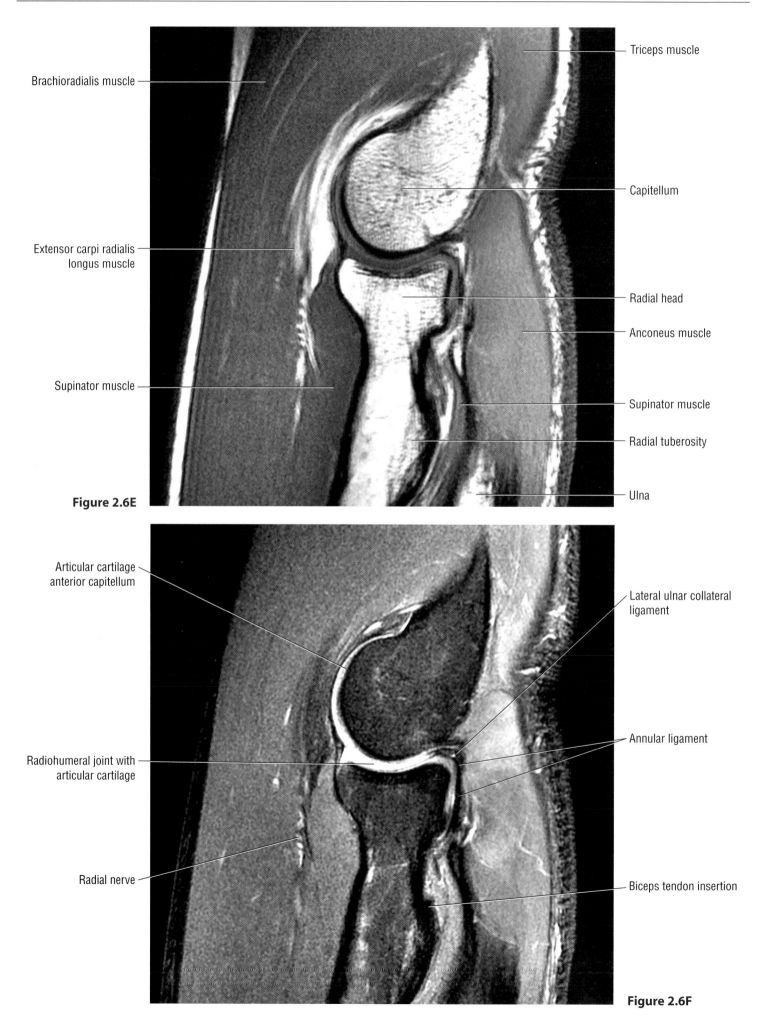

Brachioradialis muscle

Triceps muscle

Capitellum

Extensor carpi radialis longus muscle

Radial head

Anconeus muscle

Supinator muscle

Supinator muscle

Radial tuberosity

Ulna

Figure 2.6E

Articular cartilage anterior capitellum

Lateral ulnar collateral ligament

Radiohumeral joint with articular cartilage

Annular ligament

Radial nerve

Biceps tendon insertion

Figure 2.6F

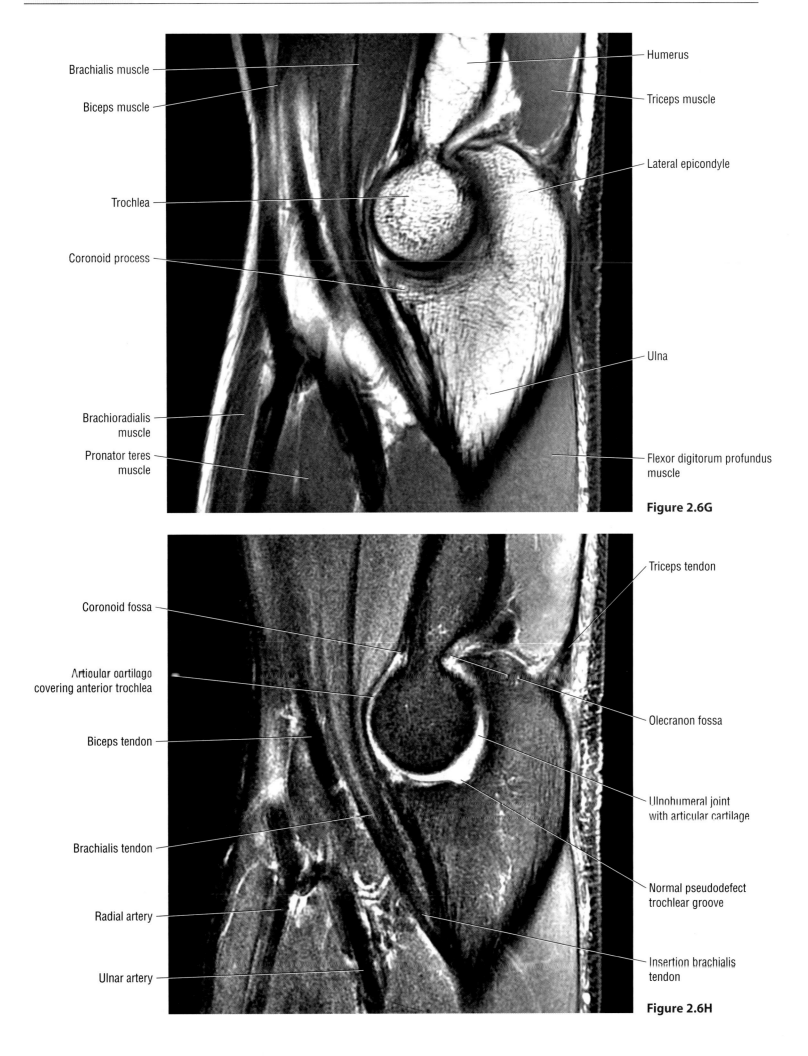

Brachialis muscle

Biceps muscle

Trochlea

Coronoid process

Brachioradialis muscle

Pronator teres muscle

Humerus

Triceps muscle

Lateral epicondyle

Ulna

Flexor digitorum profundus muscle

Figure 2.6G

Coronoid fossa

Articular cartilage covering anterior trochlea

Biceps tendon

Brachialis tendon

Radial artery

Ulnar artery

Triceps tendon

Olecranon fossa

Ulnohumeral joint with articular cartilage

Normal pseudodefect trochlear groove

Insertion brachialis tendon

Figure 2.6H

Elbow - Sagittal

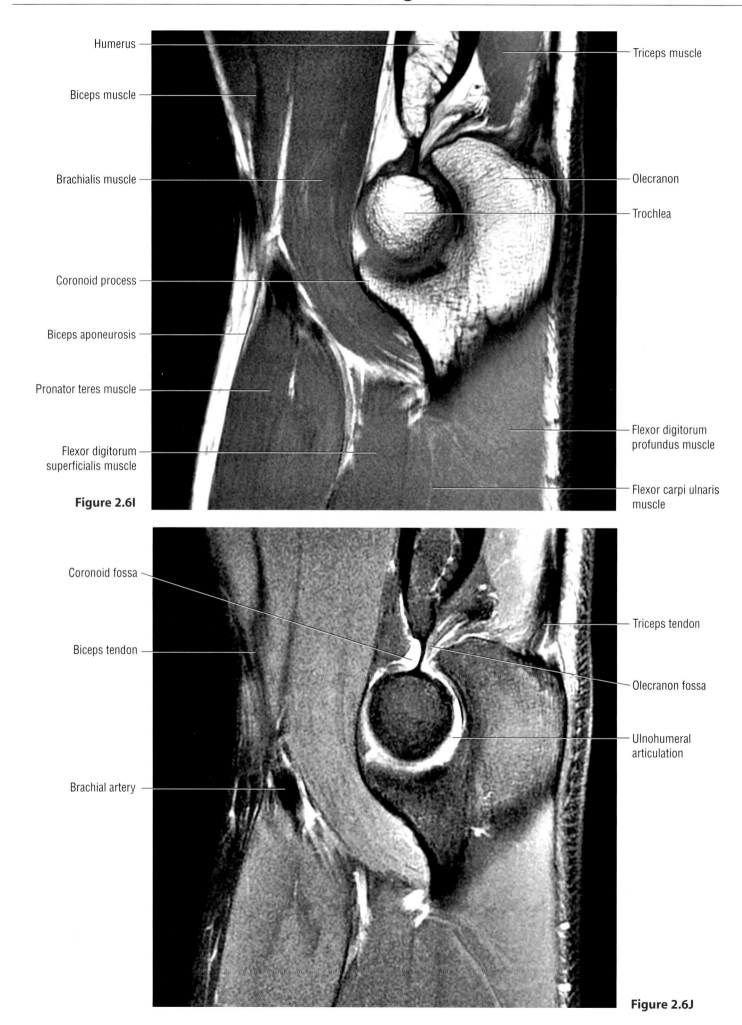

Humerus

Biceps muscle

Brachialis muscle

Coronoid process

Biceps aponeurosis

Pronator teres muscle

Flexor digitorum superficialis muscle

Figure 2.6I

Triceps muscle

Olecranon

Trochlea

Flexor digitorum profundus muscle

Flexor carpi ulnaris muscle

Coronoid fossa

Biceps tendon

Brachial artery

Triceps tendon

Olecranon fossa

Ulnohumeral articulation

Figure 2.6J

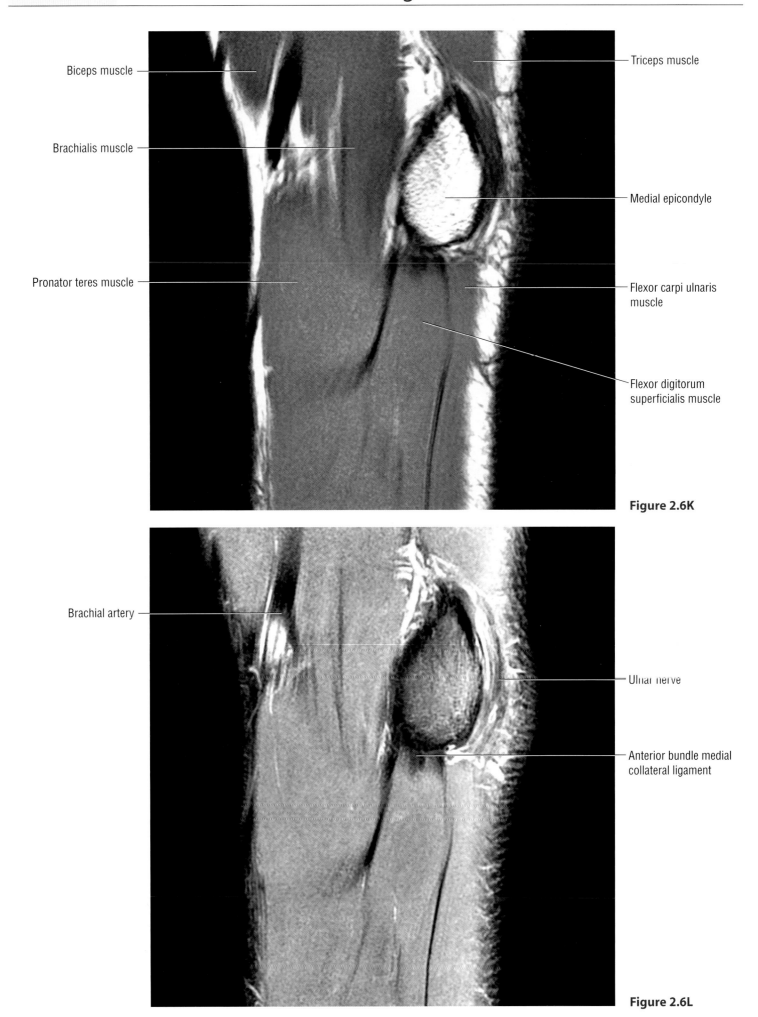

Biceps muscle

Brachialis muscle

Pronator teres muscle

Triceps muscle

Medial epicondyle

Flexor carpi ulnaris
muscle

Flexor digitorum
superficialis muscle

Figure 2.6K

Brachial artery

Ulnar nerve

Anterior bundle medial
collateral ligament

Figure 2.6L

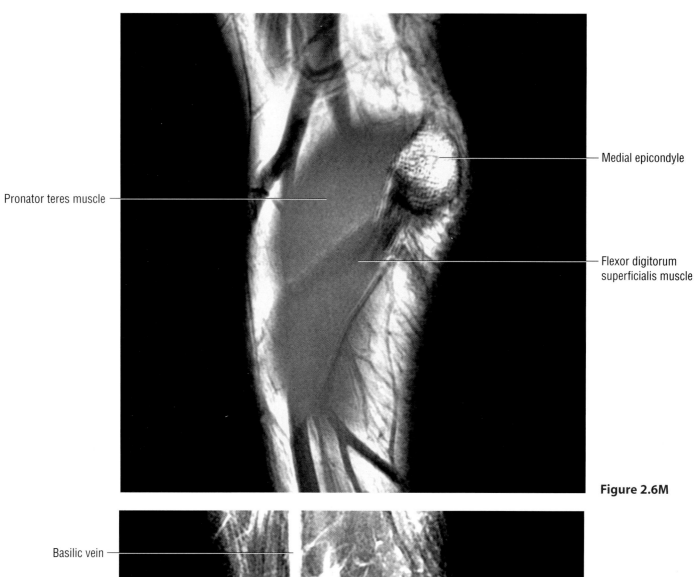

Pronator teres muscle ─────────

Medial epicondyle ─

Flexor digitorum
superficialis muscle ─

Figure 2.6M

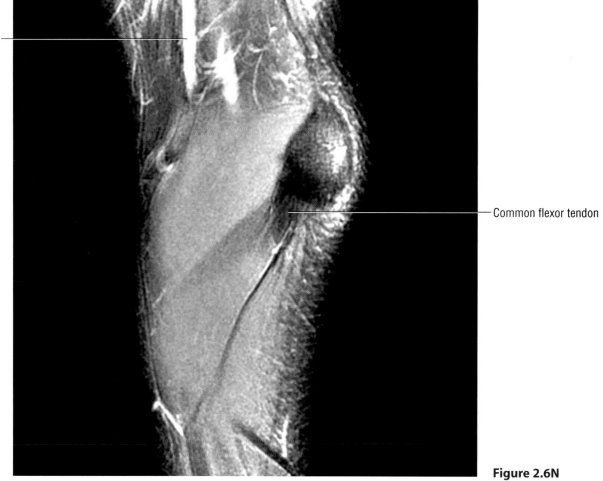

Basilic vein ─

Common flexor tendon ─

Figure 2.6N

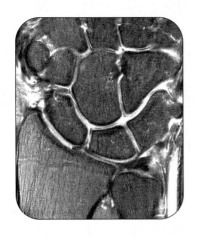

The Wrist

MR Normal Anatomy

Coronal

Axial

Sagittal

Thenar muscles

Hook of hamate

Hypothenar muscles

Trapezium

Pisiform

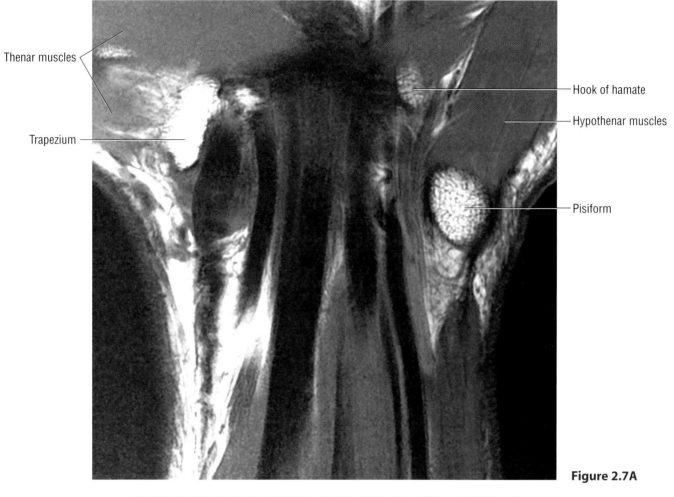

Figure 2.7A

Flexor retinaculum

Median nerve

Ulnar nerve

Flexor carpi radialis
tendon

Flexor pollicis longus
tendon

Flexor digitorum
superficialis tendons

Flexor carpi ulnaris
tendon

Ulnar artery

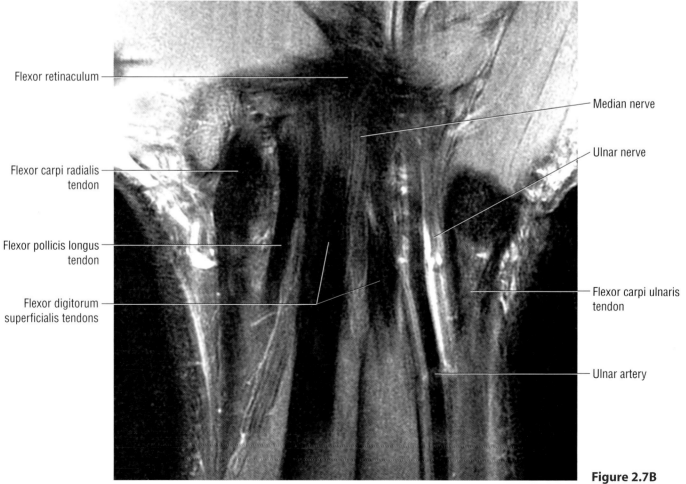

Figure 2.7B

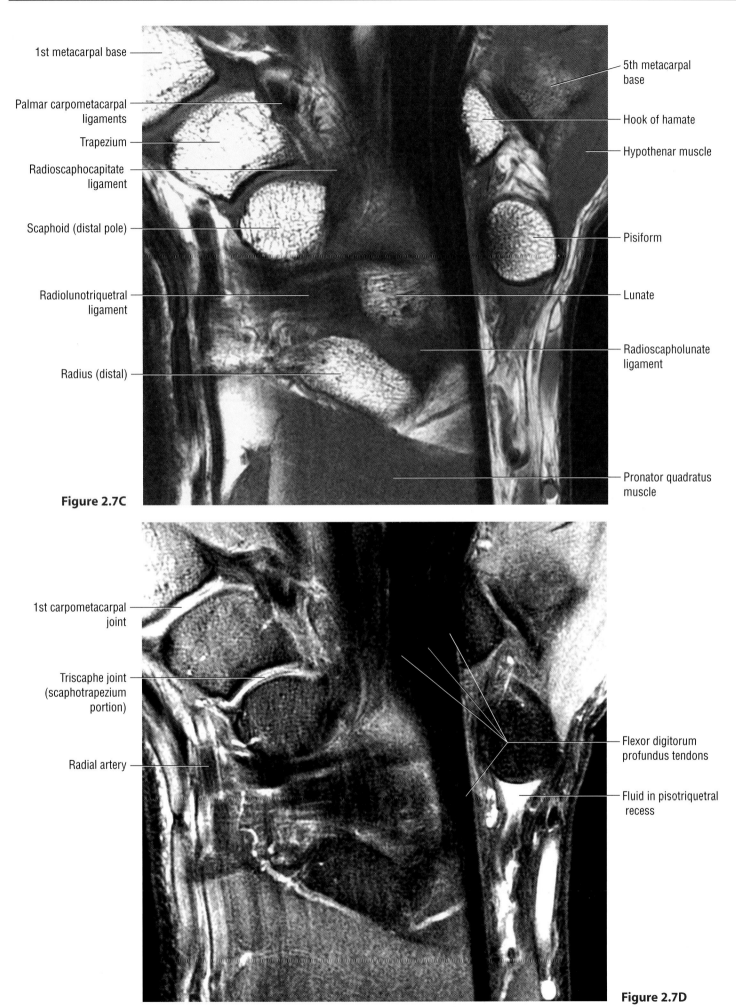

1st metacarpal base

Palmar carpometacarpal ligaments

Trapezium

Radioscaphocapitate ligament

Scaphoid (distal pole)

Radiolunotriquetral ligament

Radius (distal)

5th metacarpal base

Hook of hamate

Hypothenar muscle

Pisiform

Lunate

Radioscapholunate ligament

Pronator quadratus muscle

Figure 2.7C

1st carpometacarpal joint

Triscaphe joint (scaphotrapezium portion)

Radial artery

Flexor digitorum profundus tendons

Fluid in pisotriquetral recess

Figure 2.7D

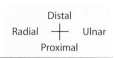

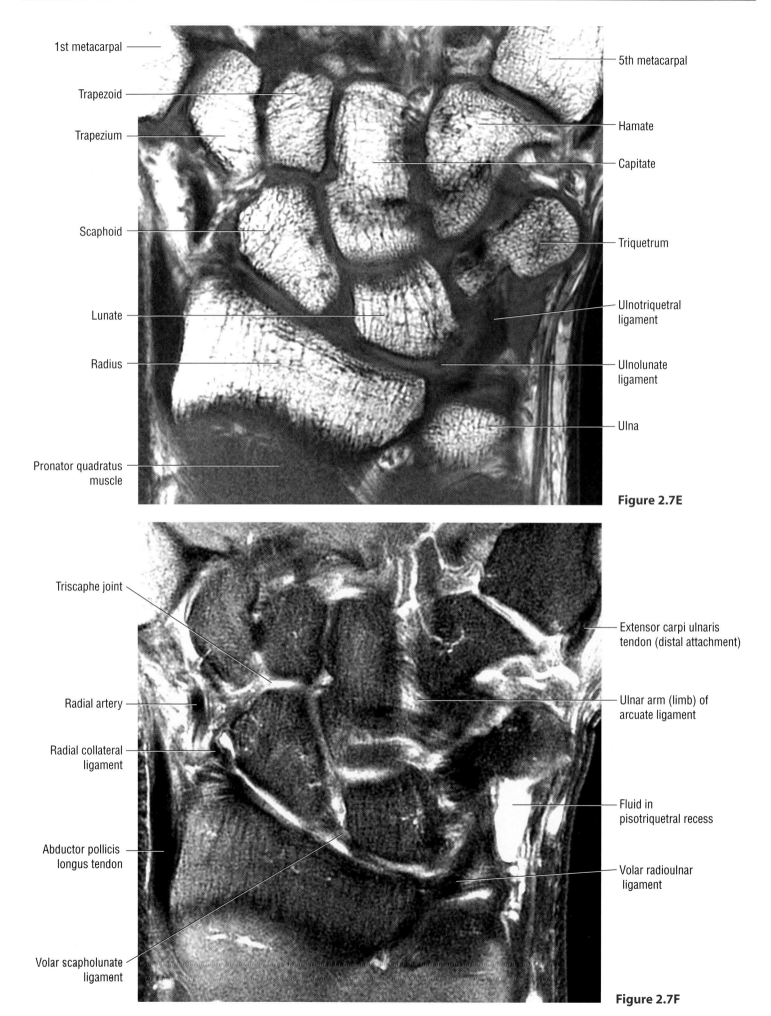

1st metacarpal

Trapezoid

Trapezium

Scaphoid

Lunate

Radius

Pronator quadratus
muscle

5th metacarpal

Hamate

Capitate

Triquetrum

Ulnotriquetral
ligament

Ulnolunate
ligament

Ulna

Figure 2.7E

Triscaphe joint

Radial artery

Radial collateral
ligament

Abductor pollicis
longus tendon

Volar scapholunate
ligament

Extensor carpi ulnaris
tendon (distal attachment)

Ulnar arm (limb) of
arcuate ligament

Fluid in
pisotriquetral recess

Volar radioulnar
ligament

Figure 2.7F

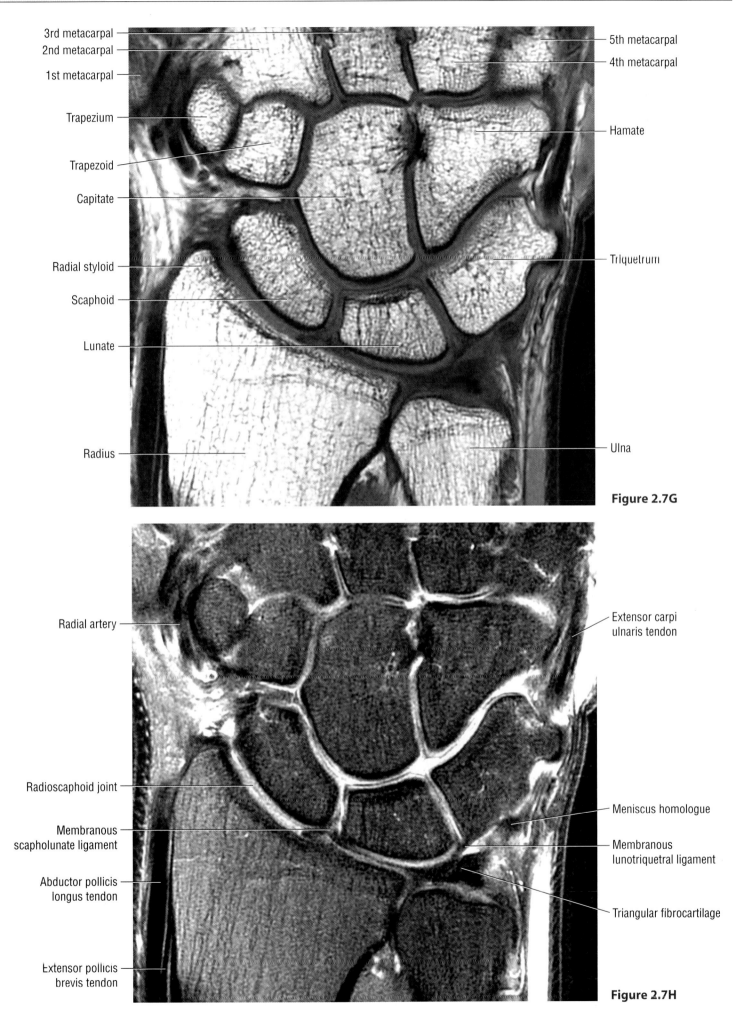

3rd metacarpal
2nd metacarpal
1st metacarpal

Trapezium

Trapezoid

Capitate

Radial styloid

Scaphoid

Lunate

Radius

5th metacarpal
4th metacarpal

Hamate

Triquetrum

Ulna

Figure 2.7G

Radial artery

Radioscaphoid joint

Membranous
scapholunate ligament

Abductor pollicis
longus tendon

Extensor pollicis
brevis tendon

Extensor carpi
ulnaris tendon

Meniscus homologue

Membranous
lunotriquetral ligament

Triangular fibrocartilage

Figure 2.7H

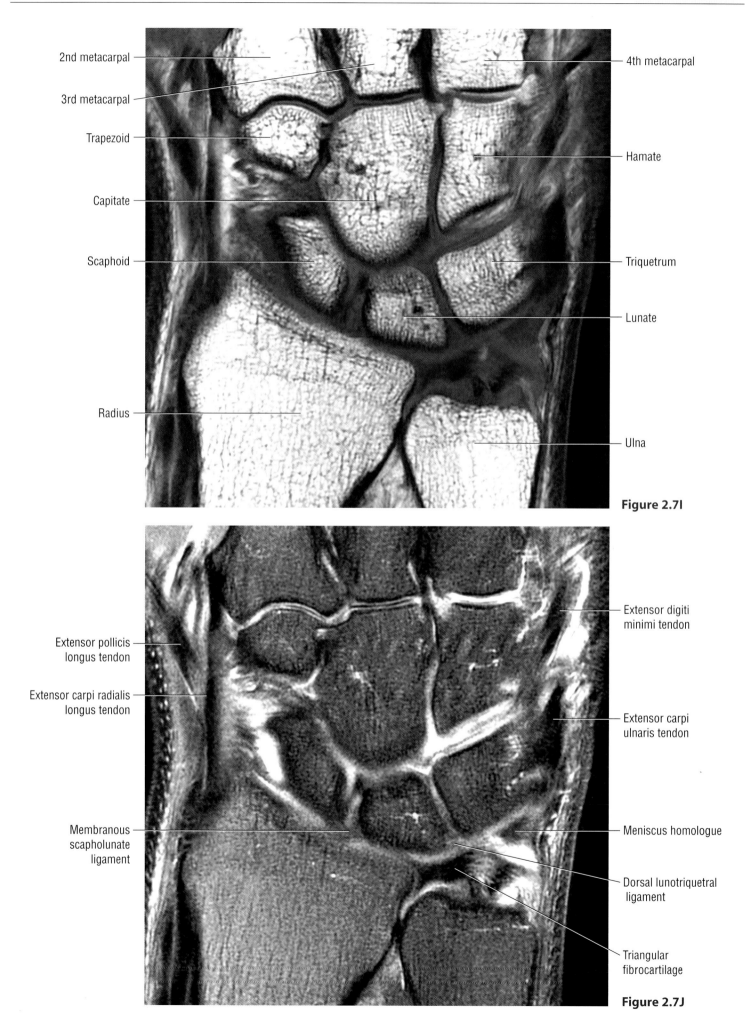

2nd metacarpal

3rd metacarpal

Trapezoid

Capitate

Scaphoid

Radius

4th metacarpal

Hamate

Triquetrum

Lunate

Ulna

Figure 2.7I

Extensor pollicis
longus tendon

Extensor carpi radialis
longus tendon

Membranous
scapholunate
ligament

Extensor digiti
minimi tendon

Extensor carpi
ulnaris tendon

Meniscus homologue

Dorsal lunotriquetral
ligament

Triangular
fibrocartilage

Figure 2.7J

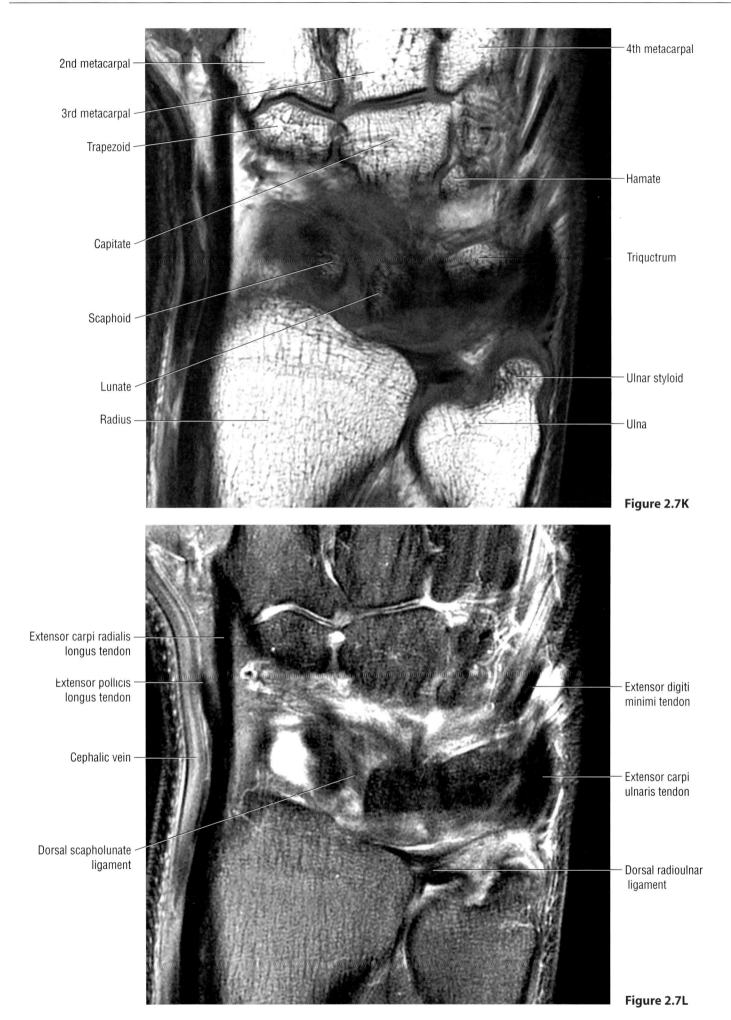

2nd metacarpal

3rd metacarpal

Trapezoid

Capitate

Scaphoid

Lunate

Radius

4th metacarpal

Hamate

Triquetrum

Ulnar styloid

Ulna

Figure 2.7K

Extensor carpi radialis longus tendon

Extensor pollicis longus tendon

Cephalic vein

Dorsal scapholunate ligament

Extensor digiti minimi tendon

Extensor carpi ulnaris tendon

Dorsal radioulnar ligament

Figure 2.7L

Wrist - Coronal

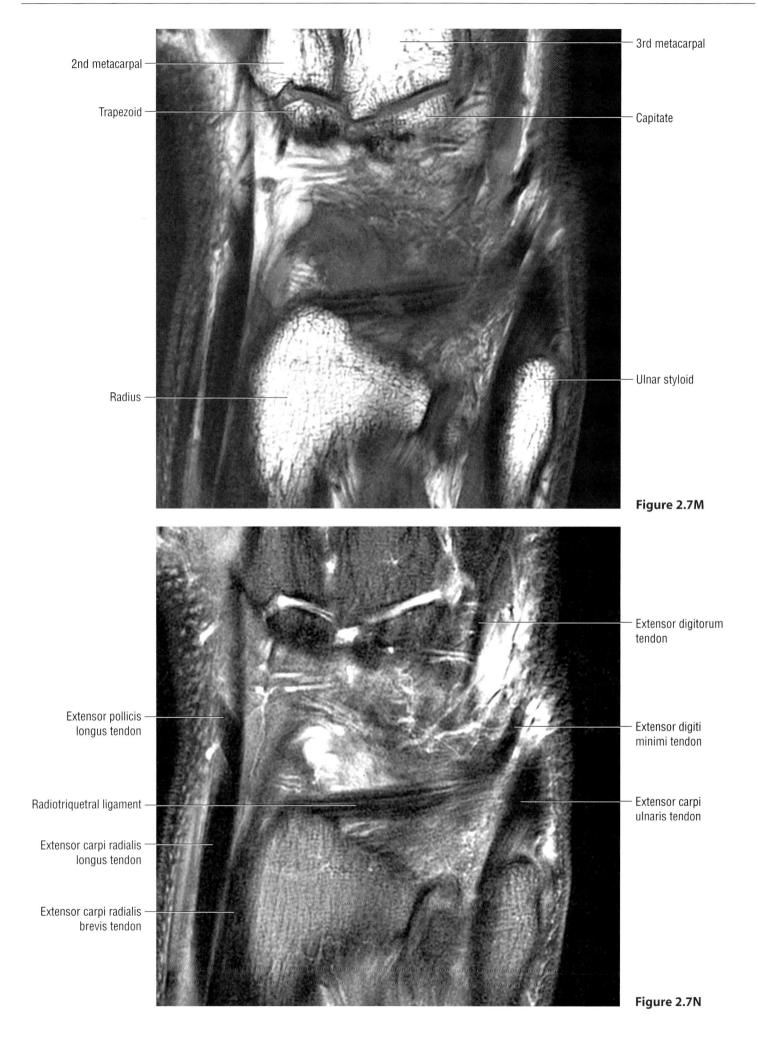

2nd metacarpal

Trapezoid

Radius

3rd metacarpal

Capitate

Ulnar styloid

Figure 2.7M

Extensor pollicis
longus tendon

Radiotriquetral ligament

Extensor carpi radialis
longus tendon

Extensor carpi radialis
brevis tendon

Extensor digitorum
tendon

Extensor digiti
minimi tendon

Extensor carpi
ulnaris tendon

Figure 2.7N

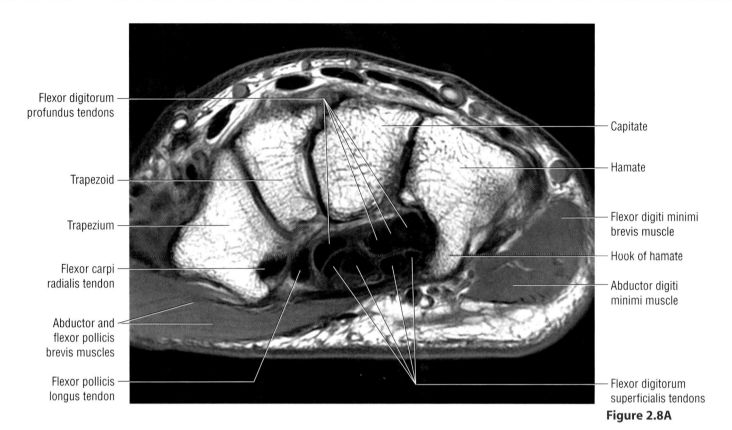

Flexor digitorum profundus tendons

Trapezoid

Trapezium

Flexor carpi radialis tendon

Abductor and flexor pollicis brevis muscles

Flexor pollicis longus tendon

Capitate

Hamate

Flexor digiti minimi brevis muscle

Hook of hamate

Abductor digiti minimi muscle

Flexor digitorum superficialis tendons

Figure 2.8A

Extensor carpi radialis brevis tendon

Extensor carpi radialis longus tendon

Extensor pollicis longus tendon

Extensor pollicis brevis tendon

Abductor pollicis longus tendon insertion

Flexor retinaculum

Palmar aponeurosis

Extensor digitorum and indicis tendons

Extensor digiti minimi tendon

Extensor carpi ulnaris tendon

Median nerve

Superficial ulnar nerve branches

Ulnar artery

Figure 2.8B

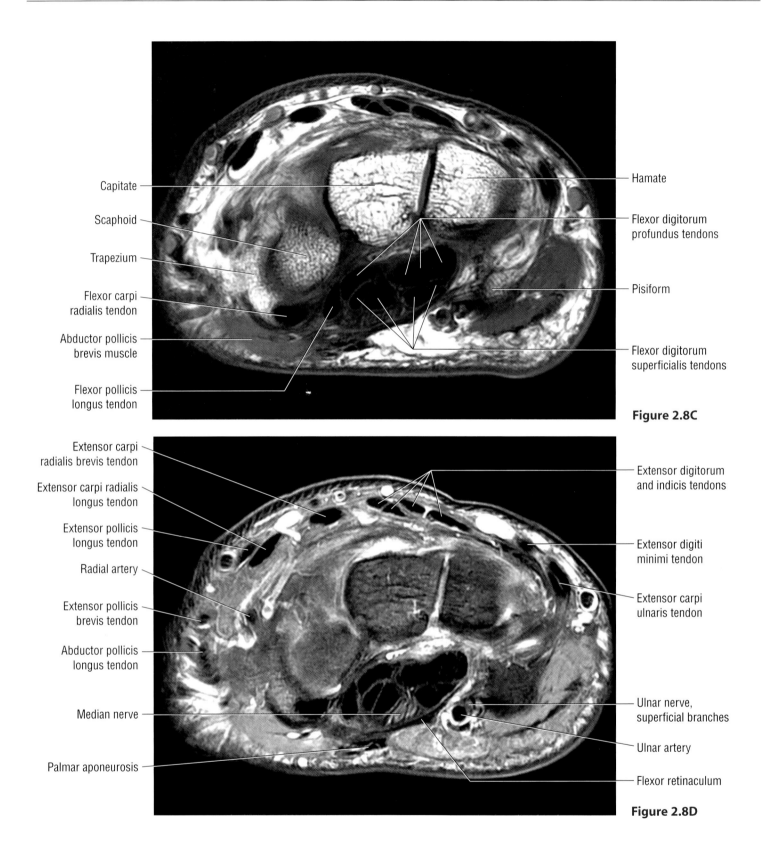

Capitate

Scaphoid

Trapezium

Flexor carpi
radialis tendon

Abductor pollicis
brevis muscle

Flexor pollicis
longus tendon

Hamate

Flexor digitorum
profundus tendons

Pisiform

Flexor digitorum
superficialis tendons

Figure 2.8C

Extensor carpi
radialis brevis tendon

Extensor carpi radialis
longus tendon

Extensor pollicis
longus tendon

Radial artery

Extensor pollicis
brevis tendon

Abductor pollicis
longus tendon

Median nerve

Palmar aponeurosis

Extensor digitorum
and indicis tendons

Extensor digiti
minimi tendon

Extensor carpi
ulnaris tendon

Ulnar nerve,
superficial branches

Ulnar artery

Flexor retinaculum

Figure 2.8D

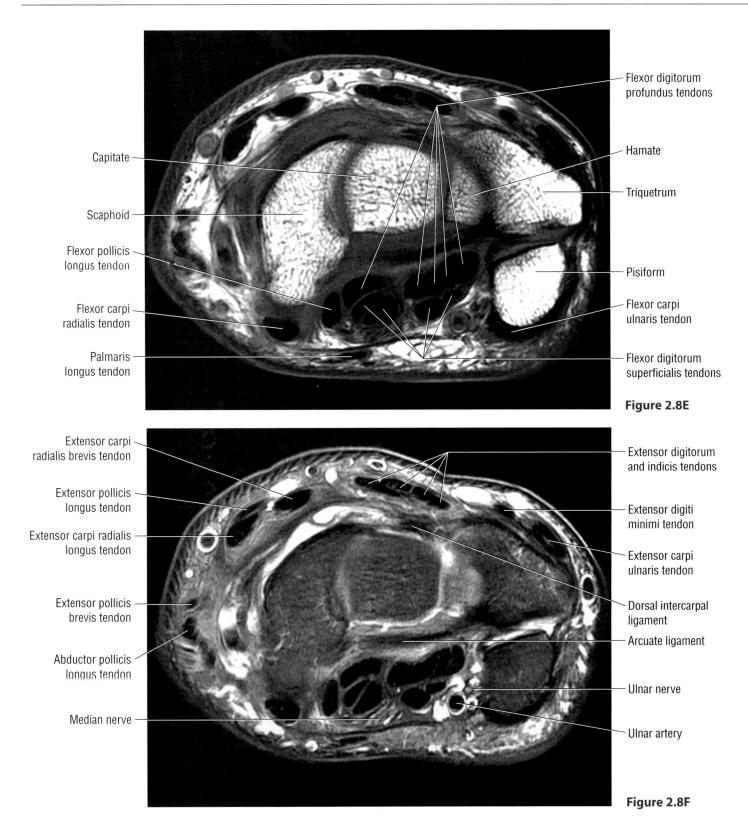

Capitate

Scaphoid

Flexor pollicis
longus tendon

Flexor carpi
radialis tendon

Palmaris
longus tendon

Flexor digitorum
profundus tendons

Hamate

Triquetrum

Pisiform

Flexor carpi
ulnaris tendon

Flexor digitorum
superficialis tendons

Figure 2.8E

Extensor carpi
radialis brevis tendon

Extensor pollicis
longus tendon

Extensor carpi radialis
longus tendon

Extensor pollicis
brevis tendon

Abductor pollicis
longus tendon

Median nerve

Extensor digitorum
and indicis tendons

Extensor digiti
minimi tendon

Extensor carpi
ulnaris tendon

Dorsal intercarpal
ligament

Arcuate ligament

Ulnar nerve

Ulnar artery

Figure 2.8F

Dorsal
Radial + Ulnar
Volar

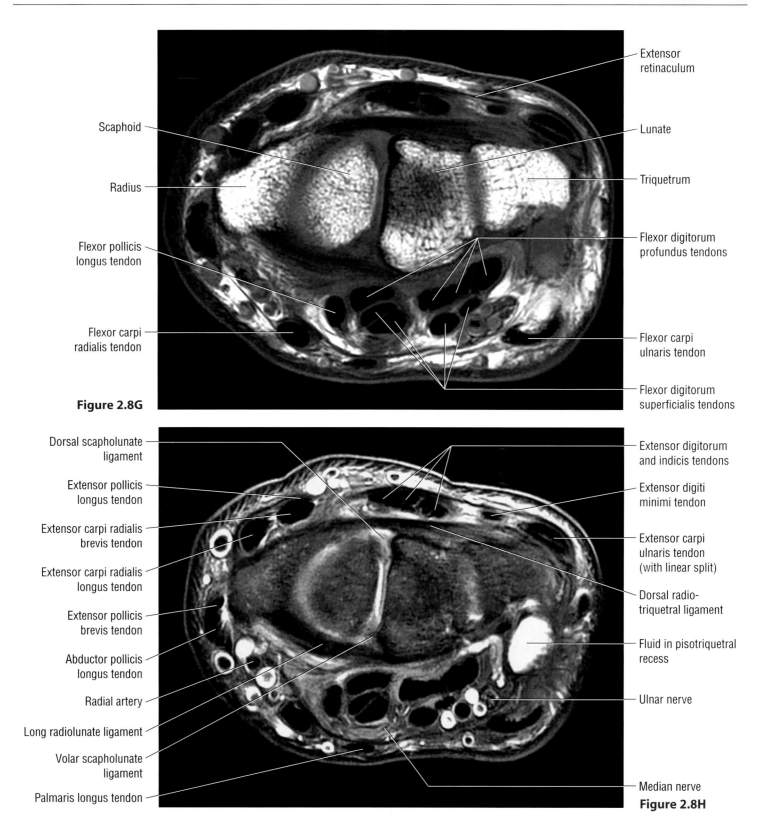

Extensor
retinaculum

Scaphoid

Lunate

Radius

Triquetrum

Flexor pollicis
longus tendon

Flexor digitorum
profundus tendons

Flexor carpi
radialis tendon

Flexor carpi
ulnaris tendon

Flexor digitorum
superficialis tendons

Figure 2.8G

Dorsal scapholunate
ligament

Extensor digitorum
and indicis tendons

Extensor pollicis
longus tendon

Extensor digiti
minimi tendon

Extensor carpi radialis
brevis tendon

Extensor carpi
ulnaris tendon
(with linear split)

Extensor carpi radialis
longus tendon

Dorsal radio-
triquetral ligament

Extensor pollicis
brevis tendon

Fluid in pisotriquetral
recess

Abductor pollicis
longus tendon

Radial artery

Ulnar nerve

Long radiolunate ligament

Volar scapholunate
ligament

Palmaris longus tendon

Median nerve

Figure 2.8H

Dorsal
Radial — + — Ulnar
Volar

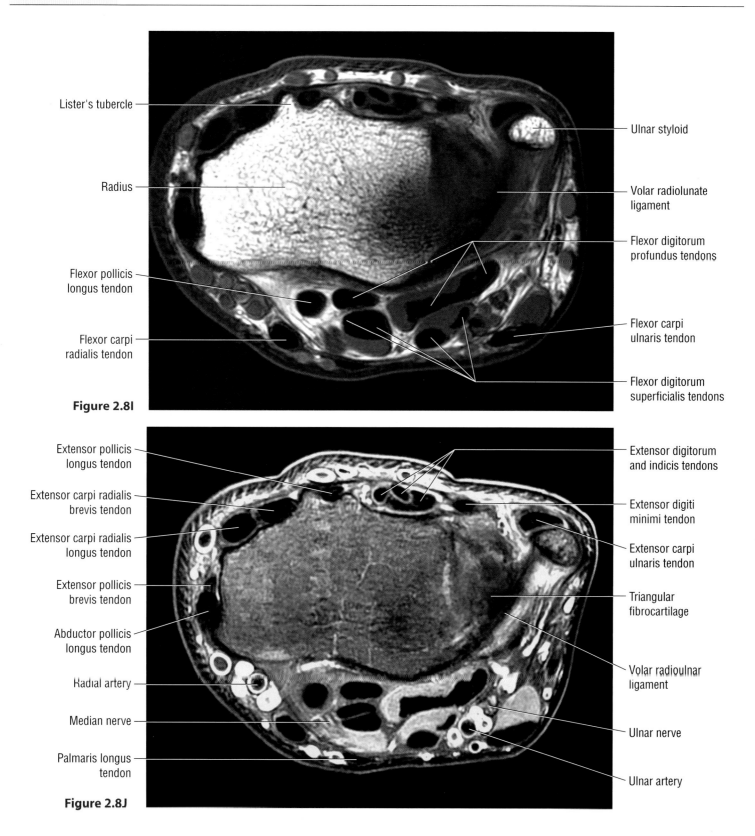

Lister's tubercle

Ulnar styloid

Radius

Volar radiolunate ligament

Flexor digitorum profundus tendons

Flexor pollicis longus tendon

Flexor carpi ulnaris tendon

Flexor carpi radialis tendon

Flexor digitorum superficialis tendons

Figure 2.8I

Extensor pollicis longus tendon

Extensor digitorum and indicis tendons

Extensor carpi radialis brevis tendon

Extensor digiti minimi tendon

Extensor carpi radialis longus tendon

Extensor carpi ulnaris tendon

Extensor pollicis brevis tendon

Triangular fibrocartilage

Abductor pollicis longus tendon

Radial artery

Volar radioulnar ligament

Median nerve

Ulnar nerve

Palmaris longus tendon

Ulnar artery

Figure 2.8J

Dorsal
Radial ━┼━ Ulnar
Volar

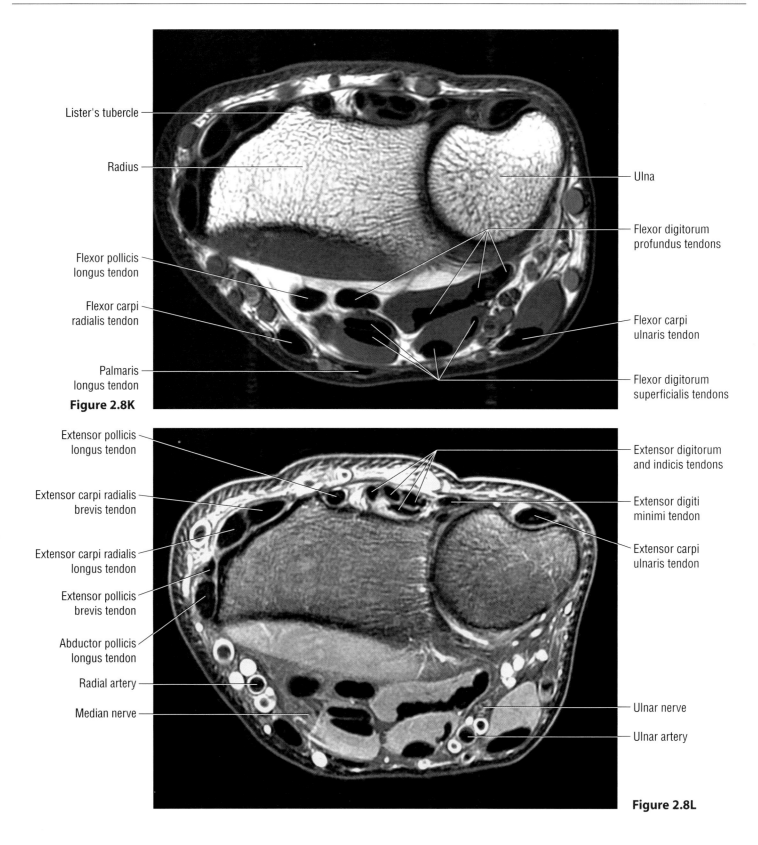

Lister's tubercle

Radius

Ulna

Flexor digitorum
profundus tendons

Flexor pollicis
longus tendon

Flexor carpi
radialis tendon

Flexor carpi
ulnaris tendon

Palmaris
longus tendon

Flexor digitorum
superficialis tendons

Figure 2.8K

Extensor pollicis
longus tendon

Extensor digitorum
and indicis tendons

Extensor carpi radialis
brevis tendon

Extensor digiti
minimi tendon

Extensor carpi radialis
longus tendon

Extensor carpi
ulnaris tendon

Extensor pollicis
brevis tendon

Abductor pollicis
longus tendon

Radial artery

Median nerve

Ulnar nerve

Ulnar artery

Figure 2.8L

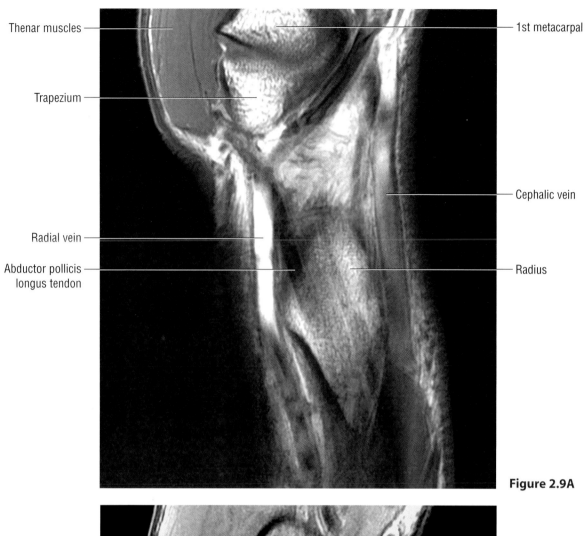

Thenar muscles —

Trapezium —

Radial vein —

Abductor pollicis
longus tendon —

— 1st metacarpal

— Cephalic vein

— Radius

Figure 2.9A

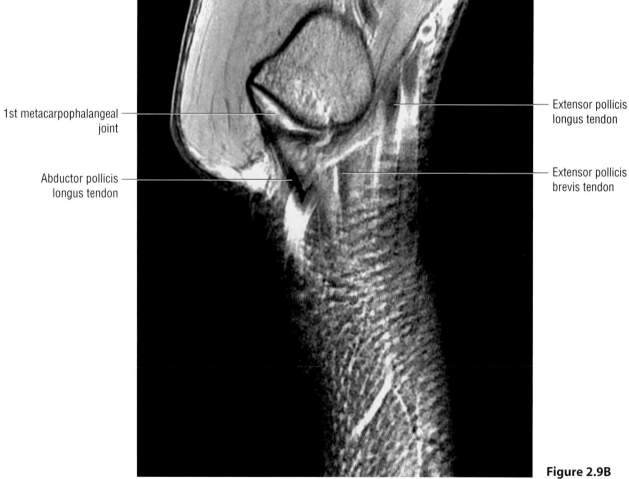

1st metacarpophalangeal
joint —

Abductor pollicis
longus tendon —

— Extensor pollicis
longus tendon

— Extensor pollicis
brevis tendon

Figure 2.9B

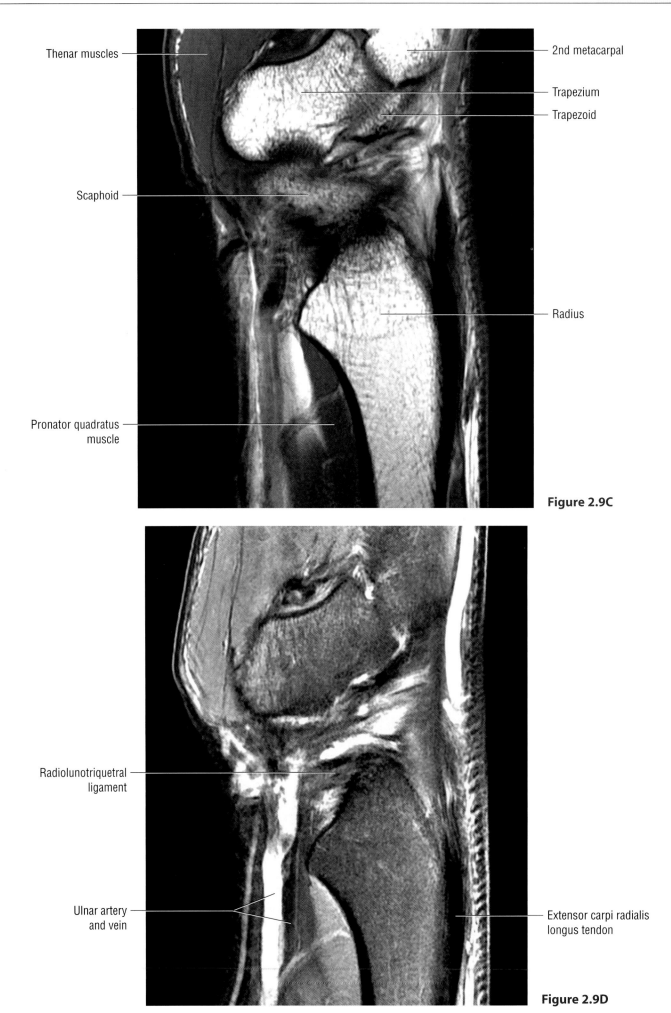

Thenar muscles

Scaphoid

Pronator quadratus muscle

2nd metacarpal

Trapezium

Trapezoid

Radius

Figure 2.9C

Radiolunotriquetral ligament

Ulnar artery and vein

Extensor carpi radialis longus tendon

Figure 2.9D

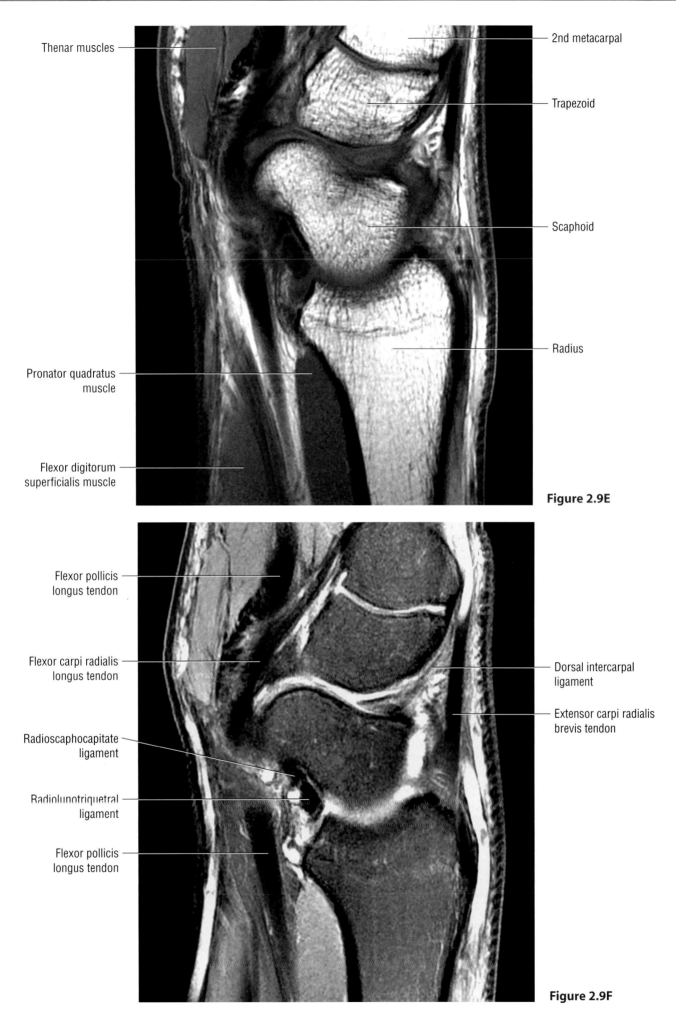

Thenar muscles

Pronator quadratus muscle

Flexor digitorum superficialis muscle

2nd metacarpal

Trapezoid

Scaphoid

Radius

Figure 2.9E

Flexor pollicis longus tendon

Flexor carpi radialis longus tendon

Radioscaphocapitate ligament

Radiolunotriquetral ligament

Flexor pollicis longus tendon

Dorsal intercarpal ligament

Extensor carpi radialis brevis tendon

Figure 2.9F

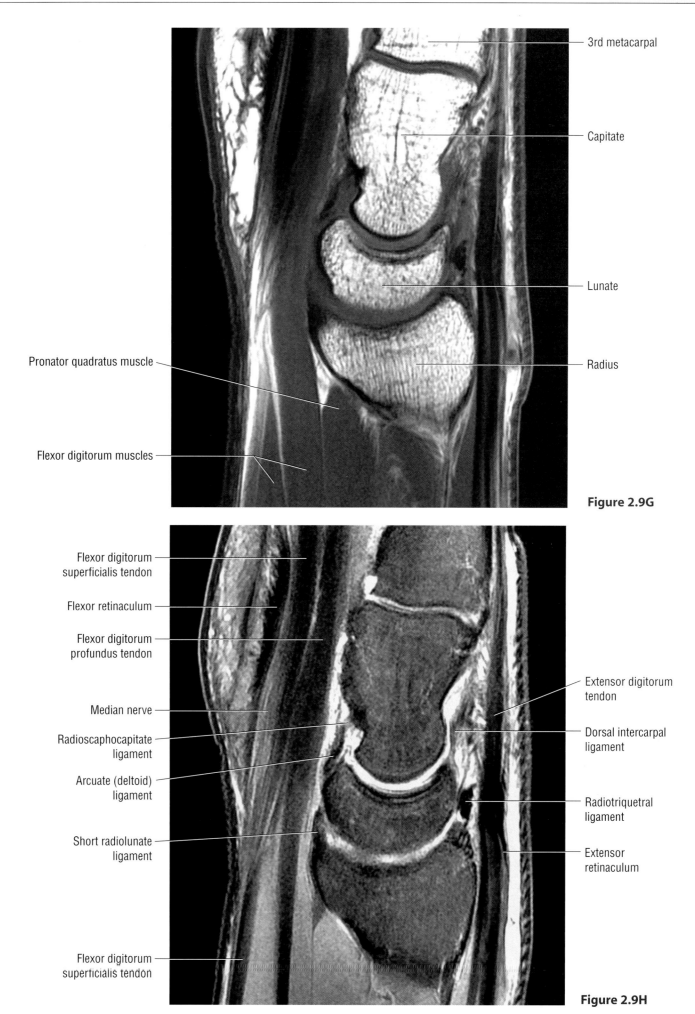

3rd metacarpal

Capitate

Lunate

Pronator quadratus muscle

Radius

Flexor digitorum muscles

Figure 2.9G

Flexor digitorum
superficialis tendon

Flexor retinaculum

Flexor digitorum
profundus tendon

Extensor digitorum
tendon

Median nerve

Radioscaphocapitate
ligament

Dorsal intercarpal
ligament

Arcuate (deltoid)
ligament

Radiotriquetral
ligament

Short radiolunate
ligament

Extensor
retinaculum

Flexor digitorum
superficialis tendon

Figure 2.9H

Distal
Volar ─┼─ Dorsal
Proximal

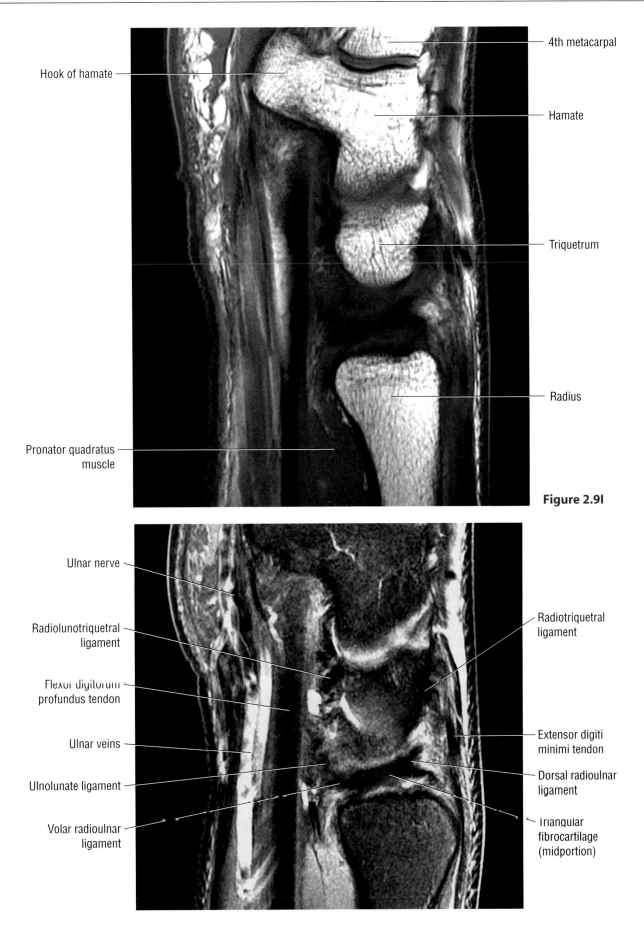

Hook of hamate

4th metacarpal

Hamate

Triquetrum

Radius

Pronator quadratus muscle

Figure 2.9I

Ulnar nerve

Radiolunotriquetral ligament

Flexor digitorum profundus tendon

Ulnar veins

Ulnolunate ligament

Volar radioulnar ligament

Radiotriquetral ligament

Extensor digiti minimi tendon

Dorsal radioulnar ligament

Triangular fibrocartilage (midportion)

Figure 2.9J

Wrist - Sagittal

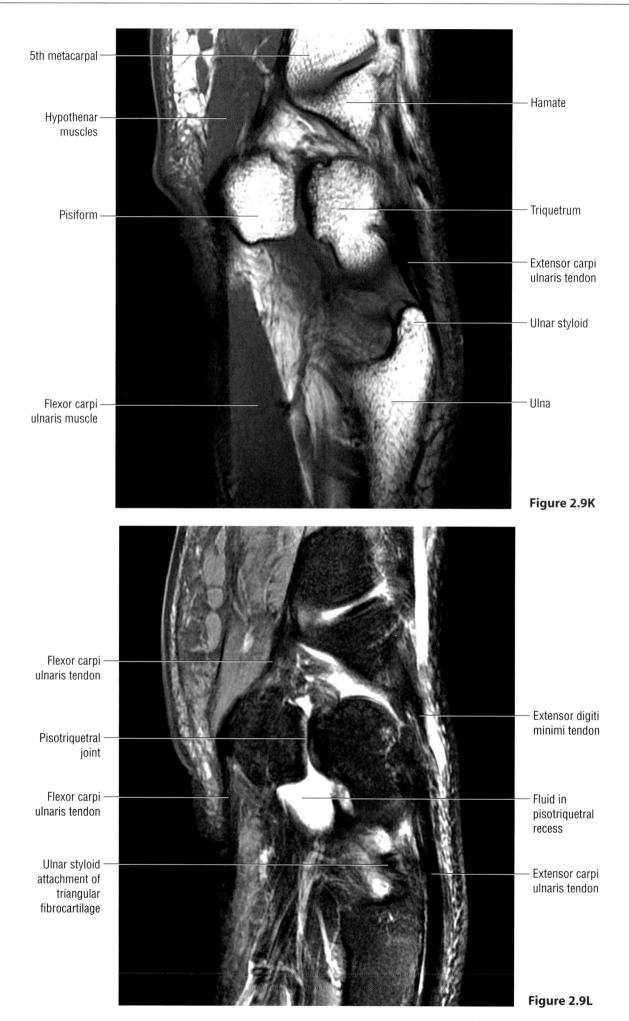

5th metacarpal

Hypothenar muscles

Pisiform

Flexor carpi ulnaris muscle

Hamate

Triquetrum

Extensor carpi ulnaris tendon

Ulnar styloid

Ulna

Figure 2.9K

Flexor carpi ulnaris tendon

Pisotriquetral joint

Flexor carpi ulnaris tendon

Ulnar styloid attachment of triangular fibrocartilage

Extensor digiti minimi tendon

Fluid in pisotriquetral recess

Extensor carpi ulnaris tendon

Figure 2.9L

Chapter

3

The Hip

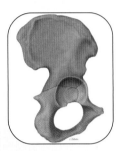

Pearls and Pitfalls & Color Illustrations

Pearls and Pitfalls

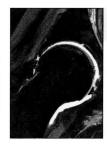

IMAGING PROTOCOLS

- A phased array torso, cardiac, or dedicated hip coil is required to evaluate femoroacetabular impingement using high-resolution images.
- FS PD FSE images in the coronal axial and sagittal planes are used to identify anterior and lateral acetabular labral tears.

- Axial oblique images are used to estimate the alpha angle in the nonspherical femoral head in cam-type femoroacetabular impingement.
- MR arthrography is an optional adjunct and is not a replacement for routine FS PD FSE imaging.

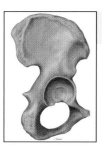

NORMAL ANATOMY AND VARIANTS
(See Figures 3.29–3.53)

- The stellate lesion or crease represents a normal bare area superior to the acetabular fossa.
- The transverse acetabular ligament bridges the incomplete acetabular ring inferiorly. The acetabular labrum ends at the anterior and posterior margins of the inferior aspect of the acetabulum.

- Normal labral variants are visualized posteroinferiorly, anterosuperiorly, at the junction of the transverse ligament and labrum, and between the capsule and labrum lateral to the acetabular rim.
- In DDH, the labrum may be hypertrophic and associated with a femoral head chondral crease.
- The sciatic nerve sheath contains two peripheral nerves: the tibial and common peroneal nerves.

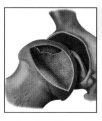

AVASCULAR NECROSIS
(See Figures 3.54–3.56)

- AVN usually involves the anterolateral aspect of the femoral head.
- Articular cartilage is intact at the initial presentation of ischemia.

- Sagittal images are the most accurate in assessing the femoral head changes that occur with subchondral fracture.
- The double line sign may be absent in 20% of cases.
- Loss of the spherical shape of the femoral head corresponds to Ficat stage 3.
- Many cases of previously diagnosed transient osteoporosis of the hip are, in fact, subchondral femoral head stress fractures.

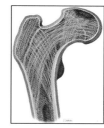

LEGG-CALVÉ-PERTHES DISEASE
(See Figure 3.57)

- Results in infarction of the bony capital epiphysis.
- Catterall classification estimates the amount of femoral head involvement.
- Hypointense irregularity of the periphery of the ossific nucleus and linear hypointensity traversing the femoral ossification center are early findings on T1- or PD-weighted images.

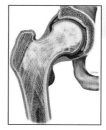

TRANSIENT OSTEOPOROSIS
(See Figure 3.58)

- Most cases actually represent subchondral femoral head stress fractures, which can be appreciated on small-FOV images.
- There is marrow sparing in the medial femoral head and greater trochanter.

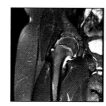

SLIPPED CAPITAL FEMORAL EPIPHYSIS

- Characterized by posterior inferior displacement of the proximal femoral epiphysis.
- MR demonstrates a widened growth plate and epiphyseal slippage.

- Arthroscopy is used to evaluate articular cartilage and labral injury and to decompress hematoma caused by physeal fracture.

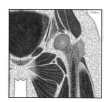

DEVELOPMENTAL DYSPLASIA OF THE HIP
(See Figures 3.59–3.61)

- Classification of DDH is based on the configuration of the acetabulum and labrum.

- Identification of the capital epiphysis location requires both coronal and axial images.
- In mild DDH, anterior coronal MR images display an increased slope of the acetabulum.
- DDH in the young adult may be associated with acetabular labral pathology and acetabular rim syndrome.

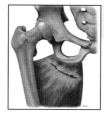

MUSCLE STRAINS
(See Figures 3.62–3.64, 3.75)

- The MTU is the weakest biomechanical link and therefore is most often the location of muscle fiber failure.
- Infection or deep venous thrombosis may be mistaken for a muscle strain.

- Grade I muscle injuries are associated with a feathery edema pattern of muscle fibers.

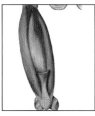

MUSCLE CONTUSIONS
(See Figures 3.65–3.67, 3.74)

- Contusions are caused by compressive or concussive forms of direct trauma.
- Contusions involve the deep muscle belly fibers.

- Muscle edema and hematoma contribute to an increase in muscle girth without architectural disruption.
- Myositis ossificans is associated with both myonecrosis and hematoma.

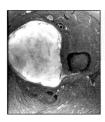

INTERSTITIAL HEMORRHAGE AND HEMATOMA

- Interstitial hemorrhage occurs between the damaged connective tissues.
- Hematomas may demonstrate susceptibility with gradient echo imaging.

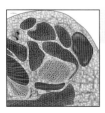

MOREL-LAVALLÉE LESION
(See Figure 3.68)

- Morel-Lavallée lesions are posttraumatic fluid collections deep to the subcutaneous tissue and superficial to the fascia lata and iliotibial band in the trochanteric region and proximal thigh.

- Types II and III Morel-Lavallée lesions demonstrate signal inhomogeneity on FS PD FSE images, reflecting nonacute hematomas.

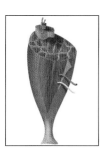

DELAYED ONSET MUSCLE SORENESS

- Symptoms peak 24 to 72 hours after nonacute injury.
- Regeneration begins 3 days after exertion.
- MR findings are similar to muscle strains.
- Delayed-onset muscle soreness is often associated with excessive eccentric muscle activity.

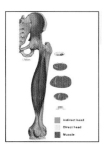

RECTUS FEMORIS MUSCLE STRAIN
(See Figures 3.69–3.73)

- Injuries to the deep intramuscular tendon of the indirect head are usually seen in track and field, football, soccer, and basketball injuries.
- Distal musculotendinous junction tears occur distally at the knee, whereas proximal injuries involve the deep indirect head.

- Fibrous encasement of the deep tendon is hypointense on FS PD FSE images and is a complication of deep indirect head injuries.

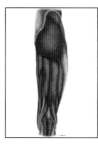

HAMSTRING TENDINOSIS AND MUSCLE INJURIES
(See Figures 3.76–3.78)

- The hamstring group consists of the biceps femoris and the semimembranosus and semitendinosus.
- Grade I strains are visualized with a feathery pattern of edema.

- Grade II strains are associated with hyperintense hematoma and intramuscular and extramuscular fluid collections.
- Grade III strains are associated with a hemorrhage-filled gap and a retracted MTU.

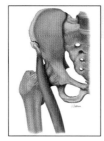

AVULSION FRACTURES
(See Figures 3.79–3.85)

- ASIS avulsion involves the origin of the sartorius.
- AIIS avulsion involves the origin of the direct head of the rectus femoris.
- Acetabular rim avulsion involves the origin of reflected (indirect) head.

- Ischial tuberosity avulsion involves the origin of the hamstring muscles.
- Lesser trochanter avulsion involves the insertion of the iliopsoas.
- The iliac crest is the attachment of the tensor fascia lata, the gluteus medius, the transverse abdominis, and the internal and external obliques.
- The symphysis pubis and pubic ramus are the site of origin of the adductor longus, adductor brevis, and gracilis.

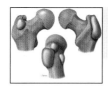

HIP ABDUCTOR INJURIES AND TROCHANTERIC BURSITIS
(See Figures 3.86–3.91)

- The anterior facet of the greater trochanter is the attachment site of the gluteus minimus.

- The lateral facet of the greater trochanter is the attachment site of the gluteus medius muscle, and the superoposterior facet is the attachment of the gluteus medius tendon.
- The trochanteric bursa is the subgluteus maximus bursa.
- The subgluteus medius bursa is deep to the gluteus medius tendon and the subgluteus minimus bursa is deep to the gluteus minimus tendon.
- Adductor tendon pathology includes tendinosis, partial tears, and full-thickness tears.

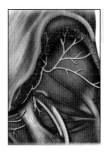

PIRIFORMIS SYNDROME
(See Figures 3.92–3.94)

- Neuritis of the proximal sciatic nerve is associated with trauma to the gluteal region.
- Pathology is related to hypertrophy of the piriformis, compression of the sciatic nerve, myositis ossificans, and mass lesion.

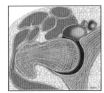

ILIOPSOAS BURSITIS
(See Figures 3.95–3.96)

- The iliopsoas bursa is medial to the iliopsoas muscle.
- Bursitis may be associated with overuse, rheumatoid arthritis, trauma, and the snapping hip syndrome.

- MR appearance is hyperintense on FS PD FSE images; heterogeneity is associated with synovitis or infection.
- There is communication with the hip joint through the tail-like extension.

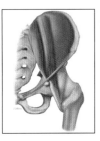

SNAPPING HIP SYNDROME
(See Figures 3.97–3.100)

- May be classified as intra-articular, external, or internal.
- Snapping occurs during hip flexion and extension.
- External type occurs as the proximal iliotibial band slides over the greater trochanter.

- Internal type occurs as the iliopsoas snaps over the iliopectineal eminence.
- Fluid signal intensity or edema associated with the iliopsoas tendon can be identified on FS PD FSE images.

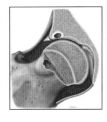

FEMOROACETABULAR IMPINGEMENT
(See Figures 3.101–3.121)

- Caused by an abnormal abutment between the proximal femur and the acetabular rim.
- Cam, pincer, and mixed cam-pincer (most common).

- Cam impingement is associated with a dysplastic femoral bump and posterior osteophytes (posterior to the bump on the lateral aspect of the femoral head-neck junction), as well as shearing of the articular cartilage from the anterolateral acetabular rim.
- The pincer type is associated with overcoverage or retroversion of the acetabulum.

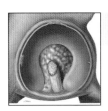

LABRAL TEARS
(See Figures 3.122–3.129)

- Labral tears are part of the FAI syndrome.
- Identification of labral tear morphology, including chondrolabral separation and cleavage tears.

- Adjacent paralabral cysts communicate with areas of lateral degradation and tears.

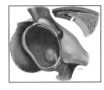

PARALABRAL CYSTS
(See Figure 3.130)

- Paralabral cysts may occur adjacent to any portion of the fibrocartilaginous labrum.

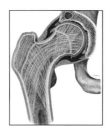

OSTEOARTHRITIS (OA)
(See Figure 3.131)

- Inflammatory OA presents with reactive subchondral edema involving both sides of the joint.
- Younger patients may present with FAI as a precursor to OA.

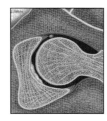

LOOSE BODIES
(See Figures 3.132–3.134)

- Loose bodies may be found in the acetabular fossa and anterior capsule.
- Loose bodies are associated with trauma, OA, and synovial chondromatosis/osteochondromatosis.

- Loose bodies usually demonstrate intermediate cartilage signal or sclerotic calcified cartilage that is hypointense on T1 and FS PD FSE images.

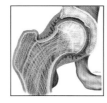

RHEUMATOID ARTHRITIS
(See Figure 3.135)

- Associated with concentric loss of hip joint space.
- Characterized by intermediate-signal-intensity synovial hypertrophy and intermediate to hyperintense pannus.

- Marrow edema of subchondral bone is hyperintense.
- Capsular distention is usually identified.

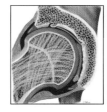

STELLATE LESION AND PLICA
(See Figure 3.138)

- The stellate lesion is located superior to the acetabular fossa and is best visualized superiorly on coronal and sagittal images opposite the femoral head convexity.

- The stellate lesion represents a normal area of chondral thinning.
- The stellate lesion is associated with a plica or fibrous cord attached to both the lesion and acetabular fossa.

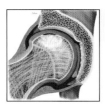

FEMORAL HEAD FRACTURES
(See Figures 3.139–3.140)

- Fractures are associated with posterior hip dislocation.
- There is an increased risk of AVN if hip dislocation is not reduced.

- The Pipkin classification is based on whether the fracture is below or above the ligamentum teres.
- Subchondral femoral head stress fractures mimic transient osteoporosis of the hip.

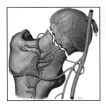

FEMORAL NECK FRACTURES
(See Figures 3.141–3.147)

- Subcapital fractures are more common than transcervical and basicervical fractures.
- Transverse or distraction fractures are insufficiency fractures that are seen in older patients and are unstable.

- Compression stress fractures in the inferomedial cortex occur in younger patients and are stable.
- Extracapsular fractures are either intertrochanteric or subtrochanteric.

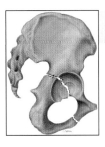

ACETABULAR FRACTURES
(See Figures 3.148–3.150)

- Acetabular fractures are divided into anterior column, posterior column, transverse, and complex fractures.
- Fracture involves the posterior wall and the anterior wall in isolation or in combination with a column injury.

- Fractures are related to high-energy trauma, with the femoral force transferred to the acetabulum.
- Complications include Morel-Lavallée lesion as an internal degloving injury.

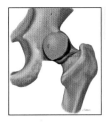

HIP DISLOCATION
(See Figures 3.151–3.152)

- Posterior dislocation is the most common type (90%) and is associated with femoral head fractures.
- The sciatic nerve is at risk, and rupture of the ligament teres is a potential complication.

- AVN is a delayed finding, and repeat MR should be performed within 2 months.

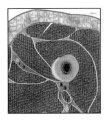

THIGH SPLINTS
(See Figure 3.153)

- Thigh splints involve the posteromedial adductor insertion.
- There is hyperintense periosteum, cortex, or a medullary cavity of the proximal to mid-femoral diaphysis.

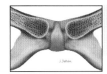

PUBIC RAMI STRESS FRACTURES AND OSTEITIS PUBIS
(See Figures 3.154–3.155)

- Inferior pubic ramus stress fractures are seen in athletes; superior ramus insufficiency fractures are seen in older patients.

- Osteitis pubis occurs as a clinical subtype in sports-related endeavors and is characterized by subchondral superior pubic ramus hyperintensity immediately adjacent to the pubic symphysis.

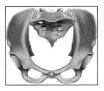

SACRAL INSUFFICIENCY FRACTURES
(See Figures 3.156–3.157)

- Unilateral or bilateral vertical sacral alar insufficiency fractures are parallel to the SI joints and appear hyperintense on FS PD FSE images.

- Fractures most commonly occur in postmenopausal osteoporosis.

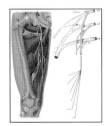

MUSCLE DENERVATION PATTERNS
(See Figures 3.160–3.162)

- **Sciatic nerve distribution**
  - □ Tibial
  - □ Peroneal
  - □ Injury associated with total hip arthroplasty
- **Femoral nerve distribution**
  - ❑ Injury associated with total hip arthroplasty or tumor
- **Obturator nerve distribution**
  - □ Pelvic tumors
  - □ Entrapment neuropathy (fascial or vascular structures as the source of hip and groin pain)

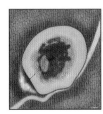

OSTEOMYELITIS
(See Figures 3.163–3.166)

- Acute hematogenous osteomyelitis is seen more often in pediatric patients, and post-traumatic osteomyelitis is seen more often in the adult population.

- Staphylococcus aureus is the most common infecting organism.
- The sinus tract is hyperintense on FS PD FSE images.
- The involucrum is a periosteal reaction.
- The sequestrum is hypointense on T1- and PD-weighted and FS PD FSE images.

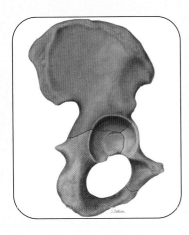

The Hip
Muscle

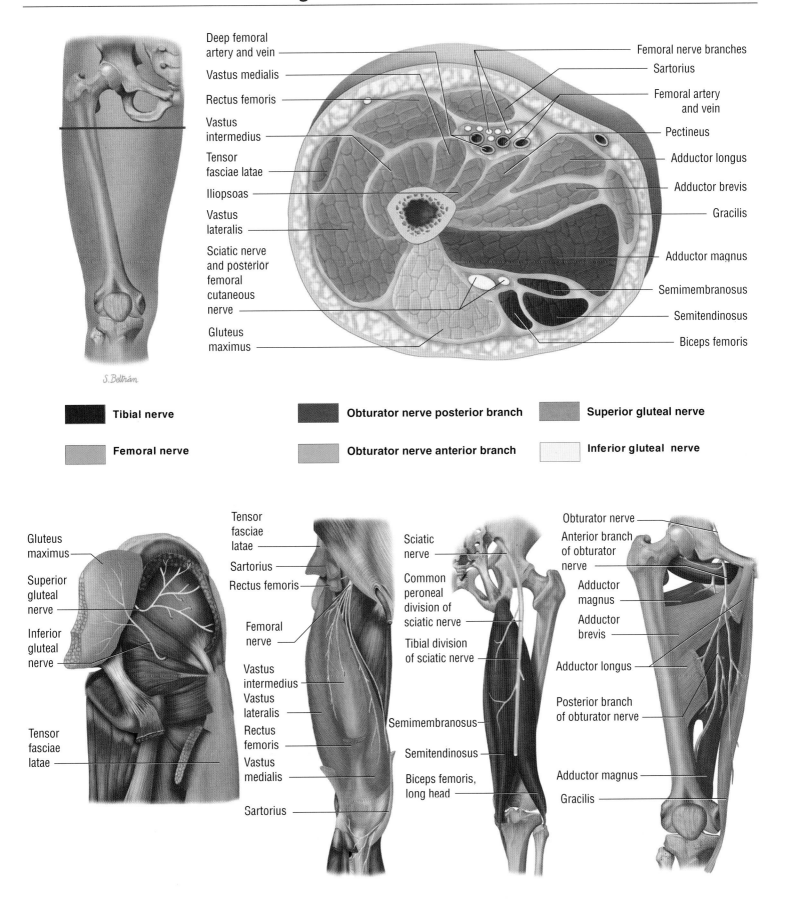

Tibial nerve

Femoral nerve

Obturator nerve posterior branch

Obturator nerve anterior branch

Superior gluteal nerve

Inferior gluteal nerve

Figure 3.1 ■ Proximal thigh muscle innervation. *Cross section based on Vahlensiech M, Genant HK, and Reiter M. MRI of the Musculoskeletal System. New York/Stuttgart: Thieme, 2000. (See Related Muscles pg. 42 and Neurovascular Structures pg. 104, in Stoller's 3rd Edition.)*

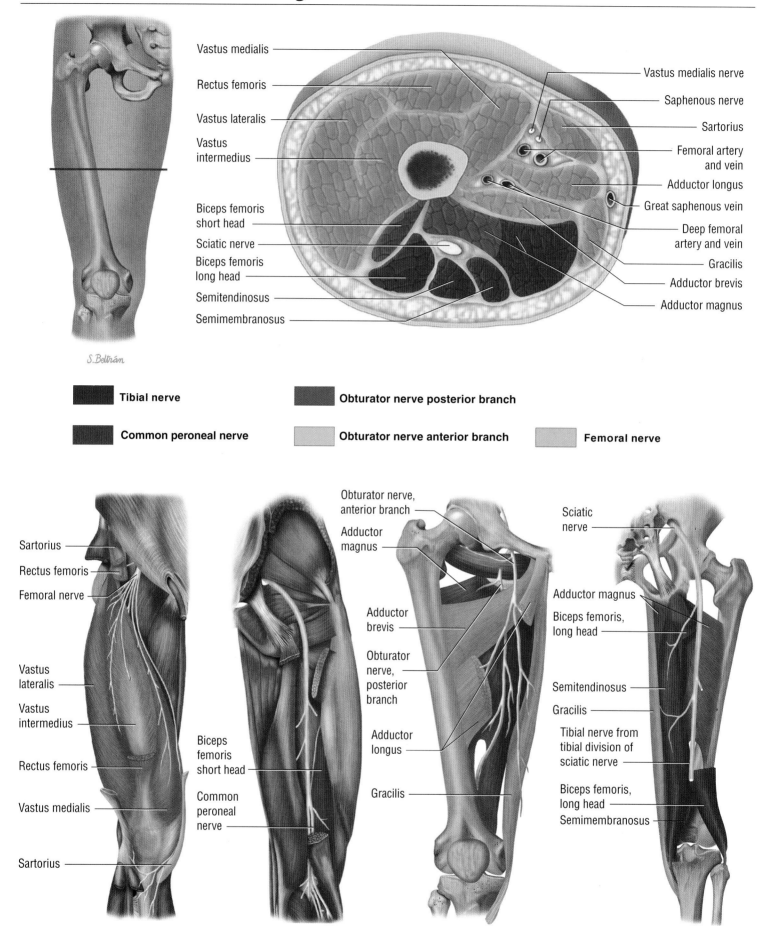

S. Beltrán

Tibial nerve

Common peroneal nerve

Obturator nerve posterior branch

Obturator nerve anterior branch

Femoral nerve

Figure 3.2 ■ Mid-thigh muscle innervation. *Cross section based on Vahlensiech M, Genant HK, and Reiter M. MRI of the Musculoskeletal System. New York/Stuttgart: Thieme, 2000. (See Related Muscles pg. 42 and Neurovascular Structures pg. 104, in Stoller's 3rd Edition.)*

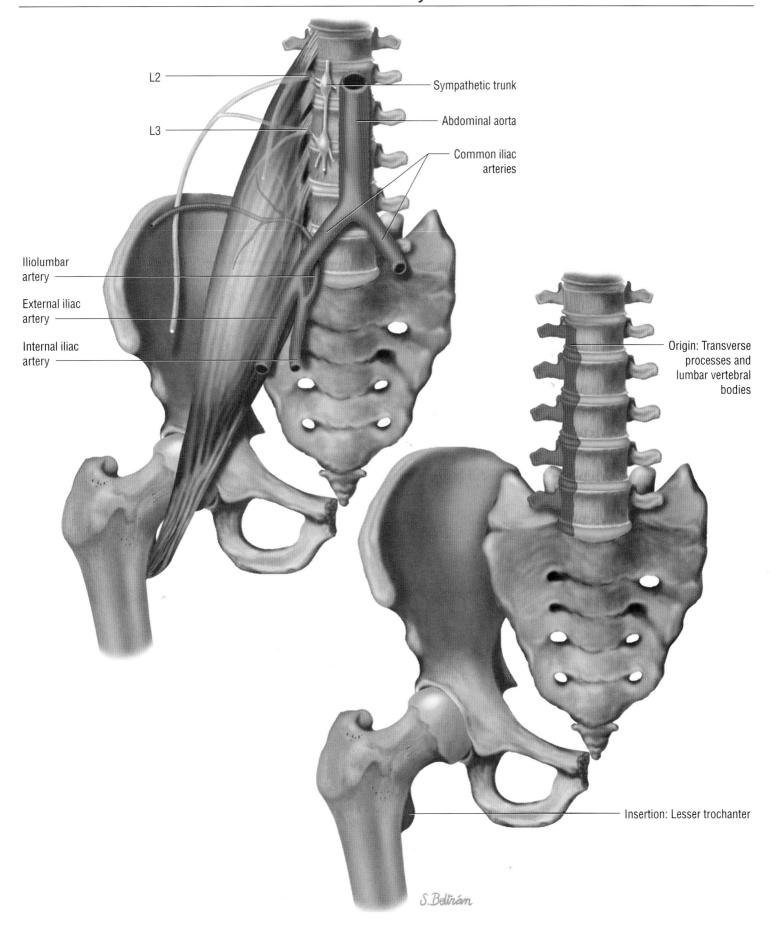

L2

L3

Iliolumbar
artery

External iliac
artery

Internal iliac
artery

Sympathetic trunk

Abdominal aorta

Common iliac
arteries

Origin: Transverse
processes and
lumbar vertebral
bodies

Insertion: Lesser trochanter

S.Beltrán

Figure 3.3 ▪ **PSOAS MAJOR.** The psoas major flexes the femur (thigh) and vertebral spine on the pelvis when the leg is fixed. The psoas major and iliacus form the iliopsoas muscle group. Iliopsoas muscle tendon strain is the result of forceful contraction of the iliopsoas when the thigh is fixed or in the extended position. *(See Related Muscles pg. 44, in Stoller's 3rd Edition.)*

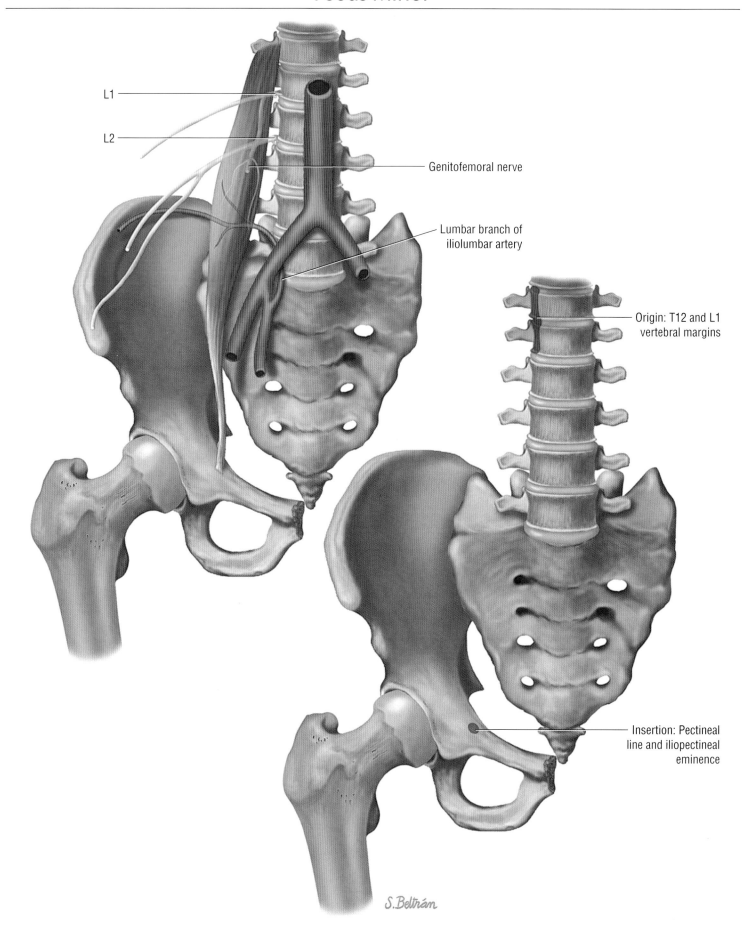

L1

L2

Genitofemoral nerve

Lumbar branch of
iliolumbar artery

Origin: T12 and L1
vertebral margins

Insertion: Pectineal
line and iliopectineal
eminence

S.Beltrán

Figure 3.4 ■ PSOAS MINOR. The psoas minor flexes the pelvis on the spine and assists the psoas major in flexing the spine. The psoas minor may be absent in 40% of
individuals. *(See Related Muscles pg. 45, in Stoller's 3rd Edition.)*

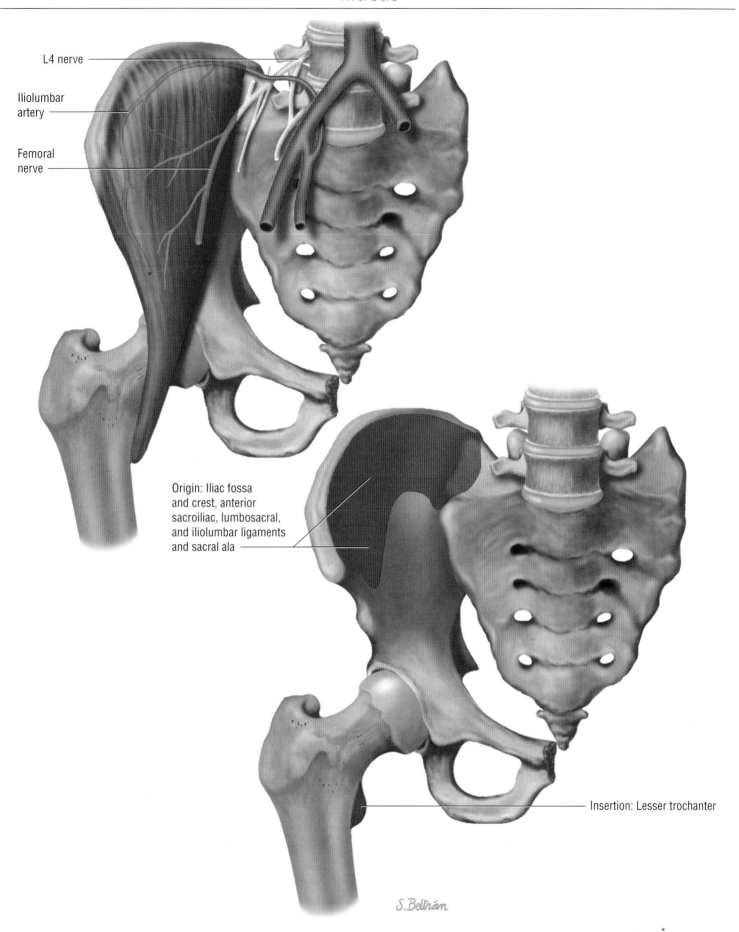

L4 nerve

Iliolumbar artery

Femoral nerve

Origin: Iliac fossa and crest, anterior sacroiliac, lumbosacral, and iliolumbar ligaments and sacral ala

Insertion: Lesser trochanter

S.Beltrán

Figure 3.5 ■ ILIACUS. The iliacus muscle flexes the femur (thigh) and tilts the pelvis anteriorly when the leg is fixed. *(See Related Muscles pg. 46, in Stoller's 3rd Edition.)*

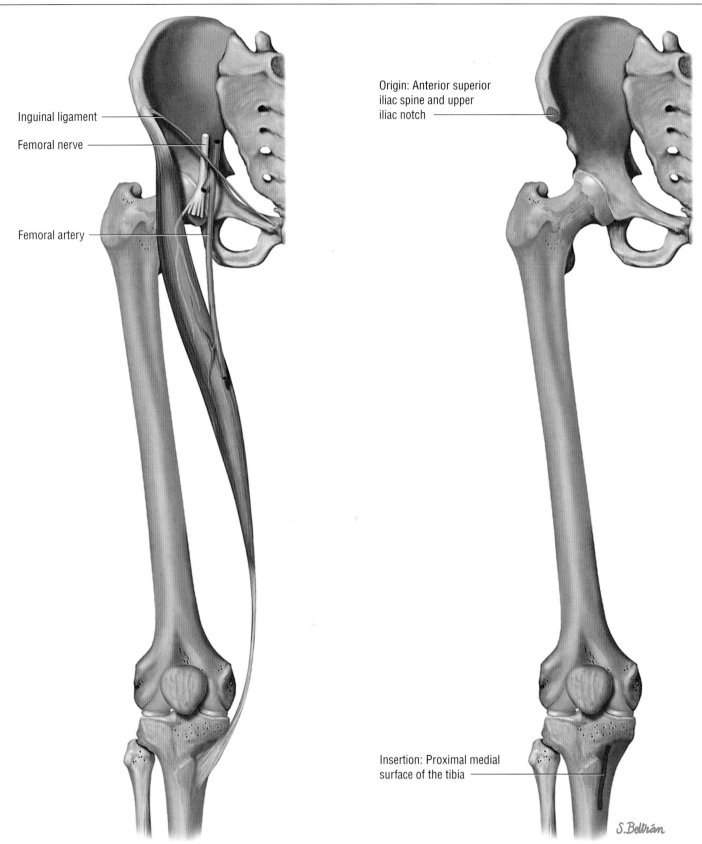

Inguinal ligament

Femoral nerve

Femoral artery

Origin: Anterior superior
iliac spine and upper
iliac notch

Insertion: Proximal medial
surface of the tibia

S.Beltrán

Figure 3.6 ▪ SARTORIUS. The sartorius flexes and externally rotates the hip and flexes the leg on the thigh. The anterior superior iliac spine at the origin of the sartorius is a common location for an avulsion fracture. These injuries are usually seen in athletes (sprinters, jumpers, soccer players, and football players). *(See Related Muscles pg. 47, in Stoller's 3rd Edition.)*

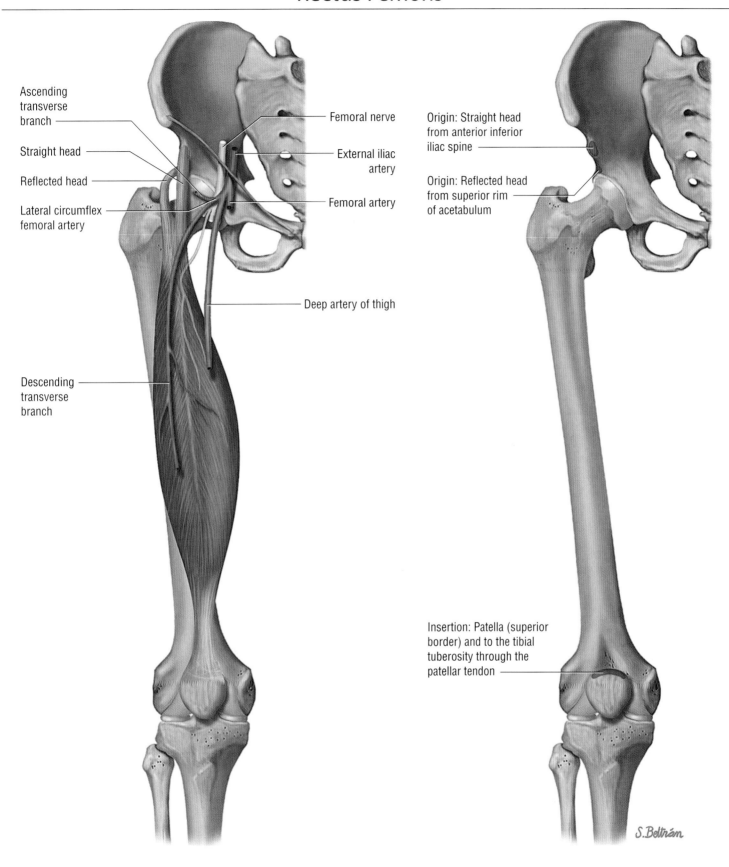

Ascending transverse branch

Straight head

Reflected head

Lateral circumflex femoral artery

Descending transverse branch

Femoral nerve

External iliac artery

Femoral artery

Deep artery of thigh

Origin: Straight head from anterior inferior iliac spine

Origin: Reflected head from superior rim of acetabulum

Insertion: Patella (superior border) and to the tibial tuberosity through the patellar tendon

S. Beltrán

Figure 3.7 ▪ RECTUS FEMORIS. The rectus femoris flexes the thigh (hip) and extends the leg (knee). Of the four quadriceps muscles (the vastus lateralis, vastus medialis, vastus intermedius, and rectus femoris), only the rectus femoris has an origin that crosses the hip joint. Soccer, football, and basketball players and track and field athletes are at risk for distal musculotendinous junction injuries and proximal intrasubstance tears of the musculotendinous junction of the indirect (reflected) head of the rectus. *(See Related Muscles pg. 48, in Stoller's 3rd Edition.)*

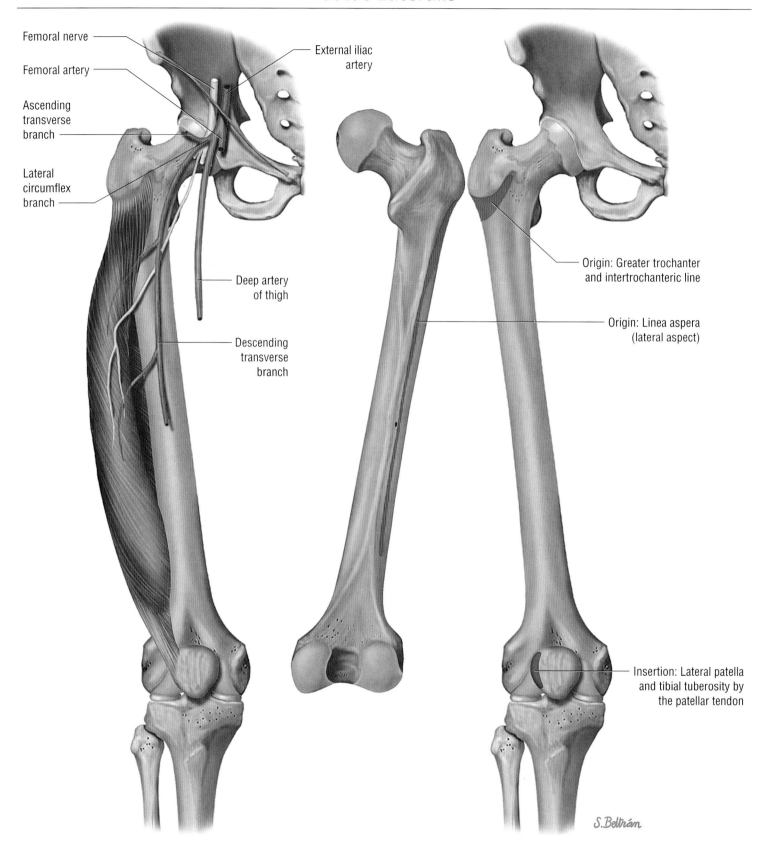

Femoral nerve

Femoral artery

Ascending
transverse
branch

Lateral
circumflex
branch

External iliac
artery

Deep artery
of thigh

Descending
transverse
branch

Origin: Greater trochanter
and intertrochanteric line

Origin: Linea aspera
(lateral aspect)

Insertion: Lateral patella
and tibial tuberosity by
the patellar tendon

S.Beltrán

Figure 3.8 ▪ VASTUS LATERALIS. The vastus lateralis extends the leg and flexes the
thigh (hip) and is one of the quadriceps muscles (vastus lateralis, vastus medialis,
vastus intermedius, and rectus femoris). Quadriceps muscle fibers are predominantly
type II and are adapted for rapid forceful activity. The vastus lateralis obliquus (VLO)
fibers of the vastus lateralis muscle interdigitate with the lateral intermuscular septum and insert onto the patella. In a lateral retinacular release, the VLO may be selectively sectioned without involving the main vastus lateralis tendon proper. *(See
Related Muscles pg. 49, in Stoller's 3rd Edition.)*

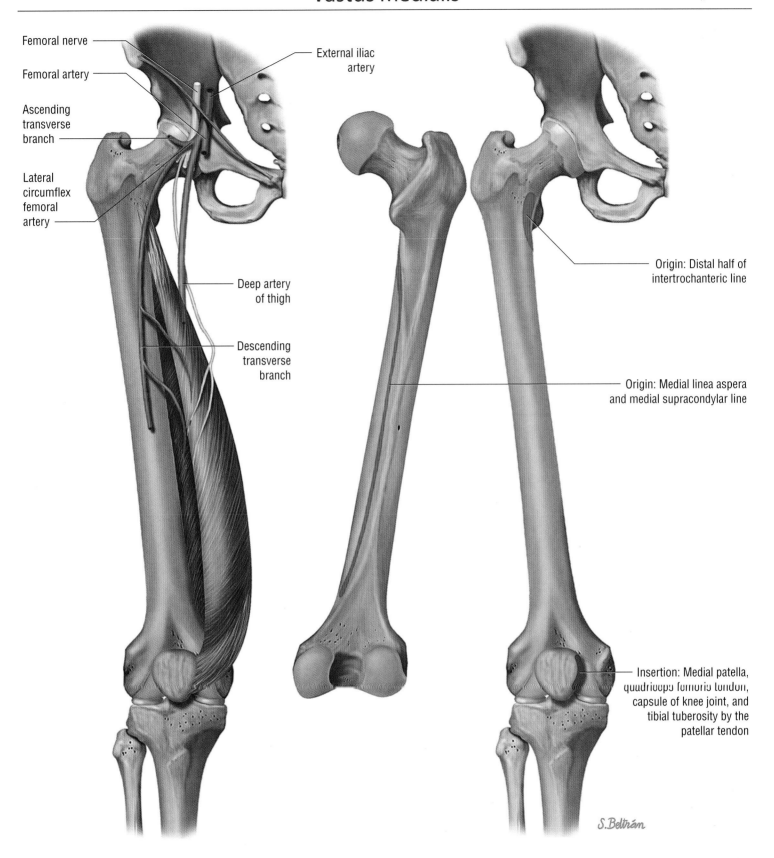

Femoral nerve

Femoral artery

Ascending transverse branch

Lateral circumflex femoral artery

External iliac artery

Deep artery of thigh

Descending transverse branch

Origin: Distal half of intertrochanteric line

Origin: Medial linea aspera and medial supracondylar line

Insertion: Medial patella, quadriceps femoris tendon, capsule of knee joint, and tibial tuberosity by the patellar tendon

S.Beltrán

Figure 3.9 ▪ VASTUS MEDIALIS. The vastus medialis extends the leg and pulls the patella medially. The quadriceps muscle group includes the vastus lateralis, the vastus medialis, the vastus intermedius, and the rectus femoris. The quadriceps muscles converge distally, forming the quadriceps tendon, which inserts on the proximal pole of the patella. The vastus medialis assists in preventing patellar dislocations and may be weak in patellofemoral disorders. Therefore, vastus medialis obliquus injuries are frequently associated with transient patellar dislocation. *(See See Related Muscles pg. 50, in Stoller's 3rd Edition.)*

Vastus Intermedius

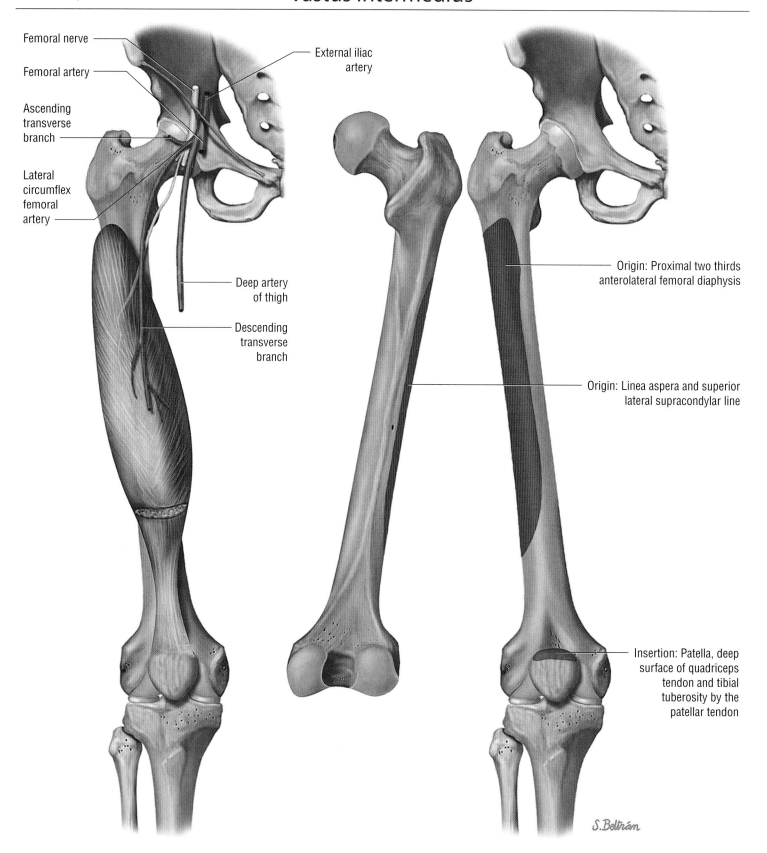

Femoral nerve

Femoral artery

Ascending transverse branch

Lateral circumflex femoral artery

External iliac artery

Deep artery of thigh

Descending transverse branch

Origin: Proximal two thirds anterolateral femoral diaphysis

Origin: Linea aspera and superior lateral supracondylar line

Insertion: Patella, deep surface of quadriceps tendon and tibial tuberosity by the patellar tendon

S.Beltrán

Figure 3.10 ▪ VASTUS INTERMEDIUS. The vastus intermedius extends the leg and covers the articularis genu. Quadriceps (vastus lateralis, vastus medialis, vastus intermedius, and rectus femoris) injuries, including strains and tendon ruptures, result from eccentric muscle contractions. The articularis genu muscle represents a few separate muscle fibers deep to the vastus intermedius and is responsible for contracting the knee joint capsule superiorly in extension. *(See Related Muscles pg. 51, in Stoller's 3rd Edition.)*

Gracilis

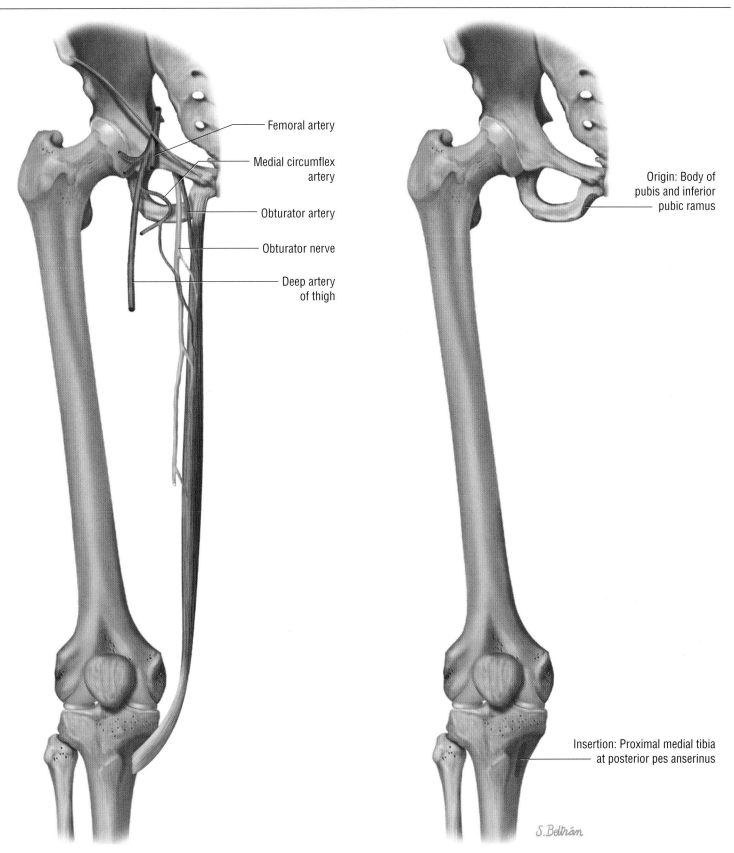

Femoral artery

Medial circumflex artery

Obturator artery

Obturator nerve

Deep artery of thigh

Origin: Body of pubis and inferior pubic ramus

Insertion: Proximal medial tibia at posterior pes anserinus

S.Beltrán

Figure 3.11 ▪ GRACILIS. The gracilis muscle adducts the thigh and flexes and internally rotates the leg and can be used for anterior cruciate ligament reconstructions. The gracilis is the one muscle of the medial aspect adductors of the thigh that does not attach to the linea aspera of the femur (as opposed to the adductor longus, magnus, and brevis and pectineus muscles). *(See Related Muscles pg. 52, in Stoller's 3rd Edition.)*

Pectineus

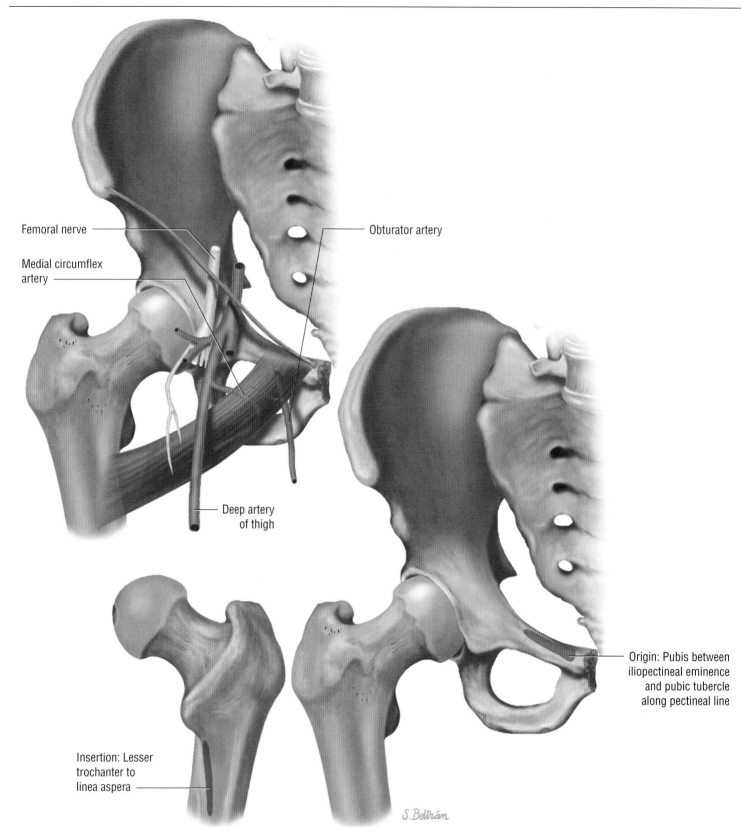

Femoral nerve

Medial circumflex
artery

Obturator artery

Deep artery
of thigh

Origin: Pubis between
iliopectineal eminence
and pubic tubercle
along pectineal line

Insertion: Lesser
trochanter to
linea aspera

S.Beltrán

Figure 3.12 ▪ **PECTINEUS.** The pectineus muscle adducts, flexes, and medially rotates the thigh. The adductor muscles, the pectineus, and the gracilis represent the
muscles of the medial aspect of the thigh. *(See Related Muscles pg. 53, in Stoller's
3rd Edition.)*

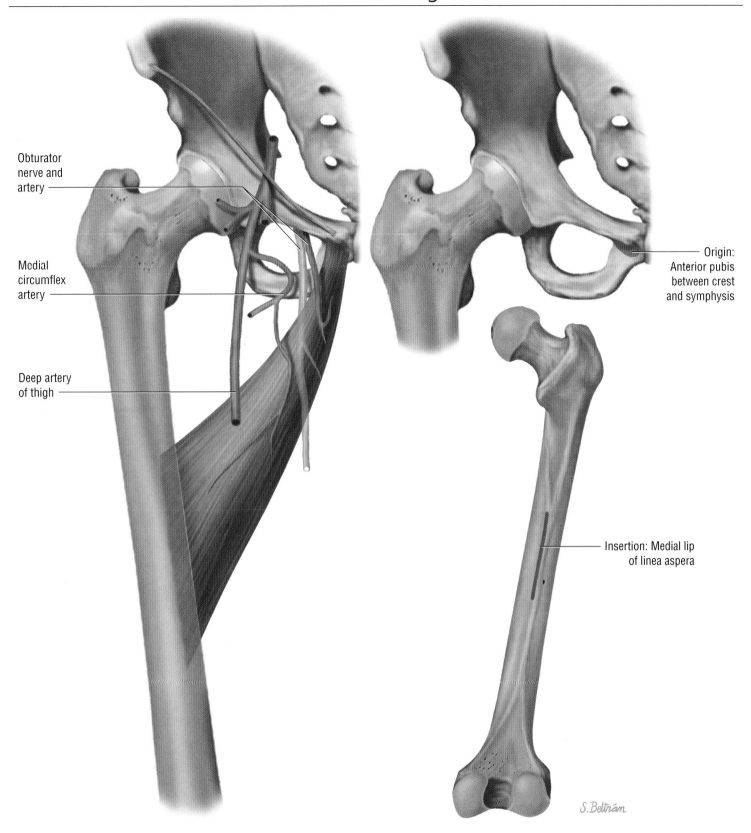

Obturator nerve and artery

Medial circumflex artery

Deep artery of thigh

Origin: Anterior pubis between crest and symphysis

Insertion: Medial lip of linea aspera

S. Beltrán

Figure 3.13 ■ ADDUCTOR LONGUS. The adductor longus adducts and assists in the flexion of the thigh. The adductor group muscles (longus, magnus, and brevis) originate at the symphysis pubis and inferior pubic ramus and insert on the linea aspera of the femur. *(See Related Muscles pg. 54, in Stoller's 3rd Edition.)*

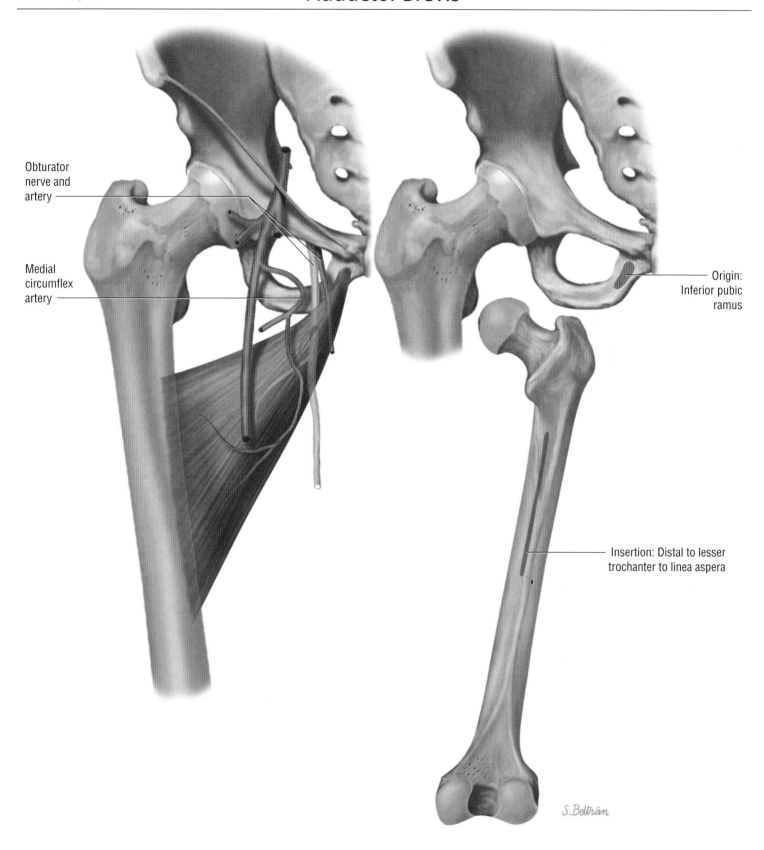

Obturator
nerve and
artery

Medial
circumflex
artery

Origin:
Inferior pubic
ramus

Insertion: Distal to lesser
trochanter to linea aspera

S.Beltrán

Figure 3.14 ▪ ADDUCTOR BREVIS. The adductor brevis muscle adducts and assists
in flexing the thigh. *(See Related Muscles pg. 55, in Stoller's 3rd Edition.)*

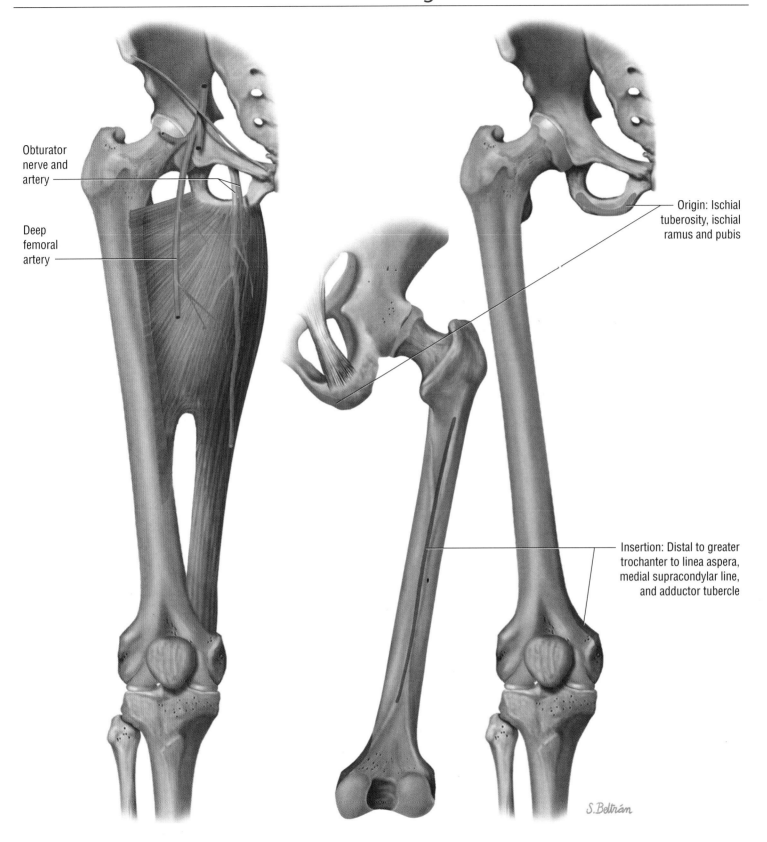

Obturator nerve and artery

Deep femoral artery

Origin: Ischial tuberosity, ischial ramus and pubis

Insertion: Distal to greater trochanter to linea aspera, medial supracondylar line, and adductor tubercle

S. Beltrán

Figure 3.15 ▪ ADDUCTOR MAGNUS. The adductor magnus adducts the femur (thigh). The proximal portion flexes the thigh and the distal portion extends it. *(See See Related Muscles pg. 56, in Stoller's 3rd Edition.)*

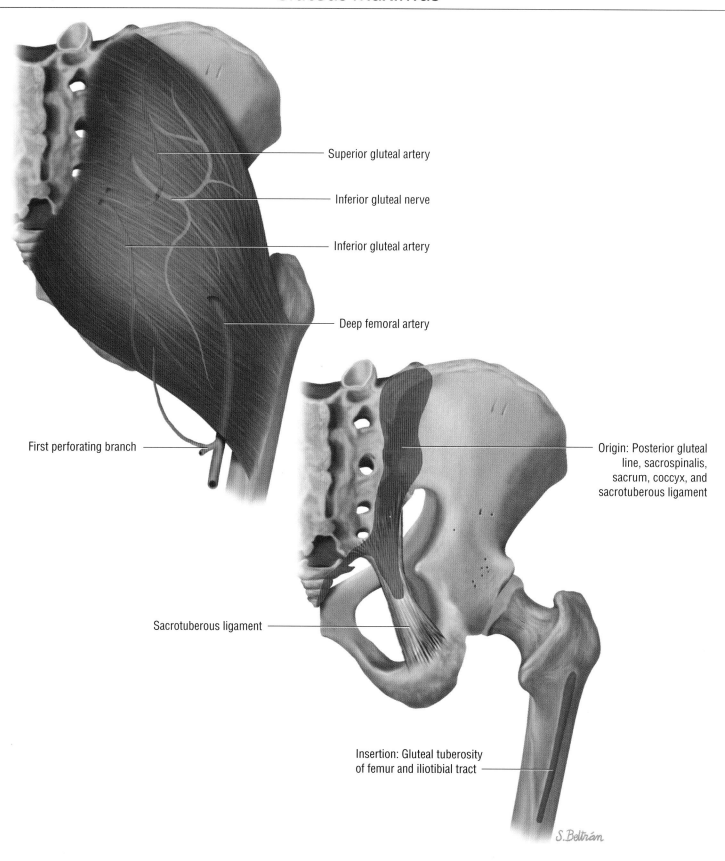

Superior gluteal artery

Inferior gluteal nerve

Inferior gluteal artery

Deep femoral artery

First perforating branch

Origin: Posterior gluteal
line, sacrospinalis,
sacrum, coccyx, and
sacrotuberous ligament

Sacrotuberous ligament

Insertion: Gluteal tuberosity
of femur and iliotibial tract

S. Beltrán

Figure 3.16 ■ **GLUTEUS MAXIMUS.** The gluteus maximus extends the thigh and assists in adduction and lateral rotation of the femur (thigh). Trunk extension is accom-
plished by action on its insertion. *(See Related Muscles pg. 57, in Stoller's 3rd
Edition.)*

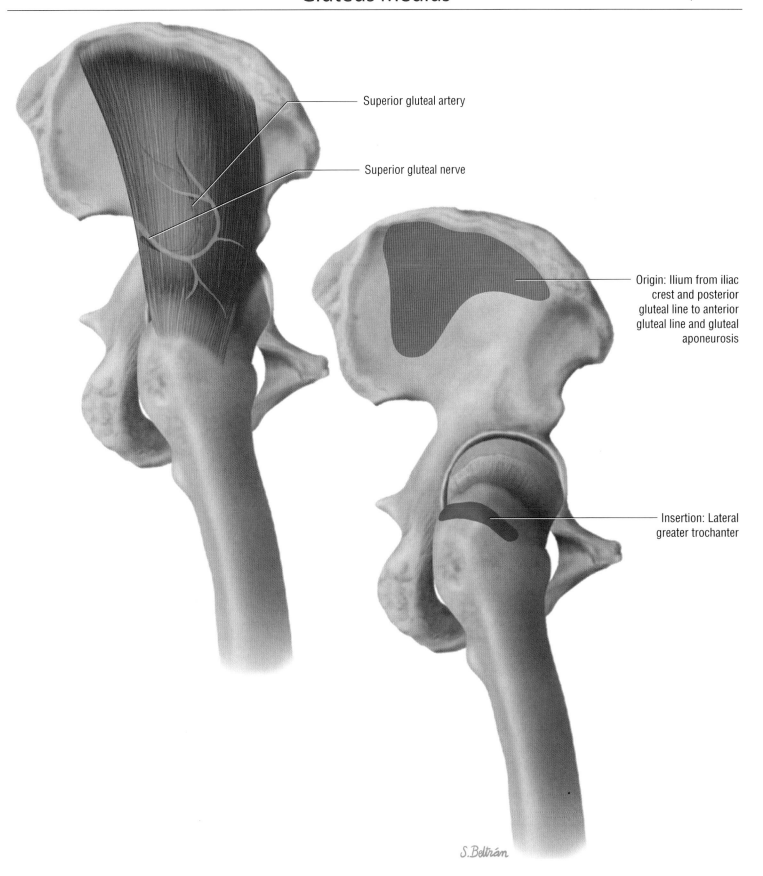

Superior gluteal artery

Superior gluteal nerve

Origin: Ilium from iliac crest and posterior gluteal line to anterior gluteal line and gluteal aponeurosis

Insertion: Lateral greater trochanter

S.Beltrán

Figure 3.17 ■ GLUTEUS MEDIUS. The gluteus medius abducts and medially rotates the thigh when the extremity is extended. *(See Related Muscles pg. 58, in Stoller's 3rd Edition.)*

Gluteus Minimus

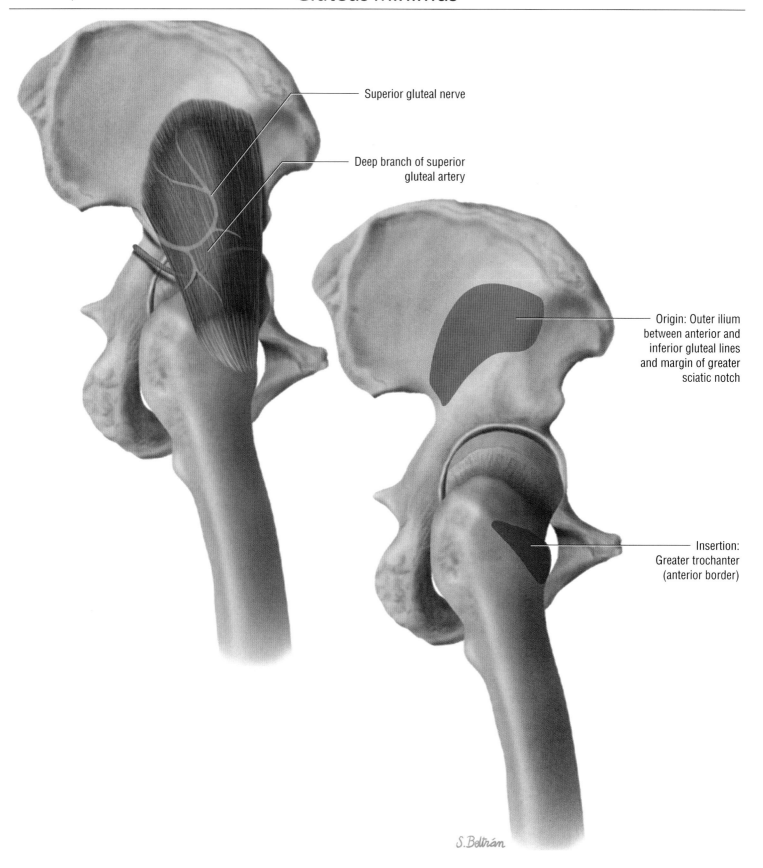

Superior gluteal nerve

Deep branch of superior
gluteal artery

Origin: Outer ilium
between anterior and
inferior gluteal lines
and margin of greater
sciatic notch

Insertion:
Greater trochanter
(anterior border)

S.Beltrán

Figure 3.18 ■ **GLUTEUS MINUMUS.** The gluteus minimus abducts and medially rotates the thigh when the extremity is extended. *(See Related Muscles pg. 59, in
Stoller's 3rd Edition.)*

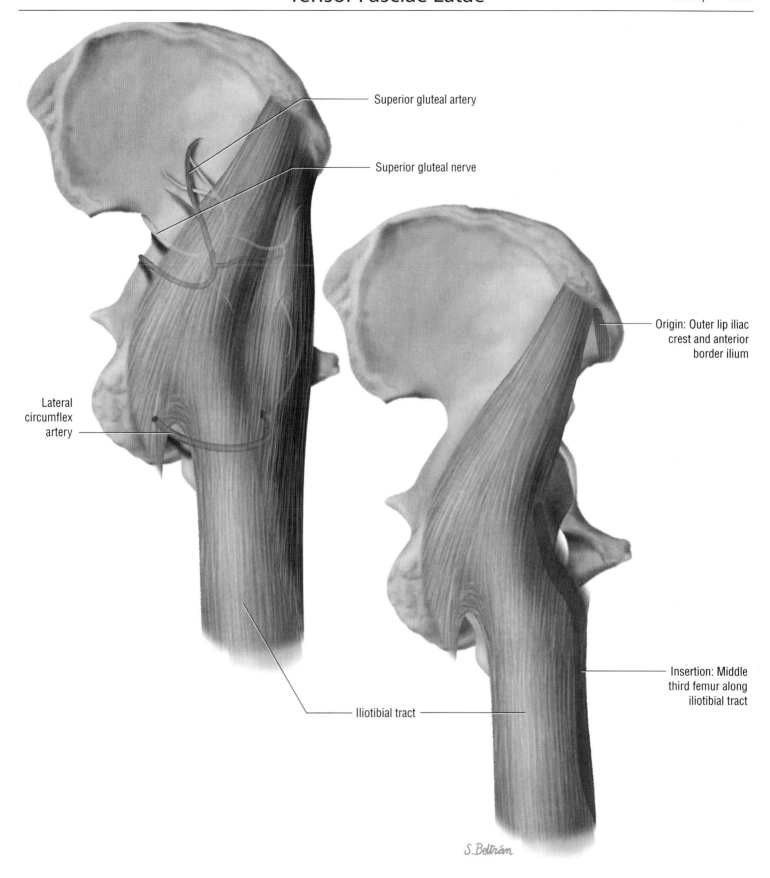

Superior gluteal artery

Superior gluteal nerve

Origin: Outer lip iliac crest and anterior border ilium

Lateral circumflex artery

Insertion: Middle third femur along iliotibial tract

Iliotibial tract

S. Beltrán

Figure 3.19 ■ TENSOR FASCIAE LATAE. The tensor fasciae latae assists in flexion, abduction, and medial rotation of the femur (thigh) and counteracts the posterior pull of the gluteus maximus on the iliotibial tract. *(See Related Muscles pg. 60, in Stoller's 3rd Edition.)*

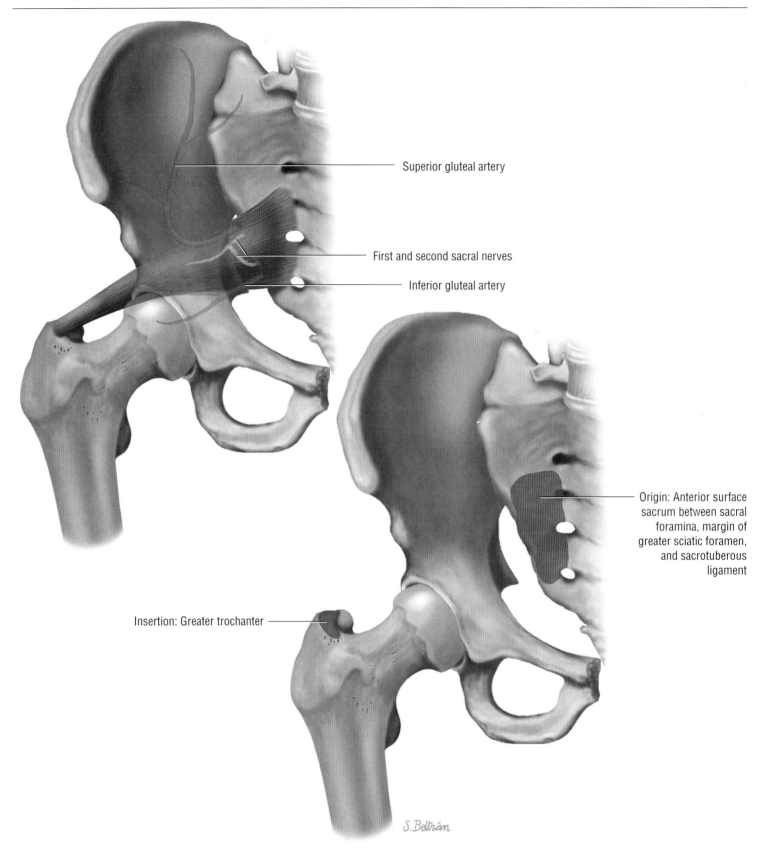

Superior gluteal artery

First and second sacral nerves

Inferior gluteal artery

Origin: Anterior surface sacrum between sacral foramina, margin of greater sciatic foramen, and sacrotuberous ligament

Insertion: Greater trochanter

S. Beltrán

Figure 3.20 ▪ PIRIFORMIS. The piriformis rotates the femur (thigh) laterally and abducts the thigh in flexion. *(See Related Muscles pg. 61, in Stoller's 3rd Edition.)*

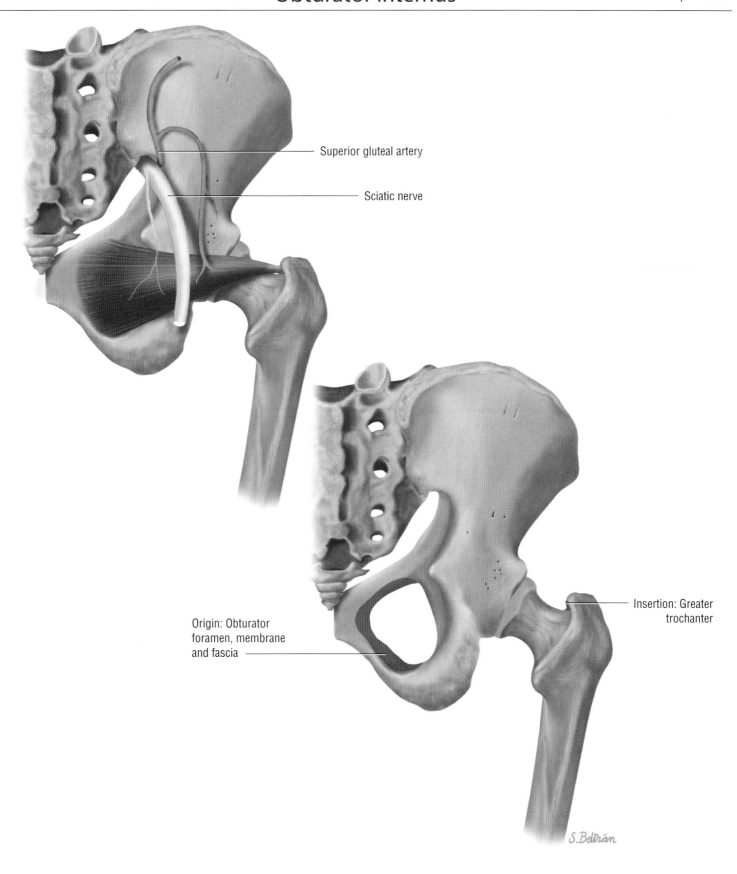

Superior gluteal artery

Sciatic nerve

Origin: Obturator
foramen, membrane
and fascia

Insertion: Greater
trochanter

S. Beltrán

Figure 3.21 ▪ OBTURATOR INTERNUS. The obturator internus rotates the femur (thigh) laterally and abducts the femur in flexion. *(See Related Muscles pg. 62, in Stoller's 3rd Edition.)*

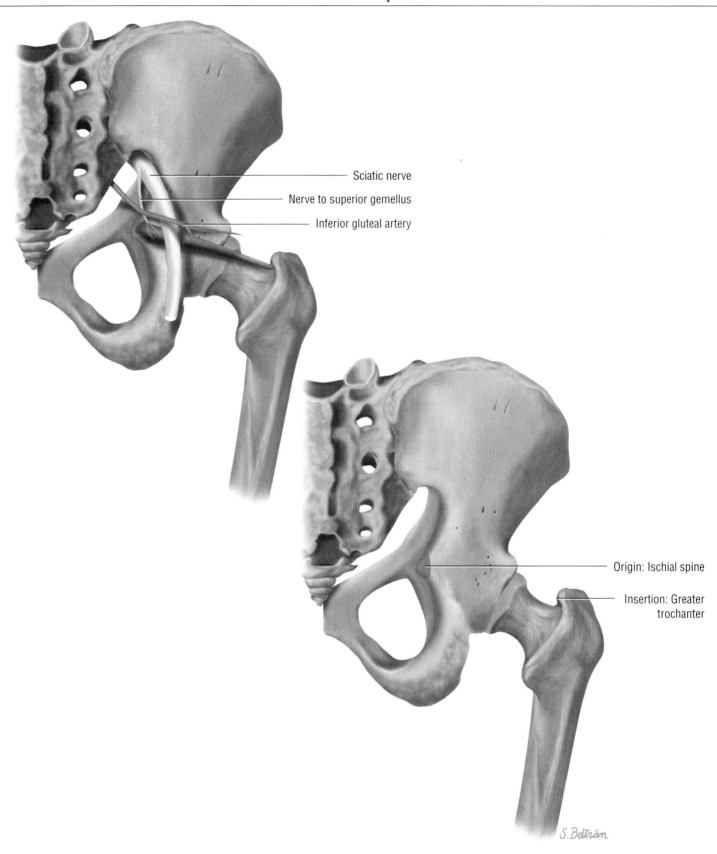

Sciatic nerve

Nerve to superior gemellus

Inferior gluteal artery

Origin: Ischial spine

Insertion: Greater trochanter

S. Beltrán

Figure 3.22 ▪ GEMELLUS SUPERIOR. The gemellus superior rotates the femur (thigh) laterally. *(See Related Muscles pg. 63, in Stoller's 3rd Edition.)*

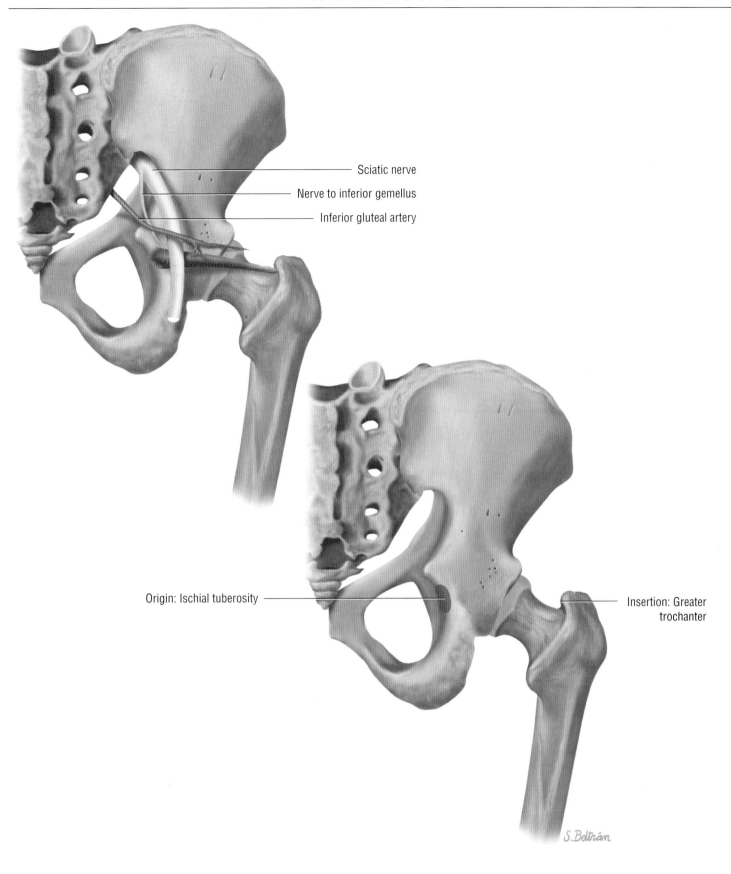

Sciatic nerve

Nerve to inferior gemellus

Inferior gluteal artery

Origin: Ischial tuberosity

Insertion: Greater trochanter

S.Beltrán

Figure 3.23 ▪ GEMELLUS INFERIOR. The gemellus inferior rotates the femur (thigh) laterally. *(See Related Muscles pg. 64, in Stoller's 3rd Edition.)*

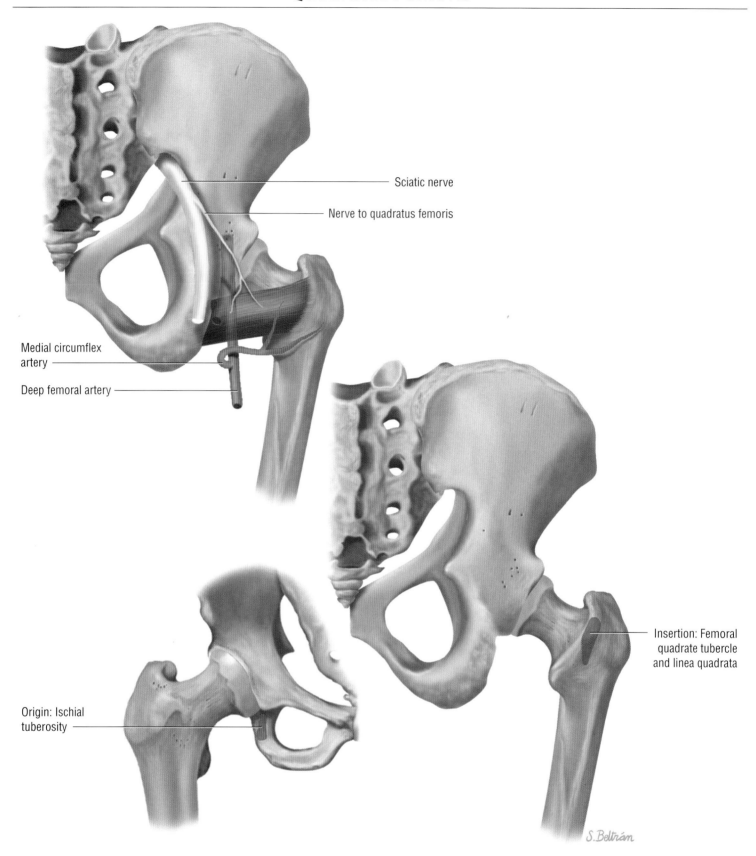

Figure 3.24 ■ QUADRATUS FEMORIS. The quadratus femoris adducts and rotates the femur (thigh) laterally. *(See Related Muscles pg. 65, in Stoller's 3rd Edition.)*

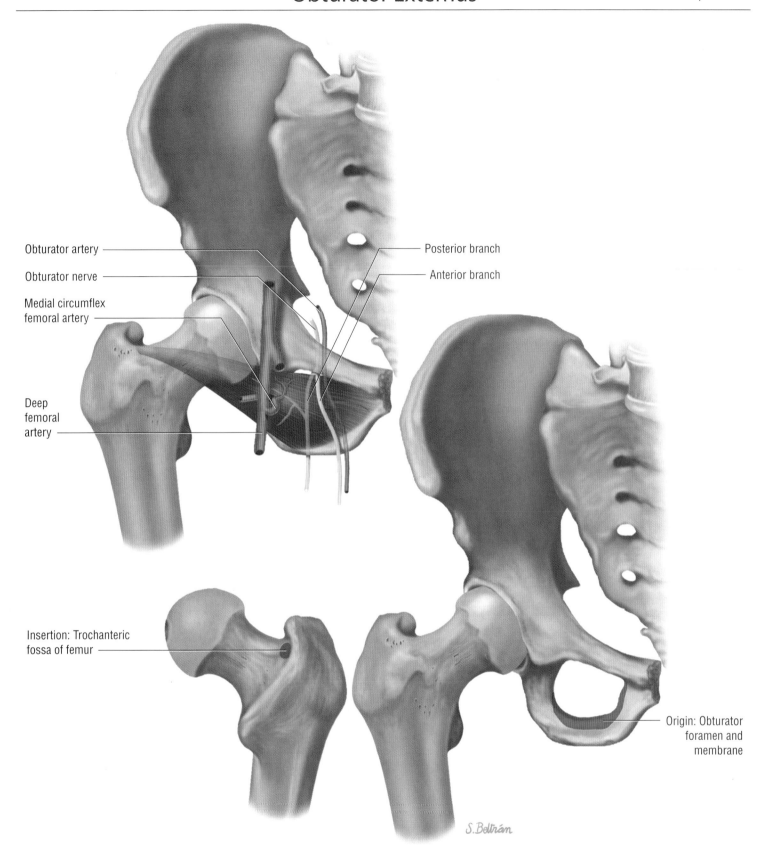

Obturator artery

Obturator nerve

Medial circumflex femoral artery

Deep femoral artery

Posterior branch

Anterior branch

Insertion: Trochanteric fossa of femur

Origin: Obturator foramen and membrane

S. Beltrán

Figure 3.25 ■ **OBTURATOR EXTERNUS.** The obturator externus adducts and rotates the femur (thigh) laterally. *(See Related Muscles pg. 66, in Stoller's 3rd Edition.)*

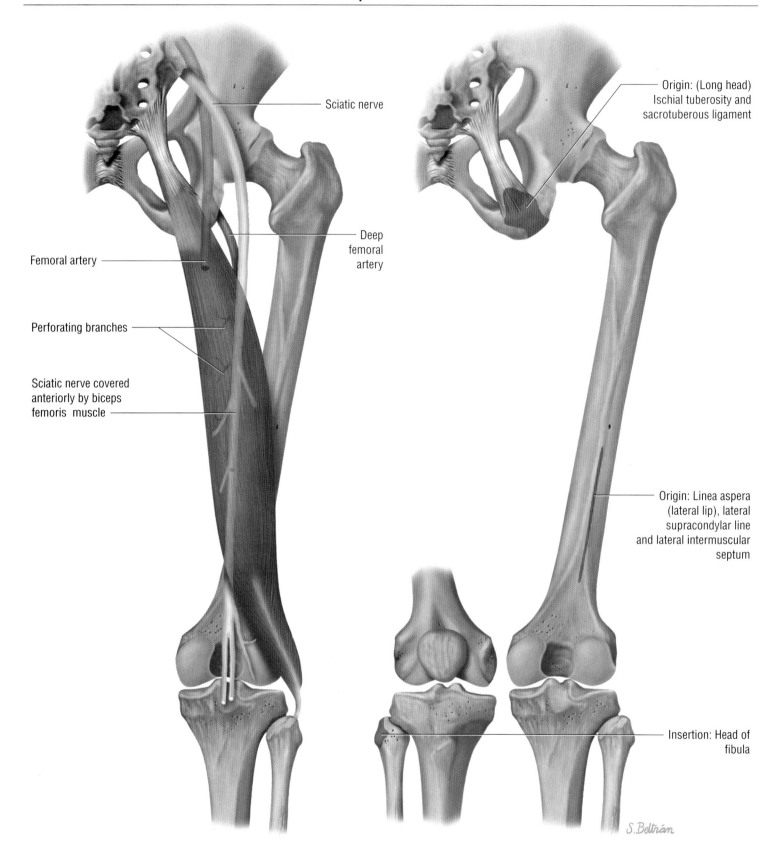

Sciatic nerve

Deep femoral artery

Origin: (Long head) Ischial tuberosity and sacrotuberous ligament

Femoral artery

Perforating branches

Sciatic nerve covered anteriorly by biceps femoris muscle

Origin: Linea aspera (lateral lip), lateral supracondylar line and lateral intermuscular septum

Insertion: Head of fibula

S. Beltrán

Figure 3.26 ▪ BICEPS FEMORIS. The biceps femoris extends the thigh and flexes the leg in external rotation of the tibia, contributing to lateral stability of the knee. The muscles of the hamstring group (biceps femoris, semimembranosus, and semitendinosus), except for the short head of the biceps femoris, all cross the hip and knee joints. Musculotendinous junctions extend the entire length of the muscle and serve as potential sites for strains. The short head is innervated by the peroneal branch of the sciatic nerve; the other hamstring muscles derive innervation from the tibial branch of the sciatic nerve. *(See Related Muscles pg. 67, in Stoller's 3rd Edition.)*

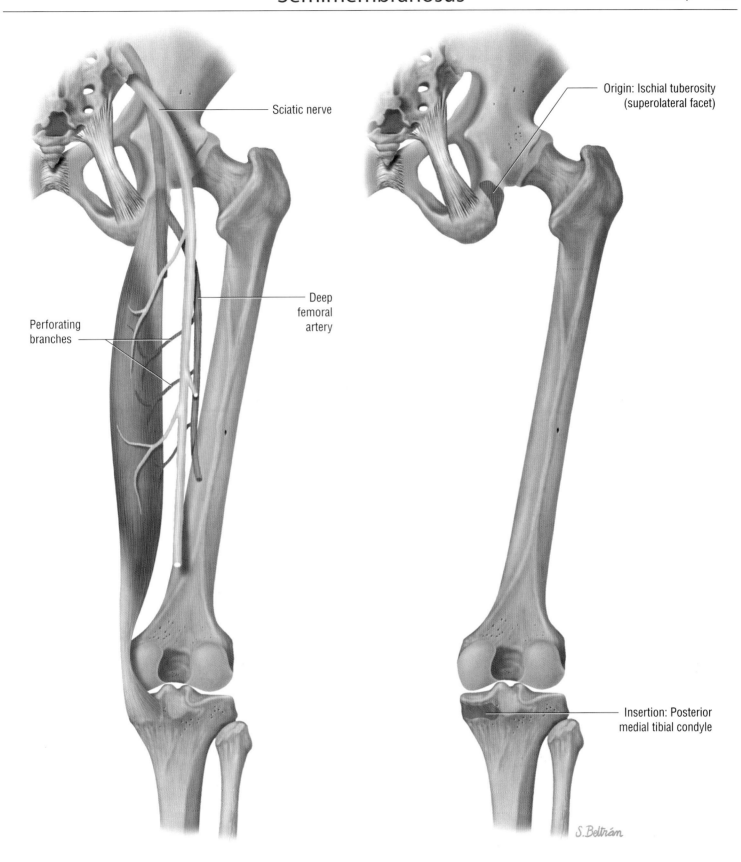

Sciatic nerve

Origin: Ischial tuberosity
(superolateral facet)

Deep
femoral
artery

Perforating
branches

Insertion: Posterior
medial tibial condyle

S. Beltrán

Figure 3.27 ■ **SEMIMEMBRANOSUS.** The semimembranosus extends the thigh and
flexes the leg. It is part of the hamstring muscle group (biceps femoris, semimembranosus, and semitendinosus) in the posterior thigh. Except for the short head of the
biceps, the origins of the hamstring tendons are from the ischial tuberosity and are
involved in ischial avulsion fractures in the young athlete. *(See Related Muscles pg.
68, in Stoller's 3rd Edition.)*

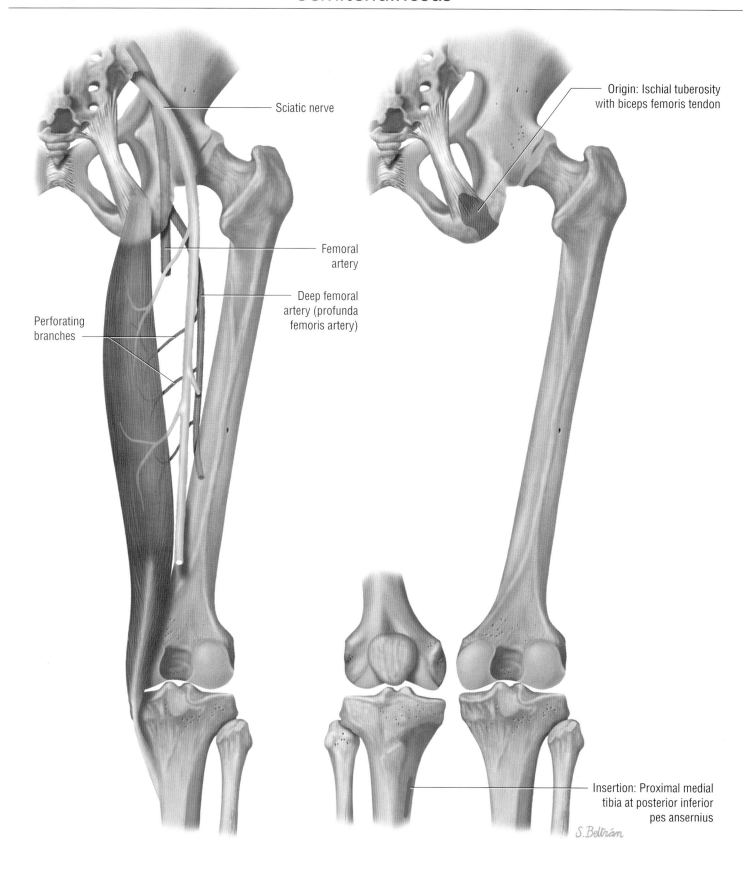

Sciatic nerve

Femoral artery

Deep femoral artery (profunda femoris artery)

Perforating branches

Origin: Ischial tuberosity with biceps femoris tendon

Insertion: Proximal medial tibia at posterior inferior pes ansernius

S.Beltrán

Figure 3.28 ■ **SEMITENDINOSUS.** The semitendinosus, which is part of the hamstring muscle group, extends the thigh and flexes the leg. It may be used for anterior cruciate ligament reconstructions, posterolateral knee reconstructions, and tenodesis for patellar subluxation. It is the most posteromedial tendon on axial knee images at the joint line. Hip hyperflexion and simultaneous knee extension is a mechanism of injury for proximal hamstring injuries in adults and apophyseal avulsions in young skeletally immature athletes. *(See Related Muscles pg. 69, in Stoller's 3rd Edition.)*

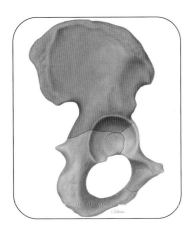

The Hip
Anatomy and Pathology

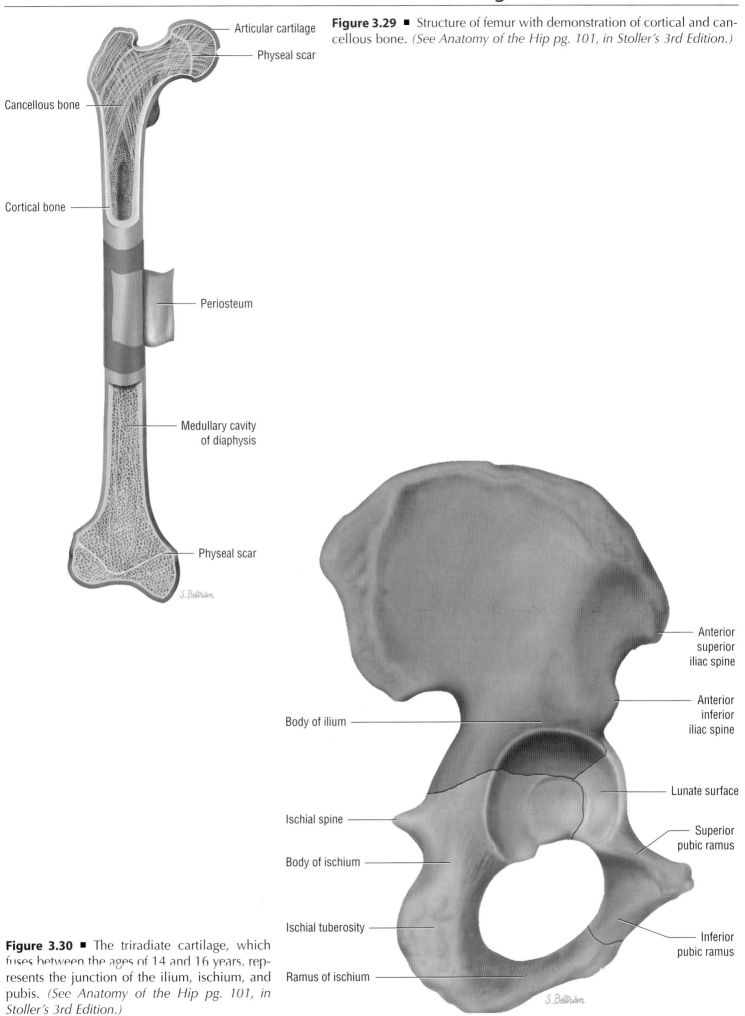

Articular cartilage

Physeal scar

Cancellous bone

Cortical bone

Periosteum

Medullary cavity
of diaphysis

Physeal scar

S. Beltrán

Figure 3.29 ■ Structure of femur with demonstration of cortical and cancellous bone. *(See Anatomy of the Hip pg. 101, in Stoller's 3rd Edition.)*

Anterior
superior
iliac spine

Anterior
inferior
iliac spine

Body of ilium

Lunate surface

Ischial spine

Superior
pubic ramus

Body of ischium

Ischial tuberosity

Inferior
pubic ramus

Ramus of ischium

S. Beltrán

Figure 3.30 ■ The triradiate cartilage, which fuses between the ages of 14 and 16 years, represents the junction of the ilium, ischium, and pubis. *(See Anatomy of the Hip pg. 101, in Stoller's 3rd Edition.)*

Coronal Section of Hip Joint and Adductors

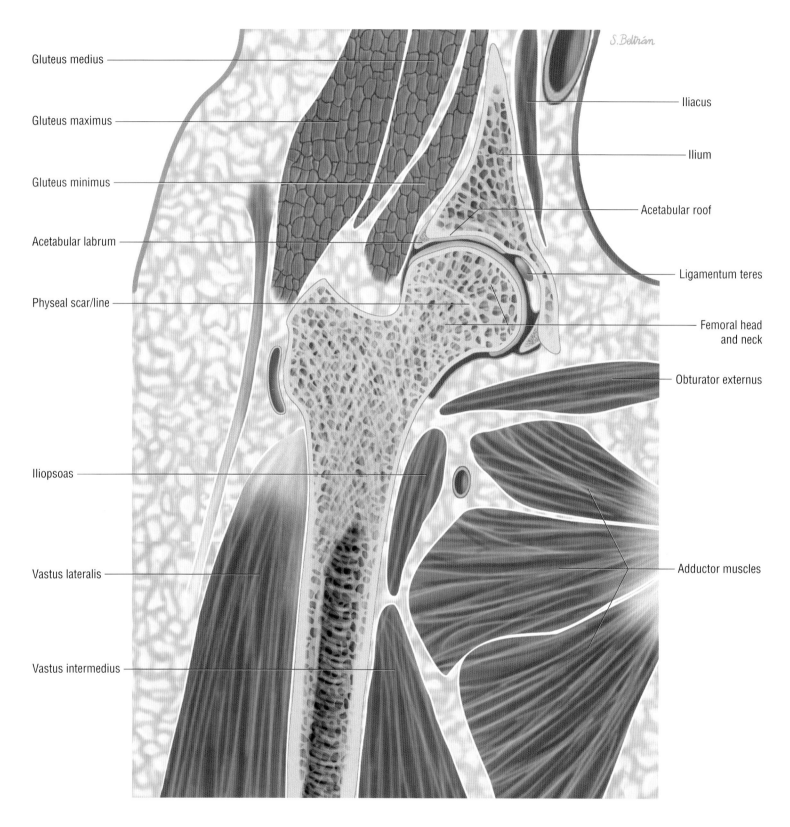

Gluteus medius

Gluteus maximus

Gluteus minimus

Acetabular labrum

Physeal scar/line

Iliopsoas

Vastus lateralis

Vastus intermedius

Iliacus

Ilium

Acetabular roof

Ligamentum teres

Femoral head and neck

Obturator externus

Adductor muscles

S. Beltrán

Figure 3.31 ■ Coronal plane of section of the hip joint and hip abductors. *(See Anatomy of the Hip pg. 101, in Stoller's 3rd Edition.)*

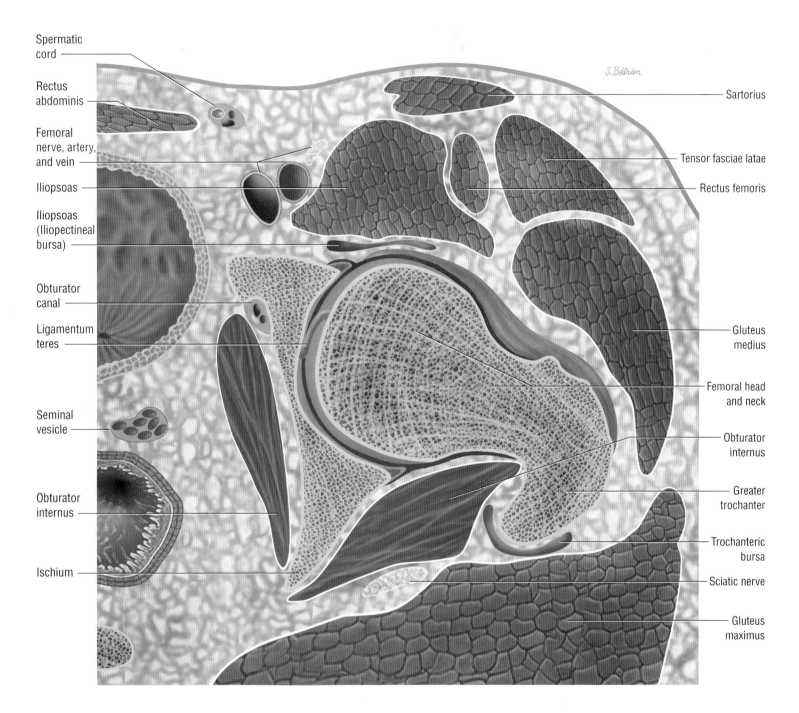

Spermatic cord

Rectus abdominis

Femoral nerve, artery, and vein

Iliopsoas

Iliopsoas (Iliopectineal bursa)

Obturator canal

Ligamentum teres

Seminal vesicle

Obturator internus

Ischium

Sartorius

Tensor fasciae latae

Rectus femoris

Gluteus medius

Femoral head and neck

Obturator internus

Greater trochanter

Trochanteric bursa

Sciatic nerve

Gluteus maximus

S. Beltrán

Figure 3.32 ▪ **Axial or transverse section of hip joint.** Plane of section is at the level of the ligamentum teres. *(See Anatomy of the Hip pg. 101, in Stoller's 3rd Edition.)*

Adductors

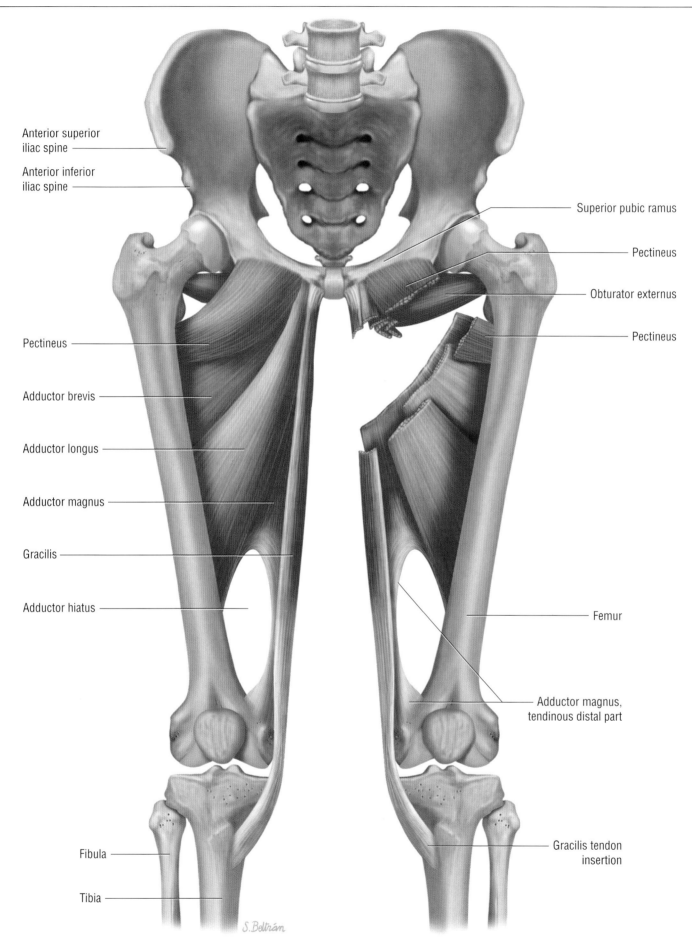

Anterior superior
iliac spine

Anterior inferior
iliac spine

Pectineus

Adductor brevis

Adductor longus

Adductor magnus

Gracilis

Adductor hiatus

Fibula

Tibia

Superior pubic ramus

Pectineus

Obturator externus

Pectineus

Femur

Adductor magnus,
tendinous distal part

Gracilis tendon
insertion

S. Beltrán

Figure 3.33 ▪ The adductors include the obturator externus, pectineus, the adductor longus, brevis, magnus, and gracilis. *(See Related Muscles pg. 42, in Stoller's 3rd Edition.)*

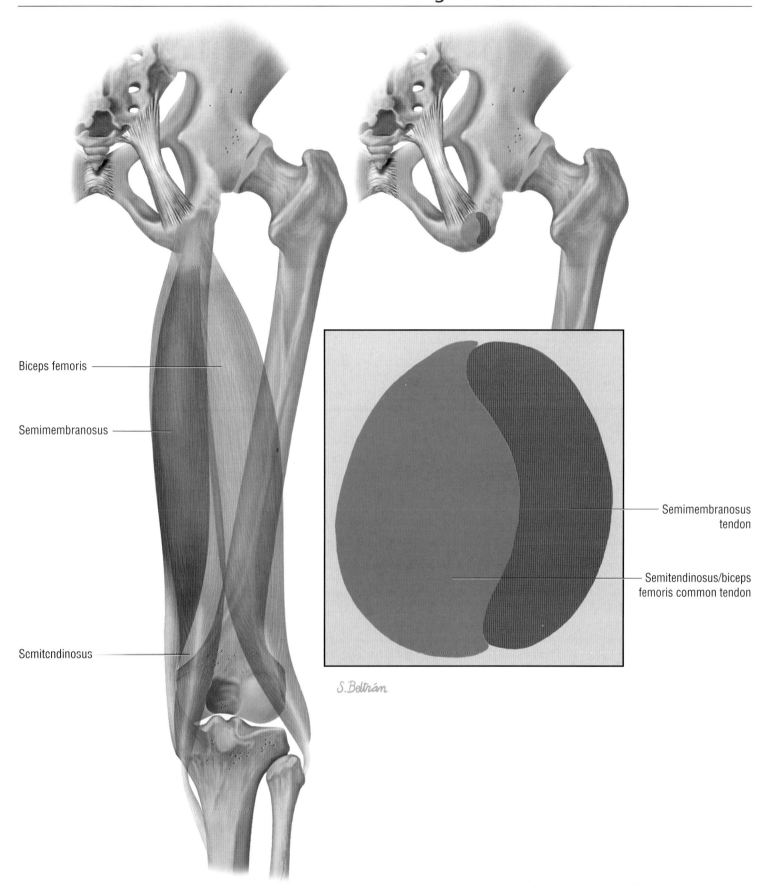

Biceps femoris

Semimembranosus

Semitendinosus

Semimembranosus tendon

Semitendinosus/biceps femoris common tendon

S. Beltrán

Figure 3.34 ■ Posterior view with inset of the medial origin of the common tendon of semitendinosus/biceps femoris (green) and the lateral origin of the semimembranosus tendon (red). *Based on Miller SL, Gil J, Webb GR. The Proximal Origin of the Hastrings and Surrounding Anatomy Encountered During Repair. A Cadaveric Study. J Bone Joint Surg [AM] 2007; 89:44–48. (See Related Muscles pg. 58, in Stoller's 3rd Edition.)*

Spaces Between Hip Capsular Ligaments

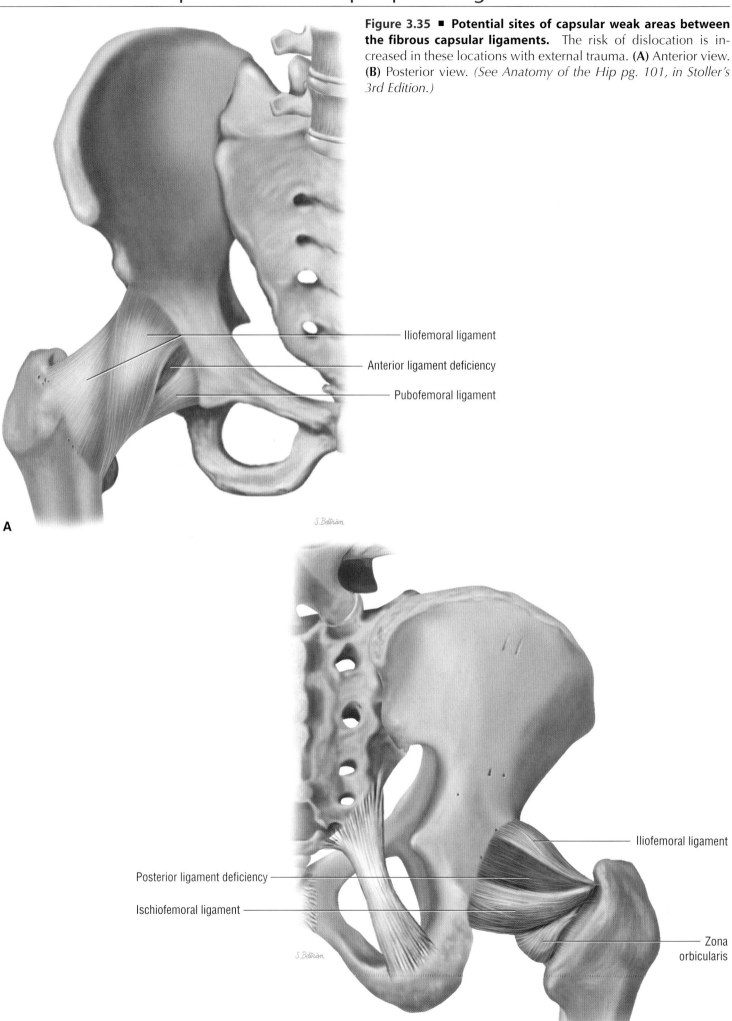

Figure 3.35 ■ **Potential sites of capsular weak areas between the fibrous capsular ligaments.** The risk of dislocation is increased in these locations with external trauma. **(A)** Anterior view. **(B)** Posterior view. *(See Anatomy of the Hip pg. 101, in Stoller's 3rd Edition.)*

Iliofemoral ligament

Anterior ligament deficiency

Pubofemoral ligament

A

Iliofemoral ligament

Posterior ligament deficiency

Ischiofemoral ligament

Zona orbicularis

B

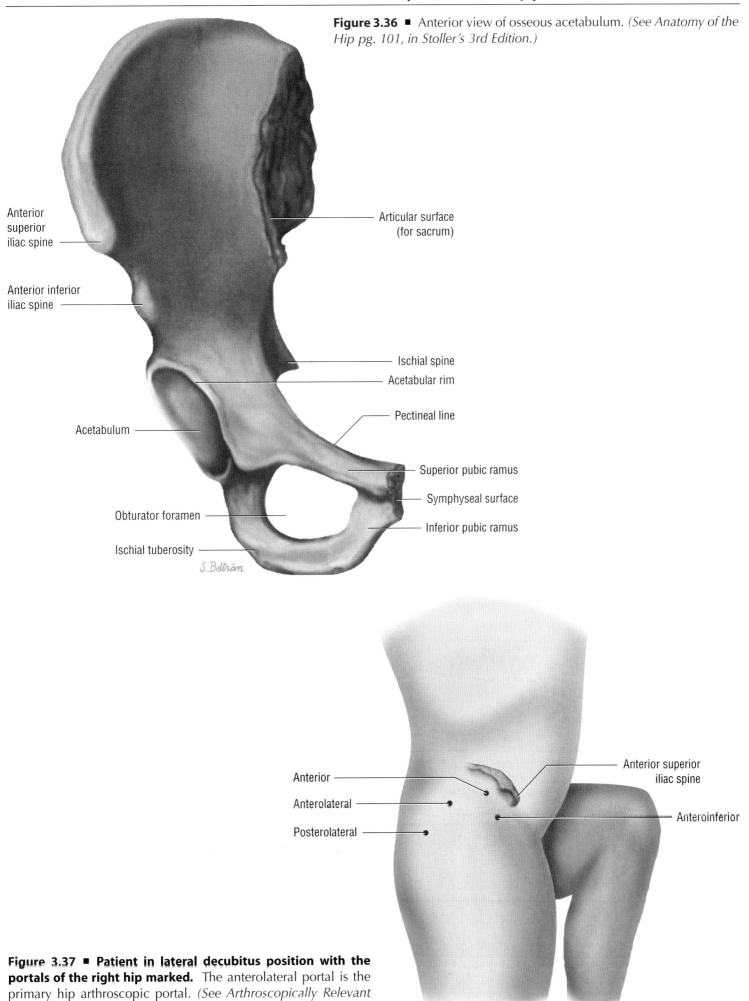

Figure 3.36 ■ Anterior view of osseous acetabulum. *(See Anatomy of the Hip pg. 101, in Stoller's 3rd Edition.)*

Anterior superior iliac spine

Articular surface (for sacrum)

Anterior inferior iliac spine

Ischial spine

Acetabular rim

Pectineal line

Acetabulum

Superior pubic ramus

Symphyseal surface

Obturator foramen

Inferior pubic ramus

Ischial tuberosity

S. Beltrán

Anterior

Anterolateral

Posterolateral

Anterior superior iliac spine

Anteroinferior

Figure 3.37 ■ **Patient in lateral decubitus position with the portals of the right hip marked.** The anterolateral portal is the primary hip arthroscopic portal. *(See Arthroscopically Relevant Anatomy pg. 118, in Stoller's 3rd Edition.)*

S. Beltrán

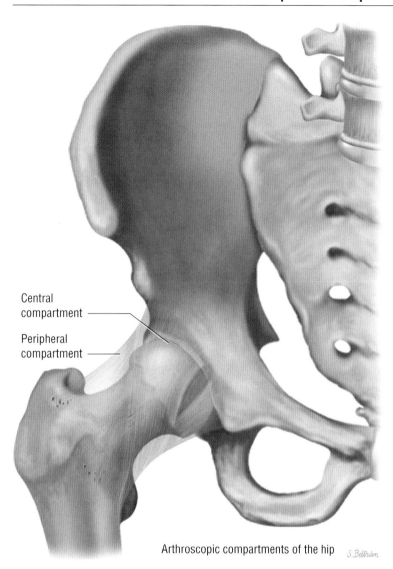

Central compartment

Peripheral compartment

Arthroscopic compartments of the hip   *S.Beltrán*

Figure 3.38 ▪ Arthroscopic compartments of the hip. *Based on Byrd JWT. Operative Hip Arthroscopy, 2nd ed. New York: Stuttgart, Springer, 2005. (See Anatomy of the Hip pg. 101 and Arthroscopically Relevant Anatomy pg. 118, in Stoller's 3rd Edition.)*

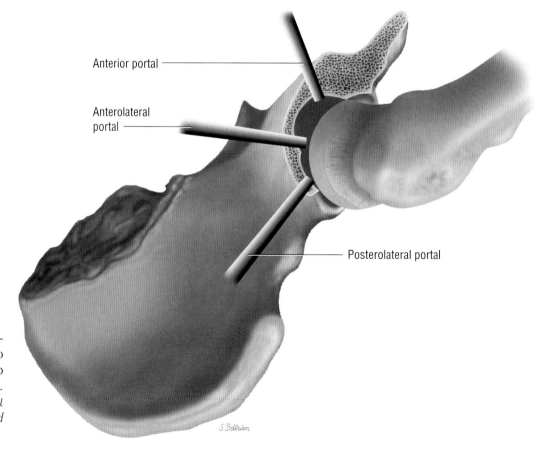

Anterior portal

Anterolateral portal

Posterolateral portal

S.Beltrán

Figure 3.39 ▪ Anterior, anterolateral, and posterolateral portals to the central compartment of the hip joint. *(See Anatomy of the Hip pg. 101 and Arthroscopically Relevant Anatomy pg. 118, in Stoller's 3rd Edition.)*

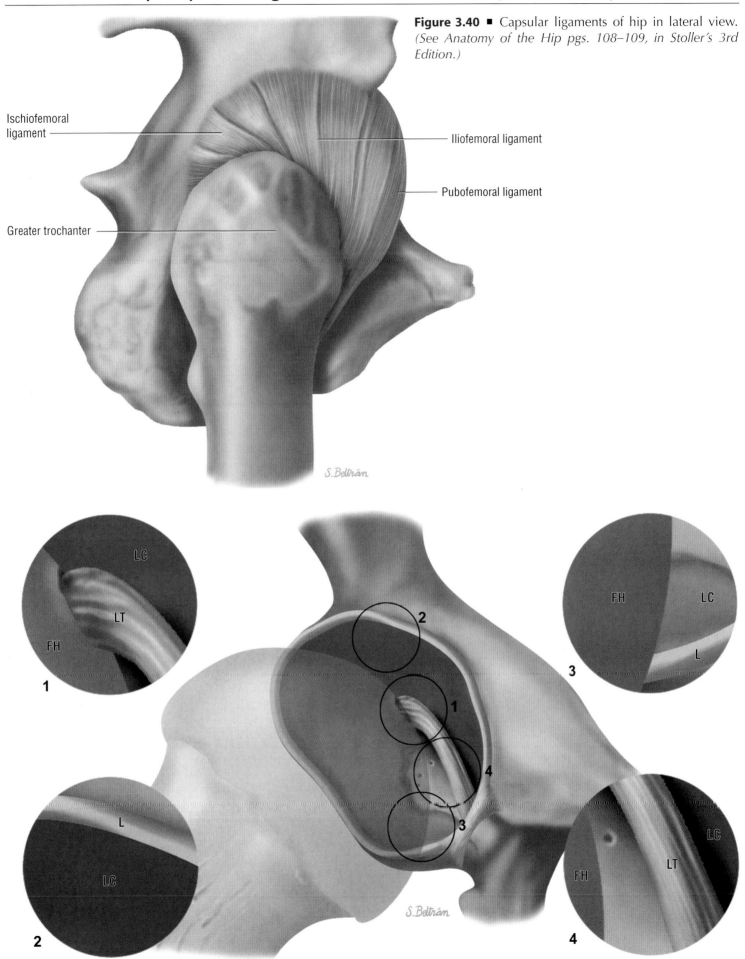

Figure 3.40 ■ Capsular ligaments of hip in lateral view. *(See Anatomy of the Hip pgs. 108–109, in Stoller's 3rd Edition.)*

Ischiofemoral ligament

Iliofemoral ligament

Pubofemoral ligament

Greater trochanter

S. Beltrán

Figure 3.41 ■ Arthroscopic anatomy demonstrating the labrum, ligamentum teres, and articular cartilage of the lunate surface of the acetabulum. *(See Anatomy of the Hip pg. 103, in Stoller's 3rd Edition.)*

LC: Lunate cartilage
FH: Femoral head

L: Acetabular labrum
LT: Ligamentum teres

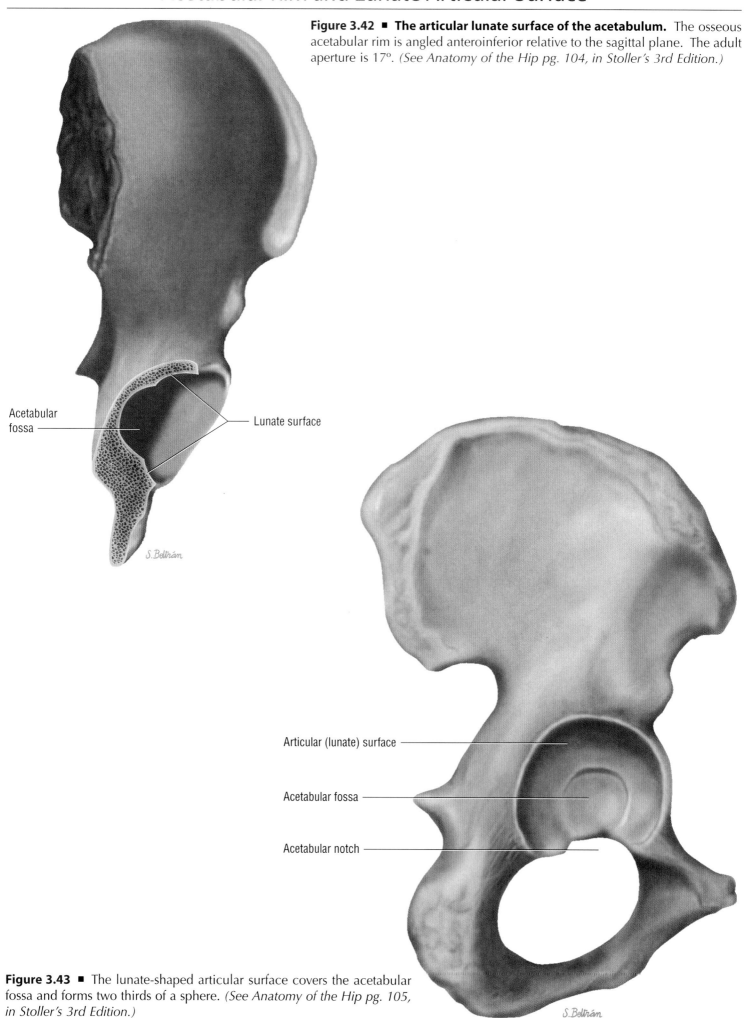

Figure 3.42 ■ The articular lunate surface of the acetabulum. The osseous acetabular rim is angled anteroinferior relative to the sagittal plane. The adult aperture is 17°. *(See Anatomy of the Hip pg. 104, in Stoller's 3rd Edition.)*

Acetabular fossa

Lunate surface

Articular (lunate) surface

Acetabular fossa

Acetabular notch

Figure 3.43 ■ The lunate-shaped articular surface covers the acetabular fossa and forms two thirds of a sphere. *(See Anatomy of the Hip pg. 105, in Stoller's 3rd Edition.)*

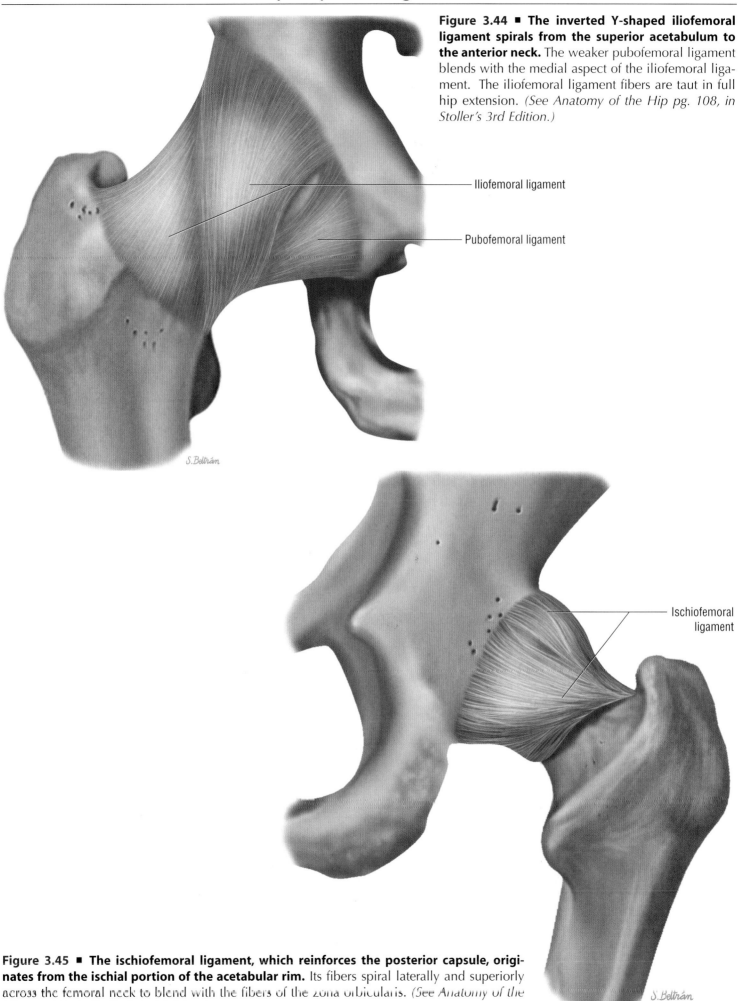

Figure 3.44 ▪ The inverted Y-shaped iliofemoral ligament spirals from the superior acetabulum to the anterior neck. The weaker pubofemoral ligament blends with the medial aspect of the iliofemoral ligament. The iliofemoral ligament fibers are taut in full hip extension. *(See Anatomy of the Hip pg. 108, in Stoller's 3rd Edition.)*

Iliofemoral ligament

Pubofemoral ligament

Ischiofemoral ligament

Figure 3.45 ▪ The ischiofemoral ligament, which reinforces the posterior capsule, originates from the ischial portion of the acetabular rim. Its fibers spiral laterally and superiorly across the femoral neck to blend with the fibers of the zona orbicularis. *(See Anatomy of the Hip pg. 109, in Stoller's 3rd Edition.)*

Sublabral Sulcus

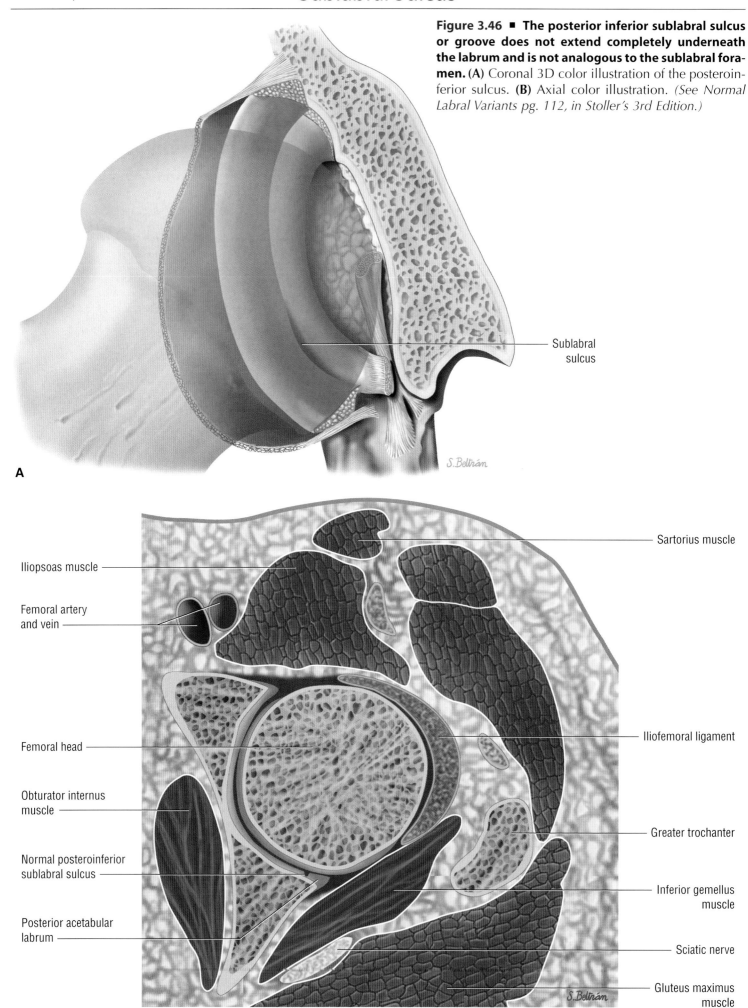

Figure 3.46 ■ The posterior inferior sublabral sulcus or groove does not extend completely underneath the labrum and is not analogous to the sublabral foramen. (A) Coronal 3D color illustration of the posteroinferior sulcus. **(B)** Axial color illustration. *(See Normal Labral Variants pg. 112, in Stoller's 3rd Edition.)*

Sublabral sulcus

Sartorius muscle

Iliopsoas muscle

Femoral artery and vein

Iliofemoral ligament

Femoral head

Obturator internus muscle

Greater trochanter

Normal posteroinferior sublabral sulcus

Inferior gemellus muscle

Posterior acetabular labrum

Sciatic nerve

Gluteus maximus muscle

A

B

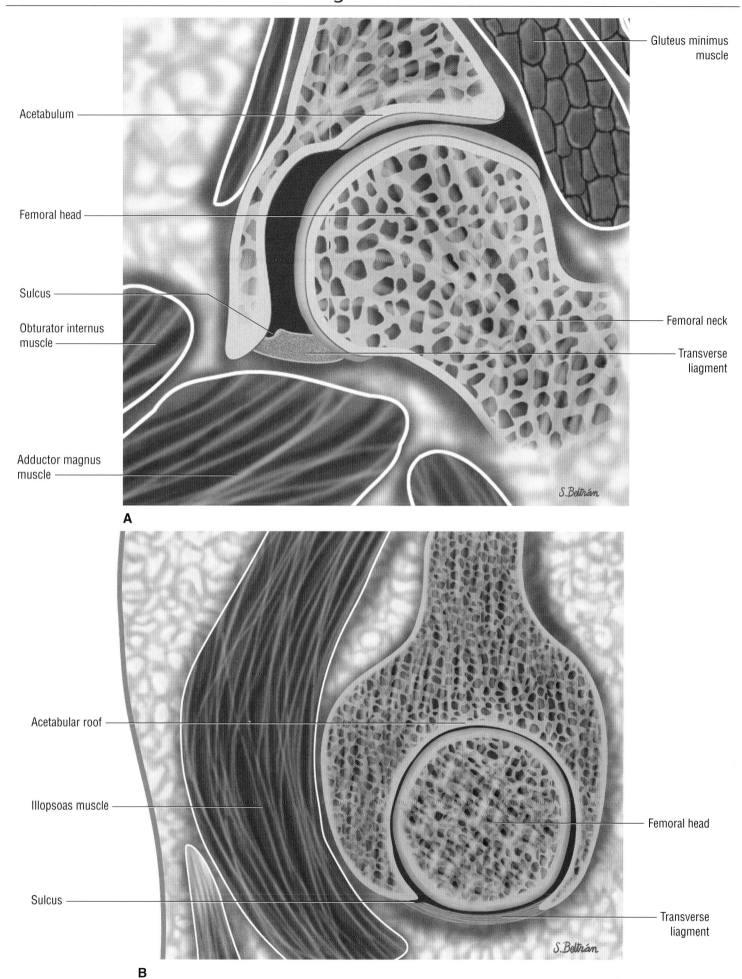

Figure 3.47 ■ Normal transverse ligament labral sulcus. (A) Coronal color illustration. **(B)** Sagittal (lateral) color illustration. *(See Normal Labral Variants pgs. 113–114, in Stoller's 3rd Edition.)*

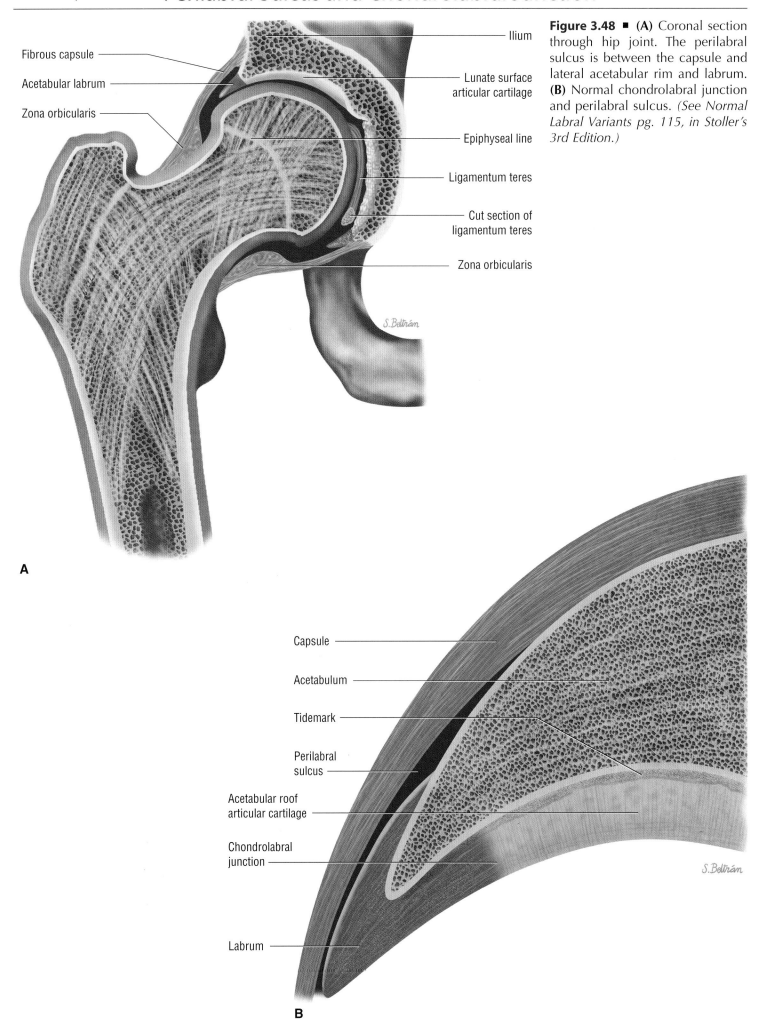

Fibrous capsule

Acetabular labrum

Zona orbicularis

Ilium

Lunate surface articular cartilage

Epiphyseal line

Ligamentum teres

Cut section of ligamentum teres

Zona orbicularis

Figure 3.48 ■ **(A)** Coronal section through hip joint. The perilabral sulcus is between the capsule and lateral acetabular rim and labrum. **(B)** Normal chondrolabral junction and perilabral sulcus. *(See Normal Labral Variants pg. 115, in Stoller's 3rd Edition.)*

A

Capsule

Acetabulum

Tidemark

Perilabral sulcus

Acetabular roof articular cartilage

Chondrolabral junction

Labrum

B

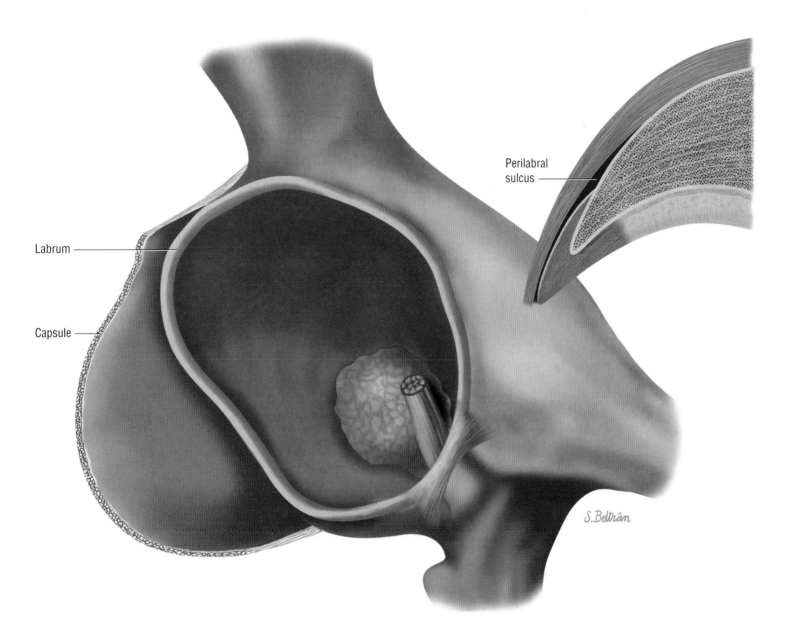

Labrum

Capsule

Perilabral
sulcus

S.Beltrán

Figure 3.49 ■ 3D image showing correlation between capsule and labrum and a corresponding coronal section of the perilabral sulcus lateral to the acetabular rim and labrum. *(See Normal Labral Variants pg. 116, in Stoller's 3rd Edition.)*

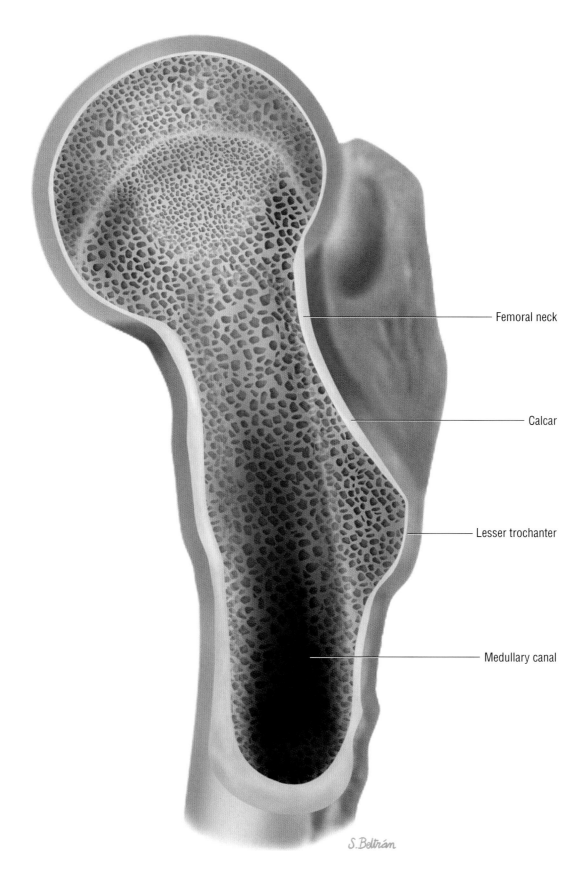

Femoral neck

Calcar

Lesser trochanter

Medullary canal

S. Beltrán

Figure 3.50 ▪ Relationship of the femoral neck and calcar. *(See Osseous Components pgs. 104 and 117, in Stoller's 3rd Edition.)*

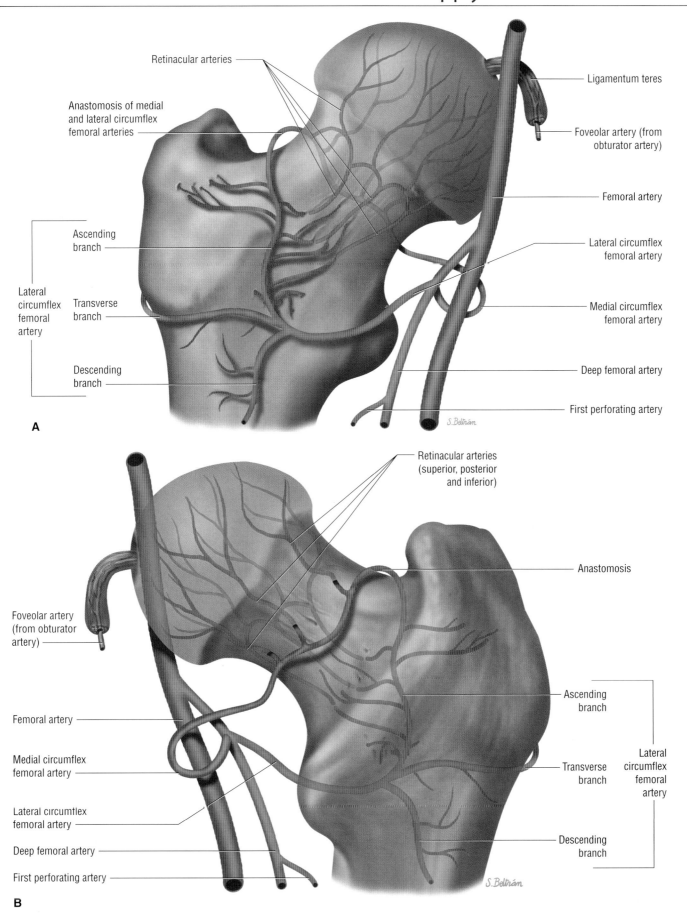

Figure 3.51 ■ Anterior (A) and posterior (B) perspectives of femoral head arterial supply. The arteries are derived from an anastomosis of three sets of vessels: the retinacular vessels (from the medial circumflex femoral artery and, to a lesser extent, the lateral circumflex femoral artery); the terminal branches of the medullary artery of the femoral shaft; and the artery of the ligamentum teres from the posterior division of the obturator artery. *(See Neurovascular Structures pgs. 104 and 117, in Stoller's 3rd Edition.)*

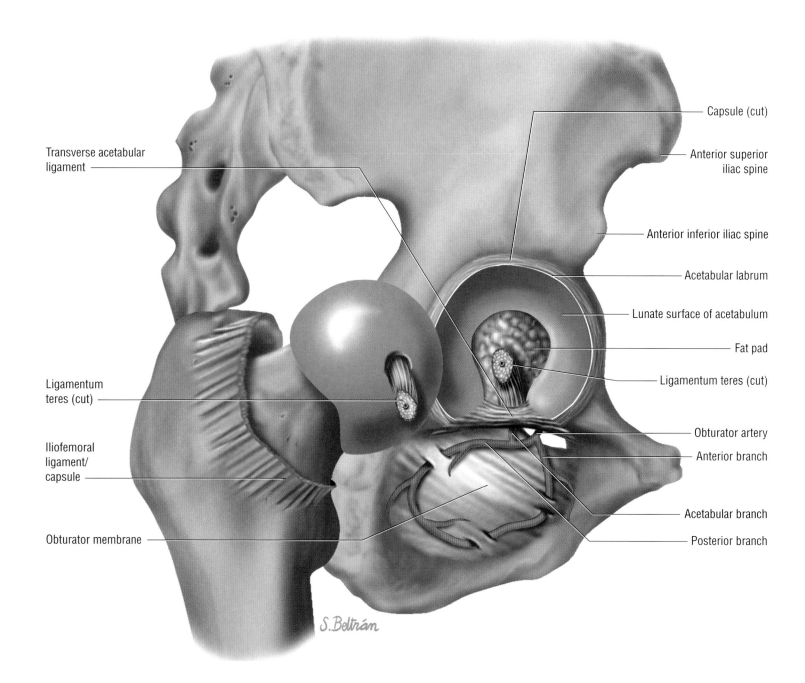

Transverse acetabular ligament

Capsule (cut)

Anterior superior iliac spine

Anterior inferior iliac spine

Acetabular labrum

Lunate surface of acetabulum

Fat pad

Ligamentum teres (cut)

Ligamentum teres (cut)

Iliofemoral ligament/ capsule

Obturator artery

Anterior branch

Acetabular branch

Posterior branch

Obturator membrane

S. Beltrán

Figure 3.52 ▪ Vascular supply of the hip joint. The relationship of the obturator artery and the small foveolar artery contained within the ligamentum teres is shown. *(See Neurovascular Structures pgs. 104 and 118, in Stoller's 3rd Edition.)*

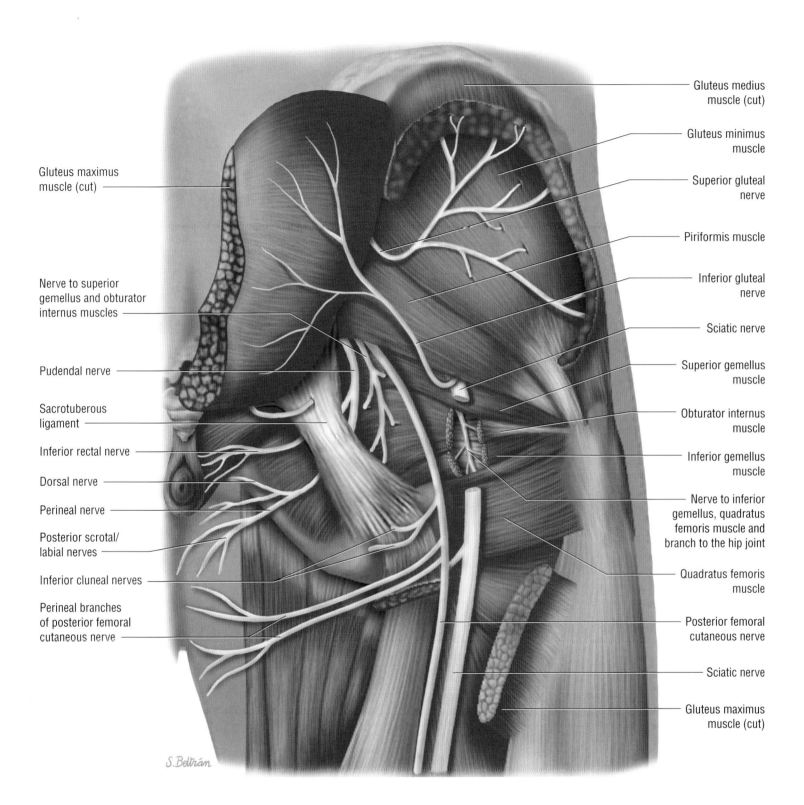

Gluteus maximus muscle (cut)

Nerve to superior gemellus and obturator internus muscles

Pudendal nerve

Sacrotuberous ligament

Inferior rectal nerve

Dorsal nerve

Perineal nerve

Posterior scrotal/ labial nerves

Inferior cluneal nerves

Perineal branches of posterior femoral cutaneous nerve

Gluteus medius muscle (cut)

Gluteus minimus muscle

Superior gluteal nerve

Piriformis muscle

Inferior gluteal nerve

Sciatic nerve

Superior gemellus muscle

Obturator internus muscle

Inferior gemellus muscle

Nerve to inferior gemellus, quadratus femoris muscle and branch to the hip joint

Quadratus femoris muscle

Posterior femoral cutaneous nerve

Sciatic nerve

Gluteus maximus muscle (cut)

S. Beltrán

Figure 3.53 ■ Posterior color illustration of the neural structures of the posterior proximal thigh. The sciatic nerve is sectioned. The sciatic nerve arises from the lumbosacral plexus and is composed of the ventral rami of the fourth and fifth lumbar roots and the first, second, and third sacral roots. It is shown exiting the pelvis through the sciatic notch inferior to the piriformis muscle. The sciatic nerve is completely motor in function. *(See Neurovascular Structures pgs. 104 and 119, in Stoller's 3rd Edition.)*

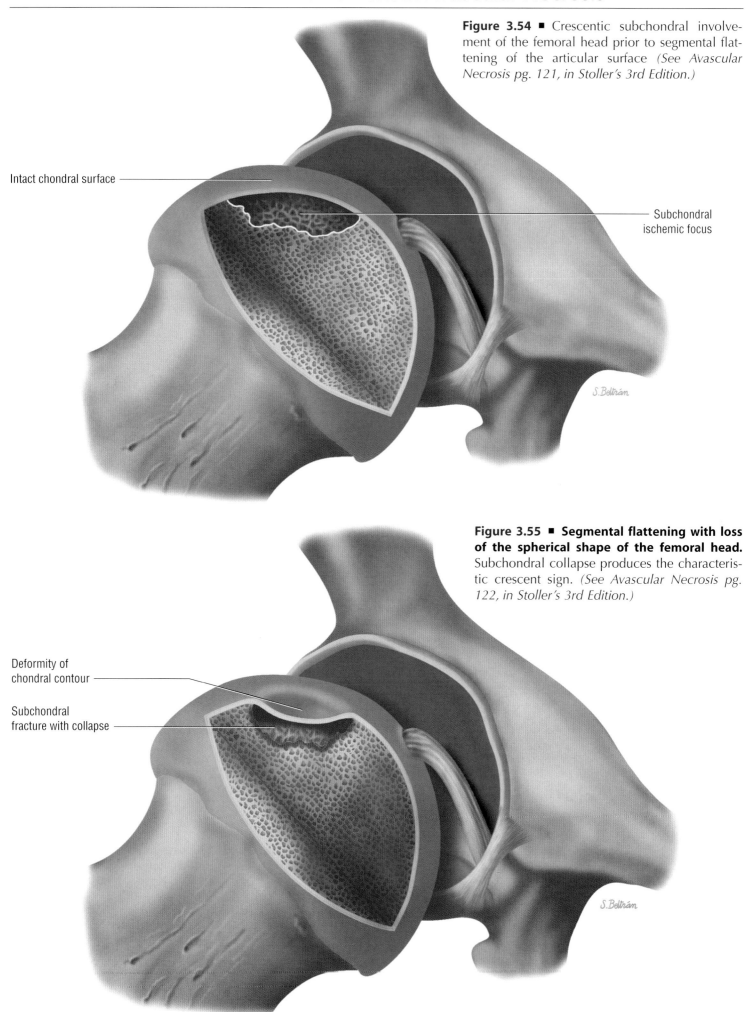

Figure 3.54 ■ Crescentic subchondral involvement of the femoral head prior to segmental flattening of the articular surface *(See Avascular Necrosis pg. 121, in Stoller's 3rd Edition.)*

Intact chondral surface

Subchondral ischemic focus

Figure 3.55 ■ **Segmental flattening with loss of the spherical shape of the femoral head.** Subchondral collapse produces the characteristic crescent sign. *(See Avascular Necrosis pg. 122, in Stoller's 3rd Edition.)*

Deformity of chondral contour

Subchondral fracture with collapse

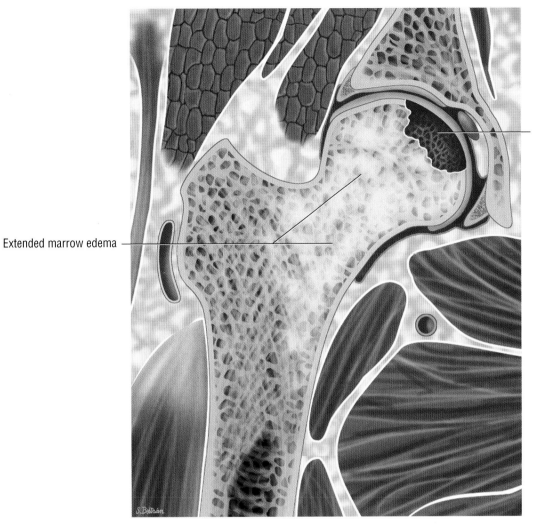

Osteonecrosis

Extended marrow edema

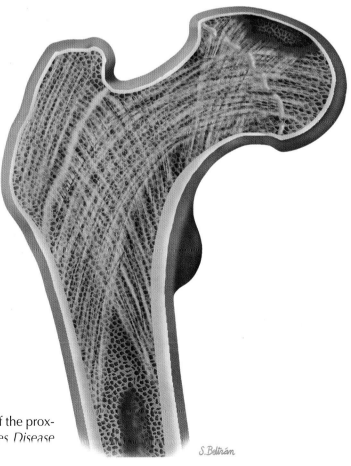

Figure 3.57 ■ Color coronal section showing subchondral necrosis of the proximal femoral epiphyses in Legg-Calvé-Perthes. *(See Legg-Calvé-Perthes Disease pgs. 134–135, in Stoller's 3rd Edition.)*

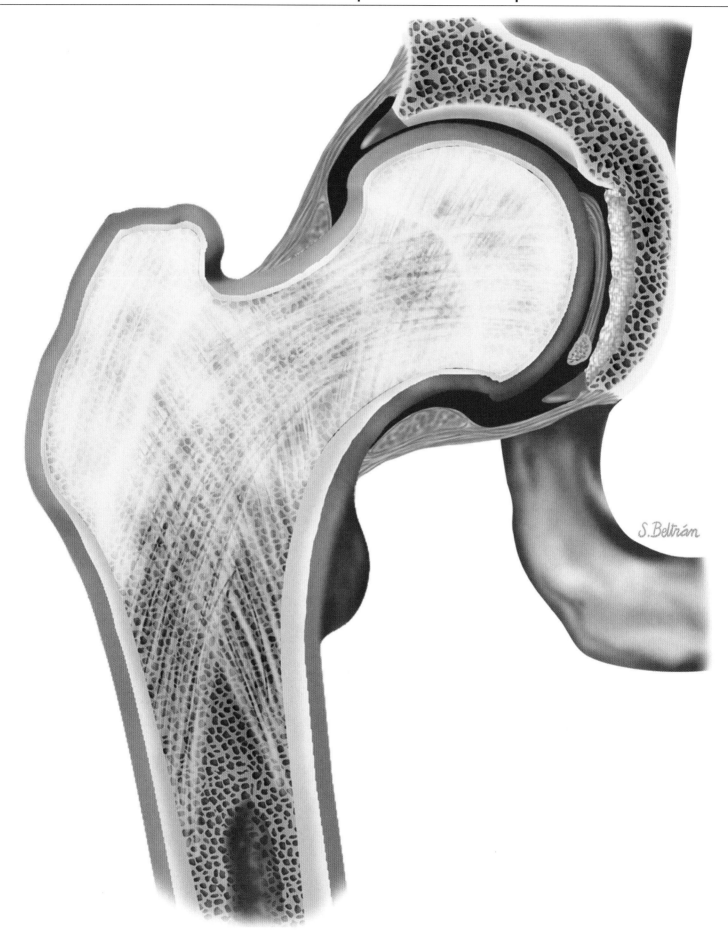

Figure 3.58 ■ **Transient osteoporosis of the hip with partial marrow-sparing of the greater trochanter and medial femoral head.** No subchondral fracture is identified. Coronal color section. *(See Transient Osteoporosis of the Hip pgs. 140–141, in Stoller's 3rd Edition.)*

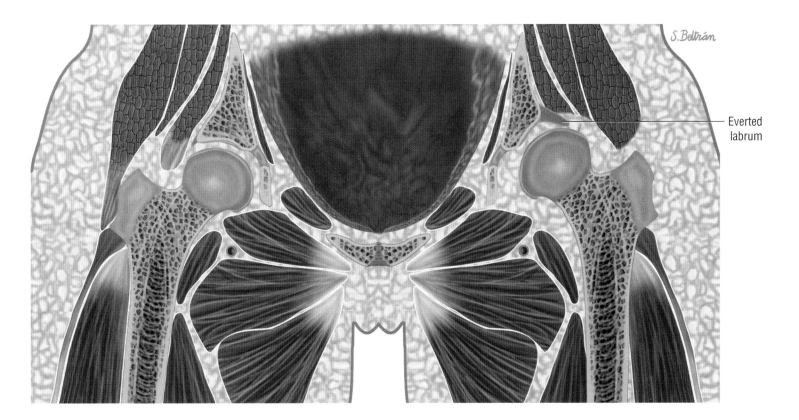

Everted
labrum

Figure 3.59 ■ **Developmental dysplasia of the hip (DDH).** Pseudo-coverage of the capital epiphysis by an everted labrum. *(See Developmental Dysplasia of the Hip pgs. 146–147, in Stoller's 3rd Edition.)*

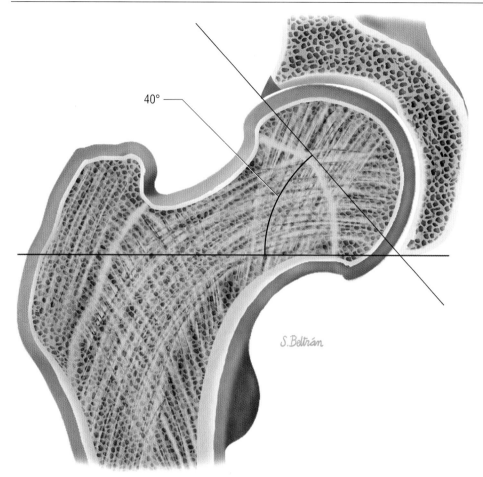

40°

S. Beltrán

Figure 3.60 ■ **The transverse angle of the osseous acetabular rim affects the degree of lateral coverage.** The normal angle of 40° is shown. *(See Developmental Dysplasia of the Hip pg. 148, in Stoller's 3rd Edition.)*

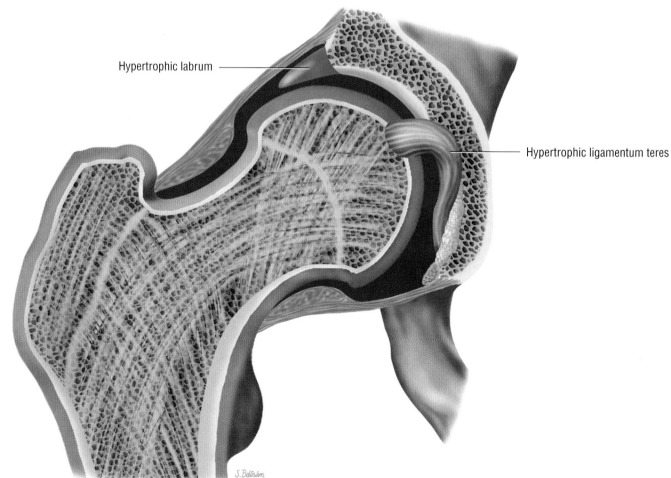

Hypertrophic labrum

Hypertrophic ligamentum teres

S. Beltrán

Figure 3.61 ■ Labral hypertrophy and hypertrophy of the ligamentum teres in DDH. *(See Developmental Dysplasia of the Hip pg. 148, in Stoller's 3rd Edition.)*

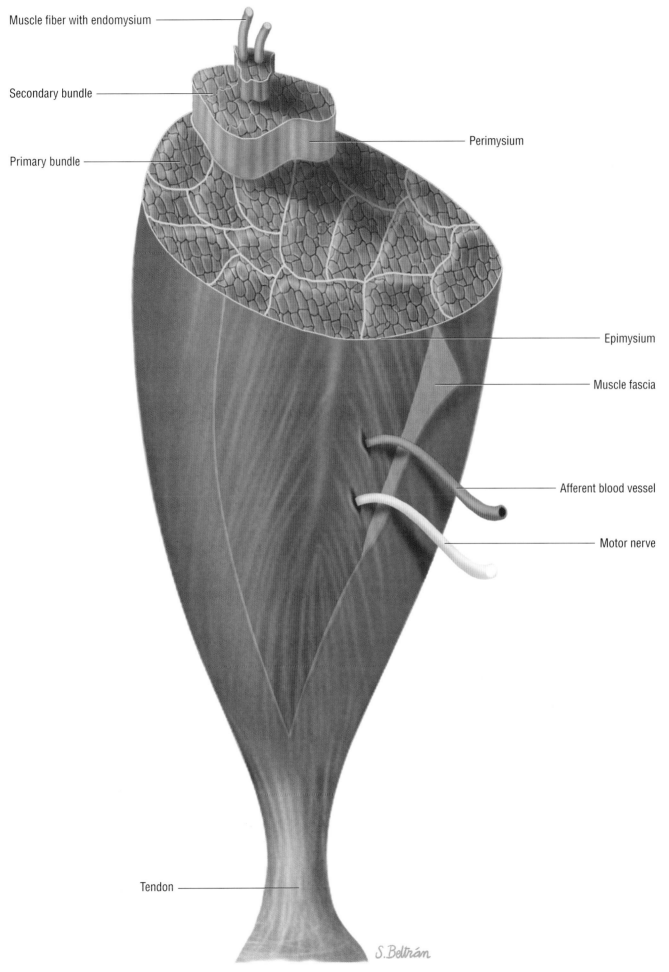

Muscle fiber with endomysium

Secondary bundle

Primary bundle

Perimysium

Epimysium

Muscle fascia

Afferent blood vessel

Motor nerve

Tendon

S. Beltrán

Figure 3.62 ■ **The structure of skeletal muscle.** The endomysium surrounds the individual muscle fibers. The perimysium surrounds groups of fascicles made up of fibers. The epimysium surrounds the entire muscle. *(See Structure of Skeletal Muscle pgs. 149–150, in Stoller's 3rd Edition.)*

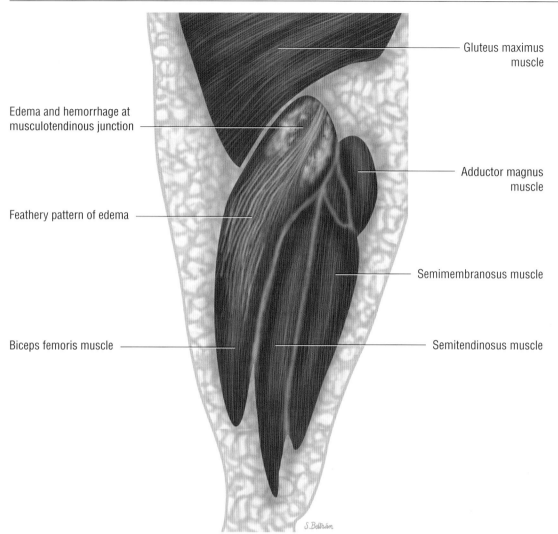

Gluteus maximus
muscle

Edema and hemorrhage at
musculotendinous junction

Feathery pattern of edema

Adductor magnus
muscle

Semimembranosus muscle

Biceps femoris muscle

Semitendinosus muscle

Figure 3.63 ■ Feathery edema pattern and intramuscular fluid (a grade 2 characteristic) in a grade 1 to 2 biceps femoris muscle strain. *(See Muscle Strains pg. 153, in Stoller's 3rd Edition.)*

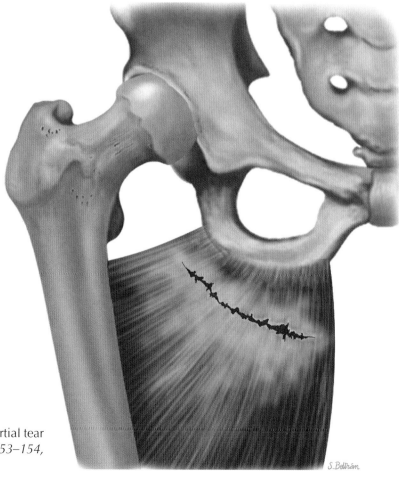

Figure 3.64 ■ Coronal color illustration anterior view of a partial tear of the proximal adductor magnus. *(See Muscle Strains pgs. 153–154, in Stoller's 3rd Edition.)*

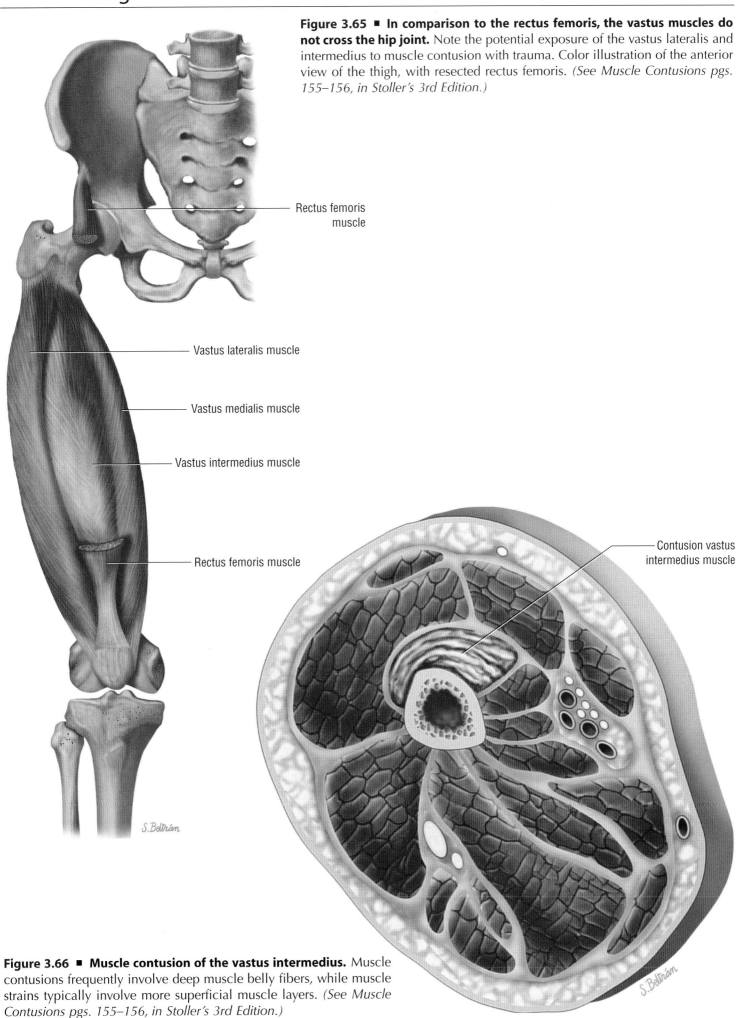

Figure 3.65 ■ **In comparison to the rectus femoris, the vastus muscles do not cross the hip joint.** Note the potential exposure of the vastus lateralis and intermedius to muscle contusion with trauma. Color illustration of the anterior view of the thigh, with resected rectus femoris. *(See Muscle Contusions pgs. 155–156, in Stoller's 3rd Edition.)*

Rectus femoris muscle

Vastus lateralis muscle

Vastus medialis muscle

Vastus intermedius muscle

Rectus femoris muscle

Contusion vastus intermedius muscle

Figure 3.66 ■ **Muscle contusion of the vastus intermedius.** Muscle contusions frequently involve deep muscle belly fibers, while muscle strains typically involve more superficial muscle layers. *(See Muscle Contusions pgs. 155–156, in Stoller's 3rd Edition.)*

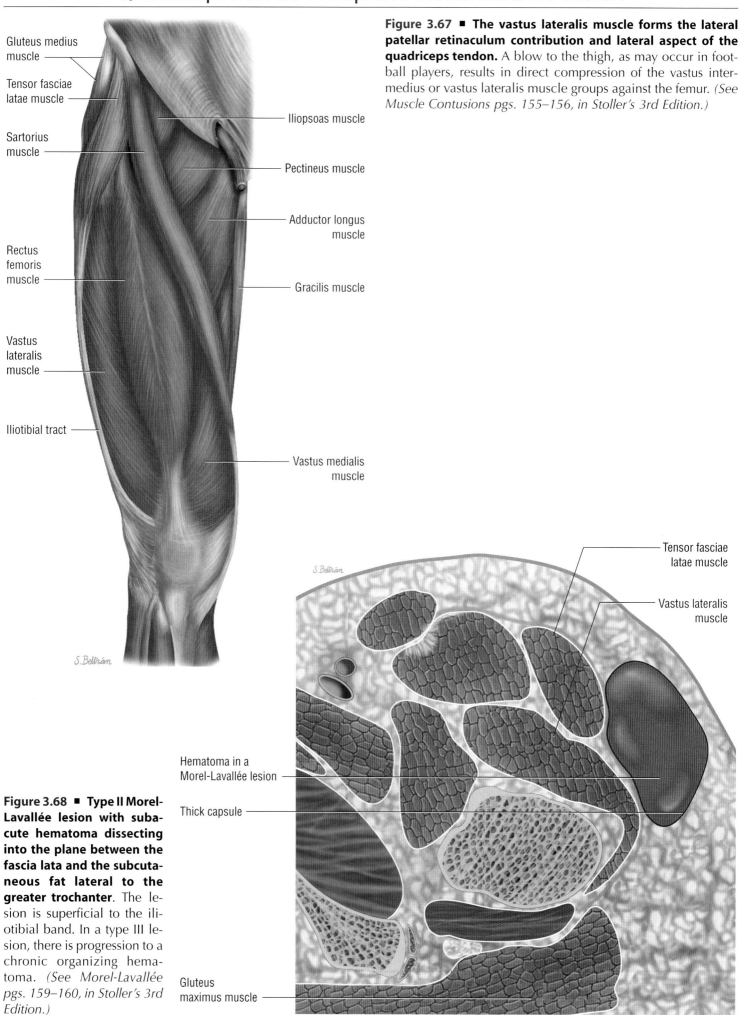

Gluteus medius muscle

Tensor fasciae latae muscle

Sartorius muscle

Rectus femoris muscle

Vastus lateralis muscle

Iliotibial tract

Iliopsoas muscle

Pectineus muscle

Adductor longus muscle

Gracilis muscle

Vastus medialis muscle

S.Beltrán

Figure 3.67 ▪ **The vastus lateralis muscle forms the lateral patellar retinaculum contribution and lateral aspect of the quadriceps tendon.** A blow to the thigh, as may occur in football players, results in direct compression of the vastus intermedius or vastus lateralis muscle groups against the femur. *(See Muscle Contusions pgs. 155–156, in Stoller's 3rd Edition.)*

Tensor fasciae latae muscle

Vastus lateralis muscle

Hematoma in a Morel-Lavallée lesion

Thick capsule

Gluteus maximus muscle

S.Beltrán

Figure 3.68 ▪ **Type II Morel-Lavallée lesion with subacute hematoma dissecting into the plane between the fascia lata and the subcutaneous fat lateral to the greater trochanter**. The lesion is superficial to the iliotibial band. In a type III lesion, there is progression to a chronic organizing hematoma. *(See Morel-Lavallée pgs. 159–160, in Stoller's 3rd Edition.)*

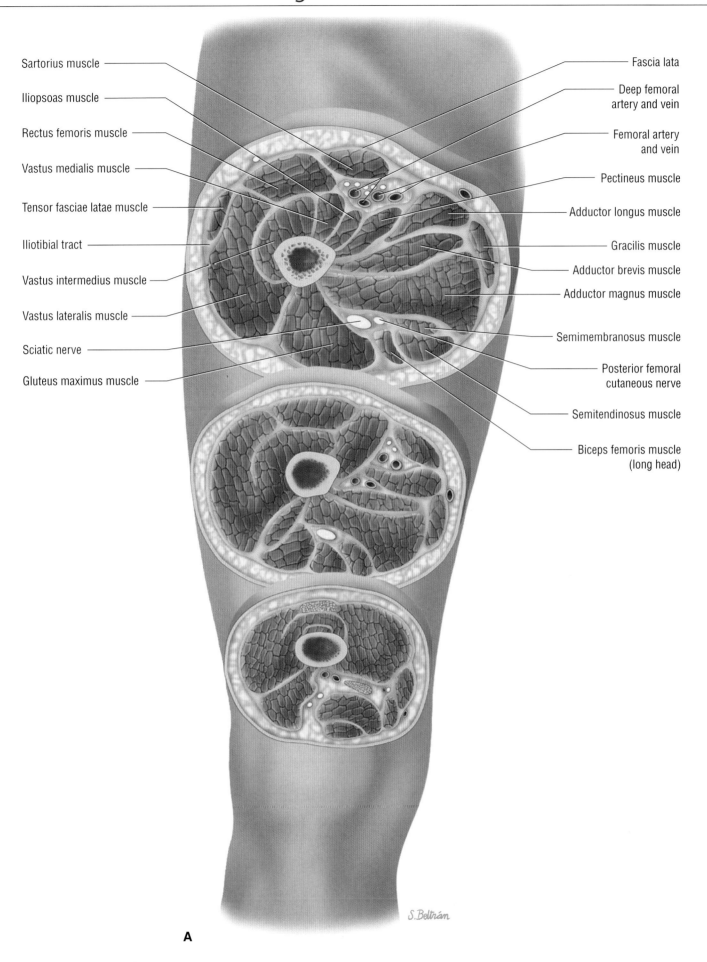

Sartorius muscle

Iliopsoas muscle

Rectus femoris muscle

Vastus medialis muscle

Tensor fasciae latae muscle

Iliotibial tract

Vastus intermedius muscle

Vastus lateralis muscle

Sciatic nerve

Gluteus maximus muscle

Fascia lata

Deep femoral artery and vein

Femoral artery and vein

Pectineus muscle

Adductor longus muscle

Gracilis muscle

Adductor brevis muscle

Adductor magnus muscle

Semimembranosus muscle

Posterior femoral cutaneous nerve

Semitendinosus muscle

Biceps femoris muscle (long head)

S. Beltrán

A

Figure 3.69 ■ (A) Proximal (B) mid-, and (C) distal muscle cross sections of the thigh. Distal rectus femoris injuries involve the distal musculotendinous junction and are associated with retraction of the rectus contribution to the quadriceps tendon *(See Rectus Femoris Muscle Strain pgs. 164–167, in Stoller's 3rd Edition.)*

(continued)

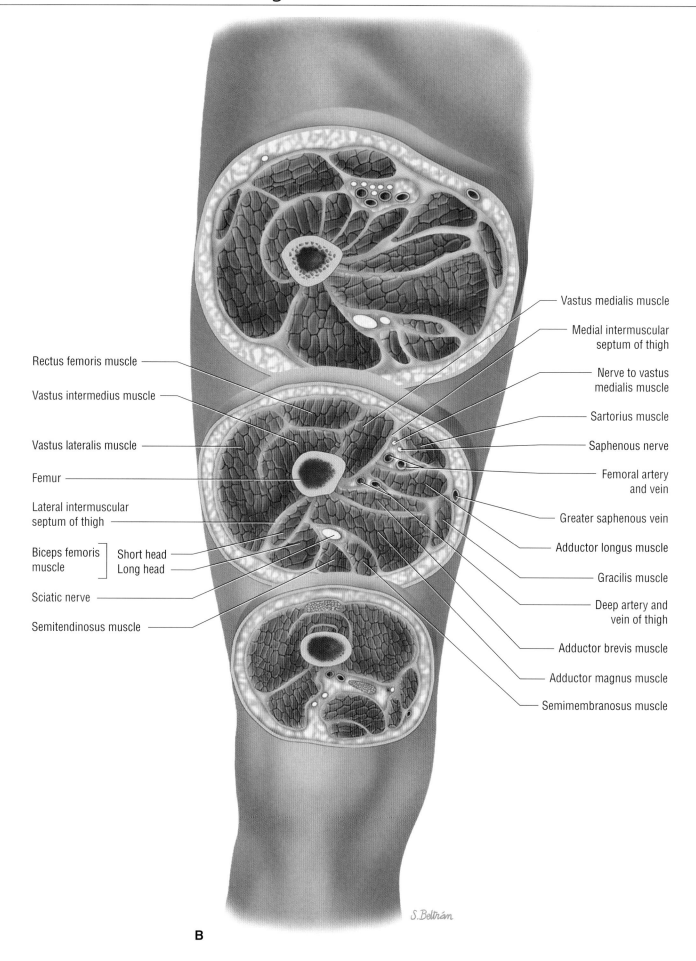

Rectus femoris muscle

Vastus intermedius muscle

Vastus lateralis muscle

Femur

Lateral intermuscular
septum of thigh

Biceps femoris   Short head
muscle   Long head

Sciatic nerve

Semitendinosus muscle

Vastus medialis muscle

Medial intermuscular
septum of thigh

Nerve to vastus
medialis muscle

Sartorius muscle

Saphenous nerve

Femoral artery
and vein

Greater saphenous vein

Adductor longus muscle

Gracilis muscle

Deep artery and
vein of thigh

Adductor brevis muscle

Adductor magnus muscle

Semimembranosus muscle

B

S.Beltrán

Figure 3.69 ■ *Continued.*

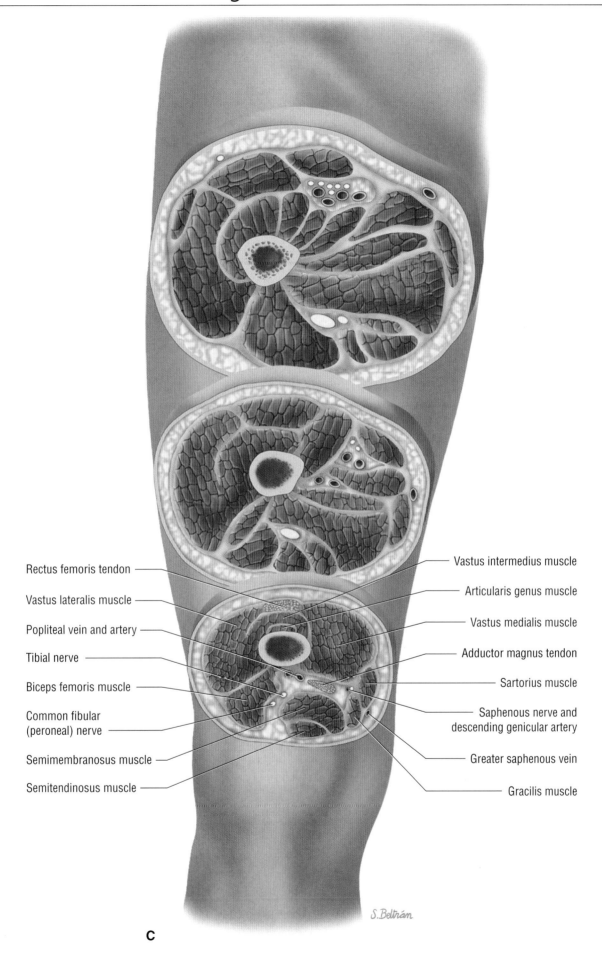

Rectus femoris tendon

Vastus lateralis muscle

Popliteal vein and artery

Tibial nerve

Biceps femoris muscle

Common fibular (peroneal) nerve

Semimembranosus muscle

Semitendinosus muscle

Vastus intermedius muscle

Articularis genus muscle

Vastus medialis muscle

Adductor magnus tendon

Sartorius muscle

Saphenous nerve and descending genicular artery

Greater saphenous vein

Gracilis muscle

C

Figure 3.69 ■ *Continued.*

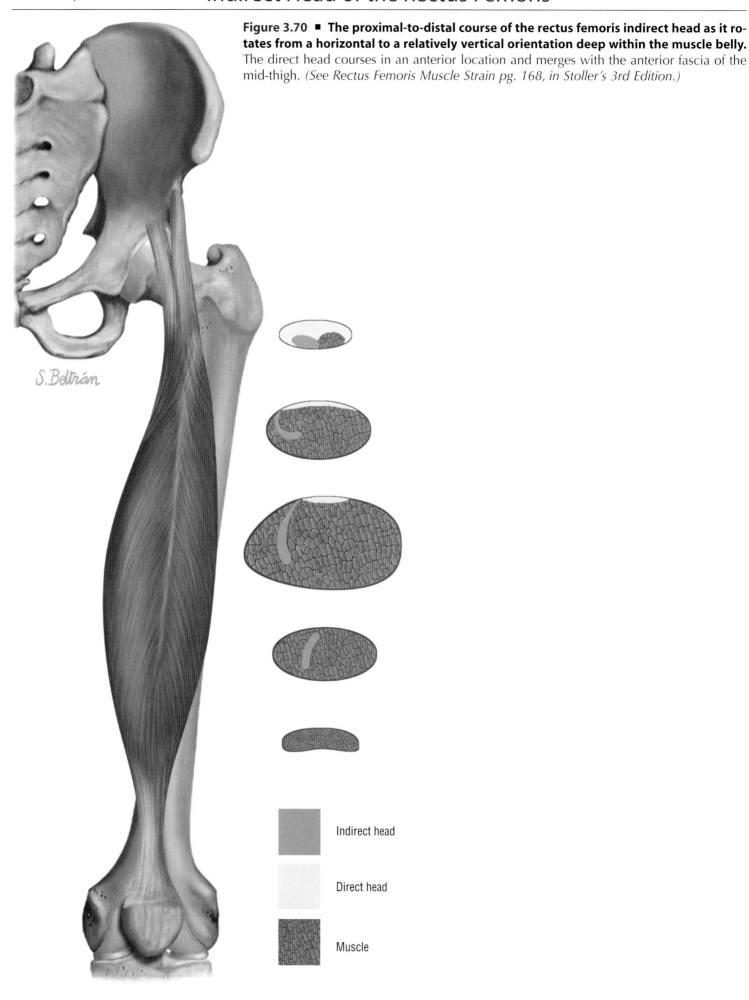

Figure 3.70 ▪ **The proximal-to-distal course of the rectus femoris indirect head as it ro-tates from a horizontal to a relatively vertical orientation deep within the muscle belly.** The direct head courses in an anterior location and merges with the anterior fascia of the mid-thigh. *(See Rectus Femoris Muscle Strain pg. 168, in Stoller's 3rd Edition.)*

S. Beltrán

Indirect head

Direct head

Muscle

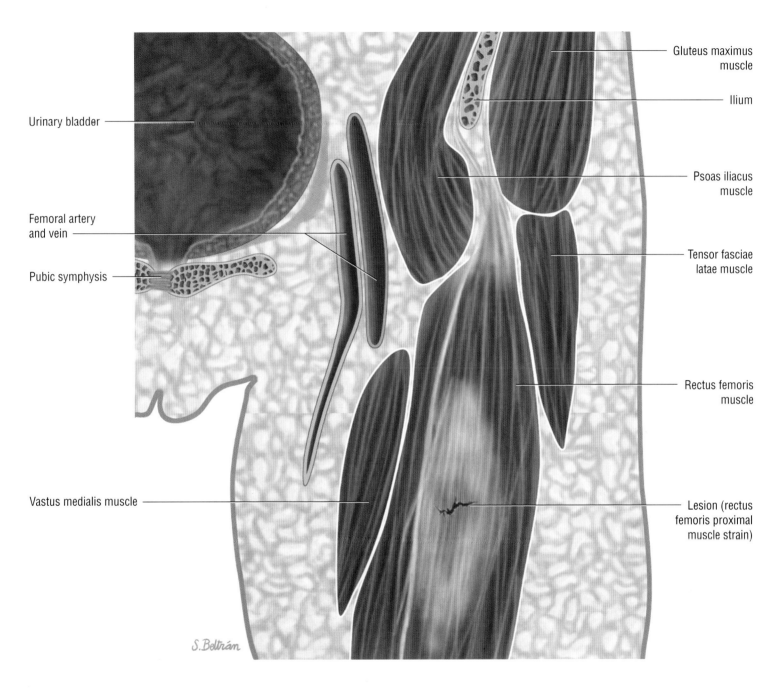

Urinary bladder

Femoral artery
and vein

Pubic symphysis

Vastus medialis muscle

Gluteus maximus
muscle

Ilium

Psoas iliacus
muscle

Tensor fasciae
latae muscle

Rectus femoris
muscle

Lesion (rectus
femoris proximal
muscle strain)

S. Beltrán

Figure 3.71 ■ Coronal color illustration of a grade 2 rectus femoris strain. *(See Rectus Femoris Muscle Strain pg. 169, in Stoller's 3rd Edition.)*

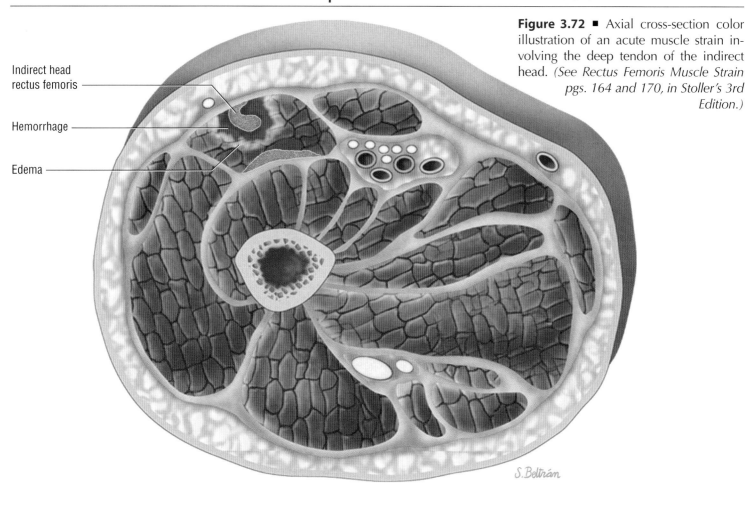

Indirect head
rectus femoris

Hemorrhage

Edema

Figure 3.72 ■ Axial cross-section color illustration of an acute muscle strain involving the deep tendon of the indirect head. *(See Rectus Femoris Muscle Strain pgs. 164 and 170, in Stoller's 3rd Edition.)*

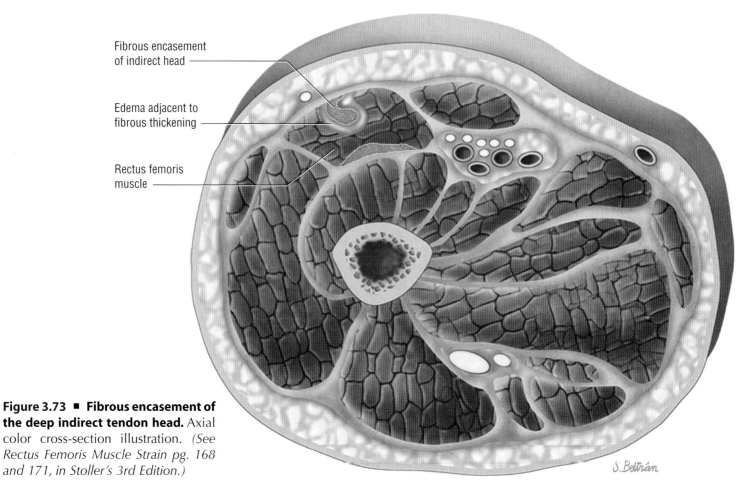

Fibrous encasement
of indirect head

Edema adjacent to
fibrous thickening

Rectus femoris
muscle

Figure 3.73 ■ **Fibrous encasement of the deep indirect tendon head.** Axial color cross-section illustration. *(See Rectus Femoris Muscle Strain pg. 168 and 171, in Stoller's 3rd Edition.)*

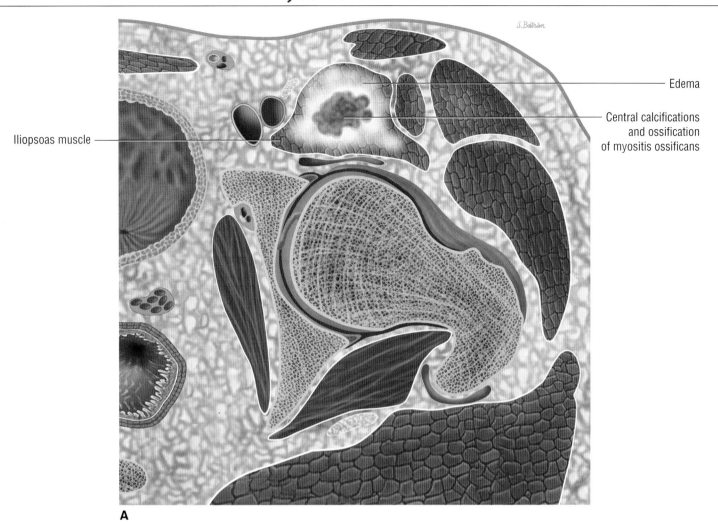

Iliopsoas muscle

Edema

Central calcifications
and ossification
of myositis ossificans

A

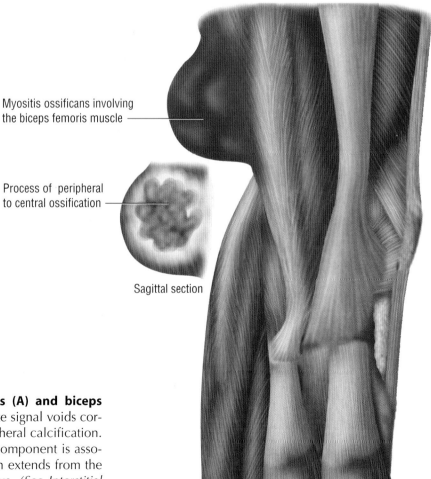

Myositis ossificans involving
the biceps femoris muscle

Process of peripheral
to central ossification

Sagittal section

Figure 3.74 ▪ Myositis ossificans of the iliopsoas (A) and biceps femoris (B) muscles. An MR image would demonstrate signal voids corresponding to areas of more mature osteoid and peripheral calcification. A hypointense periphery and heterogeneous central component is associated with the maturation process, where ossification extends from the periphery to the center of the myositis ossificans focus. *(See Interstitial Hemorrhage and Hematoma pg. 158, in Stoller's 3rd Edition.)*

B

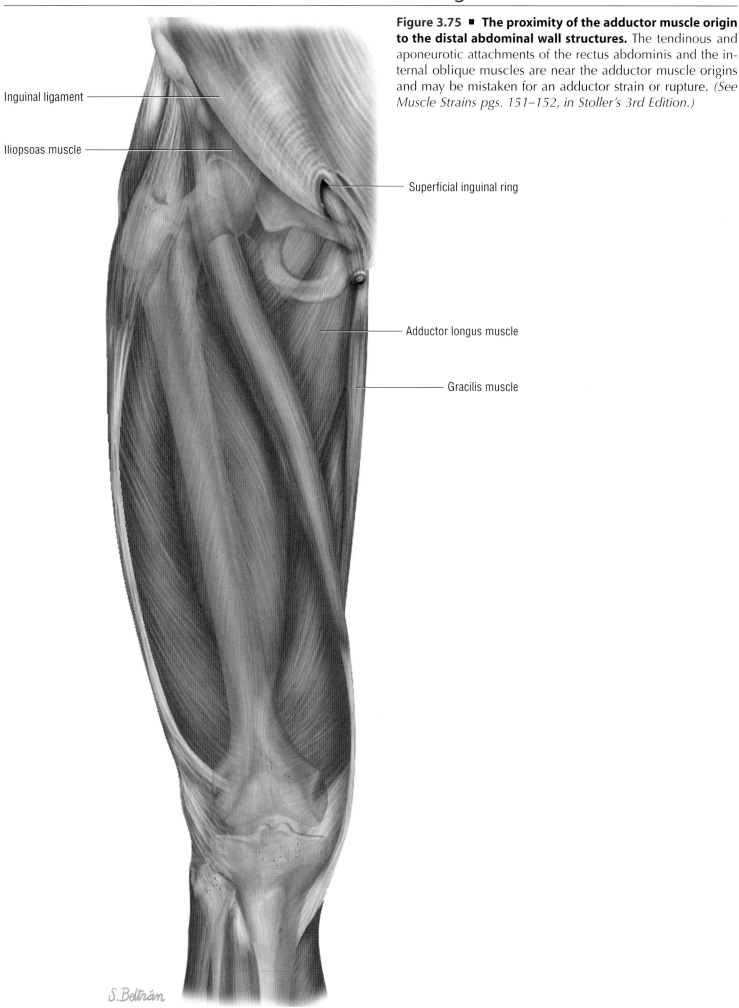

Inguinal ligament

Iliopsoas muscle

Superficial inguinal ring

Adductor longus muscle

Gracilis muscle

S.Beltrán

Figure 3.75 ■ The proximity of the adductor muscle origin to the distal abdominal wall structures. The tendinous and aponeurotic attachments of the rectus abdominis and the internal oblique muscles are near the adductor muscle origins and may be mistaken for an adductor strain or rupture. *(See Muscle Strains pgs. 151–152, in Stoller's 3rd Edition.)*

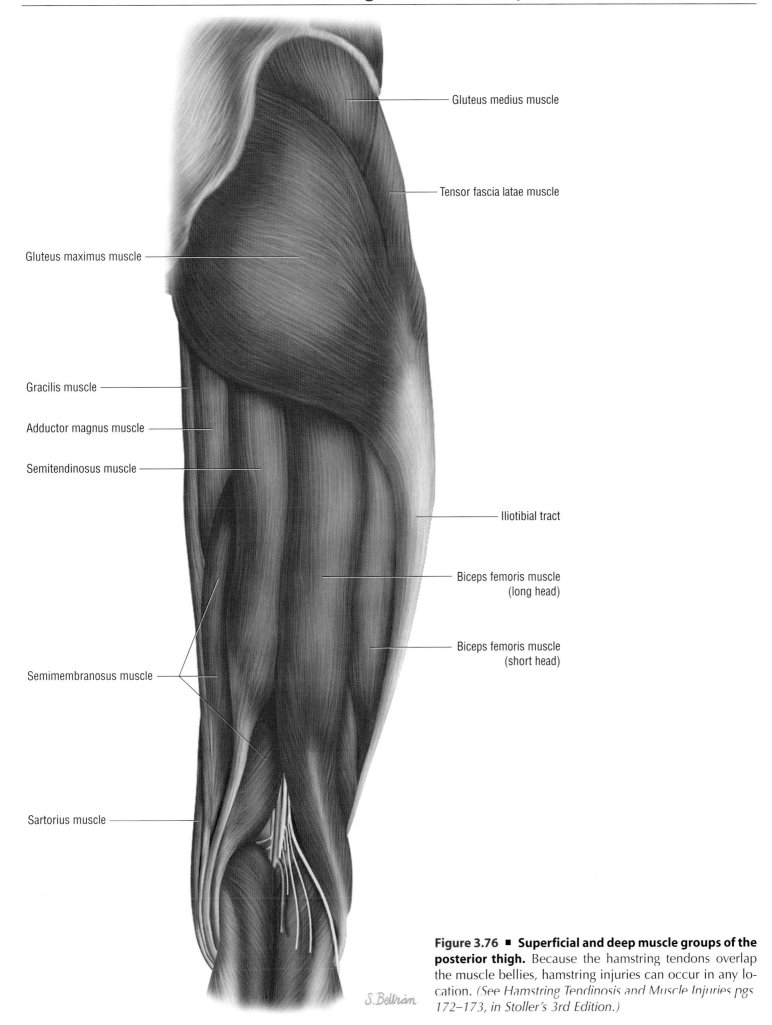

Gluteus medius muscle

Tensor fascia latae muscle

Gluteus maximus muscle

Gracilis muscle

Adductor magnus muscle

Semitendinosus muscle

Iliotibial tract

Biceps femoris muscle
(long head)

Biceps femoris muscle
(short head)

Semimembranosus muscle

Sartorius muscle

S.Beltran

Figure 3.76 ■ Superficial and deep muscle groups of the posterior thigh. Because the hamstring tendons overlap the muscle bellies, hamstring injuries can occur in any location. *(See Hamstring Tendinosis and Muscle Injuries pgs 172–173, in Stoller's 3rd Edition.)*

Figure 3.77 ■ The musculotendinous junctions of the biceps femoris muscle overlap and effectively extend over the entire longitudinal axis of the muscle as potential sites of injury. Unlike the rest of the hamstring group, including the biceps long head, the short head of the biceps does not cross the hip joint and receives its innervation from the peroneal branch of the sciatic nerve and not the tibial branch. *(See Hamstring Tendinosis and Muscle Injuries pgs. 173–175 , in Stoller's 3rd Edition.)*

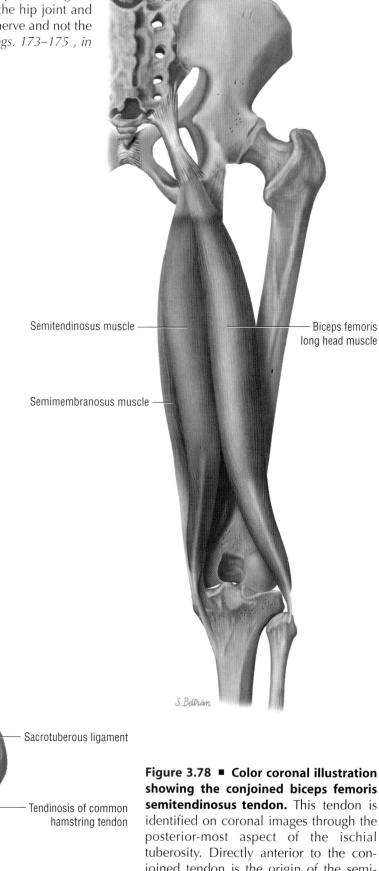

Semitendinosus muscle

Semimembranosus muscle

Biceps femoris long head muscle

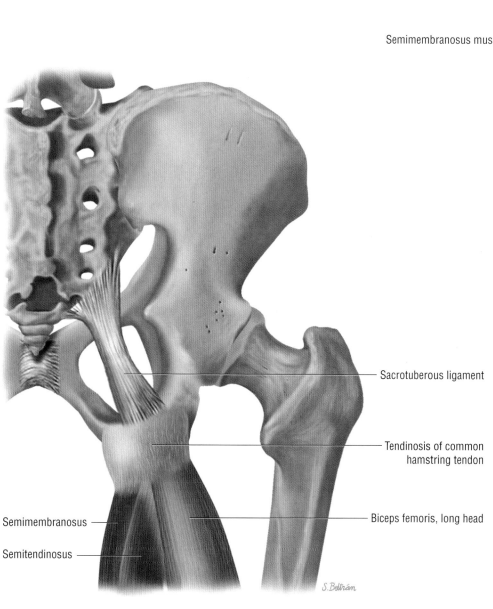

Sacrotuberous ligament

Tendinosis of common hamstring tendon

Biceps femoris, long head

Semimembranosus

Semitendinosus

Figure 3.78 ■ Color coronal illustration showing the conjoined biceps femoris semitendinosus tendon. This tendon is identified on coronal images through the posterior-most aspect of the ischial tuberosity. Directly anterior to the conjoined tendon is the origin of the semimembranosus tendon. Common hamstring tendon degeneration is illustrated. *(See Hamstring and Tendinosis and Muscle Injuries pgs. 173 and 176, in Stoller's 3rd Edition.)*

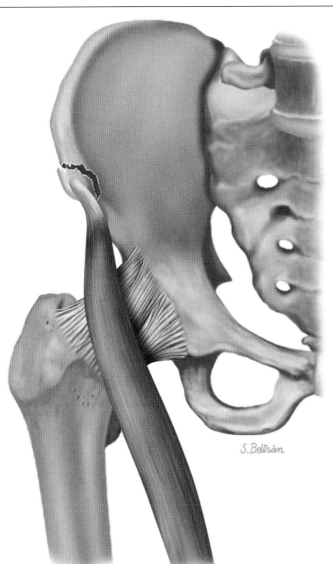

Figure 3.79 ▪ SARTORIUS AVULSION. Sartorius avulsion occurs with the hip in extension and the knee flexed, as occurs in sports involving kicking and running. *(See ASIS Avulsion pg. 178, in Stoller's 3rd Edition.)*

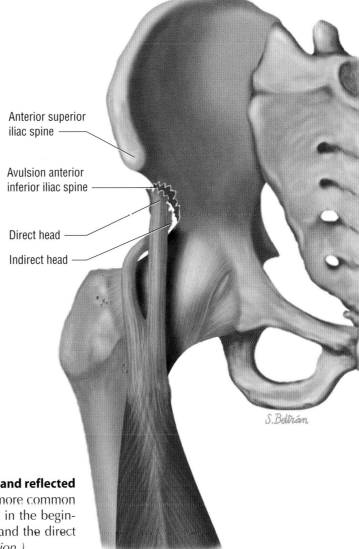

Anterior superior iliac spine

Avulsion anterior inferior iliac spine

Direct head

Indirect head

Figure 3.80 ▪ Coronal color illustration of avulsion of the direct and reflected head origins of the rectus femoris. Avulsion of the direct head is more common than avulsion of the indirect head because the direct head is taut in the beginning of hip flexion. In increased flexion the indirect head is taut and the direct head becomes lax. *(See AIIS Avulsion pg. 179, in Stoller's 3rd Edition.)*

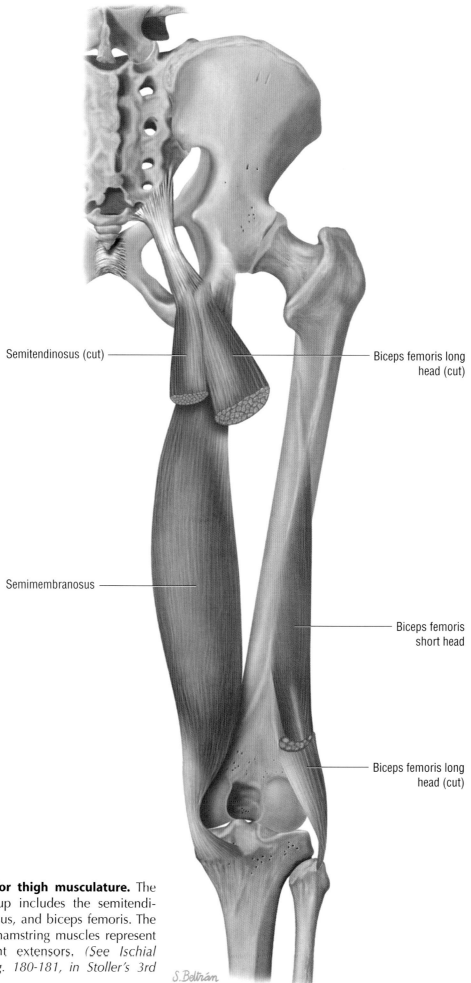

Semitendinosus (cut)

Biceps femoris long
head (cut)

Semimembranosus

Biceps femoris
short head

Biceps femoris long
head (cut)

S. Beltrán

Figure 3.81 ▪ Posterior thigh musculature. The hamstring muscle group includes the semitendinosus, semimembranosus, and biceps femoris. The gluteus maximus and hamstring muscles represent the primary hip joint extensors. *(See Ischial Tuberosity Avulsion pg. 180-181, in Stoller's 3rd Edition.)*

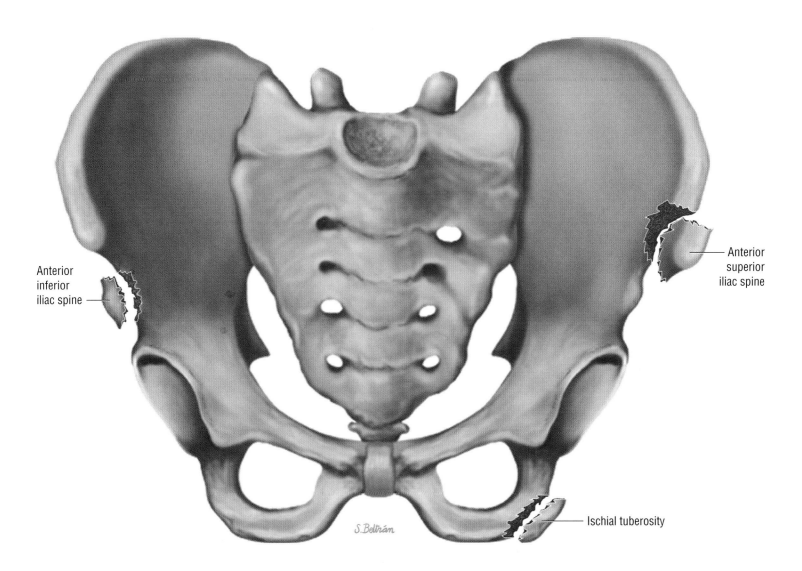

Figure 3.82 ■ Coronal color illustration of avulsion injury sites with correlation of ischial tuberosity avulsion side. *(See Ischial Tuberosity Avulsion pgs. 180–182, in Stoller's 3rd Edition.)*

Adductor Muscles

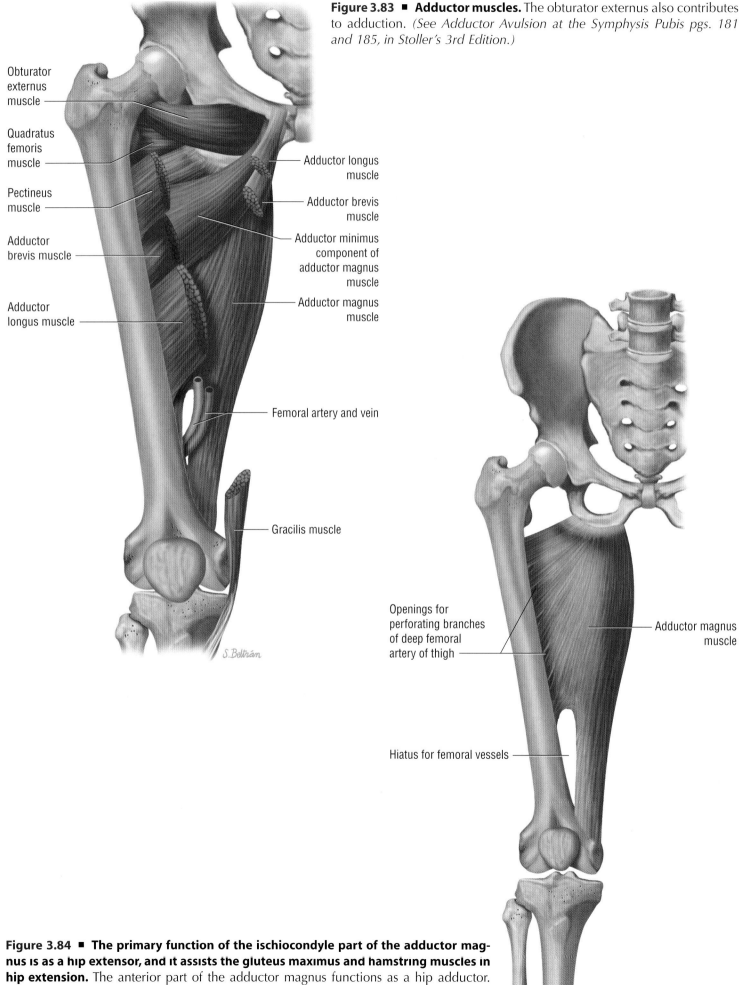

Figure 3.83 ■ Adductor muscles. The obturator externus also contributes to adduction. *(See Adductor Avulsion at the Symphysis Pubis pgs. 181 and 185, in Stoller's 3rd Edition.)*

Obturator externus muscle

Quadratus femoris muscle

Pectineus muscle

Adductor brevis muscle

Adductor longus muscle

Adductor longus muscle

Adductor brevis muscle

Adductor minimus component of adductor magnus muscle

Adductor magnus muscle

Femoral artery and vein

Gracilis muscle

Openings for perforating branches of deep femoral artery of thigh

Adductor magnus muscle

Hiatus for femoral vessels

Figure 3.84 ■ The primary function of the ischiocondyle part of the adductor magnus is as a hip extensor, and it assists the gluteus maximus and hamstring muscles in hip extension. The anterior part of the adductor magnus functions as a hip adductor. *(See Adductor Avulsion at the Symphysis Pubis pgs. 181 and 186, in Stoller's 3rd Edition.)*

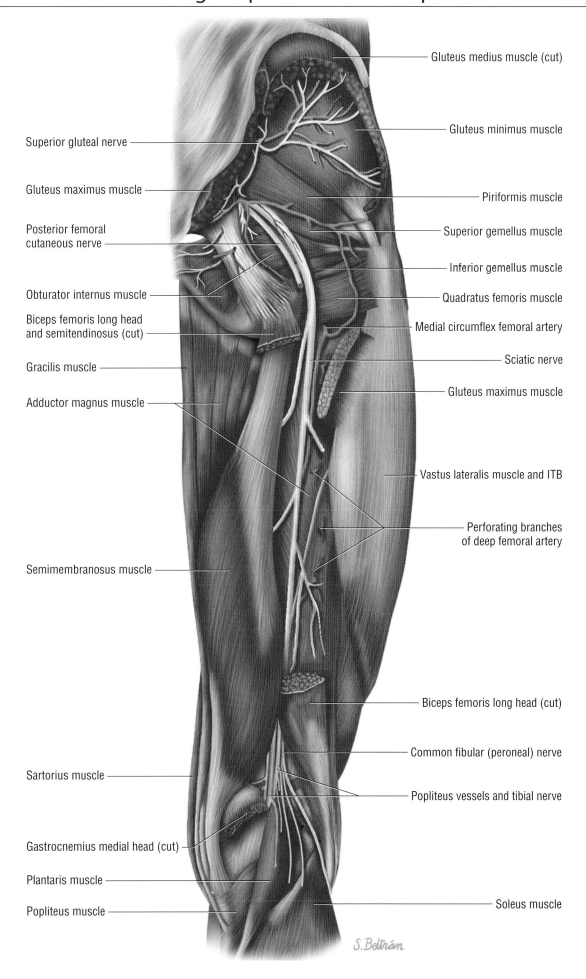

Gluteus medius muscle (cut)

Gluteus minimus muscle

Superior gluteal nerve

Gluteus maximus muscle

Piriformis muscle

Posterior femoral
cutaneous nerve

Superior gemellus muscle

Inferior gemellus muscle

Obturator internus muscle

Quadratus femoris muscle

Biceps femoris long head
and semitendinosus (cut)

Medial circumflex femoral artery

Gracilis muscle

Sciatic nerve

Gluteus maximus muscle

Adductor magnus muscle

Vastus lateralis muscle and ITB

Perforating branches
of deep femoral artery

Semimembranosus muscle

Biceps femoris long head (cut)

Common fibular (peroneal) nerve

Sartorius muscle

Popliteus vessels and tibial nerve

Gastrocnemius medial head (cut)

Plantaris muscle

Popliteus muscle

Soleus muscle

S. Beltrán

Figure 3.85 ■ Deep muscles of the posterior thigh. *(See Adductor Avulsion of the Symphysis Pubis pgs. 181, 186, and 187, in Stoller's 3rd Edition.)*

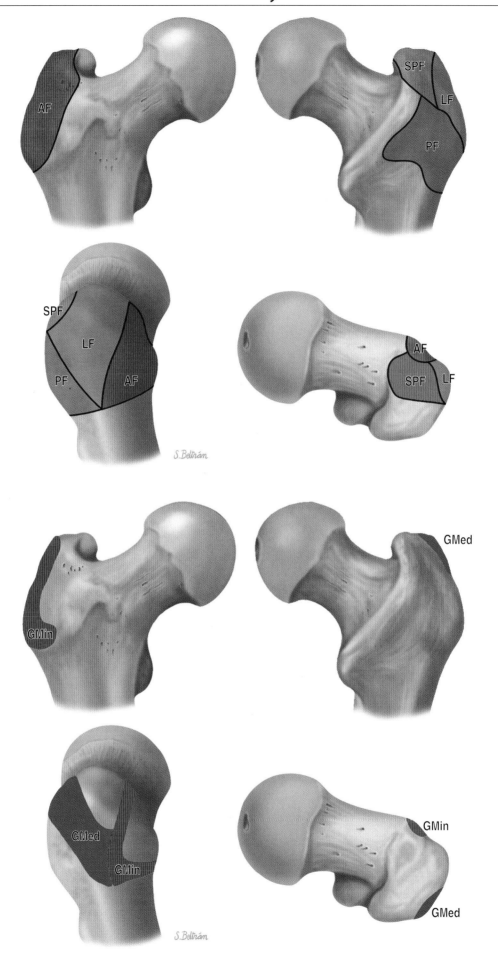

Figure 3.86 ■ Greater trochanter facet anatomy. AF, anterior facet; LF, lateral facet; SPF, superoposterior facet; PF, posterior facet. *(See Hip Abductor (Gluteus Muscle) Injuries and Trochanteric Bursitis pgs. 188–189, in Stoller's 3rd Edition.)*

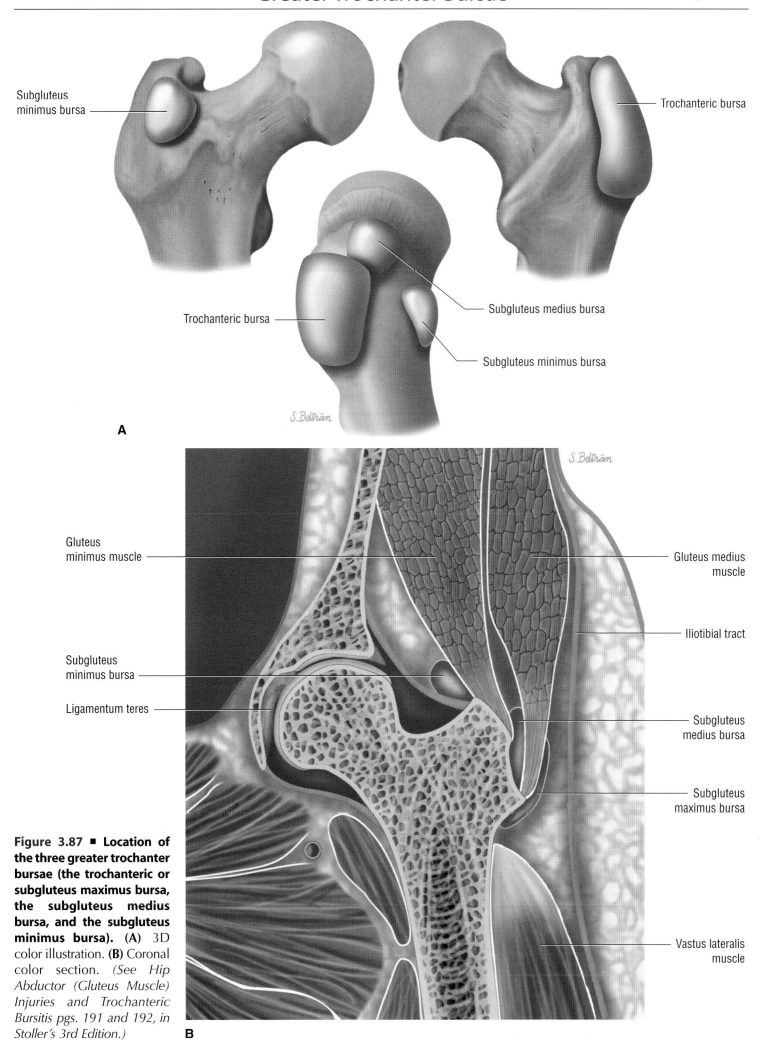

Subgluteus minimus bursa

Trochanteric bursa

Trochanteric bursa

Subgluteus medius bursa

Subgluteus minimus bursa

S. Beltrán

A

S. Beltrán

Gluteus minimus muscle

Gluteus medius muscle

Iliotibial tract

Subgluteus minimus bursa

Ligamentum teres

Subgluteus medius bursa

Subgluteus maximus bursa

Vastus lateralis muscle

Figure 3.87 ▪ Location of the three greater trochanter bursae (the trochanteric or subgluteus maximus bursa, the subgluteus medius bursa, and the subgluteus minimus bursa). (A) 3D color illustration. **(B)** Coronal color section. *(See Hip Abductor (Gluteus Muscle) Injuries and Trochanteric Bursitis pgs. 191 and 192, in Stoller's 3rd Edition.)*

B

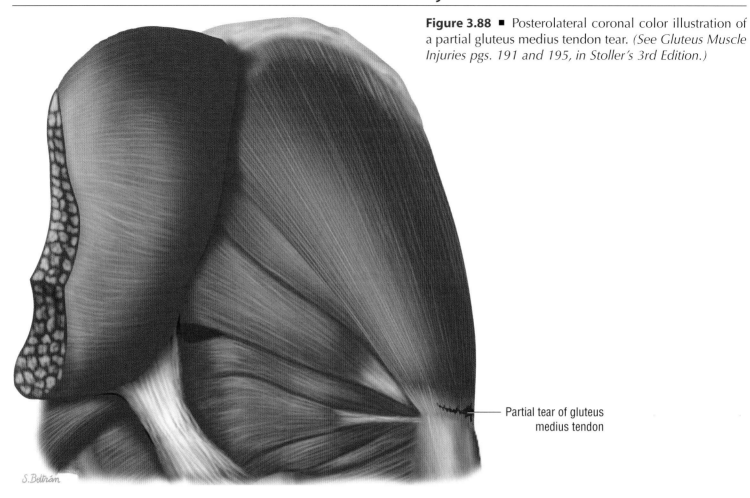

Figure 3.88 ▪ Posterolateral coronal color illustration of a partial gluteus medius tendon tear. *(See Gluteus Muscle Injuries pgs. 191 and 195, in Stoller's 3rd Edition.)*

Partial tear of gluteus medius tendon

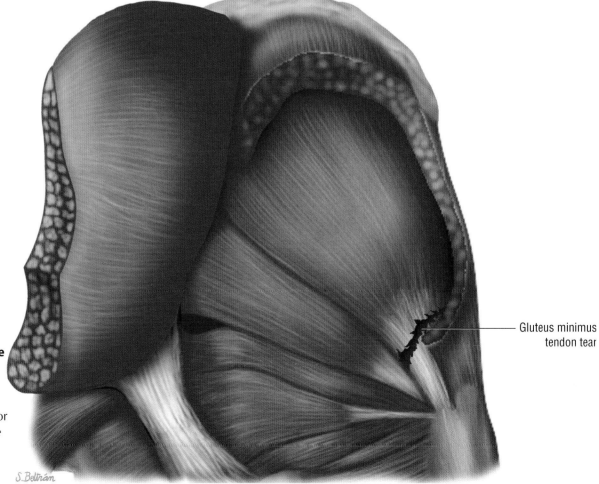

Figure 3.89 ▪ **Complete full-thickness tear of the gluteus minimus tendon.** The gluteus medius is intact. Posterior coronal illustration. *(See Gluteus Muscle Injuries pgs. 191 and 196, in Stoller's 3rd Edition.)*

Gluteus minimus tendon tear

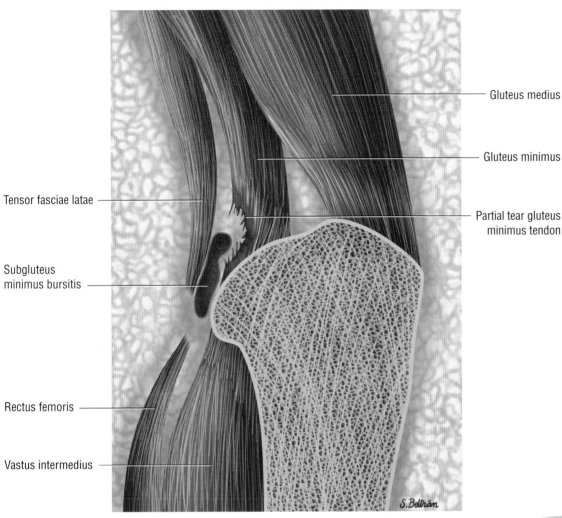

Tensor fasciae latae

Subgluteus minimus bursitis

Rectus femoris

Vastus intermedius

Gluteus medius

Gluteus minimus

Partial tear gluteus minimus tendon

Figure 3.90 ■ Partial tear and tendinosis of the gluteus minimus tendon with adjacent bursal inflammation. *(See Gluteus Muscle Injuries pgs. 191, 193, and 194, in Stoller's 3rd Edition.)*

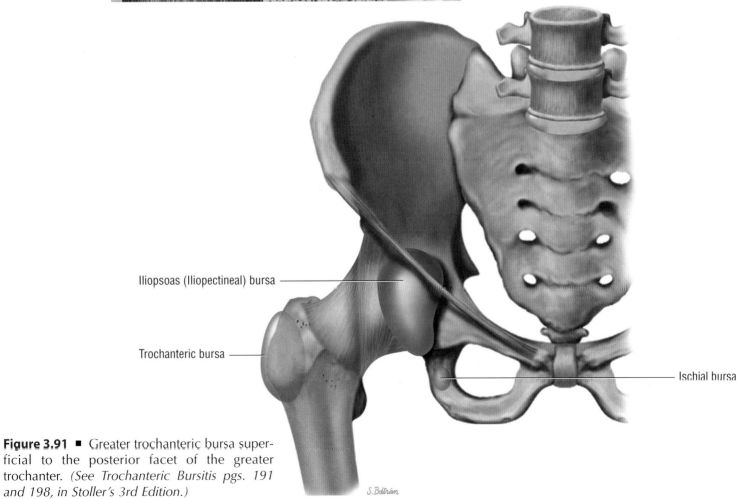

Iliopsoas (Iliopectineal) bursa

Trochanteric bursa

Ischial bursa

Figure 3.91 ■ Greater trochanteric bursa superficial to the posterior facet of the greater trochanter. *(See Trochanteric Bursitis pgs. 191 and 198, in Stoller's 3rd Edition.)*

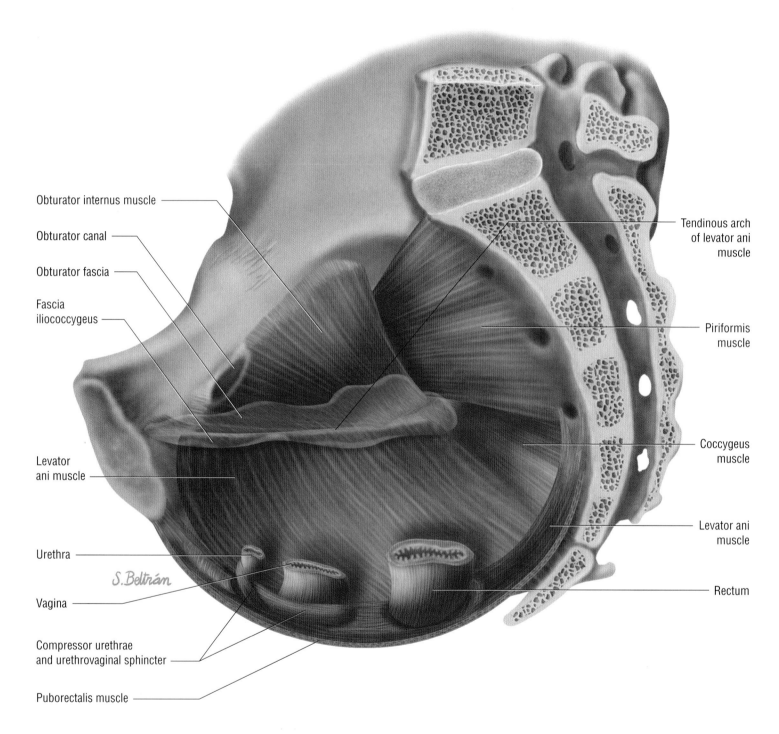

Obturator internus muscle

Obturator canal

Obturator fascia

Fascia
iliococcygeus

Levator
ani muscle

Urethra

S. Beltrán

Vagina

Compressor urethrae
and urethrovaginal sphincter

Puborectalis muscle

Tendinous arch
of levator ani
muscle

Piriformis
muscle

Coccygeus
muscle

Levator ani
muscle

Rectum

Figure 3.92 ■ Obturator internus and piriformis as viewed from the pelvis. *(See Piriformis Syndrome pg. 200, in Stoller's 3rd Edition.)*

Piriformis Syndrome

Figure 3.93 ■ **Entrapment of the sciatic nerve as it courses through the sciatic notch.** Trauma to the posterior thigh may result in irritation, inflammation, spasm, adhesion, and hypertrophy of the piriformis muscle and secondary dysfunction of the sciatic nerve. *(See Piriformis Syndrome pgs. 200 and 201, in Stoller's 3rd Edition.)*

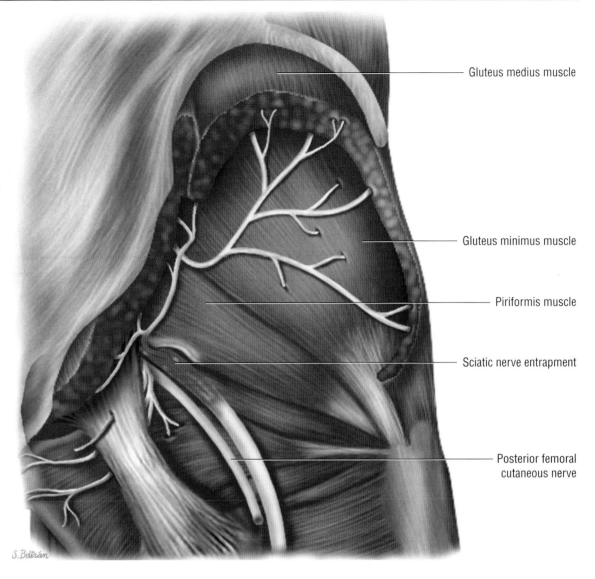

- Gluteus medius muscle
- Gluteus minimus muscle
- Piriformis muscle
- Sciatic nerve entrapment
- Posterior femoral cutaneous nerve

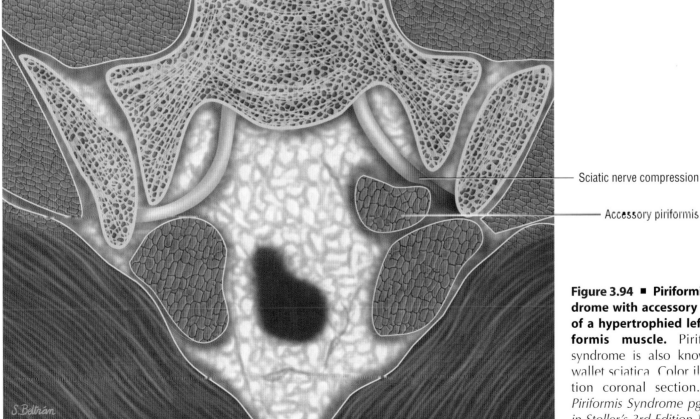

- Sciatic nerve compression
- Accessory piriformis

Figure 3.94 ■ **Piriformis syndrome with accessory fibers of a hypertrophied left piriformis muscle.** Piriformis syndrome is also known as wallet sciatica. Color illustration coronal section. *(See Piriformis Syndrome pg. 202, in Stoller's 3rd Edition.)*

Figure 3.95 ▪ **Distention and communication of the iliopsoas bursa with the hip joint.** Transverse section color illustration. *(See Iliopsoas Bursitis pg. 203, in Stoller's 3rd Edition.)*

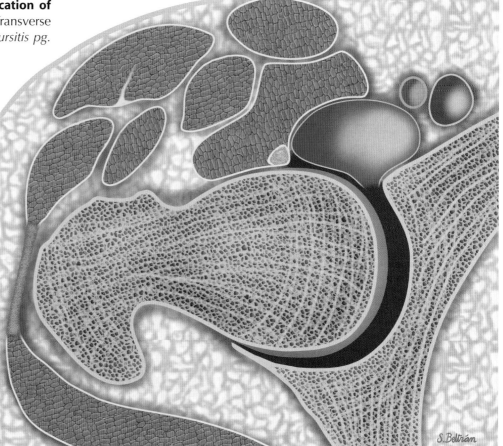

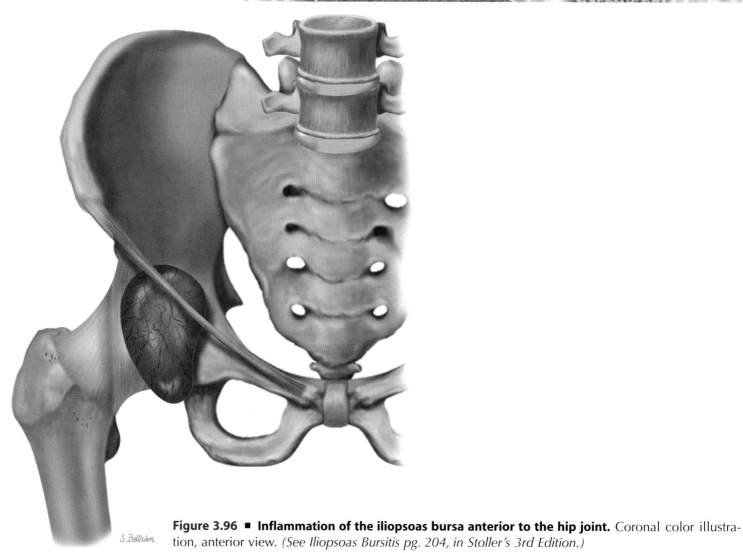

Figure 3.96 ▪ **Inflammation of the iliopsoas bursa anterior to the hip joint.** Coronal color illustration, anterior view. *(See Iliopsoas Bursitis pg. 204, in Stoller's 3rd Edition.)*

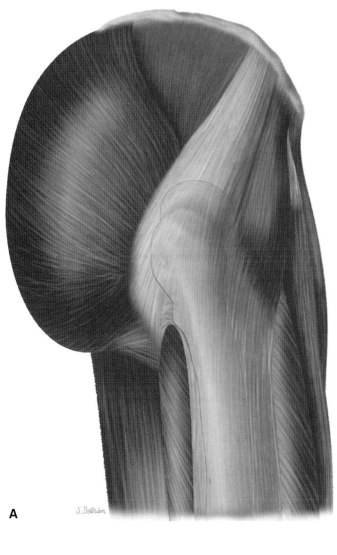

A

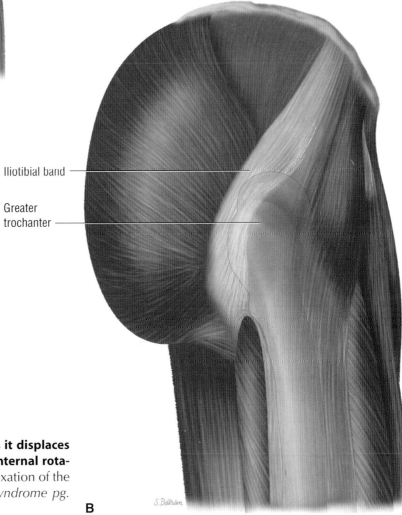

Iliotibial band

Greater
trochanter

B

**Figure 3.97 ■ Snapping of the iliotibial band occurs as it displaces
or subluxes posteriorly over the greater trochanter in internal rotation. (A)** The iliotibial band in a neutral position. **(B)** Subluxation of the
iliotibial band in internal rotation. *(See Snapping Hip Syndrome pg.
205, in Stoller's 3rd Edition.)*

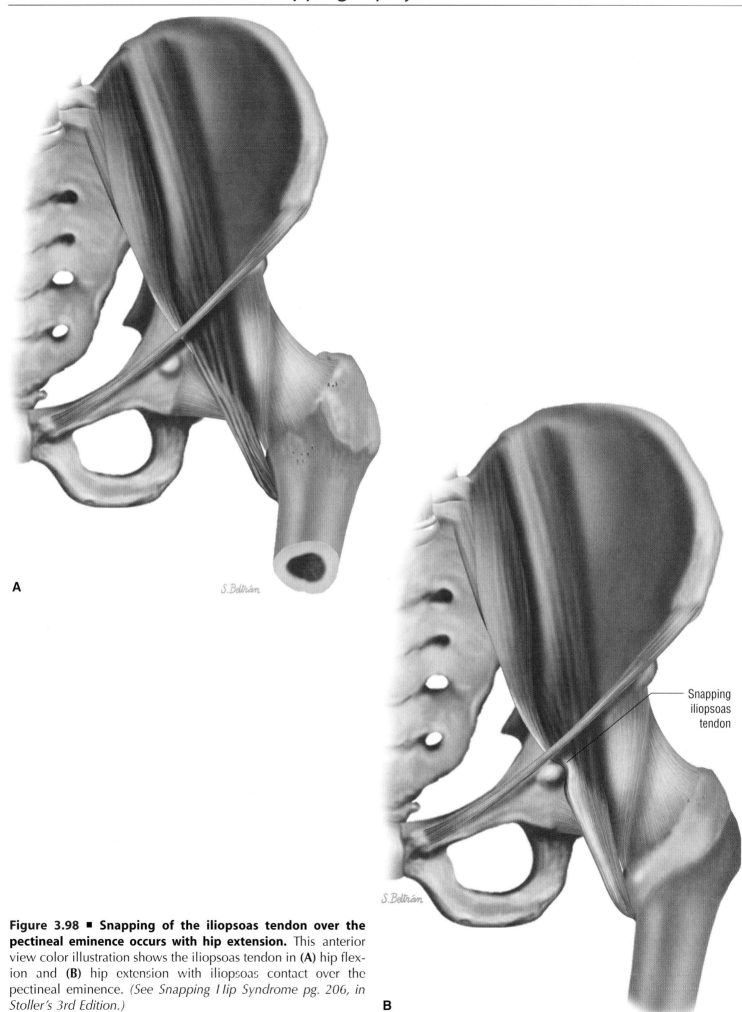

A

B

Snapping
iliopsoas
tendon

Figure 3.98 ▪ Snapping of the iliopsoas tendon over the pectineal eminence occurs with hip extension. This anterior view color illustration shows the iliopsoas tendon in **(A)** hip flexion and **(B)** hip extension with iliopsoas contact over the pectineal eminence. *(See Snapping Hip Syndrome pg. 206, in Stoller's 3rd Edition.)*

Figure 3.99 ■ Proximity of the iliopsoas (iliopectineal) eminence to the iliopsoas bursa. *(See Snapping Hip Syndrome pg. 206, in Stoller's 3rd Edition.)*

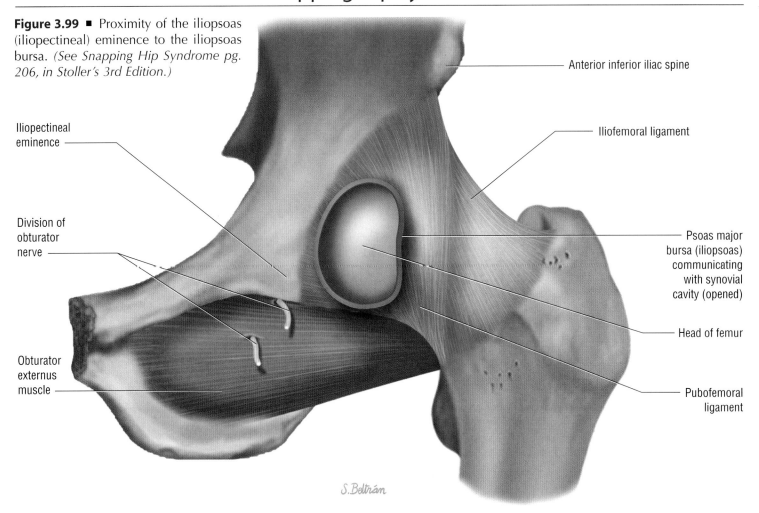

Iliopectineal eminence

Division of obturator nerve

Obturator externus muscle

Anterior inferior iliac spine

Iliofemoral ligament

Psoas major bursa (iliopsoas) communicating with synovial cavity (opened)

Head of femur

Pubofemoral ligament

S.Beltrán

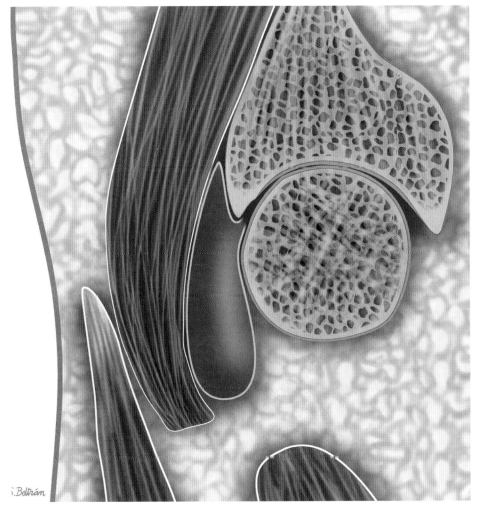

i.Beltrán

Figure 3.100 ■ Sagittal color illustration showing longitudinal extension of iliopsoas bursal fluid deep to the muscle and muscle-tendon-unit (MTU) as a cause of snapping hip syndrome. *(See Snapping Hip Syndrome pgs. 206 and 208, in Stoller's 3rd Edition.)*

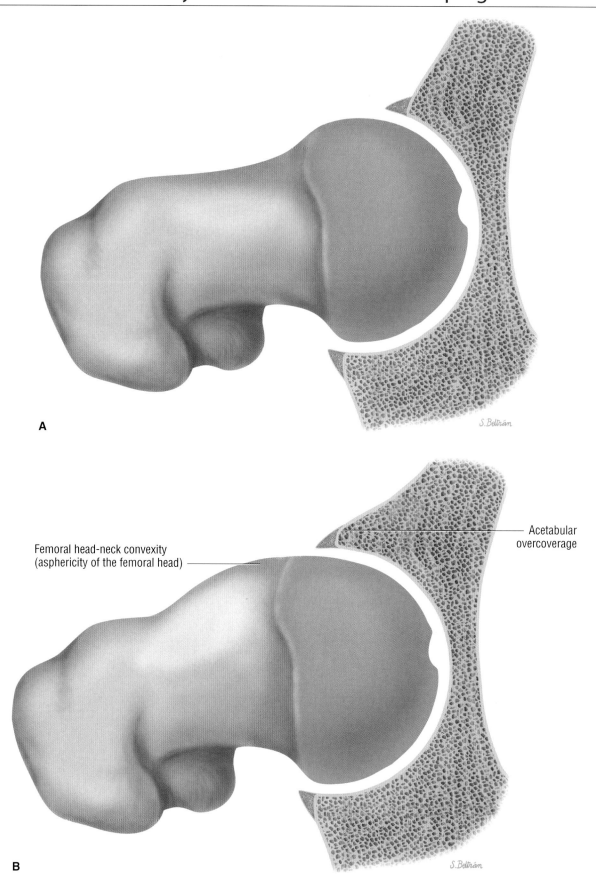

A

Femoral head-neck convexity
(asphericity of the femoral head)

Acetabular
overcoverage

B

Figure 3.101 ■ **(A)** Normal morphology of the femur and acetabulum with normal clearance of the hip. **(B)** Combination of reduced head-neck offset (cam mechanism) and excessive anterior overcoverage (pincer mechanism). Mixed cam-pincer impingement is the most common mechanism of FAI, although cam findings usually predominate on MR studies. (See *Femoroacetabular Impingement pg. 210, in Stoller's 3rd Edition.*)

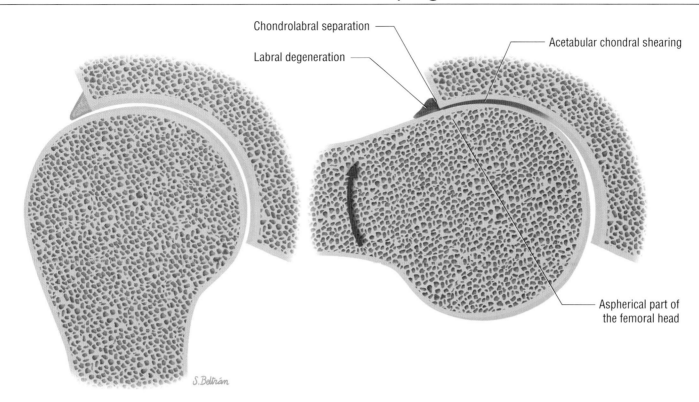

Chondrolabral separation

Labral degeneration

Acetabular chondral shearing

Aspherical part of
the femoral head

S.Beltrán

Figure 3.102 ■ Cam impingement demonstrated from the sagittal perspective.
During flexion the dysplastic convex or aspherical portion of the femoral head is
jammed against the anterolateral acetabular roof. The acetabular articular cartilage is
sheared off, and there is chondrolabral separation. Internal rotation serves to further increase impingement. *(See Cam Impingement pgs. 210 and 211, in Stoller's 3rd Edition.)*

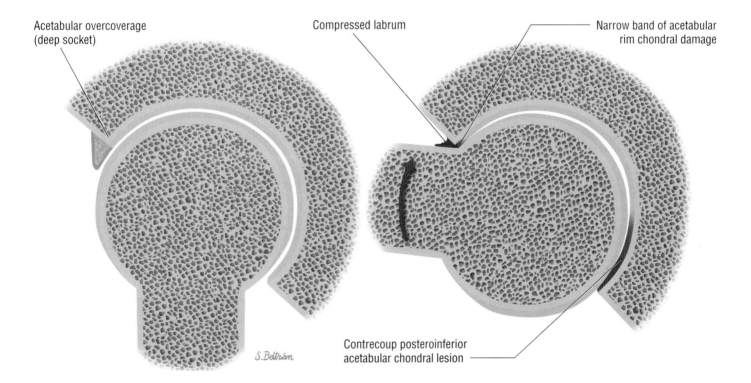

Acetabular overcoverage
(deep socket)

Compressed labrum

Narrow band of acetabular
rim chondral damage

Contrecoup posteroinferior
acetabular chondral lesion

S.Beltrán

Figure 3.103 ■ Pincer impingement from the sagittal perspective. During flexion,
the labrum is damaged because it functions as the buffer between the femoral neck
and the acetabulum, which has excessive anterior coverage. A contrecoup posteroinferior acetabular chondral lesion results as the femoral head subluxes posteriorly, creating increased pressure between the posteromedial femoral head and posteroinferior
acetabulum. *(See Pincer Impingement pgs. 212 and 214, in Stoller's 3rd Edition.)*

Figure 3.104 ■ Reduced femoral head-neck offset with dysplastic convex femoral bump. *(See Cam Impingement pgs. 211 and 212, in Stoller's 3rd Edition.)*

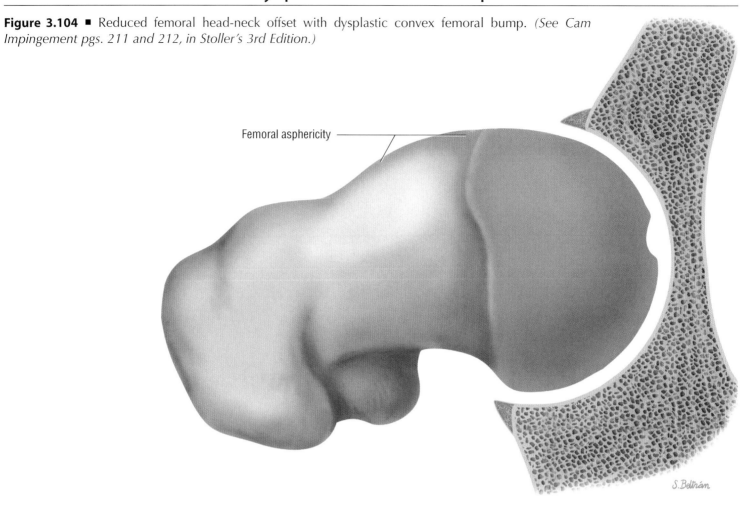

Femoral asphericity

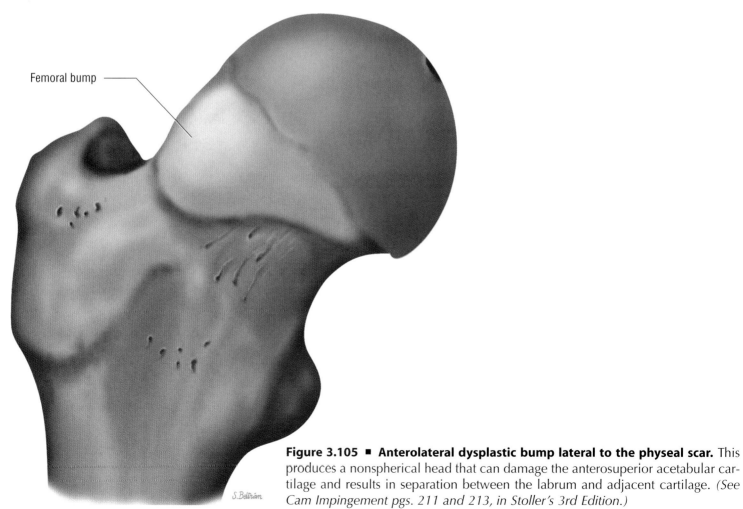

Femoral bump

Figure 3.105 ■ **Anterolateral dysplastic bump lateral to the physeal scar.** This produces a nonspherical head that can damage the anterosuperior acetabular cartilage and results in separation between the labrum and adjacent cartilage. *(See Cam Impingement pgs. 211 and 213, in Stoller's 3rd Edition.)*

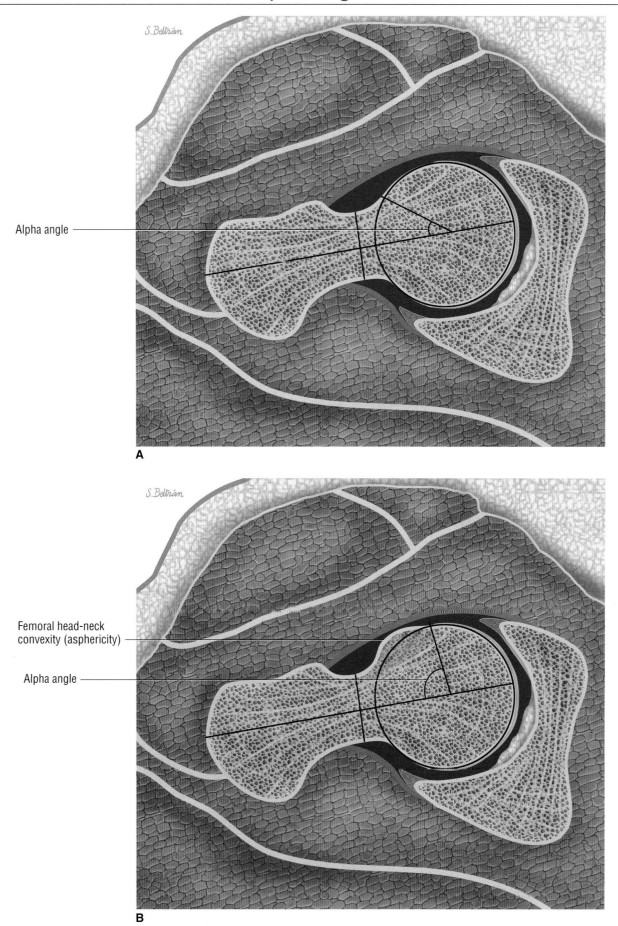

Figure 3.106 ■ **(A)** Normal alpha angle used to evaluate the femoral head-neck junction in a spherical femoral head. **(B)** Increased alpha angle in a nonspherical femoral head with a dysplastic femoral bump *(See Cam Impingement pg. 214, in Stoller's 3rd Edition.)*

Femoral Bump Resection Osteoplasty

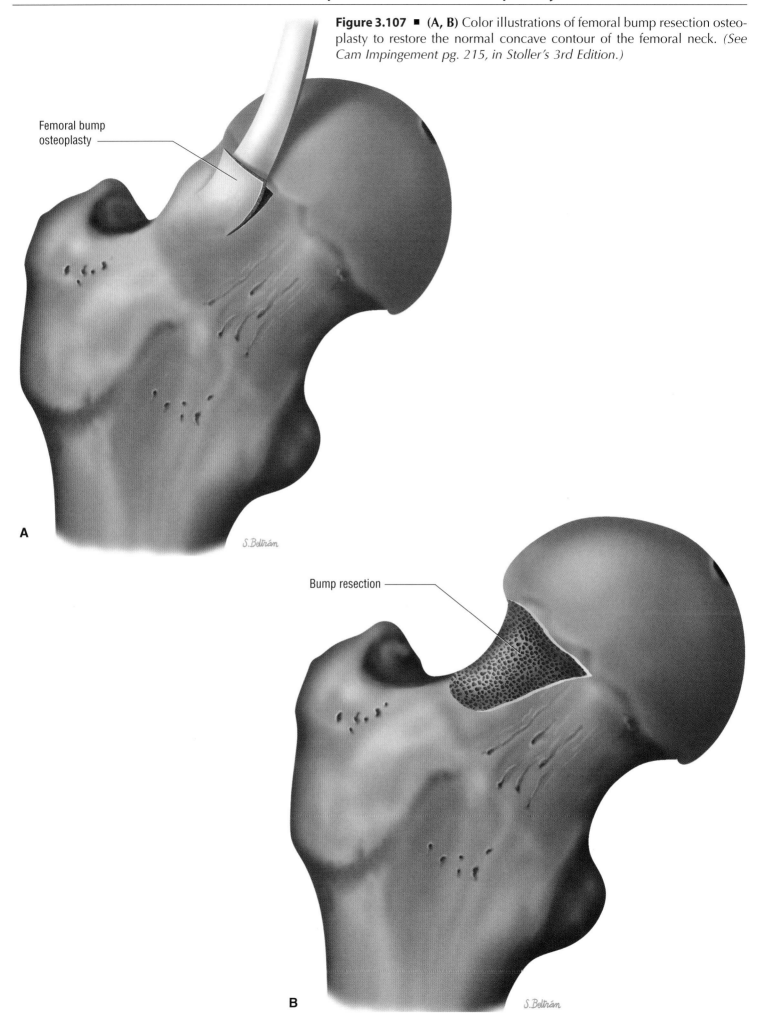

Figure 3.107 ▪ **(A, B)** Color illustrations of femoral bump resection osteoplasty to restore the normal concave contour of the femoral neck. *(See Cam Impingement pg. 215, in Stoller's 3rd Edition.)*

Femoral bump osteoplasty

A

S.Beltrán

Bump resection

B

S.Beltrán

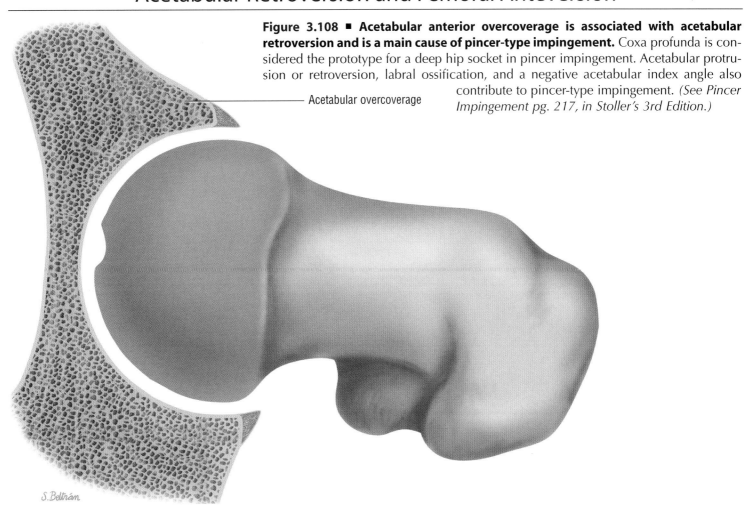

Figure 3.108 ■ **Acetabular anterior overcoverage is associated with acetabular retroversion and is a main cause of pincer-type impingement.** Coxa profunda is considered the prototype for a deep hip socket in pincer impingement. Acetabular protrusion or retroversion, labral ossification, and a negative acetabular index angle also contribute to pincer-type impingement. *(See Pincer Impingement pg. 217, in Stoller's 3rd Edition.)*

Acetabular overcoverage

S.Beltrán

Figure 3.109 ■ **Femoral anteversion of the femoral neck with the knee directed anteriorly.** Femoral anteversion and retroversion (which are associated with toeing in or toeing out) are separate from, and should not be confused with, acetabular anteversion and retroversion. *(See Pincer Impingement pg. 217, in Stoller's 3rd Edition.)*

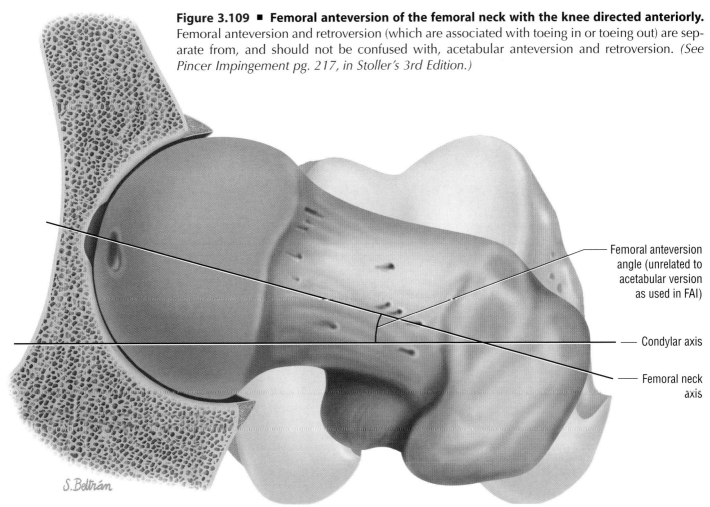

Femoral anteversion angle (unrelated to acetabular version as used in FAI)

Condylar axis

Femoral neck axis

S.Beltrán

Figure 3.110 ■ **(A)** Cross section showing normal acetabular anteversion. **(B)** Retroversion of the normal acetabulum effectively results in anterior overcoverage as the anterior lip extends more laterally compared with normal. *(See Pincer Impingement pg. 217, in Stoller's 3rd Edition.)*

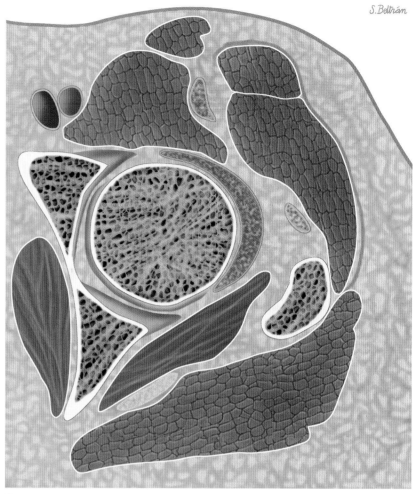

A

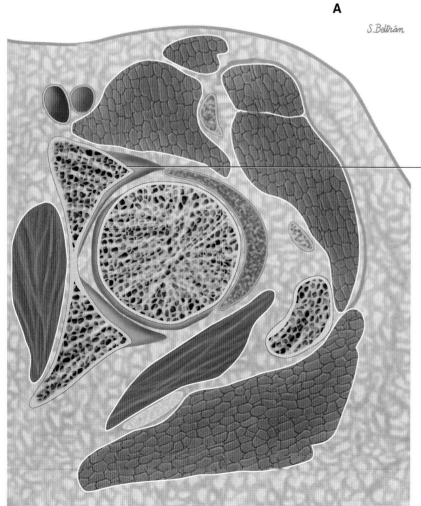

Lateral extension
of anterior lip in
acetabular retroversion

B

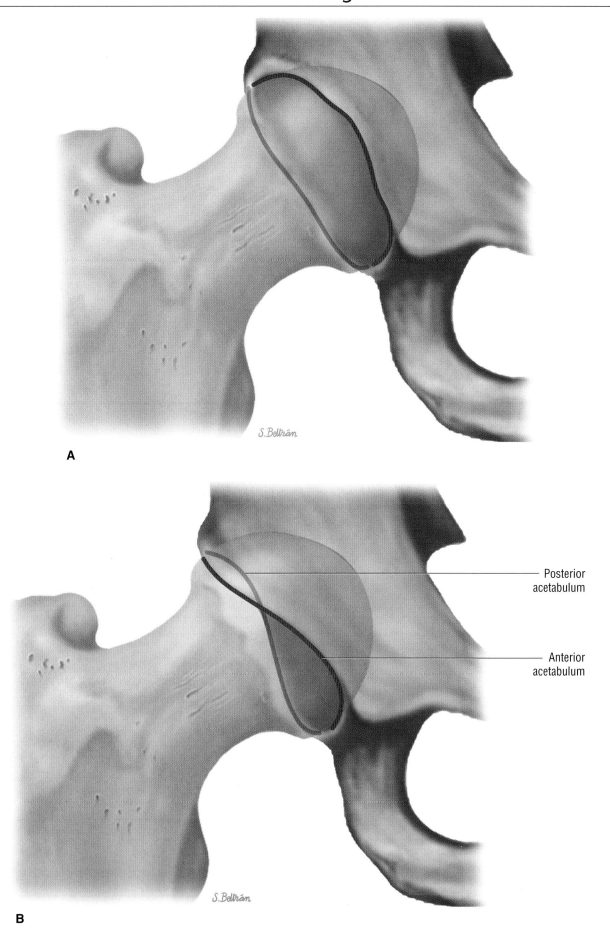

Figure 3.111 ▪ Crossover sign in acetabular retroversion. (A) The normal acetabulum. **(B)** The crossover sign in which the anterior rim crosses over the posterior acetabular rim (transparent red line) *(See Pincer Impingement pg. 218, in Stoller's 3rd Edition.)*

Cam Impingement

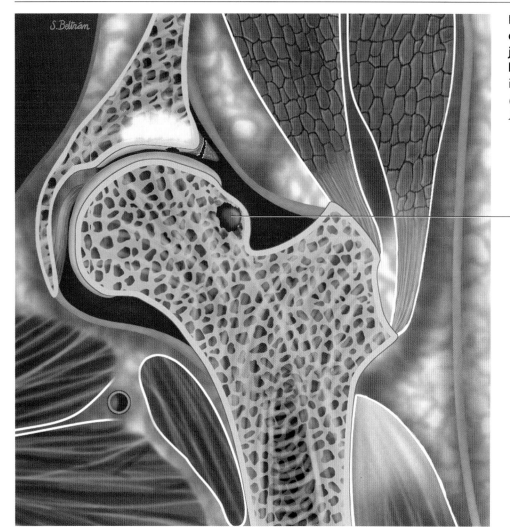

Figure 3.112 ■ Cam impingement with dysplastic (aspherical) femoral head-neck junction and fibrocystic change located lateral to the physeal scar. Coronal color illustration of femoral bump-cyst complex. *(See Femoroacetabular Impingement pg. 219, in Stoller's 3rd Edition.)*

Femoral bump-cyst complex

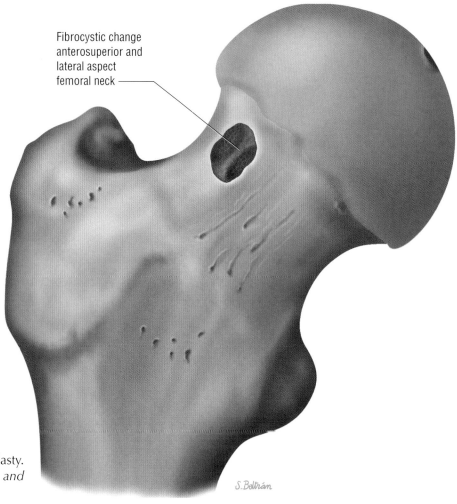

Fibrocystic change anterosuperior and lateral aspect femoral neck

Figure 3.113 ■ Femoral cyst after bump osteoplasty. *(See Femoroacetabular Impingement pgs. 221 and 222, in Stoller's 3rd Edition.)*

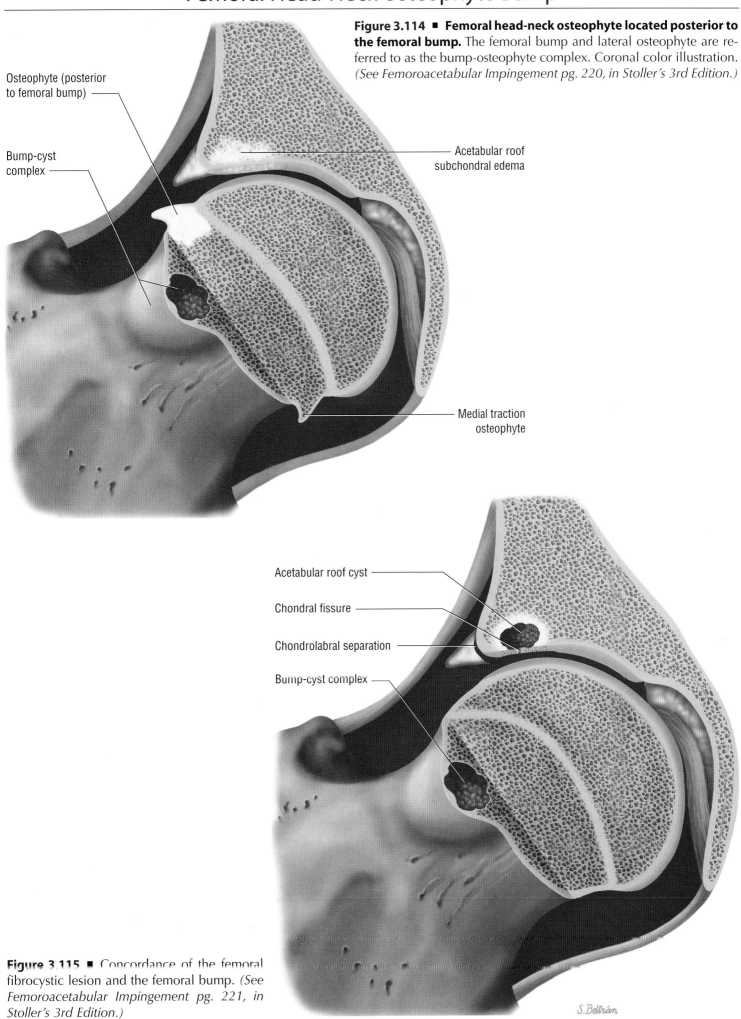

Osteophyte (posterior to femoral bump)

Bump-cyst complex

Figure 3.114 ▪ Femoral head-neck osteophyte located posterior to the femoral bump. The femoral bump and lateral osteophyte are referred to as the bump-osteophyte complex. Coronal color illustration. *(See Femoroacetabular Impingement pg. 220, in Stoller's 3rd Edition.)*

Acetabular roof subchondral edema

Medial traction osteophyte

Acetabular roof cyst

Chondral fissure

Chondrolabral separation

Bump-cyst complex

Figure 3.115 ▪ Concordance of the femoral fibrocystic lesion and the femoral bump. *(See Femoroacetabular Impingement pg. 221, in Stoller's 3rd Edition.)*

S. Beltrán

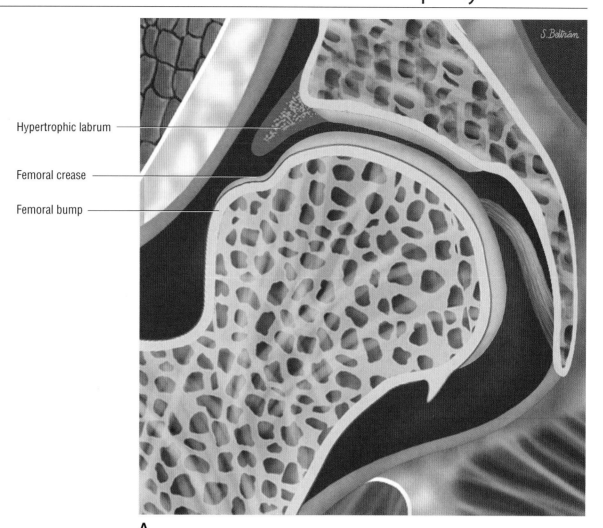

Hypertrophic labrum

Femoral crease

Femoral bump

A

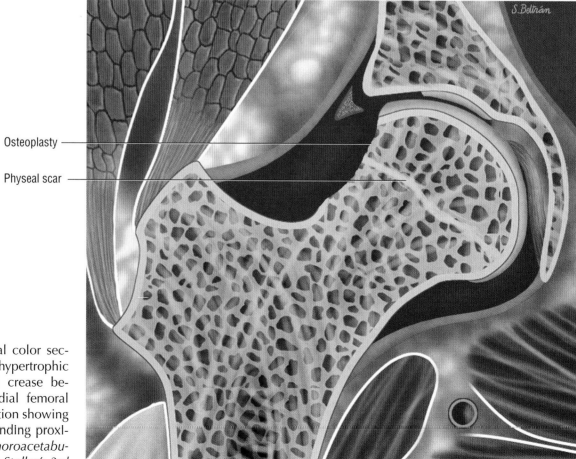

Osteoplasty

Physeal scar

Figure 3.116 ■ **(A)** Coronal color section depicting DDH with hypertrophic labrum and femoral head crease between the bump and medial femoral head. **(B)** Coronal color section showing resection of the bump extending proximal to the physis. *(See Femoroacetabular Impingement pg. 224, in Stoller's 3rd Edition.)*

B

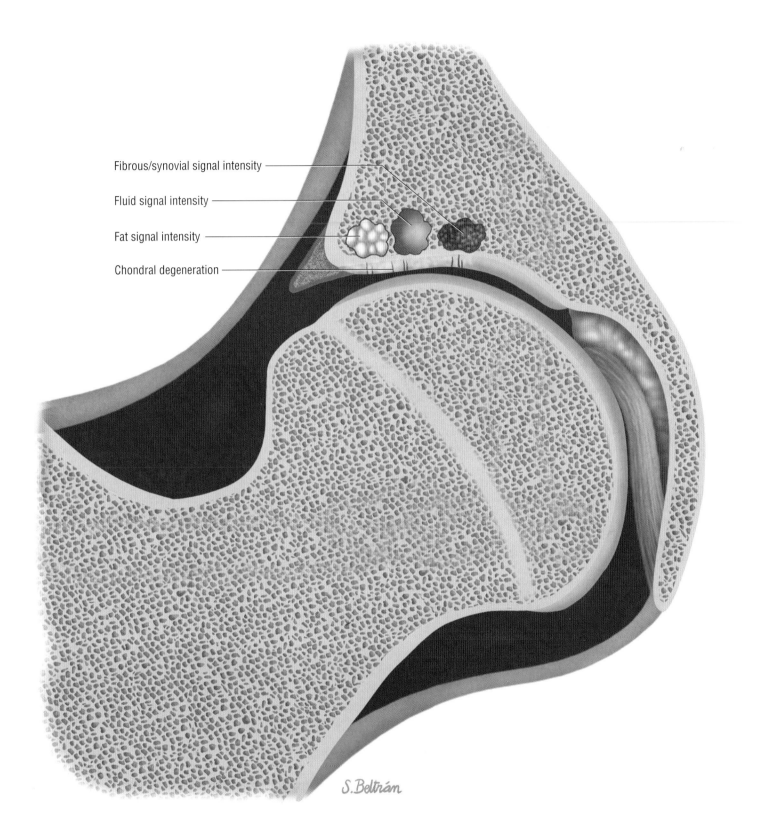

Fibrous/synovial signal intensity

Fluid signal intensity

Fat signal intensity

Chondral degeneration

S. Beltrán

Figure 3.117 ▪ Coronal section depicting types of acetabular roof cysts seen in FAI. Fat signal intensity represents a quiescent stage indicative of reparative maturation of the cyst. Fluid or fibrous/synovial signal intensity is associated with ongoing symptoms of hip pain. *(See Femoroacetabular Impingement pg. 229, in Stoller's 3rd Edition.)*

Acetabular Chondral Lesions

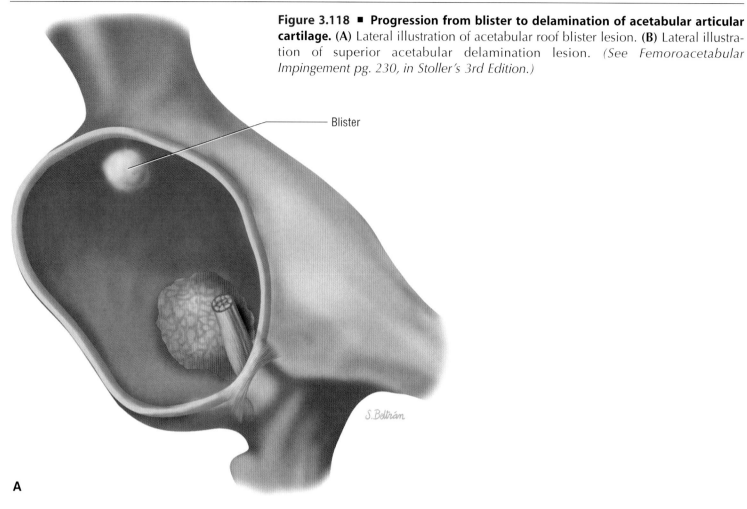

Figure 3.118 ■ Progression from blister to delamination of acetabular articular cartilage. (A) Lateral illustration of acetabular roof blister lesion. **(B)** Lateral illustration of superior acetabular delamination lesion. *(See Femoroacetabular Impingement pg. 230, in Stoller's 3rd Edition.)*

Blister

A

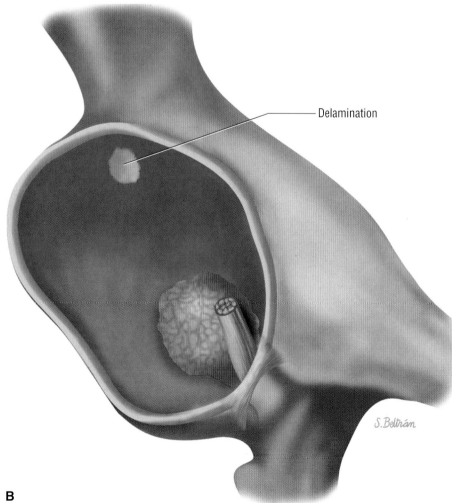

Delamination

B

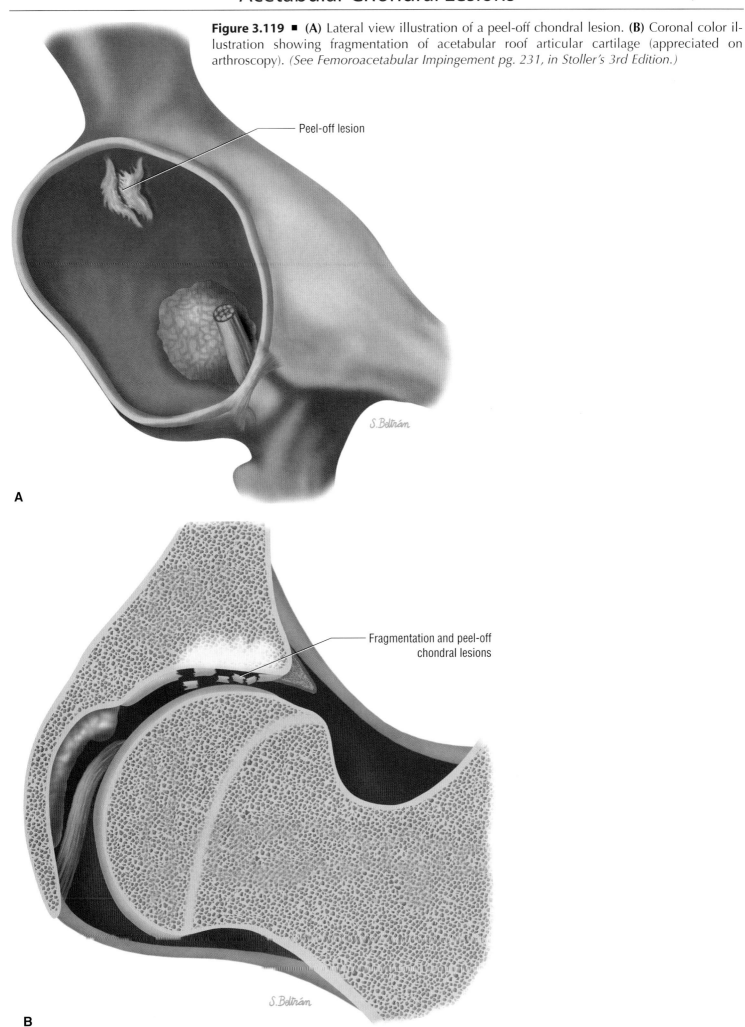

Figure 3.119 ■ **(A)** Lateral view illustration of a peel-off chondral lesion. **(B)** Coronal color illustration showing fragmentation of acetabular roof articular cartilage (appreciated on arthroscopy). *(See Femoroacetabular Impingement pg. 231, in Stoller's 3rd Edition.)*

Peel-off lesion

Fragmentation and peel-off chondral lesions

A

B

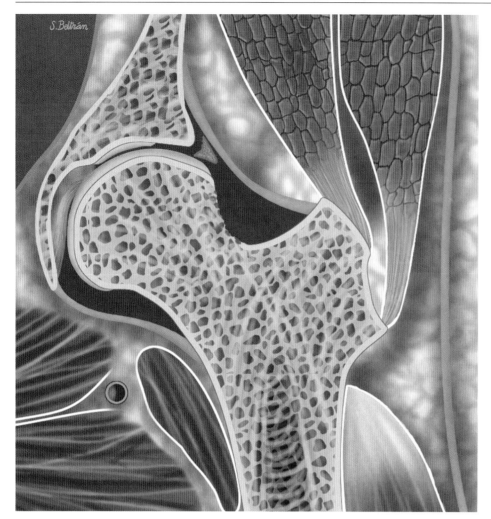

Figure 3.120 ■ Postresection osteoplasty of the acetabular bump. *(See Femoroacetabular Impingement pg. 232, in Stoller's 3rd Edition.)*

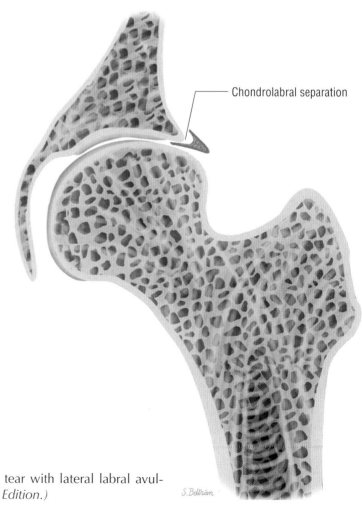

Chondrolabral separation

Figure 3.121 ■ Coronal color section of persistent chondrolabral tear with lateral labral avulsion. *(See Femoroacetabular Impingement pg. 233, in Stoller's 3rd Edition.)*

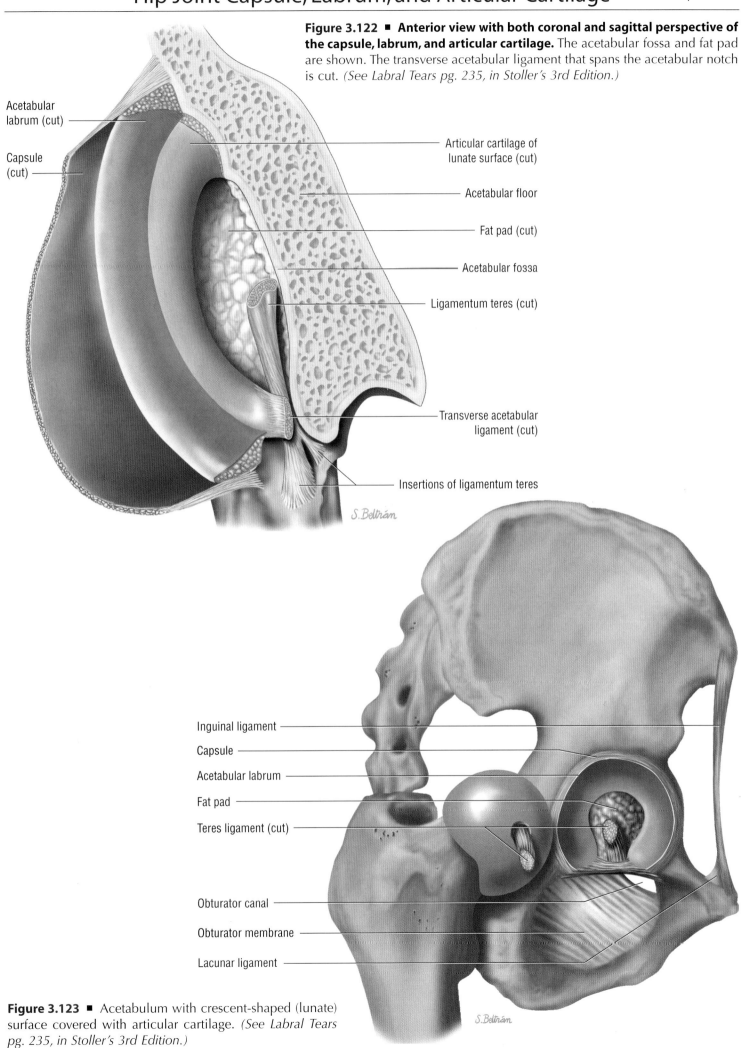

Figure 3.122 ■ **Anterior view with both coronal and sagittal perspective of the capsule, labrum, and articular cartilage.** The acetabular fossa and fat pad are shown. The transverse acetabular ligament that spans the acetabular notch is cut. (*See Labral Tears pg. 235, in Stoller's 3rd Edition.*)

Acetabular labrum (cut)

Capsule (cut)

Articular cartilage of lunate surface (cut)

Acetabular floor

Fat pad (cut)

Acetabular fossa

Ligamentum teres (cut)

Transverse acetabular ligament (cut)

Insertions of ligamentum teres

Inguinal ligament

Capsule

Acetabular labrum

Fat pad

Teres ligament (cut)

Obturator canal

Obturator membrane

Lacunar ligament

Figure 3.123 ■ Acetabulum with crescent-shaped (lunate) surface covered with articular cartilage. (*See Labral Tears pg. 235, in Stoller's 3rd Edition.*)

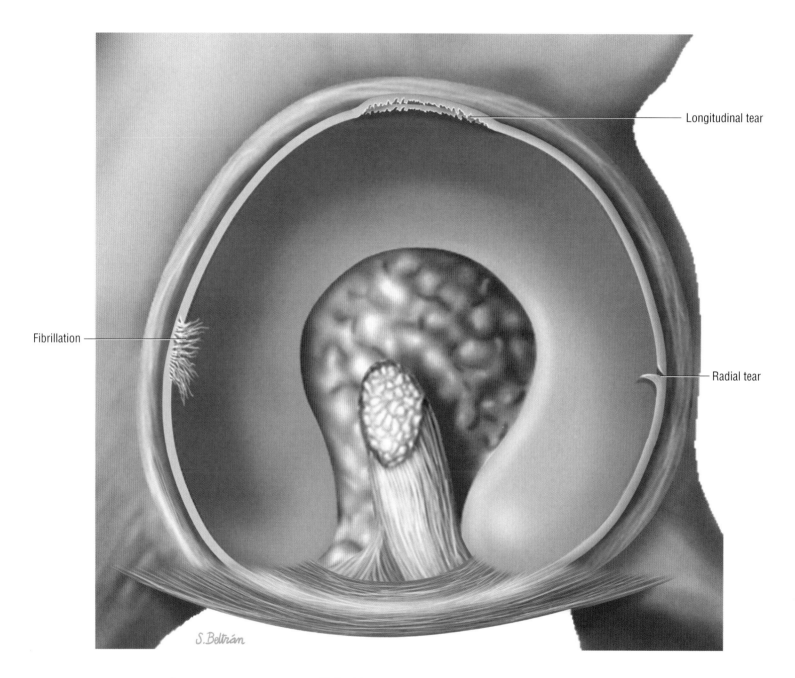

Figure 3.124 ■ Spectrum of labral lesions with fibrillation and radial and longitudinal morphology. *(See Labral Tears pg. 236, in Stoller's 3rd Edition.)*

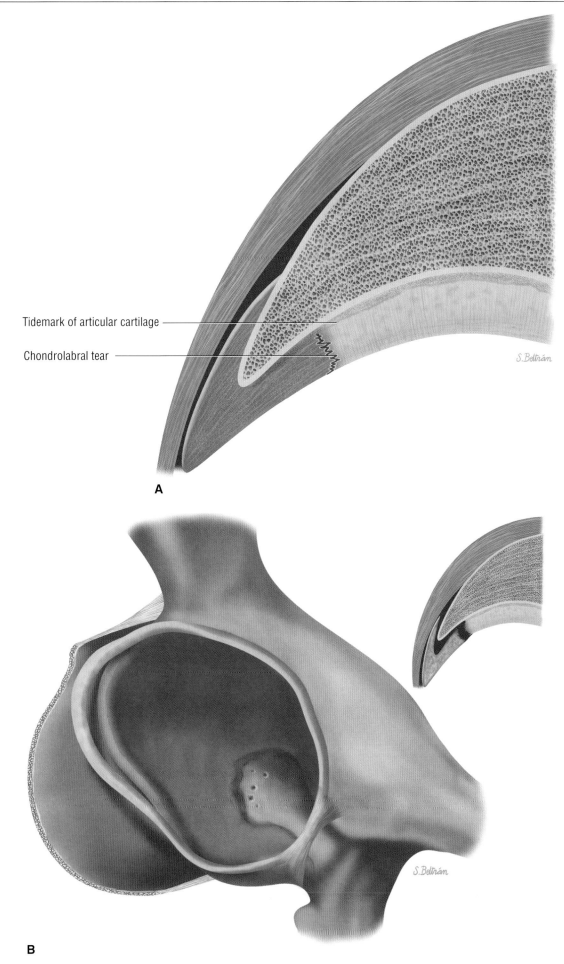

Tidemark of articular cartilage

Chondrolabral tear

A

B

Figure 3.125 ■ **(A)** Chondrolabral tear perpendicular to the long axis of the labrum. Coronal color section. **(B)** Progression of chondral labral tear to separation. Coronal color section. *(See Labral Tears pg. 239, in Stoller's 3rd Edition.)*

Labral Cleavage Tear

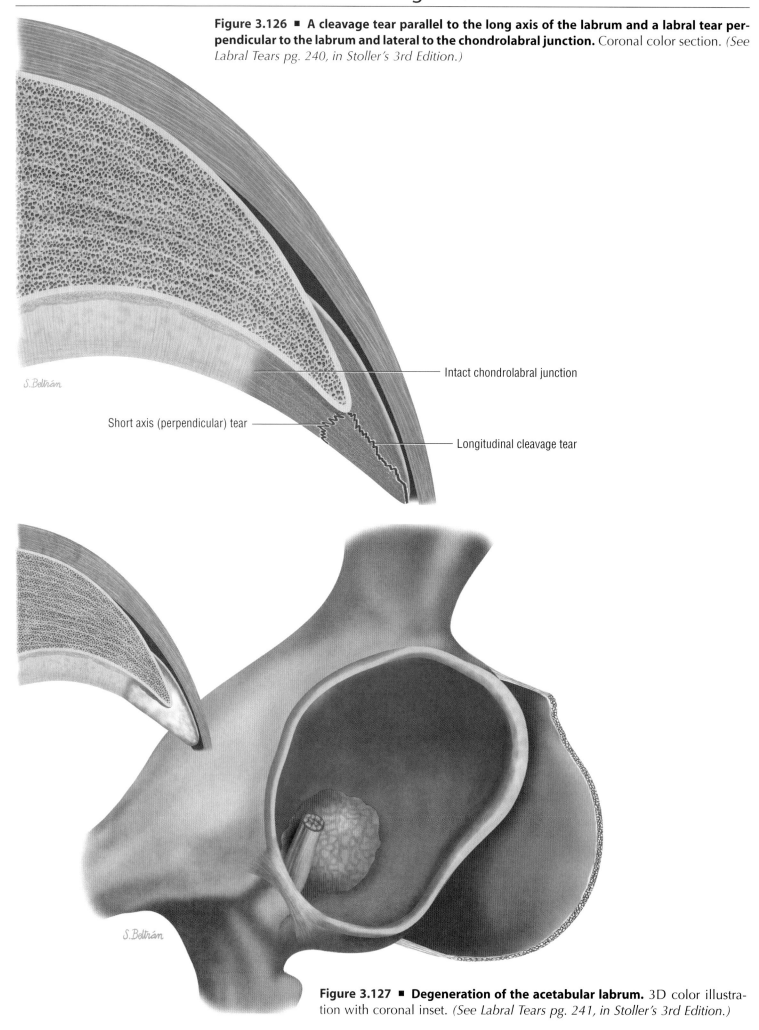

Figure 3.126 ■ **A cleavage tear parallel to the long axis of the labrum and a labral tear perpendicular to the labrum and lateral to the chondrolabral junction.** Coronal color section. *(See Labral Tears pg. 240, in Stoller's 3rd Edition.)*

Intact chondrolabral junction

Short axis (perpendicular) tear

Longitudinal cleavage tear

S.Beltrán

Figure 3.127 ■ **Degeneration of the acetabular labrum.** 3D color illustration with coronal inset. *(See Labral Tears pg. 241, in Stoller's 3rd Edition.)*

Figure 3.128 ■ Anterior labral tear on lateral color illustration. *(See Labral Tears pg. 243, in Stoller's 3rd Edition.)*

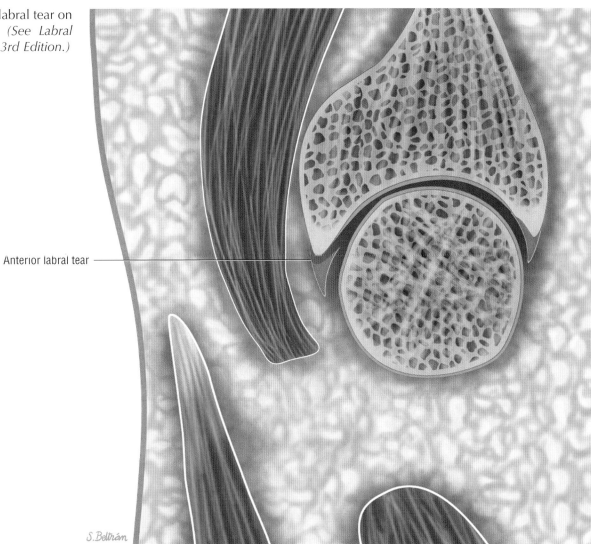

Anterior labral tear

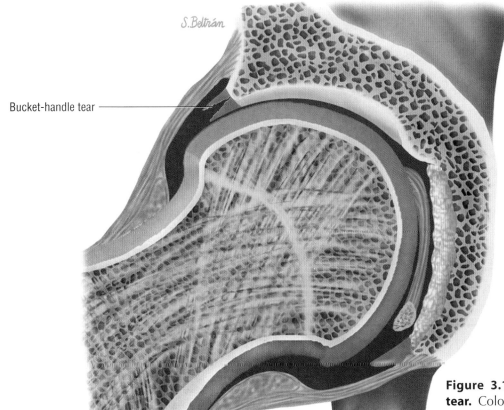

Bucket-handle tear

Figure 3.129 ■ **Bucket-handle acetabular labral tear.** Color coronal section showing a longitudinal tear of the lateral labrum. *(See Labral Tears pg. 246, in Stoller's 3rd Edition.)*

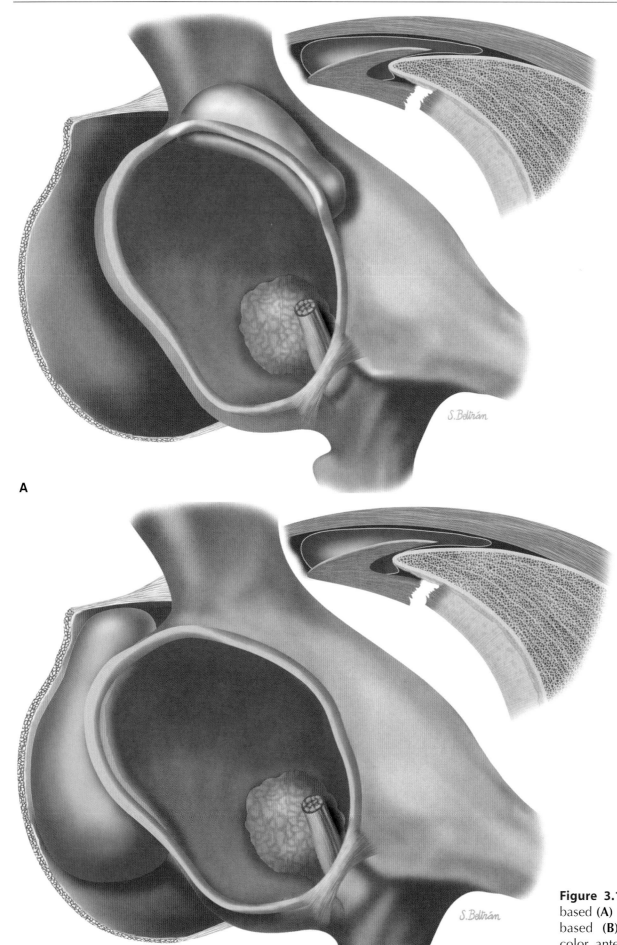

A

B

Figure 3.130 ▪ Anterosuperior-based **(A)** versus posterosuperior-based **(B)** paralabral cysts on color anterolateral views of the acetabular fossa and labrum. *(See Paralabral Cysts pgs. 242 and 247, in Stoller's 3rd Edition.)*

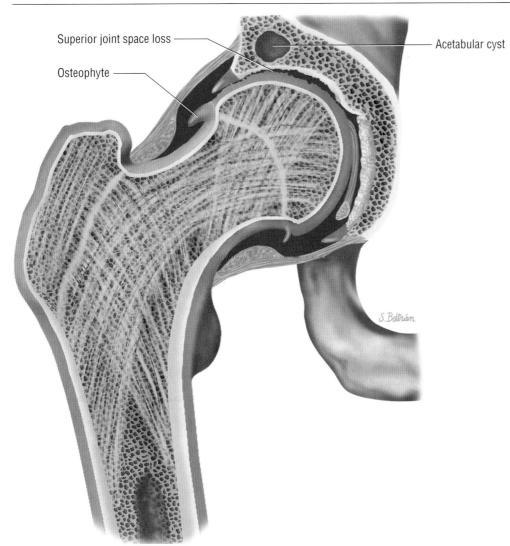

Superior joint space loss

Osteophyte

Acetabular cyst

Figure 3.131 ▪ **Advanced osteoarthritis (OA) with osteophytosis, joint space narrowing, and denuded chondral surfaces.** Coronal color illustration of OA. *(See Osteoarthritis pg. 253, in Stoller's 3rd Edition.)*

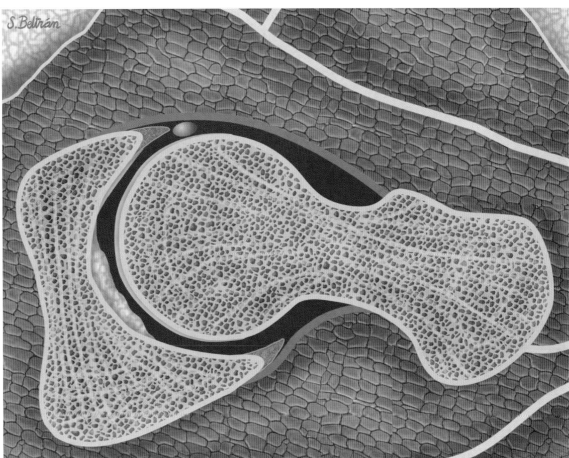

Figure 3.132 ▪ Color axial section showing anterior capsule loose body. *(See Loose Bodies pgs. 252 and 256, in Stoller's 3rd Edition.)*

Chondral Lesion and Loose Bodies

Figure 3.133 ■ Chondral flap lesion of the femoral head (FH). *(See Loose Bodies pgs. 252 and 257, in Stoller's 3rd Edition.)*

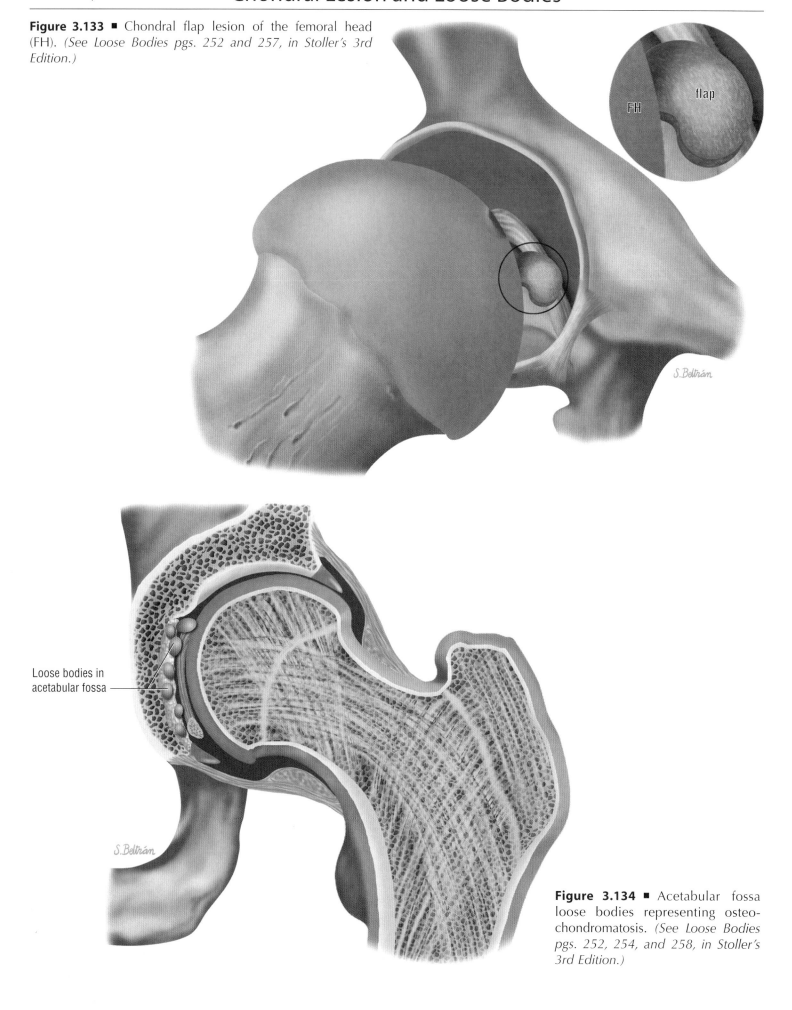

Loose bodies in acetabular fossa

Figure 3.134 ■ Acetabular fossa loose bodies representing osteochondromatosis. *(See Loose Bodies pgs. 252, 254, and 258, in Stoller's 3rd Edition.)*

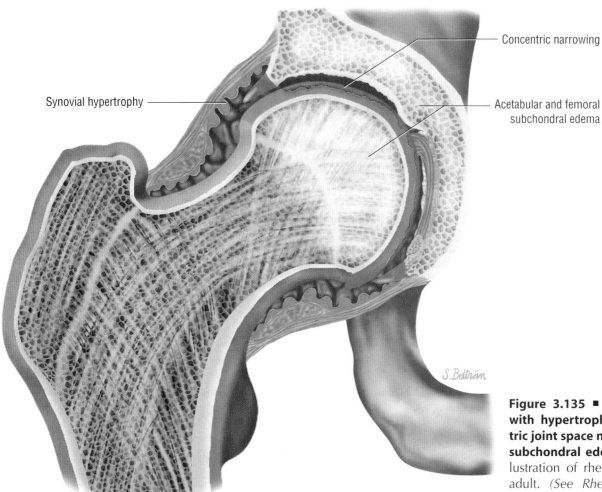

Synovial hypertrophy

Concentric narrowing

Acetabular and femoral subchondral edema

Figure 3.135 ■ **Rheumatoid arthritis with hypertrophic synovium, concentric joint space narrowing, and reactive subchondral edema.** Coronal color illustration of rheumatoid arthritis in an adult. *(See Rheumatoid Arthritis pgs. 255 and 259, in Stoller's 3rd Edition.)*

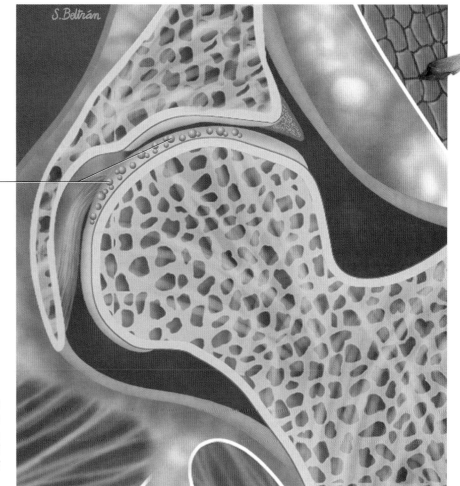

CPPD crystal deposition

Figure 3.136 ■ **CPPD crystal deposition disease with hypointense crystal deposits throughout the chondral surfaces.** Color coronal section. *(See Calcium Pyrophosphate Dihydrate Crystal Deposition (CPPD) Disease pg. 262, in Stoller's 3rd Edition.)*

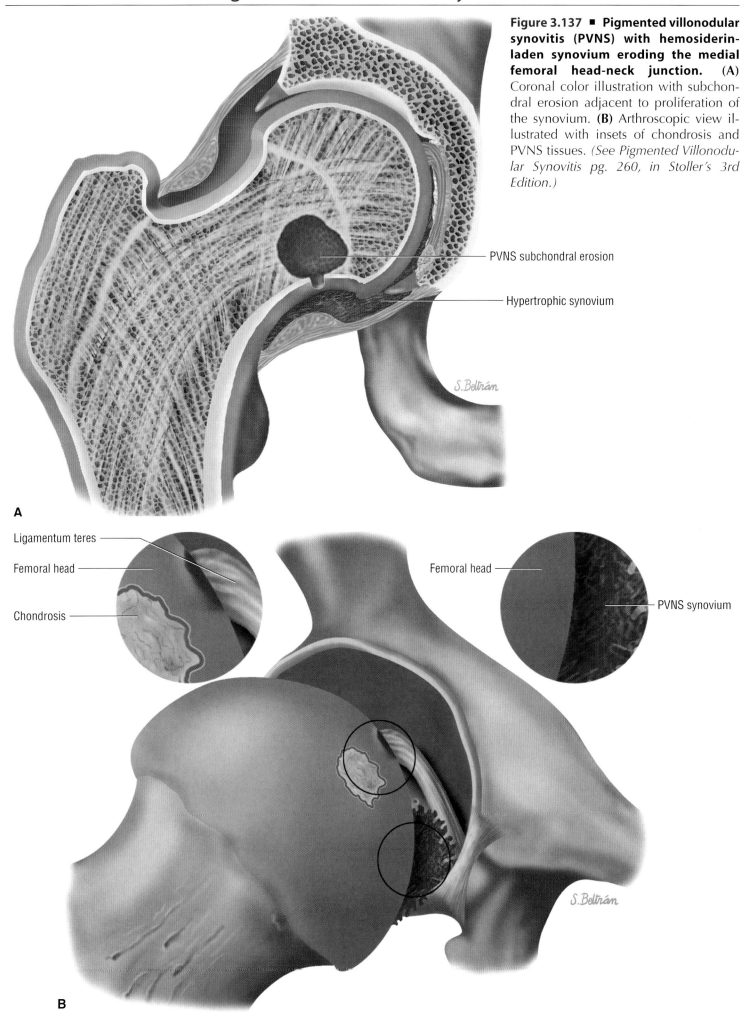

Figure 3.137 ▪ **Pigmented villonodular synovitis (PVNS) with hemosiderin-laden synovium eroding the medial femoral head-neck junction.** **(A)** Coronal color illustration with subchondral erosion adjacent to proliferation of the synovium. **(B)** Arthroscopic view illustrated with insets of chondrosis and PVNS tissues. *(See Pigmented Villonodular Synovitis pg. 260, in Stoller's 3rd Edition.)*

PVNS subchondral erosion

Hypertrophic synovium

A

Ligamentum teres

Femoral head

Chondrosis

Femoral head

PVNS synovium

B

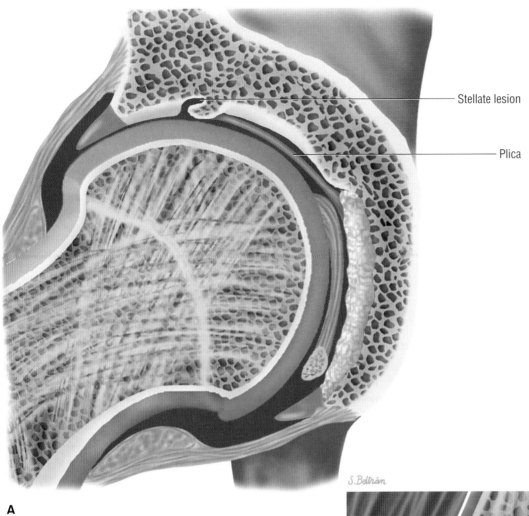

Stellate lesion

Plica

A

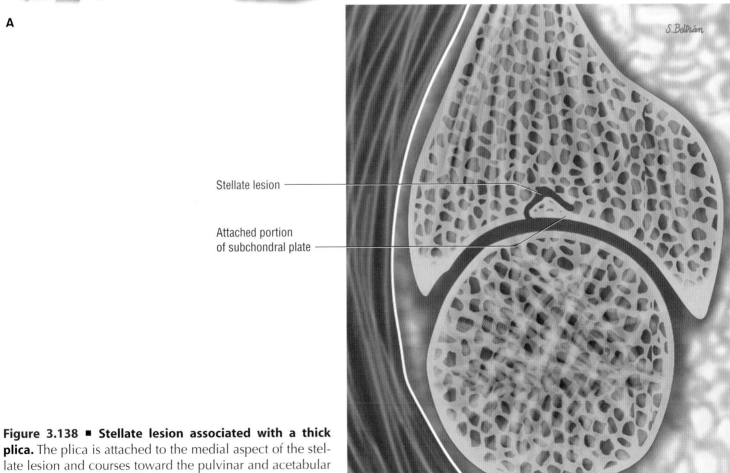

Stellate lesion

Attached portion
of subchondral plate

Figure 3.138 ■ Stellate lesion associated with a thick plica. The plica is attached to the medial aspect of the stellate lesion and courses toward the pulvinar and acetabular fossa. **(A)** Coronal color section. **(B)** Lateral color illustration. *(See Stellate Lesion and Plica pgs. 262, 263, and 264, in Stoller's 3rd Edition.)*

B

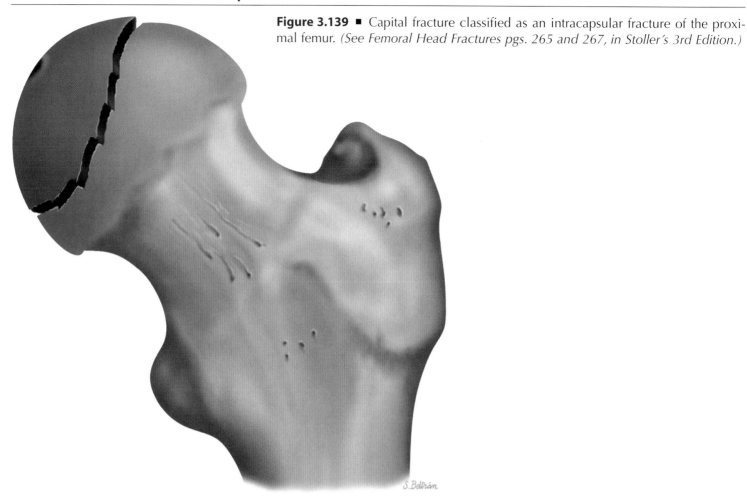

Figure 3.139 ■ Capital fracture classified as an intracapsular fracture of the proximal femur. *(See Femoral Head Fractures pgs. 265 and 267, in Stoller's 3rd Edition.)*

Figure 3.140 ■ **Subchondral stress fracture with subtle subarticular hypointense fracture line and edema that is most hyperintense adjacent to the involved subchondral trabecular microfracture.** Color coronal illustration. *(See Subchondral Femoral Head Fractures pgs. 267 and 268, in Stoller's 3rd Edition.)*

Subchondral fracture

Subchondral edema

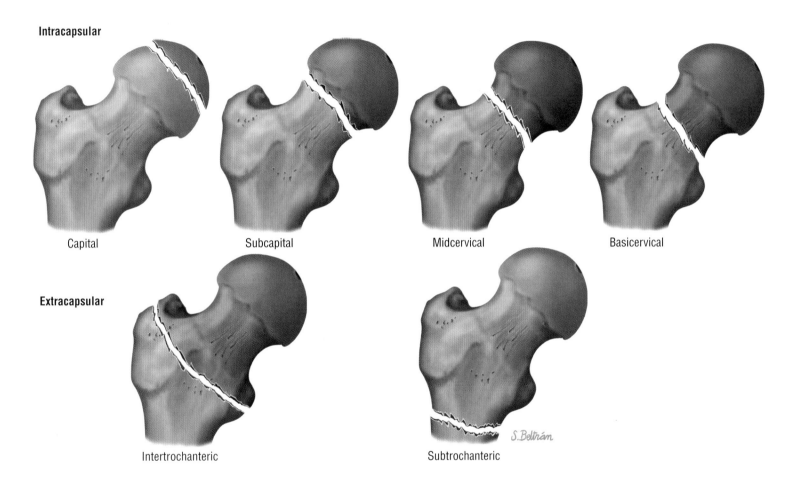

Intracapsular

Capital   Subcapital   Midcervical   Basicervical

Extracapsular

Intertrochanteric   Subtrochanteric

Figure 3.141 ■ **Fractures of the proximal femur are divided into intracapsular and extracapsular types.** Subcapital fractures are common intracapsular fractures; the capital, mid-, or transcervical and basicervical are uncommon. *(See Femoral Neck Fractures pgs. 268 and 270, in Stoller's 3rd Edition.)*

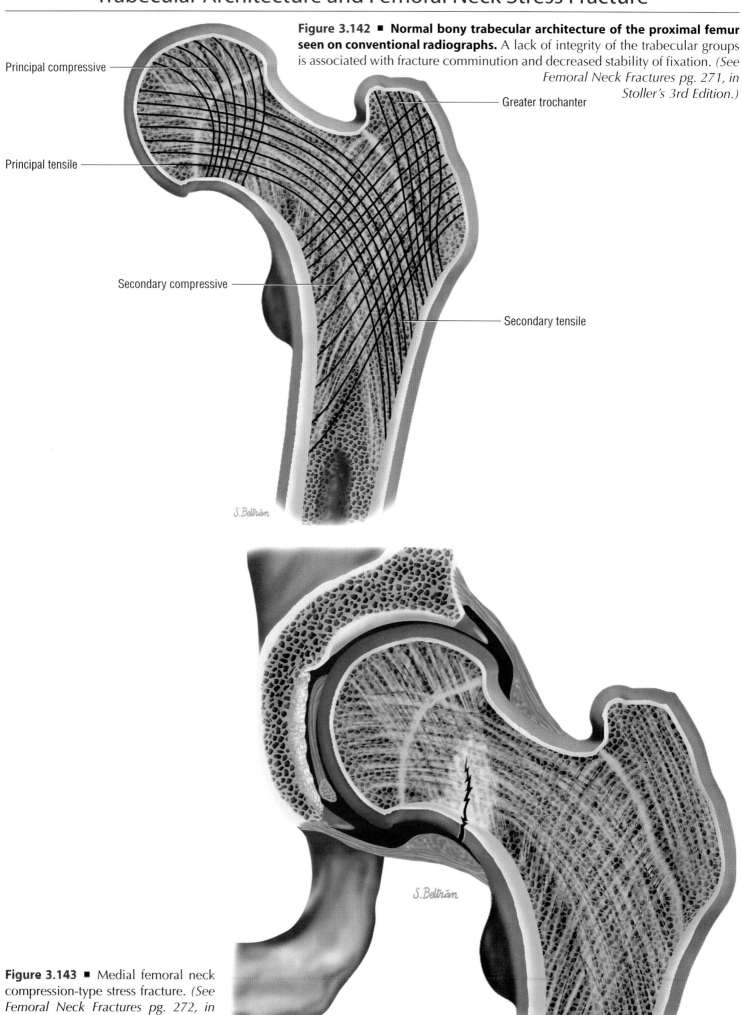

Principal compressive

Principal tensile

Secondary compressive

Figure 3.142 ■ **Normal bony trabecular architecture of the proximal femur seen on conventional radiographs.** A lack of integrity of the trabecular groups is associated with fracture comminution and decreased stability of fixation. *(See Femoral Neck Fractures pg. 271, in Stoller's 3rd Edition.)*

Greater trochanter

Secondary tensile

S. Beltrán

Figure 3.143 ■ Medial femoral neck compression-type stress fracture. *(See Femoral Neck Fractures pg. 272, in Stoller's 3rd Edition.)*

S. Beltrán

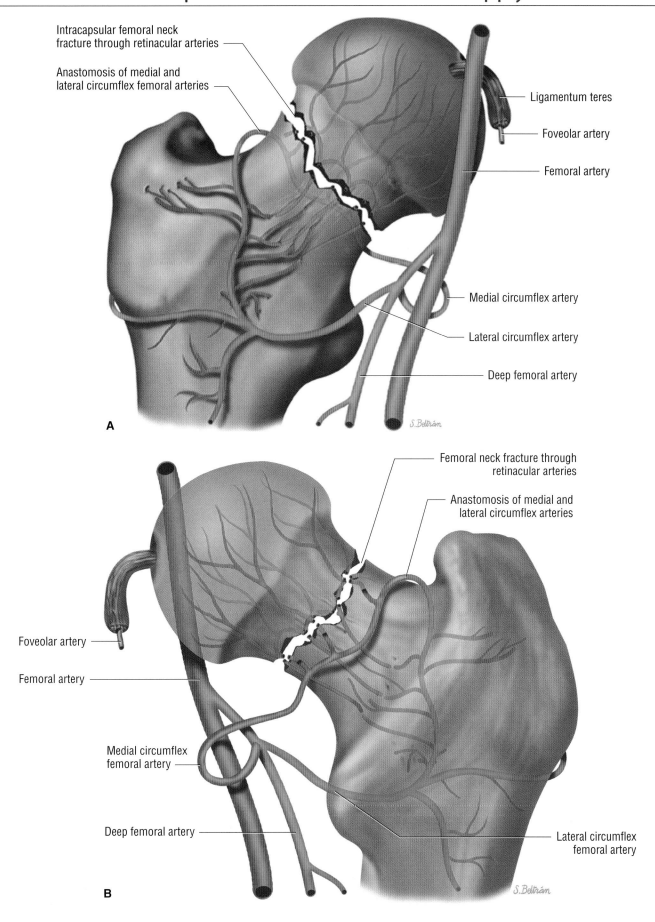

Figure 3.144 ■ **Vascular supply to the proximal femur with primary contribution from the circumflex femoral arteries.** AVN of the femoral head is associated with intracapsular fractures. The tenuous blood supply to the femoral head derives from branches of the medial femoral circumflex artery. **(A)** Anterior perspective. **(B)** Posterior perspective. *(See Femoral Neck Fractures pg. 273, in Stoller's 3rd Edition.)*

Femoral Neck Fracture

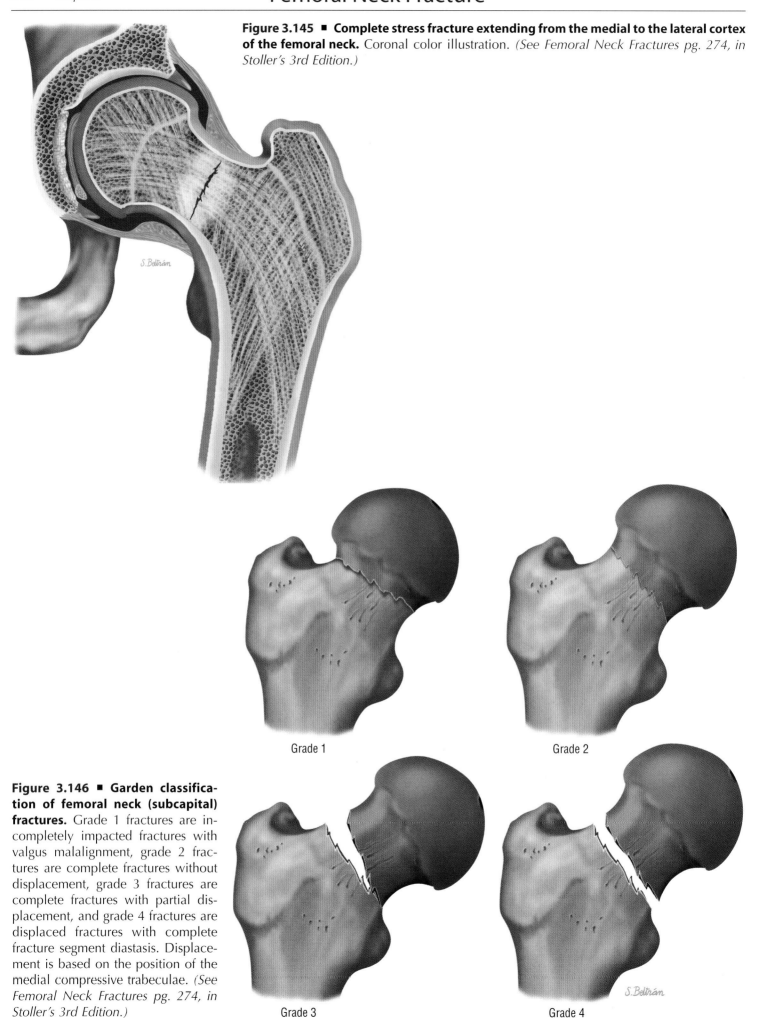

Figure 3.145 ▪ **Complete stress fracture extending from the medial to the lateral cortex of the femoral neck.** Coronal color illustration. *(See Femoral Neck Fractures pg. 274, in Stoller's 3rd Edition.)*

Figure 3.146 ▪ **Garden classification of femoral neck (subcapital) fractures.** Grade 1 fractures are incompletely impacted fractures with valgus malalignment, grade 2 fractures are complete fractures without displacement, grade 3 fractures are complete fractures with partial displacement, and grade 4 fractures are displaced fractures with complete fracture segment diastasis. Displacement is based on the position of the medial compressive trabeculae. *(See Femoral Neck Fractures pg. 274, in Stoller's 3rd Edition.)*

Grade 1

Grade 2

Grade 3

Grade 4

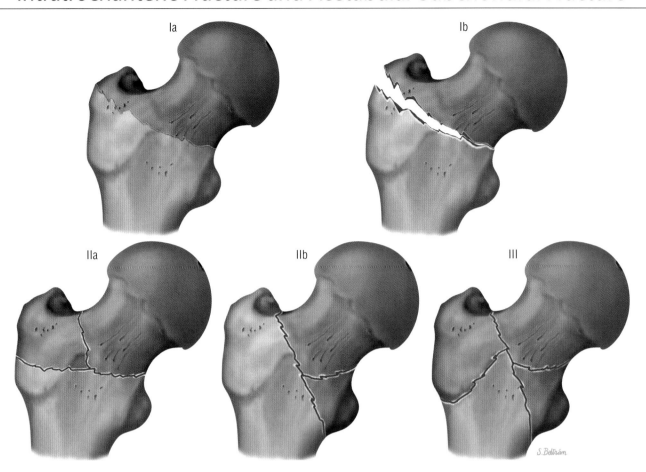

Figure 3.147 ■ **The modified Evans classification of intratrochanteric fractures divides them into three main types.** Type I fractures are two-part fractures, classified as either type Ia (not displaced) or type Ib (displaced). Type II fractures are three-part fractures and are classified as either IIa (involving the greater trochanter) or type IIb (involving the lesser trochanter). Type III fractures involve the greater and lesser trochanters and are unstable and difficult to reduce. *(See Femoral Neck Fractures pg. 277, in Stoller's 3rd Edition.)*

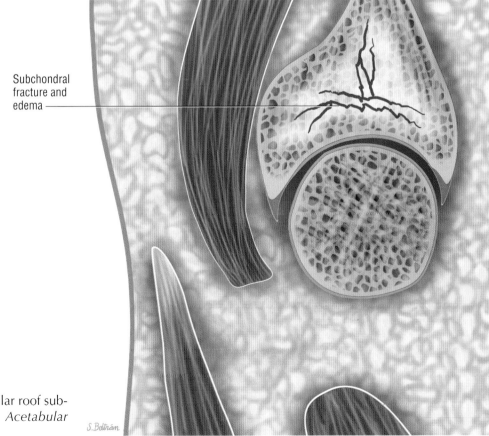

Subchondral fracture and edema

Figure 3.148 ■ Sagittal section of acetabular roof subchondral insufficiency fracture. *(See Acetabular Fractures pg. 279, in Stoller's 3rd Edition.)*

Acetabular Fractures

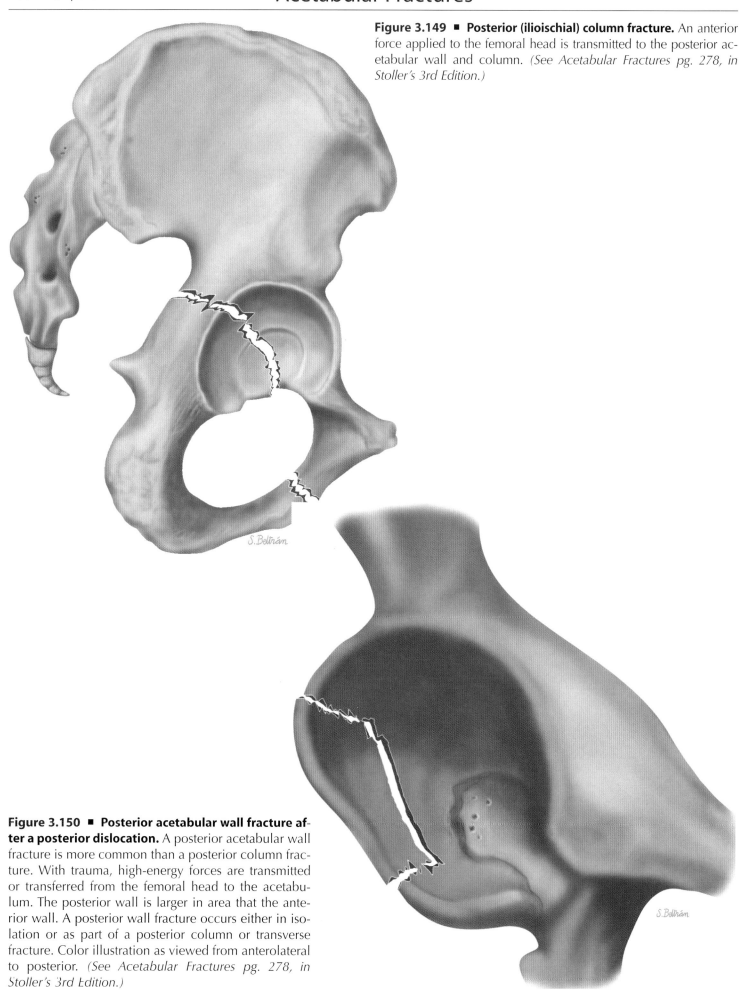

Figure 3.149 ▪ Posterior (ilioischial) column fracture. An anterior force applied to the femoral head is transmitted to the posterior acetabular wall and column. *(See Acetabular Fractures pg. 278, in Stoller's 3rd Edition.)*

Figure 3.150 ▪ Posterior acetabular wall fracture after a posterior dislocation. A posterior acetabular wall fracture is more common than a posterior column fracture. With trauma, high-energy forces are transmitted or transferred from the femoral head to the acetabulum. The posterior wall is larger in area that the anterior wall. A posterior wall fracture occurs either in isolation or as part of a posterior column or transverse fracture. Color illustration as viewed from anterolateral to posterior. *(See Acetabular Fractures pg. 278, in Stoller's 3rd Edition.)*

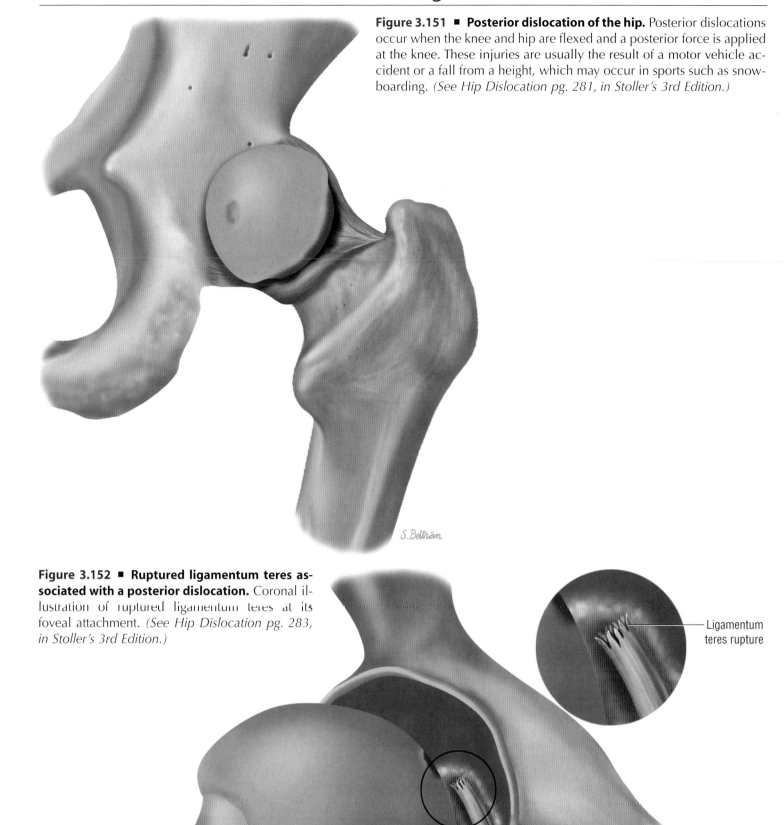

Figure 3.151 ■ **Posterior dislocation of the hip.** Posterior dislocations occur when the knee and hip are flexed and a posterior force is applied at the knee. These injuries are usually the result of a motor vehicle accident or a fall from a height, which may occur in sports such as snowboarding. *(See Hip Dislocation pg. 281, in Stoller's 3rd Edition.)*

Figure 3.152 ■ **Ruptured ligamentum teres associated with a posterior dislocation.** Coronal illustration of ruptured ligamentum teres at its foveal attachment. *(See Hip Dislocation pg. 283, in Stoller's 3rd Edition.)*

Ligamentum teres rupture

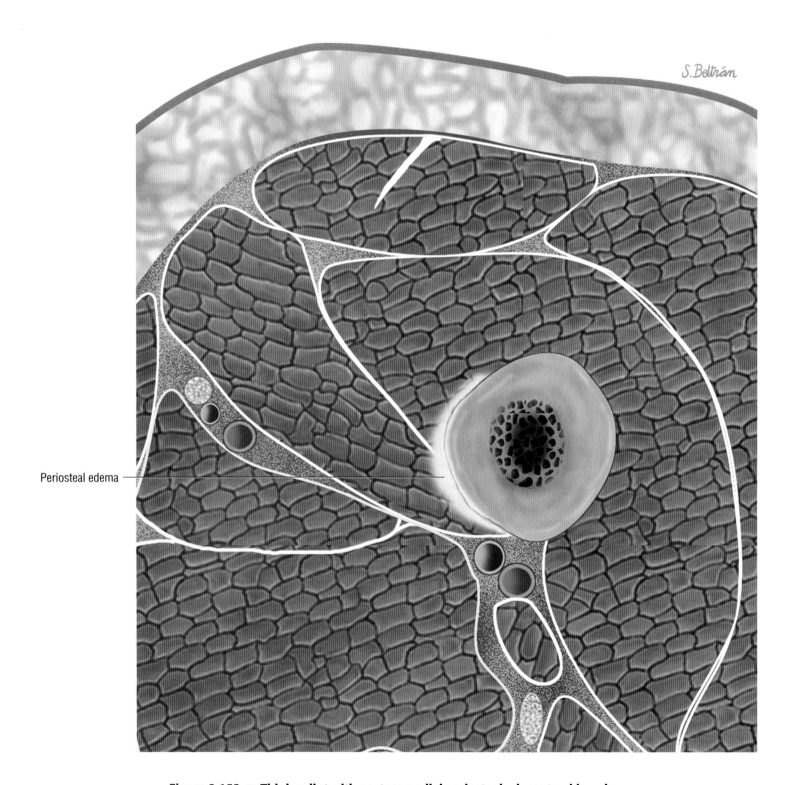

Periosteal edema

Figure 3.153 ■ Thigh splint with posteromedial periosteal edema tracking along the adductor insertion. Color axial cross section through the affected periosteum. *(See Thigh Splints pg. 284, in Stoller's 3rd Edition.)*

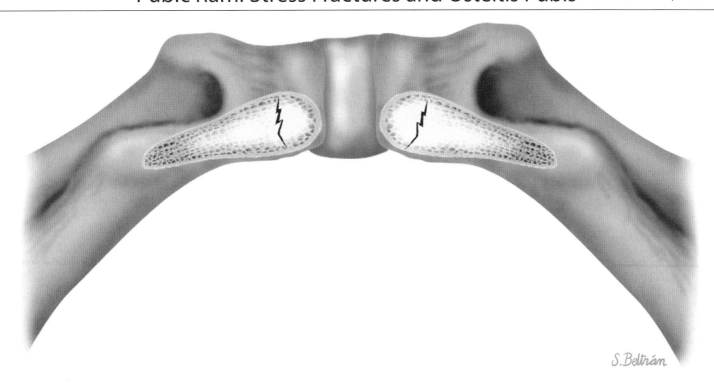

Figure 3.154 ■ Color illustration of bilateral inferior pubic rami stress fractures, inferior perspective. *(See Pubic Rami Stress Fractures and Osteitis Pubis pg. 285, in Stoller's 3rd Edition.)*

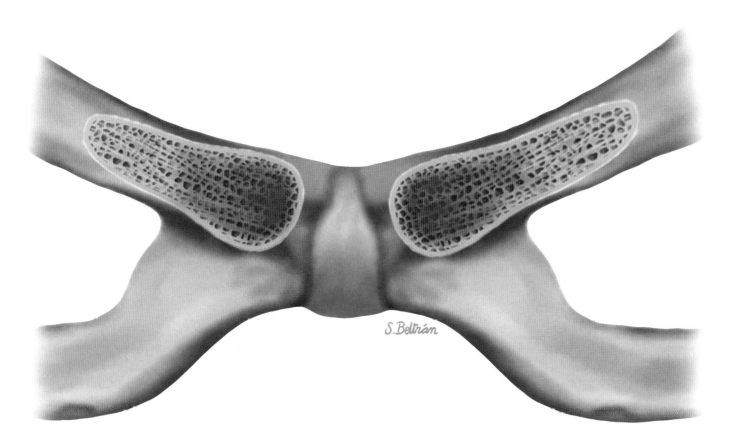

Figure 3.155 ■ **Osteitis pubis directly adjacent to the pubic symphysis may occur in sports requiring excessive twisting and turning (such as soccer) or from repetitive shear stress with excessive side-to-side motion, as occurs in runners.** Coronal color illustration illustrates parasymphyseal edema. *(See Pubic Rami Stress Fractures and Osteitis Pubis pg. 285, in Stoller's 3rd Edition.)*

Figure 3.156 ▪ Bilateral sacral alar insufficiency fractures with associated edema. *(See Sacral Insufficiency Fractures pg. 288, in Stoller's 3rd Edition.)*

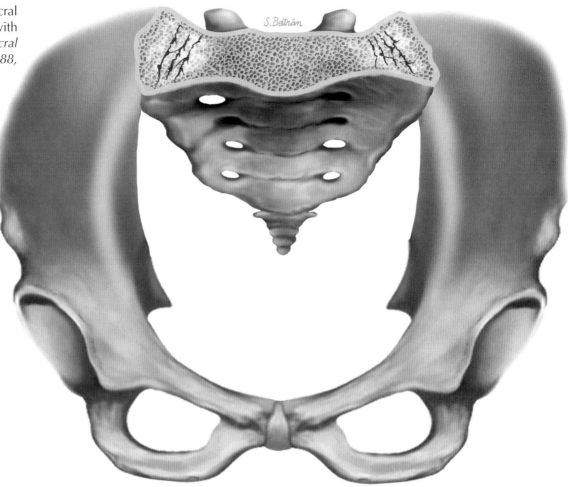

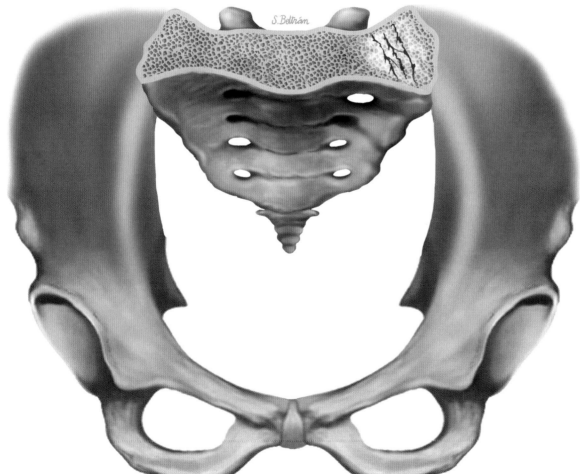

Figure 3.157 ▪ **Unilateral sacral insufficiency fractures of the left sacral alar.** The majority of patients affected with pelvic insufficiency fractures are 60 years of age or older, with a female predominance. Anterior perspective color illustration. *(See Sacral Insufficiency Fractures pg. 290, in Stoller's 3rd Edition.)*

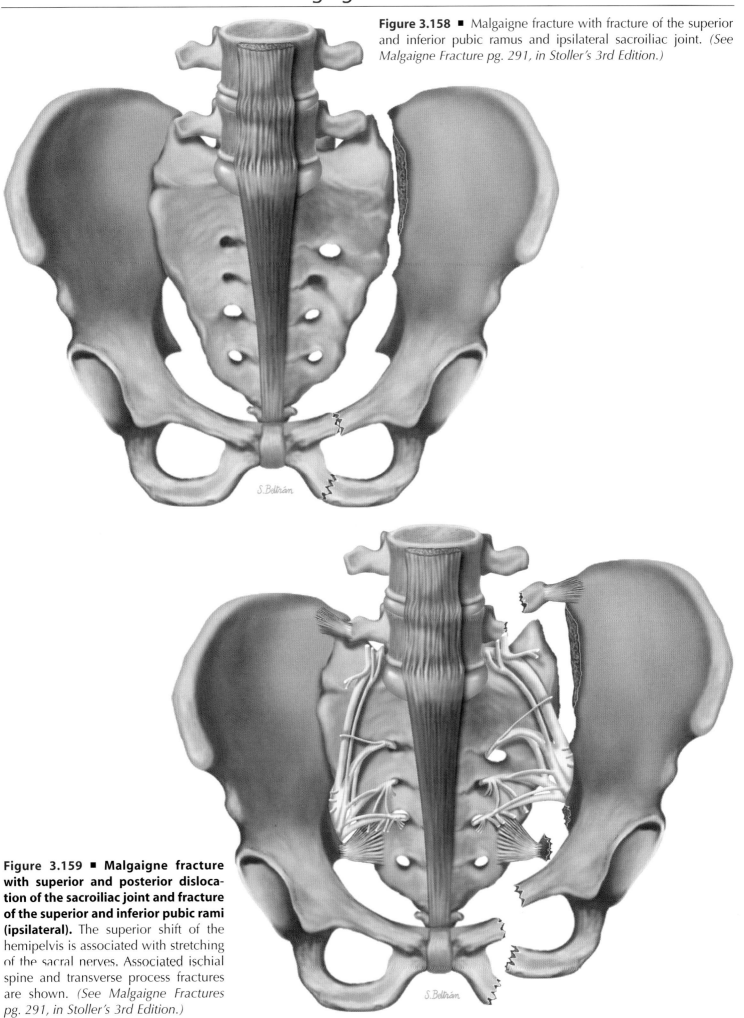

Figure 3.158 ■ Malgaigne fracture with fracture of the superior and inferior pubic ramus and ipsilateral sacroiliac joint. *(See Malgaigne Fracture pg. 291, in Stoller's 3rd Edition.)*

Figure 3.159 ■ **Malgaigne fracture with superior and posterior dislocation of the sacroiliac joint and fracture of the superior and inferior pubic rami (ipsilateral).** The superior shift of the hemipelvis is associated with stretching of the sacral nerves. Associated ischial spine and transverse process fractures are shown. *(See Malgaigne Fractures pg. 291, in Stoller's 3rd Edition.)*

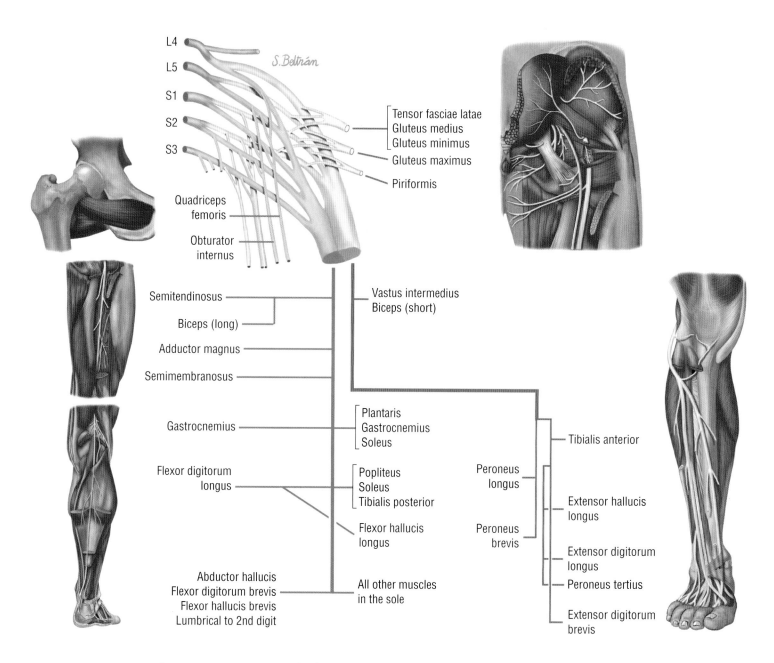

Figure 3.160 ■ Sciatic (tibial and peroneal) motor nerve distribution. *(See Muscle Denervation Patterns pg. 293, in Stoller's 3rd Edition.)*

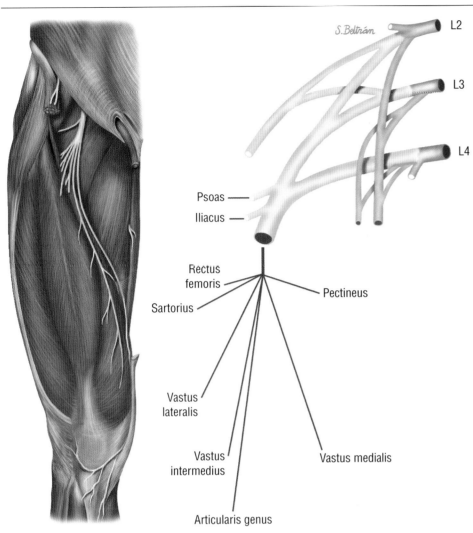

S.Beltrán

L2

L3

L4

Psoas

Iliacus

Rectus femoris

Pectineus

Sartorius

Vastus lateralis

Vastus intermedius

Vastus medialis

Articularis genus

Figure 3.161 ■ Femoral nerve distribution. *(See Muscle Denervation Patterns pg. 294, in Stoller's 3rd Edition.)*

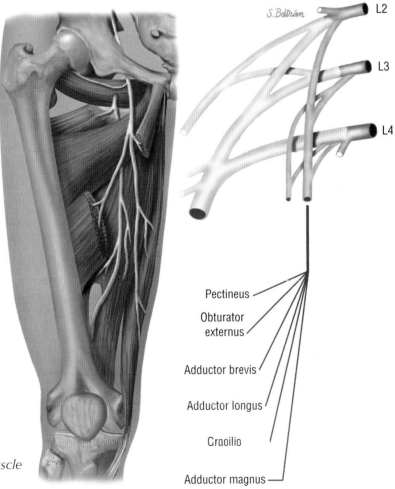

S.Beltrán

L2

L3

L4

Pectineus

Obturator externus

Adductor brevis

Adductor longus

Craoilio

Adductor magnus

Figure 3.162 ■ Obturator nerve motor distribution. *(See Muscle Denervation Patterns pg. 295, in Stoller's 3rd Edition.)*

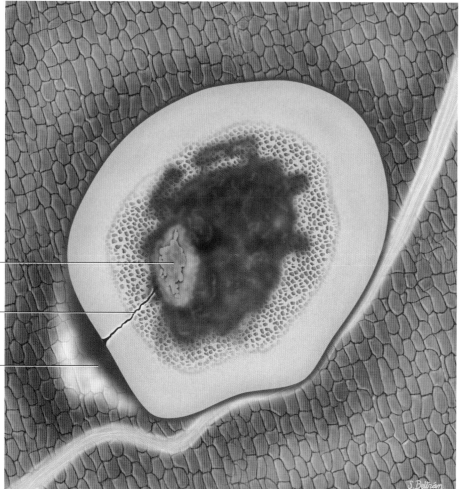

Figure 3.163 ■ Osteomyelitis of the femoral diaphysis with sequestrum, sinus tract, and periosteal reaction. *(See Osteomyelitis pg. 296, in Stoller's 3rd Edition.)*

Sequestration

Sinus tract

Periosteal reaction and edema

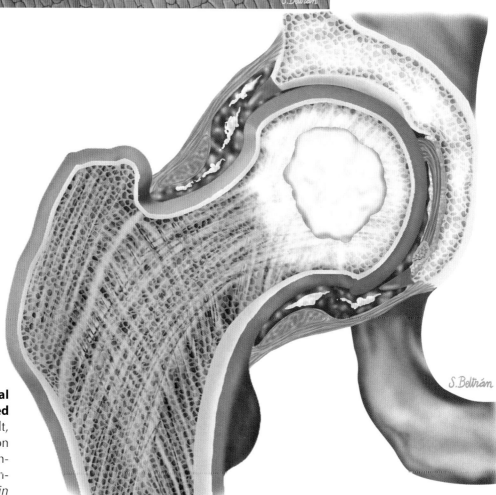

Figure 3.164 ■ **Synovitis and femoral head nidus of infection that has extended to involve the acetabulum.** In the adult, contiguous spread and direct implantation of infection from an adjacent soft tissue infection or wound are more common mechanisms. *(See Osteomyelitis pg. 297, in Stoller's 3rd Edition.)*

Osteomyelitis

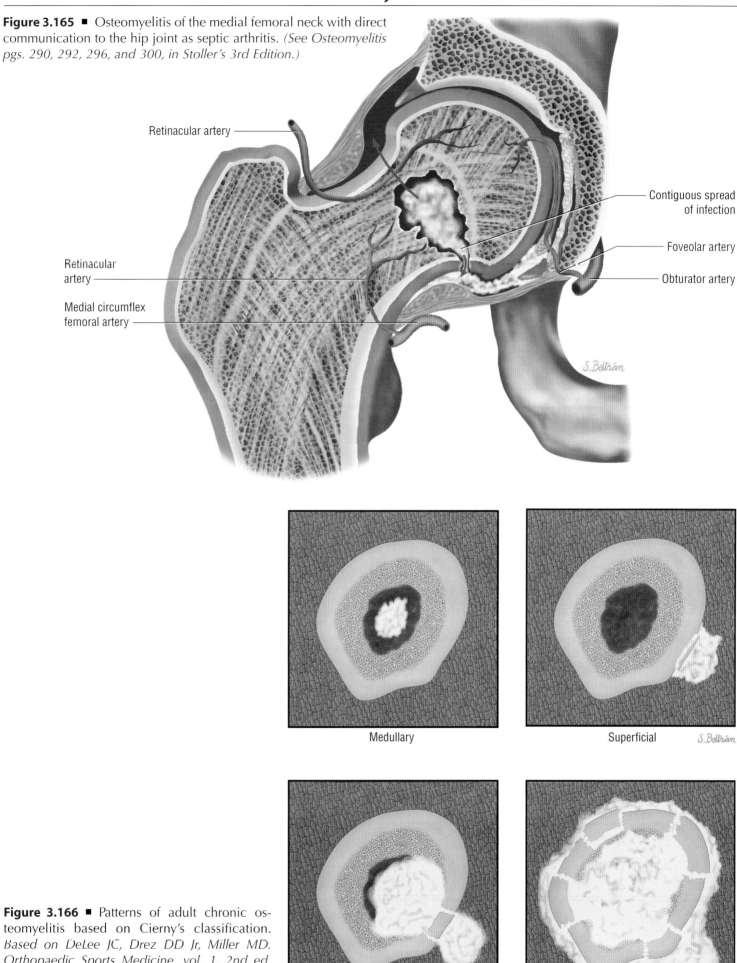

Figure 3.165 ▪ Osteomyelitis of the medial femoral neck with direct communication to the hip joint as septic arthritis. *(See Osteomyelitis pgs. 290, 292, 296, and 300, in Stoller's 3rd Edition.)*

Retinacular artery

Retinacular artery

Medial circumflex femoral artery

Contiguous spread of infection

Foveolar artery

Obturator artery

Medullary

Superficial

Localized

Diffuse

Figure 3.166 ▪ Patterns of adult chronic osteomyelitis based on Cierny's classification. *Based on DeLee JC, Drez DD Jr, Miller MD. Orthopaedic Sports Medicine, vol. 1, 2nd ed. Philadelphia: Saunders, 2003. (See Osteomyelitis pgs. 290, 292, 296, and 300, in Stoller's 3rd Edition.)*

4 The Knee

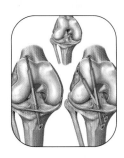

Pearls and Pitfalls & Color Illustrations

Pearls and Pitfalls

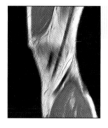

IMAGING PROTOCOLS

- FS PD FSE is a fluid-, articular cartilage-, and marrow-sensitive sequence (TR ≥ 3,000 msec and TE 40-50 msec) that should be performed in the coronal, sagittal, and axial planes.
- Sagittal T2* GRE images are helpful for identifying meniscal degeneration, patellar tendinosis, and chondrocalcinosis.
- Incorporate a T1-weighted image in at least one imaging plane to obtain an accurate assessment of marrow fat signal intensity changes in sclerosis or edema in cases of trauma, infection, and neoplasia.
- Trochlear groove chondral lesions are best evaluated with sagittal images, whereas patellar facet chondromalacia is best assessed on axial images.

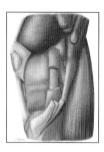

ROUTINE PROTOCOLS

- **Axial T1 or PD FSE**
  - Subchondral sclerosis in chronic patellofemoral conditions
- **Axial FS PD FSE**
  - Patellofemoral articular cartilage
- **Sagittal FS PD FSE (fluid-sensitive sequence)**
  - Chondral lesions, ligament (cruciate) tears, and meniscal morphology (meniscal fluid interface)
- **Sagittal T2* GRE**
  - Spectrum of meniscal injuries from degeneration to tear
  - Patellar tendinosis
  - Chondrocalcinosis
  - Hemosiderin deposition
- **Sagittal PD FSE (often used in place of T2* GRE)**
  - Meniscal degeneration or tear. Provides improved intrameniscal signal visualization relative to FS PD FSE but is inferior to T2* GRE or FS PD conventional spin-echo
- **Coronal T1 or PD FSE**
  - Sclerosis
  - Femoral condylar erosions
  - Subchondral marrow visualization in trauma, infection, or tumor
  - ACL sprain or scarring
- **Coronal FS PD FSE**
  - Collateral ligaments
  - Meniscal root attachments
  - Confirm continuity of ACL in cases of grade 2 vs. grade 3 ligament injuries

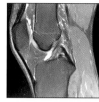

APPLICATION AND TECHNIQUES FOR ROUTINE PROTOCOLS

- **Echo Time (TE)**
  - Time at which receiver "listens" for signal (sampling)
  - Dephasing after the RF pulse ends represents T2 effect
  - Increased TE = increased dephasing (increased T2 effects)
  - Increasing the TE decreases SNR. However, resolution increases because the center of k-space is moved to later echoes. Early echoes exhibit dephasing at a faster rate, which results in increased blurring of the image
  - Fat saturation decreases the overall SNR of the image by suppressing the signal contribution from fat (FS PD FSE images should not use long TE values [e.g., >50 msec]; otherwise the SNR decreases)
  - Fat suppressed PD FSE with TE 31, 47, 78 msec. BW, TR, FOV, Matrix unchanged (see below images)

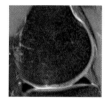 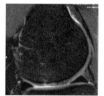 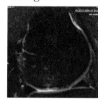

- **Repetition Time (TR)**
  - TR controls the amount of saturation (T1 effects)
  - In PD and T2-weighted imaging, the TR must be at least 3 (and preferably 5) times as long as the longest T1 of the tissue being imaged; otherwise T1 contribution will change the overall image contrast
  - TR values <3,000 msec on FS PD FSE images may result in decreased contrast and signal between fluid and articular cartilage
  - TR 2500, 3000, 3500 msec respectively. BW, TE, FOV, Matrix unchanged (see below images)

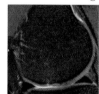 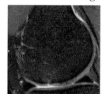 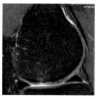

- **Receiver Bandwidth (RBW)**
  - RBW increases SNR because the amplitude of the readout gradient is reduced. However, it can also result in blurring, increased flow pulsation, and decreased number of slices. Data sampling takes longer with lower RBWs
  - Blurring in FSE images occurs with lower bandwidth values because of the increase in space between echoes in the echo train length (ETL)

□ Chemical shift increases with shorter RBWs because of a similar range of frequencies sampled across the field of view

□ To minimize image blurring, recommended bandwidths for PD FSE images are 15 to 30 kHz. With bandwidths of 15 to 20 kHz, there is greater SNR

□ BW 10, 15, 30 kHz; TR, TE, FOV, and Matrix unchanged

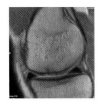 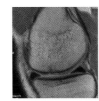 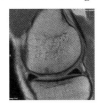

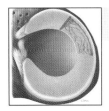

MENISCAL MICROSTRUCTURE
(See Figure 4.23)

■ Circumferential collagen fibers create normal meniscal hoop tension.

■ Radial (radial tie) fibers stabilize longitudinally oriented circumferential collagen fibers and also help resist meniscal extrusion.

■ Middle perforating collagen fibers represent a concentration of radially oriented collagen fibers in the central plane of the meniscus.

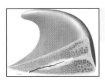

MENISCAL DEGENERATIONS AND TEARS
(See Figures 4.26–4.29)

■ Grade 1 and grade 2 signal intensity represent intrasubstance degeneration and not fibrocartilaginous tearing.

■ Grade 3 signal intensity represents a meniscal tear (the term "tear" should not be used in conjunction with grade 1 or grade 2 signal).

■ A closed meniscal tear is characterized by grade 3 signal intensity that weakens or attenuates as it approaches an articular surface of the meniscus.

■ The articular surface of the meniscus is defined as an inferior or superior surface or the free edge apex of the meniscal fibrocartilage.

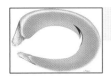

CLASSIFICATION
(See Figures 4.30–4.33)

■ **Based on MR sagittal sections:**
 □ Vertical
 □ Horizontal (includes the pure horizontal cleavage type)

■ **Based on circumferential or surface anatomy:**
 □ Longitudinal (vertical or horizontal on corresponding meniscal sections)
 □ Flap (vertical or horizontal)
 □ Radial (vertical)

■ Longitudinal and flap tears can have either a primary vertical or horizontal tear pattern on corresponding sagittal images. Confusion exists because longitudinal and flap tears have been previously classified only as vertical tear types.

■ Radial tears, including classic radial tears and root tears, are vertical tears.

HORIZONTAL TEARS
(See Figures 4.34–4.35)

■ A pure horizontal cleavage tear extends to the apex of the meniscus and results from excessive shear stress.

■ Longitudinal and flap tears may have a relative (not pure) horizontal orientation as viewed in the sagittal plane. These tear patterns, however, occur only in association with superior or inferior leaf extension.

■ Horizontal cleavage tears are less common than flap tears.

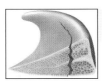

LONGITUDINAL TEARS
(See Figures 4.36–4.37)

■ Longitudinal tears occur in the peripheral aspect of the meniscus and are identified by peripheral grade 3 signal intensity on either coronal or sagittal images.

■ Longitudinal tears correspond to the long or longitudinal axis of the meniscus in the axial plane.

■ Longitudinal tears are not restricted to exclusively vertical tear patterns on sagittal images and may present with oblique or horizontally oriented signal (not parallel to the tibial plateau) that extends to an articular surface.

■ Statistically, most obliquely oriented signal intensity in the sagittal plane corresponds to flap tears, although longitudinal tears may also present with sagittal plane oblique grade 3 signal intensity. Thus, the term "oblique signal intensity" may be misleading unless used in the context of a specific circumferential or surface tear type. In practice, orthopaedic surgeons equate the term "oblique" with flap tear.

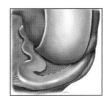

BUCKET-HANDLE TEARS
(See Figures 4.38–4.42)

■ Common tear in young patients with trauma.

■ Associated with ACL injury.

■ An unstable meniscal fragment locks into the intercondylar notch and involves at least two thirds of the meniscal circumference.

■ Diagnosis of a bucket-handle tear requires identification of displaced meniscal tissue from posterior to a relative anterior coronal location. If displaced meniscal tissue is restricted to posterior coronal images, consider a displaced flap tear pattern.

■ A double delta sign and/or a double PCL sign are sagittal MR findings of a displaced bucket-handle tear.

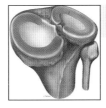

RADIAL OR TRANSVERSE TEARS
(See Figures 4.43–4.48)

■ **There are three subtypes of classic radial tears (more common in lateral meniscus):**
 □ Anterior horn-body junction
 □ Body
 □ Posterior horn-body junction

■ Root tears are more common in the posterior horn of the medial meniscus.

- Classic radial tears are commonly associated with horizontal tears in the lateral meniscus and flap tears in the medial meniscus.

- MR findings in classic radial tears include: (1) a blunted anterior horn and elongated posterior horn body segment; (2) a blunted posterior horn in association with an elongated anterior horn body segment; or (3) free edge increased signal intensity or blunting restricted to the middle third of the meniscus that does not involve blunting of the anterior or posterior horns or elongation of the body segment.

- Root tears are defined by abrupt loss or blunting of posterior horn meniscal tissue on posterior coronal images adjacent to the root meniscal insertion. A ghost meniscus or relative absence of posterior horn meniscal fibrocartilangeous tissue is characteristic of root tears on sagittal images located adjacent to the intercondylar notch.

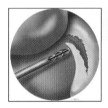

FLAP TEARS
(See Figures 4.49–4.61)

- Flap tears usually result from extensions of radial or horizontal cleavage tears and represent the most common clinical tear type.

- Vertical grade 3 signal intensity in the inner one third to one half of the meniscus or relative deficiency of the inferior surface of the meniscus are the most common findings in flap tears.

- Flap tears may demonstrate meniscal extrusion into the coronary recess of a meniscotibial ligament on coronal images. Reactive tibial plateau marrow edema is associated with these extrusions.

- Oblique meniscal signal intensity on sagittal images does not necessarily equate with flap tear morphology (see criteria for flap tear diagnosis).

- Flap tears, large radial tears (including root tears), and complex tears are associated with major (>3 mm) meniscal extrusion.

- Displaced flap tears of the posterior horn of lateral meniscus are associated with ACL tears.

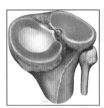

DISCOID MENISCUS
(See Figures 4.62–4.64)

- Incomplete discoid menisci can be differentiated from complete discoid types by the degree of discoid morphology. No anterior or posterior horn equivalents are identified in the complete discoid meniscus (type A).

- Prominent or cavitary grade 2 signal intensity in a discoid meniscus may be associated with positive clinical signs and symptoms related to the lateral compartment.

- The popping or snapping knee syndrome is associated with the Wrisberg variant (absence of the posterior coronary ligament).

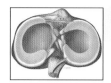

MENISCAL TEARS (PITFALLS)
(See Figures 4.65–4.68)

- Attenuation of grade 3 signal intensity extension to an articular surface is associated with a closed meniscal tear.

- External rotation of the knee may accentuate the course of the meniscofemoral ligaments. The ligament of Wrisberg is often mistaken for a peripheral tear of the posterior horn of the lateral meniscus.

- Meniscal flounce does not indicate the existence of or increased association with a meniscal tear.

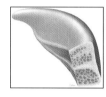

POSTOPERATIVE MENISCUS
(See Figures 4.69–4.75)

- Grade 3 signal intensity should not be mistaken for residual tear or retear in a stable meniscal remnant after partial menisectomy.

- Selective blunting of the inferior surface (leaf) is associated with partial meniscectomy of tears extending to the inferior articular surface of the meniscus.

- Stable meniscal fibrovascular scars are intermediate in signal intensity on FS PD FSE images. Direct linear extension of hyperintense fluid or intra-articular contrast, however, represents retear of the meniscal repair or extension of the tear into an unstable meniscal remnant.

- MR arthrography primarily is used to evaluate post-primary repair menisci as well as cases of more extensive partial menisecectomies.

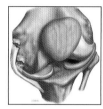

MENISCOCAPSULAR SEPARATIONS
(See Figure 4.76)

- The meniscocapsular ligaments consist of meniscofemoral and meniscotibial ligaments and are defined in layer 3 of the knee joint capsule.

- Tears of the proximal MCL are associated with meniscofemoral ligament injuries.

- Fluid interposed between the meniscus and capsular periphery posterolateral to the superficial MCL and deep MCL represents a form of meniscocapsular tearing and may be associated with a posterior medial meniscal corner tear in acute ACL injuries.

- Meniscal avulsions involving the meniscotibial attachment occur in both the medial and lateral meniscus.

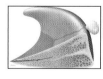

MENISCAL CYSTS
(See Figure 4.77)

- Meniscal cysts are related to either microscopic or macroscopic tears in meniscal fibrocartilage.

- Horizontal cleavage tears or complex meniscal tears with a horizontal component are associated with the development of meniscal cysts.

- Loculations, septations, and dissection of the cyst from the site of origin are common findings.

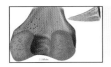

CALCIUM PYROPHOSPHATE DEHYDRATE DEPOSITION DISEASE
(See Figures 4.78–4.79)

- T2* GRE images are recommended for detection of punctate hypointense CPPD crystal depositions.

- High contrast settings help identify meniscal tissue involvement.

- Meniscal degeneration and tears may be underestimated secondary to localized susceptibility effects induced by crystal deposition, especially on T2* GRE images.

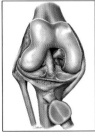

ANTERIOR CRUCIATE LIGAMENT
(See Figures 4.80–4.82)

- The ACL is a two bundle ligament with a small anteromedial and a larger posterolateral (tight in extension) bundle. Functional ACL fiber recruitment, however, is more complicated than assignment to one of two fiber bundles.

- The ACL is the primary restraint to anterior tibial displacement, with the posterolateral bundle providing the principal resistance to hyperextension forces.

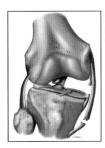

ACL INJURY
(See Figures 4.83–4.84)

- **Pivot Shift Injury**
  - Non-contact injury in skiers or American football players
  - Valgus load, flexion, and external rotation of the tibia or internal rotation of the femur
  - ACL rupture and lateral compartment contusions

- **Dashboard Injury**
  - Applied force to anterior proximal tibia with knee in flexion
  - Associated with anterior tibial and posterior patellar edema with rupture of the PCL and posterior joint capsule

- **Hyperextension Injury**
  - Direct force applied to the anterior tibia with a planted foot
  - Direct injury secondary to car bumper impacting on the anterior tibia of a pedestrian
  - Indirect force as caused by a forceful kicking motion
  - Kissing contusions of anterior femoral condyle and anterior tibial plateau (hyperextension with an applied valgus force shifts the kissing or opposing bone contusions medially)
  - Associated soft tissue injuries include ACL or PCL and a meniscal injury
  - Knee dislocation with at-risk structures, including ACL, PCL, popliteal neurovasular structures, and posterolateral complex injuries

- **Clip Injury**
  - Contact injury secondary to pure valgus stress to a partially flexed (10° to 30°) knee
  - Seen in American football players
  - Ossesous contusion of lateral femoral condyle from a direct blow with medial femoral epicondylar edema related to MCL avulsion stress

- Associated soft tissue structures at risk include the proximal MCL and ACL as a function of increased knee flexion (O'Donoghue's triad includes the medial meniscus)

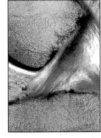

ACL APPEARANCE

- Sagittal images are oriented parallel to the lateral femoral condylar wall to optimize ligament visualization in the sagittal plane. An axial image is used as a landmark to prescribe the sagittal oblique plane.

- Elongation of the anterior-to-posterior aspect of the lateral femoral condyle is associated with excessive external rotation of the knee and may compromise accurate interpretation of the lateral meniscus.

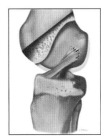

ACL TEARS
(See Figures 4.85–4.93)

- **Primary Signs**
  - Abnormal ligament course (abnormal Blumensaat angle)
  - Abnormal ligament signal intensity (coronal images should be used in conjunction with sagittal images to compensate for segmental visualization in the sagittal plane)
  - Ligament discontinuity

- **Secondary Signs**
  - Lateral compartment osseous contusions (posterolateral tibial plateau is most specific)
  - Posteromedial tibial plateau contusion or fracture
  - Anterior tibial displacement (assessed in the lateral aspect of the lateral compartment)
  - Uncovered posterior horn lateral meniscus
  - Posterior cruciate line and angle

- Coronal T1- and PD FSE images identify increased signal intensity within an ACL sprain or complete tear.

- An intact ligament remains hypointense and maintains ligamentous continuity on corresponding FS PD FSE coronal images on at least one image posterior to and including the plane of the MCL.

- Chronic ACL tears demonstrate resolution of the osseous contusions, effusions, synovitis, and ligamentous hyperintensity that are characteristic of acute injuries unless seen in the setting of an acute injury.

- Mucoid degeneration and ACL or intercondylar notch cysts may be symptomatic with associated restricted range of motion without direct evidence of an ACL sprain or partial tear.

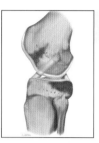

POSTEROLATERAL CORNER INJURIES
(See Figures 4.94–4.95)

- **The posterolateral corner is also referred to as the posterolateral or arcuate complex. It includes the following structures:**
  - ☐ Lateral collateral ligament
  - ☐ Popliteus muscle and tendon
  - ☐ Arcuate ligament (medial and lateral limb)
- Medial limb-courses over the popliteus muscle and tendon and joins the oblique popliteal ligament
- Lateral limb-blends with the capsule near the condylar insertion of the lateral head of the gastrocnemius muscle
- Popliteofibular ligament
- Popliteomeniscal fascicles
- Fabellofibular ligament
- Lateral head of gastrocnemius muscle
- The biceps femoris tendon and iliotibial band, although not usually listed as components of the posterolateral complex, contribute to the stability of the lateral and posterolateral knee.

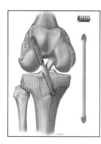

OSSEOUS INJURIES
(See Figures 4.96–4.98)

- Posteromedial tibial plateau contusions or fractures represent contre-coup injuries associated with lateral compartment osseous impaction with ACL ruptures.
- Posterior peripheral medial meniscus tears and meniscocapsular separations occur in conjunction with posteromedial tibial plateau injuries.
- The Segond fracture is visualized on anterior coronal images at the location of the lateral compartment of the meniscotibial ligament. It is associated with avulsion forces directed by the posterior fibers of the iliotibial tract.
- The arcuate sign (associated with posterolateral corner injury) represents an avulsion fracture of the fibular styloid process that may involve the popliteofibular ligament or arcuate and fabellofibular ligaments.
- Avulsion fractures of the fibular head are associated with PCL tears.

ACL RECONSTRUCTION
(See Figures 4.99–4.108)

- **Isometry**
  - ☐ Success is related to the position of the femoral tunnel. Proper tunnel placement is at the intersection of the posterior femoral cortex and the posterior aspect of the distal femoral physeal scar on sagittal images. The position of the femoral tunnel is at the 10 o'clock and 2 o'clock positions in the right and left knees respectively
  - ☐ Successful repair allows for constant length and tension of the ACL graft throughout flexion and extension
  - ☐ An anteriorly placed femoral tunnel is associated with graft elongation and instability

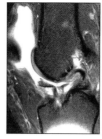

ACL RECONSTRUCTION (MRI)

- **MR is useful for assessing the following after ACL reconstruction:**
  - ☐ Graft failure
  - ☐ Graft placement
  - ☐ Impingement
  - ☐ Arthrofibrosis (cyclops lesion)
  - ☐ ACL graft ganglia (related to graft tunnel)
  - ☐ Hardware placement
- Increased signal intensity may be seen in ACL grafts for 1 to 2 years after reconstruction with the bone-patellar tendon-bone construct.
- Uniform hypointensity of the graft is demonstrated after 2 years.

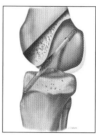

GRAFT IMPINGEMENT
(See Figure 4.109)

- **Potential sites of bone impingement**
  - ☐ Intercondylar roof
  - ☐ Side walls of intercondylar fossa
  - ☐ Intraarticular exits of osseous tunnels
- **Roof impingement**
  - ☐ Lateral or excessively anterior placement of the tibial tunnel (posterior placement of tibial tunnel or anterior placement of femoral tunnel produces instability)
  - ☐ Placement of the tibial tunnel parallel and posterior to the Blumensaat line (slope of the intercondylar roof) on sagittal images avoids roof impingement. The tibial tunnel opens on the intercondylar eminence on coronal MR images
  - ☐ Intermediate graft signal may be caused by vascularized periligamentous tissue, graft revascularization (seen up to 2 years after graft placement), or graft impingement

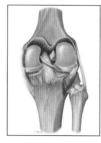

POSTERIOR CRUCIATE LIGAMENT
(See Figures 4.112–4.123)

- PCL injuries include reverse Segond fractures, an arcuate sign, and anterior compartment osseous contusions.
- MR findings of partial or interstitial tears of the PCL are more common than complete ligament ruptures.

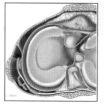

MEDIAL COLLATERAL LIGAMENT
(See Figures 4.124–4.139)

- The superficial MCL represents layer 2 of the medial supporting structures. Layer 3 is formed by the deep MCL (meniscofemoral and meniscotibial attachments), found deep to the superficial MCL.
- Laxity of the MCL is associated with distal MCL tears.
- The MCL heals with scar formation, which is visualized as a thickened hypointense structure.
- Medial meniscal injuries may be associated with MCL tears and should be looked for carefully.

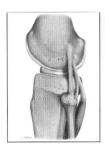

LATERAL COLLATERAL LIGAMENT AND POSTEROLATERAL CORNER
(See Figures 4.140, 4.151)

- LCL tears are associated with injury to other posterolateral structures.

- Popliteus muscle or myotendinous unit strains represent extra-articular injuries. Intra-articular popliteus tears, which are less common, involve the hiatus or popliteus femoral attachment at the fossa.

- The LCL and biceps femoris attach to the lateral margin of the fibular head and not the styloid, accounting for a reduced likelihood of avulsion injury compared to the popliteofibular, fabellofibular, and arcuate ligaments.

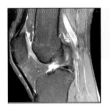

PATELLOFEMORAL JOINT AND EXTENSOR MECHANISM

- The medial patellar facet has a convex articular surface, whereas the lateral patellar facet has a concave articular surface.

- The medial facet of the patella is divided into a medial odd facet and a lateral middle facet. The lateral middle facet is located between the lateral and odd patellar facets.

- The excessive lateral pressure syndrome is associated with lateral patellar facet chondromalacia and edema of the proximal lateral aspect of Hoffa's fat pad.

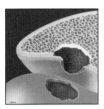

CHONDROMALACIA
(See Figures 4.152–4.156)

- Chondromalacia is commonly associated with patellofemoral overload or malalignment.

- FS PD FSE images identify basal, intrasubstance, and surface chondral defects.

- The patellar facets are evaluated on axial images, whereas trochlear groove articular cartilage is assessed on sagittal images. Patellar subchondral sclerosis is associated with chronic chondral injuries.

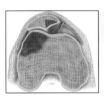

TRAUMATIC DISLOCATIONS
(See Figures 4.158–4.165)

- FS PD FSE axial images define medial patellofemoral ligament disruption tears of the adductor tubercle or medial retinaculum tearing from the medial patellar facet.

- Osteochondral injuries of the medial patellar facet and lateral femoral condyle may be seen in addition to strain of the vastus medialis obliquus, sprains of the MCL, and disruption of the medial patellofemoral ligaments.

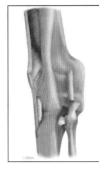

ILIOTIBIAL BAND SYNDROME
(See Figures 4.173–4.176)

- Chronic functional trauma occurs when the ITB rubs on the outer aspect of the lateral femoral condyle.

- FS PD FSE is used to identify thickened synovium with variable degrees of inflammation within the lateral synovial recess.

- Thickening and signal heterogeneity of the ITB is visualized on anterior coronal images.

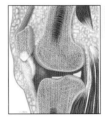

PATELLAR TENDINITIS
(See Figures 4.177–4.178)

- Most commonly affects the proximal posterior (deep) fibers of the patellar tendon.

- The constellation of MRI findings includes thickening or expansion of the medial to central tendon fibers and hyperintensity of the tendon, adjacent proximal infrapatellar fat pad, and inferior pole of the patella.

- T2* GRE sagittal images are sensitive and specific for identifying patellar tendon collagen degeneration.

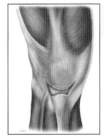

PATELLAR TENDON TEARS
(See Figure 4.179)

- Patellar tendon tears are less common then quadriceps tendon rupture.

- Although degeneration of tendon fibers represents a predisposing factor to rupture, the tensile and viscoelastic properties of the patellar tendon are relatively stable between younger and older age groups.

- Edema and hemorrhage are best visualized on FS PD FSE images, whereas underlying collagen degeneration is best seen on T2* GRE images.

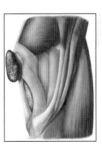

PATELLAR BURSAE
(See Figures 4.182–4.185)

- The prepatellar bursa represents one of three potential bursal spaces anterior to the patella.

- Small amounts of fluid may be found normally in the deep infrapatellar bursa.

- Bursae present as flattened synovial sacs usually are not visualized on MR unless distended with fluid.

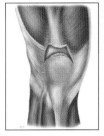

QUADRICEPS TENDON AND MUSCLE TEARS
(See Figures 4.186–4.187)

- Quadriceps tendinosis or tears are best identified on the superior aspects of sagittal images through the extension mechanism.
- Tears usually occur proximal to the patellar insertion or expansion of the quadriceps tendon and may extend through the vastus intermedius tendon.

- Inferior migration of the patella and tendon discontinuity with interposed hemorrhage at the tendon gap are common findings in complete tendon rupture.

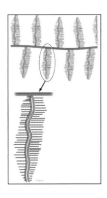

CARTILAGE EVALUATION
(See Figures 4.188–4.191)

- The articular cartilage extracellular matrix is composed primarily of type II collagen, the proteoglycan aggrecan, noncollagenous matrix proteins, and water. Type II collagen has its greatest concentration in the upper or superficial zone, where the chondral ultrastructure demonstrates a parallel arrangement of collagen fibers. Glycosaminoglycans, especially chondrotin and keratan sulfate, are associated with the swelling and water-imbibing properties of proteoglycan aggregates and have an increased distribution in the deeper zones of cartilage.

- Early changes of osteoarthritis-related chondral degeneration may be initiated in the deeper layers of cartilage rather than in the superficial zone.
- FS PD FSE and PD FSE are routinely used as morphologic imaging techniques in the evaluation of articular cartilage lesions. T2* GRE is not a chondral-sensitive imaging technique. Physiologic imaging techniques such as T2 mapping or contrast-enhanced imaging do not replace standard morphologic cartilage imaging techniques.

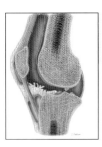

SYNOVIUM AND IRREGULAR HOFFA'S INTRAPATELLAR FAT PAD
(See Figures 4.193–4.195)

- An irregular free edge of Hoffa's infrapatellar fat pad is associated with synovitis.
- Inflammation of the synovial lining and reflection is seen in trauma (hemorrhagic effusions with ACL tears and fractures), inflammatory arthritis, pigmented villonodular synovitis, hemophilia, and infection (septic arthritis).

- Synovial hypertrophy (hypertrophic villous fronds) in thickened synovium is typically located between periarticular fat and joint fluid and is visualized as intermediate signal intensity on PD or FS PD FSE images.

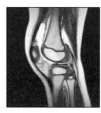

JUVENILE CHRONIC ARTHRITIS

- Juvenile chronic arthritis is divided into pauciarticular, polyarticular, and systemic-onset patterns.
- Joint effusions, synovitis (irregular fat pad sign), and low- to intermediate-signal-intensity synovial thickening are seen in early disease.

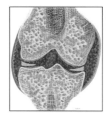

RHEUMATOID ARTHRITIS
(See Figures 4.196–4.198)

- MR imaging signs in rheumatoid arthritis include soft tissue swelling and the direct visualization of intermediate-signal-intensity pannus tissue, juxta-articular osteoporosis (marrow inhomogeneity), loss of the subchondral plate, erosion, subchondral cysts, and joint space narrowing.

- FS PD FSE images demonstrate subchondral marrow edema, and IV contrast enhances thickened synovium.

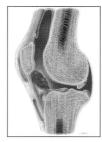

PIGMENTED VILLONODULAR SYNOVITIS
(See Figures 4.199–4.200)

- PVNS presents as either a localized or nodular type of mass posterior to Hoffa's fat pad or a diffuse type with distribution through joint recesses.
- Localized or nodular PVNS is also known as localized nodular synovitis, emphasizing its common location involving the infrapatellar fat pad, lack of diffuse frond-like projections of synovium, and decreased hemosiderin deposition compared to diffuse PVNS.

- T2* GRE images demonstrate greater susceptibility to increased hemosiderin content in diffuse PVNS than in localized or nodular PVNS.

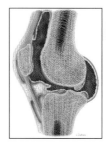

HEMOPHILIA

- Recurrent hemorrhage into the knee joint is typical in hemophilic arthropathy.
- An irregular infrapatellar fat-pad sign with hypointense hemosiderin deposited in a thickened synovial reflection is characteristic.

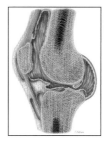

LYME ARTHRITIS

- Lyme arthritis can be identified by the finding of an irregular fat pad within the affected knee without pannus formation.

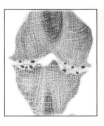

OSTEOARTHRITIS
(See Figures 4.201–4.203)

- The process of osteoarthritis begins as a fatigue fracture of the collagen meshwork followed by increased hydration of the articular cartilage, as opposed to the desiccated cartilage seen with aging.

- MR findings of early chondral erosions require FS PD FSE images.

- An irregular fat-pad sign is associated with an inflammatory component to the osteoarthritis process.

- False-positive interpretations of ACL tears increase in the presence of osteoarthritis.

- The degree of osteoarthritis-related sclerosis is underestimated on PD or FS PD FSE images. Increased accuracy in the identification of an area of sclerosis requires a T1-weighted sequence in at least one plane.

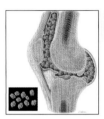

LIPOMA ARBORESCENS
(See Figure 4.206)

- Lesion consists of intra-articular fatty villonodular proliferation with well-vascularized fat covered by a uniform thickened cell lining.

- T1-weighted sequences are required to document fat signal, and FS PD FSE or STIR sequences are used to demonstrate uniform fat suppression.

- Fatty villonodular proliferation should not be mistaken for inflammatory synovitis.

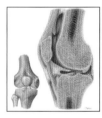

JOINT EFFUSIONS

- Modifying window level and width to the threshold of the constituents of a joint effusion increases MR sensitivity in the evaluation of synovial disorders.

- Evaluate for the contour of Hoffa's fat pad, which is irregular in synovitis.

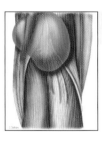

POPLITEAL AND ATYPICAL CYSTS
(See Figures 4.207–4.208)

- Atypical popliteal cysts that are not adjacent to the semimembranosus or medial head of the gastrocnemius and cysts with nonuniform signal intensity require follow-up, including IV contrast, to exclude a soft tissue sarcoma.

- A hemorrhagic popliteal cyst demonstrates characteristic susceptibility of blood product degradation.

- It is important to appreciate that the articular branch of the common peroneal nerve serves as a conduit for superior (proximal) tibiofibular joint ganglia.

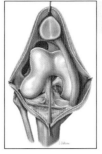

PLICAE
(See Figures 4.209–4.212)

- The suprapatellar plica can impinge on the articular cartilage of the superomedial angle of the trochlea in knee flexion. A suprapatellar septum or complete shelf may result in fluid build-up in the suprapatellar bursa and present as a soft tissue mass.

- The infrapatella plica, anterior to the ACL, may attach to the transverse ligament before coursing through Hoffa's fat pad to its inferior patellar pole attachment.

- The medial or mediopatellar plica is visualized on medial sagittal images and axial images through the patellofemoral joint. A thick or shelf-like medial plica is frequently associated with medial patellar facet chondromalacia.

- A thickened lateral patellar plica may be mistaken for lateral retinacular tissue.

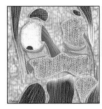

OSTEONECROSIS AND RELATED OSSEOUS DISORDERS
(See Figures 4.213–4.224)

- The subchondral fracture of spontaneous osteonecrosis of the knee (SONK) may in fact represent an insufficiency fracture without associated cellular necrosis.

- Healed or healing stages of osteochondritis dissecans may demonstrate a return to subchondral marrow fat signal intensity with varying degrees of overlying chondral degeneration.

- Epiphyseal subchondral hypointensity with overlying chondral heterogeneity can represent normal epiphyseal maturation during the ossification of the immature skeleton.

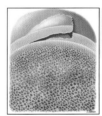

CHONDRAL AND OSTEOCHONDRAL LESIONS
(See Figures 4.225–4.231)

- FS PD FSE images are sensitive to chondral fractures, flaps, and osteochondral trauma by demonstrating the extent and location of fluid extension across the fracture segment.

- Chondral resurfacing techniques include abrasion with microfracture, osteochondral plugs (OATS), osteochondral allografts, and chondrocyte implantation.

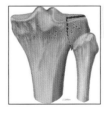

FRACTURES
(See Figures 4.232–4.234)

- Fracture morphology and associated edema may be underestimated on PD FSE or conventional T2-weighted images.

- Red marrow heterogeneity should not extend distal to the femoral physeal scar or proximal to the tibial physeal scar.

- In reflex sympathetic dystrophy, FS PD FSE or STIR images are needed to appreciate marrow hyperintensity.

INFECTION
(See Figures 4.235–4.236)

- Secondary signs of joint sepsis include intermediate-signal-intensity synovial thickening and an irregular fat-pad sign with or without fat-pad edema. Marrow edema may not be visualized until osseous extension and/or soft tissue tracts develop.

- Although GRE images are not sensitive to marrow edema, hyperintensity of subchondral bone on $T2^*$ GRE in the absence of trauma is associated with osteomyelitis in the setting of joint sepsis.

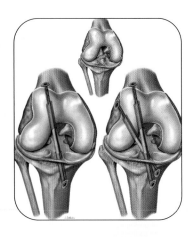

The Knee
Muscle

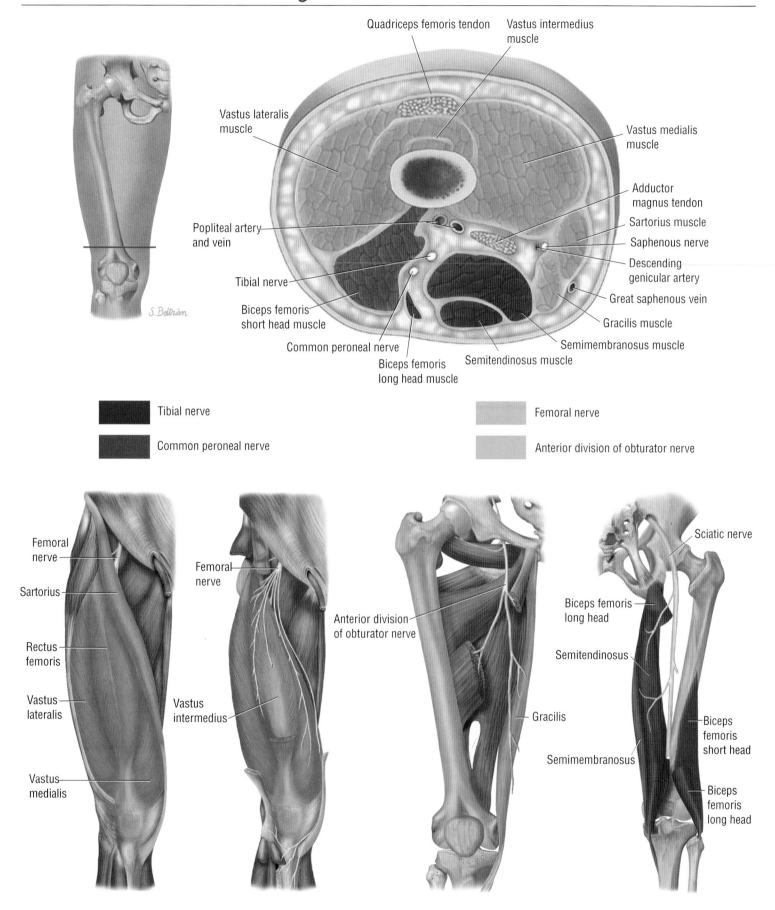

Figure 4.1 ■ Distal thigh muscle innervation. *Cross section based on Vahlensiech M, Genant HK, Reiter M. MRI of the Musculoskeletal System. New York/Stuttgart: Thieme, 2000. (See Related Muscles pg. 310, in Stoller's 3rd Edition.)*

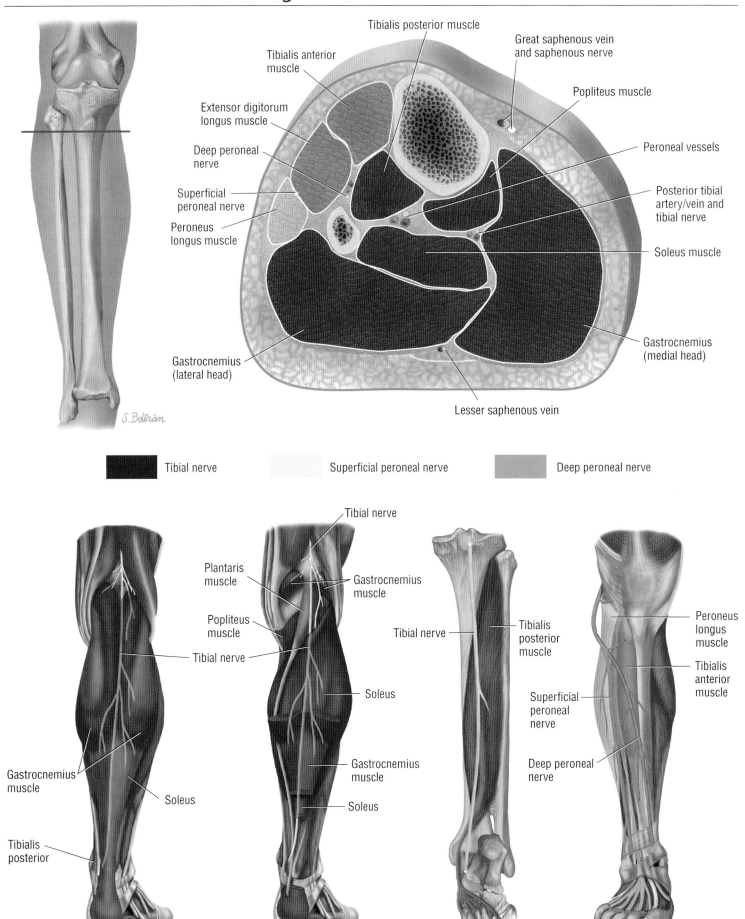

Figure 4.2 ■ Proximal leg muscle innervation. *Cross section based on Vahlensiech M, Genant HK, Reiter M. MRI of the Musculoskeletal System. New York/Stuttgart: Thieme, 2000. (See Related Muscles pg. 310, in Stoller's 3rd Edition.)*

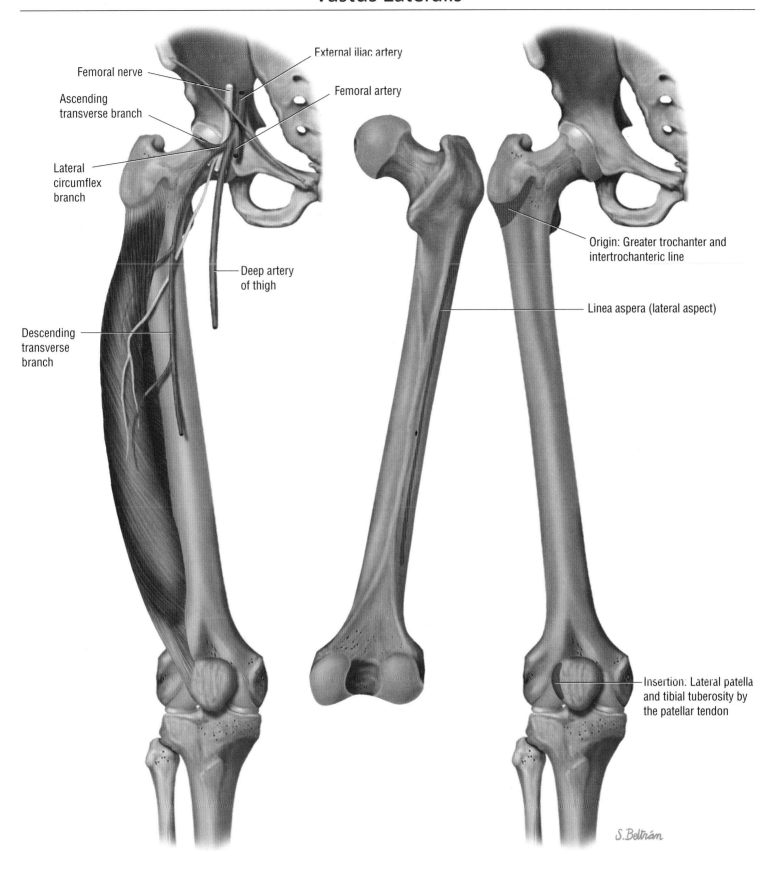

Figure 4.3 ▪ VASTUS LATERALIS. The vastus lateralis extends the leg and flexes the thigh (hip) and is one of the quadriceps muscles (the quadriceps group includes the vastus lateralis, vastus medialis, vastus intermedius, and rectus femoris). Quadriceps muscle fibers are predominantly type II, adapted for rapid forceful activity. The vastus lateralis obliquus (VLO) fibers of the vastus lateralis muscle interdigitate with the lateral intermuscular septum and insert onto the patella. The VLO may be selectively sectioned in a lateral retinacular release without involving the main vastus lateralis tendon proper. *(See Related Muscles pg. 311, in Stoller's 3rd Edition.)*

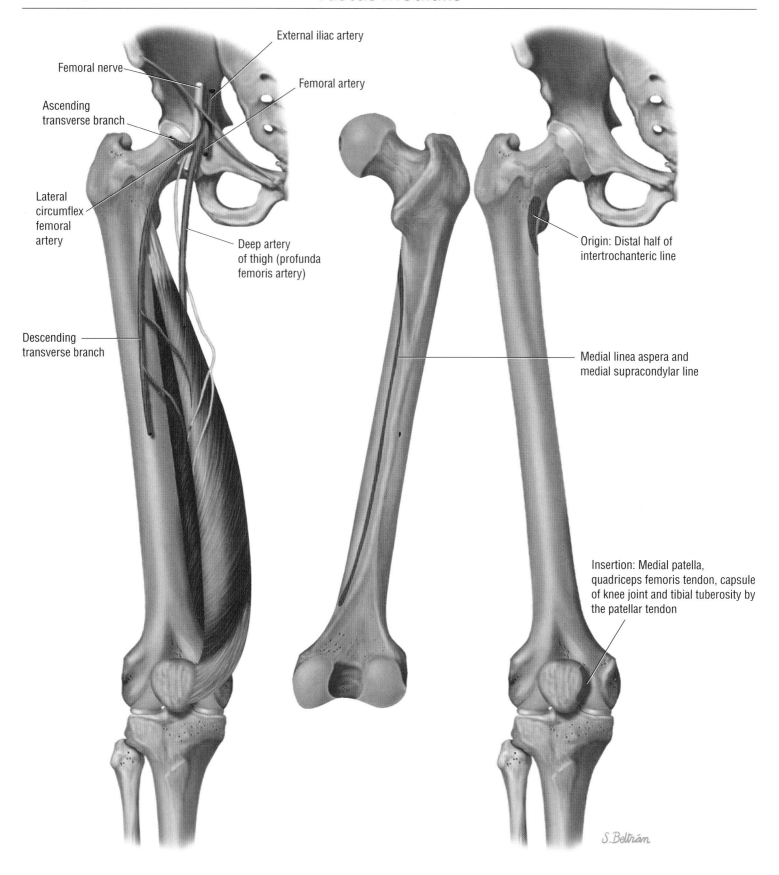

Femoral nerve

Ascending
transverse branch

Lateral
circumflex
femoral
artery

Descending
transverse branch

External iliac artery

Femoral artery

Deep artery
of thigh (profunda
femoris artery)

Origin: Distal half of
intertrochanteric line

Medial linea aspera and
medial supracondylar line

Insertion: Medial patella,
quadriceps femoris tendon, capsule
of knee joint and tibial tuberosity by
the patellar tendon

S. Beltrán

Figure 4.4 ▪ VASTUS MEDIALIS. The vastus medialis extends the leg and pulls the
patella medially. The quadriceps muscles, which include the vastus lateralis, the vastus medialis, the vastus intermedius, and the rectus femoris, converge distally, forming the quadriceps tendon, which inserts onto the proximal pole of the patella. The
vastus medialis assists in preventing patellar dislocation and may be weakened in
patellofemoral disorders. Vastus medialis obliquus injuries are associated with transient patellar dislocation. *(See Related Muscles pg. 312, in Stoller's 3rd Edition.)*

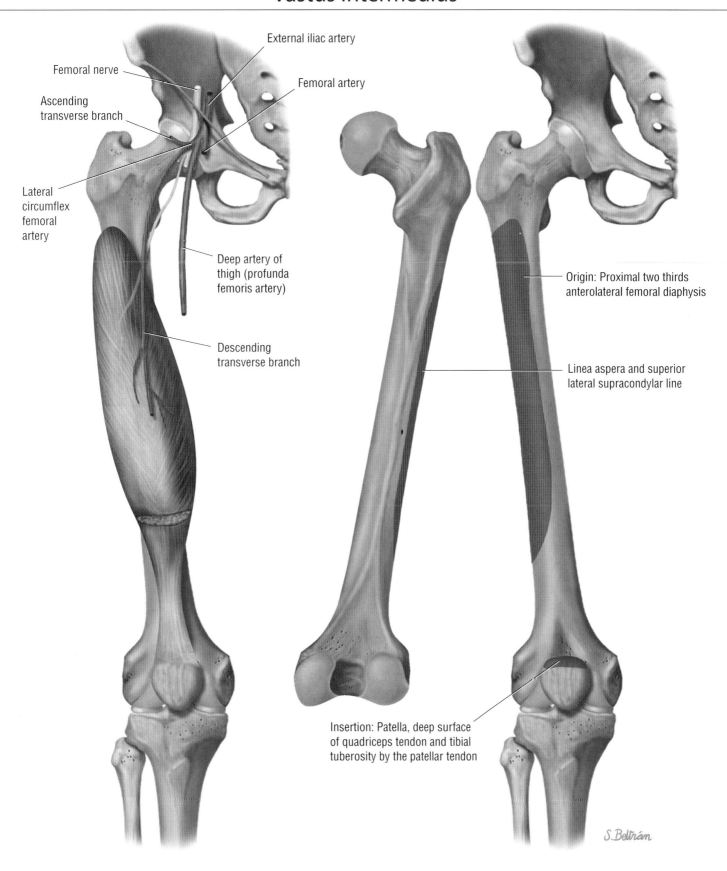

External iliac artery

Femoral nerve

Ascending transverse branch

Femoral artery

Lateral circumflex femoral artery

Deep artery of thigh (profunda femoris artery)

Descending transverse branch

Origin: Proximal two thirds anterolateral femoral diaphysis

Linea aspera and superior lateral supracondylar line

Insertion: Patella, deep surface of quadriceps tendon and tibial tuberosity by the patellar tendon

S.Beltrán

Figure 4.5 ■ VASTUS INTERMEDIUS. The vastus intermedius extends the leg and is occasionally blended with the articularis genu. Quadriceps (vastus lateralis, vastus medialis, vastus intermedius, and rectus femoris) injuries, including strains and tendon ruptures, result from eccentric muscle contractions. The articularis genu muscle is responsible for retracting the knee joint capsule superiorly in extension. *(See Related Muscles pg. 313, in Stoller's 3rd Edition.)*

Rectus Femoris

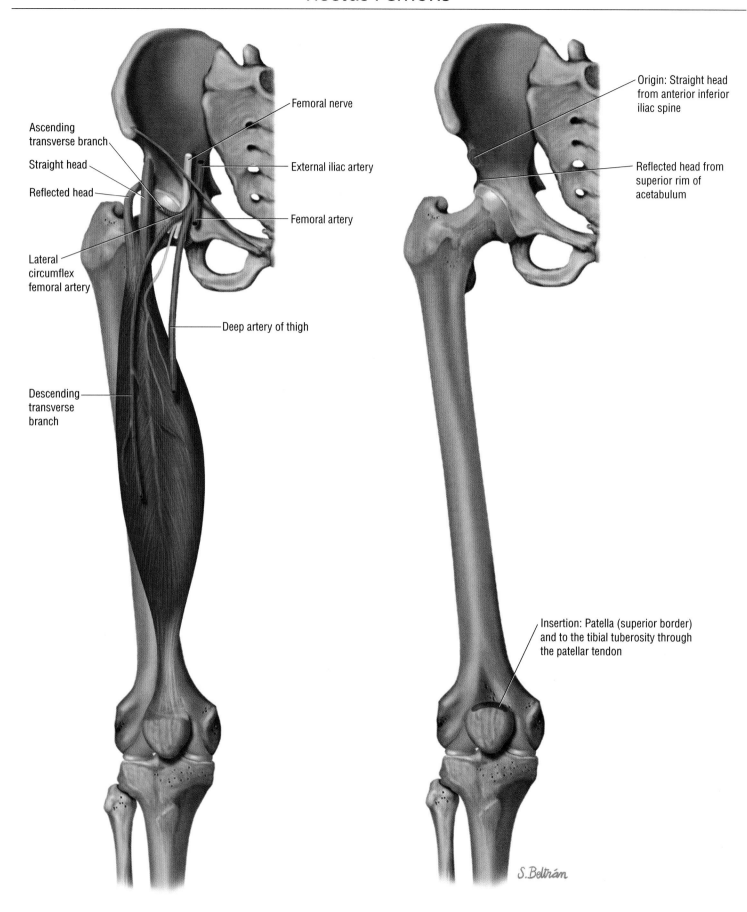

Femoral nerve

Ascending transverse branch

Straight head

Reflected head

External iliac artery

Femoral artery

Lateral circumflex femoral artery

Deep artery of thigh

Descending transverse branch

Origin: Straight head from anterior inferior iliac spine

Reflected head from superior rim of acetabulum

Insertion: Patella (superior border) and to the tibial tuberosity through the patellar tendon

S. Beltrán

Figure 4.6 ■ RECTUS FEMORIS. The rectus femoris flexes the thigh (hip) and extends the leg (knee). Of the four quadriceps muscles, only the rectus femoris has an origin that crosses the hip joint. Soccer, football, basketball, and track and field athletes are at risk for distal musculotendinous junction injuries and for proximal intrasubstance tears of the musculotendinous junction of the indirect head of the rectus femoris. *(See Related Muscles pg. 314, in Stoller's 3rd Edition.)*

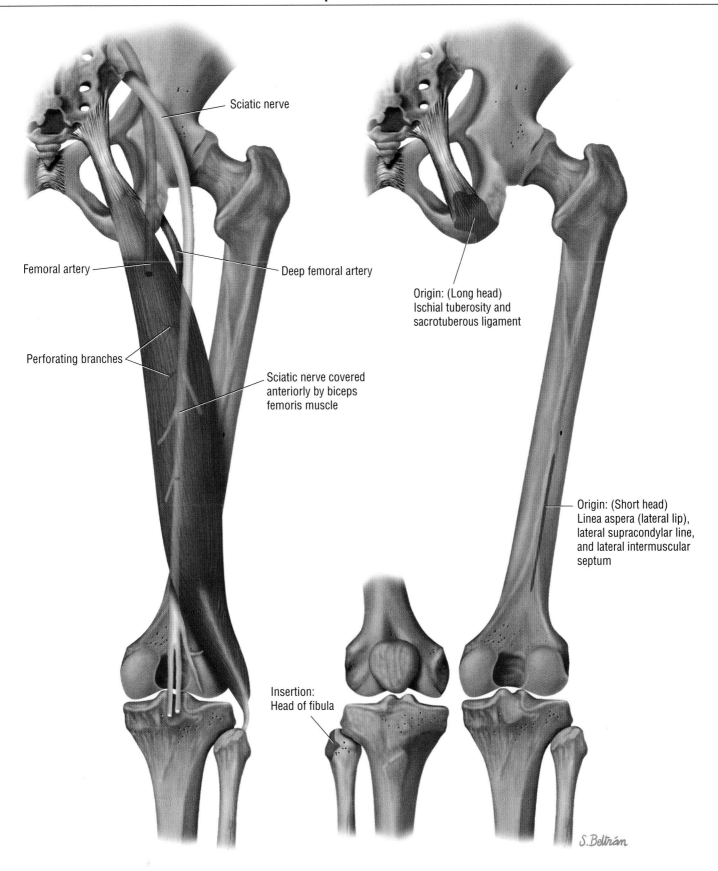

Figure 4.7 ■ BICEPS FEMORIS. The biceps femoris extends the thigh, flexes the leg, and contributes to the lateral stability of the knee as an external rotator of the tibia. The hamstring group (which includes the biceps femoris and the semimembranosus and semitendinosus muscles) all cross the hip and the knee joint, except for the short head of the biceps femoris. Musculotendinous junctions extend the entire length of the muscle and serve as potential sites for strains. The short head of the biceps femoris is innervated by the peroneal branch of the sciatic nerve. The other hamstring muscles are supplied by the tibial branch of the sciatic nerve. *(See Related Muscles pg. 315, in Stoller's 3rd Edition.)*

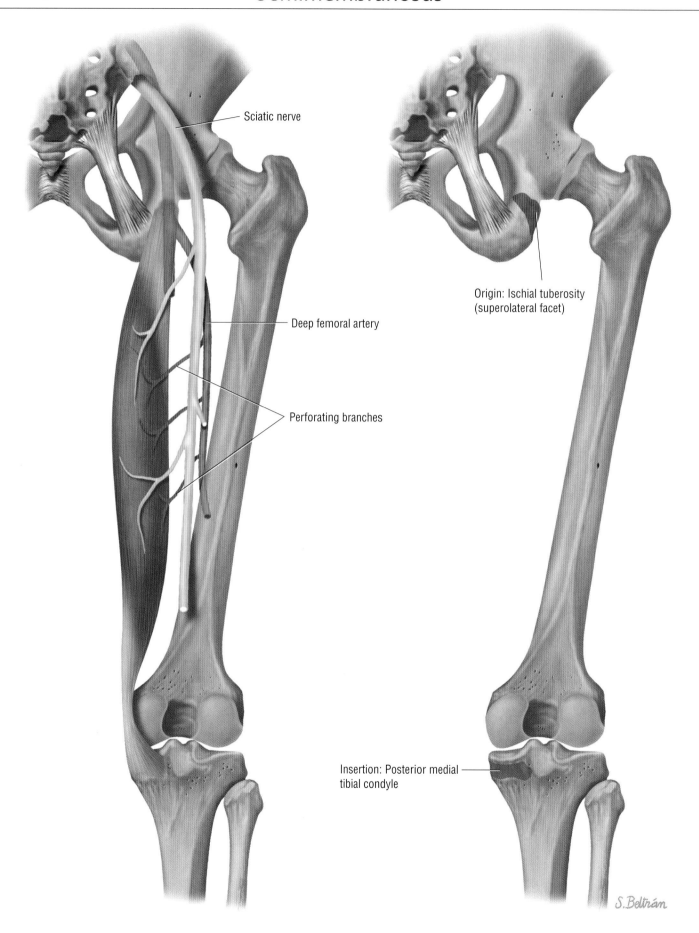

Sciatic nerve

Deep femoral artery

Perforating branches

Origin: Ischial tuberosity
(superolateral facet)

Insertion: Posterior medial
tibial condyle

S.Beltrán

Figure 4.8 ▪ SEMIMEMBRANOSUS. The semimembranosus extends the thigh and flexes the leg.
As a group, the hamstring muscle group (biceps femoris, semimembranosus, semitendinosus)
make up the posterior thigh. Except for the short head of the biceps femoris, the hamstrings arise
from the ischial tuberosity and are responsible for ischial avulsion fractures in the young athlete.
(See Related Muscles pg. 316, in Stoller's 3rd Edition.)

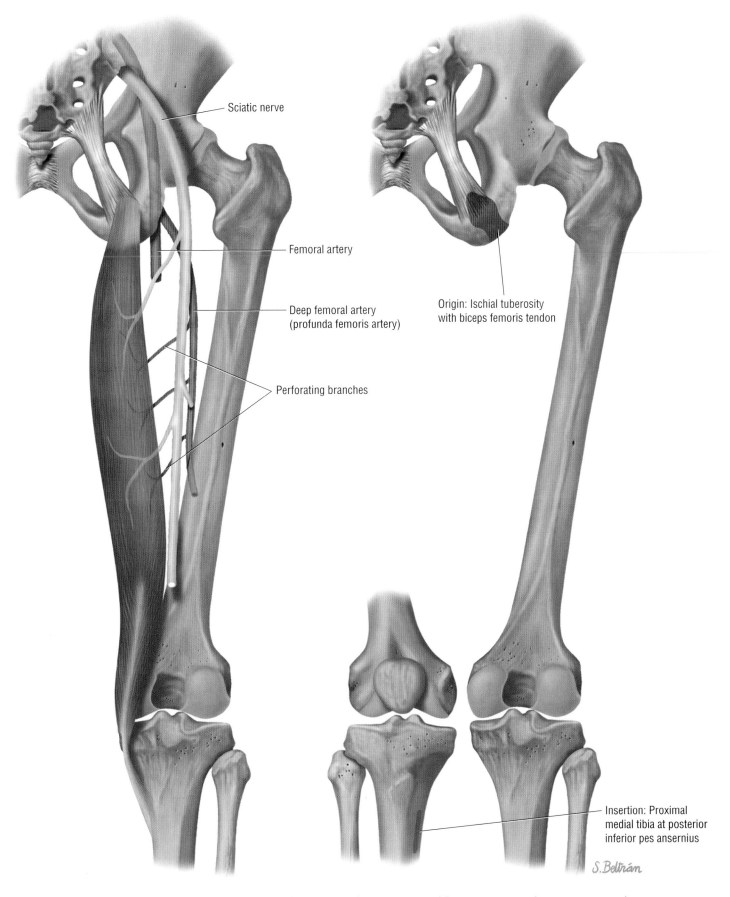

Sciatic nerve

Femoral artery

Deep femoral artery
(profunda femoris artery)

Origin: Ischial tuberosity
with biceps femoris tendon

Perforating branches

Insertion: Proximal
medial tibia at posterior
inferior pes ansernius

S. Beltrán

Figure 4.9 ■ **SEMITENDINOSUS.** The semitendinosus (part of hamstring muscle group) extends the thigh and flexes the leg. The hamstring muscles are important in anterior cruciate ligament reconstructions, in posterolateral knee reconstructions, and in tenodesis for patellar subluxation. The posteromedial tendons are seen on axial knee images at the joint line. Hip hyperflexion with simultaneous knee extension is a mechanism of injury for proximal hamstring injuries in adults and apophyseal avulsions in young skeletally immature athletes. *(See Related Muscles pg 317, in Stoller's 3rd Edition.)*

Sartorius

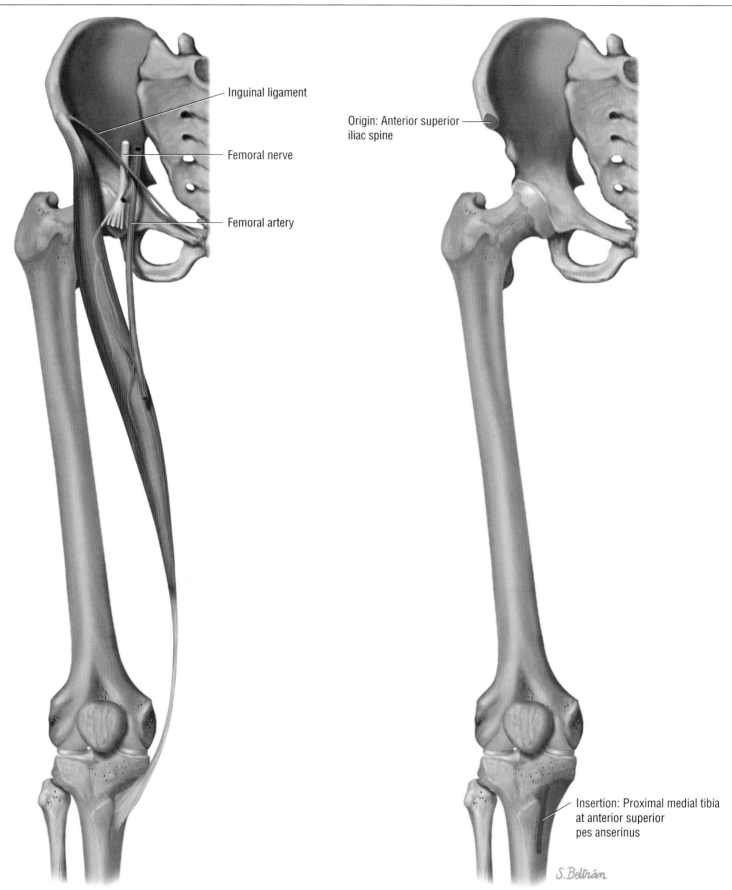

Inguinal ligament

Femoral nerve

Femoral artery

Origin: Anterior superior iliac spine

Insertion: Proximal medial tibia at anterior superior pes anserinus

S. Beltrán

Figure 4.10 ▪ SARTORIUS. The sartorius flexes and externally rotates the hip and flexes the leg on the thigh. The anterior superior iliac spine at the origin of the sartorius is a common location for an avulsion fracture. These injuries are seen in sprinters, jumpers, soccer, and football players. *(See Related Muscles pg. 318, in Stoller's 3rd Edition.)*

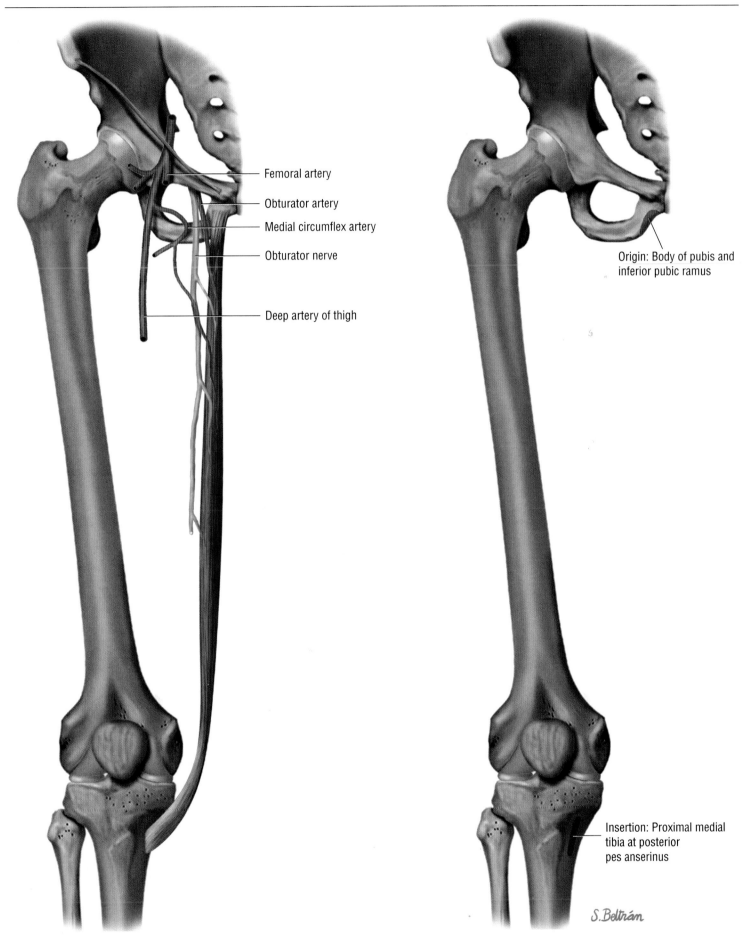

Femoral artery

Obturator artery

Medial circumflex artery

Obturator nerve

Deep artery of thigh

Origin: Body of pubis and inferior pubic ramus

Insertion: Proximal medial tibia at posterior pes anserinus

S. Beltrán

Figure 4.11 ■ GRACILIS. The gracilis adducts the thigh and flexes and internally rotates the leg. It is also used for anterior cruciate ligament reconstructions. The gracilis is the one muscle of the medial aspect adductors of the thigh (the others being the adductor longus, magnus, brevis, and the pectineus) that does not attach to the linear aspect of the femur. *(See Related Muscles pg. 319, in Stoller's 3rd Edition.)*

Popliteus

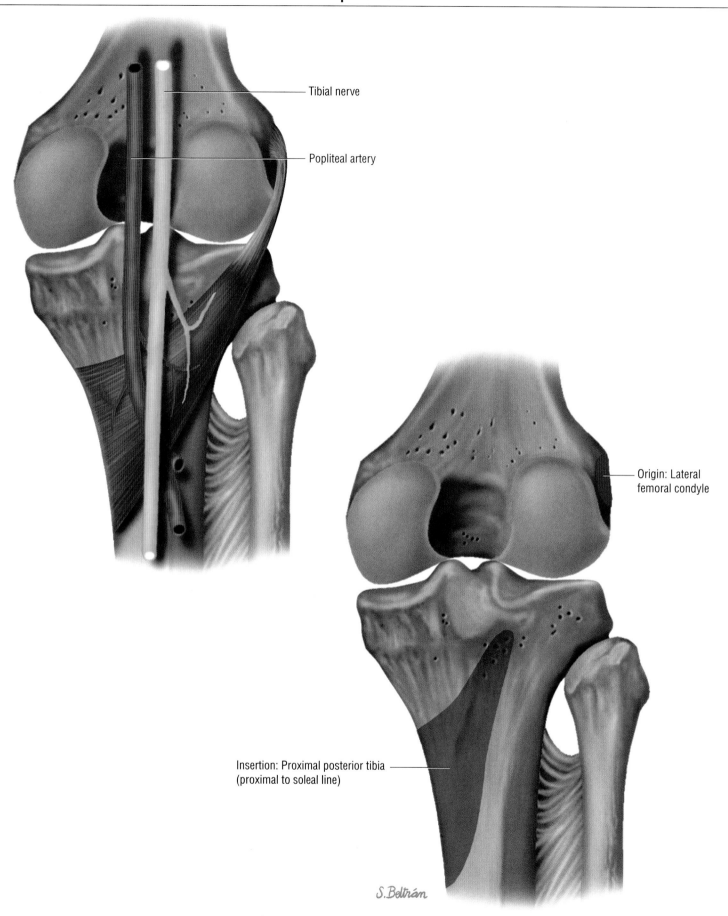

Tibial nerve

Popliteal artery

Origin: Lateral
femoral condyle

Insertion: Proximal posterior tibia
(proximal to soleal line)

S.Beltrán

Figure 4.12 ■ POPLITEUS. The popliteus flexes the knee (leg) and internally rotates the tibia at the start of flexion. It is important in injuries to the posterolateral structures. A hiatus in the coronary ligament allows passage of the popliteus tendon to its insertion on the lateral femoral epicondyle. Posterosuperior and posteroinferior popliteomeniscal fascicles attach the popliteus to the lateral meniscus. *(See Related Muscles pg. 320, in Stoller's 3rd Edition.)*

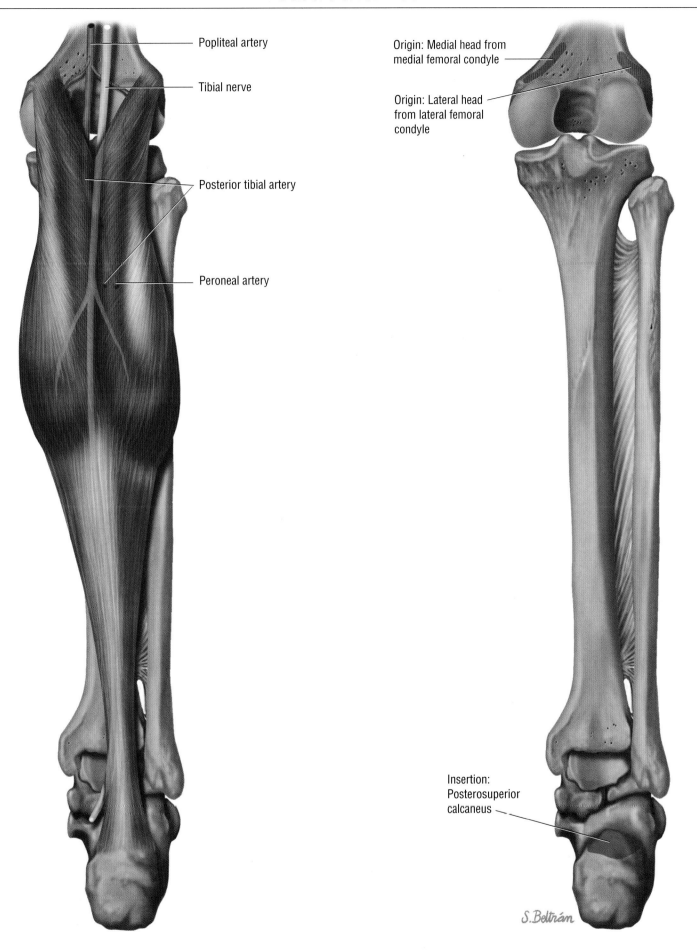

Popliteal artery

Tibial nerve

Posterior tibial artery

Peroneal artery

Origin: Medial head from medial femoral condyle

Origin: Lateral head from lateral femoral condyle

Insertion: Posterosuperior calcaneus

S.Beltrán

Figure 4.13 ■ GASTROCNEMIUS. The gastrocnemius is responsible for plantar flexion of the foot and also for flexion of the femur on the tibia. Medial head strains are frequently seen in tennis leg. Gastrocnemius fascia is used in augmentation of Achilles tendon repairs. *(See Related Muscles pg. 321, in Stoller's 3rd Edition.)*

Plantaris

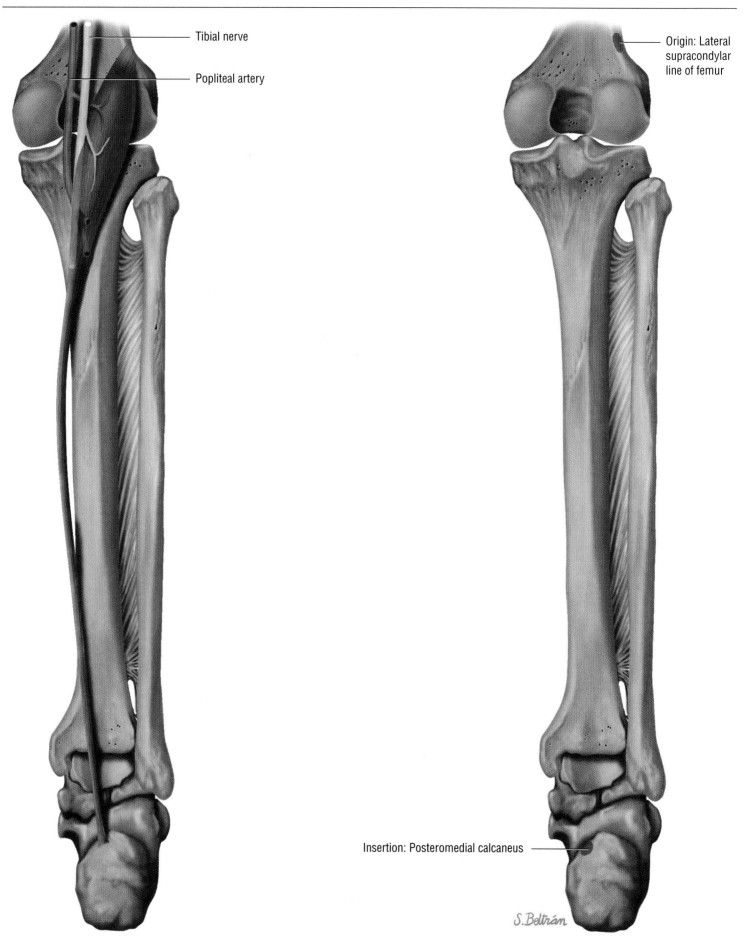

Tibial nerve

Popliteal artery

Origin: Lateral supracondylar line of femur

Insertion: Posteromedial calcaneus

S.Beltrán

Figure 4.14 ■ **PLANTARIS.** The plantaris is responsible for plantar flexion of the foot. The short muscle belly is posterolateral at the level of the knee joint and its long tendon courses between the soleus and medial head of the gastrocnemius medially. *(See Related Muscles pg. 322, in Stoller's 3rd Edition.)*

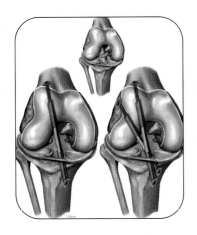

The Knee
Anatomy and Pathology

288

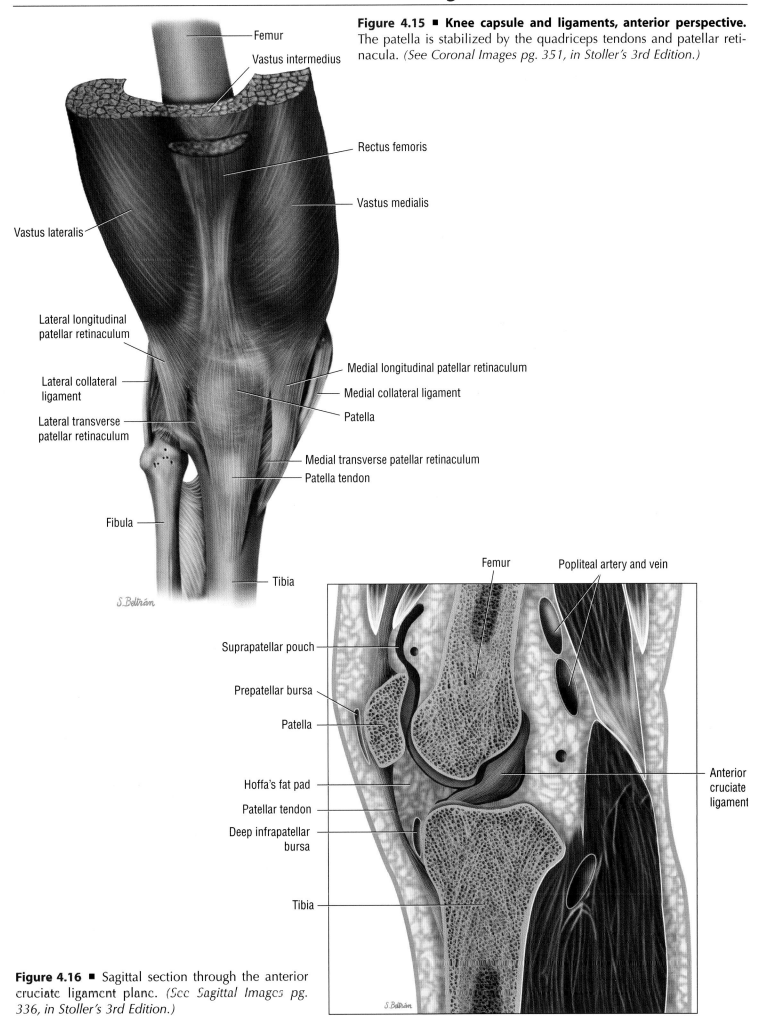

Figure 4.15 ■ Knee capsule and ligaments, anterior perspective. The patella is stabilized by the quadriceps tendons and patellar retinacula. *(See Coronal Images pg. 351, in Stoller's 3rd Edition.)*

Femur

Vastus intermedius

Rectus femoris

Vastus medialis

Vastus lateralis

Lateral longitudinal patellar retinaculum

Medial longitudinal patellar retinaculum

Lateral collateral ligament

Medial collateral ligament

Lateral transverse patellar retinaculum

Patella

Medial transverse patellar retinaculum

Patella tendon

Fibula

Tibia

Femur

Popliteal artery and vein

Suprapatellar pouch

Prepatellar bursa

Patella

Hoffa's fat pad

Patellar tendon

Deep infrapatellar bursa

Anterior cruciate ligament

Tibia

Figure 4.16 ■ Sagittal section through the anterior cruciate ligament plane. *(See Sagittal Images pg. 336, in Stoller's 3rd Edition.)*

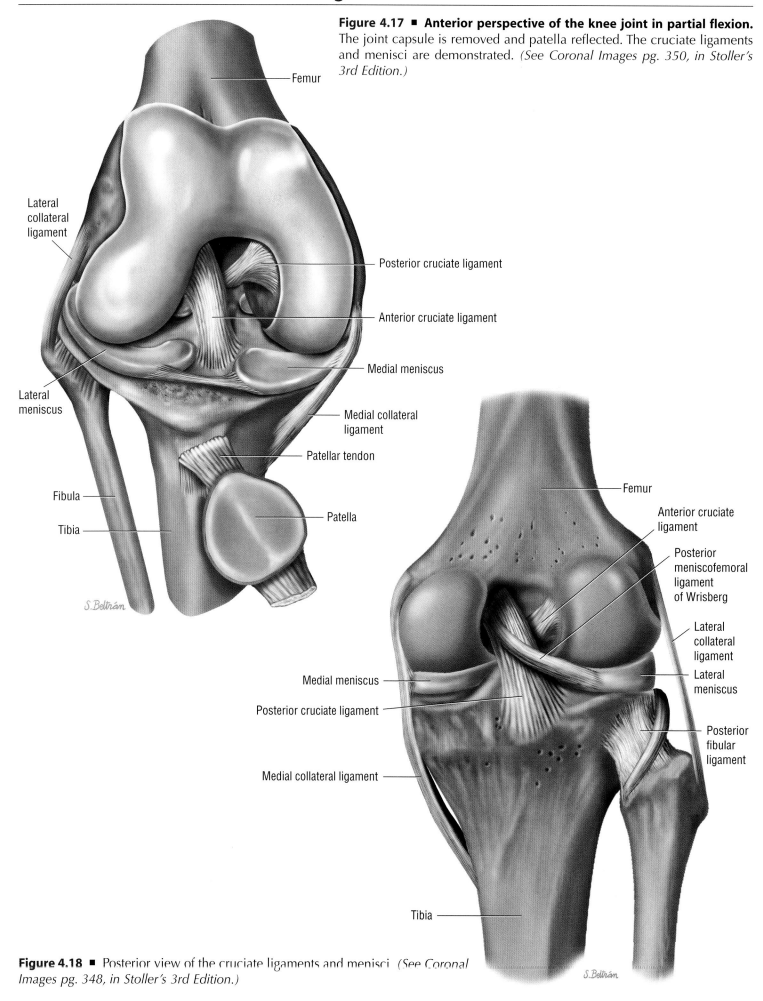

Figure 4.17 ▪ Anterior perspective of the knee joint in partial flexion. The joint capsule is removed and patella reflected. The cruciate ligaments and menisci are demonstrated. *(See Coronal Images pg. 350, in Stoller's 3rd Edition.)*

Femur

Lateral collateral ligament

Posterior cruciate ligament

Anterior cruciate ligament

Medial meniscus

Lateral meniscus

Medial collateral ligament

Patellar tendon

Fibula

Patella

Tibia

S. Beltrán

Femur

Anterior cruciate ligament

Posterior meniscofemoral ligament of Wrisberg

Medial meniscus

Lateral collateral ligament

Posterior cruciate ligament

Lateral meniscus

Medial collateral ligament

Posterior fibular ligament

Tibia

S. Beltrán

Figure 4.18 ▪ Posterior view of the cruciate ligaments and menisci *(See Coronal Images pg. 348, in Stoller's 3rd Edition.)*

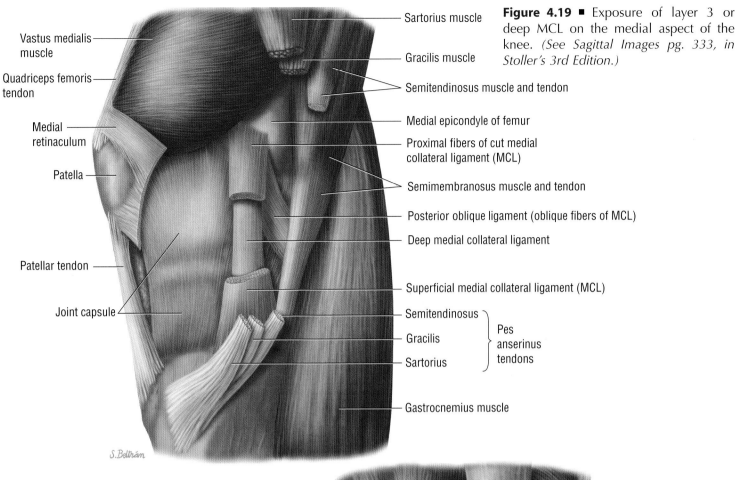

Vastus medialis muscle

Quadriceps femoris tendon

Medial retinaculum

Patella

Patellar tendon

Joint capsule

S.Beltrán

Sartorius muscle

Gracilis muscle

Semitendinosus muscle and tendon

Medial epicondyle of femur

Proximal fibers of cut medial collateral ligament (MCL)

Semimembranosus muscle and tendon

Posterior oblique ligament (oblique fibers of MCL)

Deep medial collateral ligament

Superficial medial collateral ligament (MCL)

Semitendinosus ⎤
Gracilis   ⎬ Pes anserinus tendons
Sartorius   ⎦

Gastrocnemius muscle

Figure 4.19 ■ Exposure of layer 3 or deep MCL on the medial aspect of the knee. *(See Sagittal Images pg. 333, in Stoller's 3rd Edition.)*

Figure 4.20 ■ **Lateral retinaculum and related structures and attachment of the iliotibial band (also referred to as the iliotibial tract) to Gerdy's tubercle.** The thickened fascia lata forms a longitudinal fiber band referred to as the iliotibial tract. The iliotibial tract and tensor fasciae latae originate from the anterior superior iliac spine. The distal iliotibial tract divides into anterior intermediate and posterior fibers. Strong "Kaplan fibers" bind the iliotibial tract to the femoral diaphysis. *(See Sagittal Images pg. 335, in Stoller's 3rd Edition.)*

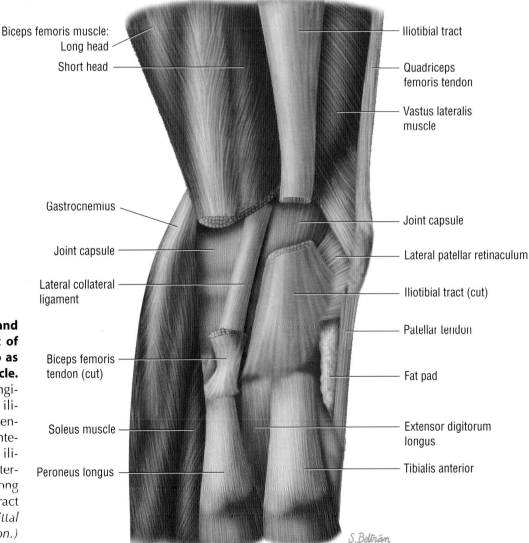

Biceps femoris muscle:
Long head

Short head

Gastrocnemius

Joint capsule

Lateral collateral ligament

Biceps femoris tendon (cut)

Soleus muscle

Peroneus longus

Iliotibial tract

Quadriceps femoris tendon

Vastus lateralis muscle

Joint capsule

Lateral patellar retinaculum

Iliotibial tract (cut)

Patellar tendon

Fat pad

Extensor digitorum longus

Tibialis anterior

S.Beltrán

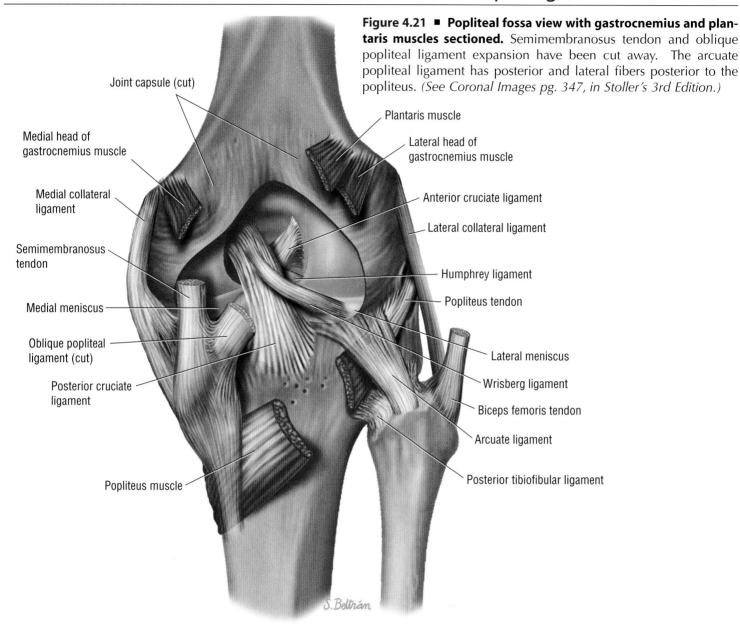

Figure 4.21 ■ **Popliteal fossa view with gastrocnemius and plantaris muscles sectioned.** Semimembranosus tendon and oblique popliteal ligament expansion have been cut away. The arcuate popliteal ligament has posterior and lateral fibers posterior to the popliteus. *(See Coronal Images pg. 347, in Stoller's 3rd Edition.)*

Joint capsule (cut)

Medial head of gastrocnemius muscle

Medial collateral ligament

Semimembranosus tendon

Medial meniscus

Oblique popliteal ligament (cut)

Posterior cruciate ligament

Popliteus muscle

Plantaris muscle

Lateral head of gastrocnemius muscle

Anterior cruciate ligament

Lateral collateral ligament

Humphrey ligament

Popliteus tendon

Lateral meniscus

Wrisberg ligament

Biceps femoris tendon

Arcuate ligament

Posterior tibiofibular ligament

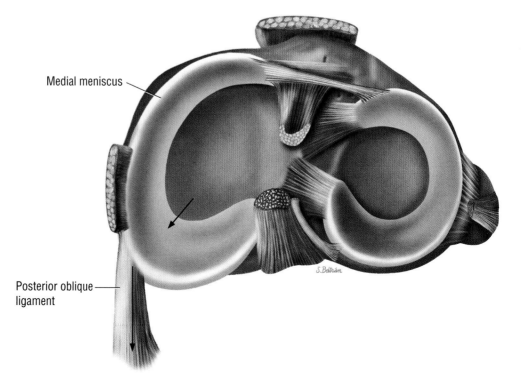

Medial meniscus

Posterior oblique ligament

Figure 4.22 ■ **Superior view of the menisci showing the dynamic stabilizing action of the semimembranosus pull on the posterior oblique ligament.** Tension of the posterior oblique ligament assists in posterior meniscal retraction. *(See See Coronal Images pgs. 346–347 and Axial Images pg. 325, in Stoller's 3rd Edition.)*

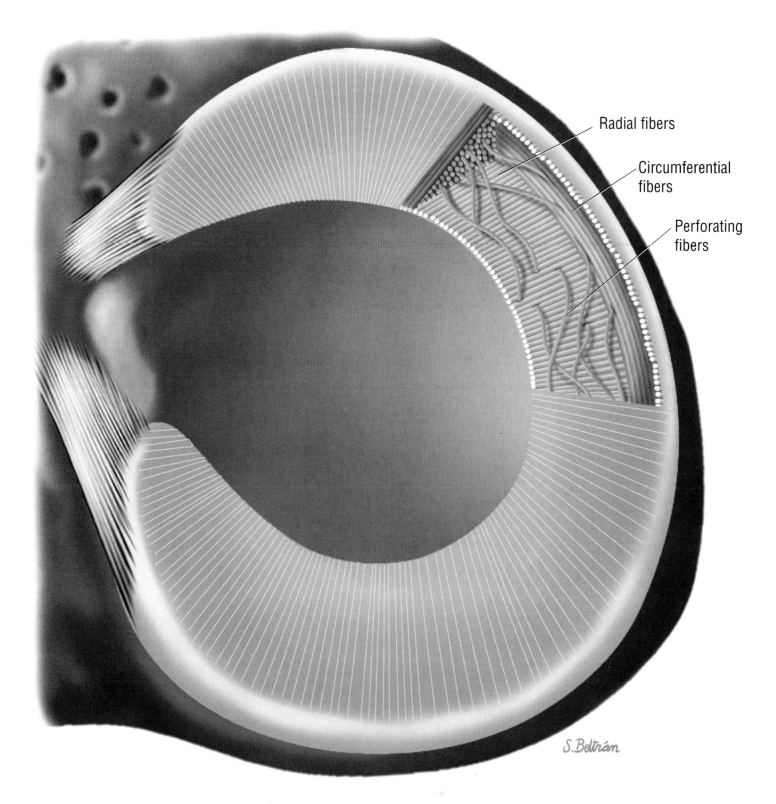

Radial fibers

Circumferential fibers

Perforating fibers

S.Beltrán

Figure 4.23 ■ **Idealized structure of meniscal fibrocartilage with peripheral circumferential fibers, radial fibers, and perforating fibers.** The middle layer of the meniscus functions in load transmission across the knee joint. Prominent and coarse collagen fibers directed in a parallel and circumferential direction to the meniscal periphery allow this middle layer to resist tensile forces. (Based on Miller RH. Knee injuries. In: Canale ST, ed. Operative Orthopaedics, 10th ed. Philadelphia: Mosby, 2003; 2184.) *(See Microstructure of the Meniscus pg. 380, in Stoller's 3rd Edition.)*

Geniculate Artery and Perimeniscal Capillary Plexus

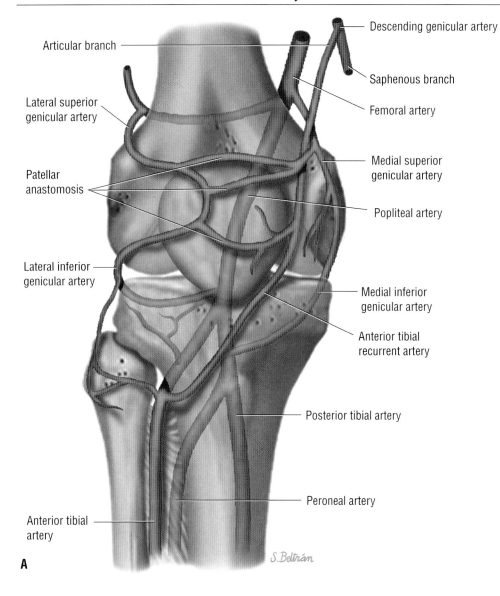

Articular branch

Lateral superior genicular artery

Patellar anastomosis

Lateral inferior genicular artery

Anterior tibial artery

Descending genicular artery

Saphenous branch

Femoral artery

Medial superior genicular artery

Popliteal artery

Medial inferior genicular artery

Anterior tibial recurrent artery

Posterior tibial artery

Peroneal artery

A

Figure 4.24 ■ **(A)** The geniculate (genicular) artery anatomy, anterior anastomosis, and branches of the popliteal artery (in transparency). The vascular circle of the patellar anastomosis supplies the patella through nutrient arteries that enter at the inferior pole. The menisci receive their vascular supply primarily from the medial and lateral geniculate arteries, with the inferior and superior branches forming the perimeniscal capillary plexus within the synovium and capsular tissues. **(B)** Peripheral blood supply to the meniscus through vascular branches of the perimeniscal capillary plexus. This plexus receives terminal branches of all four medial and lateral geniculate arteries. *(See Vascular Supply of the Meniscus pg. 383, in Stoller's 3rd Edition.)*

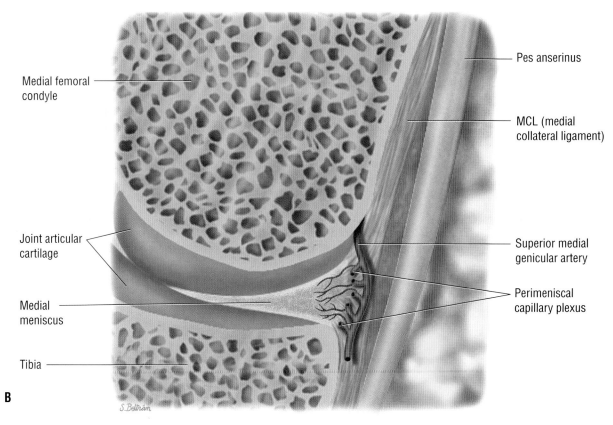

Medial femoral condyle

Joint articular cartilage

Medial meniscus

Tibia

Pes anserinus

MCL (medial collateral ligament)

Superior medial genicular artery

Perimeniscal capillary plexus

B

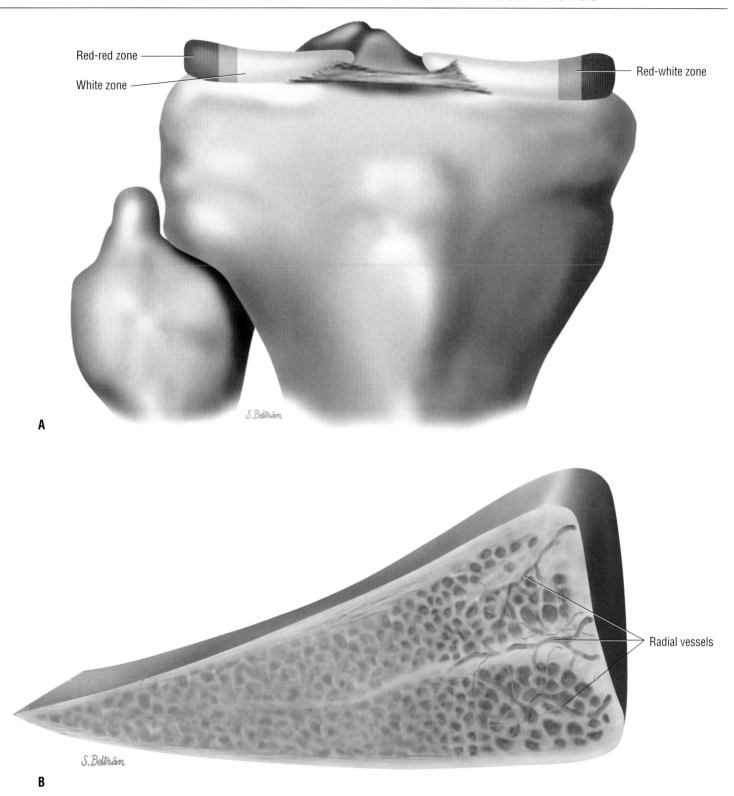

Red-red zone

White zone

Red-white zone

A

Radial vessels

B

Figure 4.25 ■ **(A)** The meniscal vascular supply is divided into zones of vascularity to help determine feasibility or success of repair. The red/red zone, the peripheral 3 mm of the meniscus, maintains an excellent blood supply. The centrally located red/white zone demonstrates variable vascularity. The white/white zone extends beyond 5mm from the periphery and represents the avascular inner portion (including the free edge) of the meniscus. **(B)** Corresponding sagittal cross-section of the meniscus. The perimeniscal capillary plexus supplies the branching radial vessels, which penetrate the peripheral or outer border of the meniscus. A circumferential pattern of perimeniscal vessels is formed with the radial branches directed centrally. Peripheral vascular penetration is 10% to 30% of the width of the medial meniscus, and 10% to 25% of the width of the lateral meniscus. *(See Vascular Supply of the Meniscus pgs. 382 and 385, in Stoller's 3rd Edition.)*

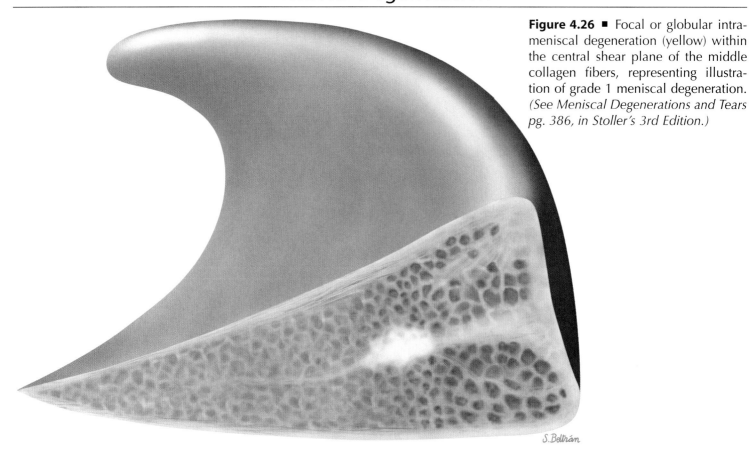

Figure 4.26 ■ Focal or globular intrameniscal degeneration (yellow) within the central shear plane of the middle collagen fibers, representing illustration of grade 1 meniscal degeneration. *(See Meniscal Degenerations and Tears pg. 386, in Stoller's 3rd Edition.)*

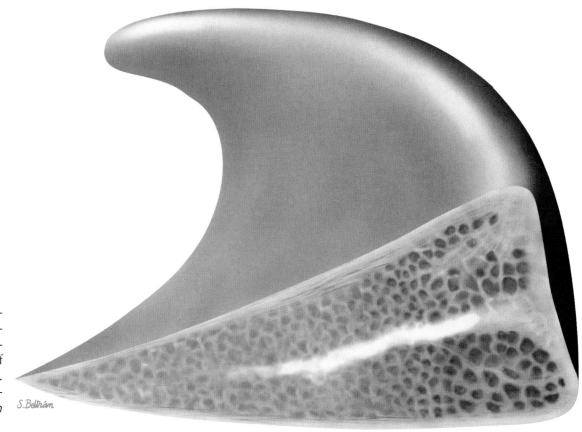

Figure 4.27 ■ Linear orientation of grade 2 intrasubstance degeneration (yellow) in the middle layer of the meniscal fibrocartilage. *(See Meniscal Degenerations and Tears pg. 388, in Stoller's 3rd Edition.)*

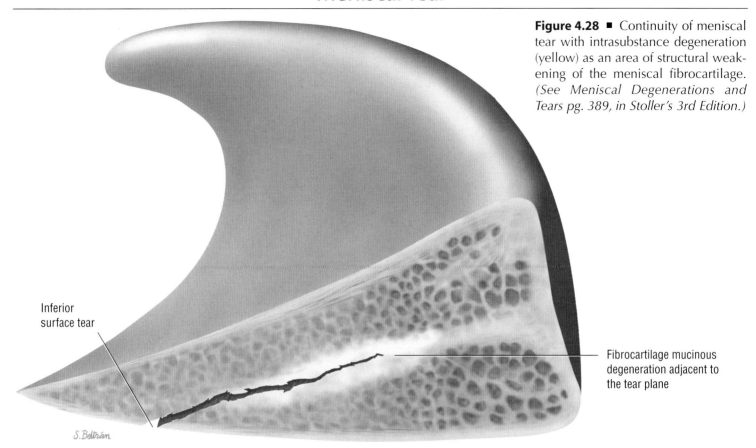

Figure 4.28 ■ Continuity of meniscal tear with intrasubstance degeneration (yellow) as an area of structural weakening of the meniscal fibrocartilage. *(See Meniscal Degenerations and Tears pg. 389, in Stoller's 3rd Edition.)*

Inferior surface tear

Fibrocartilage mucinous degeneration adjacent to the tear plane

S.Beltrán

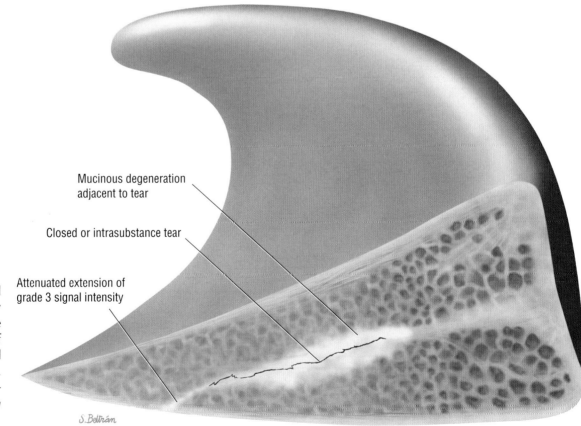

Mucinous degeneration adjacent to tear

Closed or intrasubstance tear

Attenuated extension of grade 3 signal intensity

Figure 4.29 ■ Attenuated grade 3 signal intensity that weakens toward the inferior articular surface of the meniscus in a closed tear (sagittal perspective). *(See Meniscal Degenerations and Tears pg. 391, in Stoller's 3rd Edition.)*

S.Beltrán

Meniscal Tear Patterns

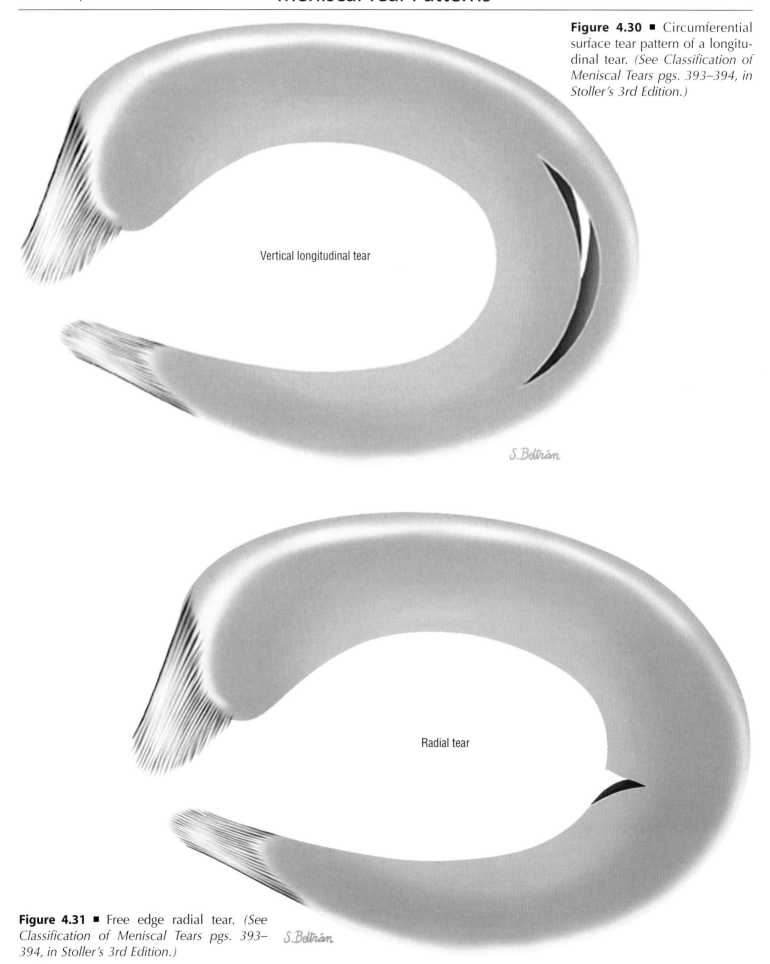

Vertical longitudinal tear

Radial tear

S.Beltrán

S.Beltrán

Figure 4.30 ■ Circumferential surface tear pattern of a longitudinal tear. *(See Classification of Meniscal Tears pgs. 393–394, in Stoller's 3rd Edition.)*

Figure 4.31 ■ Free edge radial tear. *(See Classification of Meniscal Tears pgs. 393–394, in Stoller's 3rd Edition.)*

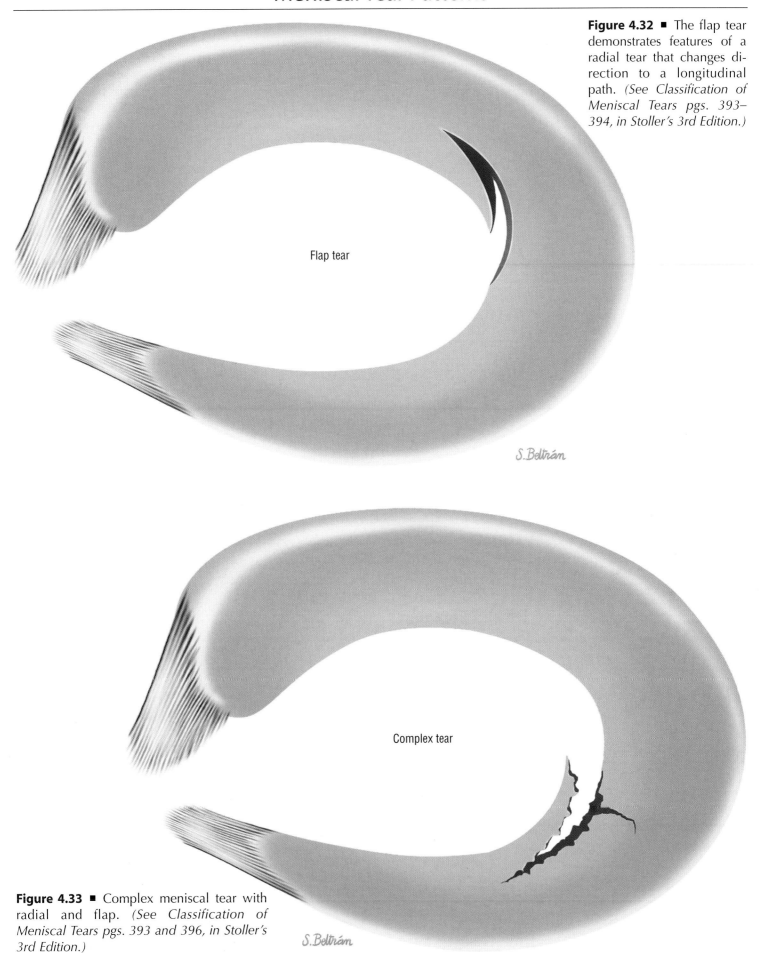

Figure 4.32 ■ The flap tear demonstrates features of a radial tear that changes direction to a longitudinal path. *(See Classification of Meniscal Tears pgs. 393–394, in Stoller's 3rd Edition.)*

Flap tear

S. Beltrán

Complex tear

Figure 4.33 ■ Complex meniscal tear with radial and flap. *(See Classification of Meniscal Tears pgs. 393 and 396, in Stoller's 3rd Edition.)*

S. Beltrán

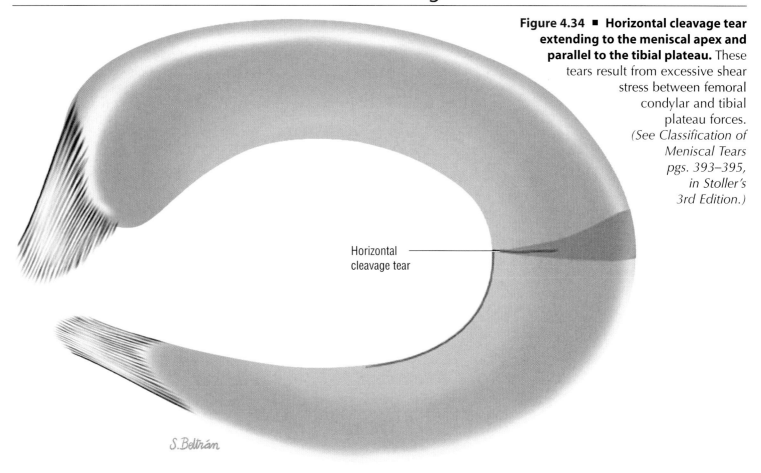

Figure 4.34 ■ **Horizontal cleavage tear extending to the meniscal apex and parallel to the tibial plateau.** These tears result from excessive shear stress between femoral condylar and tibial plateau forces. *(See Classification of Meniscal Tears pgs. 393–395, in Stoller's 3rd Edition.)*

Horizontal cleavage tear

S.Beltrán

Figure 4.35 ■ Horizontal cleavage tear divides the meniscus into superior and inferior leaflets. *(See Classification of Meniscal Tears pg. 396, in Stoller's 3rd Edition.)*

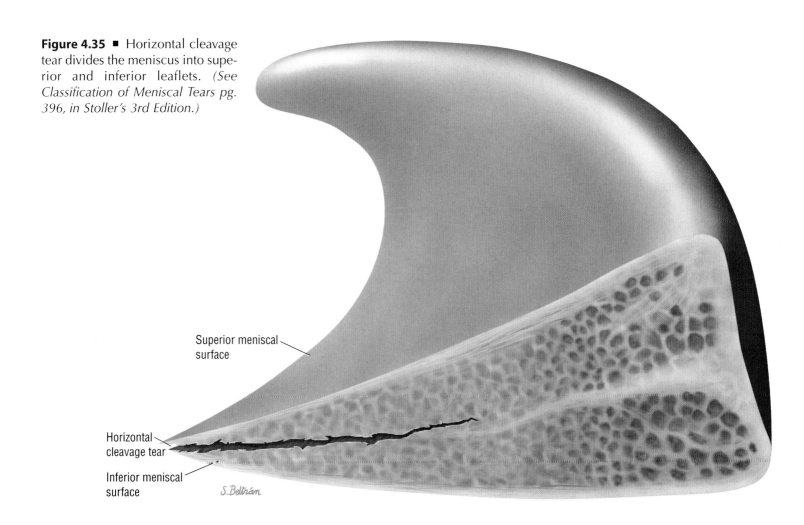

Superior meniscal surface

Horizontal cleavage tear

Inferior meniscal surface

S.Beltrán

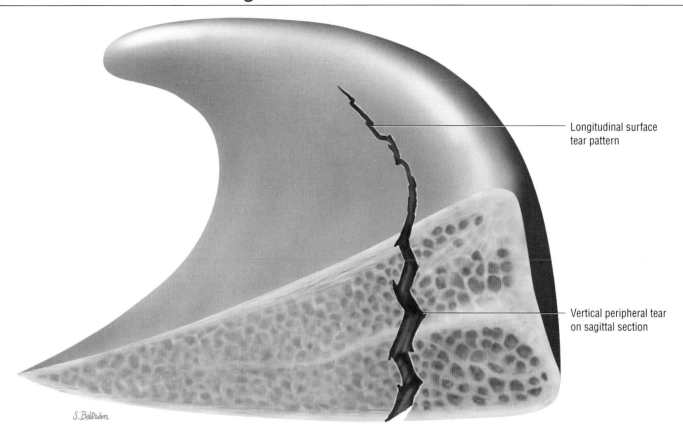

Figure 4.36 ■ **Longitudinal tear with peripheral vertical orientation through the circumferential collagen fibers.** These tears result from excessive axial loads that produce radial strain that exceeds the capacity of the radial tie fibers to resist plastic deformation. Longitudinal tears are associated with ACL injuries because the meniscus may become trapped between the distal femoral condyle and the tibial plateau. Sagittal cross-section of a vertical longitudinal tear pattern. *(See Longitudinal Tears pg. 399, in Stoller's 3rd Edition.)*

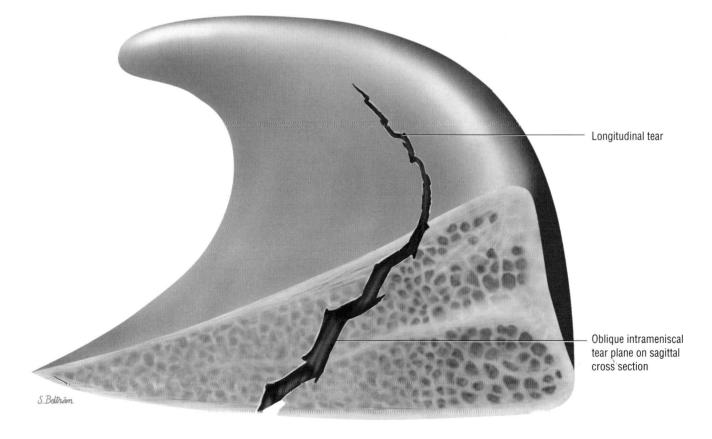

Figure 4.37 ■ Surface longitudinal tear created by a cross-sectional pattern of vertical and horizontal forces, producing an oblique tear plane. *(See Longitudinal Tears pg. 399, in Stoller's 3rd Edition.)*

Figure 4.38 ■ Displaced fragment of a medial meniscus bucket-handle tear lodged within the intercondylar notch. The intercondylar notch fragments are identified anterior to the PCL. *(See Bucket-Handle Tears pg. 403, in Stoller's 3rd Edition.)*

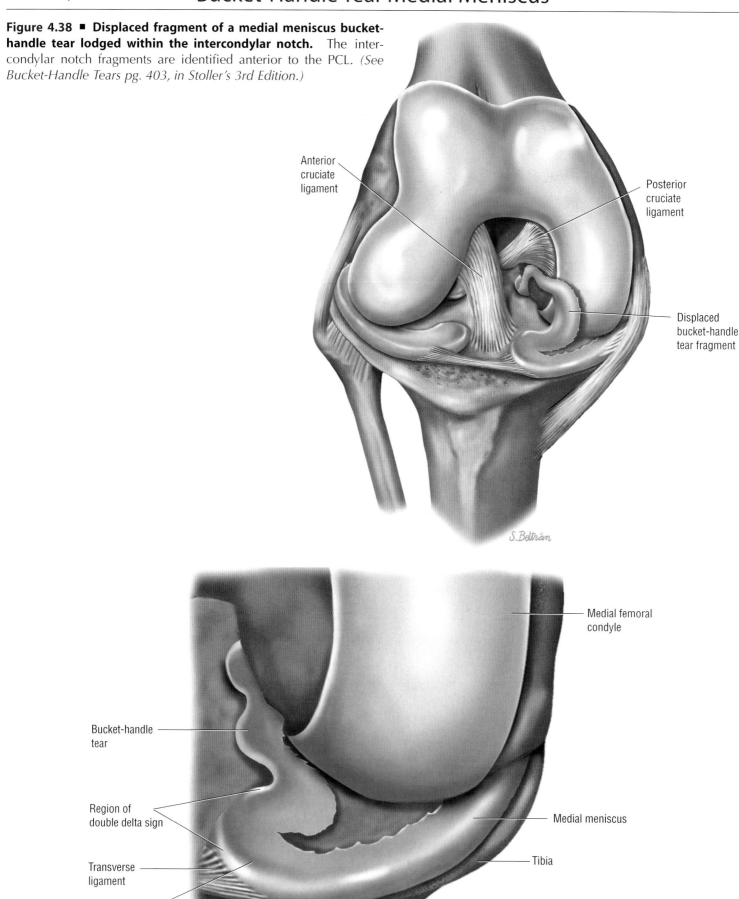

Figure 4.39 ■ Bucket-handle tear with the peripheral meniscus shown as the source of the bucket-handle fragment. The anterior double delta sign is created by the location of the anterior portion of the displaced fragment adjacent (posterior) to the native anterior horn of the meniscus. *(See Bucket-Handle Tears pg. 404, in Stoller's 3rd Edition.)*

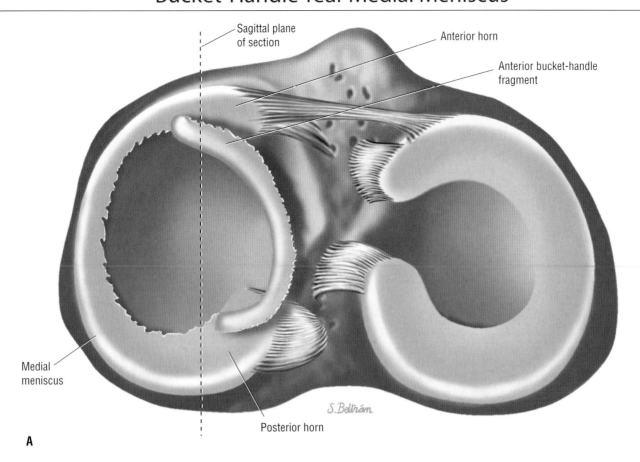

Sagittal plane of section

Anterior horn

Anterior bucket-handle fragment

Medial meniscus

Posterior horn

A

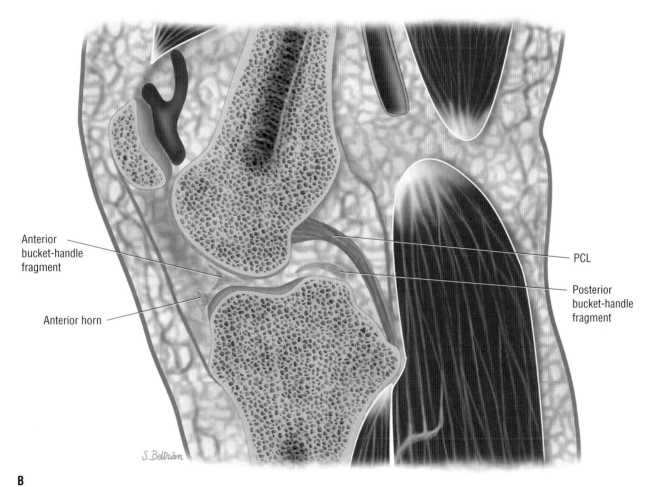

Anterior bucket-handle fragment

Anterior horn

PCL

Posterior bucket-handle fragment

B

Figure 4.40 ■ Double delta and double PCL signs. (A) Axial perspective color illustration showing the displaced fragment in proximity and posterior to the anterior horn segment. The central portion of the bucket fragment is responsible for the double PCL sign. (B) Corresponding sagittal section with double delta and double PCL fragments. *(See Bucket-Handle Tears pg. 405, in Stoller's 3rd Edition.)*

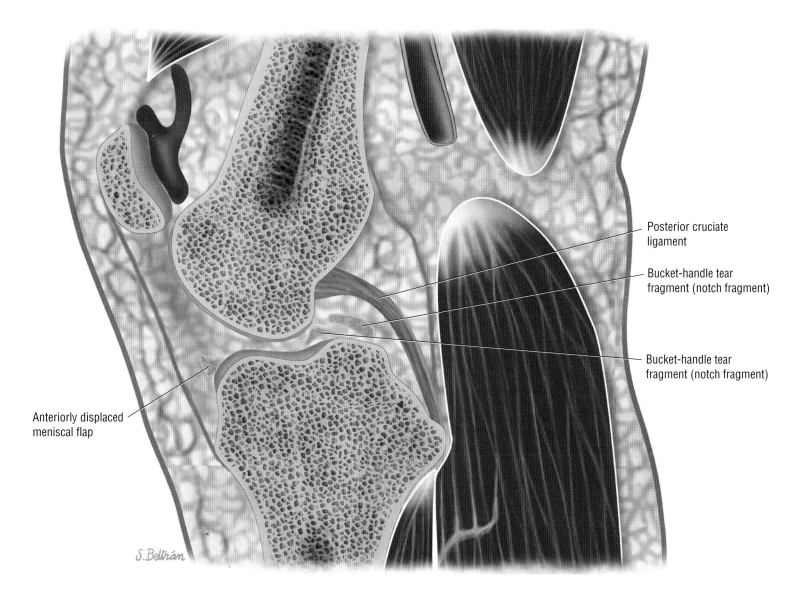

Posterior cruciate
ligament

Bucket-handle tear
fragment (notch fragment)

Bucket-handle tear
fragment (notch fragment)

Anteriorly displaced
meniscal flap

S.Beltrán

Figure 4.41 ▪ Increased gap between anterior horn and bucket-handle fragments in complex bucket-handle tear. *(See Bucket-Handle Tears pg. 407, in Stoller's 3rd Edition.)*

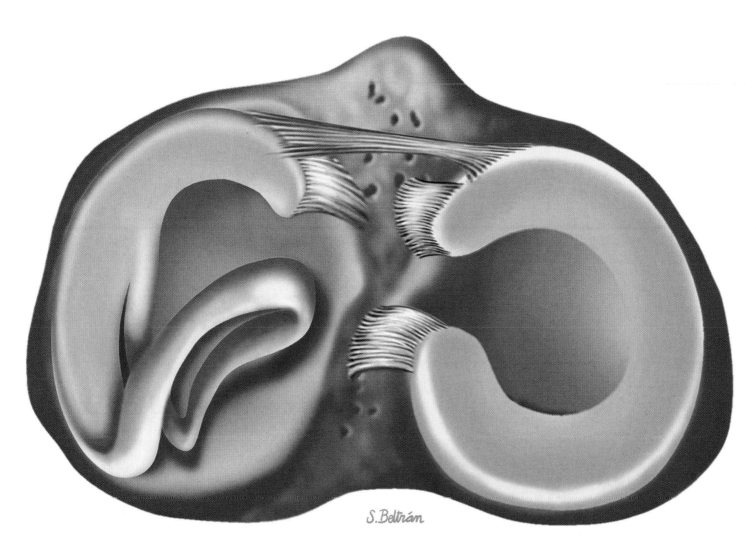

Figure 4.42 ■ Axial view, complex bucket-handle tear with greater posterior horn body involvement. *(See Bucket-Handle Tears pg. 411, in Stoller's 3rd Edition.)*

Radial Tear

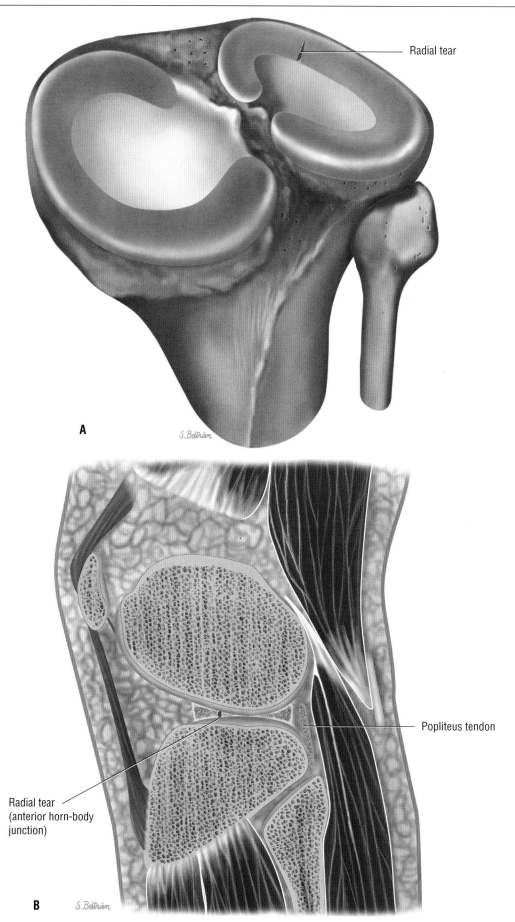

Radial tear

Popliteus tendon

Radial tear
(anterior horn-body
junction)

A

B

Figure 4.43 ▪ **(A)** Free edge radial tear at the junction of the anterior horn and body of the lateral meniscus. **(B)** Corresponding sagittal section produces the characteristic blunted foreshortened anterior horn and elongated components of the meniscal body and posterior horn. *(See Radial or Transverse Tears pgs. 409 and 414, in Stoller's 3rd Edition.)*

Radial Tear

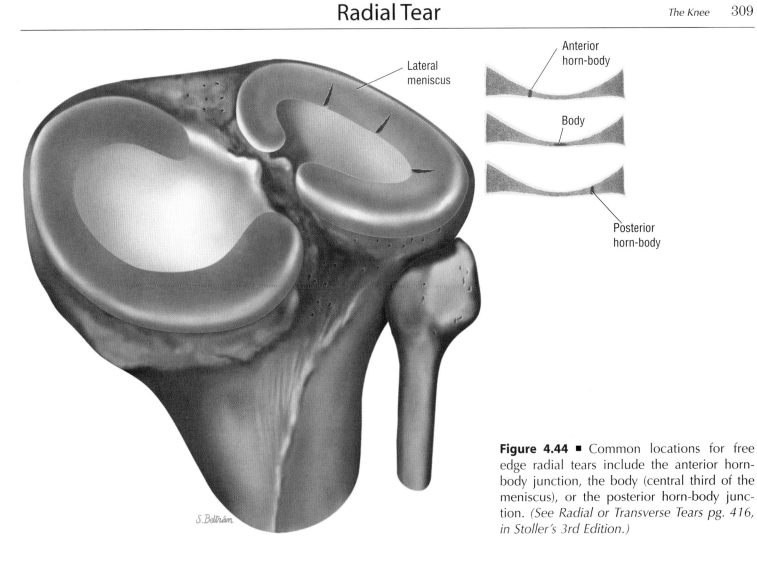

Lateral
meniscus

Anterior
horn-body

Body

Posterior
horn-body

Figure 4.44 ■ Common locations for free edge radial tears include the anterior horn-body junction, the body (central third of the meniscus), or the posterior horn-body junction. *(See Radial or Transverse Tears pg. 416, in Stoller's 3rd Edition.)*

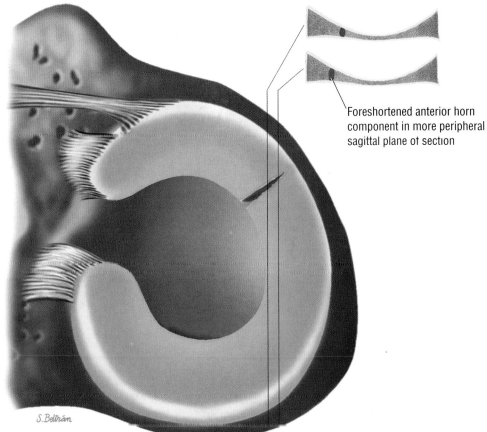

Foreshortened anterior horn
component in more peripheral
sagittal plane of section

Figure 4.45 ■ **The size of the anterior component of a classic radial tear varies depending on the location of the sagittal plane of section.** Further foreshortening of the anterior horn-body junction occurs with a more peripheral plane of section *(See Radial or Transverse Tears pg. 417, in Stoller's 3rd Edition.)*

Root Tear

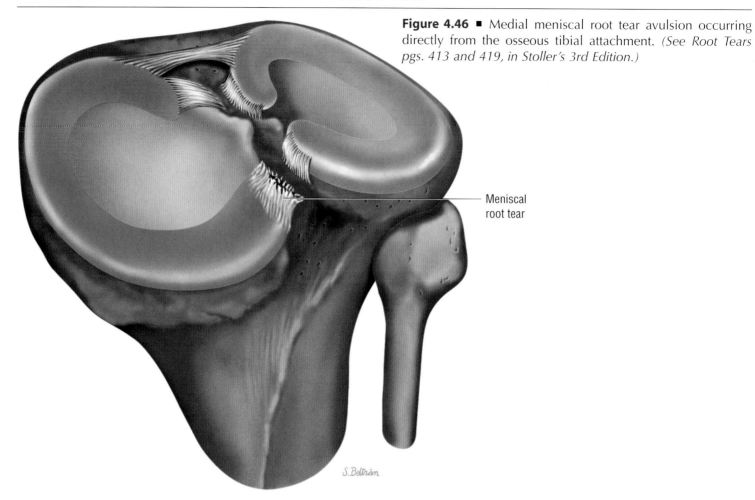

Figure 4.46 ■ Medial meniscal root tear avulsion occurring directly from the osseous tibial attachment. *(See Root Tears pgs. 413 and 419, in Stoller's 3rd Edition.)*

Meniscal root tear

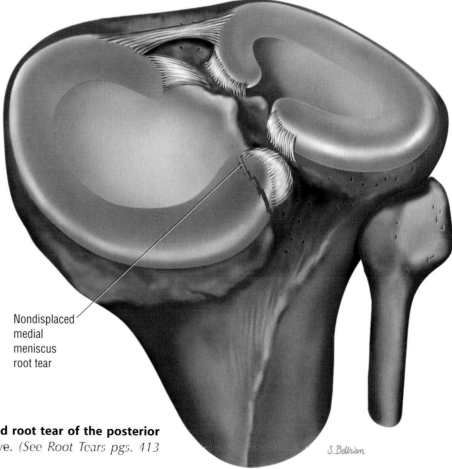

Nondisplaced medial meniscus root tear

Figure 4.47 ■ **Color illustration of non-displaced root tear of the posterior horn medial meniscus.** Posterosuperior perspective. *(See Root Tears pgs. 413 and 420, in Stoller's 3rd Edition.)*

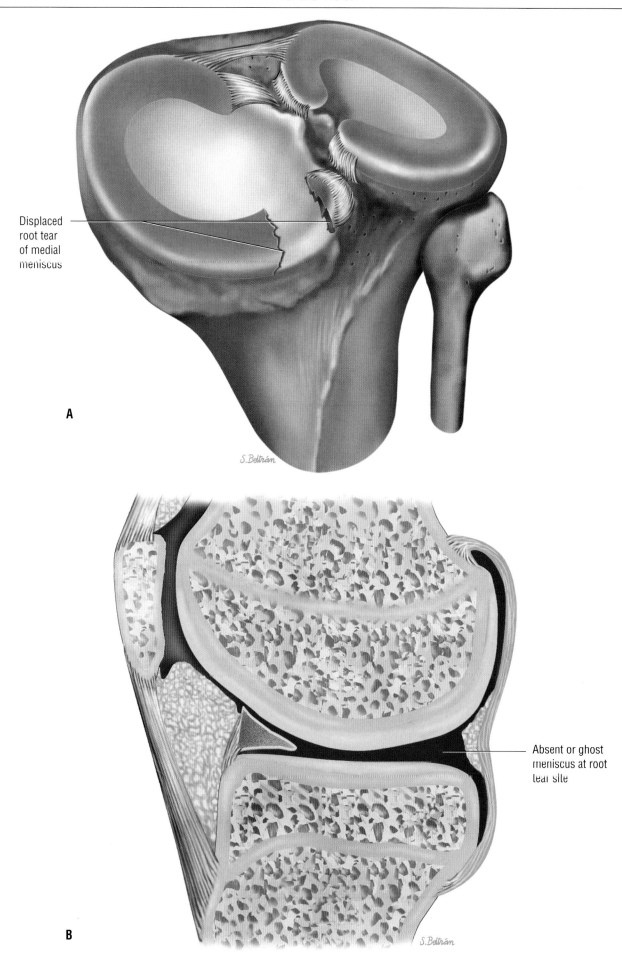

Displaced
root tear
of medial
meniscus

A

S.Beltrán

Absent or ghost
meniscus at root
tear site

B

S.Beltrán

Figure 4.48 ■ **(A)** Displaced posterior horn root tear of the medial meniscus on axial illustration. **(B)** "Ghost" meniscus is demonstrated on a corresponding sagittal illustration. *(See Root Tears pgs. 413 and 421, in Stoller's 3rd Edition.)*

Flap Tear

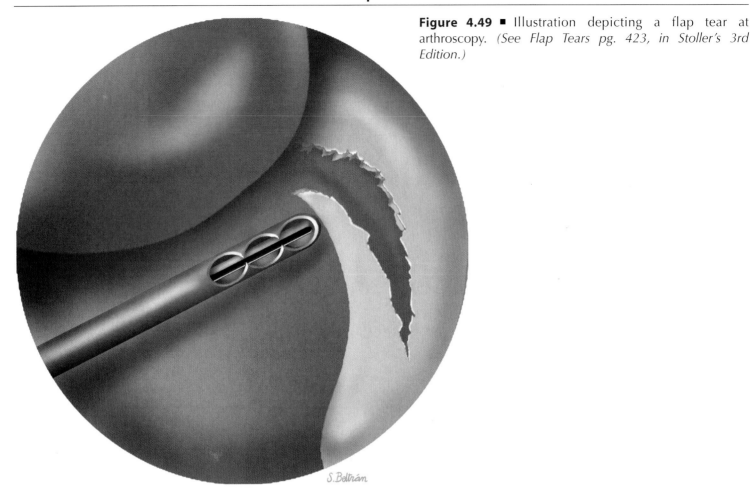

Figure 4.49 ■ Illustration depicting a flap tear at arthroscopy. *(See Flap Tears pg. 423, in Stoller's 3rd Edition.)*

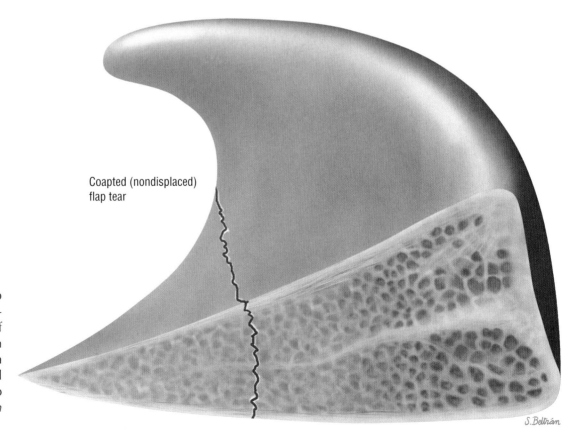

Coapted (nondisplaced) flap tear

Figure 4.50 ■ Coapted flap tear with vertical tear morphology involving the inner third of the medial meniscus as seen on a sagittal color illustration with superior and cross-sectional view of the meniscus and flap tear. *(See Flap Tears pg. 424, in Stoller's 3rd Edition.)*

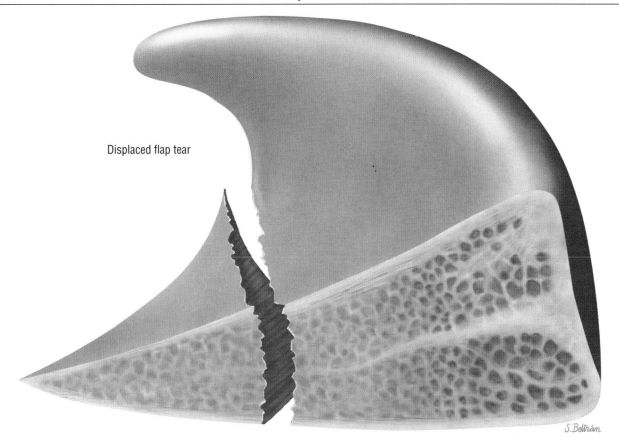

Displaced flap tear

Figure 4.51 ■ Color sagittal illustration of the superior view of a displaced non-coapted flap tear of the posterior horn of the medial meniscus. *(See Flap Tears pg. 425, in Stoller's 3rd Edition.)*

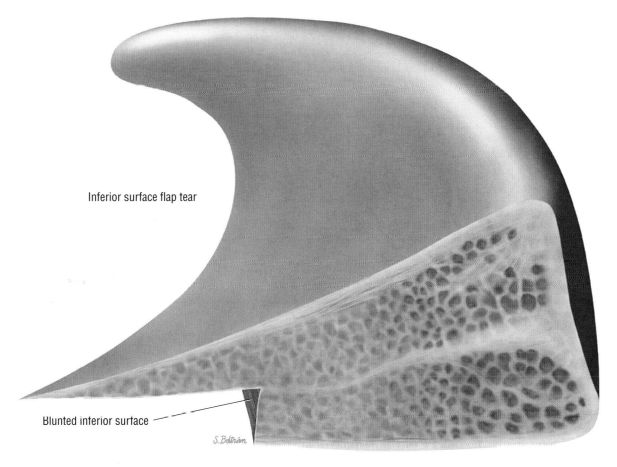

Inferior surface flap tear

Blunted interior surface

Figure 4.52 ■ Illustration of inferior surface flap tear subtype. *(See Flap Tears pg. 426, in Stoller's 3rd Edition.)*

Flap Tear

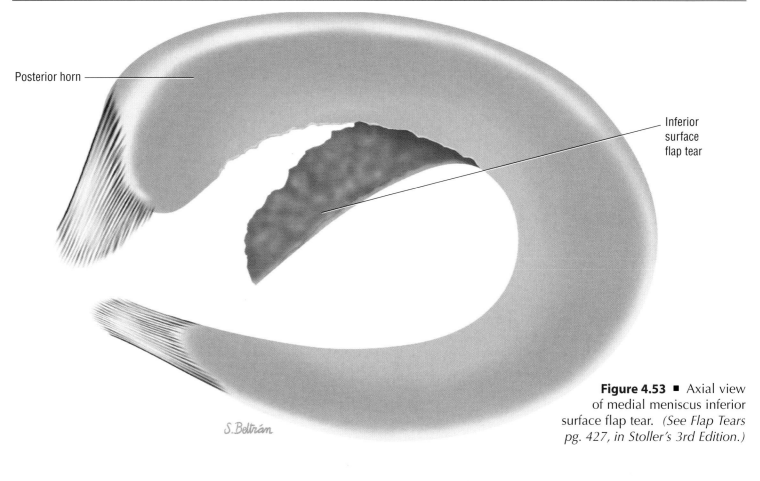

Posterior horn

Inferior
surface
flap tear

S. Beltrán

Figure 4.53 ■ Axial view
of medial meniscus inferior
surface flap tear. *(See Flap Tears
pg. 427, in Stoller's 3rd Edition.)*

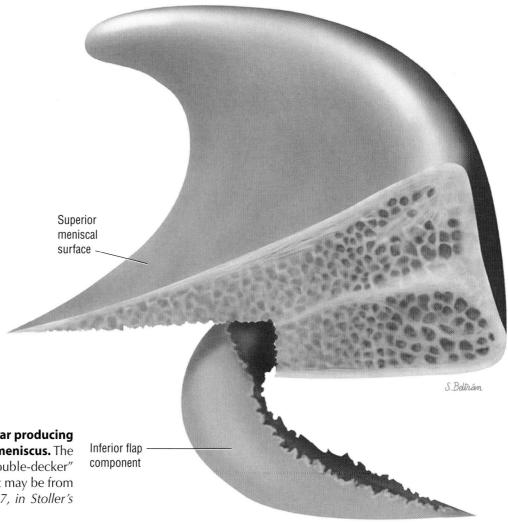

Superior
meniscal
surface

S. Beltrán

Figure 4.54 ■ **Inferior displaced flap tear producing
a blunted posterior horn of the medial meniscus.** The
stacked meniscal leaflets create a "double-decker"
pattern. Rotation of the flap tear fragment may be from
the inferior leaf. *(See Flap Tears pg. 427, in Stoller's
3rd Edition.)*

Inferior flap
component

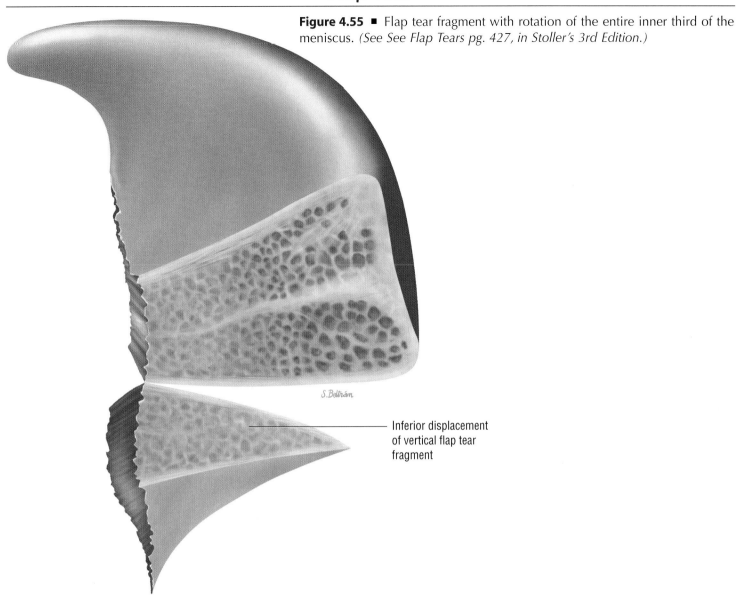

Figure 4.55 ■ Flap tear fragment with rotation of the entire inner third of the meniscus. *(See See Flap Tears pg. 427, in Stoller's 3rd Edition.)*

Inferior displacement of vertical flap tear fragment

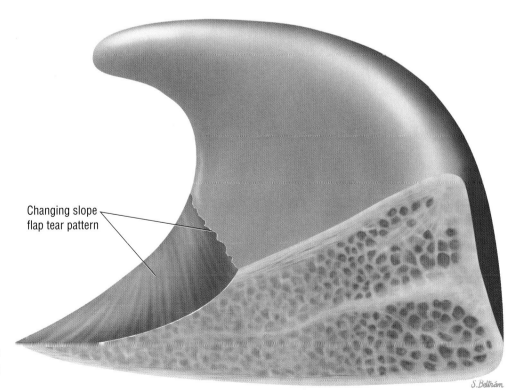

Changing slope flap tear pattern

Figure 4.56 ■ Changing slope sign of a flap tear. *(See Flap Tears pg. 427, in Stoller's 3rd Edition.)*

Flap Tear

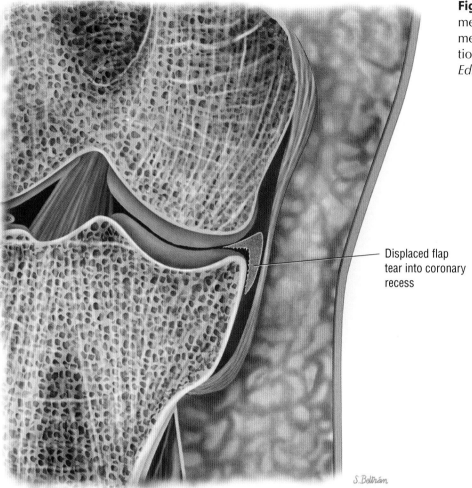

Figure 4.57 ■ Separation of displaced medial meniscus flap fragment with inferior displacement into coronary recess on color coronal section. *(See Flap Tears pg. 429, in Stoller's 3rd Edition.)*

Displaced flap tear into coronary recess

S. Beltrán

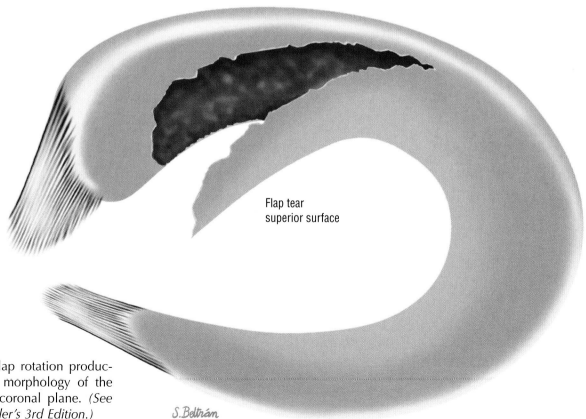

Flap tear superior surface

Figure 4.58 ■ Superior flap rotation producing the "double-decker" morphology of the medial meniscus in the coronal plane. *(See Flap Tears pg. 430, in Stoller's 3rd Edition.)*

S. Beltrán

Figure 4.59 ■ Displaced flap tear into the meniscotibial or coronary recess on sagittal (lateral) color illustration. *(See Flap Tears pg. 431, in Stoller's 3rd Edition.)*

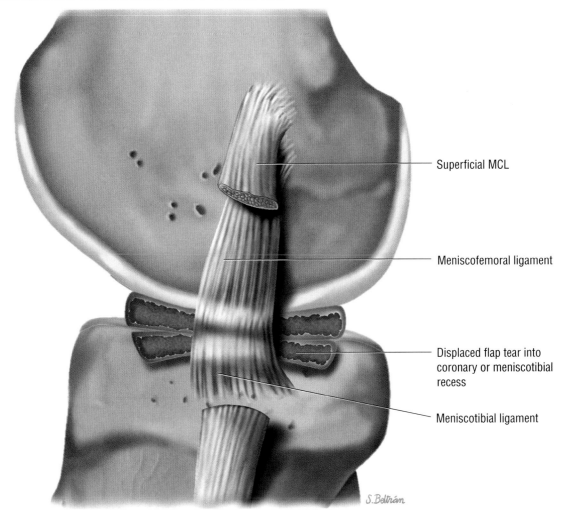

Superficial MCL

Meniscofemoral ligament

Displaced flap tear into coronary or meniscotibial recess

Meniscotibial ligament

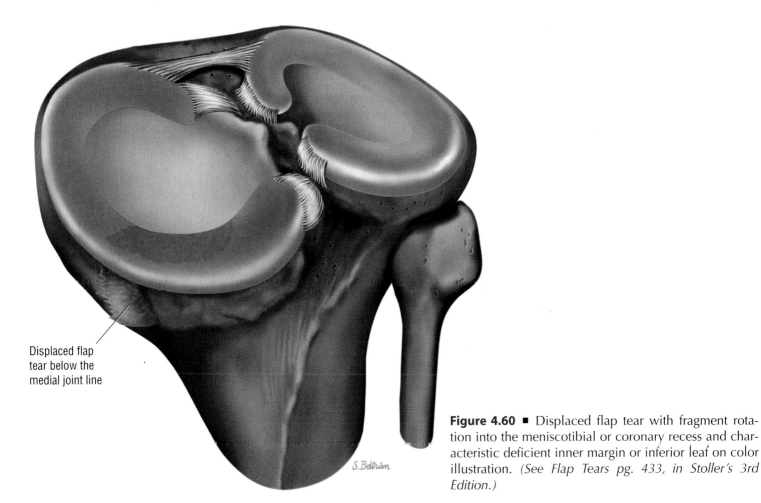

Displaced flap tear below the medial joint line

Figure 4.60 ■ Displaced flap tear with fragment rotation into the meniscotibial or coronary recess and characteristic deficient inner margin or inferior leaf on color illustration. *(See Flap Tears pg. 433, in Stoller's 3rd Edition.)*

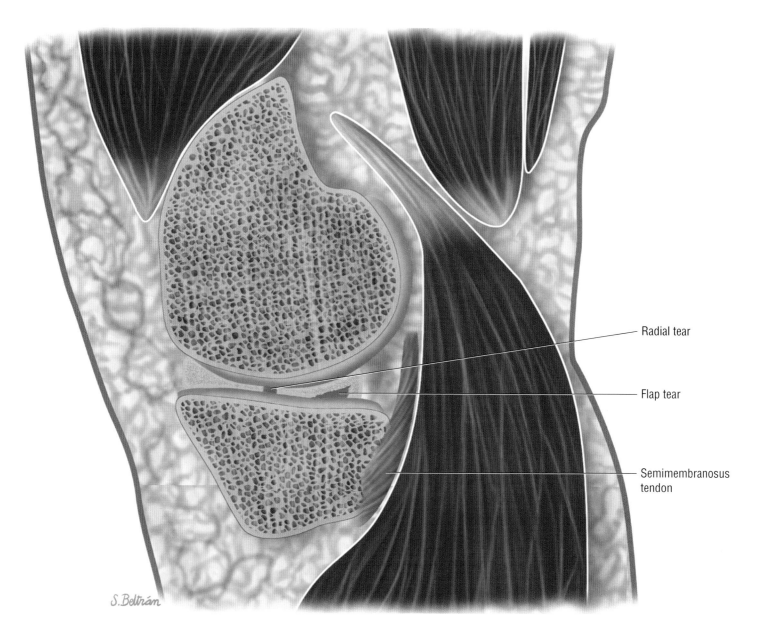

Figure 4.61 ■ **Continuity of a radial tear and flap tear pattern in the medial meniscus.** The tear initiates as a radial tear, which changes direction with a longitudinal component to create the flap pattern. The relative deficiency of the inner margin of the inferior leaf with blunting of the remaining inferior leaf is characteristic of a flap tear. *(See Flap Tears pg. 436, in Stoller's 3rd Edition.)*

Discoid Lateral Meniscus

Figure 4.62 ▪ Incomplete discoid lateral meniscus illustrated on superior view. *(See Discoid Meniscus pg. 441, in Stoller's 3rd Edition.)*

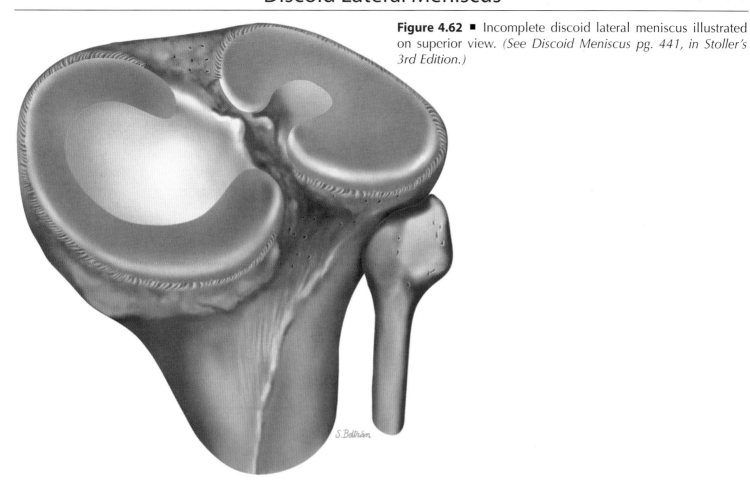

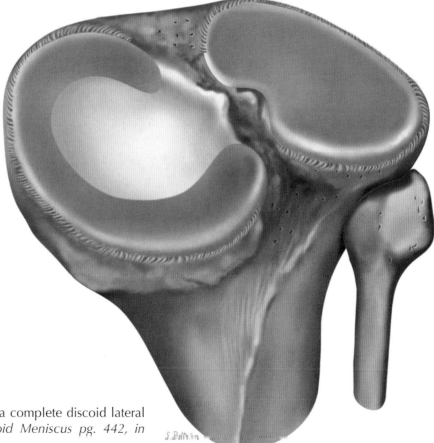

Figure 4.63 ▪ Color illustration of superior view of a complete discoid lateral meniscus from a posterior perspective. *(See Discoid Meniscus pg. 442, in Stoller's 3rd Edition.)*

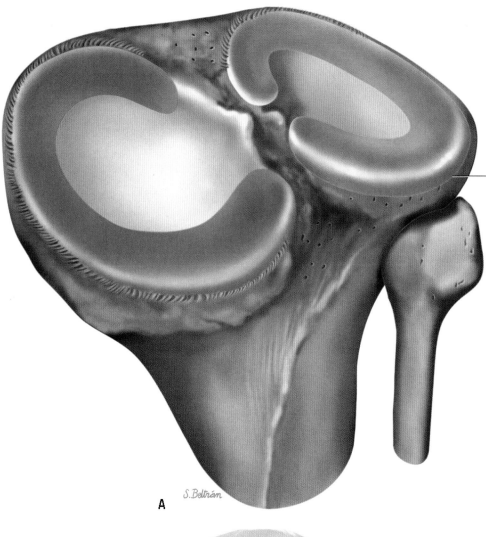

A

Figure 4.64 ▪ **(A)** Wrisberg variant with absence of the posterior coronary ligament on posterior superior view. **(B)** Without meniscotibial restraint, there is potential for entrapment of the posterior aspect of the fibrocartilage. In extension, the attached Wrisberg ligament pulls and displaces the posterior aspect of the meniscus into the intercondylar notch. *(See Discoid Meniscus pg. 443, in Stoller's 3rd Edition.)*

— Absent posterior coronary ligament

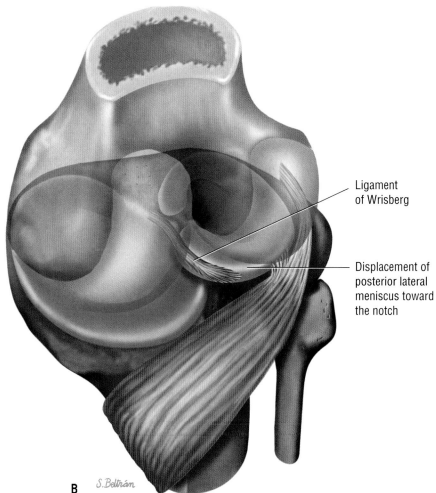

B

Ligament of Wrisberg

Displacement of posterior lateral meniscus toward the notch

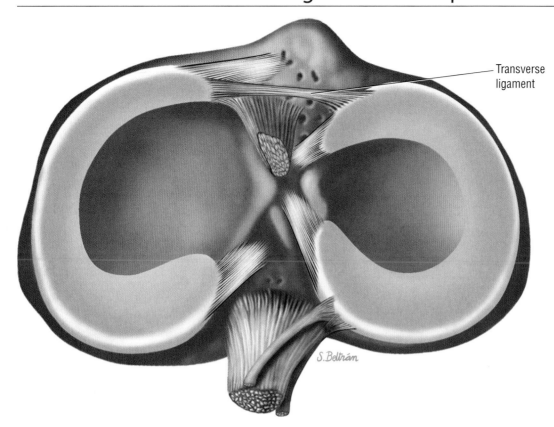

Figure 4.65 ■ **The transverse ligament of the knee connects the anterior horns of the medial and lateral menisci.** Axial superior view color illustration showing the transverse ligament coursing anterior to the anterior horn of the lateral meniscus. In the medial compartment anterior horn fibrocartilage extends anterior to the transverse ligament attachment. *(See Transverse Ligament pgs. 445 and 446, in Stoller's 3rd Edition.)*

Transverse ligament

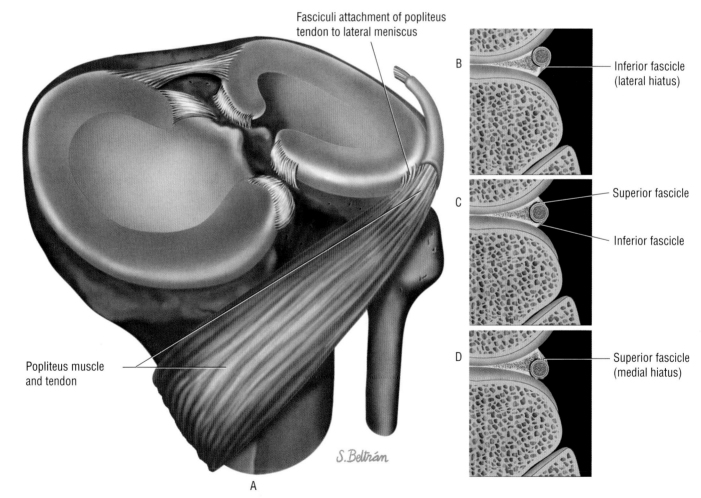

Fasciculi attachment of popliteus tendon to lateral meniscus

B — Inferior fascicle (lateral hiatus)

C — Superior fascicle / Inferior fascicle

D — Superior fascicle (medial hiatus)

Popliteus muscle and tendon

A

Figure 4.66 ■ **(A)** The popliteus tendon is extra-articular but intracapsular and susceptible in posterolateral corner injuries. It is covered by a synovial membrane on its medial aspect. The popliteal hiatus is bound anteroinferiorly by the superior fascicle. These fascicles are also referred to as popliteomeniscal ligaments. Normal deficiencies of the fascicle allow passage of the popliteus tendon from the lateral **(B)** to the medial **(D)** aspect of the hiatus. Both superior and inferior fascicles are shown at the midportion of the hiatus **(C)**. *(See Popliteus Tendon pgs. 447 and 451, in Stoller's 3rd Edition.)*

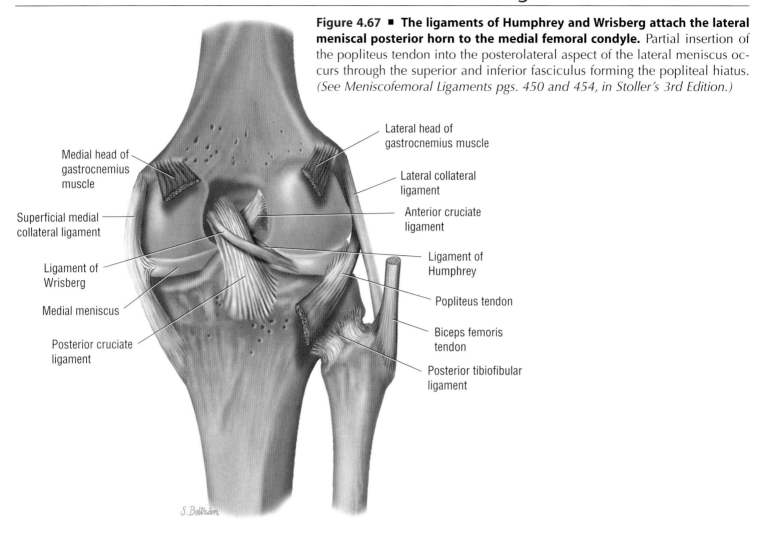

Figure 4.67 ▪ The ligaments of Humphrey and Wrisberg attach the lateral meniscal posterior horn to the medial femoral condyle. Partial insertion of the popliteus tendon into the posterolateral aspect of the lateral meniscus occurs through the superior and inferior fasciculus forming the popliteal hiatus. *(See Meniscofemoral Ligaments pgs. 450 and 454, in Stoller's 3rd Edition.)*

Medial head of gastrocnemius muscle

Lateral head of gastrocnemius muscle

Superficial medial collateral ligament

Lateral collateral ligament

Anterior cruciate ligament

Ligament of Wrisberg

Ligament of Humphrey

Medial meniscus

Popliteus tendon

Posterior cruciate ligament

Biceps femoris tendon

Posterior tibiofibular ligament

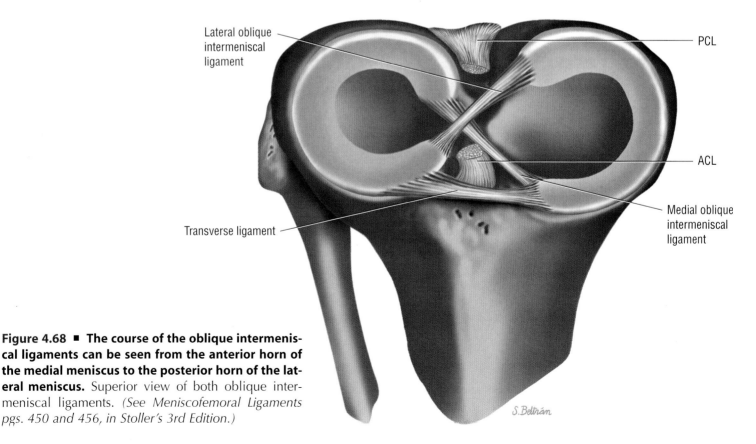

Lateral oblique intermeniscal ligament

PCL

Transverse ligament

ACL

Medial oblique intermeniscal ligament

Figure 4.68 ▪ The course of the oblique intermeniscal ligaments can be seen from the anterior horn of the medial meniscus to the posterior horn of the lateral meniscus. Superior view of both oblique intermeniscal ligaments. *(See Meniscofemoral Ligaments pgs. 450 and 456, in Stoller's 3rd Edition.)*

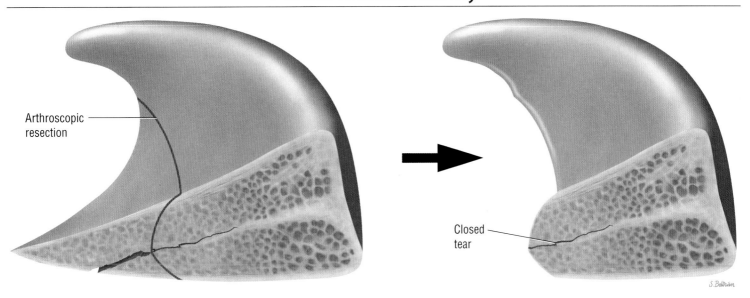

Arthroscopic resection

Closed tear

Figure 4.69 ■ **Boundary of partial meniscectomy to a stable meniscal rim.** Residual degeneration or a closed tear is left to preserve the surrounding meniscal tissue. *(See Postoperative Appearance of the Meniscus pg. 459, in Stoller's 3rd Edition.)*

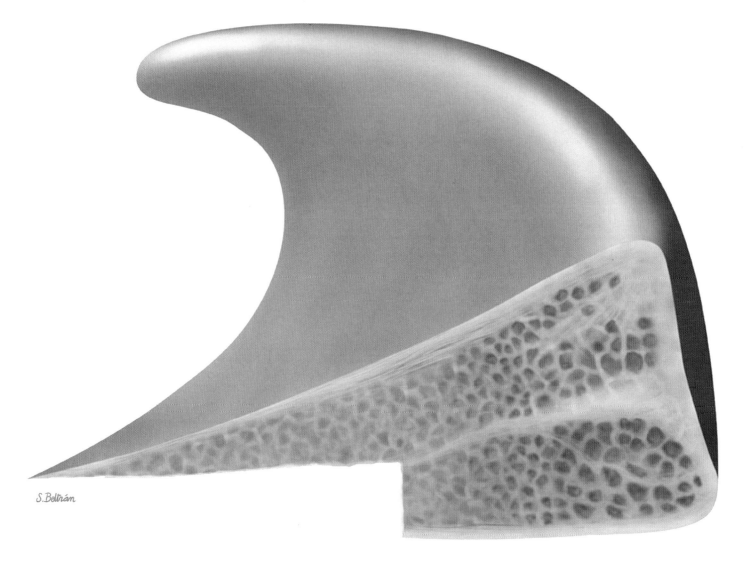

Figure 4.70 ■ Preferential resection of inner margin of inferior leaf (leaflet) in partial meniscectomy. *(See Postoperative Appearance of the Meniscus pg. 460, in Stoller's 3rd Edition.)*

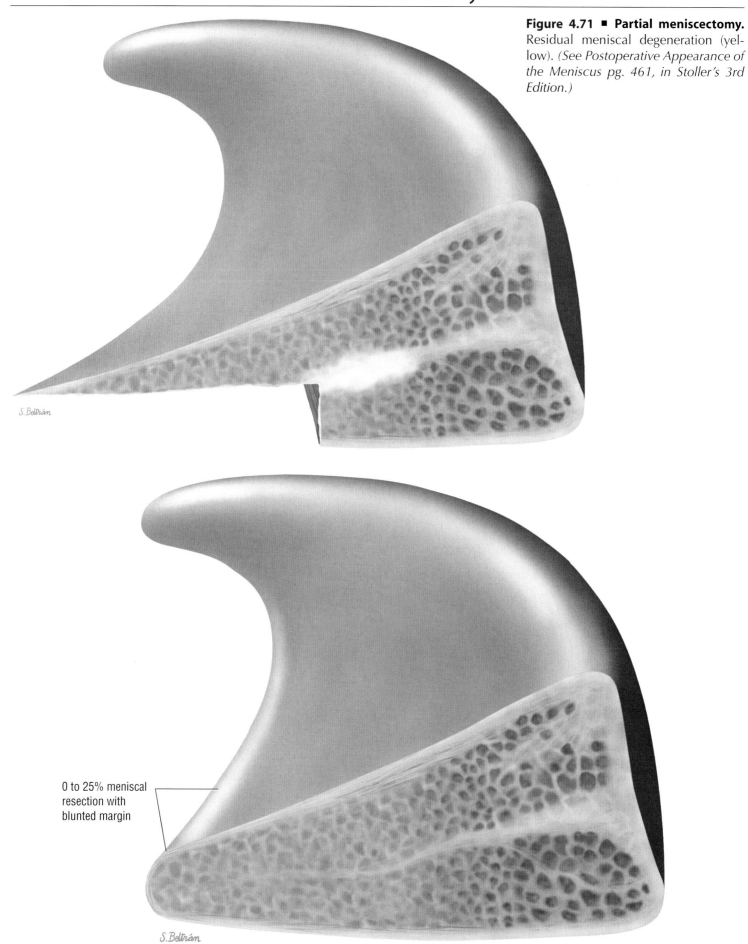

S.Beltrán

Figure 4.71 ▪ Partial meniscectomy. Residual meniscal degeneration (yellow). *(See Postoperative Appearance of the Meniscus pg. 461, in Stoller's 3rd Edition.)*

0 to 25% meniscal resection with blunted margin

S.Beltrán

Figure 4.72 ▪ Mild free edge blunting after a minimal or micro-partial meniscectomy. Sagittal cross-sectional illustration. *(See Postoperative Appearance of the Meniscus pg. 463, in Stoller's 3rd Edition.)*

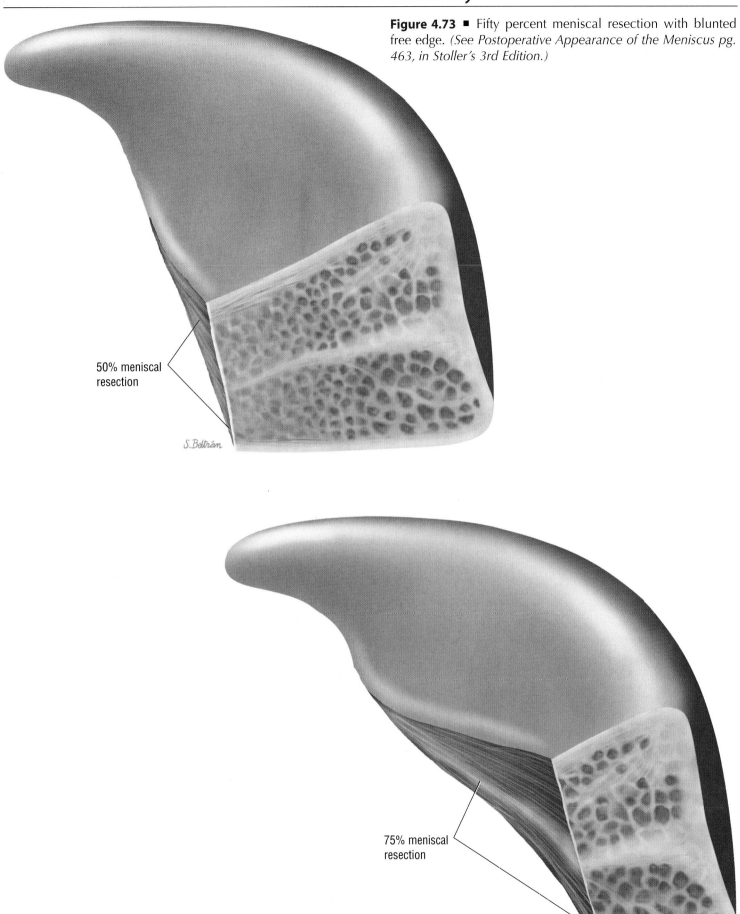

Figure 4.73 ■ Fifty percent meniscal resection with blunted free edge. *(See Postoperative Appearance of the Meniscus pg. 463, in Stoller's 3rd Edition.)*

50% meniscal resection

75% meniscal resection

Figure 4.74 ■ Cross-sectional sagittal illustration of 75% resection of posterior horn lateral meniscus with a thick rim of meniscal remnant. *(See Postoperative Appearance of the Meniscus pg. 464, in Stoller's 3rd Edition.)*

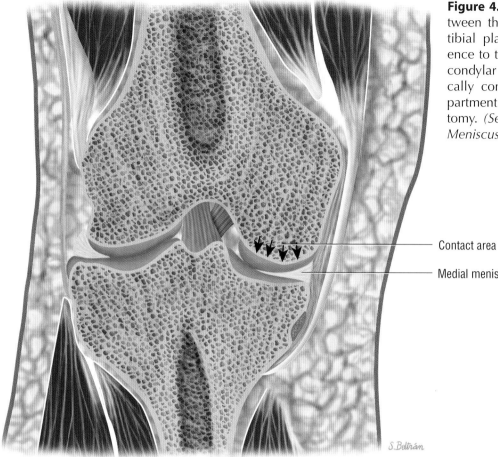

Contact area

Medial meniscus

A

Figure 4.75 ■ **(A)** A large contact area between the medial femoral condyle and the tibial plateau allows normal load transference to the intact meniscus. **(B)** Loss of the condylar meniscus contact area results in focally concentrated stress and medial compartment arthrosis after a partial meniscotomy. *(See Postoperative Appearance of the Meniscus pg. 465, in Stoller's 3rd Edition.)*

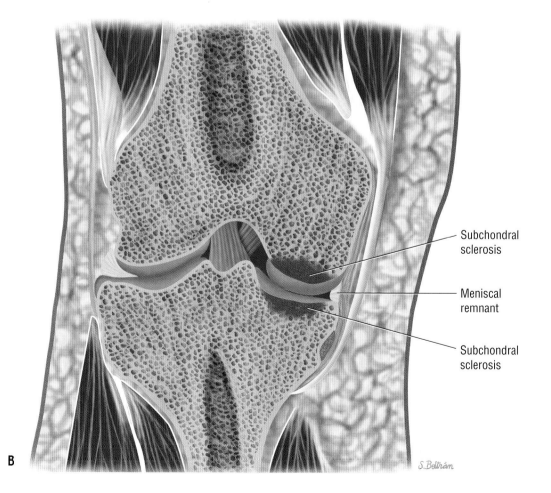

Subchondral sclerosis

Meniscal remnant

Subchondral sclerosis

B

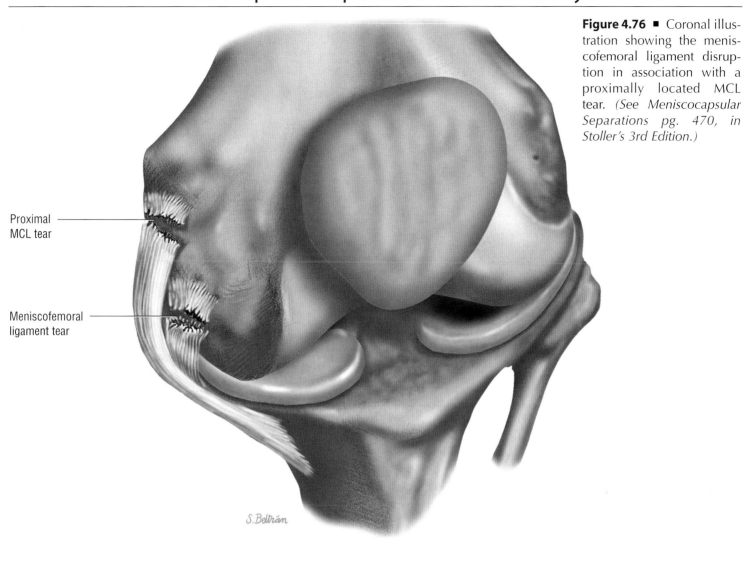

Proximal
MCL tear

Meniscofemoral
ligament tear

S.Beltrán

Figure 4.76 ■ Coronal illustration showing the meniscofemoral ligament disruption in association with a proximally located MCL tear. *(See Meniscocapsular Separations pg. 470, in Stoller's 3rd Edition.)*

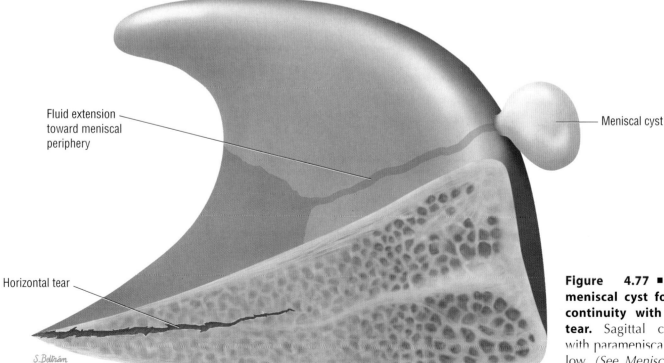

Fluid extension
toward meniscal
periphery

Meniscal cyst

Horizontal tear

S.Beltrán

Figure 4.77 ■ **Peripheral meniscal cyst formation in continuity with horizontal tear.** Sagittal cross-section with parameniscal cyst in yellow. *(See Meniscal Cysts pg. 474, in Stoller's 3rd Edition.)*

Chondrocalcinosis

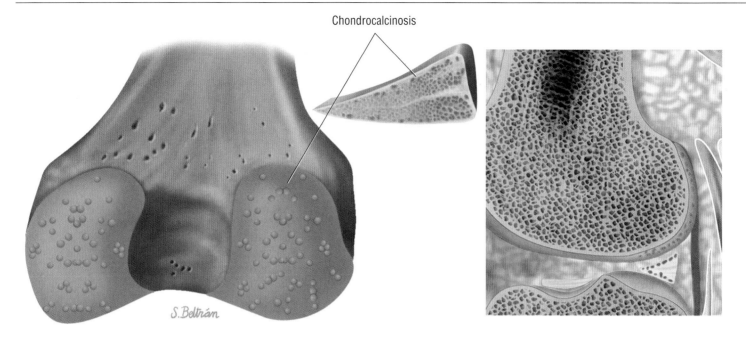

Figure 4.78 ■ **Chondrocalcinosis affecting both the articular cartilage and meniscus.** Posterior coronal and sagittal (lateral) cross-section illustration. *(See Calcium Pyrophosphate Dehydrate Depositions Disease pg. 476, in Stoller's 3rd Edition.)*

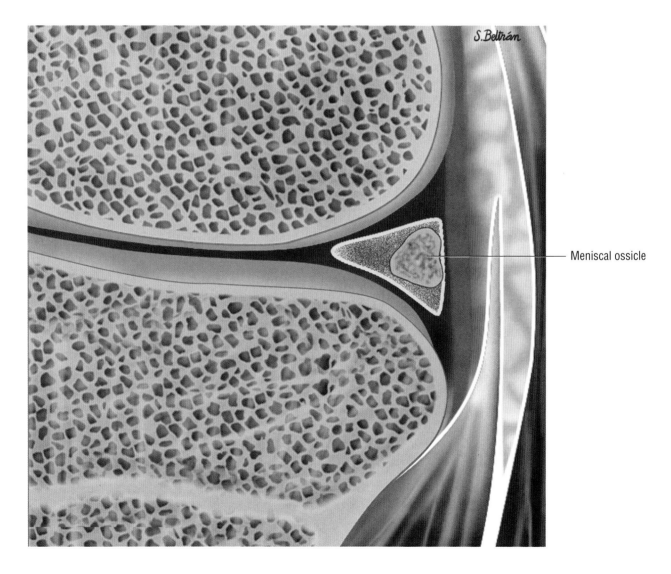

Meniscal ossicle

Figure 4.79 ■ Meniscal ossicle associated with the posterior horn of the medial meniscus. *(See Miscellaneous Meniscal Pathology pg. 478, in Stoller's 3rd Edition.)*

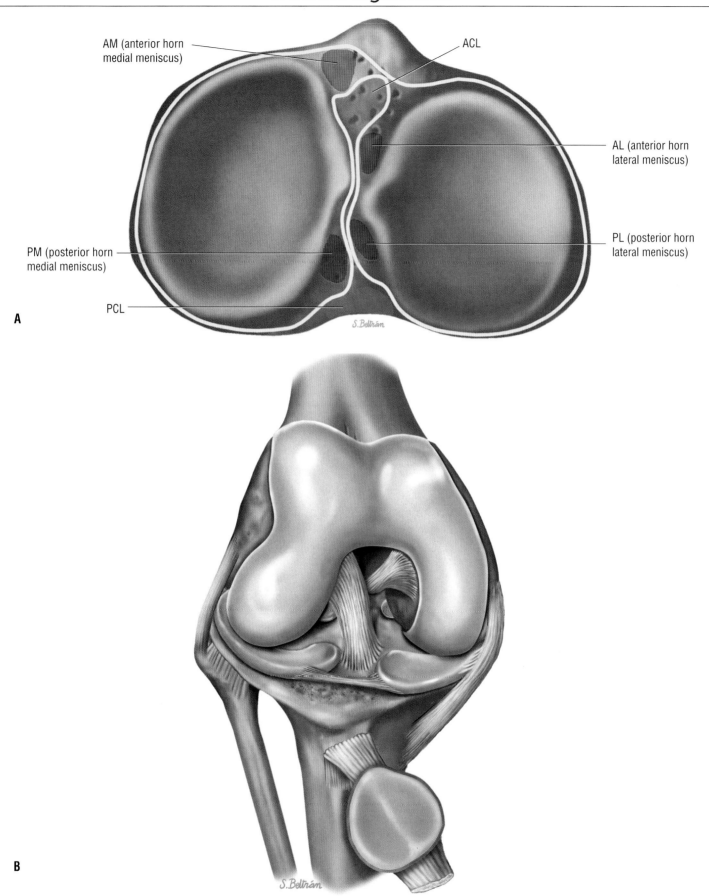

Figure 4.80 ■ **(A)** Tibial insertion sites for the anterior cruciate ligament (ACL) and posterior cruciate ligament (PCL). Insertions are also indicated for the meniscal fibrocartilage. The ACL inserts between the anterior attachments of the menisci. The PCL attaches to the posterior intercondylar area and posterior tibial surface. **(B)** Anterior tibial insertion sites of the ACL and menisci on anterior coronal perspective. *(See Anterior Cruciate Ligament pg. 479, in Stoller's 3rd Edition.)*

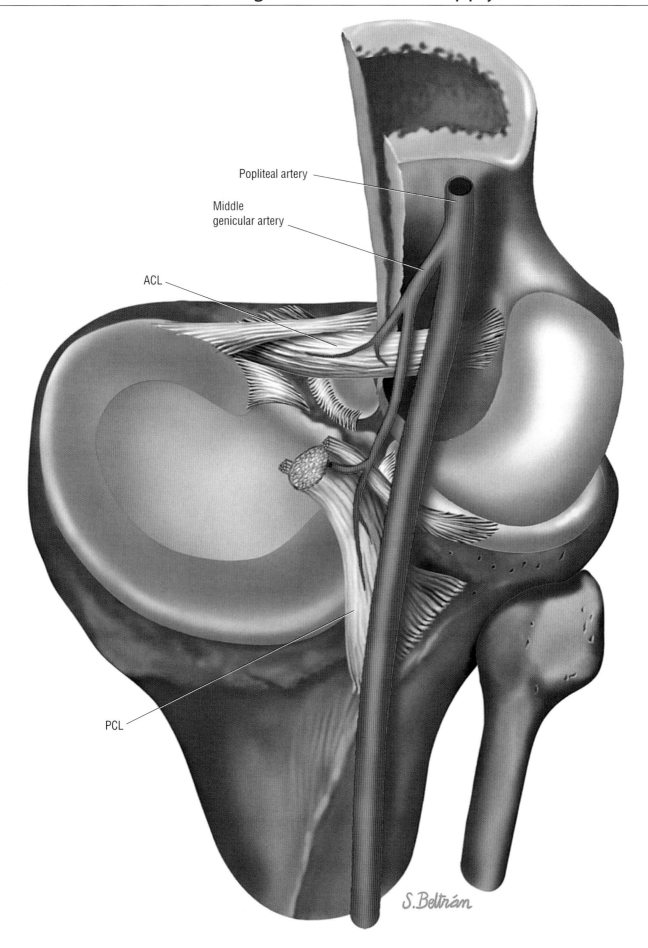

Popliteal artery

Middle
genicular artery

ACL

PCL

S.Beltrán

Figure 4.81 ■ **The vascular supply to the cruciate ligaments via the middle genic-ulate (genicular) arterial branch of the anterior popliteal artery.** There is no blood supply derived from the ACL ligament to the bone insertion site. *(See Anterior Cruciate Ligament pg. 480, in Stoller's 3rd Edition.)*

Figure 4.82 ■ Anteromedial and posterolateral fibers of the ACL in extension **(A)** and flexion **(B)**. In extension the longer anteromedial fibers are identified anterior to the shorter posteriorly located posterolateral fibers. In flexion the ACL ligament twists and the posterolateral fibers rotate beneath the anteromedial fibers. The ACL, therefore, is more cord-like in flexion, with the anterior superior portion comprising posterolateral fibers. *(See Anterior Cruciate Ligament pg. 481, in Stoller's 3rd Edition.)*

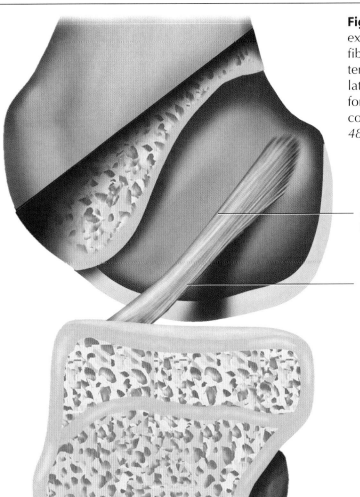

Anteromedial portion

Posterolateral portion

A

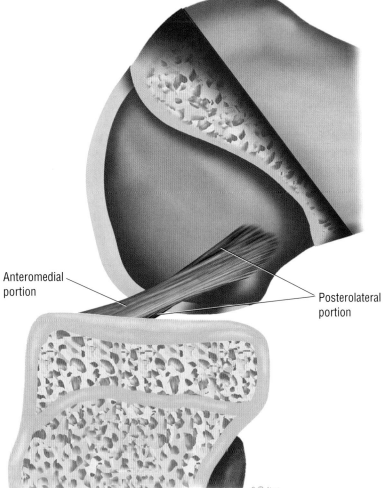

Anteromedial portion

Posterolateral portion

B

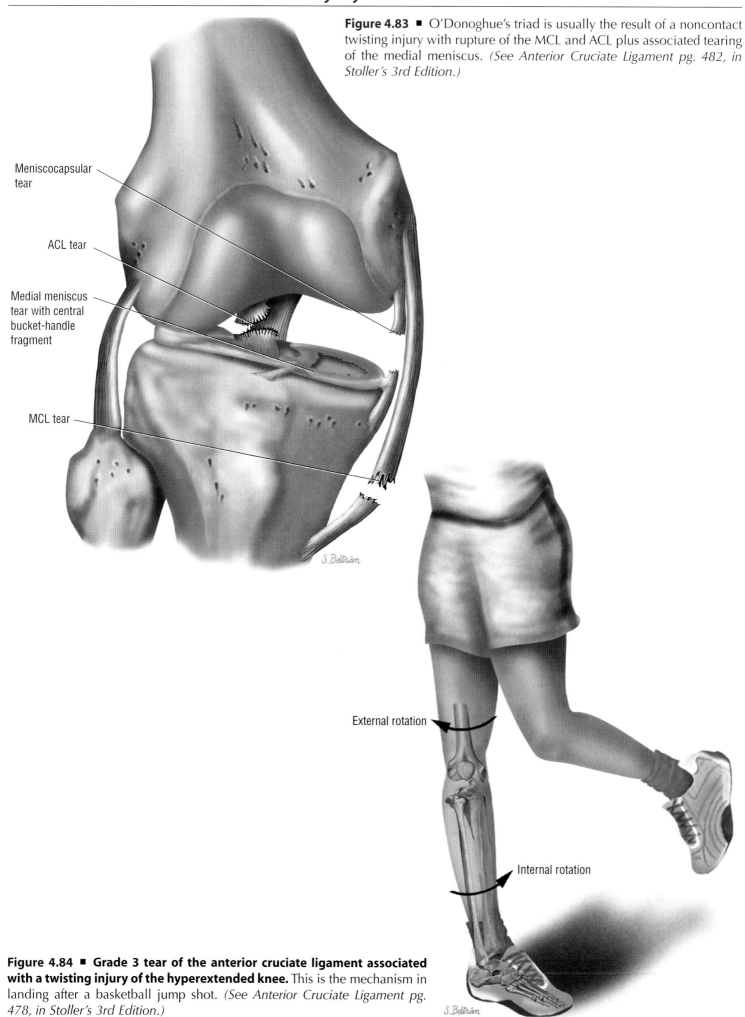

Figure 4.83 ■ O'Donoghue's triad is usually the result of a noncontact twisting injury with rupture of the MCL and ACL plus associated tearing of the medial meniscus. *(See Anterior Cruciate Ligament pg. 482, in Stoller's 3rd Edition.)*

Meniscocapsular tear

ACL tear

Medial meniscus tear with central bucket-handle fragment

MCL tear

External rotation

Internal rotation

Figure 4.84 ■ **Grade 3 tear of the anterior cruciate ligament associated with a twisting injury of the hyperextended knee.** This is the mechanism in landing after a basketball jump shot. *(See Anterior Cruciate Ligament pg. 478, in Stoller's 3rd Edition.)*

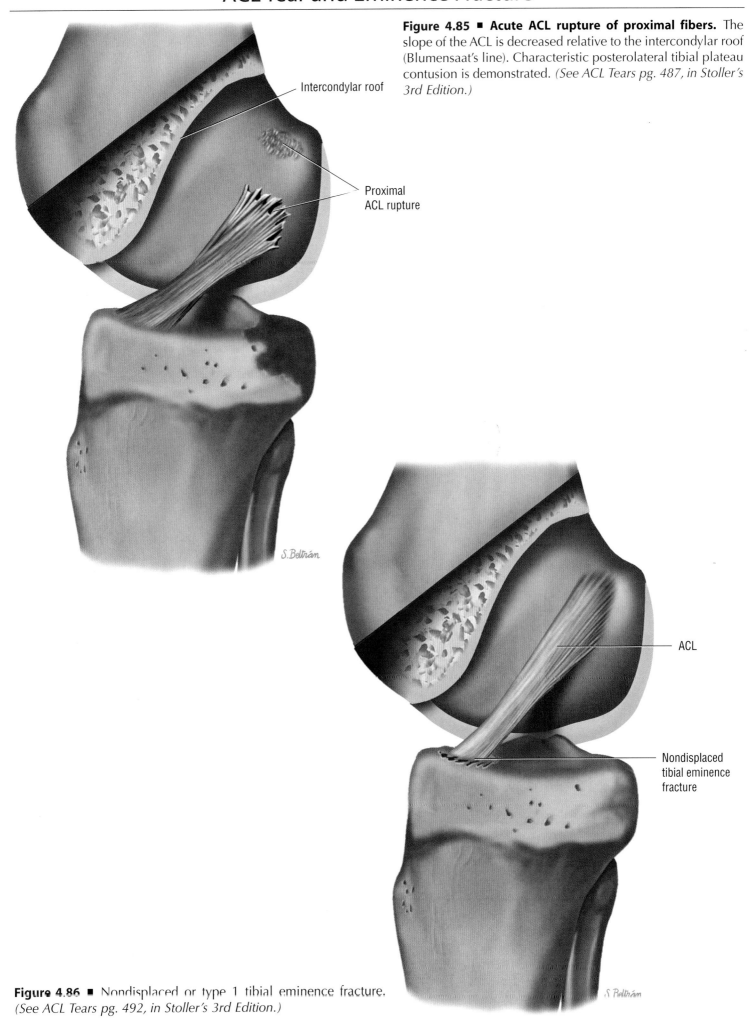

Figure 4.85 ■ **Acute ACL rupture of proximal fibers.** The slope of the ACL is decreased relative to the intercondylar roof (Blumensaat's line). Characteristic posterolateral tibial plateau contusion is demonstrated. *(See ACL Tears pg. 487, in Stoller's 3rd Edition.)*

Intercondylar roof

Proximal ACL rupture

ACL

Nondisplaced tibial eminence fracture

Figure 4.86 ■ Nondisplaced or type 1 tibial eminence fracture. *(See ACL Tears pg. 492, in Stoller's 3rd Edition.)*

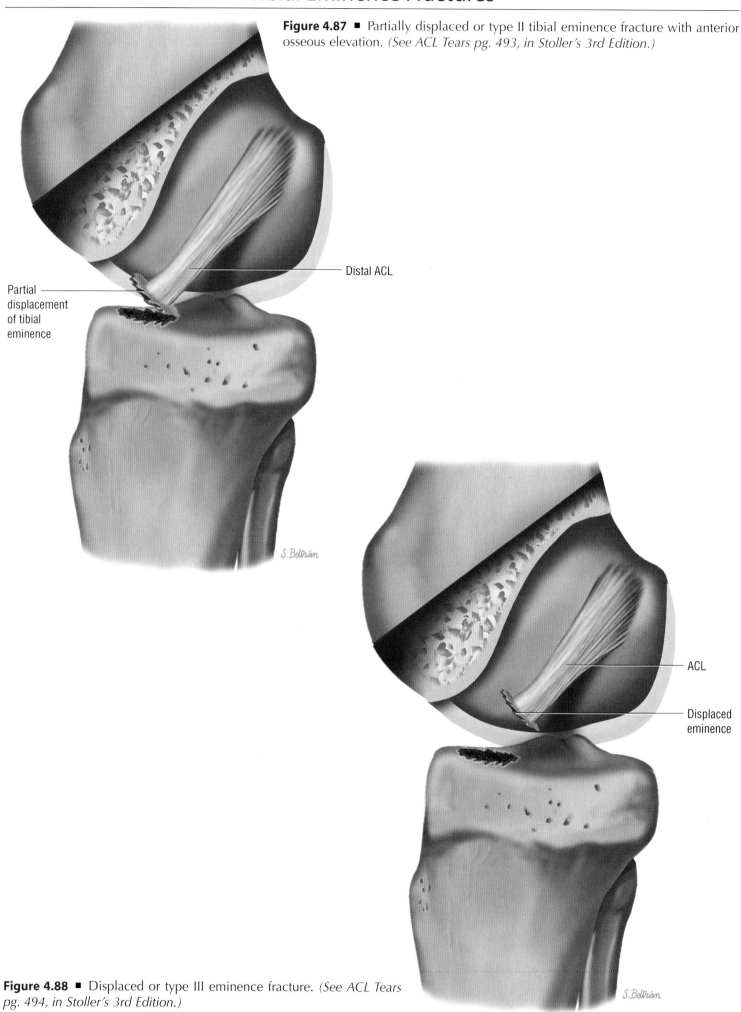

Figure 4.87 ■ Partially displaced or type II tibial eminence fracture with anterior osseous elevation. *(See ACL Tears pg. 493, in Stoller's 3rd Edition.)*

Distal ACL

Partial displacement of tibial eminence

ACL

Displaced eminence

Figure 4.88 ■ Displaced or type III eminence fracture. *(See ACL Tears pg. 494, in Stoller's 3rd Edition.)*

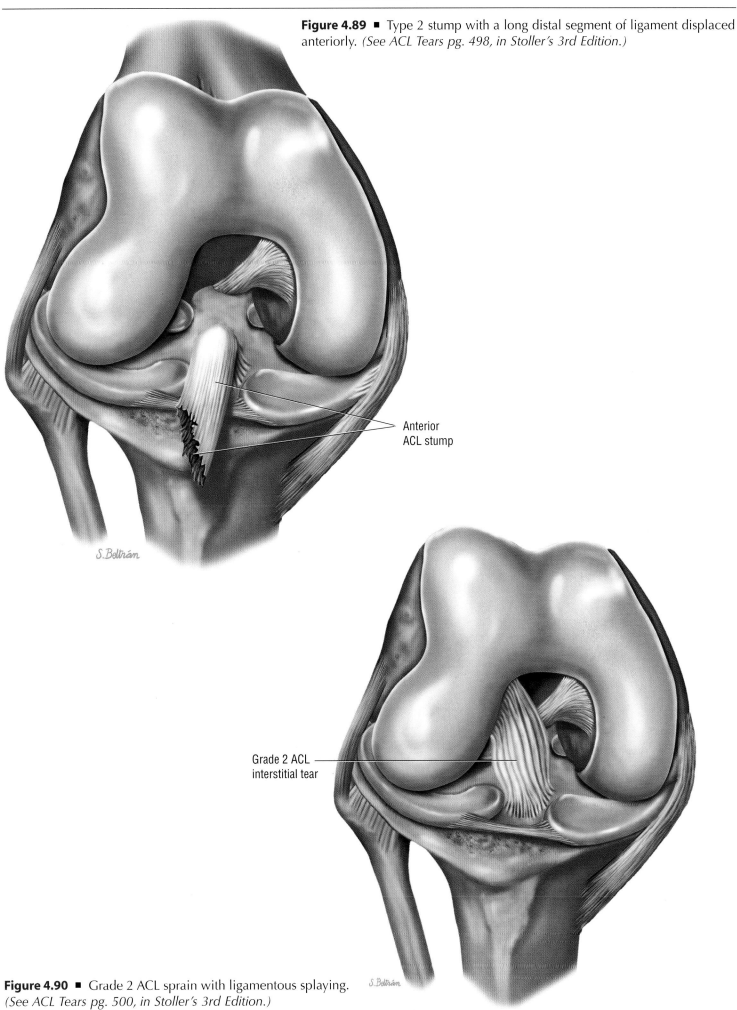

Figure 4.89 ▪ Type 2 stump with a long distal segment of ligament displaced anteriorly. *(See ACL Tears pg. 498, in Stoller's 3rd Edition.)*

Anterior
ACL stump

Grade 2 ACL
interstitial tear

Figure 4.90 ▪ Grade 2 ACL sprain with ligamentous splaying.
(See ACL Tears pg. 500, in Stoller's 3rd Edition.)

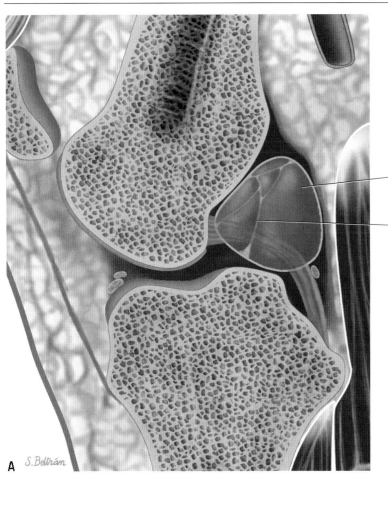

Intercondylar notch cyst

Internal cyst septations

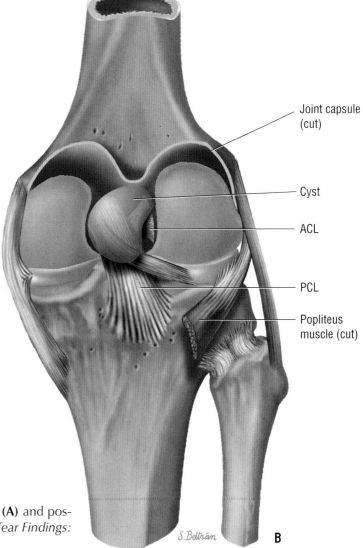

Joint capsule (cut)

Cyst

ACL

PCL

Popliteus muscle (cut)

Figure 4.91 ■ Intercondylar notch cyst or ganglion from a sagittal **(A)** and posterior coronal **(B)** perspective. *(See Pitfalls in Interpretations of ACL Tear Findings: ACL Ganglia pg. 503, in Stoller's 3rd Edition.)*

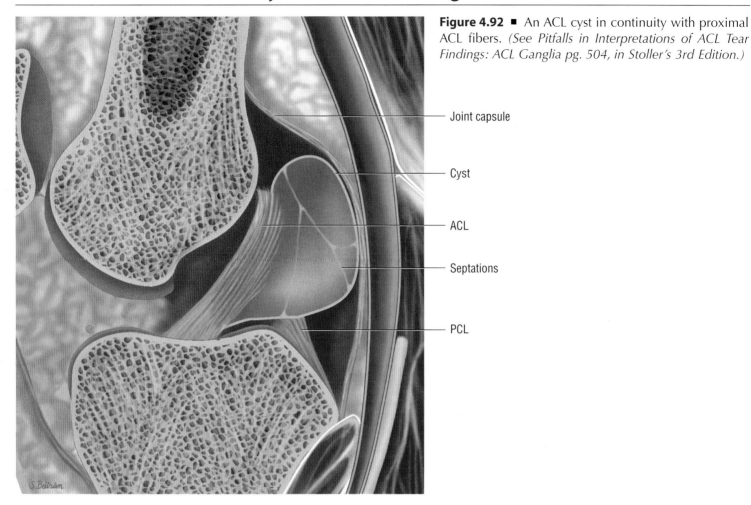

Figure 4.92 ■ An ACL cyst in continuity with proximal ACL fibers. *(See Pitfalls in Interpretations of ACL Tear Findings: ACL Ganglia pg. 504, in Stoller's 3rd Edition.)*

— Joint capsule

— Cyst

— ACL

— Septations

— PCL

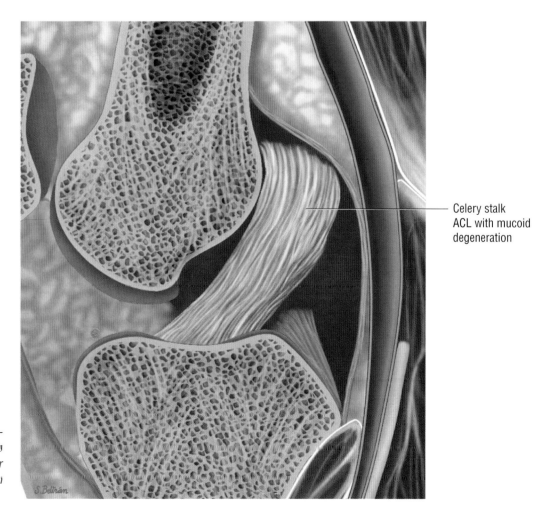

Celery stalk ACL with mucoid degeneration

Figure 4.93 ■ "Celery stalk" or mucoid ACL degeneration. *(See Pitfalls in Interpretations of ACL Tear Findings: ACL Ganglia pg. 506, in Stoller's 3rd Edition.)*

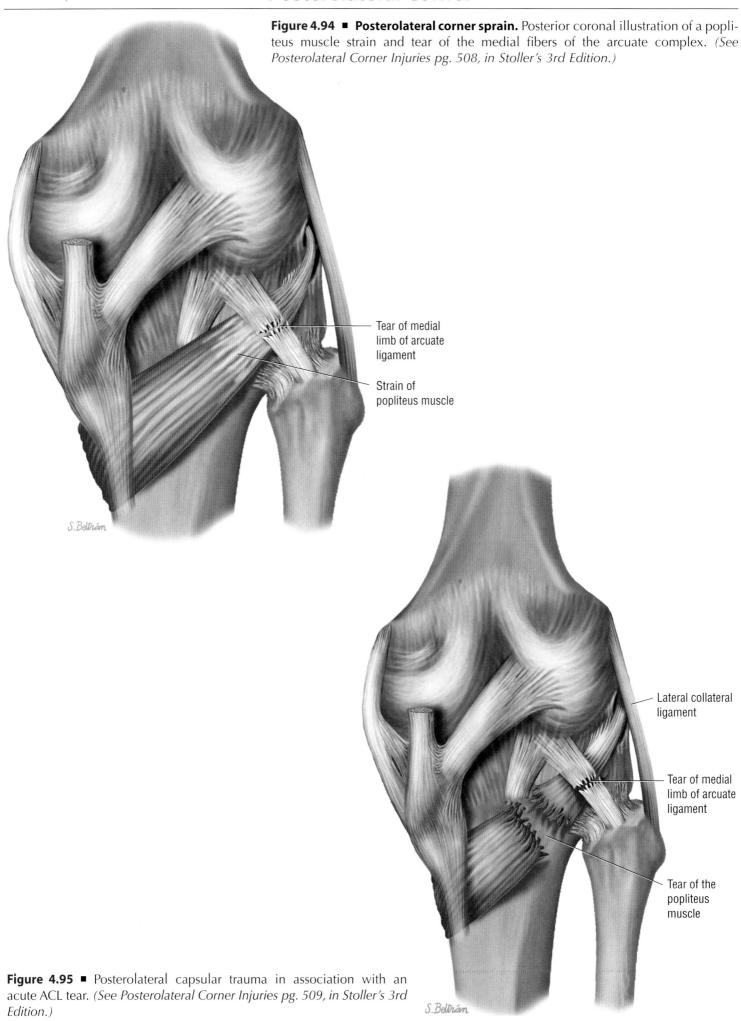

Figure 4.94 ■ Posterolateral corner sprain. Posterior coronal illustration of a popliteus muscle strain and tear of the medial fibers of the arcuate complex. *(See Posterolateral Corner Injuries pg. 508, in Stoller's 3rd Edition.)*

Tear of medial limb of arcuate ligament

Strain of popliteus muscle

Lateral collateral ligament

Tear of medial limb of arcuate ligament

Tear of the popliteus muscle

Figure 4.95 ■ Posterolateral capsular trauma in association with an acute ACL tear. *(See Posterolateral Corner Injuries pg. 509, in Stoller's 3rd Edition.)*

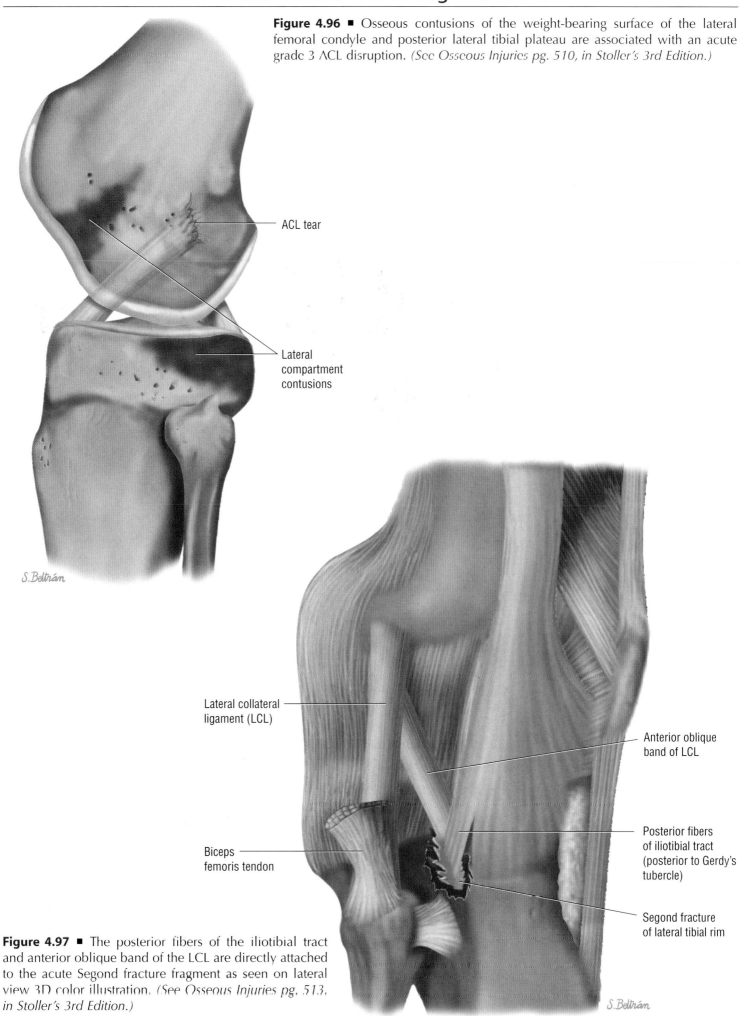

Figure 4.96 ■ Osseous contusions of the weight-bearing surface of the lateral femoral condyle and posterior lateral tibial plateau are associated with an acute grade 3 ACL disruption. *(See Osseous Injuries pg. 510, in Stoller's 3rd Edition.)*

ACL tear

Lateral compartment contusions

S.Beltrán

Lateral collateral ligament (LCL)

Biceps femoris tendon

Anterior oblique band of LCL

Posterior fibers of iliotibial tract (posterior to Gerdy's tubercle)

Segond fracture of lateral tibial rim

Figure 4.97 ■ The posterior fibers of the iliotibial tract and anterior oblique band of the LCL are directly attached to the acute Segond fracture fragment as seen on lateral view 3D color illustration. *(See Osseous Injuries pg. 513, in Stoller's 3rd Edition.)*

S.Beltrán

Figure 4.98 ■ **(A)** Meniscocapsular separation with posterior medial tibial plateau contusion caused by an ACL rupture-related contrecoup injury. **(B)** Associated ACL mid-ligament rupture, coronal perspective. *(See Osseous Injuries pg. 514, in Stoller's 3rd Edition.)*

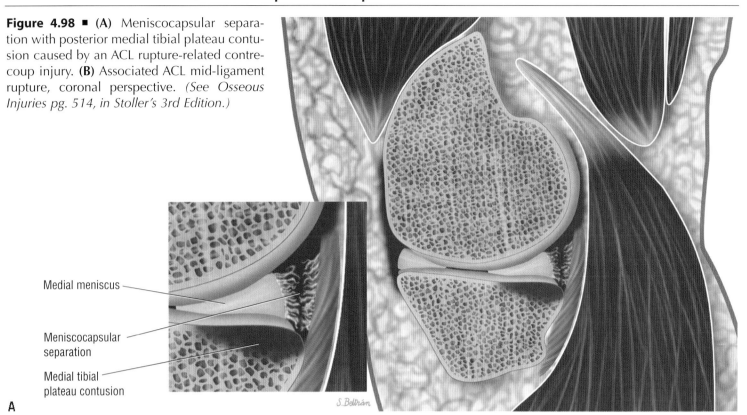

Medial meniscus

Meniscocapsular separation

Medial tibial plateau contusion

A

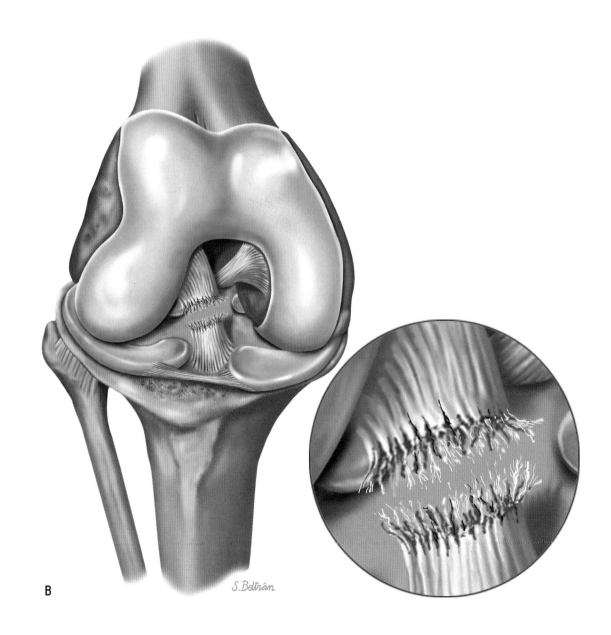

B

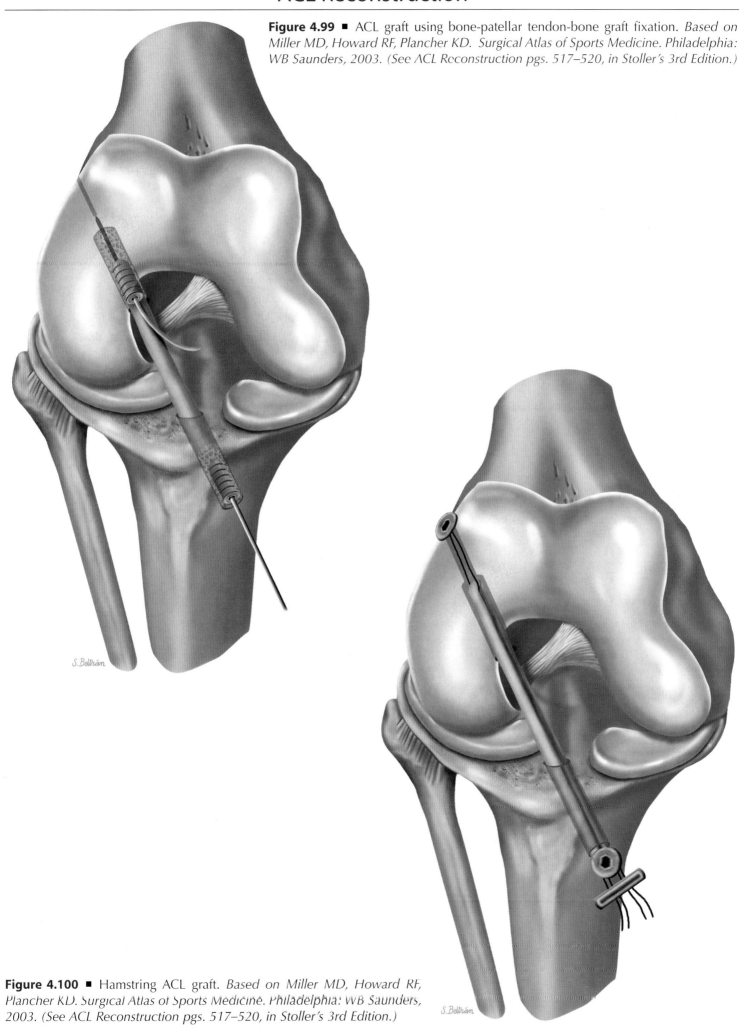

Figure 4.99 ■ ACL graft using bone-patellar tendon-bone graft fixation. *Based on Miller MD, Howard RF, Plancher KD. Surgical Atlas of Sports Medicine. Philadelphia: WB Saunders, 2003. (See ACL Reconstruction pgs. 517–520, in Stoller's 3rd Edition.)*

Figure 4.100 ■ Hamstring ACL graft. *Based on Miller MD, Howard RF, Plancher KD. Surgical Atlas of Sports Medicine. Philadelphia: WB Saunders, 2003. (See ACL Reconstruction pgs. 517–520, in Stoller's 3rd Edition.)*

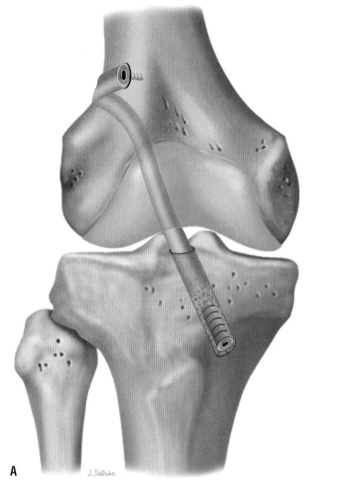

A

Anterior coronal view

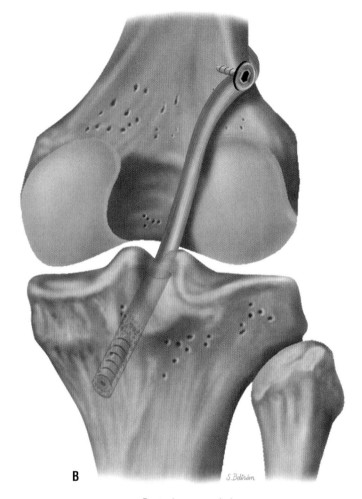

B

Posterior coronal view

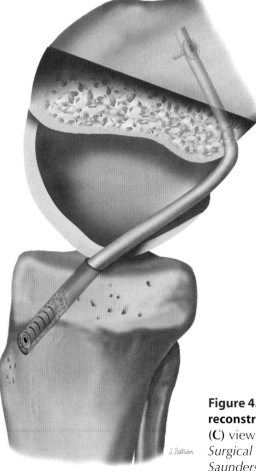

C

Sagittal view

Figure 4.101 ▪ Over-the-top anterior cruciate ligament reconstruction: Anterior **(A),** posterior **(B)**, and sagittal **(C)** views. *Based on Miller MD, Howard RF, Plancher KD. Surgical Atlas of Sports Medicine. Philadelphia: WB Saunders, 2003. (See ACL Reconstruction pgs. 517–520, in Stoller's 3rd Edition.)*

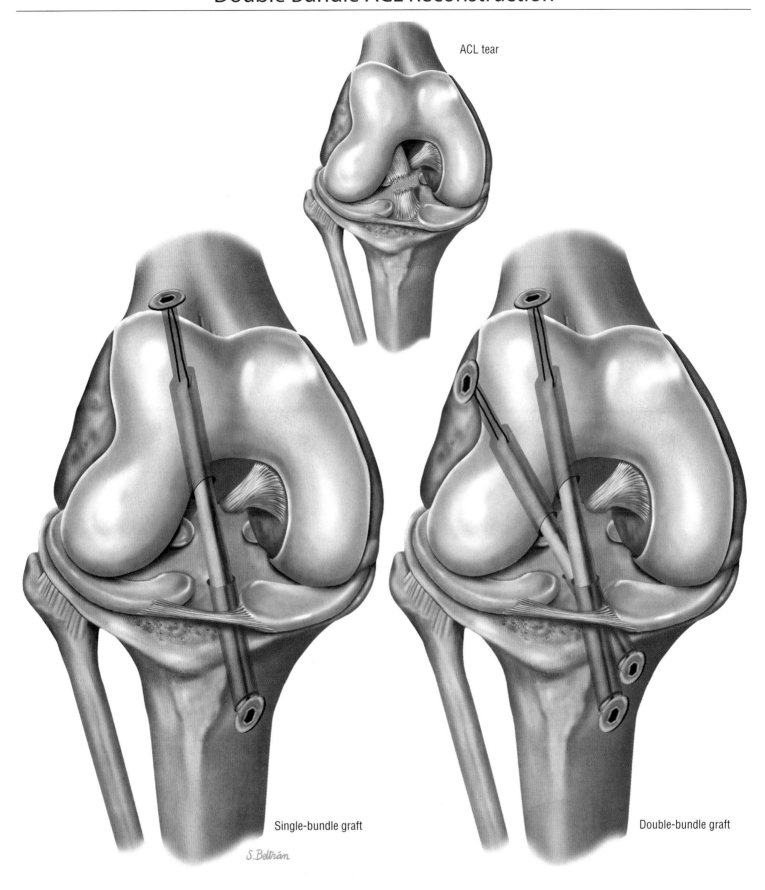

ACL tear

Single-bundle graft

Double-bundle graft

S.Beltrán

Figure 4.102 ■ Double bundle anatomic ACL reconstruction used to recreate the anteromedial and posterolateral bundles, resist combined rotatory loads, and improve anteroposterior stability. (*See ACL Reconstruction pgs. 517–520, in Stoller's 3rd Edition.*)

{AU}

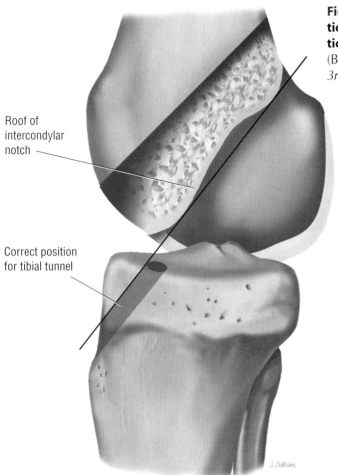

Roof of
intercondylar
notch

Correct position
for tibial tunnel

Figure 4.103 ▪ **ACL graft tibial tunnel placement at the posterior portion of the ACL tibial insertion site (near the posterolateral bundle location).** The tibial tunnel is posterior to the slope of the intercondylar roof (Blumensaat's line). *(See ACL Reconstruction pgs. 517–520, in Stoller's 3rd Edition.)*

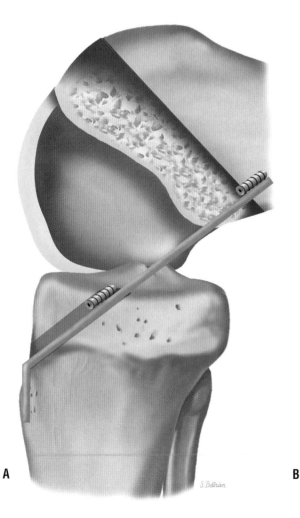

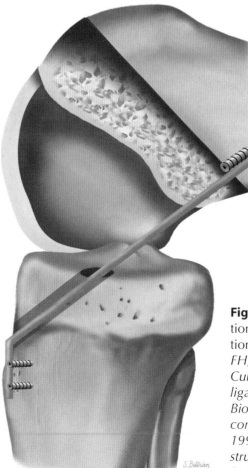

A

B

Figure 4.104 ▪ **(A)** Proximal fixation of an ACL graft. **(B)** Distal fixation of an ACL graft. *Based on Fu FH, Bennett CH, Ma CB, et al. Current trends in anterior cruciate ligament reconstruction. Part I. Biology and biomechanics of reconstruction. Am J Sports Med 1999:27,821. (See ACL Reconstruction pgs. 517–520, in Stoller's 3rd Edition.)*

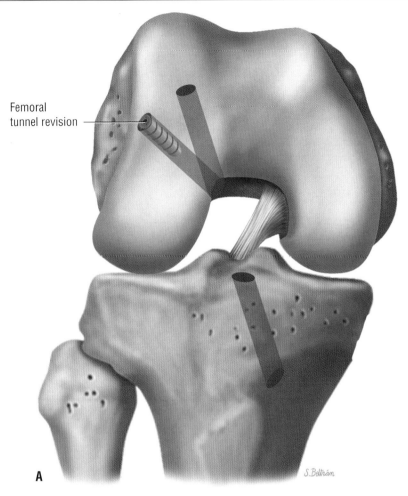

Femoral tunnel revision

A

Figure 4.105 ▪ **(A)** Revision of a vertically oriented ACL graft with a divergent tunnel technique. The femoral tunnel is realigned to the relative 10 o'clock position. **(B)** Improper anterior femoral tunnel placement in lateral perspective. **(C)** Posterior femoral tunnel revision after initial improper anterior femoral tunnel placement. *Based on Insall JN, Scott WN. Surgery of the Knee, 4 ed, vol. 2. Philadelphia: Elsevier, 2006. (See ACL Reconstruction pgs. 517–520, in Stoller's 3rd Edition.)*

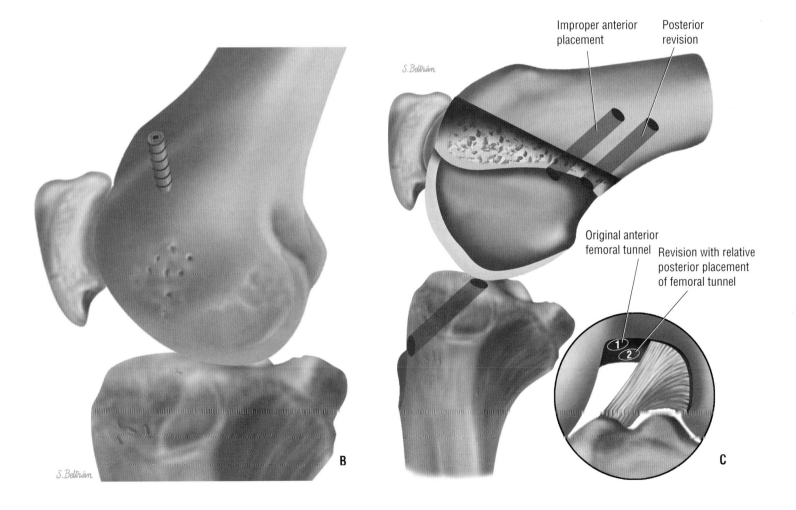

Improper anterior placement   Posterior revision

Original anterior femoral tunnel   Revision with relative posterior placement of femoral tunnel

B

C

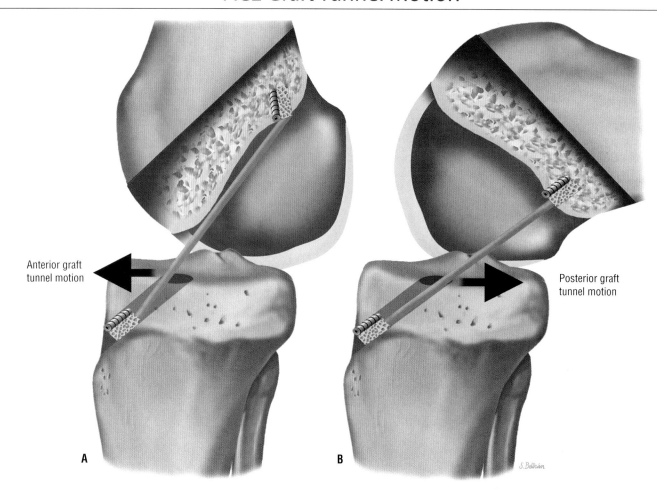

Anterior graft tunnel motion

Posterior graft tunnel motion

A

B

S.Beltrán

Figure 4.106 ■ ACL graft tunnel motion in the anteroposterior plane occurring during extension **(A)** and flexion **(B)**. A windshield wiper effect predominates at the tibial tunnel side of the ACL graft. If the bone block is placed distally the windshield wiper effect is increased as a function of increased distance of the graft fixation relative to the joint line. *Based on Fu FH, Bennett CH, Ma CB, et al. Current trends in anterior cruciate ligament reconstruction. Part I. Biology and biomechanics of reconstruction. Am J Sports Med 1999:27,821, and based on Resnick D, Kang HS, Petterklieber ML. Internal Derangements of Joints, 2 ed, vol. 2. Philadelphia: Elsevier, 2007. (See ACL Reconstruction pgs. 517–520, in Stoller's 3rd Edition.)*

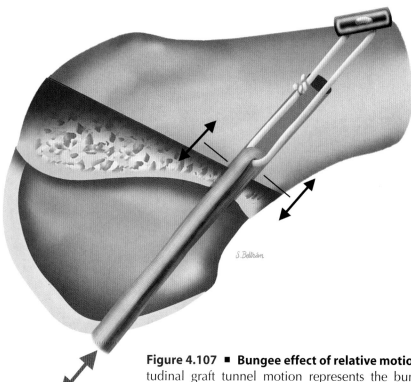

S.Beltrán

Figure 4.107 ■ **Bungee effect of relative motion between the ACL graft and femoral tunnel.** This longitudinal graft tunnel motion represents the bungee effect. *(See ACL Reconstruction pgs. 517–520, in Stoller's 3rd Edition.)*

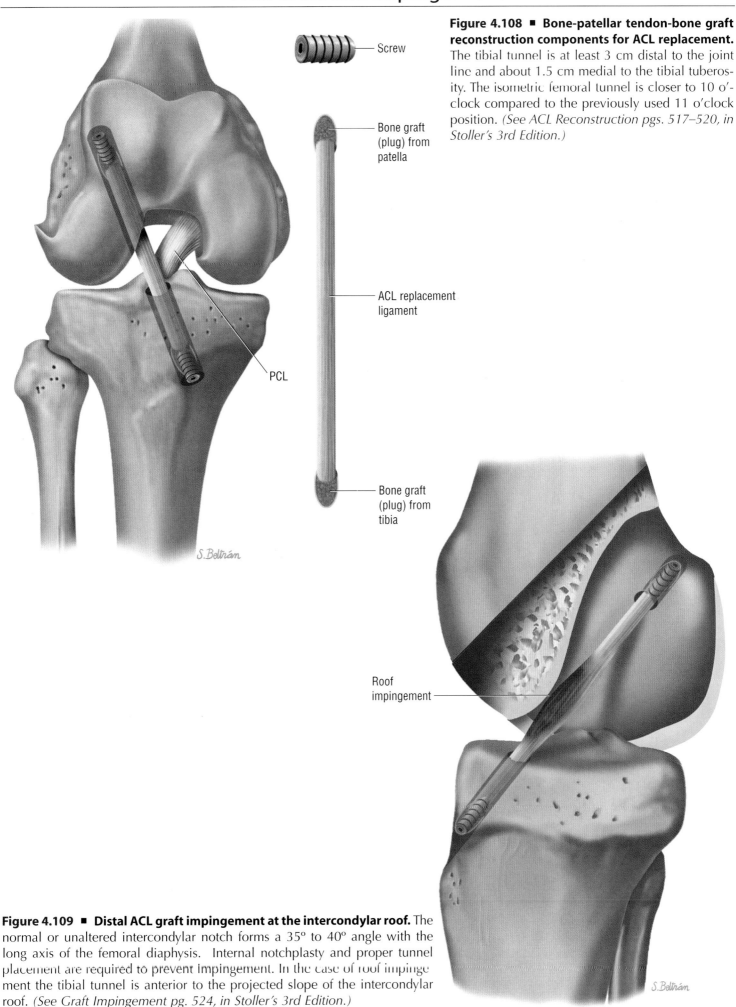

Figure 4.108 ■ Bone-patellar tendon-bone graft reconstruction components for ACL replacement. The tibial tunnel is at least 3 cm distal to the joint line and about 1.5 cm medial to the tibial tuberosity. The isometric femoral tunnel is closer to 10 o'clock compared to the previously used 11 o'clock position. *(See ACL Reconstruction pgs. 517–520, in Stoller's 3rd Edition.)*

Screw

Bone graft (plug) from patella

ACL replacement ligament

Bone graft (plug) from tibia

PCL

Roof impingement

Figure 4.109 ■ Distal ACL graft impingement at the intercondylar roof. The normal or unaltered intercondylar notch forms a 35° to 40° angle with the long axis of the femoral diaphysis. Internal notchplasty and proper tunnel placement are required to prevent impingement. In the case of roof impingement the tibial tunnel is anterior to the projected slope of the intercondylar roof. *(See Graft Impingement pg. 524, in Stoller's 3rd Edition.)*

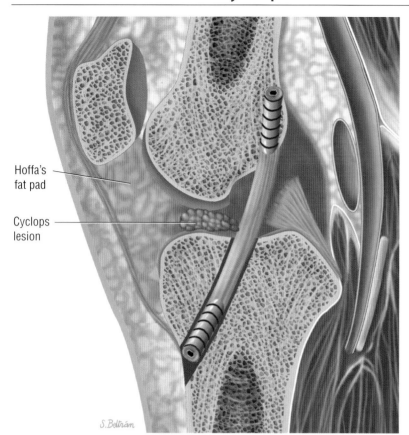

Figure 4.110 ■ Sagittal section color illustration of a cyclops lesion between the free edge of Hoffa's fat pad and the anterior surface of the distal ACL graft. *(See Graft Impingement pg. 526, in Stoller's 3rd Edition.)*

Hoffa's fat pad

Cyclops lesion

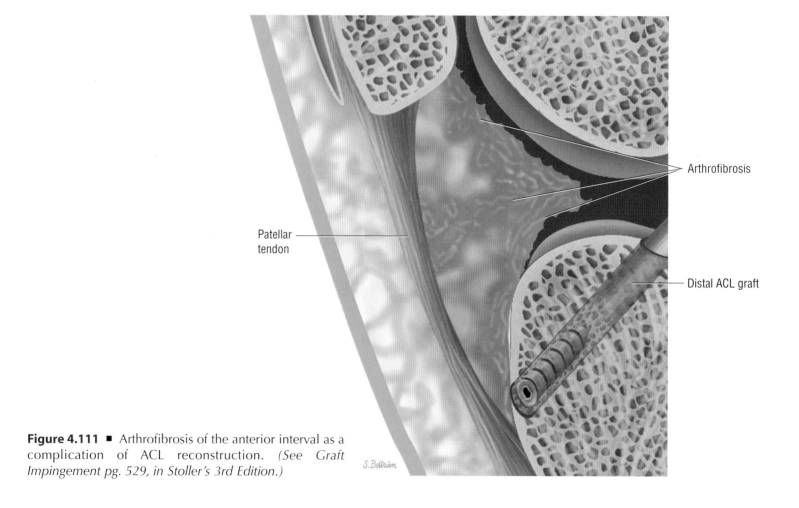

Arthrofibrosis

Patellar tendon

Distal ACL graft

Figure 4.111 ■ Arthrofibrosis of the anterior interval as a complication of ACL reconstruction. *(See Graft Impingement pg. 529, in Stoller's 3rd Edition.)*

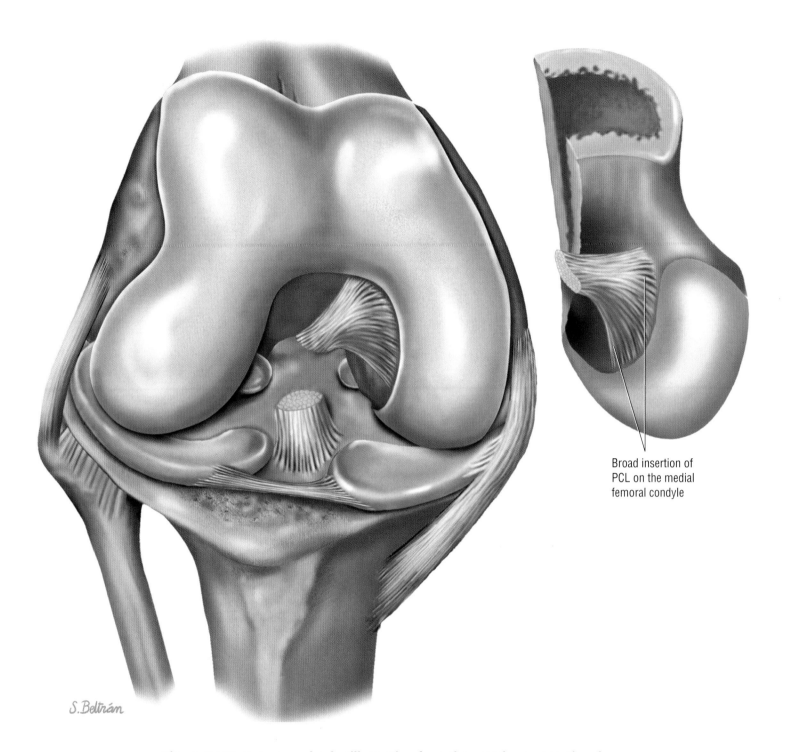

Broad insertion of
PCL on the medial
femoral condyle

S. Beltrán

Figure 4.112 ▪ A coronal color illustration from the anterior perspective shows the broad insertion of the PCL on the medial femoral condyle with horizontal orientation of fibers in extension. This contrasts to the vertical femoral attachment of the ACL. The PCL has traditionally been described as having a long, thick anterolateral bundle and a shorter posteromedial bundle. The anterolateral bundle tightens with knee flexion and the posteromedial bundle tightens with knee extension. The PCL exists as a fiber continuum and is not made up of morphologically distinct bands. The PCL has been further described as having anterior, central, posterior longitudinal, and posterior oblique fiber regions. *(See Posterior Cruciate Ligament (PCL) pg. 530, in Stoller's 3rd Edition.)*

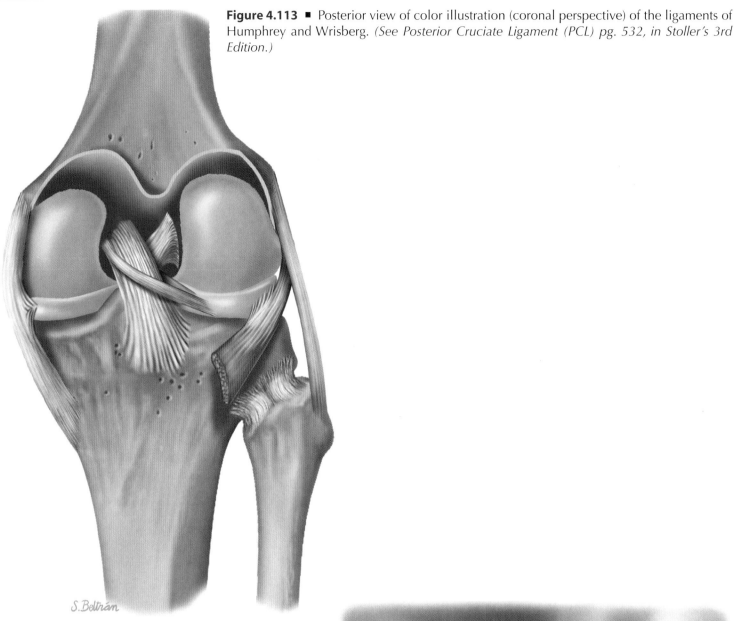

Figure 4.113 ■ Posterior view of color illustration (coronal perspective) of the ligaments of Humphrey and Wrisberg. *(See Posterior Cruciate Ligament (PCL) pg. 532, in Stoller's 3rd Edition.)*

Figure 4.114 ■ **An illustration from the anterior perspective directed posteriorly shows both meniscofemoral ligaments at their attachment to the posterior horn of the lateral meniscus.** The ligament of Humphrey course anterior to the PCL and the ligament of Wrisberg passes posterior to the PCL. *(See Posterior Cruciate Ligament (PCL) pg. 533, in Stoller's 3rd Edition.)*

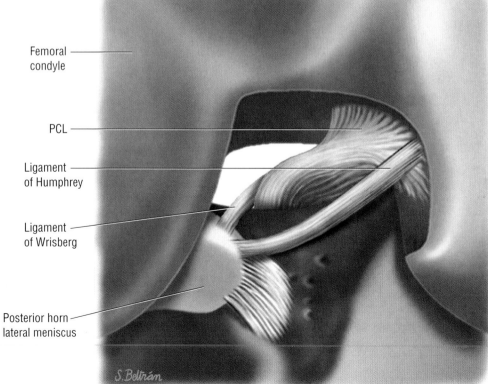

Femoral condyle

PCL

Ligament of Humphrey

Ligament of Wrisberg

Posterior horn lateral meniscus

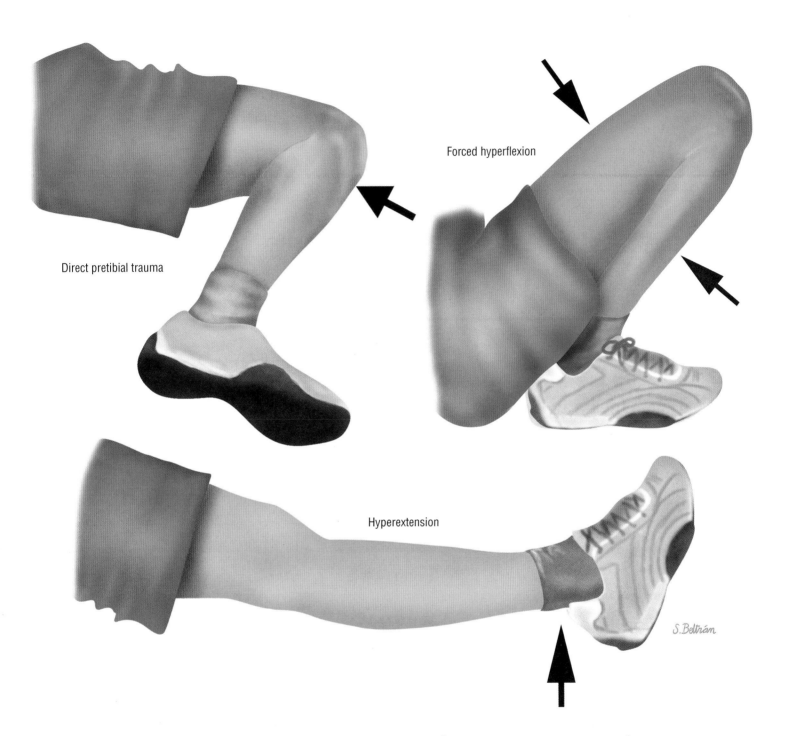

Forced hyperflexion

Direct pretibial trauma

Hyperextension

S. Beltrán

Figure 4.115 ■ Mechanisms of posterior cruciate ligament injury. *(See Location and Mechanism of Injury pgs. 534 and 537, in Stoller's 3rd Edition.)*

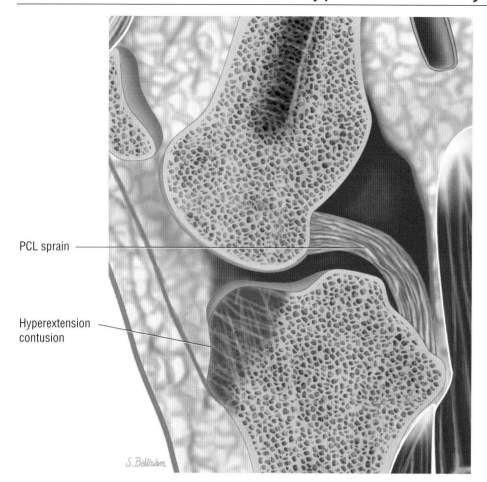

PCL sprain

Hyperextension
contusion

S. Beltrán

**Figure 4.116 ■ PCL injury with hyperexten-
sion and valgus mechanism results in contusions of the anterior compartment of the
knee.** Forced hyperextension of the knee may
tear the ACL, PCL, and posterior capsule.
Sagittal color illustration with anterior tibial hyperextension contusions. *(See Location and
Mechanism of Injury pgs. 534 and 537, in
Stoller's 3rd Edition.)*

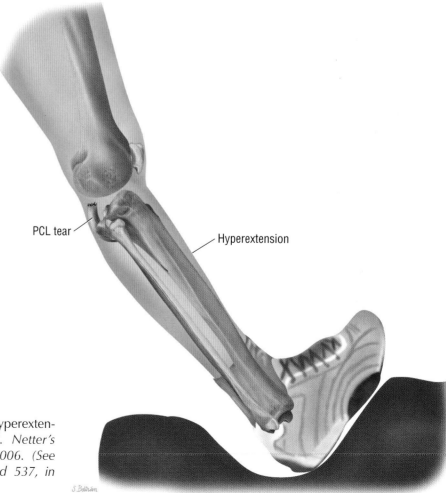

PCL tear

Hyperextension

S. Beltrán

Figure 4.117 ■ PCL rupture associated with a hyperexten-
sion injury. *Based on Green WB, Netter FH. Netter's
Orthopaedics. Philadelphia: Saunders Elsevier, 2006. (See
Location and Mechanism of Injury pgs. 534 and 537, in
Stoller's 3rd Edition.)*

Figure 4.118 ■ A fall onto a flexed knee with the foot in dorsiflexion (**A**) results in patellofemoral joint injury. In contrast, a fall landing with the foot positioned in plantarflexion (**B**) results in a PCL injury (**C**) as the posterior force vector is transmitted to the tibial tubercle. *Based on DeLee JC, Drez DD Jr, Miller MD. Orthopaedic Sports Medicine, 2 ed, vol 1. Philadelphia: Saunders, 2003. (See Location and Mechanism of Injury pgs. 534 and 537, in Stoller's 3rd Edition.)*

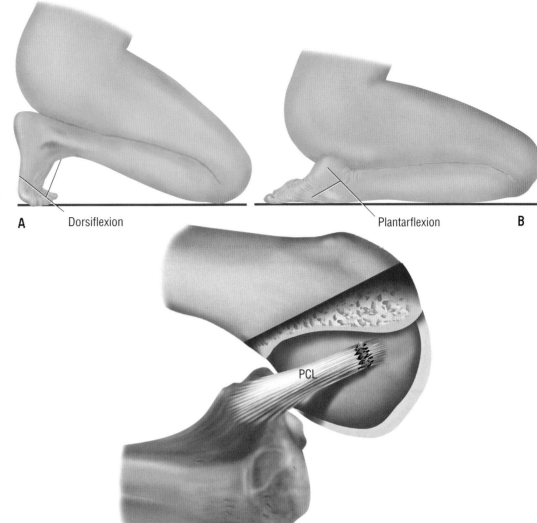

A — Dorsiflexion

B — Plantarflexion

PCL

C — S.Beltrán

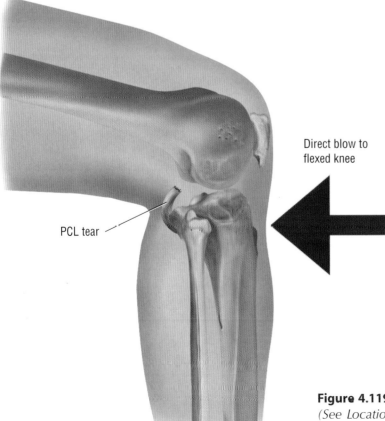

Direct blow to flexed knee

PCL tear

S.Beltrán

Figure 4.119 ■ PCL rupture secondary to a direct blow to a flexed knee. *(See Location and Mechanism of Injury pgs. 534 and 537, in Stoller's 3rd Edition.)*

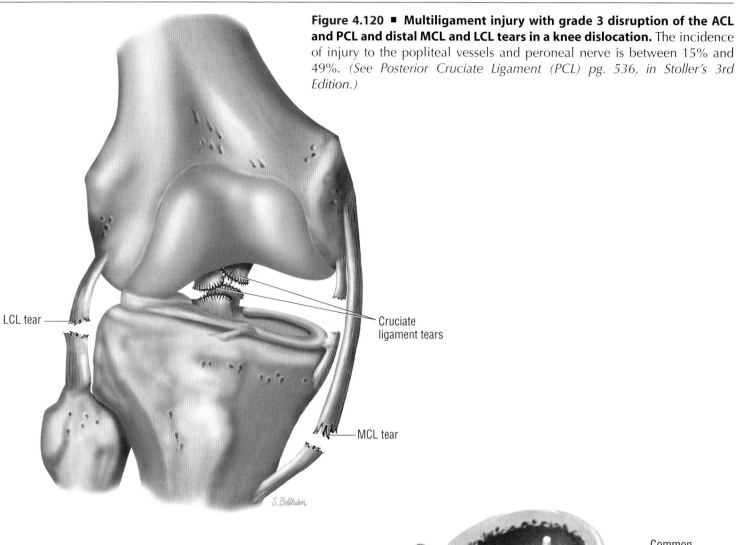

Figure 4.120 ▪ Multiligament injury with grade 3 disruption of the ACL and PCL and distal MCL and LCL tears in a knee dislocation. The incidence of injury to the popliteal vessels and peroneal nerve is between 15% and 49%. *(See Posterior Cruciate Ligament (PCL) pg. 536, in Stoller's 3rd Edition.)*

LCL tear

Cruciate ligament tears

MCL tear

S.Beltrán

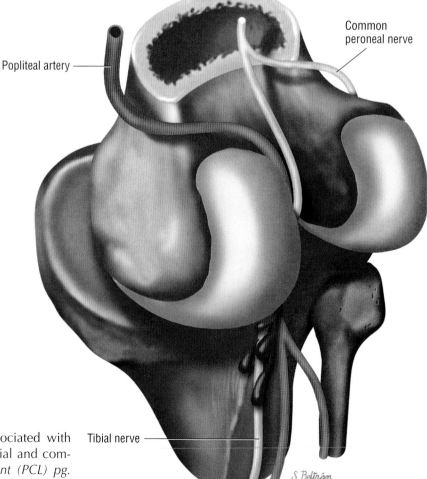

Popliteal artery

Common peroneal nerve

Tibial nerve

S.Beltrán

Figure 4.121 ▪ Posterior dislocation of the knee associated with tear of the popiteal artery and stretch injury of the tibial and common peroneal nerves. *(See Posterior Cruciate Ligament (PCL) pg. 536, in Stoller's 3rd Edition.)*

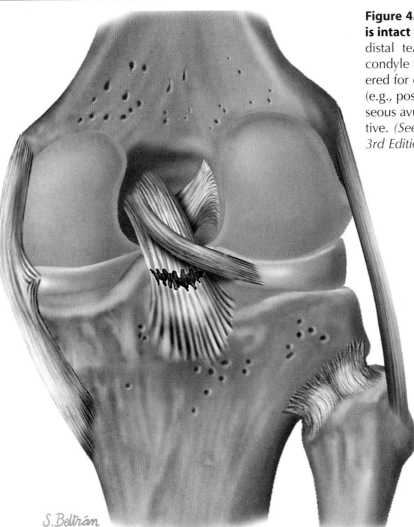

S.Beltrán

Figure 4.122 ■ At least one of the meniscofemoral ligaments is intact with either acute or chronic PCL injuries. Grade 3 PCL distal tear is shown with posteriorly located lateral femoral condyle flexion-related contusion. PCL reconstruction is considered for cases of grade 3 laxity with combined ligament injuries (e.g., posterolateral corner injuries) or meniscal, chondral, or osseous avulsion. Coronal color illustration with posterior perspective. *(See Posterior Cruciate Ligament (PCL) pg. 539, in Stoller's 3rd Edition.)*

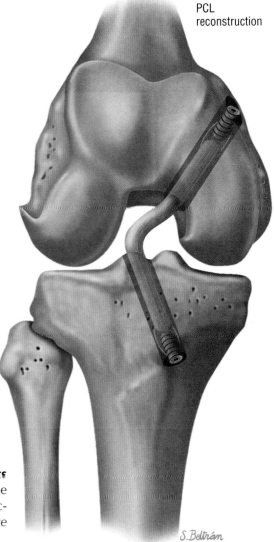

PCL reconstruction

S.Beltrán

Figure 4.123 ■ Bone-patellar tendon bone and Achilles tendon are allografts commonly used for PCL reconstruction. The double-bundle technique offers the advantage of less posterior tibial translation compared to single-bundle reconstruction (coronal color illustration anterior perspective). *(See Posterior Cruciate Ligament pg. 544, in Stoller's 3rd Edition.)*

Figure 4.124 ▪ Axial 3D section demonstrating the superficial and deep MCL as well as the popliteus tendon and lateral collateral ligament. There are three layers that stabilize the medial aspect of the knee. MCL trauma may affect any or all of these layers. Layer 1 is the deep investing fascia, which merges with the posteromedial capsule and hamstring muscle group. Layer 2 contains the superficial MCL. Layer 3 is the joint capsule, which can be divided into three parts. The anterior third is attached to the anterior horn and is reinforced by the medial retinaculum. The middle third is the deep MCL and the posterior third contains the POL and OPL. The POL component represents fused layers 2 and 3. *(See Medial Collateral Ligament pg. 545, in Stoller's 3rd Edition.)*

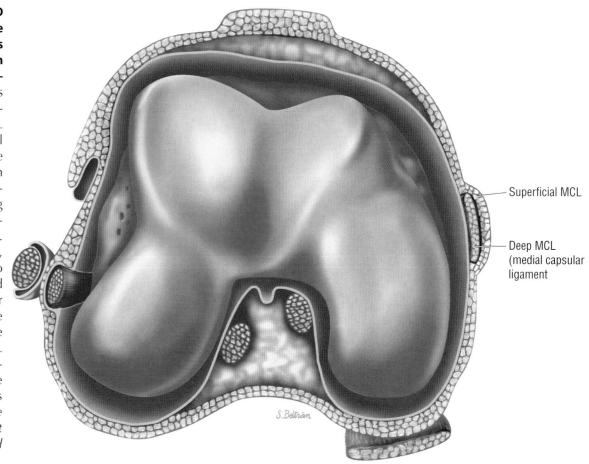

Superficial MCL

Deep MCL (medial capsular ligament

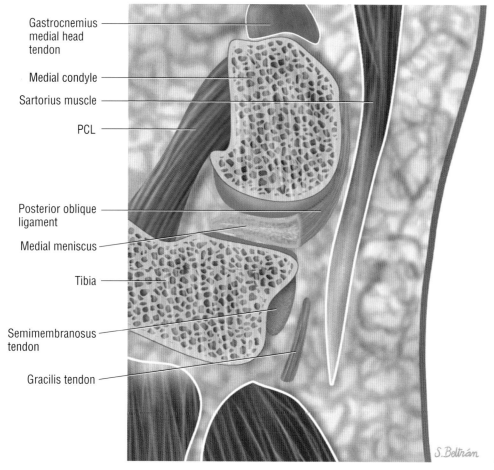

Gastrocnemius medial head tendon

Medial condyle

Sartorius muscle

PCL

Posterior oblique ligament

Medial meniscus

Tibia

Semimembranosus tendon

Gracilis tendon

Figure 4.125 ▪ Posteromedial coronal illustration showing the posterior oblique ligament (POL). The POL helps maintain medial stability and resists anteromedial tibial subluxation. It is tight in knee extension and lax in knee flexion. Sports-related injuries commonly occur between 45° and 90° of knee flexion. The semimembranosus assists in flexion by pulling the medial meniscus posteriorly to avoid entrapment and also engages the POL through its expansion below the joint line. *(See Medial Collateral Ligament pg. 547, in Stoller's 3rd Edition.)*

Medial and Posteromedial Structures

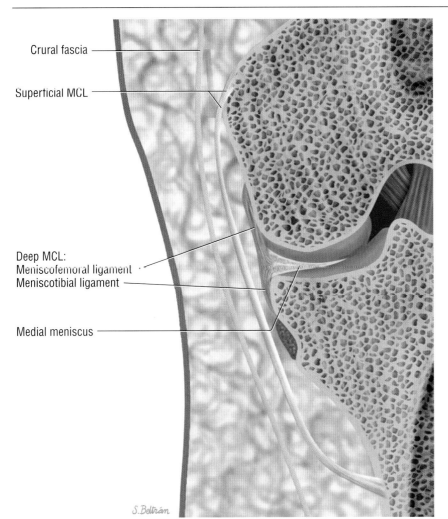

Crural fascia

Superficial MCL

Deep MCL:
Meniscofemoral ligament
Meniscotibial ligament

Medial meniscus

S.Beltrán

Figure 4.126 ■ **The static medial stabilizers include the superficial medial collateral ligament (MCL), the posterior oblique ligament, and the deep capsular (meniscofemoral and meniscotibial) ligaments.** Dynamic support is provided by the semimembranosus insertions and the vastus medialis. *(See Medial Collateral Ligament pg. 548, in Stoller's 3rd Edition.)*

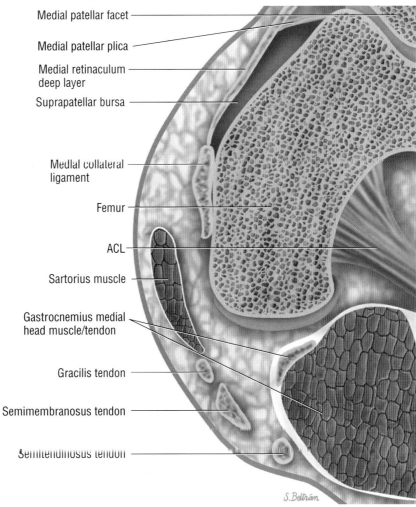

Medial patellar facet

Medial patellar plica

Medial retinaculum deep layer

Suprapatellar bursa

Medial collateral ligament

Femur

ACL

Sartorius muscle

Gastrocnemius medial head muscle/tendon

Gracilis tendon

Semimembranosus tendon

Semitendinosus tendon

S.Beltrán

Figure 4.127 ■ Posteromedial structures above the joint line on a color axial cross-section. *(See Medial Collateral Ligament pg. 549, in Stoller's 3rd Edition.)*

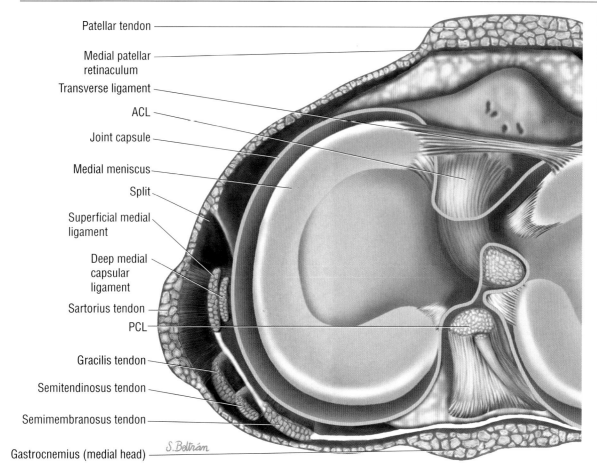

Patellar tendon
Medial patellar retinaculum
Transverse ligament
ACL
Joint capsule
Medial meniscus
Split
Superficial medial ligament
Deep medial capsular ligament
Sartorius tendon
PCL
Gracilis tendon
Semitendinosus tendon
Semimembranosus tendon
Gastrocnemius (medial head)

Figure 4.128 ■ Posteromedial corner at the level of the joint line on a superior view illustration. *(See Medial Collateral Ligament pg. 550, in Stoller's 3rd Edition.)*

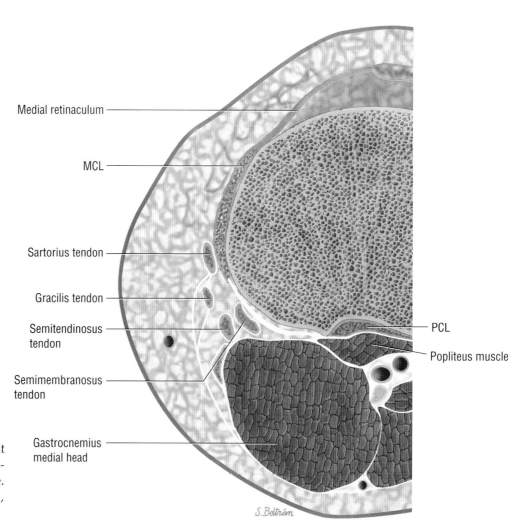

Medial retinaculum
MCL
Sartorius tendon
Gracilis tendon
Semitendinosus tendon
Semimembranosus tendon
Gastrocnemius medial head
PCL
Popliteus muscle

Figure 4.129 ■ Posteromedial corner at the level of the proximal tibia on a cross-section illustration below the joint line. *(See Medial Collateral Ligament pg. 551, in Stoller's 3rd Edition.)*

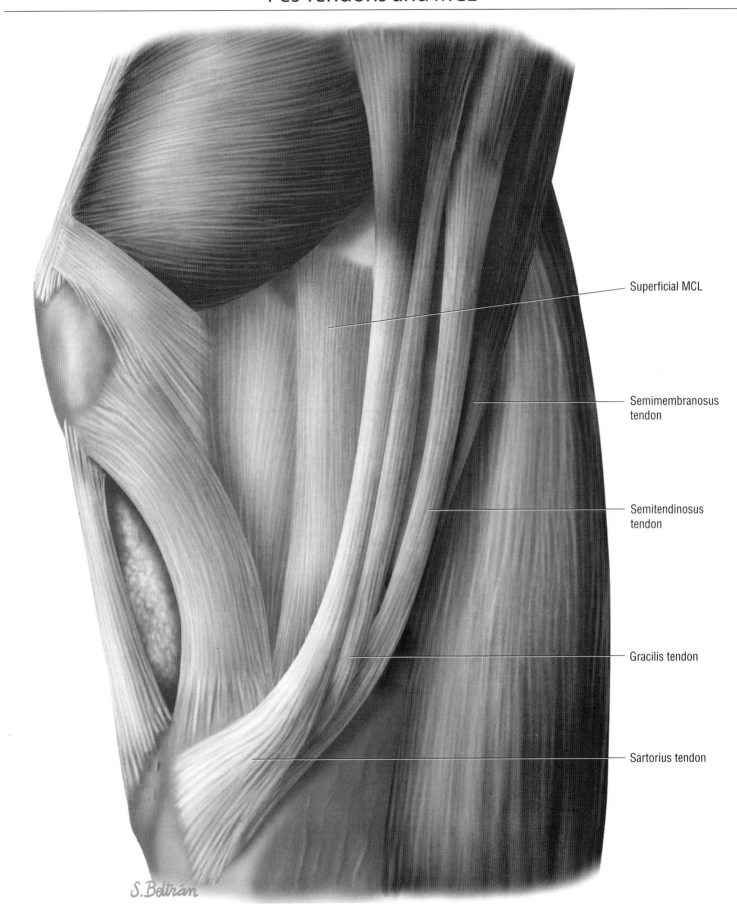

Superficial MCL

Semimembranosus tendon

Semitendinosus tendon

Gracilis tendon

Sartorius tendon

S.Beltrán

Figure 4.130 ■ Medial view of normal pes tendons and MCL on a color illustration from the sagittal perspective. *(See Medial Collateral Ligament pg. 552, in Stoller's 3rd Edition.)*

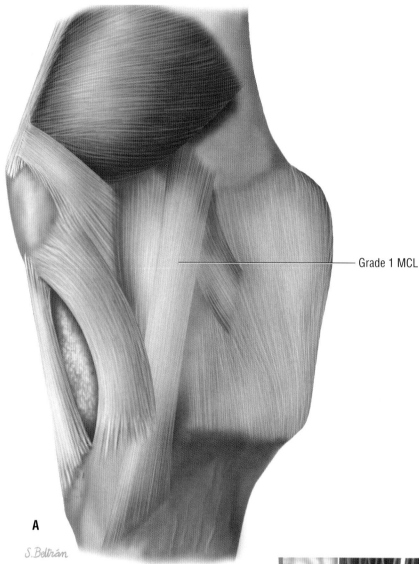

Grade 1 MCL

A

S. Beltrán

Figure 4.131 ■ **(A)** A lateral view 3D illustration and **(B)** a coronal color section showing a grade 1 MCL sprain with edema superficial to the ligament. Although there may be a few torn fibers, there is no loss of ligamentous integrity. *(See Medial Collateral Ligament pg. 553, in Stoller's 3rd Edition.)*

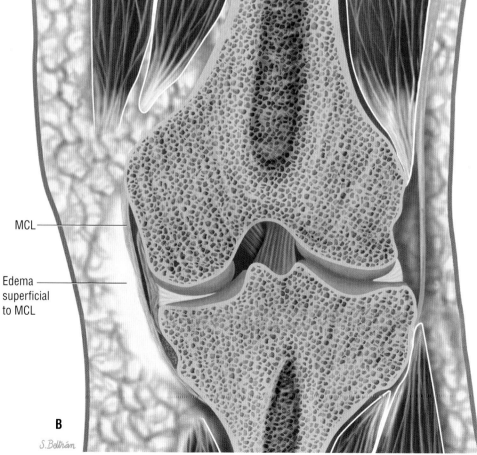

MCL

Edema superficial to MCL

B

S. Beltrán

Figure 4.132 ■ **Grade 2 MCL sprain with intraligamentous thickening and degeneration in association with fluid or edema superficial and deep to the ligament.** Grade 2 injuries are moderate sprains or incomplete tears without pathologic laxity. The MCL fibers are apposed, allowing for ligamentous healing. **(A)** Lateral 3D color illustration. **(B)** Coronal color section. *(See Medial Collateral Ligament pg. 555, in Stoller's 3rd Edition.)*

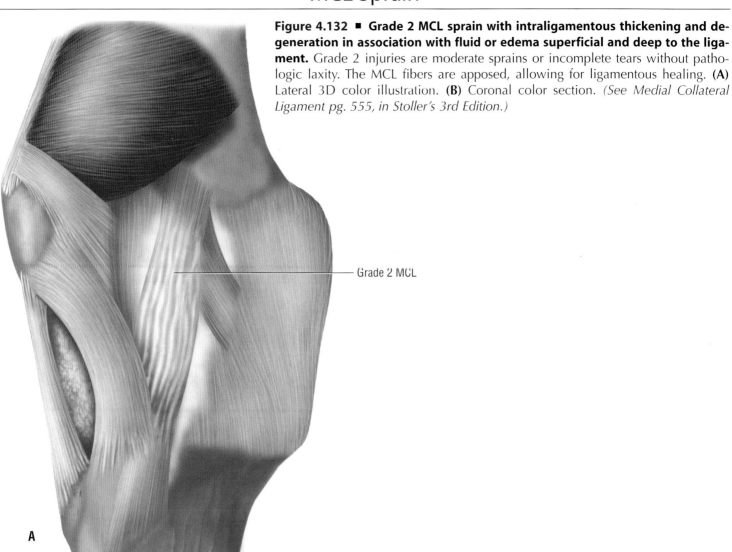

Grade 2 MCL

A

S.Beltrán

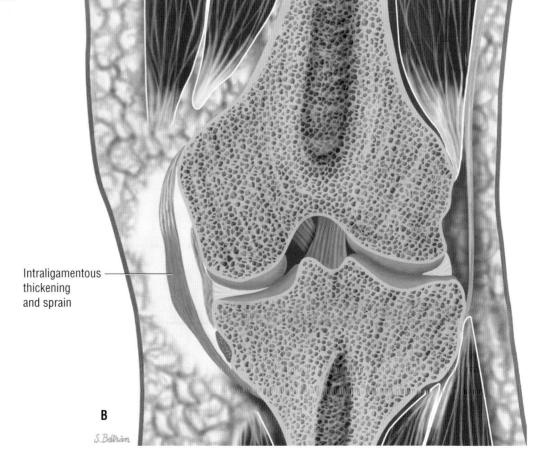

Intraligamentous thickening and sprain

B

S.Beltrán

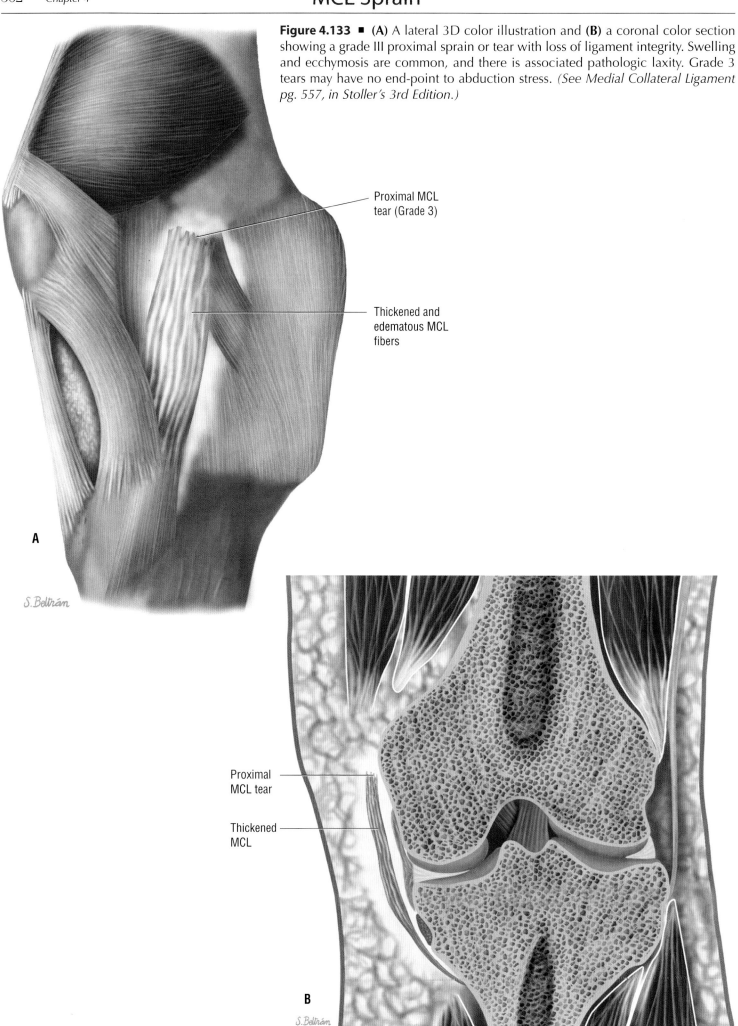

Figure 4.133 ■ **(A)** A lateral 3D color illustration and **(B)** a coronal color section showing a grade III proximal sprain or tear with loss of ligament integrity. Swelling and ecchymosis are common, and there is associated pathologic laxity. Grade 3 tears may have no end-point to abduction stress. *(See Medial Collateral Ligament pg. 557, in Stoller's 3rd Edition.)*

Proximal MCL
tear (Grade 3)

Thickened and
edematous MCL
fibers

Proximal
MCL tear

Thickened
MCL

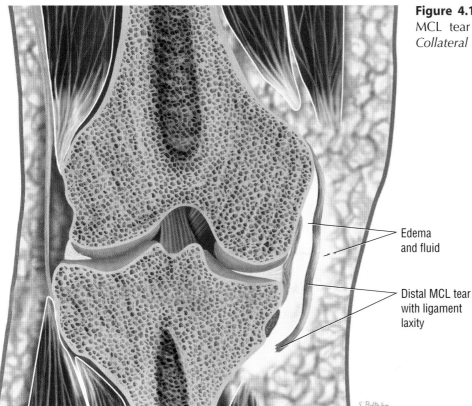

Figure 4.134 ▪ Coronal color illustration of a distal MCL tear without significant retraction. *(See Medial Collateral Ligament pg. 558, in Stoller's 3rd Edition.)*

Edema and fluid

Distal MCL tear with ligament laxity

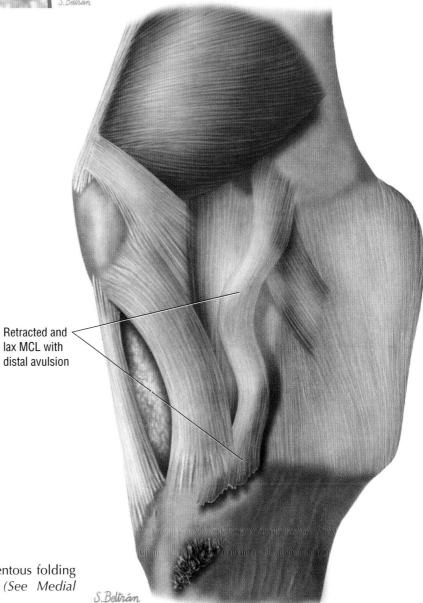

Retracted and lax MCL with distal avulsion

Figure 4.135 ▪ Retracted distal MCL tear with ligamentous folding demonstrated on a lateral 3D color illustration. *(See Medial Collateral Ligament pg. 559, in Stoller's 3rd Edition.)*

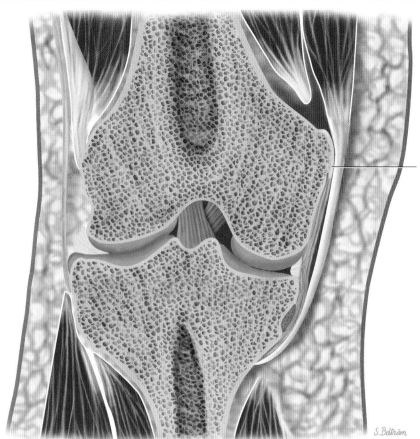

Ossification MCL
femoral attachment

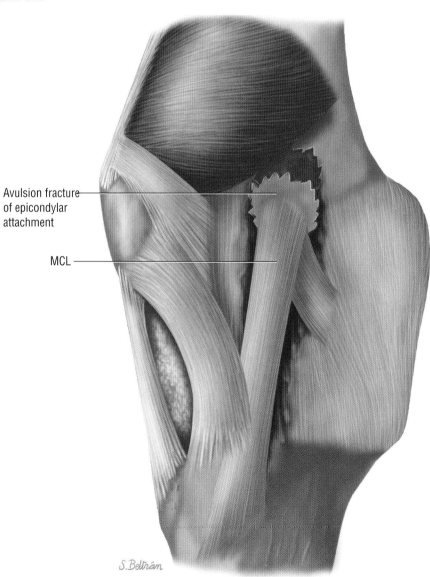

Avulsion fracture
of epicondylar
attachment

MCL

Figure 4.137 ■ Lateral view 3D color illustration of an avulsion fracture of the epicondylar attachment of the MCL. *(See Medial Collateral Ligament pg. 562, in Stoller's 3rd Edition.)*

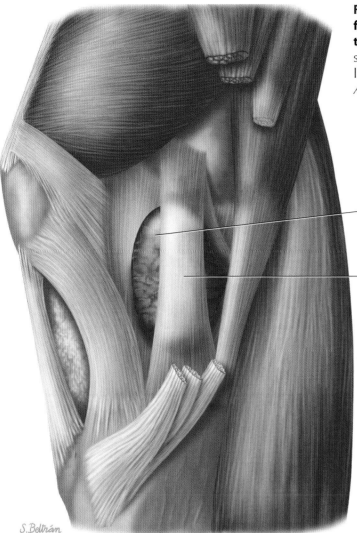

Figure 4.138 ■ **The bursa of Voshell is located between the superficial and deep MCL distally and is a potential site for inflammation.** Medial or tibial collateral ligament bursitis is seen between the superficial MCL and meniscotibial ligament of the deep capsular layer (layer 3). *(See MCL (Tibial Collateral Ligament) and Pes Anserinus Bursitis pg. 564, in Stoller's 3rd Edition.)*

Medial collateral ligament (MCL) bursitis deep to superficial MCL

MCL

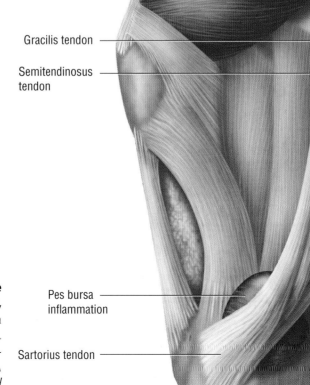

Gracilis tendon

Semitendinosus tendon

Pes bursa inflammation

Sartorius tendon

Figure 4.139 ■ **Pes anserinus bursitis at the tibial attachment site of the sartorius, gracilis, and semitendinosus tendons.** The pes bursa can be injured by direct trauma or contusion, and pes bursitis may be associated with excessive pronation (lateral 3D color illustration). *(See See MCL (Tibial Collateral Ligament) and Pes Anserinus Bursitis pg. 565, in Stoller's 3rd Edition.)*

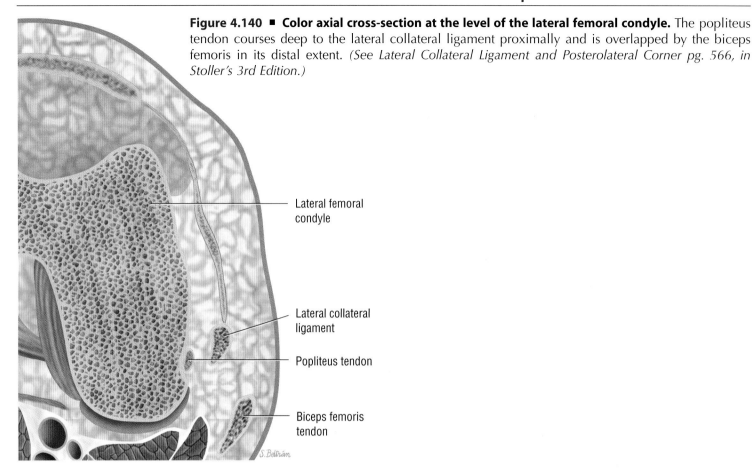

Figure 4.140 ■ **Color axial cross-section at the level of the lateral femoral condyle.** The popliteus tendon courses deep to the lateral collateral ligament proximally and is overlapped by the biceps femoris in its distal extent. *(See Lateral Collateral Ligament and Posterolateral Corner pg. 566, in Stoller's 3rd Edition.)*

Lateral femoral condyle

Lateral collateral ligament

Popliteus tendon

Biceps femoris tendon

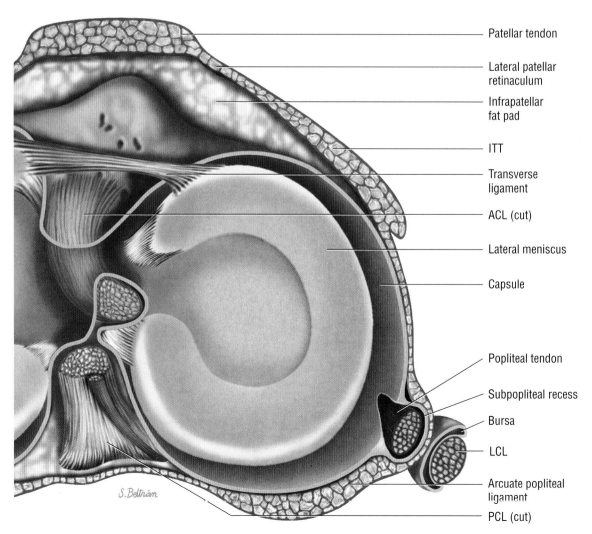

Figure 4.141 ■ Superior axial cross-section of the lateral compartment at the level of the lateral meniscus on a 3D color illustration. *(See Lateral Collateral Ligament and Posterolateral Corner pg. 567, in Stoller's 3rd Edition.)*

Patellar tendon

Lateral patellar retinaculum

Infrapatellar fat pad

ITT

Transverse ligament

ACL (cut)

Lateral meniscus

Capsule

Popliteal tendon

Subpopliteal recess

Bursa

LCL

Arcuate popliteal ligament

PCL (cut)

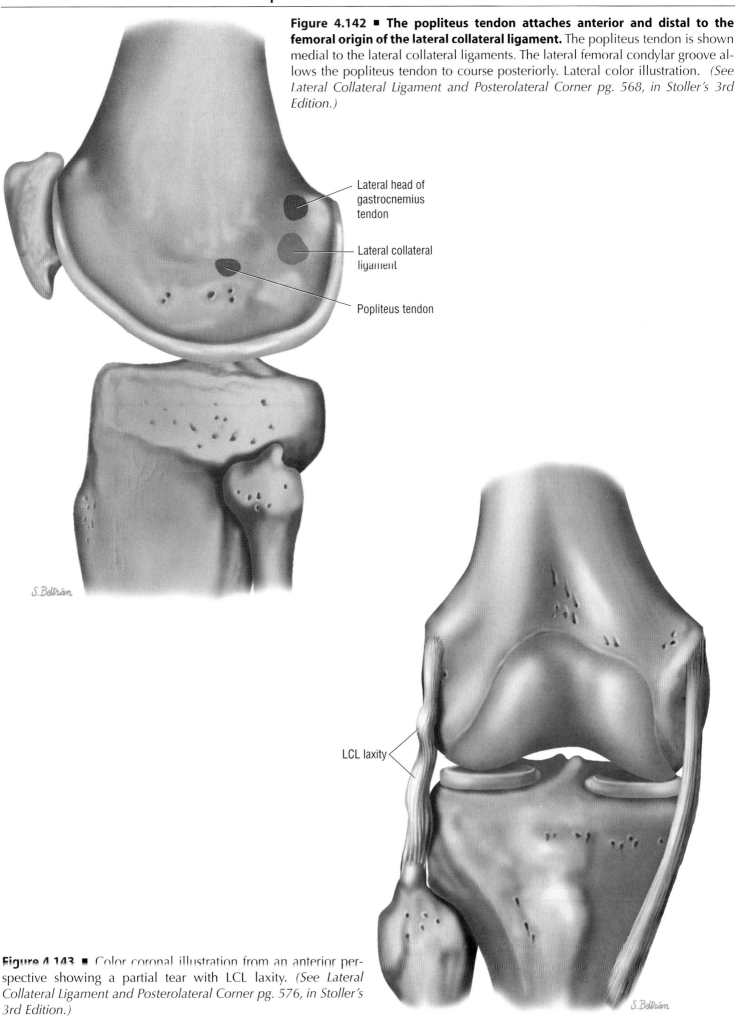

Lateral head of
gastrocnemius
tendon

Lateral collateral
ligament

Popliteus tendon

Figure 4.142 ▪ **The popliteus tendon attaches anterior and distal to the femoral origin of the lateral collateral ligament.** The popliteus tendon is shown medial to the lateral collateral ligaments. The lateral femoral condylar groove allows the popliteus tendon to course posteriorly. Lateral color illustration. *(See Lateral Collateral Ligament and Posterolateral Corner pg. 568, in Stoller's 3rd Edition.)*

LCL laxity

Figure 4.143 ▪ Color coronal illustration from an anterior perspective showing a partial tear with LCL laxity. *(See Lateral Collateral Ligament and Posterolateral Corner pg. 576, in Stoller's 3rd Edition.)*

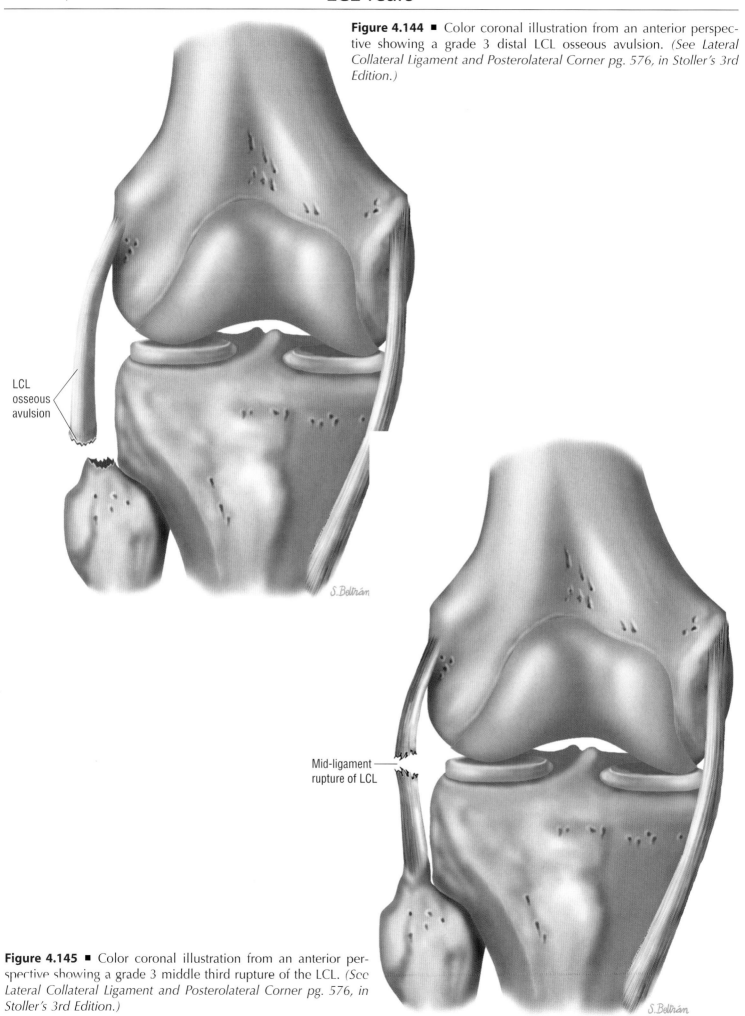

Figure 4.144 ■ Color coronal illustration from an anterior perspective showing a grade 3 distal LCL osseous avulsion. *(See Lateral Collateral Ligament and Posterolateral Corner pg. 576, in Stoller's 3rd Edition.)*

LCL osseous avulsion

Mid-ligament rupture of LCL

Figure 4.145 ■ Color coronal illustration from an anterior perspective showing a grade 3 middle third rupture of the LCL. *(See Lateral Collateral Ligament and Posterolateral Corner pg. 576, in Stoller's 3rd Edition.)*

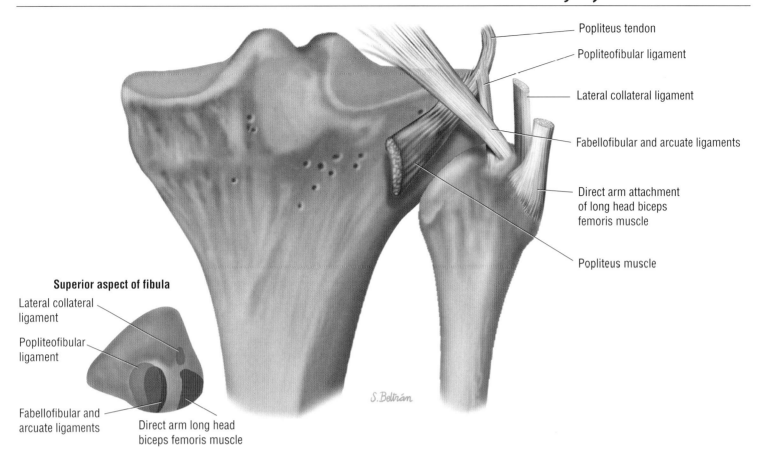

Superior aspect of fibula

Lateral collateral ligament

Popliteofibular ligament

Fabellofibular and arcuate ligaments

Direct arm long head biceps femoris muscle

Popliteus tendon

Popliteofibular ligament

Lateral collateral ligament

Fabellofibular and arcuate ligaments

Direct arm attachment of long head biceps femoris muscle

Popliteus muscle

Figure 4.146 ■ **The popliteofibular ligament attaches to the upper facet of the apex of the fibular head medial to the insertions of the fabellofibular and arcuate ligaments.** The lateral collateral ligament and the direct arm of the long head of the biceps femoris tendon are attached more peripherally to the lateral margin of the fibular head. *(See Lateral Collateral Ligament and Posterolateral Corner pg. 579, in Stoller's 3rd Edition.)*

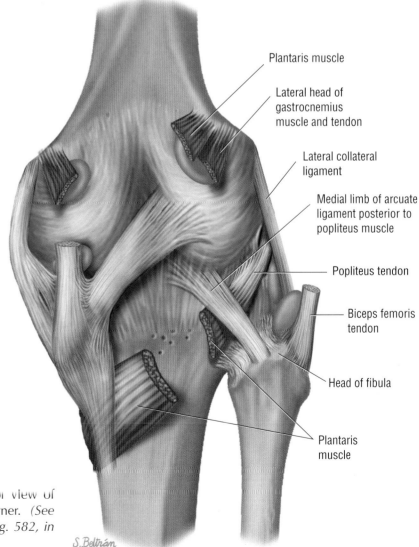

Plantaris muscle

Lateral head of gastrocnemius muscle and tendon

Lateral collateral ligament

Medial limb of arcuate ligament posterior to popliteus muscle

Popliteus tendon

Biceps femoris tendon

Head of fibula

Plantaris muscle

Figure 4.147 ■ Color illustration showing the posterior view of the normal posterior capsule and posterolateral corner. *(See Lateral Collateral Ligament and Posterolateral Corner pg. 582, in Stoller's 3rd Edition.)*

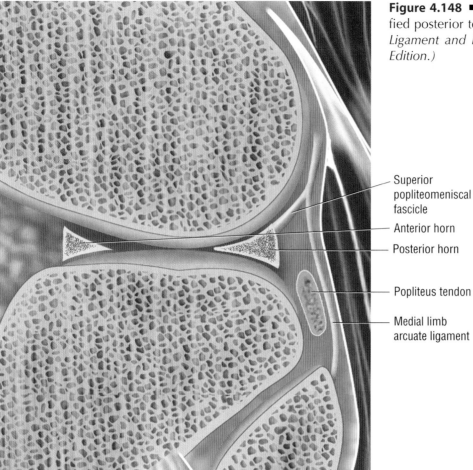

Figure 4.148 ■ Medial limb of the arcuate ligament identified posterior to the popliteus tendon. *(See Lateral Collateral Ligament and Posterolateral Corner pg. 571, in Stoller's 3rd Edition.)*

Superior popliteomeniscal fascicle

Anterior horn

Posterior horn

Popliteus tendon

Medial limb arcuate ligament

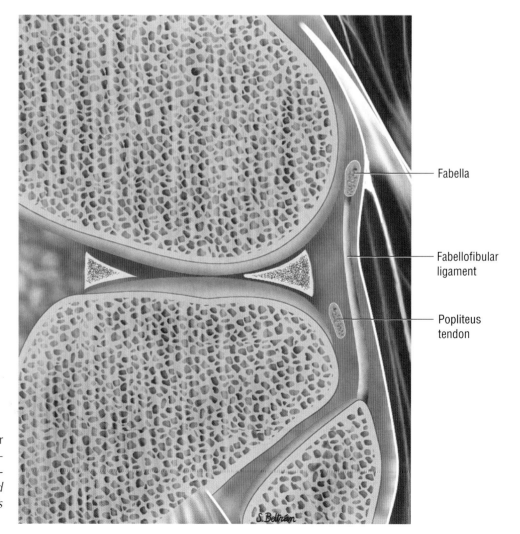

Fabella

Fabellofibular ligament

Popliteus tendon

Figure 4.149 ■ Prominent fabellofibular ligament with attachments to both the fabella proximally and the fibular styloid distally. *(See Lateral Collateral Ligament and Posterolateral Corner pg. 573, in Stoller's 3rd Edition.)*

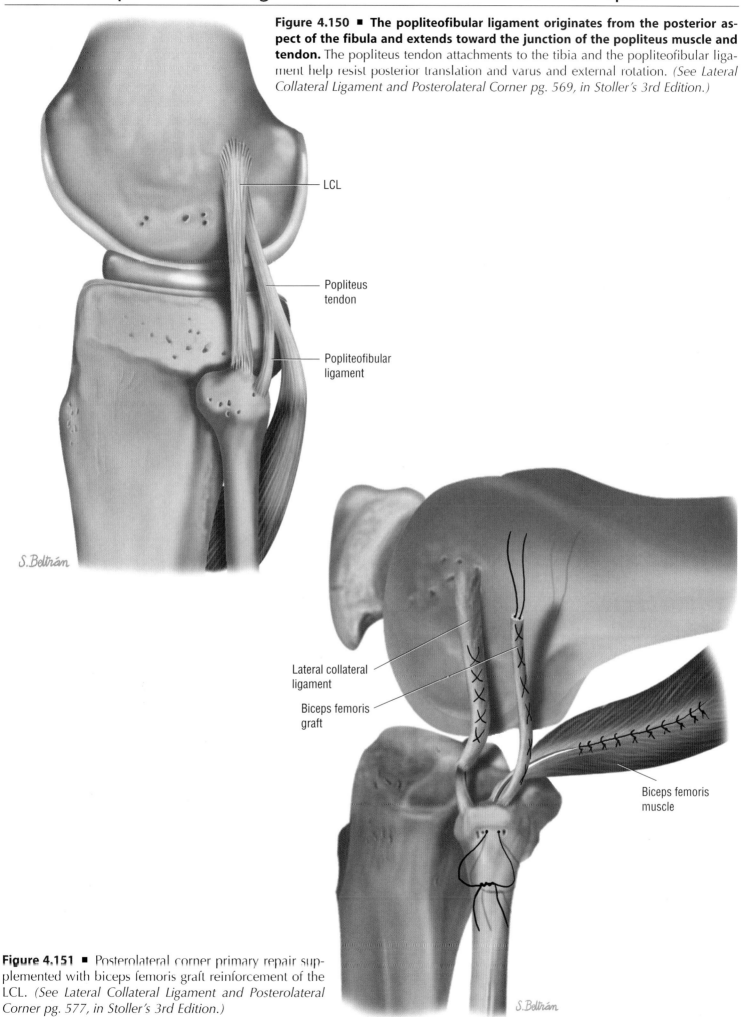

Figure 4.150 ■ **The popliteofibular ligament originates from the posterior aspect of the fibula and extends toward the junction of the popliteus muscle and tendon.** The popliteus tendon attachments to the tibia and the popliteofibular ligament help resist posterior translation and varus and external rotation. *(See Lateral Collateral Ligament and Posterolateral Corner pg. 569, in Stoller's 3rd Edition.)*

LCL

Popliteus tendon

Popliteofibular ligament

Lateral collateral ligament

Biceps femoris graft

Biceps femoris muscle

Figure 4.151 ■ Posterolateral corner primary repair supplemented with biceps femoris graft reinforcement of the LCL. *(See Lateral Collateral Ligament and Posterolateral Corner pg. 577, in Stoller's 3rd Edition.)*

Grade 1

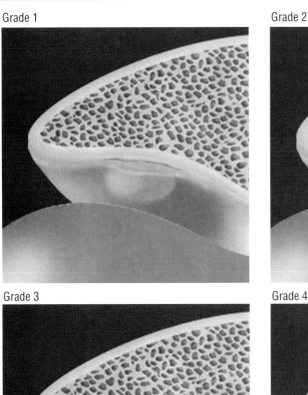

Grade 2

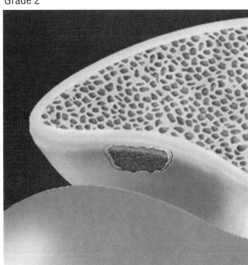

Figure 4.152 ▪ Outerbridge classification of chondromalacia. Grade 1 chondromalacia with softening of articular cartilage. Grade 1 represents closed chondromalacia, which includes softening and blistering. Grade 2 chondromalacia with fragmentation and fissuring less than 1.5 cm in diameter. Grade 3 chondromalacia with fragmentation and fissuring greater than 1.5 cm in diameter. Grade 4 with full-thickness chondral erosion to exposed subchondral bone. *(See Chondromalacia pg. 589, in Stoller's 3rd Edition.)*

Grade 3

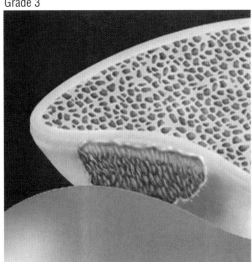

Grade 4

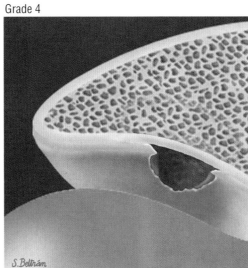

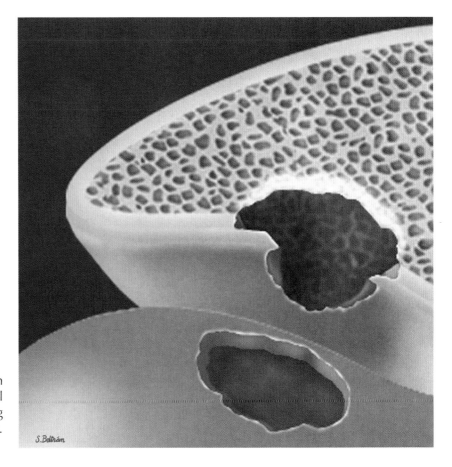

Figure 4.153 ▪ Patellofemoral arthrosis (arthritis) with progression of chondromalacia to involve subchondral erosion of the patella and erosion of the opposing femoral chondral surface. *(See Chondromalacia pg. 591, in Stoller's 3rd Edition.)*

Grade 1

Grade 2

Grade 3

Grade 4

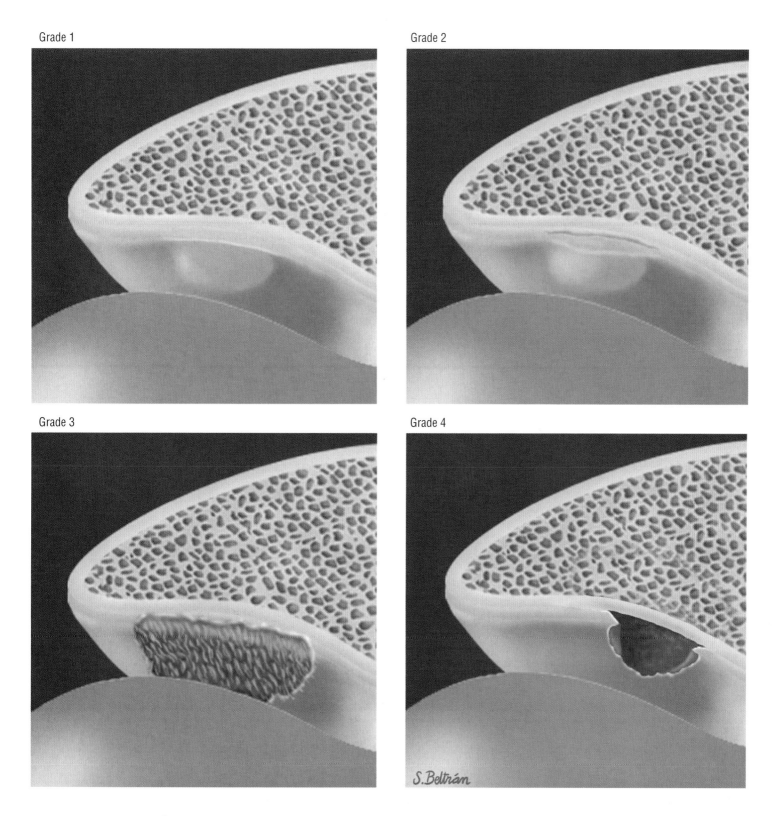

S. Beltrán

Figure 4.154 ▪ Alternative classification distinguishing between chondral softening in grade 1 and blistering in grade 2. Grade 3 still represents chondral fibrillation and grade 4 is frank cartilage ulceration. *(See Chondromalacia pg. 591, in Stoller's 3rd Edition.)*

Chondromalacia

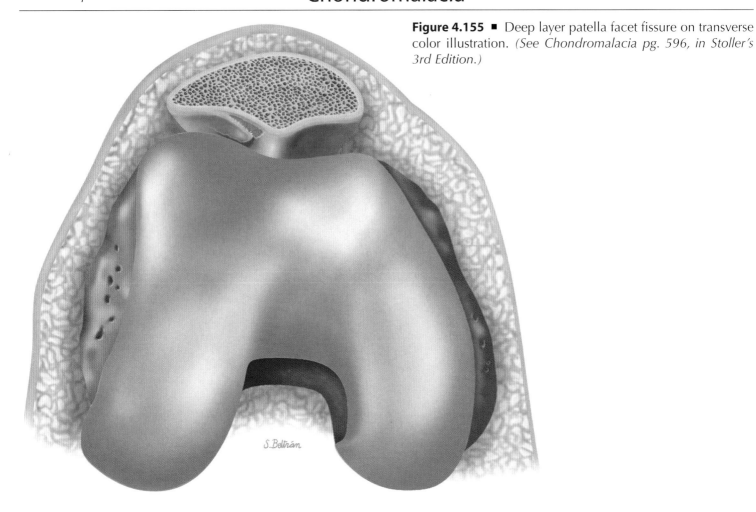

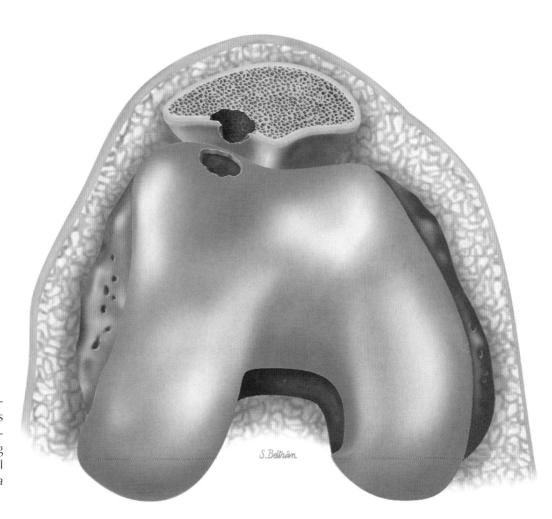

Figure 4.156 ■ Transverse color illustration of patellofemoral arthritis with lateral femoral condyle full-thickness erosion and matching subchondral erosion of the lateral patellar facet. *(See Chondromalacia pg. 600, in Stoller's 3rd Edition.)*

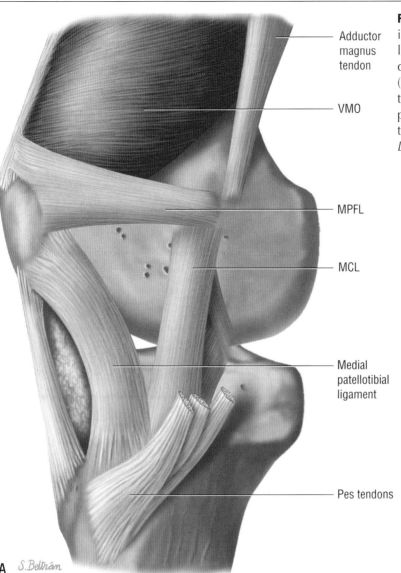

Adductor
magnus
tendon

VMO

MPFL

MCL

Medial
patellotibial
ligament

Pes tendons

A *S.Beltrán*

Figure 4.157 ■ **(A)** Sagittal view from a medial perspective illustration of the normal course of the medial patellofemoral ligament (MPFL) arising between the adductor tubercle (adductor magnus insertion site) and the medial epicondyle (medial collateral ligament origin). The MPFL fibers contribute to the medial retinaculum at their more anterior patellar attachment. **(B)** Transverse view of MPFL femoral attachment. The MPFL is a layer 2 structure. *(See Traumatic Dislocations pg. 606, in Stoller's 3rd Edition.)*

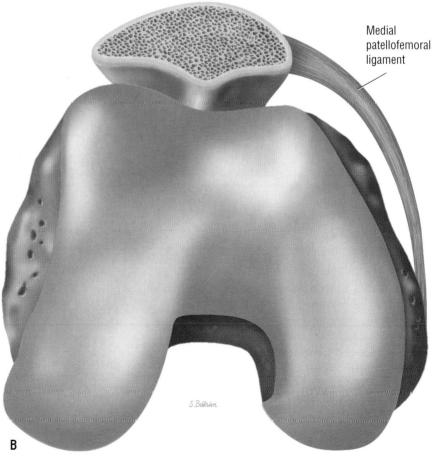

Medial
patellofemoral
ligament

B

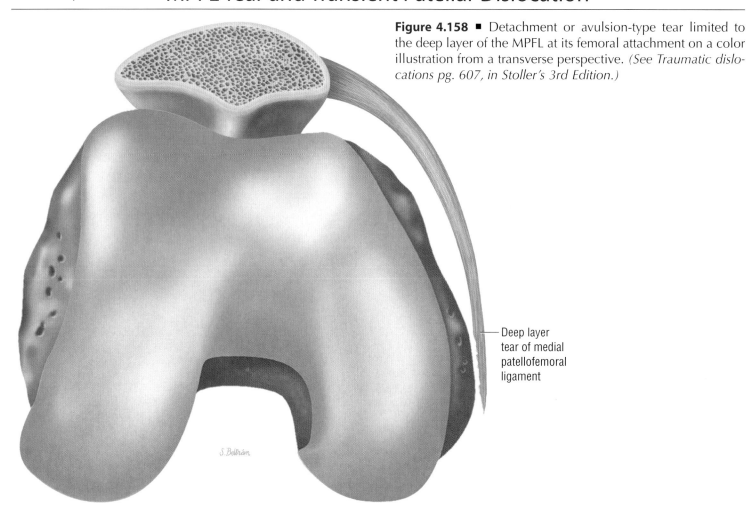

Figure 4.158 ■ Detachment or avulsion-type tear limited to the deep layer of the MPFL at its femoral attachment on a color illustration from a transverse perspective. *(See Traumatic dislocations pg. 607, in Stoller's 3rd Edition.)*

Deep layer tear of medial patellofemoral ligament

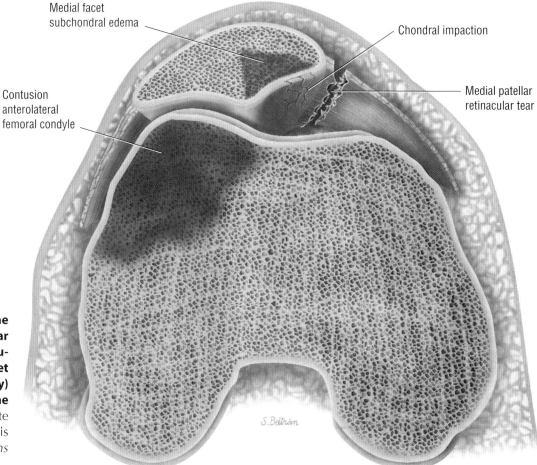

Medial facet subchondral edema

Chondral impaction

Contusion anterolateral femoral condyle

Medial patellar retinacular tear

Figure 4.159 ■ **Transverse plane illustration of a transient patellar dislocation with osseous contusions of the medial patellar facet (with associated chondral injury) and the anterolateral aspect of the lateral femoral condyle.** Complete medial retinaculum disruption is shown. *(See Traumatic Dislocations pg. 608, in Stoller's 3rd Edition.)*

Figure 4.160 ■ **(A)** 3D and **(B)** 2D transverse color illustrations of complete disruption of the femoral origin of the MPFL. Medial patellar facet chondral fragmentation and associated osseous contusion of the medial facets and lateral femoral condyle are shown on **(B)**. *(See Traumatic Dislocations pg. 609, in Stoller's 3rd Edition.)*

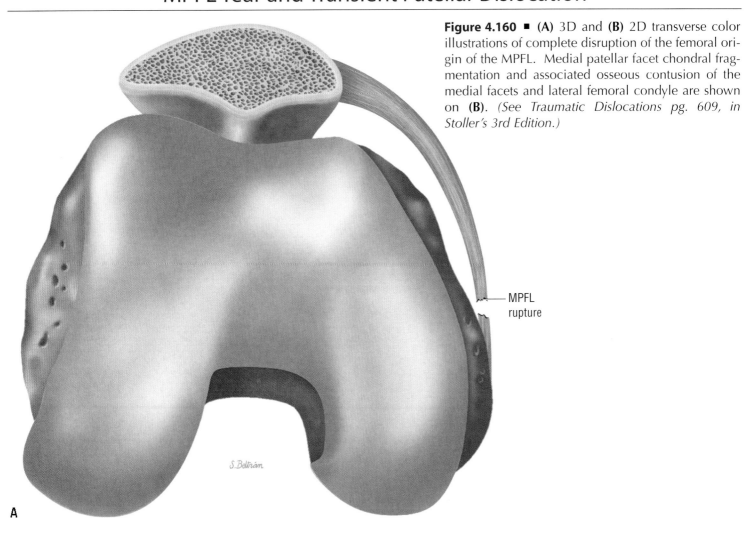

MPFL rupture

A

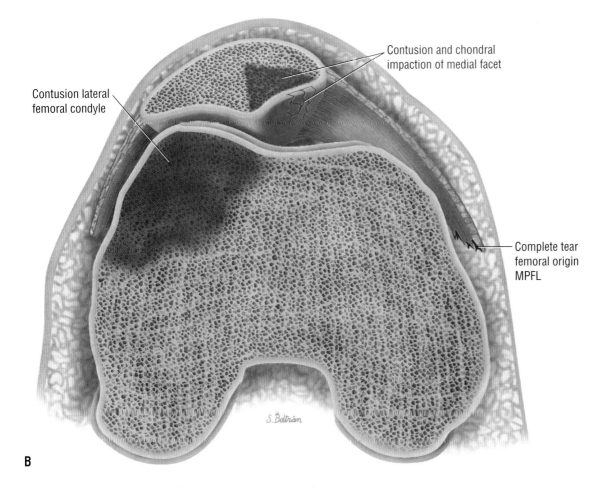

Contusion and chondral impaction of medial facet

Contusion lateral femoral condyle

Complete tear femoral origin MPFL

B

Vastus Medialis Obliquus (VMO) Injury

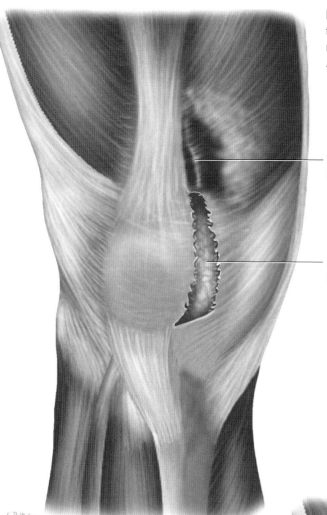

Figure 4.161 ■ Patellar dislocation with interstitial tearing of the distal vastus medialis obliquus (VMO) muscle associated with a medial retinaculum tear. *(See Traumatic Dislocations pg. 610, in Stoller's 3rd Edition.)*

VMO
interstitial tear

Medial
retinacular tear

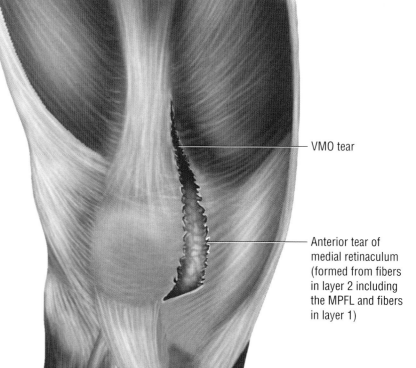

VMO tear

Anterior tear of
medial retinaculum
(formed from fibers
in layer 2 including
the MPFL and fibers
in layer 1)

Figure 4.162 ■ **The superior fibers of the medial patellofemoral ligament are confluent with distal vastus medialis deep fascia.** Associated vastus medialis obliquus (VMO) tearing is demonstrated. Interstitial tears are more frequent than discrete insertional rupture. *(See Traumatic Dislocations pg. 610, in Stoller's 3rd Edition.)*

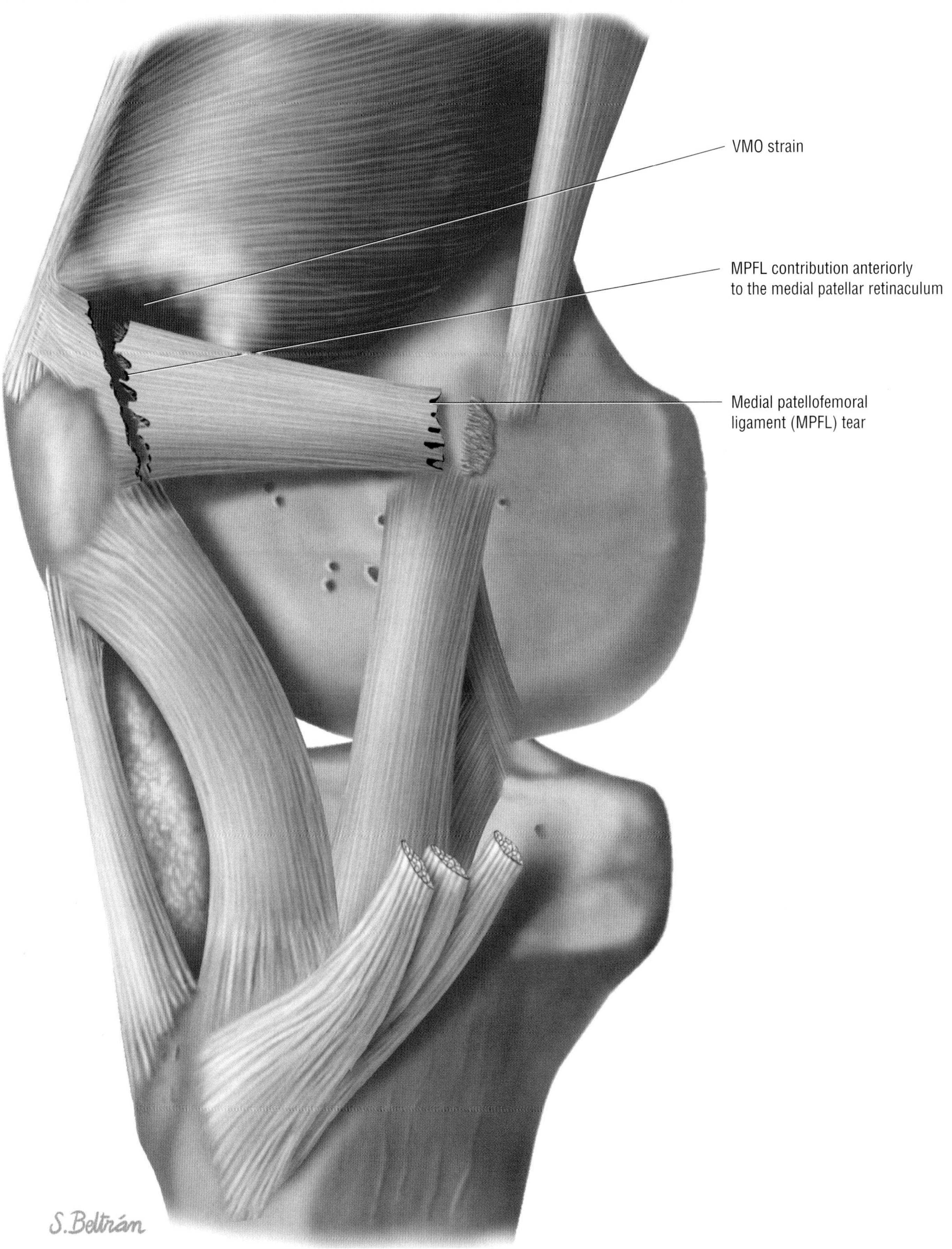

VMO strain

MPFL contribution anteriorly
to the medial patellar retinaculum

Medial patellofemoral
ligament (MPFL) tear

S.Beltrán

Figure 4.163 ■ **Sagittal view color illustration from the medial perspective of complete discontinuity of the medial patellofemoral ligament from its femoral attachment and patellar insertion through its contribution to the medial retinaculum.** Static subluxation and patellar instability result with unopposed action of the lateral retinaculum. *(See Traumatic Dislocations pg. 611, in Stoller's 3rd Edition.)*

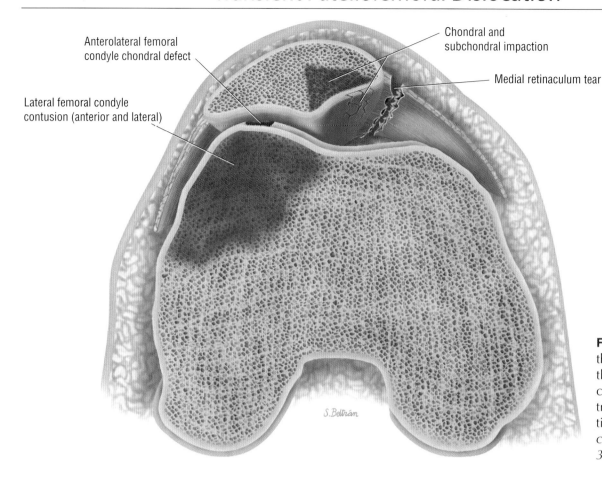

Anterolateral femoral
condyle chondral defect

Chondral and
subchondral impaction

Medial retinaculum tear

Lateral femoral condyle
contusion (anterior and lateral)

S.Beltrán

Figure 4.164 ■ Focal full-thickness chondral defect of the anterolateral femoral condyle associated with transient patellar dislocation. *(See Traumatic Dislocations pg. 612, in Stoller's 3rd Edition.)*

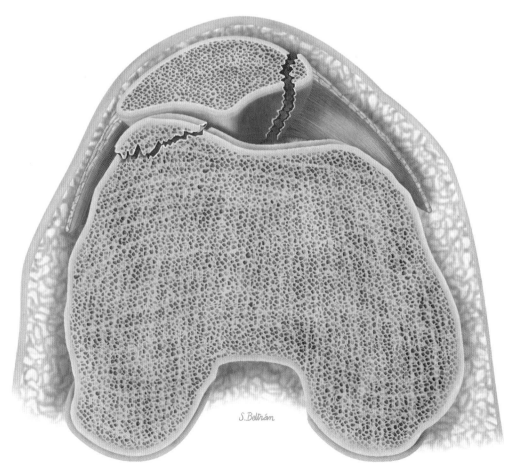

S.Beltrán

Figure 4.165 ■ An osteochondral fracture of the lateral femoral condyle and the medial patellar facet is seen in association with patellar dislocation. *(See Traumatic Dislocations pg. 614, in Stoller's 3rd Edition.)*

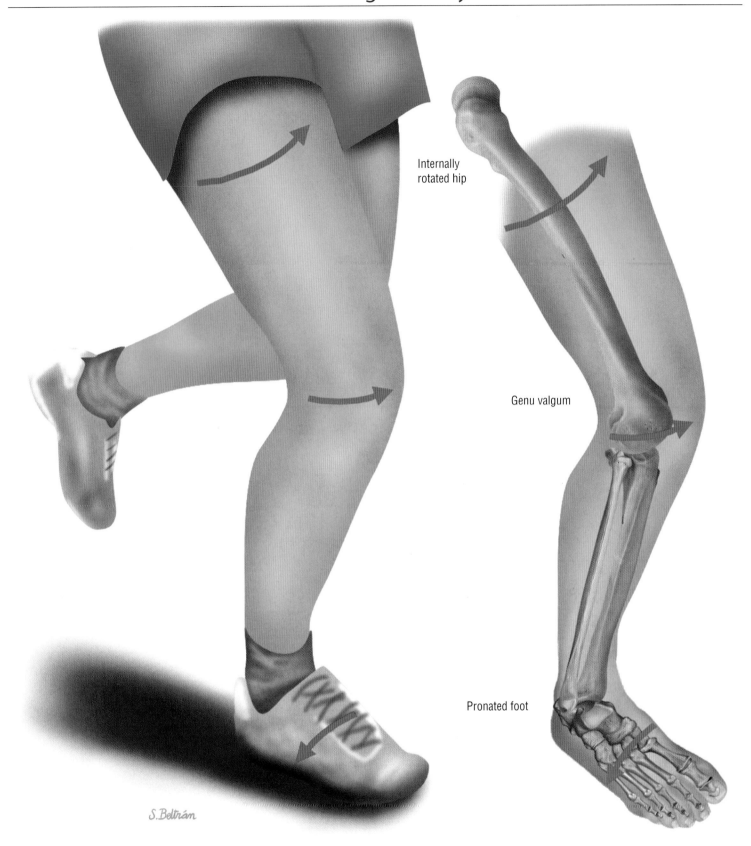

Internally rotated hip

Genu valgum

Pronated foot

S. Beltrán

Figure 4.166 ■ **Miserable malalignment as a cause of anterior knee pain is associated with internal femoral rotation, a valgus knee, and hyperpronation.** A hypermobile patella and hypoplastic vastus medialis obliquus (VMO) muscle also may be demonstrated features. *(See Patellar Tracking pgs. 577 and 579, in Stoller's 3rd Edition.)*

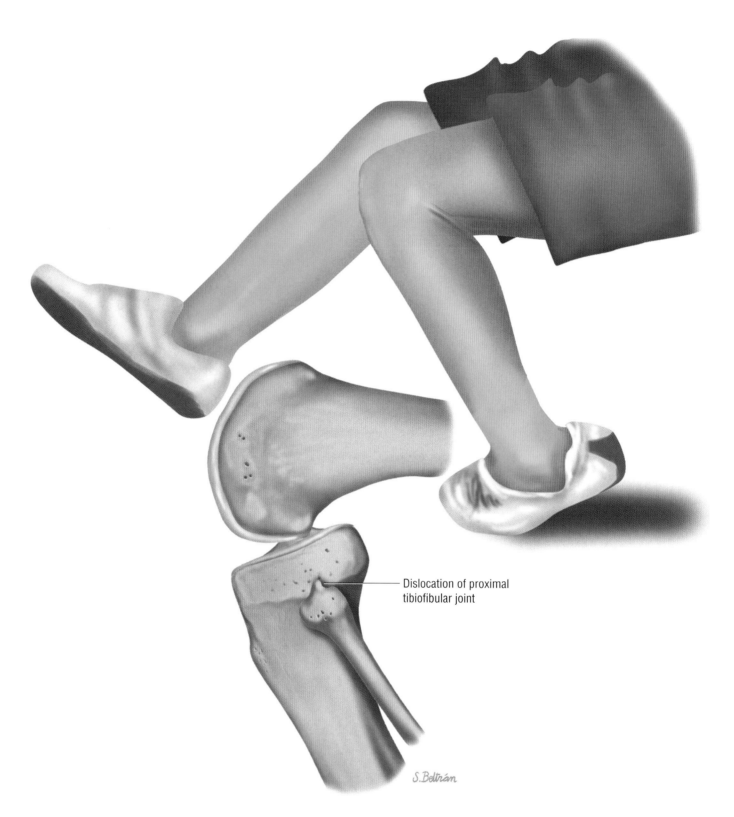

Dislocation of proximal
tibiofibular joint

S. Beltrán

Figure 4.167 ■ Dislocation of the proximal tibiofibular joint associated with adduction of the leg with the knee in flexion and a plantarflexed and inverted foot (e.g.
soccer type injury). *(See Tibiofibular Joint Arthrosis and Ganglia pg. 666, in Stoller's
3rd Edition.)*

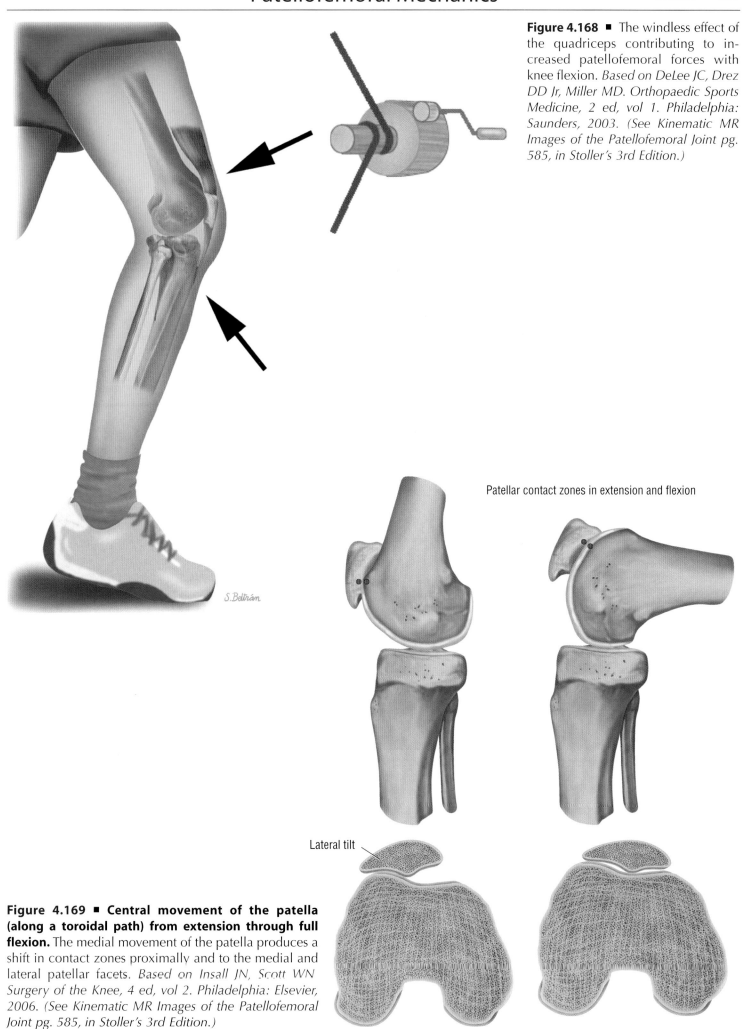

Figure 4.168 ▪ The windless effect of the quadriceps contributing to increased patellofemoral forces with knee flexion. *Based on DeLee JC, Drez DD Jr, Miller MD. Orthopaedic Sports Medicine, 2 ed, vol 1. Philadelphia: Saunders, 2003. (See Kinematic MR Images of the Patellofemoral Joint pg. 585, in Stoller's 3rd Edition.)*

Patellar contact zones in extension and flexion

Lateral tilt

Figure 4.169 ▪ **Central movement of the patella (along a toroidal path) from extension through full flexion.** The medial movement of the patella produces a shift in contact zones proximally and to the medial and lateral patellar facets. *Based on Insall JN, Scott WN Surgery of the Knee, 4 ed, vol 2. Philadelphia: Elsevier, 2006. (See Kinematic MR Images of the Patellofemoral Joint pg. 585, in Stoller's 3rd Edition.)*

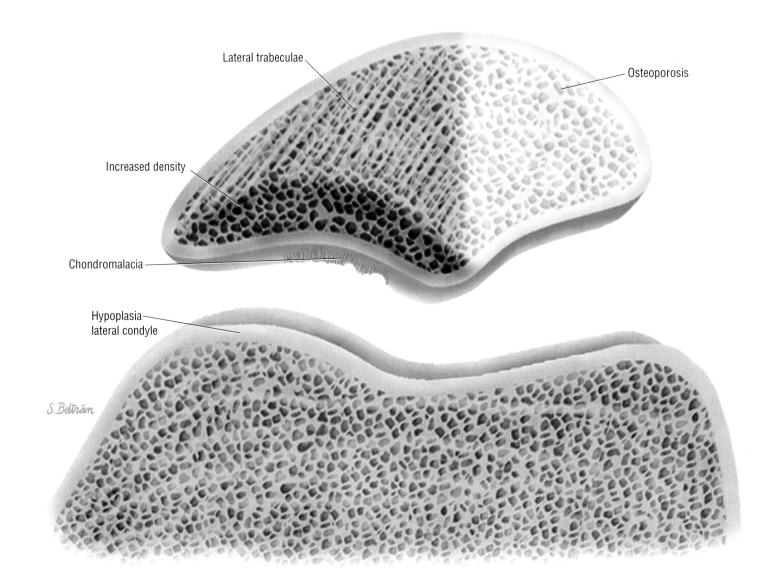

Figure 4.170 ▪ Excessive lateral pressure findings on radiographs are associated with MR findings of lateral facet subchondral edema and chondromalacia along with edema of the proximal lateral aspect of Hoffa's fat pad. *Based on DeLee JC, Drez DD Jr, Miller MD. Orthopaedic Sports Medicine, 2 ed, vol 1. Philadelphia: Saunders, 2003. (See Lateral Patellar Tilt or Excessive Lateral Pressure Syndrome pg. 587 and Retinacular Attachments pg. 616, in Stoller's 3rd Edition.)*

Lateral Retinaculum and Iliotibial Band

Figure 4.171 ■ **(A)** The superficial layer (superficial oblique retinaculum) consists of oblique fibers directed in a distal and anterior direction from the anterior aspect of the ITB to the lateral margin of the patella and the lateral border of the patellar tendon. **(B)** The deep layer of the lateral retinaculum is composed of three distinct structures. The epicondylopatellar band is the most proximal and connects the lateral epicondyle to the superolateral aspect of the patella. The midportion includes the deep transverse retinaculum, which courses from the deep surface of the ITB to the lateral border of the patella. The patellotibial band (most distal) connects the tibia (near Gerdy's tubercle) to the inferior lateral aspect of the patella. Sagittal color illustrations, lateral perspective. *(See Iliotibial Band Syndrome pg. 615, in Stoller's 3rd Edition.)*

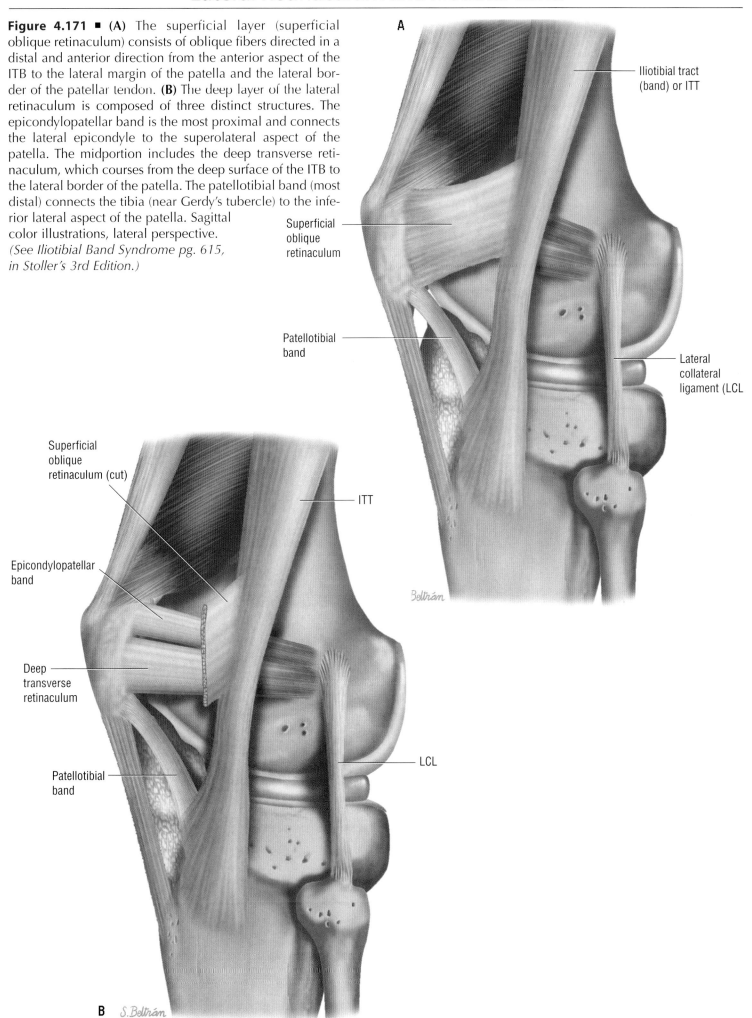

Iliotibial Band

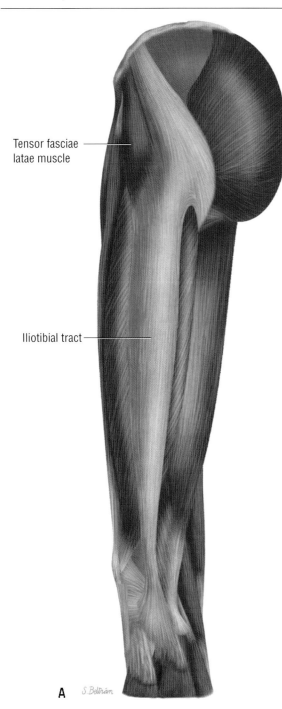

Tensor fasciae
latae muscle

Iliotibial tract

A   *S. Beltrán*

Figure 4.172 ■ **(A)** The lateral aspect of the fascia lata is thickened into a longitudinal fiber band known as the iliotibial tract (ITT) or iliotibial band (ITB). Note the ITT arises with the tensor fasciae latae from the anterior superior iliac spine. Chronic inflammation deep to the ITT may result from the formation of a secondary or adventitious bursa instead of inflammation of a primary bursa.**(B)** The distal fibers of the ITT divide into anterior intermediate and posterior portions. The anterior fibers blend with the lateral retinaculum and posterior fibers join with distal biceps femoris expansions into crural fascia. The midportion, corresponding to the intermediate fibers of the distal ITT trifurcation, extends distally to insert anterolaterally on Gerdy's tubercle. *(See Iliotibial Band Syndrome pg. 617, in Stoller's 3rd Edition.)*

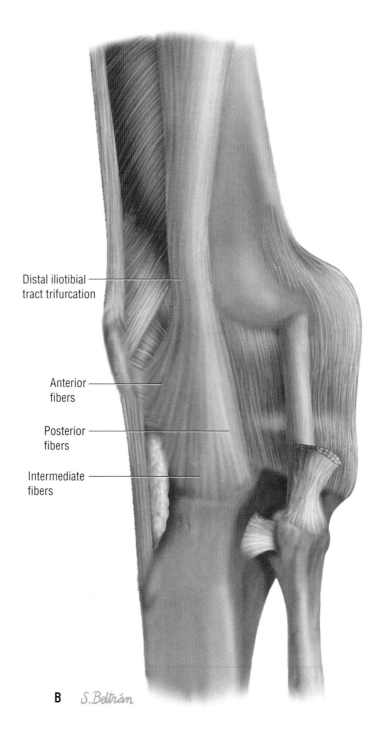

Distal iliotibial
tract trifurcation

Anterior
fibers

Posterior
fibers

Intermediate
fibers

B   *S. Beltrán*

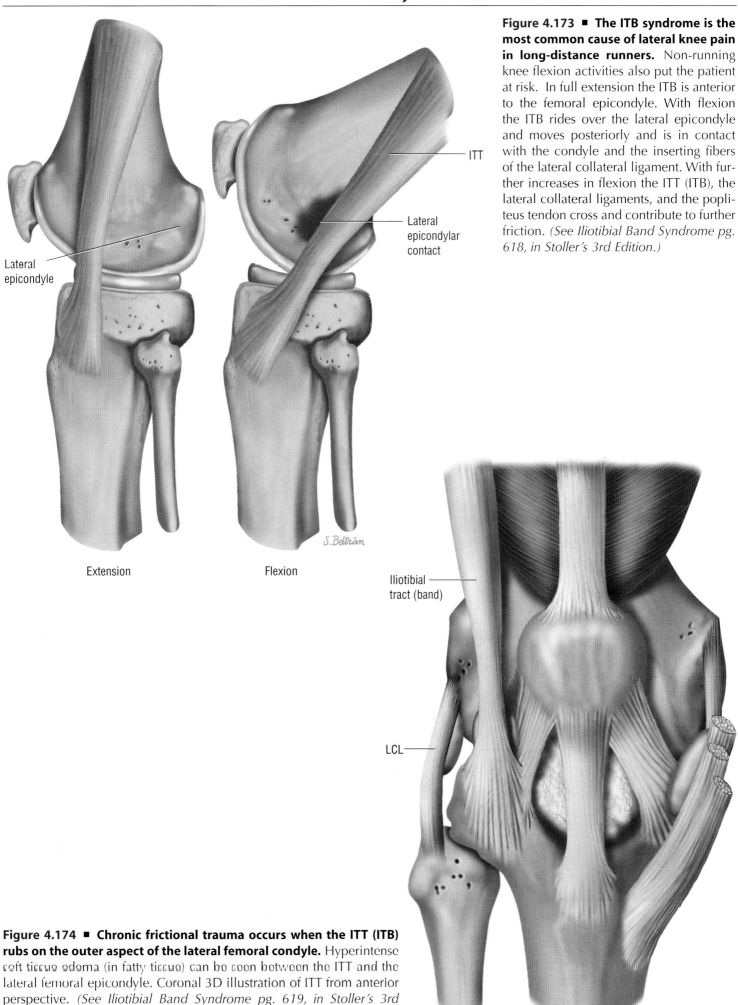

Figure 4.173 ■ The ITB syndrome is the most common cause of lateral knee pain in long-distance runners. Non-running knee flexion activities also put the patient at risk. In full extension the ITB is anterior to the femoral epicondyle. With flexion the ITB rides over the lateral epicondyle and moves posteriorly and is in contact with the condyle and the inserting fibers of the lateral collateral ligament. With further increases in flexion the ITT (ITB), the lateral collateral ligaments, and the popliteus tendon cross and contribute to further friction. *(See Iliotibial Band Syndrome pg. 618, in Stoller's 3rd Edition.)*

ITT

Lateral epicondylar contact

Lateral epicondyle

S. Beltrán

Extension

Flexion

Iliotibial tract (band)

LCL

Figure 4.174 ■ Chronic frictional trauma occurs when the ITT (ITB) rubs on the outer aspect of the lateral femoral condyle. Hyperintense soft tissue edema (in fatty tissue) can be seen between the ITT and the lateral femoral epicondyle. Coronal 3D illustration of ITT from anterior perspective. *(See Iliotibial Band Syndrome pg. 619, in Stoller's 3rd Edition.)*

S. Beltrán

Iliotibial Band Syndrome

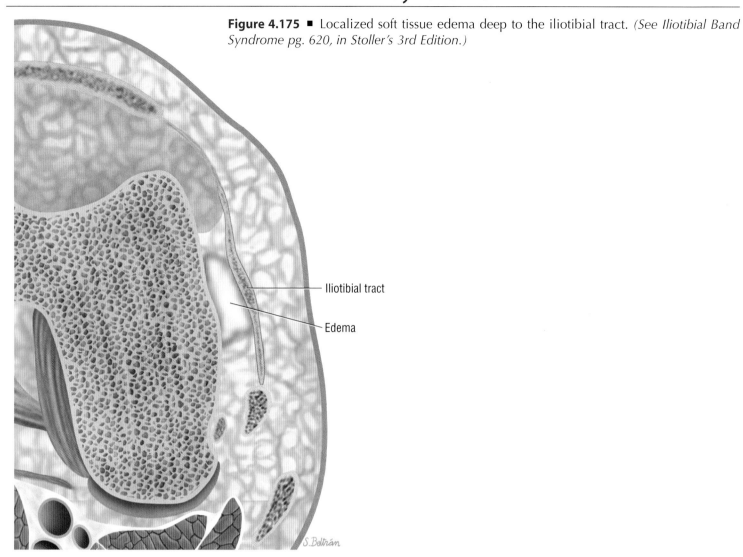

Figure 4.175 ■ Localized soft tissue edema deep to the iliotibial tract. *(See Iliotibial Band Syndrome pg. 620, in Stoller's 3rd Edition.)*

Iliotibial tract

Edema

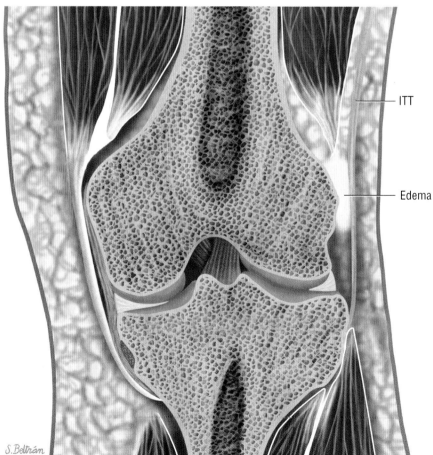

ITT

Edema

Figure 4.176 ■ **Edema shown deep to the ITT (ITB) on a color coronal section.** Newer theories of the cause of inflammation in the ITB syndrome hold that it is not invagination of the lateral recess of the knee or inflammation of a primary bursa but rather inflammation occurring as a result of dynamic changes during knee flexion. *(See Iliotibial Band Syndrome pg. 622, in Stoller's 3rd Edition.)*

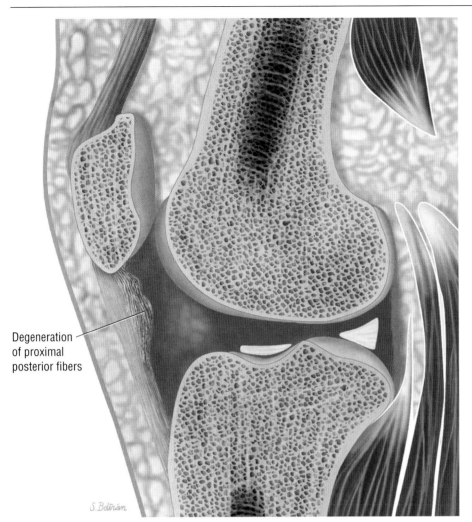

Degeneration
of proximal
posterior fibers

S. Beltrán

Figure 4.177 ■ **Patellar tendinosis involving thickening of the proximal posterior fibers.** The earliest changes manifest as edema in the peritenon with normal tendon morphology. The tendinitis is a tendinopathy with tendon degeneration and collagen breakdown. *(See Extensor Mechanism and Patellar Tendon Abnormalities pg. 623, in Stoller's 3rd Edition.)*

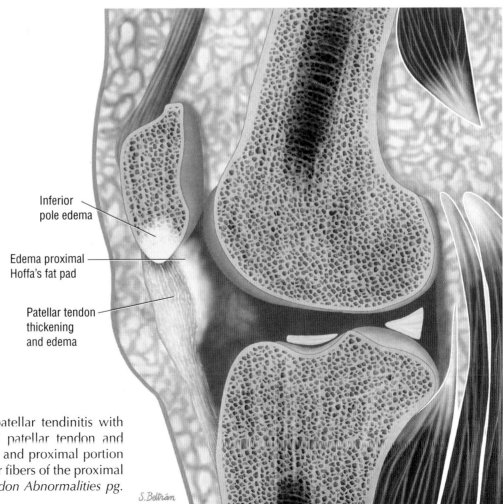

Inferior
pole edema

Edema proximal
Hoffa's fat pad

Patellar tendon
thickening
and edema

S. Beltrán

Figure 4.178 ■ Advanced changes of patellar tendinitis with edema and thickening of the proximal patellar tendon and edema of the inferior pole of the patella and proximal portion of Hoffa's fat pad adjacent to the posterior fibers of the proximal tendon. *(See Mechanism of Patellar Tendon Abnormalities pg. 626, in Stoller's 3rd Edition.)*

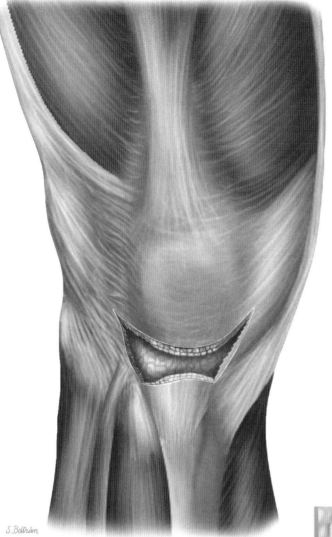

S.Beltrán

Figure 4.179 ▪ Rupture of the proximal patellar tendon at the inferior pole of the patella. Clinical examination may show a displaced patella, hemarthrosis, and an inability to extend the knee. *(See Patellar Tendon Tears pg. 628, in Stoller's 3rd Edition.)*

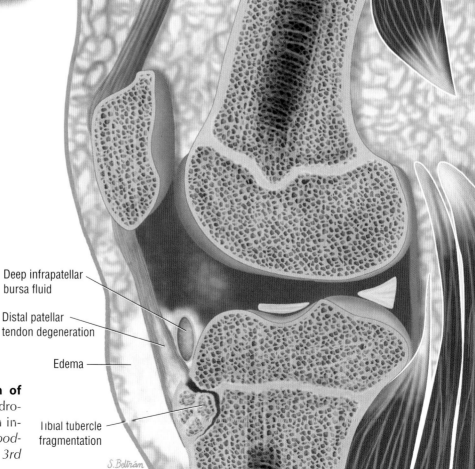

Deep infrapatellar bursa fluid

Distal patellar tendon degeneration

Edema

Tibial tubercle fragmentation

S.Beltrán

Figure 4.180 ▪ Sagittal color illustration of Osgood-Schlatter disease. Tibial osteochondrosis (apophysitis) is seen at the patellar tendon insertion on the tibial tubercle. *(See Osgood-Schlatter Disease Tears pg. 633, in Stoller's 3rd Edition.)*

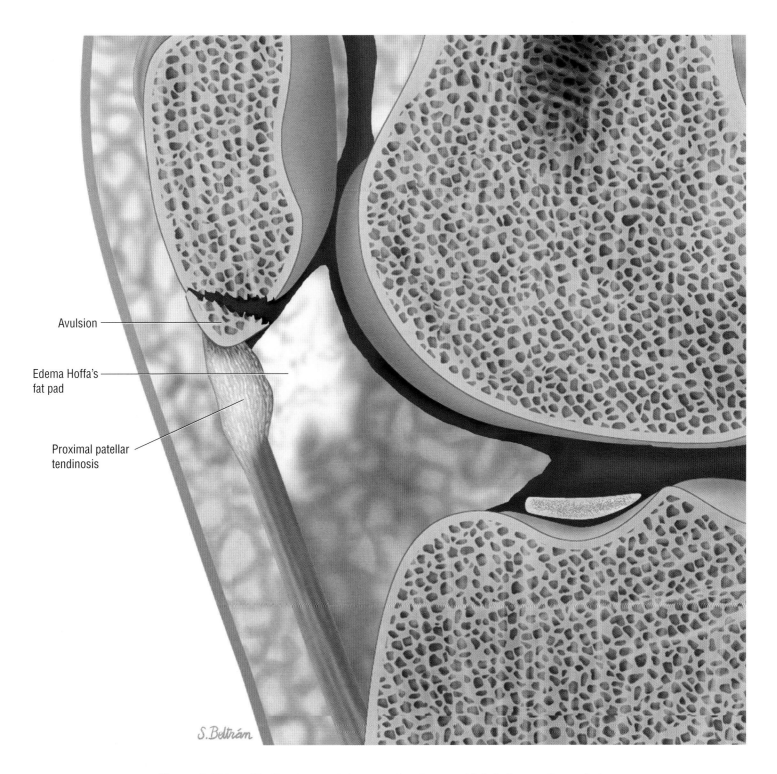

Avulsion

Edema Hoffa's
fat pad

Proximal patellar
tendinosis

S.Beltrán

Figure 4.181 ■ Sinding-Larsen-Johansson Syndrome with inferior patellar pole fragmentation, adjacent patellar tendinosis, and edema of the anterior proximal aspect of Hoffa's fat pad. *(See Sinding-Larsen-Johansson Syndrome pg. 635, in Stoller's 3rd Edition.)*

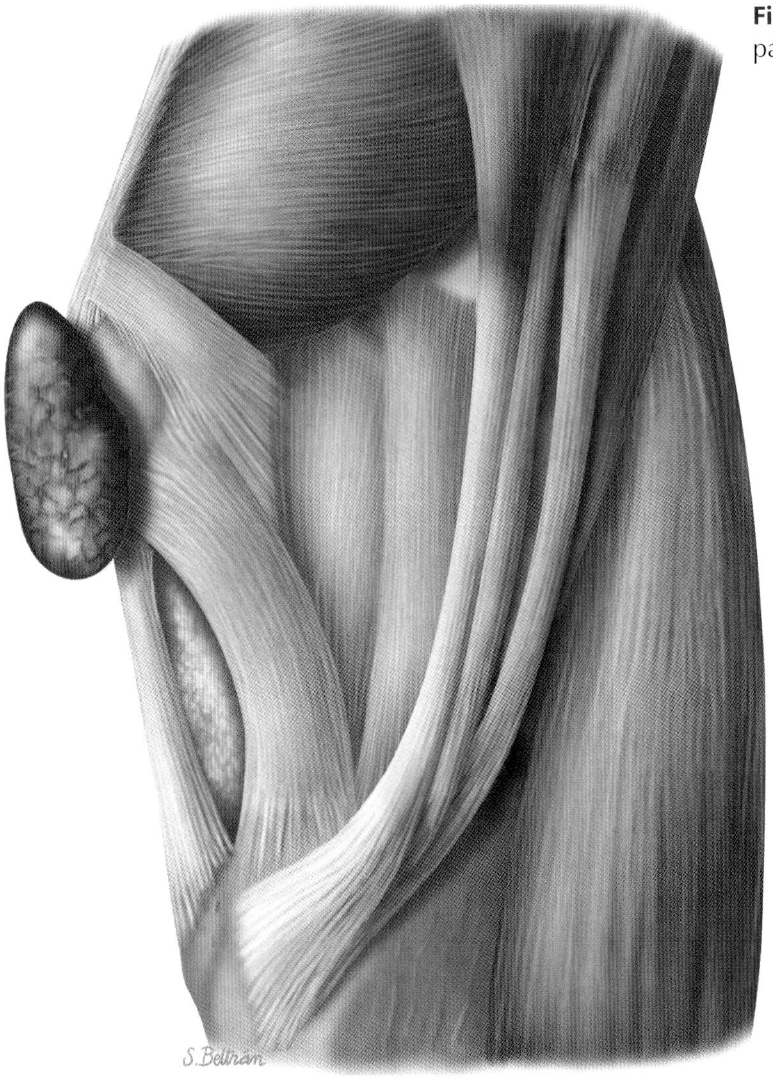

Prepatellar and Superficial Infrapatellar Bursa

Figure 4.182 ■ Subcutaneous prepatellar bursa anterior to the patella. *(See Patellar Bursae pg. 637, in Stoller's 3rd Edition.)*

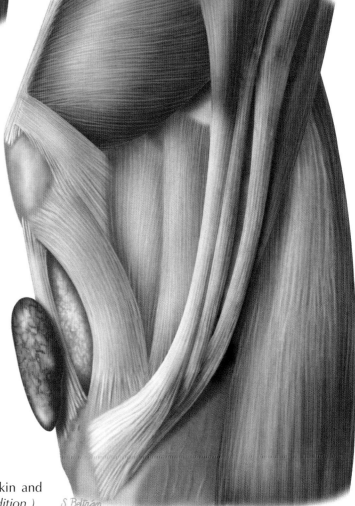

Figure 4.183 ■ The superficial infrapatellar bursa between the skin and the tibial tuberosity. *(See Patellar Bursae pg. 638, in Stoller's 3rd Edition.)*

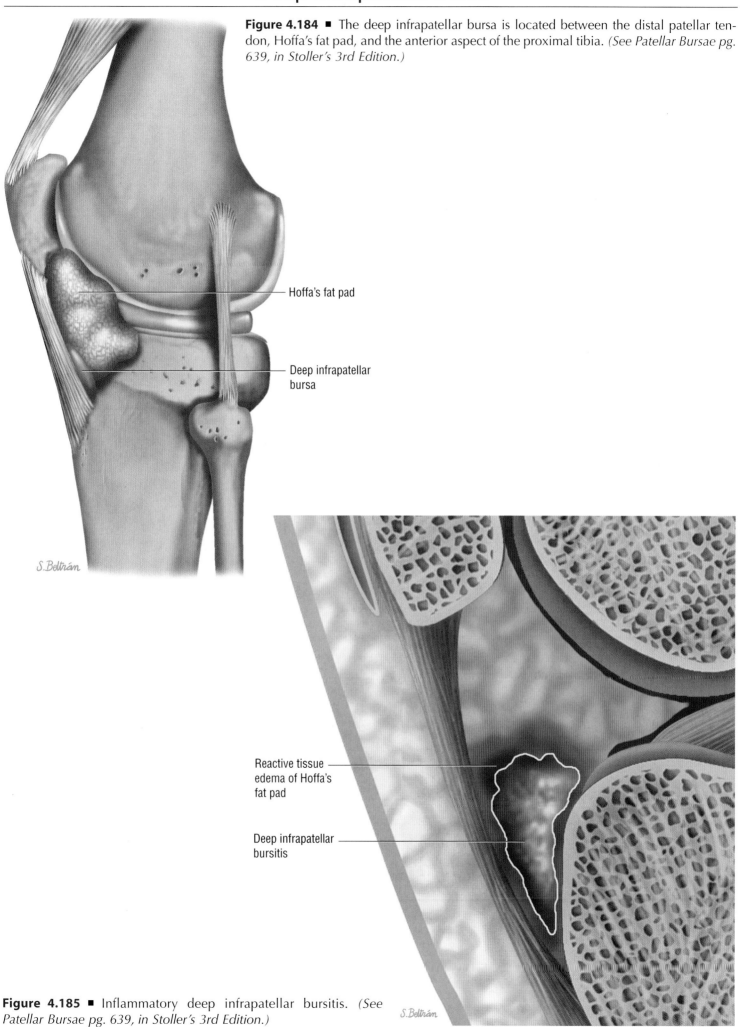

Figure 4.184 ▪ The deep infrapatellar bursa is located between the distal patellar tendon, Hoffa's fat pad, and the anterior aspect of the proximal tibia. *(See Patellar Bursae pg. 639, in Stoller's 3rd Edition.)*

Hoffa's fat pad

Deep infrapatellar bursa

S. Beltrán

Reactive tissue edema of Hoffa's fat pad

Deep infrapatellar bursitis

Figure 4.185 ▪ Inflammatory deep infrapatellar bursitis. *(See Patellar Bursae pg. 639, in Stoller's 3rd Edition.)*

S. Beltrán

Quadriceps Tendinosis and Tear

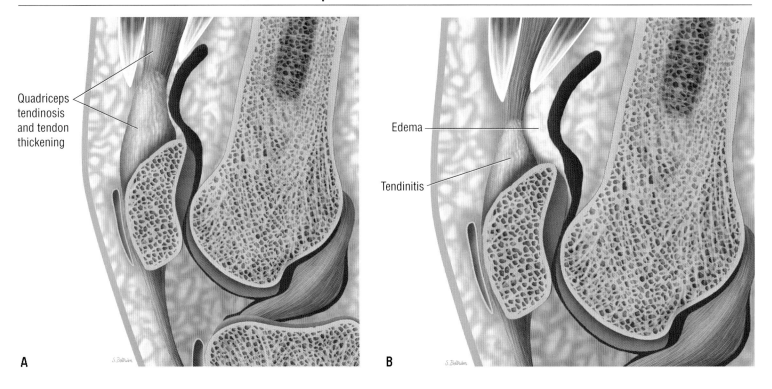

Quadriceps tendinosis and tendon thickening

Edema

Tendinitis

A   **B**

Figure 4.186 ▪ **(A)** Distal quadriceps tendinosis with diffuse tendon thickening. **(B)** Edema of the quadriceps fat pad associated with distal quadriceps tendinosis. *(See Quadriceps Tendon and Muscle Tears pg. 641, in Stoller's 3rd Edition.)*

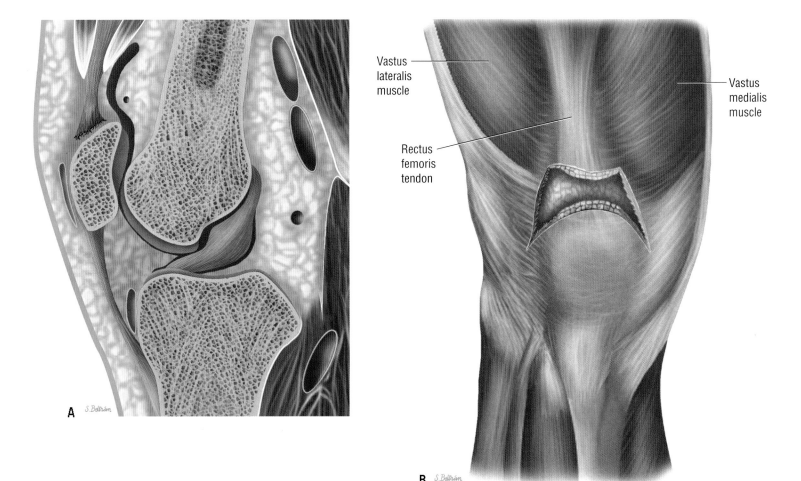

Vastus lateralis muscle

Rectus femoris tendon

Vastus medialis muscle

A   **B**

Figure 4.187 ▪ **Grade III tendon strain with disruption of the tendon unit.** A large hemarthrosis with a freely mobile patella, loss of extensor function, and a palpable defect occur with full-thickness tears. Partial tears present with an extensor lag. **(A)** Sagittal view. **(B)** Anterior view. *(See Quadriceps Tendon and Muscle Tears pg. 642, in Stoller's 3rd Edition.)*

Proteoglycan Complex and Collagen Fibers

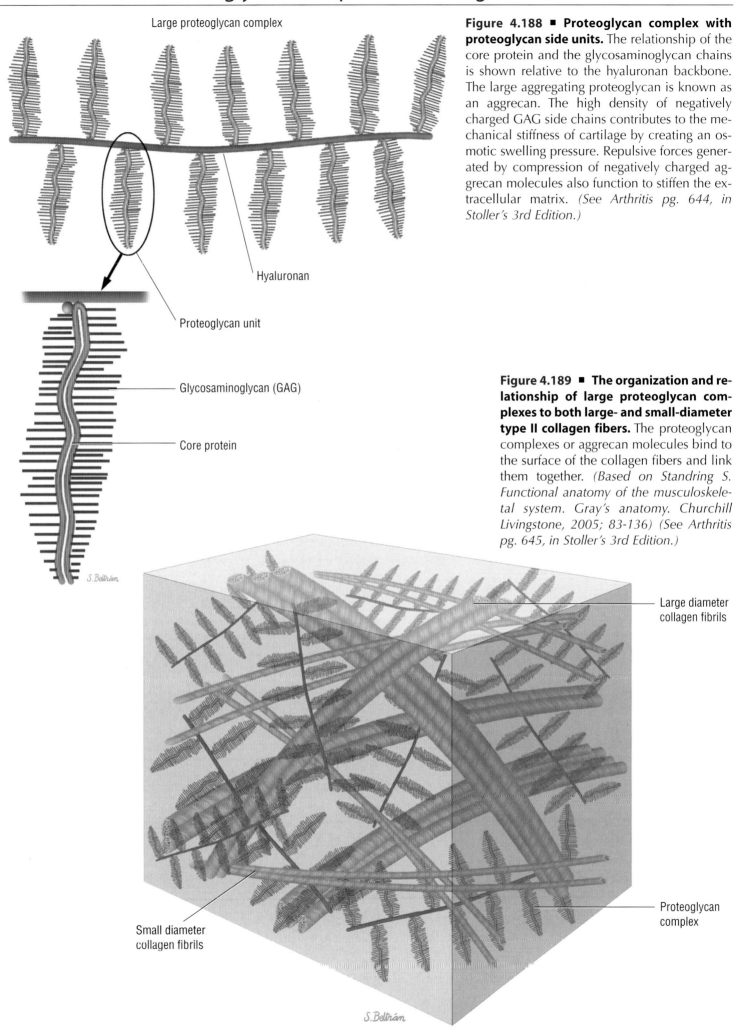

Large proteoglycan complex

Hyaluronan

Proteoglycan unit

Glycosaminoglycan (GAG)

Core protein

S.Beltrán

Figure 4.188 ▪ Proteoglycan complex with proteoglycan side units. The relationship of the core protein and the glycosaminoglycan chains is shown relative to the hyaluronan backbone. The large aggregating proteoglycan is known as an aggrecan. The high density of negatively charged GAG side chains contributes to the mechanical stiffness of cartilage by creating an osmotic swelling pressure. Repulsive forces generated by compression of negatively charged aggrecan molecules also function to stiffen the extracellular matrix. *(See Arthritis pg. 644, in Stoller's 3rd Edition.)*

Figure 4.189 ▪ The organization and relationship of large proteoglycan complexes to both large- and small-diameter type II collagen fibers. The proteoglycan complexes or aggrecan molecules bind to the surface of the collagen fibers and link them together. *(Based on Standring S. Functional anatomy of the musculoskeletal system. Gray's anatomy. Churchill Livingstone, 2005; 83-136) (See Arthritis pg. 645, in Stoller's 3rd Edition.)*

Large diameter collagen fibrils

Proteoglycan complex

Small diameter collagen fibrils

S.Beltrán

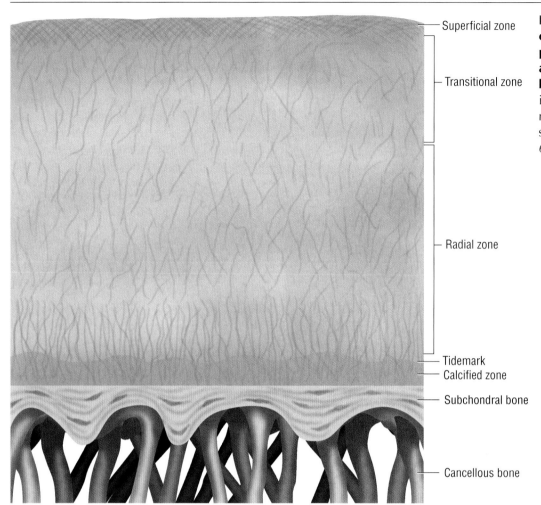

Superficial zone

Transitional zone

Radial zone

Tidemark
Calcified zone

Subchondral bone

Cancellous bone

Figure 4.190 ■ **The collagen fibers of the radial zone are oriented perpendicular to the subchondral plate and anchor articular cartilage to bone.** Collagen fibers form arcades in the transitional zone and are directed parallel to the surface in the superficial zone. *(See Arthritis pg. 646, in Stoller's 3rd Edition.)*

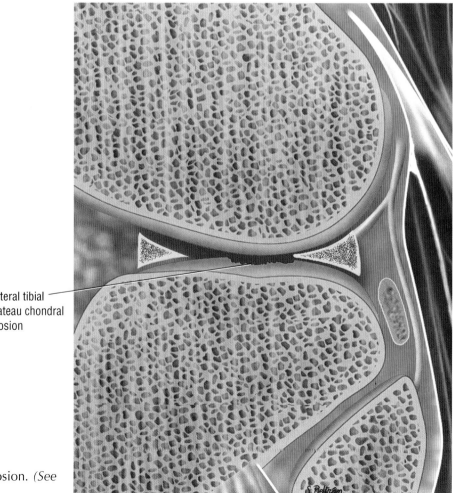

Lateral tibial plateau chondral erosion

Figure 4.191 ■ Lateral tibial plateau chondral erosion. *(See Arthritis pg. 646, in Stoller's 3rd Edition.)*

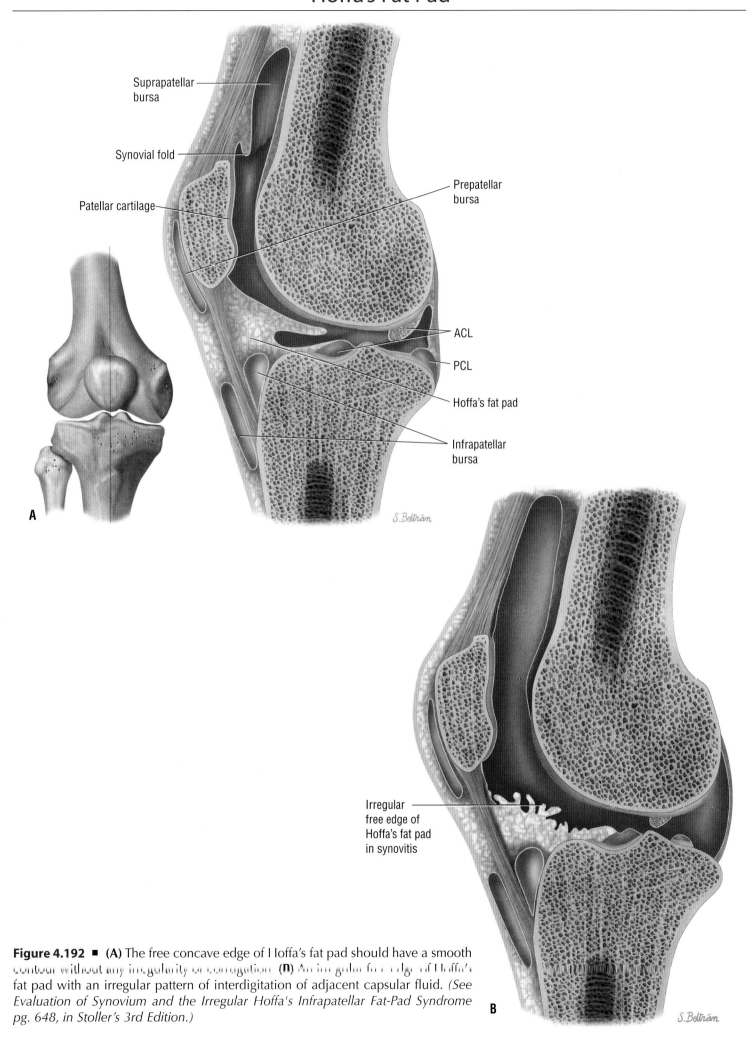

Figure 4.192 ■ **(A)** The free concave edge of Hoffa's fat pad should have a smooth contour without any irregularity or corrugation. **(B)** An irregular free edge of Hoffa's fat pad with an irregular pattern of interdigitation of adjacent capsular fluid. *(See Evaluation of Synovium and the Irregular Hoffa's Infrapatellar Fat-Pad Syndrome pg. 648, in Stoller's 3rd Edition.)*

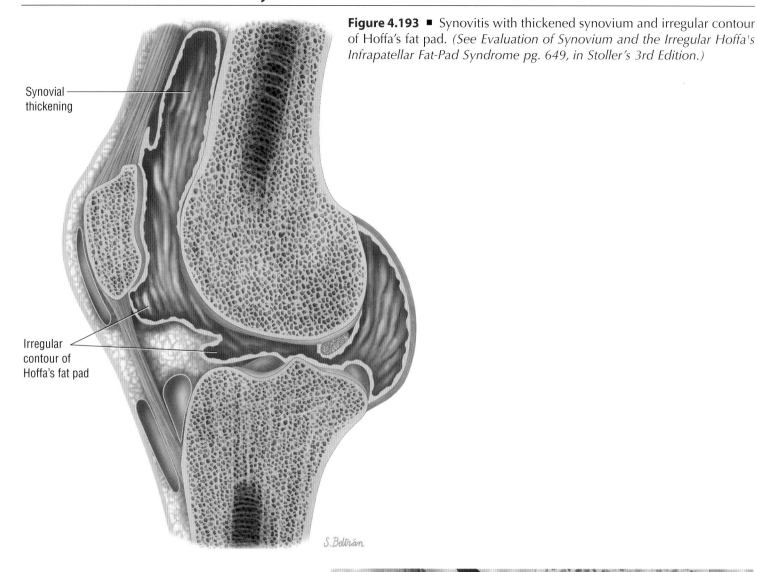

Synovial thickening

Irregular contour of Hoffa's fat pad

Figure 4.193 ■ Synovitis with thickened synovium and irregular contour of Hoffa's fat pad. *(See Evaluation of Synovium and the Irregular Hoffa's Infrapatellar Fat-Pad Syndrome pg. 649, in Stoller's 3rd Edition.)*

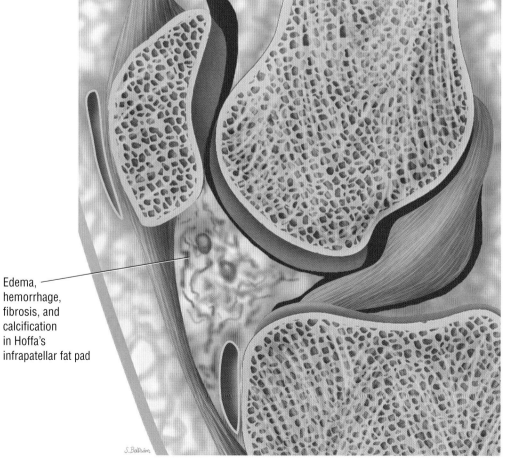

Edema, hemorrhage, fibrosis, and calcification in Hoffa's infrapatellar fat pad

Figure 4.194 ■ Hoffa's disease with enlargement of the infrapatellar fat pad associated with edema, hemorrhage, or chronic changes, including fibrosis and calcifications. *(See Evaluation of Synovium and the Irregular Hoffa's Infrapatellar Fat-Pad Syndrome pg. 652, in Stoller's 3rd Edition.)*

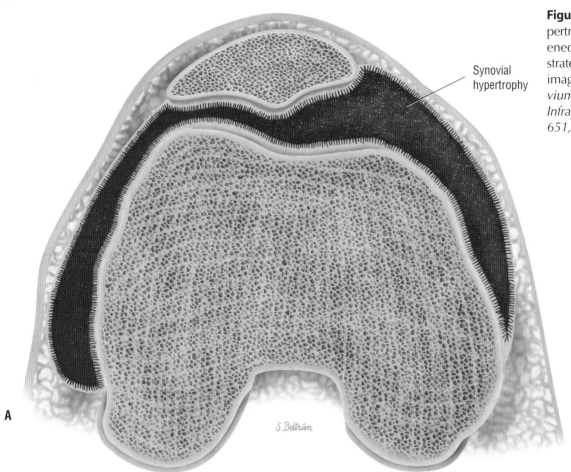

Figure 4.195 ■ **(A)** Synovial hypertrophy. **(B)** Characteristic thickened synovium that is demonstrated on contrast enhanced MR images. *(See Evaluation of Synovium and the Irregular Hoffa's Infrapatellar Fat-Pad Syndrome pg. 651, in Stoller's 3rd Edition.)*

Synovial hypertrophy

A

S.Beltrán

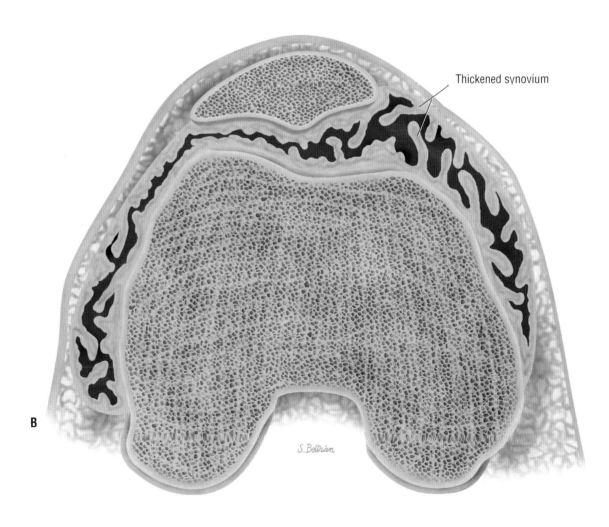

Thickened synovium

B

S.Beltrán

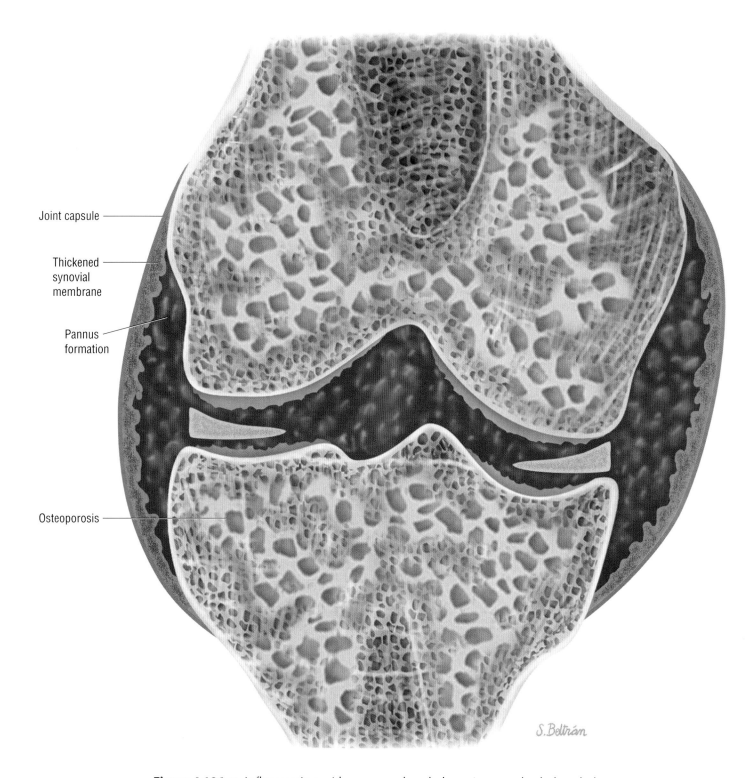

Joint capsule

Thickened
synovial
membrane

Pannus
formation

Osteoporosis

S. Beltrán

Figure 4.196 ▪ Inflammation with pannus, chondral erosions, and subchondral osteopenia (osteoporosis). *(See Rheumatoid Arthritis pg. 656, in Stoller's 3rd Edition.)*

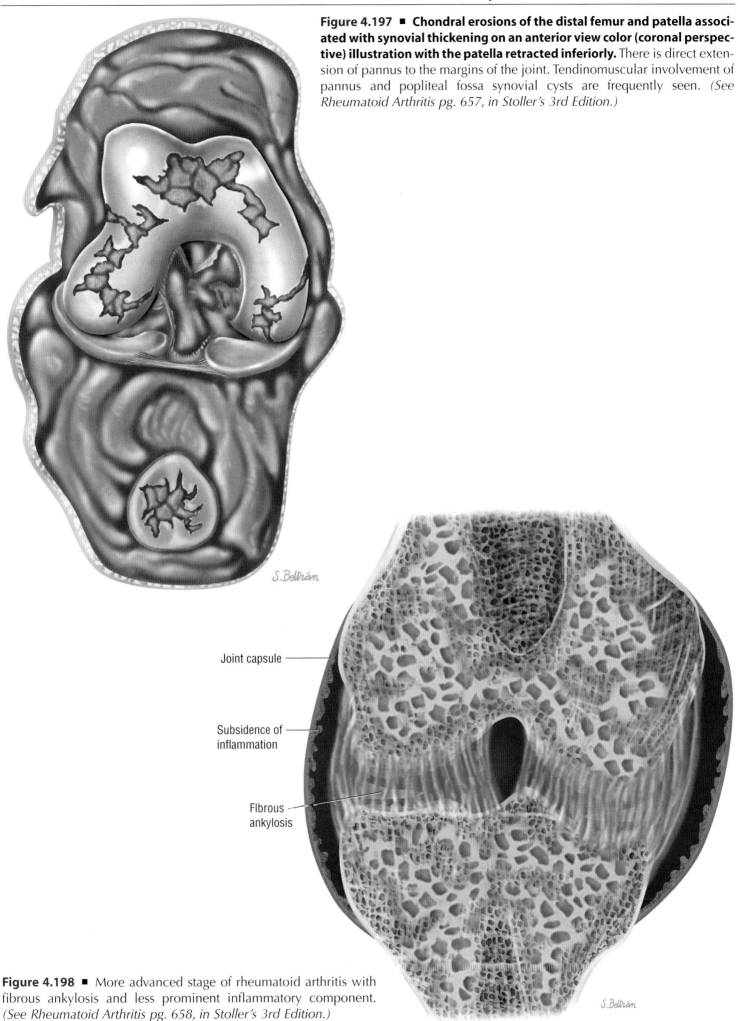

Figure 4.197 ■ **Chondral erosions of the distal femur and patella associated with synovial thickening on an anterior view color (coronal perspective) illustration with the patella retracted inferiorly.** There is direct extension of pannus to the margins of the joint. Tendinomuscular involvement of pannus and popliteal fossa synovial cysts are frequently seen. *(See Rheumatoid Arthritis pg. 657, in Stoller's 3rd Edition.)*

Joint capsule

Subsidence of inflammation

Fibrous ankylosis

Figure 4.198 ■ More advanced stage of rheumatoid arthritis with fibrous ankylosis and less prominent inflammatory component. *(See Rheumatoid Arthritis pg. 658, in Stoller's 3rd Edition.)*

Pigmented Villonodular Synovitis (PVNS)

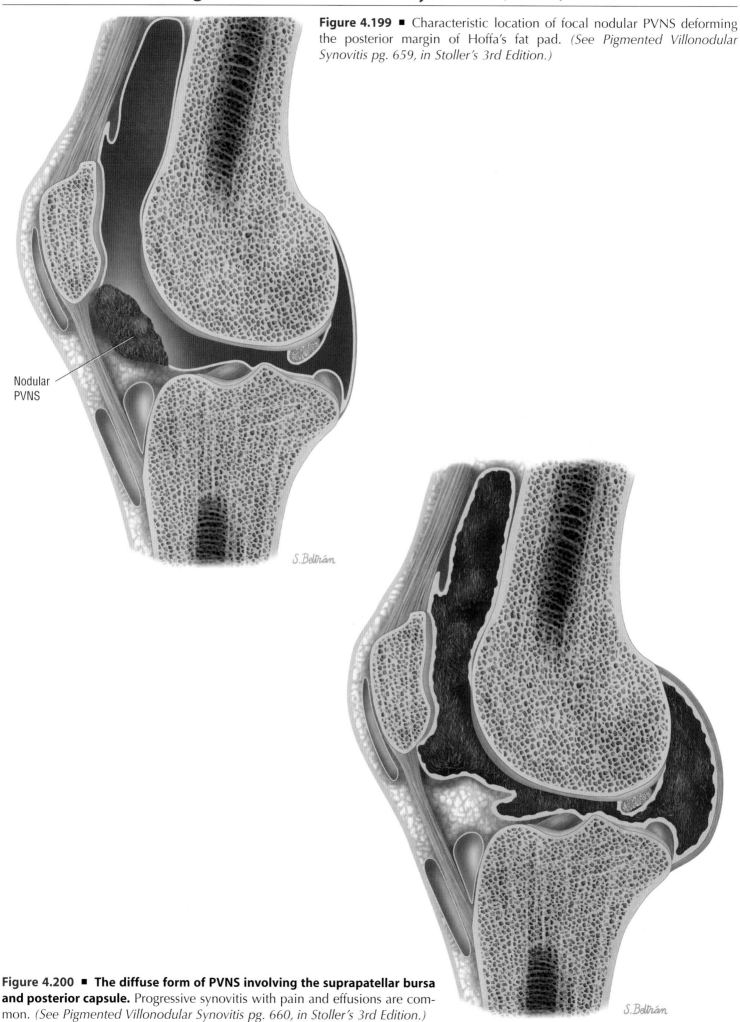

Nodular
PVNS

S.Beltrán

Figure 4.199 ■ Characteristic location of focal nodular PVNS deforming the posterior margin of Hoffa's fat pad. *(See Pigmented Villonodular Synovitis pg. 659, in Stoller's 3rd Edition.)*

Figure 4.200 ■ **The diffuse form of PVNS involving the suprapatellar bursa and posterior capsule.** Progressive synovitis with pain and effusions are common. *(See Pigmented Villonodular Synovitis pg. 660, in Stoller's 3rd Edition.)*

S.Beltrán

Osteoarthritis

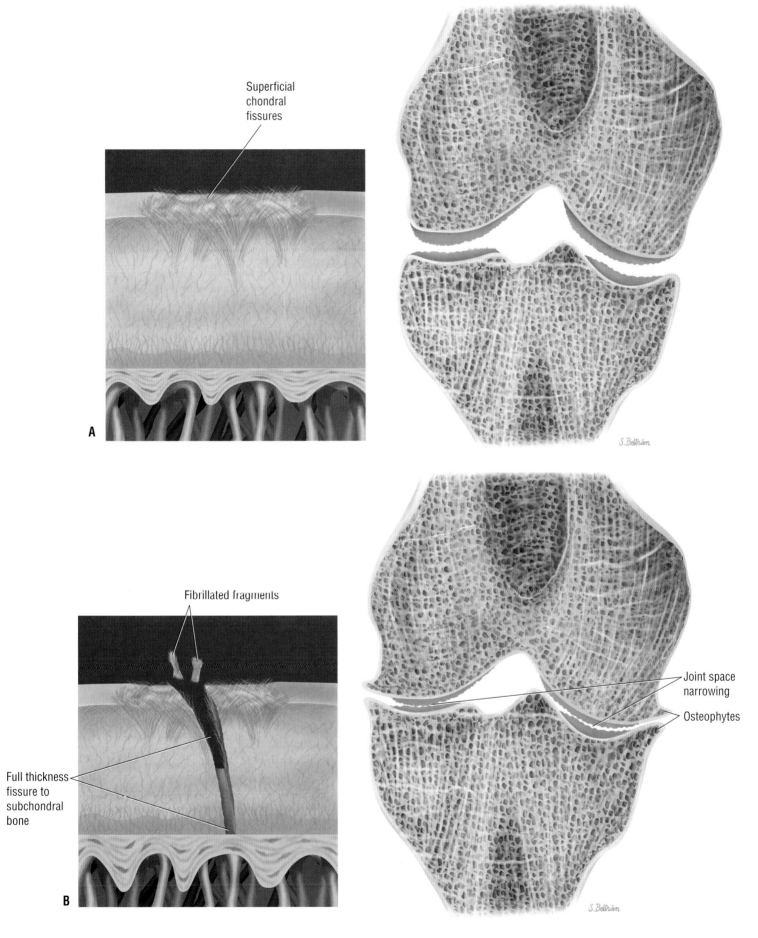

Figure 4.201 ■ **(A)** Early degenerative arthritis with superficial fissures of the articular cartilage. **(B)** Progression to more advanced degenerative arthrosis. Chondral fissures extending down to the subchondral bone, release of fibrillated cartilage debris, joint space narrowing, subchondral sclerosis, and osteophyte formation are seen. *(See Osteoarthritis pg. 667, in Stoller's 3rd Edition.)*

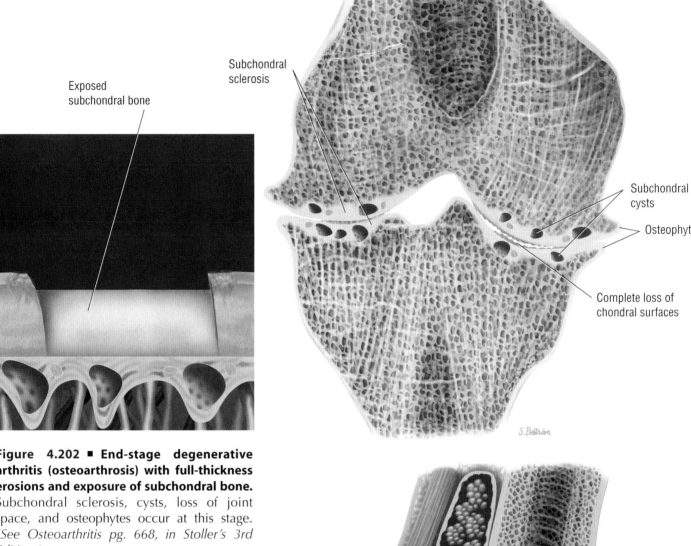

Exposed
subchondral bone

Subchondral
sclerosis

Subchondral
cysts

Osteophytes

Complete loss of
chondral surfaces

S.Beltrán

Figure   4.202 ■ End-stage   degenerative arthritis (osteoarthrosis) with full-thickness erosions and exposure of subchondral bone. Subchondral sclerosis, cysts, loss of joint space, and osteophytes occur at this stage. *(See Osteoarthritis pg. 668, in Stoller's 3rd Edition.)*

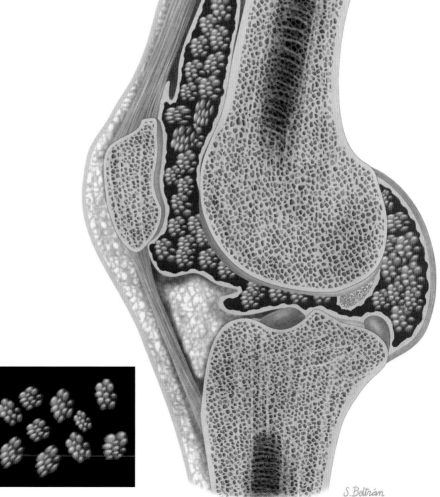

Figure 4.203 ■ Sagittal color illustration with inset of synovial chondromatosis derived from synovial metaplasia producing multiple chondromas in contact with and receiving nutrients from the joint capsule synovial lining. *(See Osteoarthritis pg. 670, in Stoller's 3rd Edition.)*

S.Beltrán

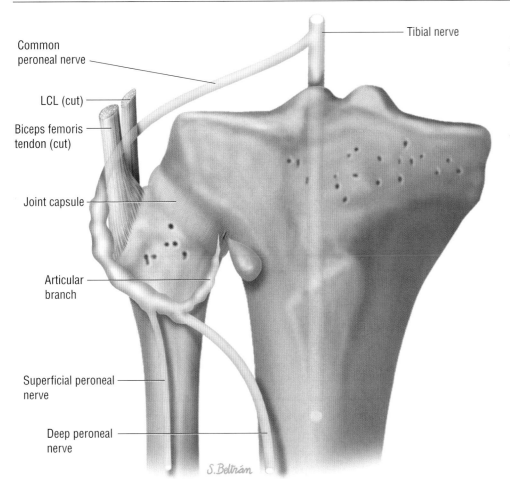

Common peroneal nerve

LCL (cut)

Biceps femoris tendon (cut)

Joint capsule

Articular branch

Superficial peroneal nerve

Deep peroneal nerve

Tibial nerve

S. Beltrán

Figure 4.204 ■ **Common peroneal nerve and its anterior branches, which include the articular branch (anterior to the tibiofibular joint), the superficial branch, and deep branch.** The common peroneal nerve separates from the sciatic nerve in the upper popliteal fossa. *(See Tibiofibular Joint Arthritis and Ganglia pg. 671, in Stoller's 3rd Edition.)*

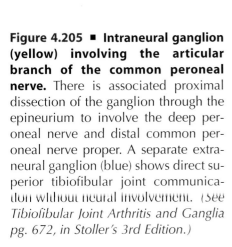

Figure 4.205 ■ **Intraneural ganglion (yellow) involving the articular branch of the common peroneal nerve.** There is associated proximal dissection of the ganglion through the epineurium to involve the deep peroneal nerve and distal common peroneal nerve proper. A separate extraneural ganglion (blue) shows direct superior tibiofibular joint communication without neural involvement. *(See Tibiofibular Joint Arthritis and Ganglia pg. 672, in Stoller's 3rd Edition.)*

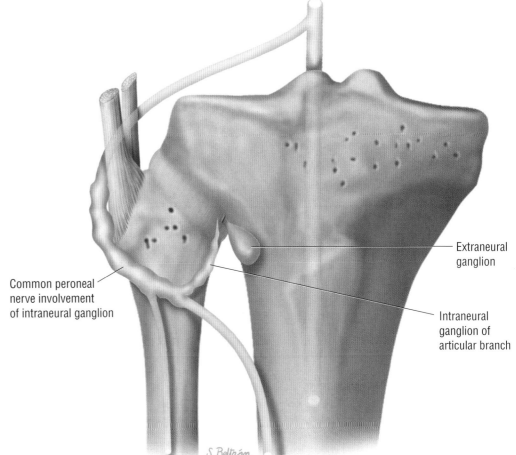

Common peroneal nerve involvement of intraneural ganglion

Extraneural ganglion

Intraneural ganglion of articular branch

S. Beltrán

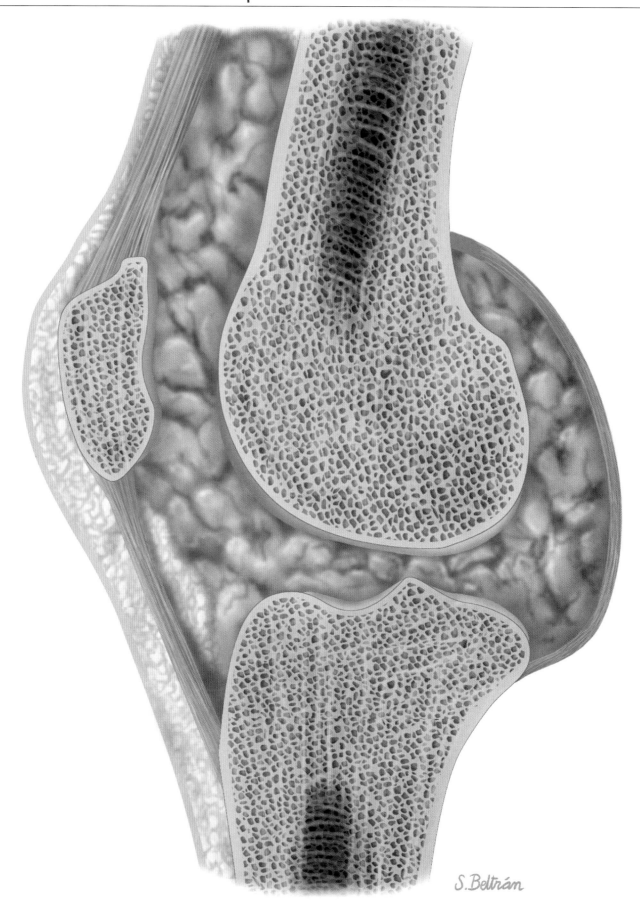

Figure 4.206 ■ Lipoma arborescens or villous lipomatous proliferation of the synovium is non-neoplastic condition. It may be associated with osteoarthritis, rheumatoid arthritis, psoriasis, or diabetes mellitus. *(See Lipoma Arborescens pg. 674, in Stoller's 3rd Edition.)*

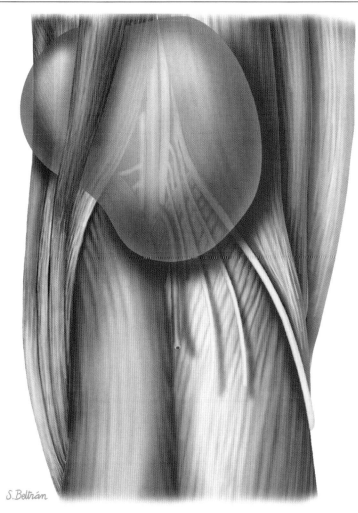

Figure 4.207 ■ **Popliteal cysts are either primary or secondary to intraarticular pathology.** Their characteristic location is adjacent to the semimembranosus or medial head of the gastrocnemius. If the cyst is located in an atypical location or cannot be aspirated, further evaluation, including IV contrast, is recommended to exclude a soft tissue sarcoma. *(See Popliteal and Atypical Cysts pg. 676, in Stoller's 3rd Edition.)*

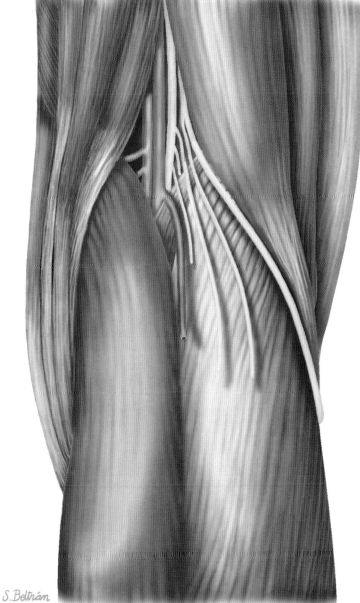

Figure 4.208 ■ **Postoperative popliteal artery entrapment with medial leaking of blood, which is in direct communication with the popliteal artery.** Popliteal artery entrapment was the result of an accessory head of the gastrocnemius muscle. A fibrous band between the medial head gastrocnemius and lateral condyle or hypertrophy of the plantaris or semimembranosus also may cause compression of the popliteal artery. Posterior view of normal neurovascular structures for reference (color illustration). *(See Popliteal and Atypical Cysts pg. 681, in Stoller's 3rd Edition.)*

Plicae

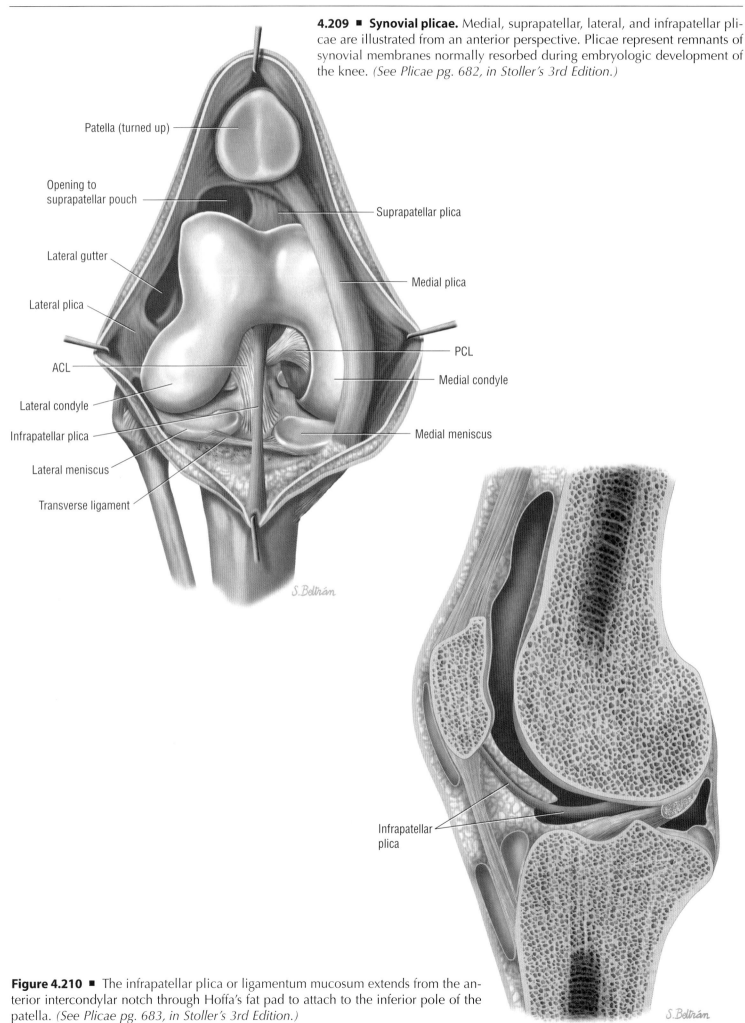

4.209 ■ Synovial plicae. Medial, suprapatellar, lateral, and infrapatellar plicae are illustrated from an anterior perspective. Plicae represent remnants of synovial membranes normally resorbed during embryologic development of the knee. *(See Plicae pg. 682, in Stoller's 3rd Edition.)*

Patella (turned up)

Opening to suprapatellar pouch

Lateral gutter

Lateral plica

ACL

Lateral condyle

Infrapatellar plica

Lateral meniscus

Transverse ligament

Suprapatellar plica

Medial plica

PCL

Medial condyle

Medial meniscus

Infrapatellar plica

Figure 4.210 ■ The infrapatellar plica or ligamentum mucosum extends from the anterior intercondylar notch through Hoffa's fat pad to attach to the inferior pole of the patella. *(See Plicae pg. 683, in Stoller's 3rd Edition.)*

Figure 4.211 ▪ Type C medial patellar plica that covers the anteromedial femoral condyle. Axial color illustration. *(See Plicae pg. 686, in Stoller's 3rd Edition.)*

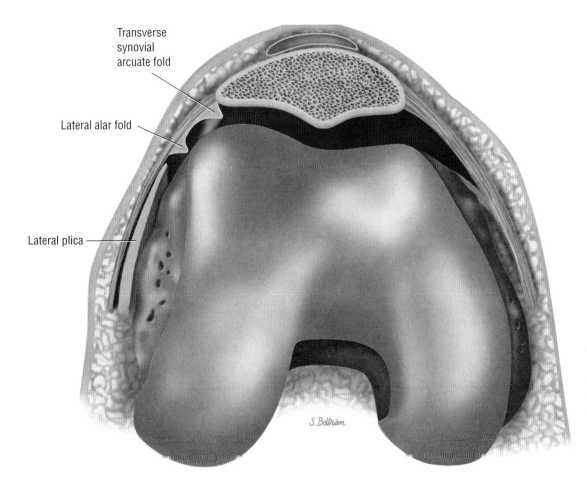

Type C medial plica

Anteromedial femoral condyle

Transverse synovial arcuate fold

Lateral alar fold

Lateral plica

Figure 4.212 ▪ Longitudinal course of a lateral patellar plica demonstrated on a cross-sectional color illustration. A lateral plica may interfere with access to the anterolateral portal at arthroscopy. *(See Plicae pg. 687, in Stoller's 3rd Edition.)*

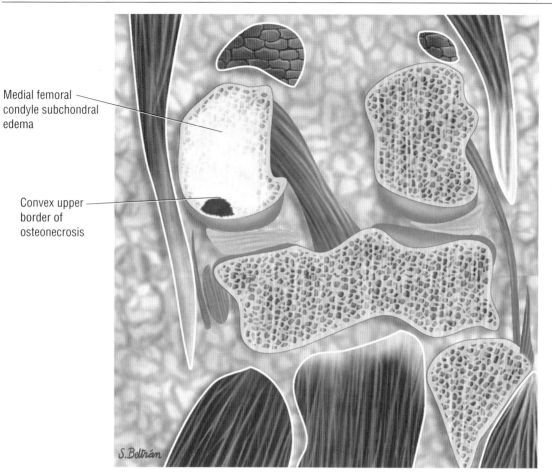

Medial femoral condyle subchondral edema

Convex upper border of osteonecrosis

Figure 4.213 ■ **The characteristic convex upper border demarcating a subchondral focus of osteonecrosis in spontaneous osteonecrosis of the knee (SONK).** This morphology would be unusual in an insufficiency or stress fracture. *(See Spontaneous Osteonecrosis and Insufficiency Fractures pg. 689, in Stoller's 3rd Edition.)*

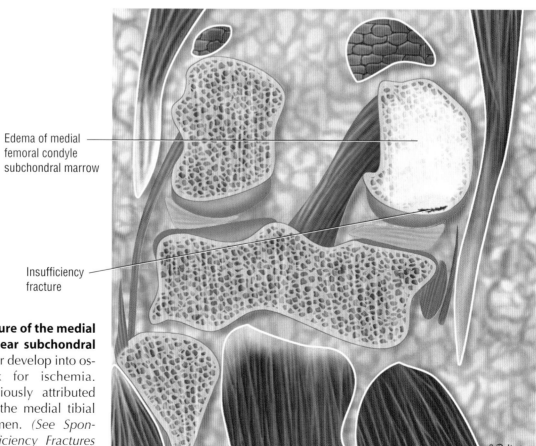

Edema of medial femoral condyle subchondral marrow

Insufficiency fracture

Figure 4.214 ■ **Insufficiency fracture of the medial femoral condyle with discrete linear subchondral fracture.** These fractures may heal or develop into osteonecrosis in marrow at risk for ischemia. Insufficiency fractures were previously attributed only to the subchondral bone of the medial tibial plateau in older osteopenic women. *(See Spontaneous Osteonecrosis and Insufficiency Fractures pg. 691, in Stoller's 3rd Edition.)*

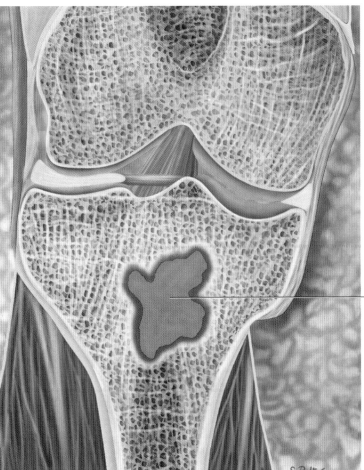

Figure 4.215 ■ Serpiginous border of medullary infarct. Metaphyseal involvement is more common than epiphyseal or diaphyseal involvement. (*See Bone Infarcts pg. 694, in Stoller's 3rd Edition.*)

Metaphyseal
bone infarct

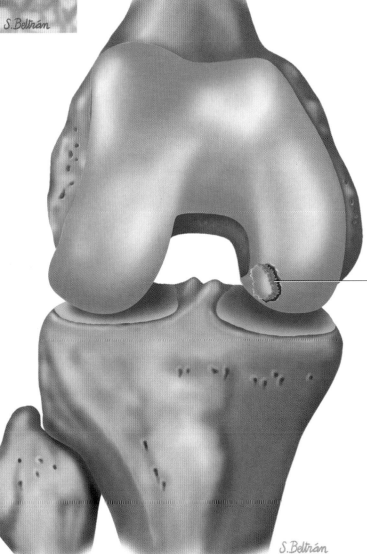

OCD lateral
aspect medial
femoral condyle
and adjacent
intercondylar
notch

Figure 4.216 ■ Classic osteochondritis dissecans of the non-weight-bearing lateral aspect of the medial femoral condyle and intercondylar notch. (*See Osteochondritis Dissecans pg. 697, in Stoller's 3rd Edition.*)

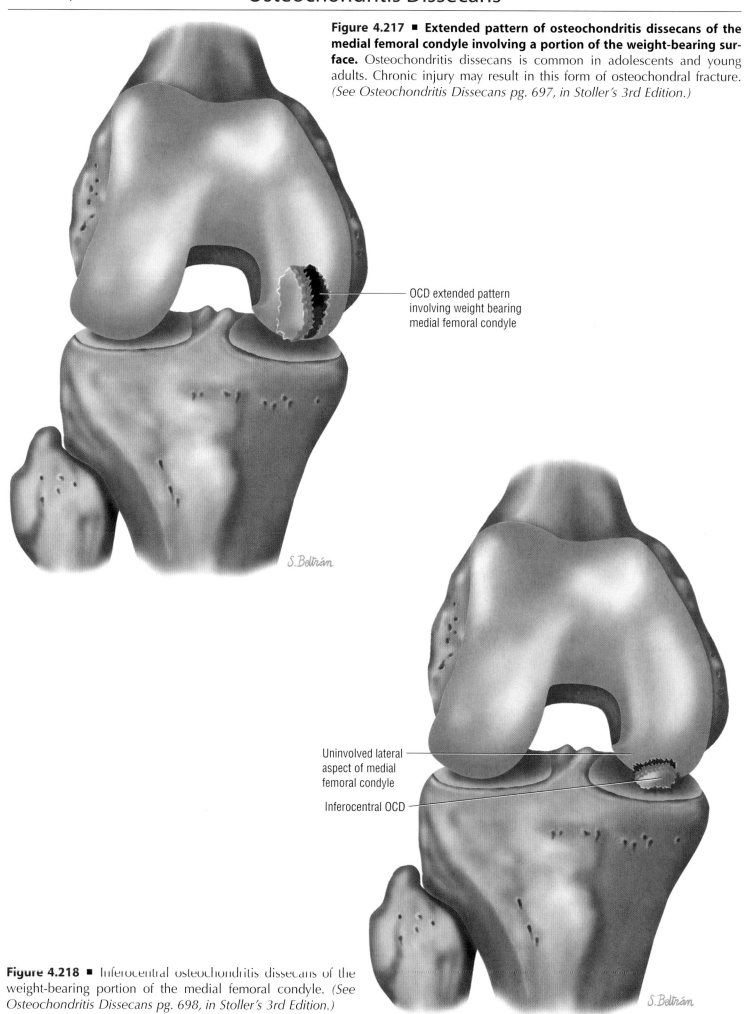

Figure 4.217 ■ **Extended pattern of osteochondritis dissecans of the medial femoral condyle involving a portion of the weight-bearing surface.** Osteochondritis dissecans is common in adolescents and young adults. Chronic injury may result in this form of osteochondral fracture. *(See Osteochondritis Dissecans pg. 697, in Stoller's 3rd Edition.)*

OCD extended pattern involving weight bearing medial femoral condyle

Uninvolved lateral aspect of medial femoral condyle

Inferocentral OCD

Figure 4.218 ■ Inferocentral osteochondritis dissecans of the weight-bearing portion of the medial femoral condyle. *(See Osteochondritis Dissecans pg. 698, in Stoller's 3rd Edition.)*

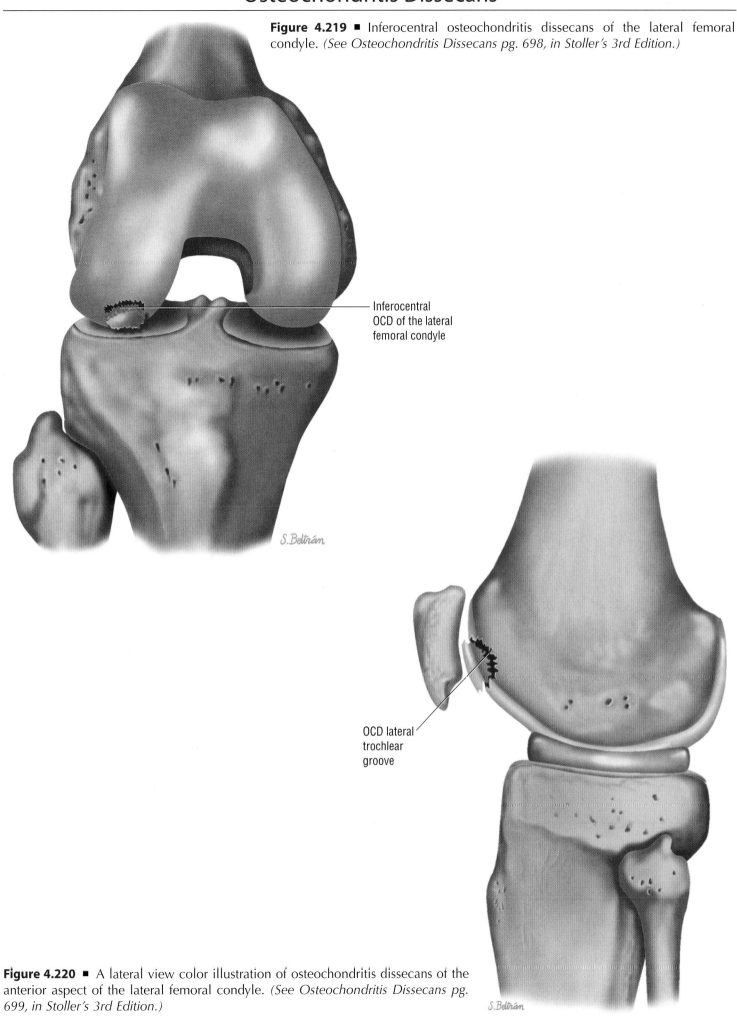

Figure 4.219 ■ Inferocentral osteochondritis dissecans of the lateral femoral condyle. *(See Osteochondritis Dissecans pg. 698, in Stoller's 3rd Edition.)*

Inferocentral OCD of the lateral femoral condyle

OCD lateral trochlear groove

Figure 4.220 ■ A lateral view color illustration of osteochondritis dissecans of the anterior aspect of the lateral femoral condyle. *(See Osteochondritis Dissecans pg. 699, in Stoller's 3rd Edition.)*

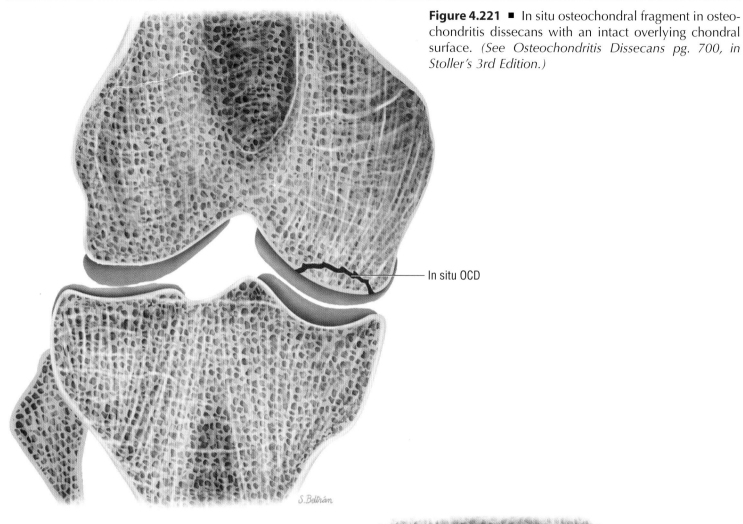

Figure 4.221 ■ In situ osteochondral fragment in osteochondritis dissecans with an intact overlying chondral surface. *(See Osteochondritis Dissecans pg. 700, in Stoller's 3rd Edition.)*

In situ OCD

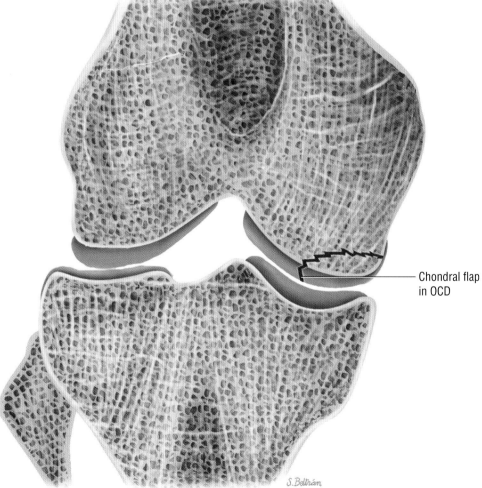

Chondral flap in OCD

Figure 4.222 ■ The development of an osteocartilaginous flap in osteochondritis dissecans. *(See Osteochondritis Dissecans pg. 700, in Stoller's 3rd Edition.)*

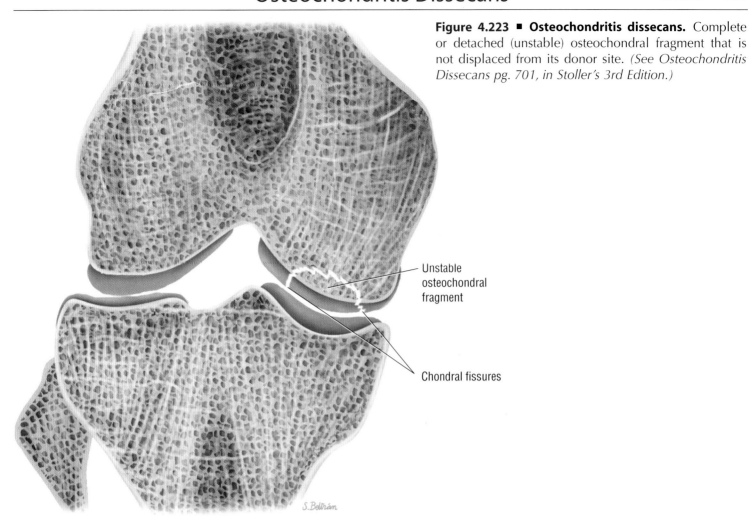

Figure 4.223 ■ **Osteochondritis dissecans.** Complete or detached (unstable) osteochondral fragment that is not displaced from its donor site. *(See Osteochondritis Dissecans pg. 701, in Stoller's 3rd Edition.)*

Unstable osteochondral fragment

Chondral fissures

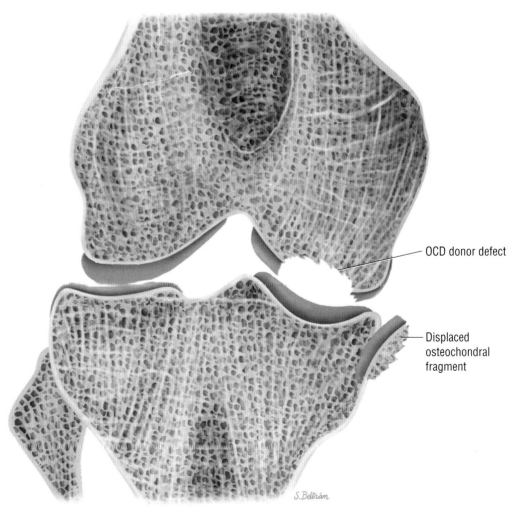

OCD donor defect

Displaced osteochondral fragment

Figure 4.224 ■ **Osteochondritis dissecans.** Displaced or dislodged osteochondral fragments leaving an osteochondral defect at the donor site. *(See Osteochondritis Dissecans pg. 701, in Stoller's 3rd Edition.)*

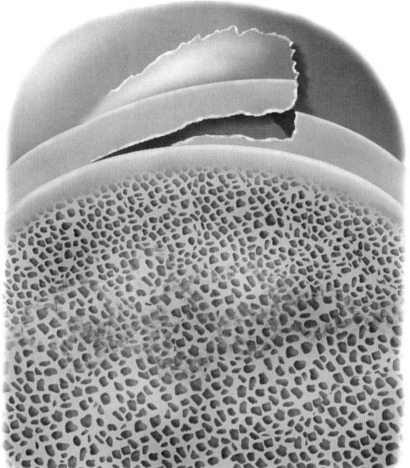

A

Figure 4.225 ■ **(A)** Chondral flaps, produced by either a twisting force or a direct blow, are often associated with ligament tears. **(B)** Chondral fractures or separations such as chondral flaps are associated with athletic injuries. The fragment either remains in situ or becomes displaced and is seen as in intra-articular loose body. *(See Chondral and Osteochondral Lesions pg. 704, in Stoller's 3rd Edition.)*

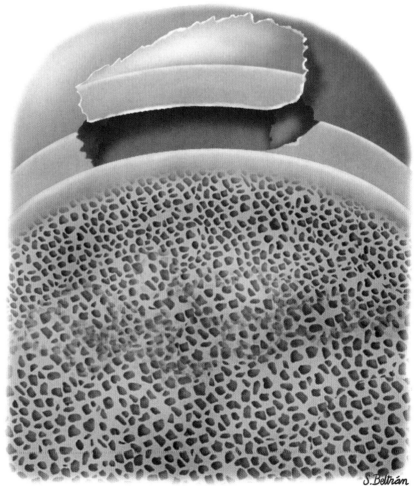

B

Figure 4.226 ■ **(A)** Chondral lesion of the lateral femoral condyle and osteochondral fracture of the medial femoral condyle. Osteochondral fractures often occur in an adolescent population, where there is no well-defined articular cartilage tidemark and stresses are transmitted directly to the subchondral bone. In the skeletally mature patient the tidemark functions as a weak transitional zone and allows the transference of forces, resulting in a chondral fracture. **(B)** Osteochondral fracture with involvement of both chondral and subchondral bone with fracture extension across the subchondral plate, presenting as osteochondritis dissecans. *(See Chondral and Osteochondral Lesions pg. 706, in Stoller's 3rd Edition.)*

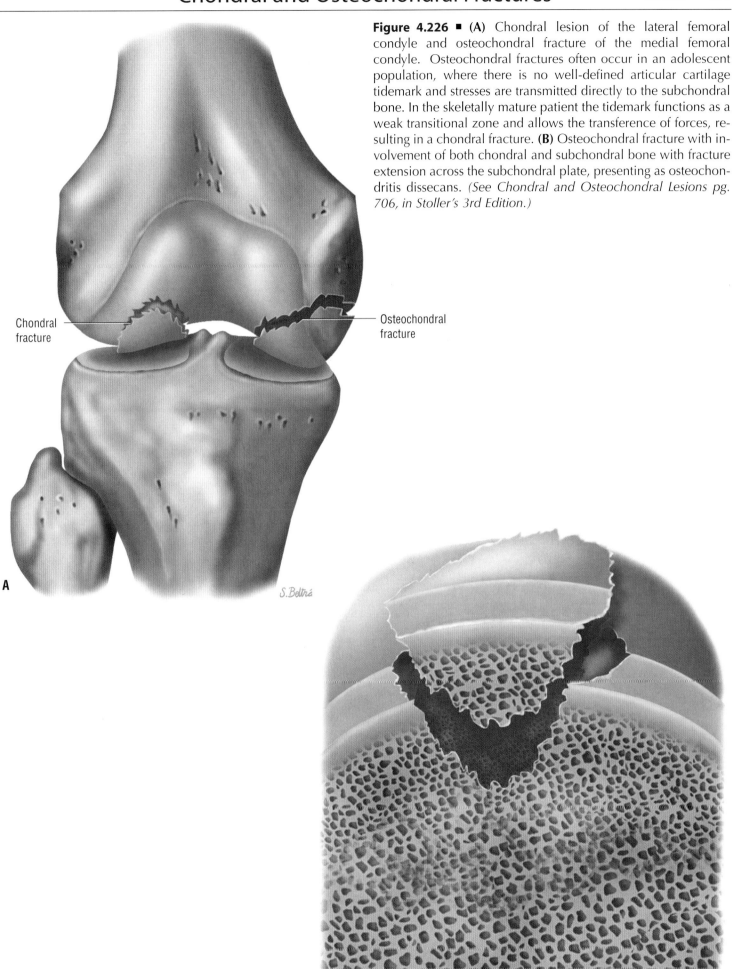

Chondral fracture

Osteochondral fracture

A

B

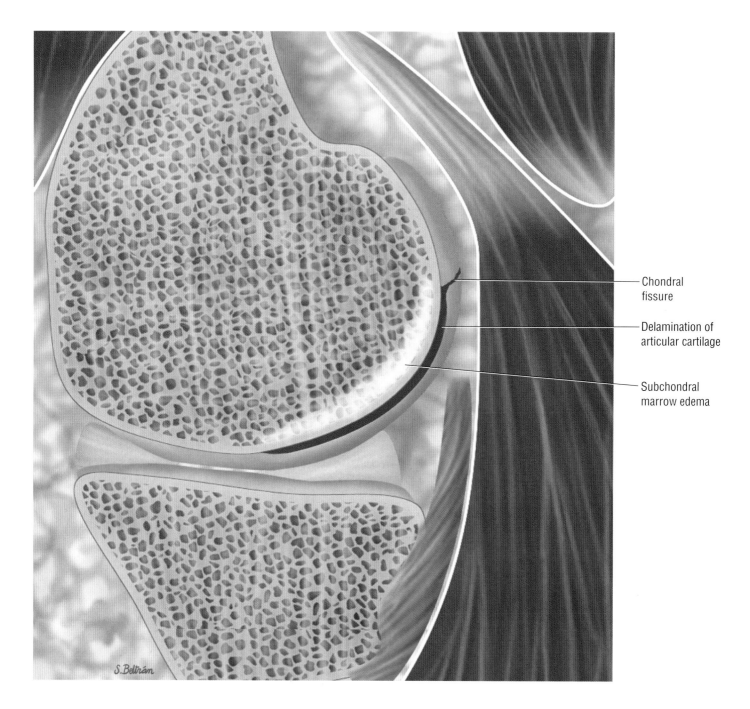

Chondral
fissure

Delamination of
articular cartilage

Subchondral
marrow edema

Figure 4.227 ▪ Delamination of articular cartilage with a fluid interface between the long-segment chondral flap of delamination and the deeper subchondral plate. *(See Chondral and Osteochondral Lesions pg. 707, in Stoller's 3rd Edition.)*

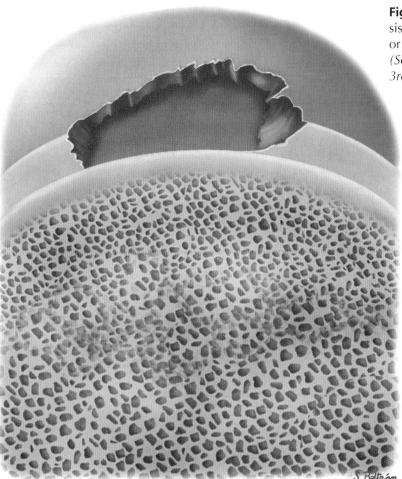

Figure 4.228 ■ In chondromalacia or degenerative chondrosis, the margins of the chondral lesion are less sharply defined or shallow than those seen in chondral flaps and fractures. *(See Chondral and Osteochondral Lesions pg. 708, in Stoller's 3rd Edition.)*

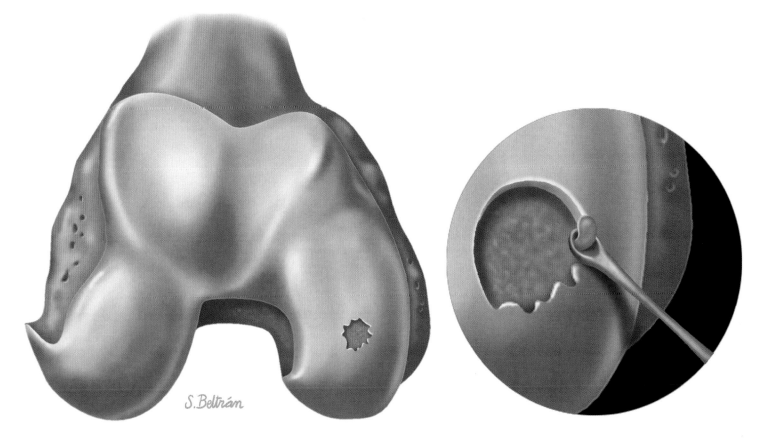

Figure 4.229 ■ Debridement of a full thickness chondral lesion without abrasion. *(See Chondral and Osteochondral Lesions pg. 709, in Stoller's 3rd Edition.)*

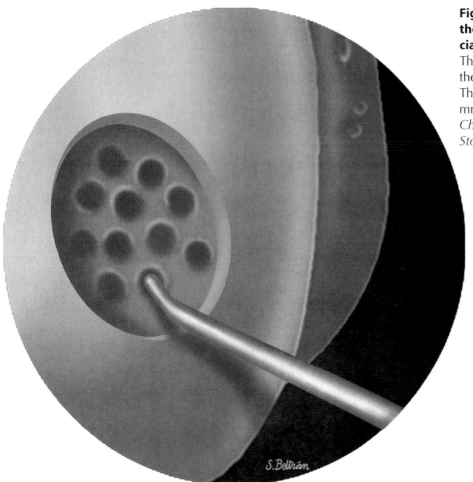

Figure 4.230 ■ **Microfracture technique with the creation of subchondral holes using a specialized awl to penetrate the subchondral plate.** This technique is performed after debridement of the lesion, including the calcified cartilage layer. The awl is inserted to a depth of approximately 4 mm to facilitate the formation of a superclot. *(See Chondral and Osteochondral Lesions pg. 710, in Stoller's 3rd Edition.)*

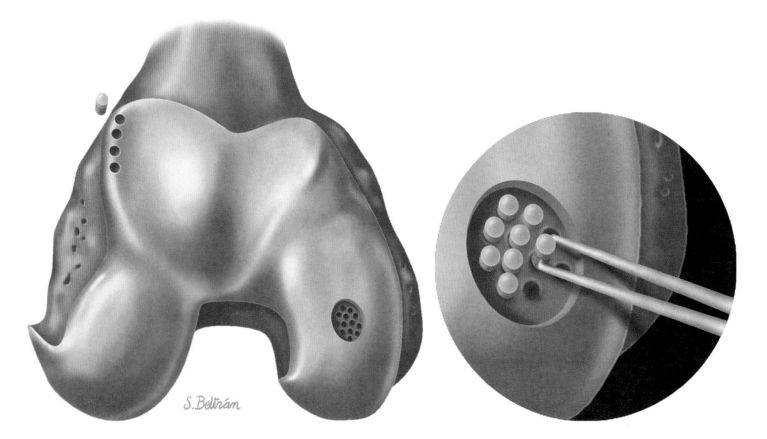

Figure 4.231 ■ **Osteochondral plugs of cartilage and subchondral bone placed into prepared recipient defects.** The superior aspect of the lateral femoral condyle is a common site for harvesting plugs. *(See Chondral and Osteochondral Lesions pg. 711, in Stoller's 3rd Edition.)*

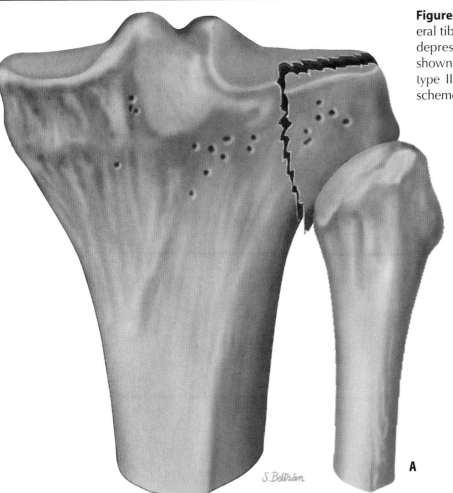

Figure 4.232 ■ **(A)** Nondisplaced split fracture of the lateral tibial plateau (Hohl type 1 fracture). **(B)** Local central depression with medial-to-lateral fracture extension shown on a coronal color section. This corresponds to a type II tibial plateau fracture in the Hohl classification scheme. *(See Fractures pg. 713, in Stoller's 3rd Edition.)*

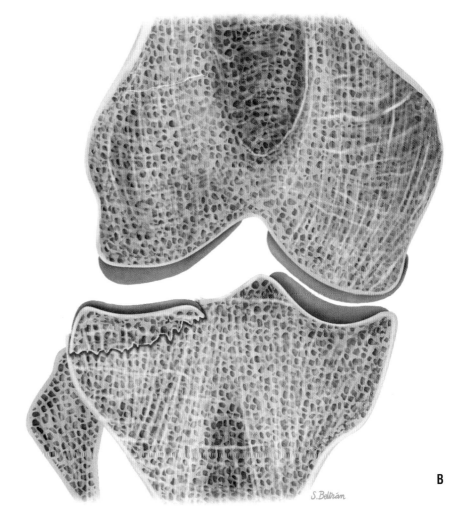

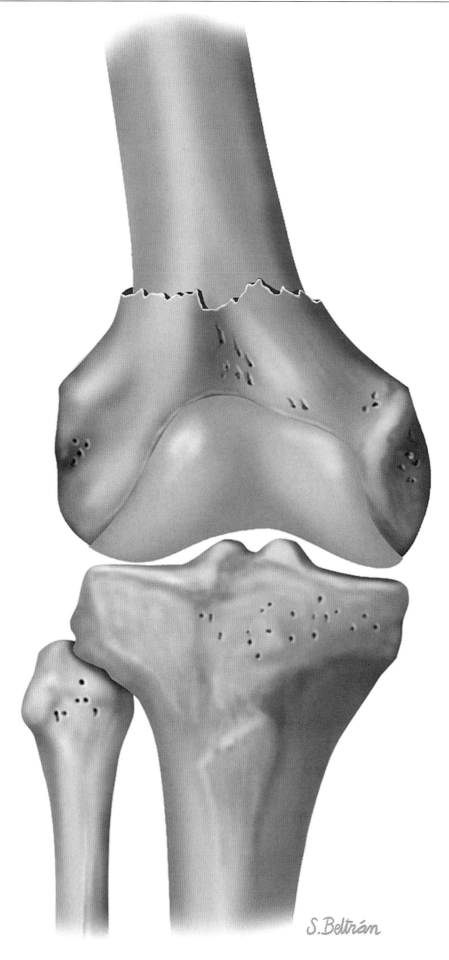

Figure 4.233 ▪ **Impacted supracondylar fracture of the distal femur.** Fractures of the distal femur are classified as supracondylar, condylar, or intercondylar. *(See Fractures pg. 720, in Stoller's 3rd Edition.)*

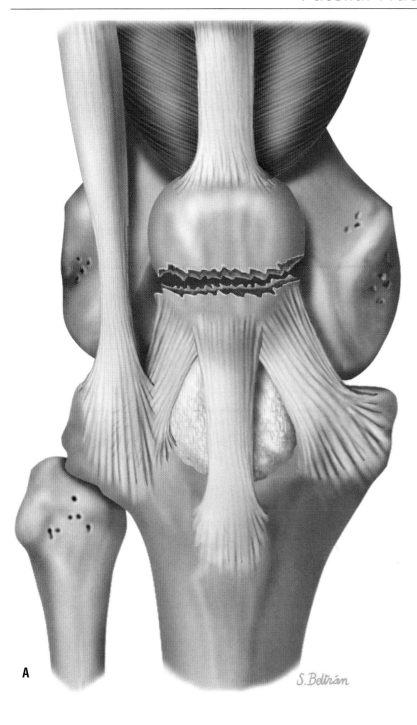

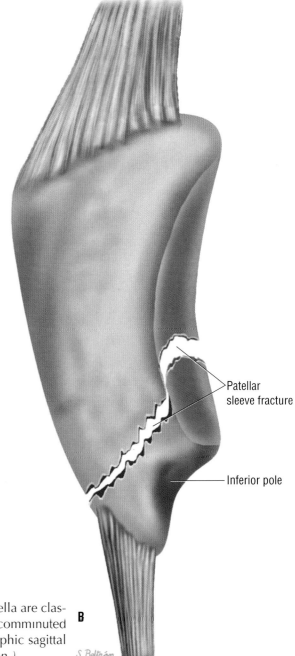

Patellar
sleeve fracture

Inferior pole

Figure 4.234 ■ **(A)** Transverse displaced patellar fracture. Fractures of the patella are classified as longitudinal (vertical), transverse (nondisplaced or displaced), comminuted (nondisplaced or displaced), and superior margin avulsion type. **(B)** Color graphic sagittal view of a patellar sleeve fracture. *(See Fractures pg. 722, in Stoller's 3rd Edition.)*

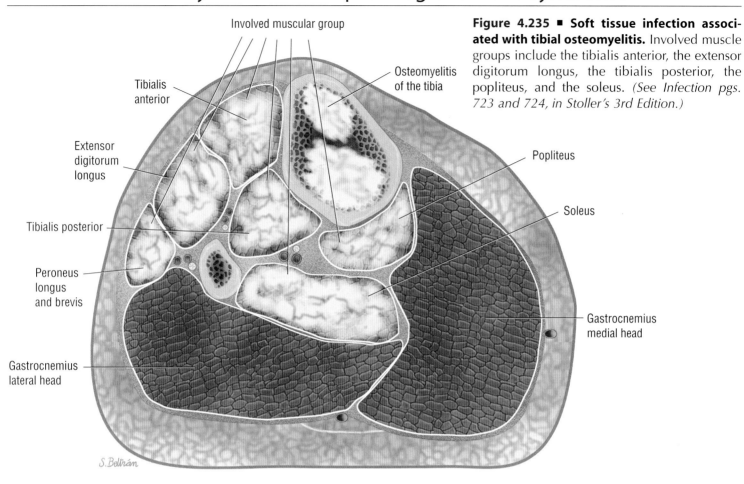

Figure 4.235 ■ **Soft tissue infection associated with tibial osteomyelitis.** Involved muscle groups include the tibialis anterior, the extensor digitorum longus, the tibialis posterior, the popliteus, and the soleus. *(See Infection pgs. 723 and 724, in Stoller's 3rd Edition.)*

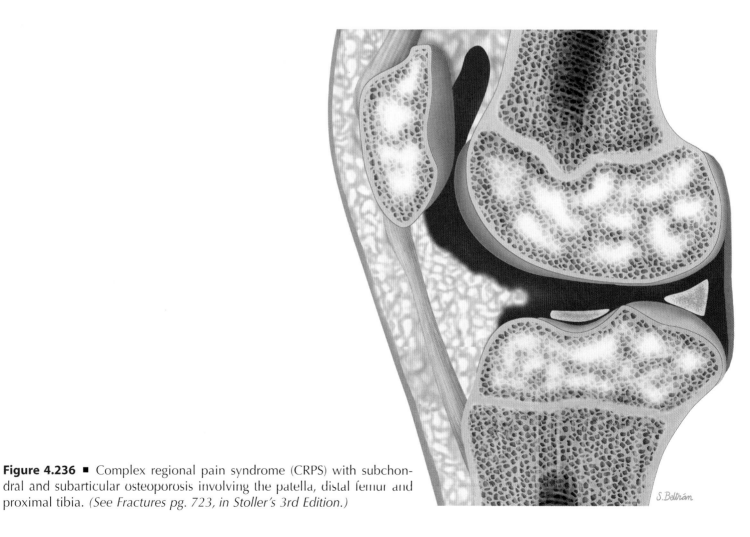

Figure 4.236 ■ Complex regional pain syndrome (CRPS) with subchondral and subarticular osteoporosis involving the patella, distal femur and proximal tibia. *(See Fractures pg. 723, in Stoller's 3rd Edition.)*

5

The Ankle and Foot

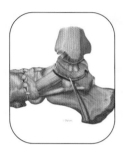

Pearls and Pitfalls & Color Illustrations

Pearls and Pitfalls

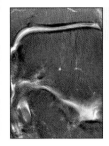

IMAGING PROTOCOLS

- FS PD FSE sequences are performed in all three orthogonal or orthogonal-oblique planes.
- Decreasing the FOV or increasing the resolution in the coronal plane allows optimal separation of the distal tibial and talar dome chondral surfaces.

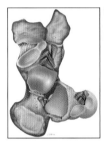

ANATOMY OF ANKLE AND FOOT
(See Figures 5.26–5.31)

- The syndesmotic ligaments consist of the anterior syndesmotic or anterior inferior tibiofibular ligament and the posterior syndesmotic or posterior inferior tibiofibular ligament, the interosseous membrane, and the transverse tibiofibular ligament.
- The transverse tibiofibular ligament represents the posterior labrum of the ankle and projects inferior to the posterior tibial margin.
- The deltoid ligament consists of superficial and deep layers.
- The ATFL is taut in plantarflexion.
- The tibial slip is the posterior intermalleolar ligament.
- The tendons of the deep calf and the neurovascular structures of the posterior compartment pass deep to the flexor retinaculum.

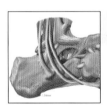

ANATOMIC VARIANTS
(See Figures 5.32–5.33)

- An accessory soleus may present as a mass in the distal calf or medial ankle.
- The flexor digitorum accessorius is an anomalous muscle posterior to the FHL.
- The peroneus quartus originates from the peroneus brevis muscle and inserts onto the peroneal tubercle of the calcaneus.

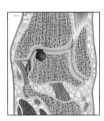

OSTEOCHONDRAL LESIONS
(See Figures 5.34–5.41)

- Osteochondral lesion of the talus (OLT) is the accepted terminology and should be used in place of transchondral fracture, osteochondral fracture, or osteochondritis dissecans.
- Osteochondral lesions may involve the posteromedial or anterolateral talus.
- An equivalent tibial lesion is also referred to as an osteochondral lesion (osteochondral lesion of the tibia).
- It is important not to overestimate the size of the lesion by including adjacent marrow edema in the dimensions of the lesion proper.

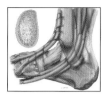

ACHILLES TENDINITIS
(See Figures 5.42–5.52)

- Tendinitis or tendinopathy represents intrasubstance tendon degeneration.
- Achilles tendinitis is subdivided into non-insertional tendinosis and insertional tendinitis.
- The Achilles tendon has no synovial sheath but is associated with a paratenon or connective tissue envelope.
- MR identifies nodular or convex tendon thickening and intratendinous mucoid degeneration.
- Haglund's deformity represents insertional tendinitis with a posterosuperior calcaneal bony prominence and retrocalcaneal and tendo-Achilles bursitis.

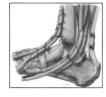

PARTIAL AND COMPLETE ACHILLES TENDON TEARS
(See Figures 5.53–5.58)

- Achilles tendon rupture usually occurs 2 to 6 cm proximal to its os calcis insertion.
- Sagittal images are used to identify the proximal and distal tendon ends.
- Axial FS PD FSE images are used to confirm complete rupture (an intact plantaris may simulate an intact tendon in the sagittal plane).

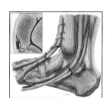

TIBIALIS POSTERIOR INJURIES
(See Figures 5.59–5.63)

- Tendinopathy and progressive tendon tear results in a collapsed pes valgus deformity.
- Tibialis posterior tendon tears occur at or just distal to the medial malleolus.
- Tears are classified as type 1 (enlarged tendon), type 2 (attenuated tendon), or type 3 (complete rupture).
- Associated medial malleolar spur may contribute to tendon degeneration.
- Subtendons are evaluated on axial images.

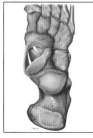

SPRING LIGAMENT COMPLEX AND PATHOLOGY
(See Figure 5.64)

- The spring ligament complex consists of three components: the lateral, intermediate, and superomedial oblique calcaneonavicular ligaments.
- Degeneration of the spring ligament complex is associated with posterior tibial (tibialis posterior) tendinopathy.

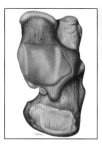

FLEXOR HALLUCIS LONGUS ABNORMALITIES
(See Figure 5.65–5.68)

- Tenosynovitis is associated with hyperintense fluid in the FHL synovial sheath disproportionate to the quantity of tibiotalar joint fluid.
- Chronic muscle changes and acute tenosynovitis are associated with hyperplantar flexion in ballet dancers.

- The distal course of the FHL should be examined on coronal images to exclude a distal rupture at its third or last fibroosseous tunnel.

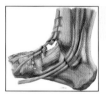

TIBIALIS ANTERIOR TENDON INJURIES
(See Figures 5.69–5.72)

- Rupture occurs between the extensor retinaculum and the insertion onto the medial first cuneiform and the adjacent base of the first metatarsal.

- It is important to differentiate between a partial and complete rupture using axial and coronal oblique images.

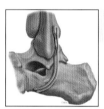

PERONEUS BREVIS TENDON TEARS
(See Figures 5.73–5.77)

- The peroneus brevis splits into two subtendons at the level of the retrofibular groove near the distal lateral malleolus.
- Lateral ligament tears and laxity of the superior peroneal retinaculum lead to peroneus brevis tendon split and tendon subluxation.

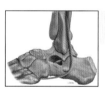

PERONEUS LONGUS TENDON TEAR
(See Figures 5.78–5.80)

- Peroneus longus tendon ruptures are associated with peroneus brevis tendon tears at the level of the malleolus.

- Isolated peroneus longus tendon tears frequently occur in the mid foot.
- The painful os peroneum syndrome (POPS) may be associated with a fracture or proximal displacement of the os perineum.

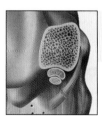

SUPERIOR PERONEAL RETINACULAR TEARS
(See Figures 5.81–5.84)

- Laxity or tear of the SPR may be associated with acute or chronic dislocation of the peroneal tendons.
- Chronic ankle instability is associated with SPR laxity.

- Stripping of the SPR produces a pouch or potential space facilitating peroneal tendon dislocation.

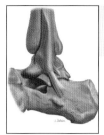

ANTERIOR TALOFIBULAR LIGAMENT TEAR
(See Figures 5.85–5.93)

- The ATFL is divided into two distinct bands and is taut in plantarflexion.
- Injury is associated with inversion, internal rotation, and plantarflexion mechanisms.

- Use T1- or PD-weighted axial imaging to appreciate increased signal intensity in a sprain with a partial tear and a corresponding FS PD FSE image to document ligament laxity, continuity, or disruption.

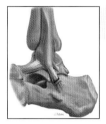

CALCANEOFIBULAR LIGAMENT SPRAIN
(See Figure 5.94)

- The CFL is crossed superficially by the peroneal tendons and stabilizes both the tibiotalar and subtalar joints.
- CFL sprains and complete tears are seen with ATFL injuries.

- CFL injuries are associated with subtalar injuries and sinus tarsi ligament pathology.

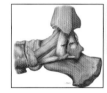

MEDIAL LIGAMENT COMPLEX INJURIES/DELTOID LIGAMENT SPRAIN
(See Figures 5.99–5.102)

- The thick deltoid or medial collateral ligament consists of two sets of fibers: superficial and deep.

- Up to 10% of deltoid injuries are associated with syndesmotic ligament pathology.
- Partial tears are more common than grade 3 ligamentous disruptions.

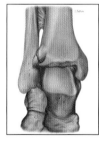

SYNDESMOSIS SPRAINS
(See Figures 5.103–5.109)

- Syndesmotic sprains or high ankle sprains may involve the anterior inferior tibiofibular (anterior syndesmotic) ligament, the posterior inferior tibiofibular (posterior syndesmotic) ligament, the transverse tibiofibular ligament, and interosseous membrane.

- Tearing is associated with bi- and trimalleolar and fibular subluxation and fractures.
- Severe syndesmosis injuries are seen with superior dislocation of the talus and an increased intermalleolar distance.
- Axial images at the level of the distal tibial plafond are used to evaluate the anterior and posterior syndesmotic ligaments.

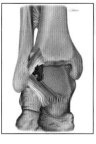

ANTEROLATERAL IMPINGEMENT
(See Figures 5.110–5.111)

- Involves synovitis and fibrosis of the AITF, the anterior talofibular ligament, and the lateral gutter
- Synovial thickening, hyalinized scar/meniscoid lesions, and chondral erosion of the lateral talar dome may all be seen.

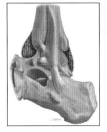

SYNDESMOTIC IMPINGEMENT
(See Figures 5.112–5.113)

- Inflamed synovium envelops the AITF and the inferior articulation of the tibia and fibula.
- Synovitis may involve the anterior and posterior aspects of the syndesmotic ligament.

- There may be associated loose bodies, chondromalacia, and osteophytes.
- Bassett's ligament is a separate distal fascicle of the AITF and may be associated with syndesmotic impingement against the lateral talus.

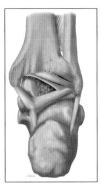

POSTERIOR IMPINGEMENT
(See Figures 5.114–5.116)

- Posterior impingement can occur alone or in combination with anterolateral and syndesmosis impingement.
- Generalized posterolateral impingement occurs with fibrosis, capsulitis, and synovial swelling involving any or a combination of the posterior ankle ligaments, including the posterior syndesmotic (inferior tibiofibular) ligament, the transverse tibiofibular ligament, the tibial slip, and the PTFL.

- Normal variations exist in the size of the tibial slip and transverse ligament. These structures should be evaluated for hypertrophy and tears.

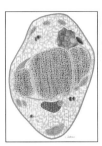

ANTEROMEDIAL AND POSTEROMEDIAL IMPINGEMENT
(See Figures 5.117– 5.118)

- Anteromedial impingement is associated with pathology of the anterior fibers of the deltoid ligament.
- Posteromedial impingement occurs as a complication of inversion injuries with injury to the deep layer of the deltoid ligament.

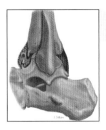

ANTERIOR IMPINGEMENT
(See Figures 5.119–5.124)

- Anterior impingement represents spur formation between the anterior inferior tibial plafond and the talar neck.
- The "door jam" effect is created by loss of dorsiflexion from opposing anterior osteophytes.

- FS PD FSE sagittal images are used to identify tibiotalar effusion, marrow edema, fragmentation of osteophytes, and associated chondral lesions.

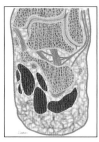

SINUS TARSI SYNDROME
(See Figures 5.125–5.132)

- Sinus tarsi syndrome is associated with sinus tarsi and lateral hindfoot pain and instability with injury to the contents of the tarsal canal and sinus.
- T1- or PD-weighted sagittal or coronal images demonstrate effacement of sinus tarsi fat.

- Synovitis, fibrosis, or ligament disruption is identified on FS PD FSE images.
- Tibialis posterior tendon dysfunction and spring ligament pathology may be associated with sinus tarsi syndrome.
- The three layers of lateral ligamentous support of the joint are the superficial or peripheral layer (e.g., the calcaneofibular ligament); the intermediate layer (e.g., the cervical ligament); and the deep layer (e.g., the interosseous talocalcaneal ligament).

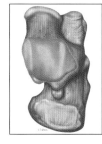

OS TRIGONUM SYNDROME
(See Figures 5.133–5.140)

- Os trigonum syndrome pain may be associated with disruption of the cartilaginous synchondrosis between the os trigonum and the lateral tubercle of the posterior process.
- Stieda's process is a prominent posterior extension of the lateral tubercle.

- Compression of the os trigonum between the FHL and posterior talofibular ligaments occurs in extreme ankle flexion. Compression of the os trigonum between the calcaneus and talus occurs in the end range of plantarflexion.

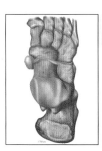

ACCESSORY NAVICULAR
(See Figure 5.141)

- The accessory navicular, also known as the os tibiale externum, is the development of a congenital navicular tuberosity from a secondary center of ossification.
- Evaluation includes determining the status of the PTT.

- FS PD FSE or STIR images in the axial plane are used to appreciate hyperintense edema across the synchondrosis.

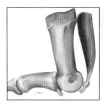

TURF TOE
(See Figures 5.142–5.149)

- The key ligaments of the capsuloligamentous complex of the first MTP joint are the metatarsosesamoid and sesamoid-phalangeal ligaments.

- The plantar plate is less substantial in the hallux relative to the lesser metatarsals. It can be visualized between the sesamoid-phalangeal ligaments extending from the sesamoids to the proximal aspect of the proximal phalanx.
- Turf toe evaluation must include assessment of tearing of the sesamoid-phalangeal ligament, plantar plate, and displacement or fracture of the sesamoids.

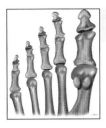

SESAMOID DYSFUNCTION
(See Figures 5.150–5.153)

- A bipartite sesamoid usually involves the medial sesamoid.
- The sesamoids may be affected by fracture, osteochondritis, sesamoiditis, and arthritis.

- FS PD FSE or STIR imaging is required to identify sesamoid edema.
- CT may be helpful if a fracture cannot be distinguished from bipartite morphology.

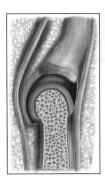

PLANTAR PLATE INJURIES OF THE LESSER METATARSOPHALANGEAL JOINTS
(See Figures 5.154–5.157)

- Pitfalls in the MR interpretation of the lesser MTP joints include the normal plantar plate recess, the capsular plantar plate attachment, and the distal phalangeal bare area.
- Intermediate-signal-intensity hyaline articular cartilage may undercut the plantar plate on sagittal images.

- Plantar plate tears occur most frequently at their distal attachment.
- MTP joint instability is associated with plantar plate degeneration and rupture.

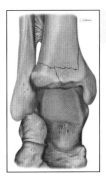

ANKLE FRACTURES
(See Figures 5.158–5.163)

- Fractures of the distal tibia include pilon, Tillaux, juvenile Tillaux, and triplanar (triplane) types.
- A triplane fracture is a combination of the juvenile Tillaux fracture (Salter-Harris type III fracture) and a Salter-Harris type II fracture and involves a fracture plane in the sagittal, axial, and coronal directions.

- Fractures of the fibula include Pott, Dupuytren, and Maisonneuve types.

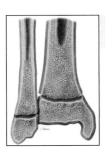

EPIPHYSEAL FRACTURES
(See Figures 5.164–5.167)

- The Salter-Harris classification is divided into five types. Salter-Harris type V represents a compression fracture through the physis.
- Trauma can also occur to the perichondrium, or there may be isolated epiphyseal or metaphyseal injuries or avulsion of the periosteum.

- Entrapment of the periosteum is associated with Salter-Harris type I injuries.

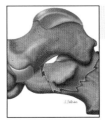

CALCANEAL FRACTURES
(See Figures 5.168–5.170)

- Fractures of the calcaneus are either extra-articular or intra-articular.
- Intra-articular fractures are divided into Essex-Lopresti type A, or tongue-type, and Essex-Lopresti type B, or joint depression type.

- 75% of calcaneal fractures extend into the subtalar joint.
- The Rowe classification of calcaneal fractures is based on five types, with type IV and V involving the subtalar joint.

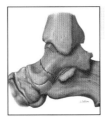

TALAR FRACTURES
(See Figures 5.171–5.173)

- Talar fractures may involve the talar head, neck, body, or lateral or posterior process.
- Talar fractures are associated with high-energy traumatic injuries, including falls and motor vehicle accidents.

- Lateral process fractures, also known as snowboarder's fractures, are associated with inversion, dorsiflexion, and compressive force.
- It is important to evaluate for AVN with talar neck fractures.

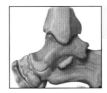

NAVICULAR FRACTURES
(See Figure 5.174)

- Navicular fractures include fractures of the tuberosity, body avulsion, and stress fractures.

- The central third of the navicular is avascular and at increased risk for stress fracture and nonunion.
- Navicular marrow edema visualized on sagittal images should be correlated with axial or coronal images to identify fracture morphology.

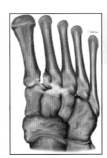

TARSOMETATARSAL OR LISFRANC FRACTURES
(See Figures 5.175–5.179)

- Lisfranc fractures may be homolateral or divergent tarsometatarsal fracture dislocations.
- Lisfranc's ligament extends from the medial cuneiform to the medial aspect of the second metatarsal base.

- Axial MR images are used to evaluate Lisfranc's ligament and to assess the lateral effect of the first metatarsal base relative to the medial cuneiform and the medial second metatarsal base relative to the intermediate cuneiform in the homolateral type of injury.
- Fractures are associated with sports-related injuries in athletes and Charcot arthropathy in diabetic patients.
- Direct coronal images are used to appreciate dorsal/plantar displacement.

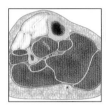

METATARSAL FRACTURES
(See Figures 5.180–5.183)

- Fracture types include stress, head, neck, midshaft, base, first, central (second through fourth), or fifth metatarsal fractures.

- The Jones fracture occurs through the proximal metatarsal diaphysis and is at risk for delayed or fibrous union.

- Stress fractures are associated with overuse, including running and dancing.

- Metatarsal marrow edema may persist after clinical resolution of stress fracture symptoms.

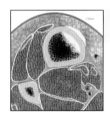

COMPARTMENT SYNDROME
(See Figures 5.184–5.187)

- Compartment syndrome may be acute or chronic (exertional).

- Anterior, lateral, superficial, and deep posterior compartments may be affected.

- Axial FS PD FSE images are used to identify diffuse muscle edema and compartmental bulging with convex deep fascial margins.

- There may be loss of normal muscle striations and muscle herniations in chronic compartment syndrome.

MEDIAL TIBIAL STRESS SYNDROME
(See Figures 5.188–5.189)

- Characterized by hyperintense signal along the anterior medial tibial border.

- Related to periosteal avulsion and periostitis at the medial soleus insertional site resulting from hyperpronation.

- Spectrum of findings is classified as grade 1 (periosteal edema) through grade IV (fracture).

- FS PD FSE or STIR images in the axial plane are used to identify subtle periosteal edema.

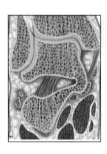

TARSAL COALITION
(See Figure 5.190)

- Coalitions can be osseous, cartilaginous, or a fibrous union of two or more bones involving the hindfoot or midfoot.

- A synostosis is a complete coalition, a synchondrosis is cartilaginous, and a syndesmosis is fibrous.

- An osseous bar is extra-articular, whereas a bridge is intra-articular.

- Talocalcaneal coalitions are best visualized on coronal images; calcaneonavicular coalitions require sagittal images.

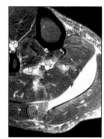

GASTROCNEMIUS-SOLEUS STRAIN
(See Figure 5.191)

- Represents a strain or tear of the medial head of the gastrocnemius muscle.

- There is diffuse hyperintense signal intensity within the medial head on FS PD FSE or STIR images.

- Soleus muscle strains should be evaluated in association with medial head gastrocnemius strains.

- Deep venous thrombosis with prominent venous collaterals should not be mistaken for a muscle strain.

- Axial images are useful in the identification of fascial tearing.

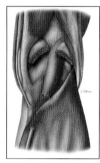

PLANTARIS RUPTURE
(See Figure 5.192)

- The term "tennis leg" has been used for injuries to the medial head of the gastrocnemius (more common presentation of tennis leg) and for plantaris tendon rupture.

- A myotendinous proximal tear is associated with distal retraction of the plantaris tendon with a hemorrhagic mass effect between the medial head of the gastrocnemius and the soleus muscle.

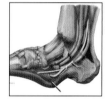

TARSAL TUNNEL SYNDROME
(See Figures 5.193–5.197)

- Tarsal tunnel syndrome is an entrapment or compression neuropathy of the posterior tibial nerve.

- A space-occupying lesion may be identified, as well as denervation or atrophy of the muscles supplied by the posterior tibial nerve or one of its branches.

- Causative factors include fracture, varicosities, ganglions, lipomas, nerve sheath tumors, and a thickened flexor retinaculum and accessory muscles.

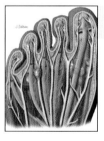

MORTON'S NEUROMA
(See Figure 5.198)

- Represents a metatarsalgia with localized enlargement of the interdigital nerve between the third and fourth metatarsal heads.

- FS PD FSE or STIR images in the coronal plane are used to distinguish between intermetatarsal bursitis and the teardrop-shaped soft-tissue plantar mass seen in Morton's neuroma.

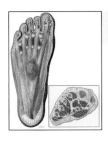

PLANTAR FIBROMATOSIS
(See Figure 5.199)

- Represents fibrous and collagenous nodules in the plantar aponeurosis.
- May present as single or multiple nodular lesions.
- Occurs in a more distal location than plantar fasciitis.

- The upper or deep border may be infiltrative.
- FS PD FSE or STIR images are used to appreciate central hyperintensity in single nodules.

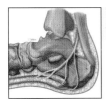

PLANTAR FASCIITIS
(See Figures 5.200–5.203)

- Plantar fasciitis also is known as heel pain syndrome or subcalcaneal pain syndrome.
- The origin of the plantar fascia from the calcaneal tuberosity is most commonly affected.

- Microtrauma of the plantar fascia or repetitive tensile overload may lead to an inflammatory response.
- There may be plantar fascial tearing, or involvement may be localized to the medial, central, or lateral portions of the aponeurosis.
- Effacement of subcutaneous fat by fibrosis and edema seen in the sagittal plane may assist in early diagnosis.

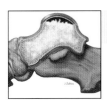

AVASCULAR NECROSIS OF THE TALUS
(See Figures 5.204–5.208)

- In acute and subacute stages, AVN of the talus is indicated by a localized subchondral ischemic focus with surrounding diffuse edema or by a more diffuse infarct pattern throughout the entire talar body.

- Posttraumatic etiologies include a talar neck fracture and talar dislocation.
- Follow-up MR studies are used to document resolution of bone marrow edema and to help define the AVN focus.

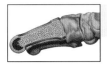

FREIBERG'S INFRACTION
(See Figure 5.209)

- Sagittal images are the most sensitive in demonstrating the initial flattening of the second metatarsal head.

- Trauma either from a single episode or from repeated injury of a metatarsal at risk (e.g., the long second metatarsal) is the primary etiology of Freiberg's infraction.

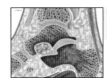

NEUROPATHIC FOOT
(See Figure 5.210)

- Osteomyelitis is associated with pressure point ulcers and marrow changes that are hypointense on T1-weighted images and hyperintense on FS PD FSE or STIR images.

- Neuropathic joint involvement is usually independent of the presence of soft-tissue ulcers and typically involves multiple joints.
- Neuropathic marrow changes are not hyperintense on T2* GRE images. Hyperintense marrow on T2* contrast indicates increased free water and, thus, has a high association with osteomyelitis.

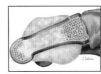

OSTEOMYELITIS
(See Figures 5.211–5.212)

- Primary signs include osseous erosion, adjacent soft-tissue mass (abscess), and a sinus tract.

- Marrow is hypointense on T1-weighted images and hyperintense on FS PD FSE or STIR images.

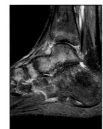

REFLEX SYMPATHETIC DYSTROPHY

- New terminology is complex regional pain syndrome (CRPS).
- Type I CRPS replaces the term *reflex sympathic dystrophy* (pain related to a noxious event or immobilization).
- Type II CRPS replaces the term causalgia (pain related to nerve injury, but not necessarily limited to the distribution of the injured nerve).

- Osteoporosis and CRPS may demonstrate similar patchy marrow patterns of hypointensity on T1-weighted images and hyperintensity on FS PD FSE images.

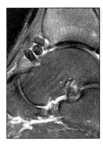

ARTHRITIS
(See Figure 5.213)

- Degenerative arthritis targets both the tibiotalar joint and the hindfoot.
- Rheumatoid arthritis frequently involves the forefoot and talonavicular joint.
- There may be associated synovitis and subchondral marrow edema in rheumatoid disease.

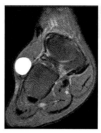

GANGLIA
(See Figure 5.214)

- Ganglia are commonly located in the dorsolateral foot, including the talonavicular joint.
- Intravenous contrast shows peripheral enhancement without central hyperintensity.
- Cyst-like structures with central intermediate signal intensity should be further evaluated with intravenous contrast to exclude a soft-tissue sarcoma.
- A medial malleolus bursa may have imaging characteristics similar to a ganglion.

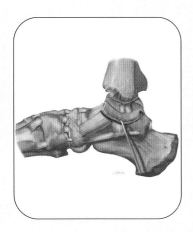

The Ankle and Foot
Muscle

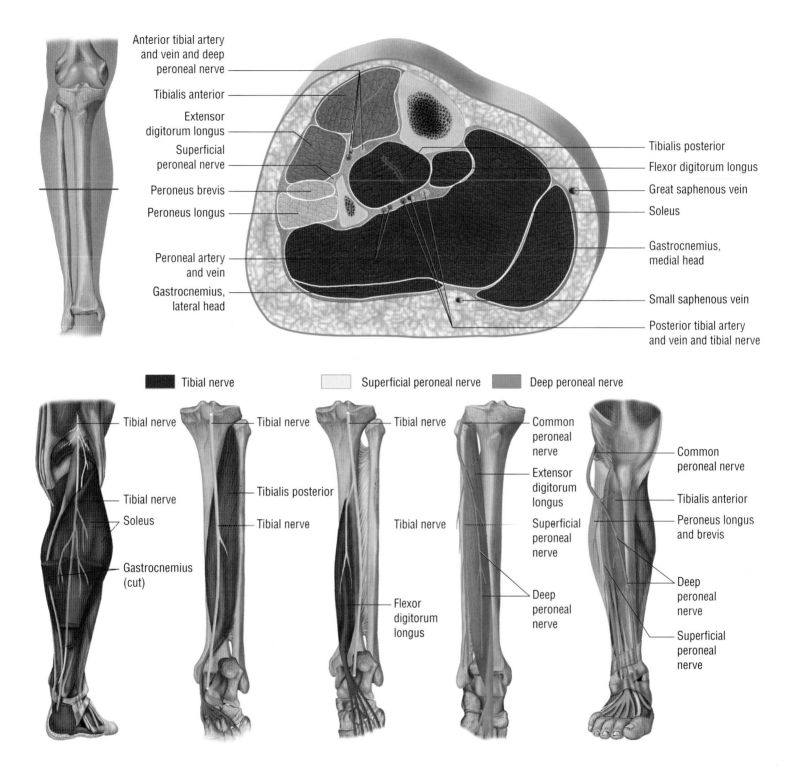

Figure 5.1 ■ Mid lower leg innervation pattern on cross section and 3D muscle display. *Cross section based on Vahlensiech M, Genant HK, Reiter M. MRI of the Musculoskeletal System. New York/Stuttgart: Thieme, 2000. (See Related Muscles pg. 734, in Stoller's 3rd Edition.)*

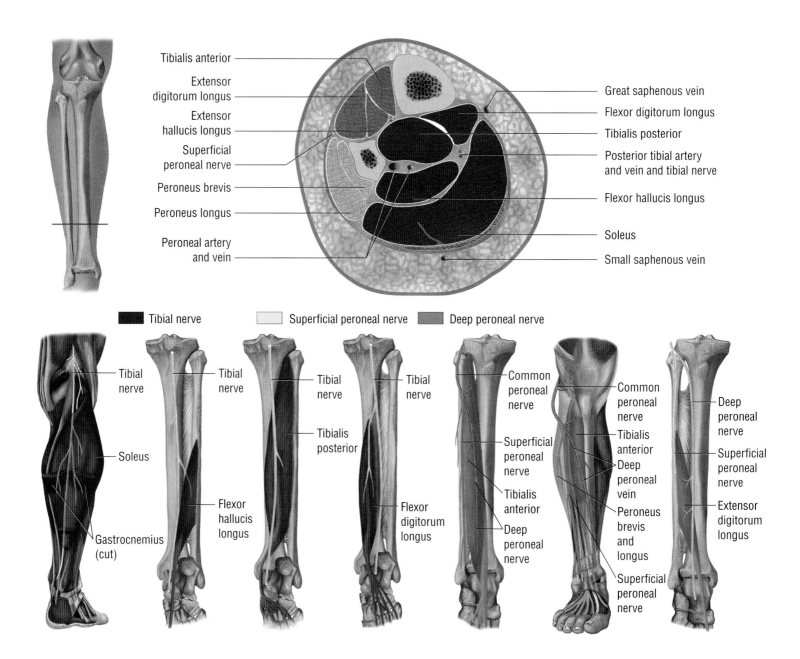

Figure 5.2 ▪ Distal lower leg innervation with cross section and 3D muscle group display. *Cross section based on Vahlensiech M, Genat HK, Reiter M. MRI of the Musculoskeletal System. New York/Stuttgart: Thieme, 2000. (See Related Muscles pg. 734, in Stoller's 3rd Edition.)*

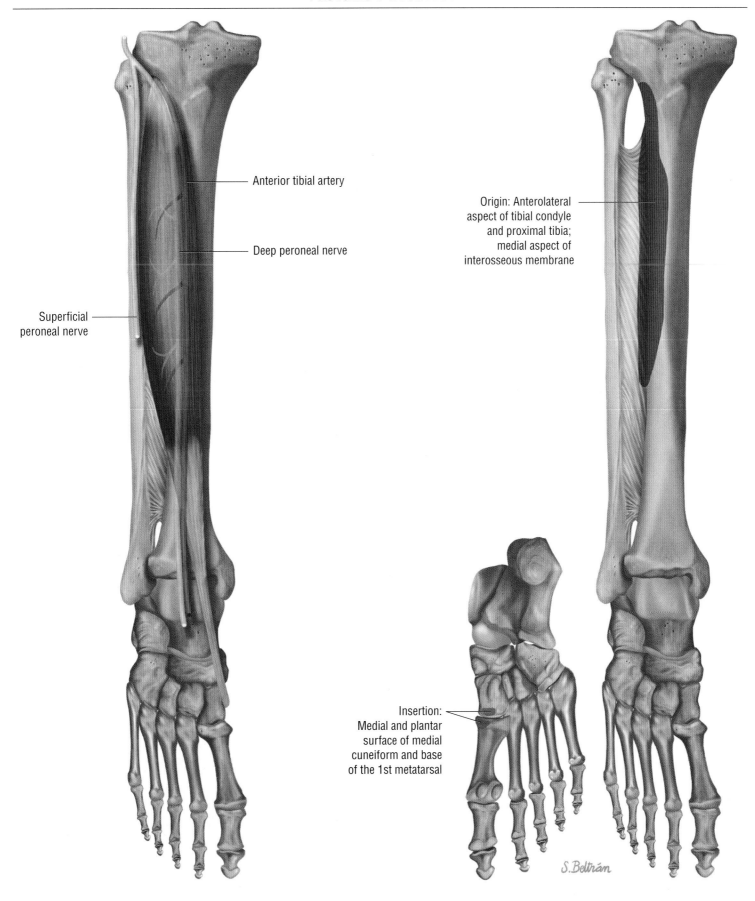

Anterior tibial artery

Deep peroneal nerve

Superficial
peroneal nerve

Origin: Anterolateral
aspect of tibial condyle
and proximal tibia;
medial aspect of
interosseous membrane

Insertion:
Medial and plantar
surface of medial
cuneiform and base
of the 1st metatarsal

S.Beltrán

Figure 5.3 ■ TIBIALIS ANTERIOR. The tibialis anterior muscle functions eccentrically after the heel strike to control deceleration of the foot and concentrically after the toe off in ankle dorsiflexion. In runners and hikers, paratenonitis is associated with the use of excessive eccentric contraction during midfoot and forefoot impact on downhill slopes. Paratenonitis is also associated with direct mechanical irritation from ski boots or hockey skates. The tibialis anterior dorsiflexes and inverts the foot. *(See Related Muscles pg. 735, in Stoller's 3rd Edition.)*

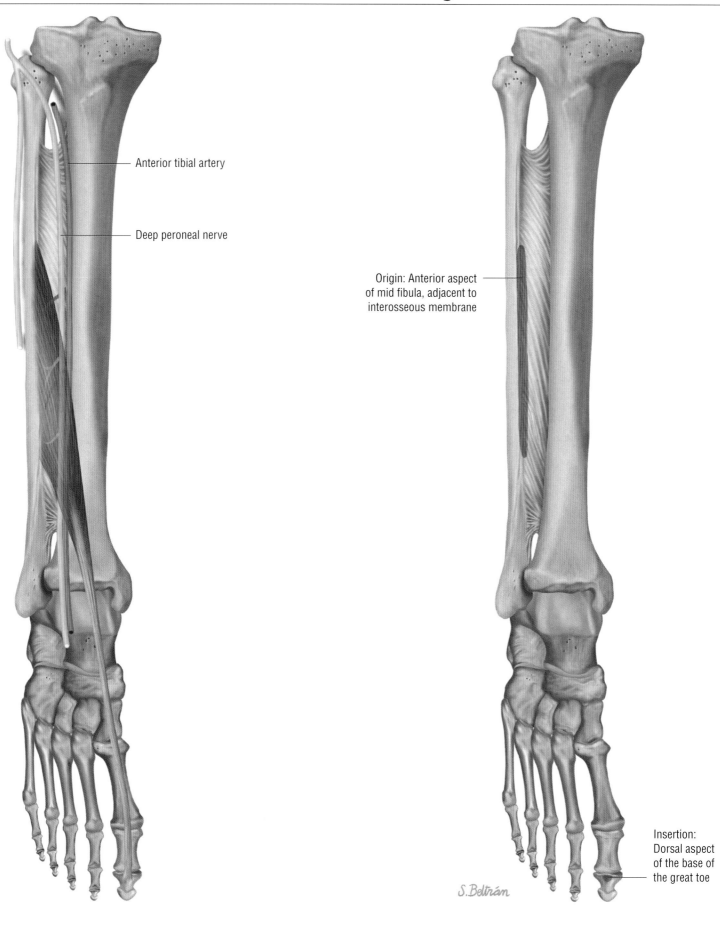

Anterior tibial artery

Deep peroneal nerve

Origin: Anterior aspect
of mid fibula, adjacent to
interosseous membrane

Insertion:
Dorsal aspect
of the base of
the great toe

S.Beltrán

Figure 5.4 ▪ EXTENSOR HALLUCIS LONGUS. Extensor hallucis (and extensor digitorum) injuries are similar in origin to injuries of the tibialis anterior tendon. Extensor hallucis longus (EHL) paratenonitis is associated with pain and swelling localized to the
ankle joint with painful resisted extension of the hallux. The EHL extends the great toe
and dorsiflexes the foot. *(See Related Muscles pg. 735, in Stoller's 3rd Edition.)*

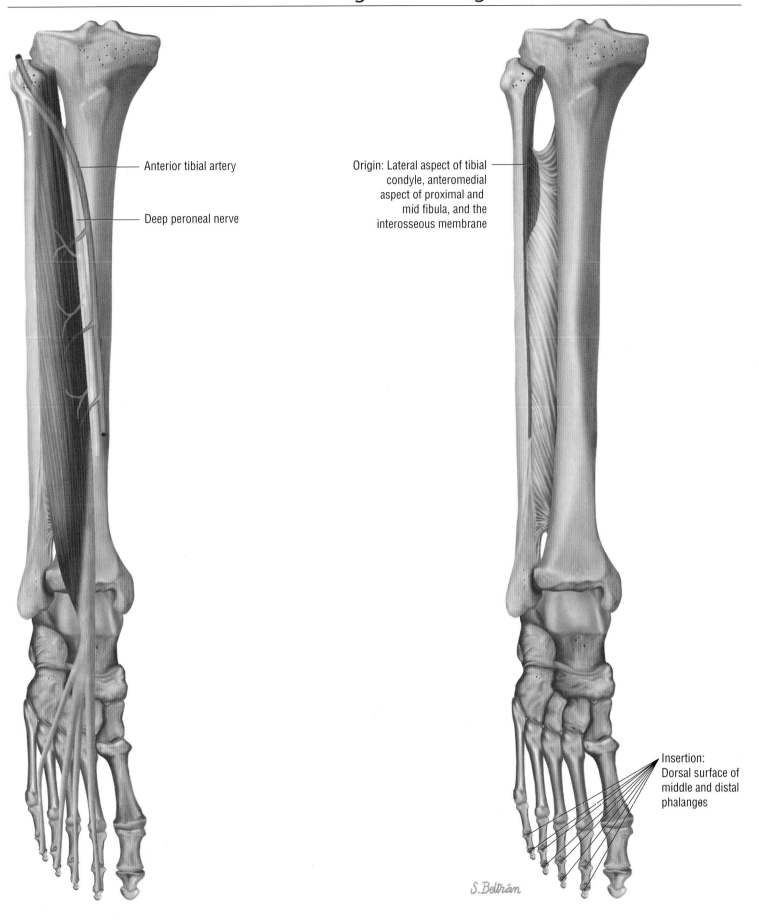

Anterior tibial artery

Deep peroneal nerve

Origin: Lateral aspect of tibial condyle, anteromedial aspect of proximal and mid fibula, and the interosseous membrane

Insertion: Dorsal surface of middle and distal phalanges

S. Beltrán

Figure 5.5 ■ EXTENSOR DIGITORUM LONGUS. Extensor digitorum longus (EDL) paratenonitis is associated with pain and swelling over the ankle joint and lateral to the extensor hallucis longus. There is pain with resisted extension of the lesser toes in paratenonitis. The EDL extends the phalanges of the lateral four toes and dorsiflexes the foot. *(See Related Muscles pg. 736, in Stoller's 3rd Edition.)*

Peroneus Tertius

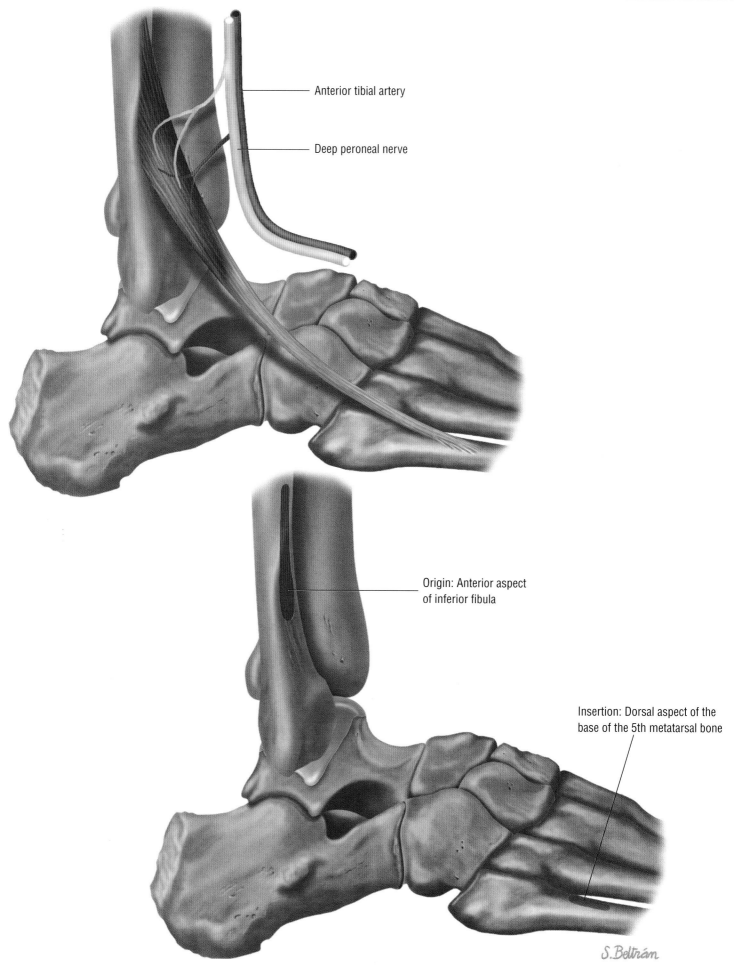

Anterior tibial artery

Deep peroneal nerve

Origin: Anterior aspect
of inferior fibula

Insertion: Dorsal aspect of the
base of the 5th metatarsal bone

S. Beltrán

Figure 5.6 ■ **PERONEUS TERTIUS.** The peroneus tertius represents a lateral slip of the extensor digitorum longus. Isolated ruptures of the peroneus tertius tendons do not occur. The peroneus tertius dorsiflexes and everts the foot. *(See Related Muscles pg. 736, in Stoller's 3rd Edition.)*

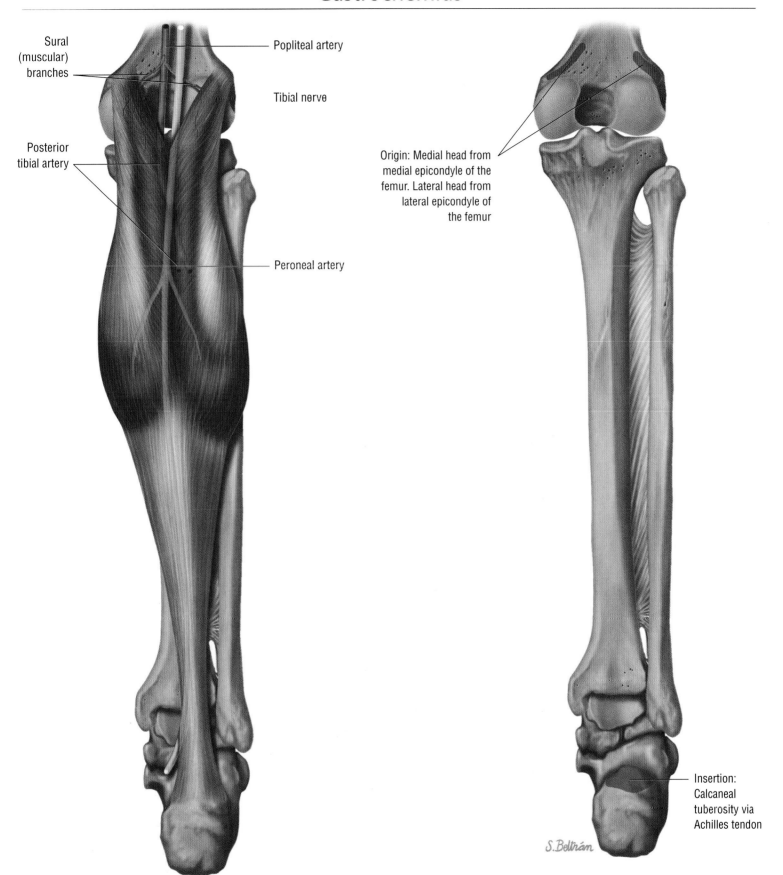

Sural (muscular) branches

Popliteal artery

Tibial nerve

Posterior tibial artery

Peroneal artery

Origin: Medial head from medial epicondyle of the femur. Lateral head from lateral epicondyle of the femur

Insertion: Calcaneal tuberosity via Achilles tendon

S. Beltrán

Figure 5.7 ▪ GASTROCNEMIUS. The gastrocnemius plantarflexes the foot and also flexes the knee joint, as its origin is on the femoral condyles. In contrast to the soleus muscle (which has a more postural function), the gastrocnemius generates the power for propulsion in walking, running, and jumping. *(See Related Muscles pg. 737, in Stoller's 3rd Edition.)*

Soleus

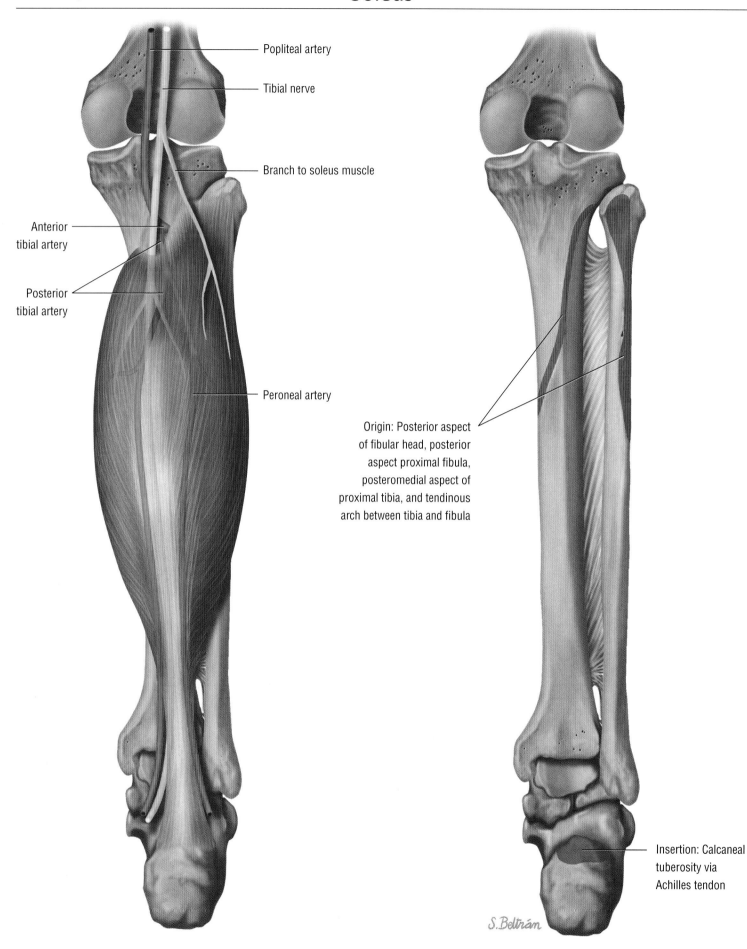

- Popliteal artery
- Tibial nerve
- Branch to soleus muscle
- Anterior tibial artery
- Posterior tibial artery
- Peroneal artery
- Origin: Posterior aspect of fibular head, posterior aspect proximal fibula, posteromedial aspect of proximal tibia, and tendinous arch between tibia and fibula
- Insertion: Calcaneal tuberosity via Achilles tendon

S. Beltrán

Figure 5.8 ▪ SOLEUS. The gastrocnemius and the soleus muscles function in plantarflexion of the foot. The soleus consists primarily of type I or slow-twitch oxidative fibers and rapidly develops disuse atrophy in response to immobilization. *(See Related Muscles pg. 737, in Stoller's 3rd Edition.)*

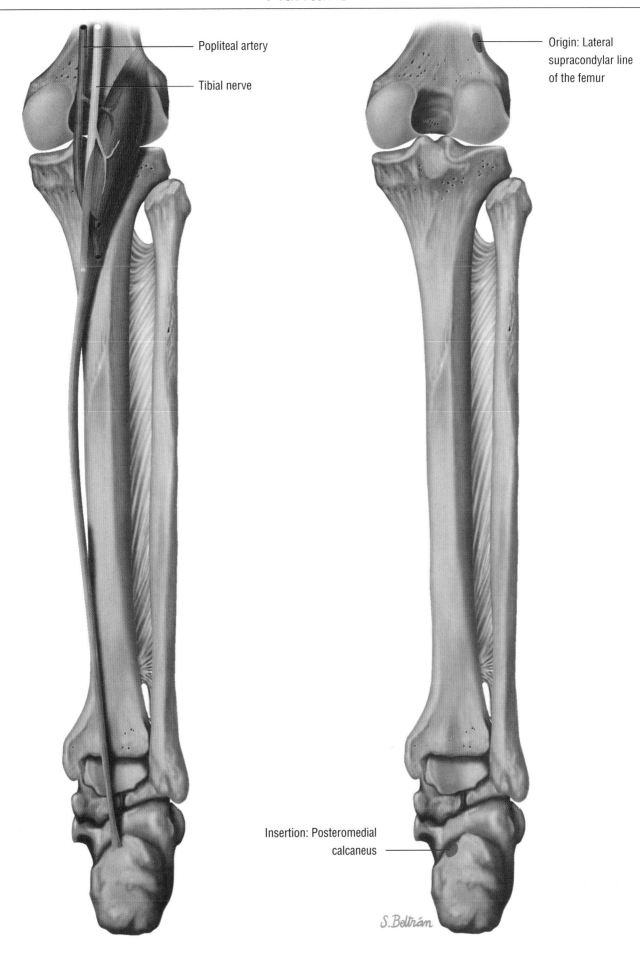

Popliteal artery

Tibial nerve

Origin: Lateral supracondylar line of the femur

Insertion: Posteromedial calcaneus

S. Beltrán

Figure 5.9 ■ PLANTARIS. The plantaris plantar flexes the foot and is visualized as a 2 to 3 mm hypointense dot-like structure on axial images anteromedial to the Achilles tendon. The plantaris tendon courses obliquely between the gastrocnemius and soleus muscles. *(See Related Muscles pg. 738, in Stoller's 3rd Edition.)*

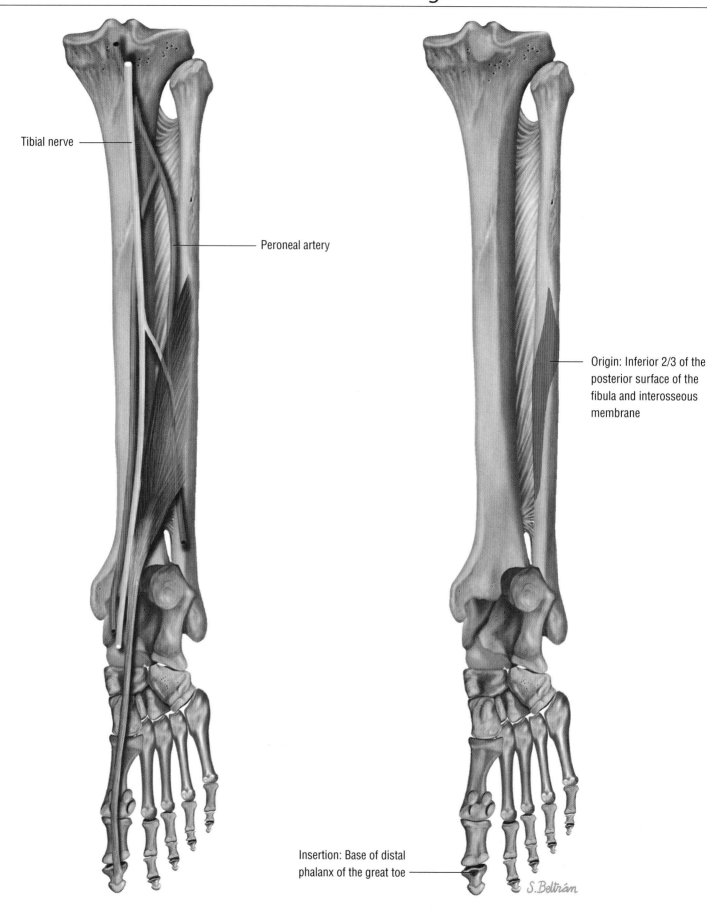

Tibial nerve

Peroneal artery

Origin: Inferior 2/3 of the posterior surface of the fibula and interosseous membrane

Insertion: Base of distal phalanx of the great toe

S. Beltrán

Figure 5.10 ▪ FLEXOR HALLUCIS LONGUS. The flexor hallucis longus (FHL) flexes the great toe and plantarflexes the foot. The FHL is susceptible to injury during extremes of ankle plantarflexion and metatarsophalangeal dorsiflexion. The proximal sheath, 10 to 12 cm in length, has no mesotenon, and may communicate with the ankle joint and the sheaths of the flexor digitorum longus and tibialis posterior. *(See Related Muscles pg. 738, in Stoller's 3rd Edition.)*

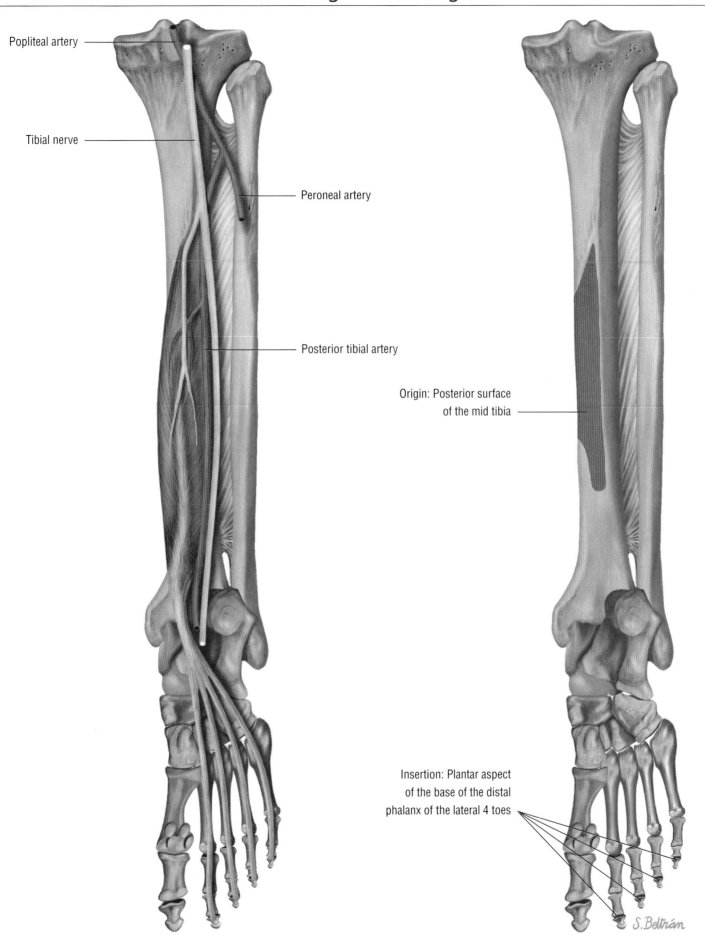

Popliteal artery

Tibial nerve

Peroneal artery

Posterior tibial artery

Origin: Posterior surface
of the mid tibia

Insertion: Plantar aspect
of the base of the distal
phalanx of the lateral 4 toes

S. Beltrán

Figure 5.11 ■ FLEXOR DIGITORUM LONGUS. The flexor digitorum longus (FDL) flexes the phalanges of the lateral four toes and plantarflexes the foot. The FDL is superficial to the flexor hallucis in the sole of the foot. Paratenonitis of the FDL is more infrequent than involvement of the flexor hallucis longus. *(See Related Muscles pg. 739, in Stoller's 3rd Edition.)*

Tibialis Posterior

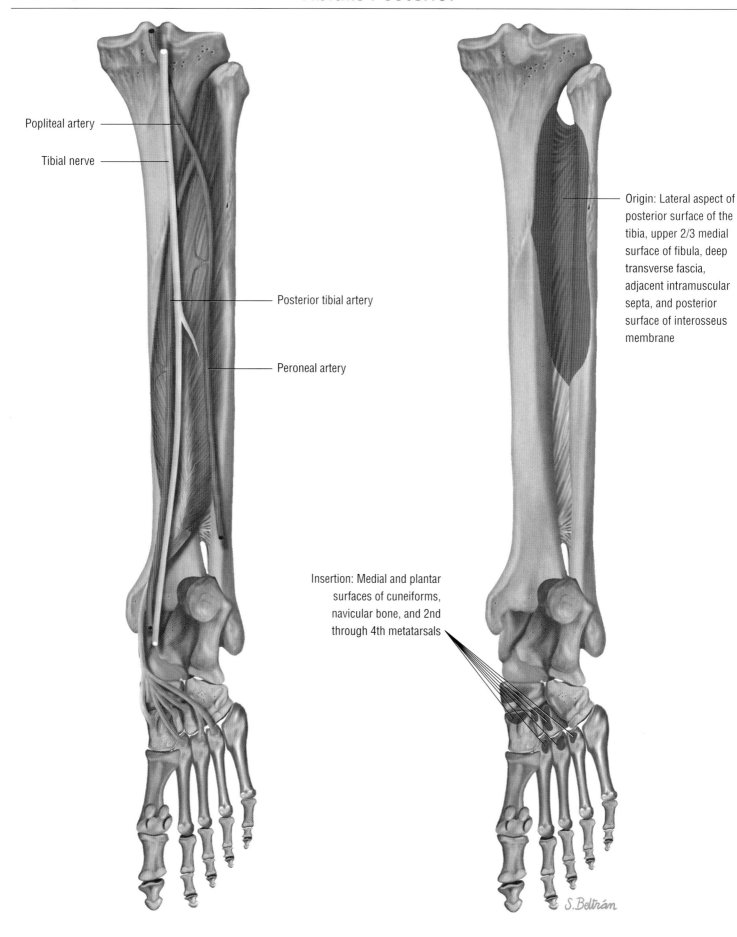

Popliteal artery

Tibial nerve

Posterior tibial artery

Peroneal artery

Origin: Lateral aspect of posterior surface of the tibia, upper 2/3 medial surface of fibula, deep transverse fascia, adjacent intramuscular septa, and posterior surface of interosseus membrane

Insertion: Medial and plantar surfaces of cuneiforms, navicular bone, and 2nd through 4th metatarsals

S. Beltrán

Figure 5.12 ■ TIBIALIS POSTERIOR. The tibialis posterior plantarflexes and inverts the foot. The tibialis posterior tendon passes over (superficial to) the deltoid and changes from a tubular tendon to a flattened structure containing a fibrocartilaginous sesamoid (under the plantar calcaneonavicular ligament). *(See Related Muscles pg. 739, in Stoller's 3rd Edition.)*

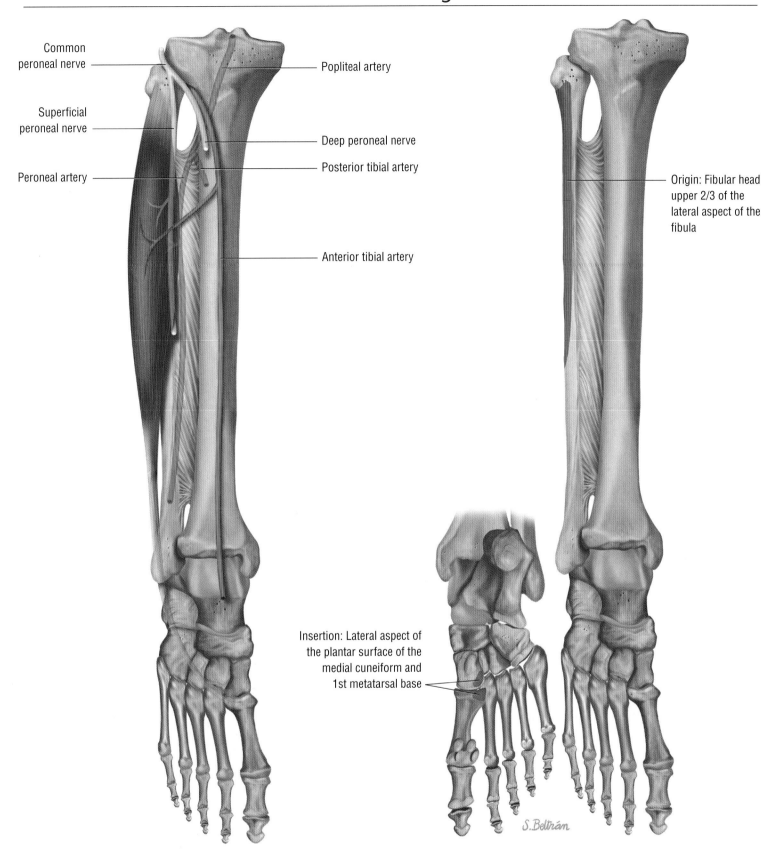

Common peroneal nerve

Superficial peroneal nerve

Peroneal artery

Popliteal artery

Deep peroneal nerve

Posterior tibial artery

Anterior tibial artery

Origin: Fibular head upper 2/3 of the lateral aspect of the fibula

Insertion: Lateral aspect of the plantar surface of the medial cuneiform and 1st metatarsal base

S. Beltrán

Figure 5.13 ■ PERONEUS LONGUS. The peroneus longus plantarflexes and everts the foot. The peroneus longus passes underneath the superior peroneal retinaculum, then runs superficial to the calcaneofibular ligament, and passes deep to the inferior peroneal retinaculum. The third turn of the peroneus longus occurs as it enters the plantar tunnel between the cuboid and fifth metatarsal base. Ossification of the fibrocartilaginous sesamoid (which protects the tendon as it glides over the cuboid tuberosity) within the peroneus longus occurs in up to 20% of cases. *(See Related Muscles pg. 740, in Stoller's 3rd Edition.)*

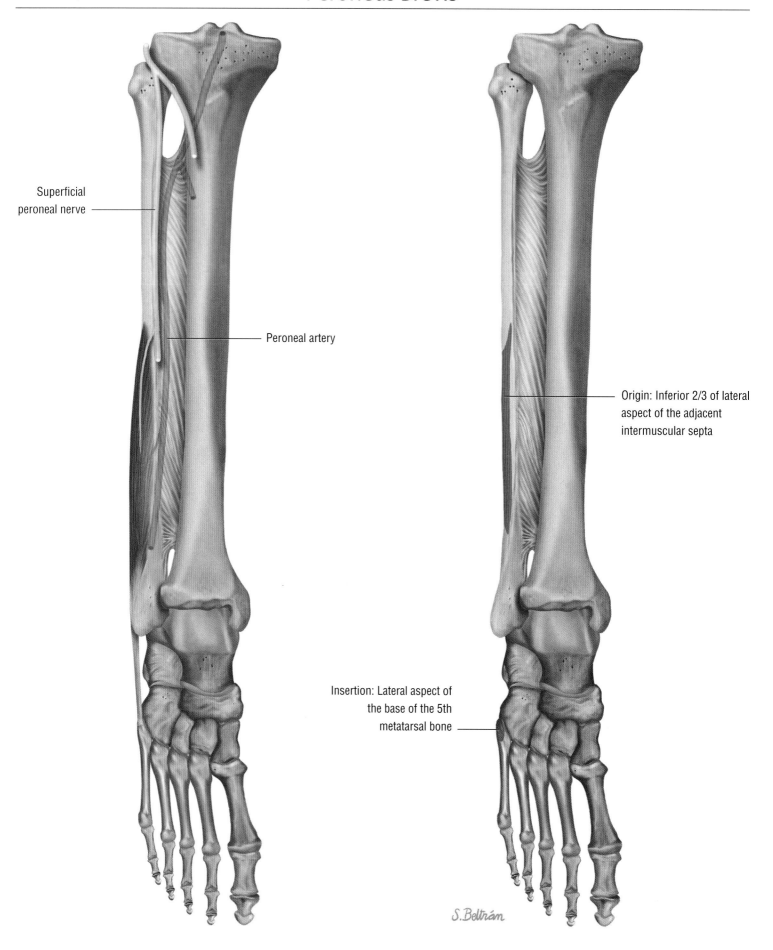

Superficial
peroneal nerve —

—— Peroneal artery

Origin: Inferior 2/3 of lateral
aspect of the adjacent
intermuscular septa

Insertion: Lateral aspect of
the base of the 5th
metatarsal bone ——

S. Beltrán

Figure 5.14 ■ PERONEUS BREVIS. The peroneus brevis plantarflexes and everts the
foot. The peroneus brevis has a shorter and smaller muscle belly than the peroneus
longus and becomes tendinous 2 to 3 cm proximal to the tip of the lateral malleolus. *(See Related Muscles pg. 740, in Stoller's 3rd Edition.)*

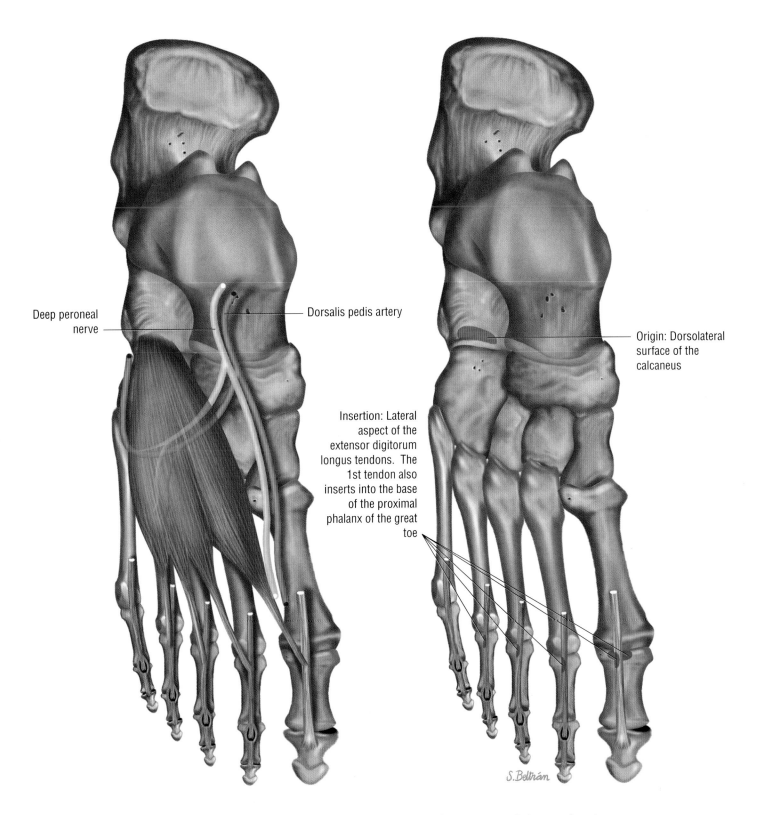

Deep peroneal nerve

Dorsalis pedis artery

Origin: Dorsolateral surface of the calcaneus

Insertion: Lateral aspect of the extensor digitorum longus tendons. The 1st tendon also inserts into the base of the proximal phalanx of the great toe

S.Beltrán

Figure 5.15 ■ EXTENSOR DIGITORUM BREVIS. The extensor digitorum brevis extends the phalanges of the four medial toes. The extensor digitorum brevis and longus tendons contribute to the metatarsophalangeal extensor expansion. *(See Related Muscles pg. 741, in Stoller's 3rd Edition.)*

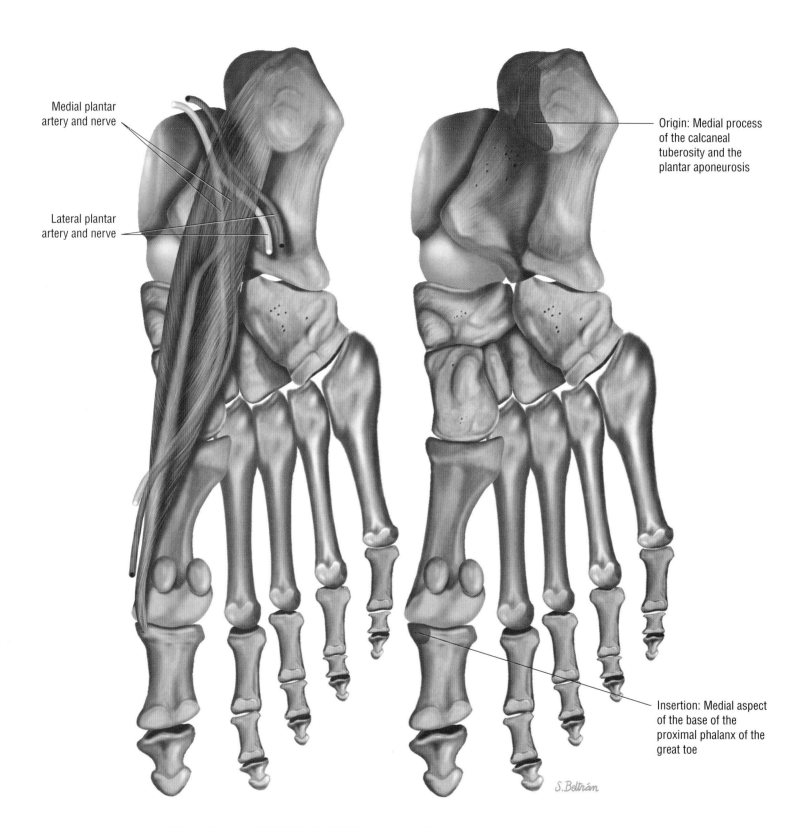

Medial plantar
artery and nerve

Lateral plantar
artery and nerve

Origin: Medial process
of the calcaneal
tuberosity and the
plantar aponeurosis

Insertion: Medial aspect
of the base of the
proximal phalanx of the
great toe

S. Beltrán

Figure 5.16 ■ ABDUCTOR HALLUCIS. The abductor hallucis functions in abduction
of the great toe. In tarsal tunnel syndrome, the medial and lateral plantar nerves may
be decompressed by releasing the fascia of the abductor hallucis muscle. *(See
Related Muscles pg. 741, in Stoller's 3rd Edition.)*

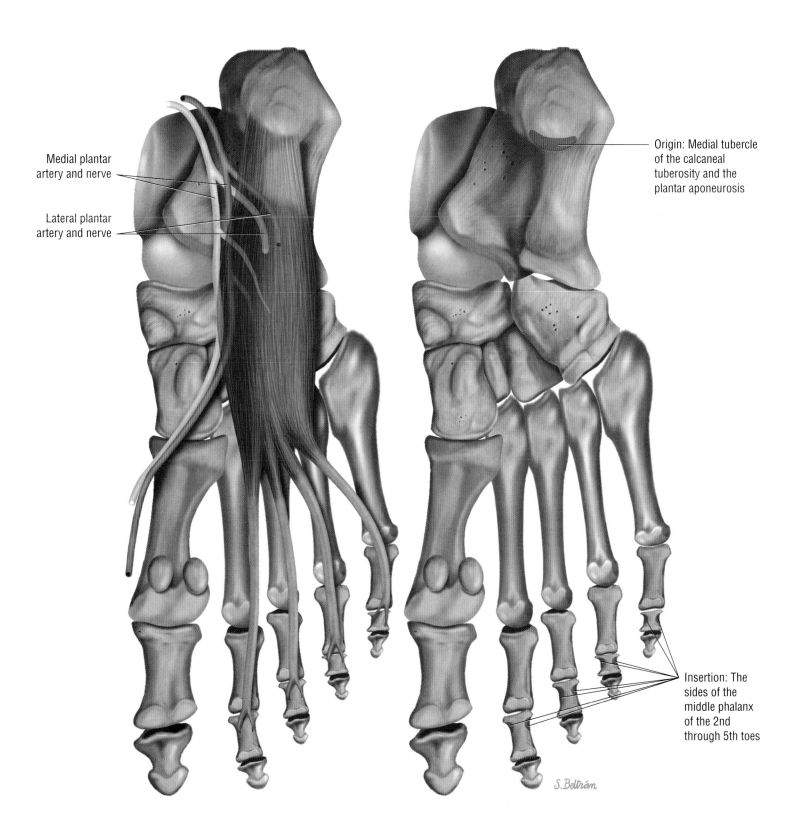

Medial plantar
artery and nerve

Lateral plantar
artery and nerve

Origin: Medial tubercle
of the calcaneal
tuberosity and the
plantar aponeurosis

Insertion: The
sides of the
middle phalanx
of the 2nd
through 5th toes

S. Beltrán

Figure 5.17 ■ **FLEXOR DIGITORUM BREVIS.** The flexor digitorum brevis (FDB) divides into two slips to allow the passage of the flexor digitorum longus tendon. The FDB flexes the middle phalanges (PIP joints) and is a weak plantarflexor of the MP joint (for the lateral four toes). *(See Related Muscles pg. 742, in Stoller's 3rd Edition.)*

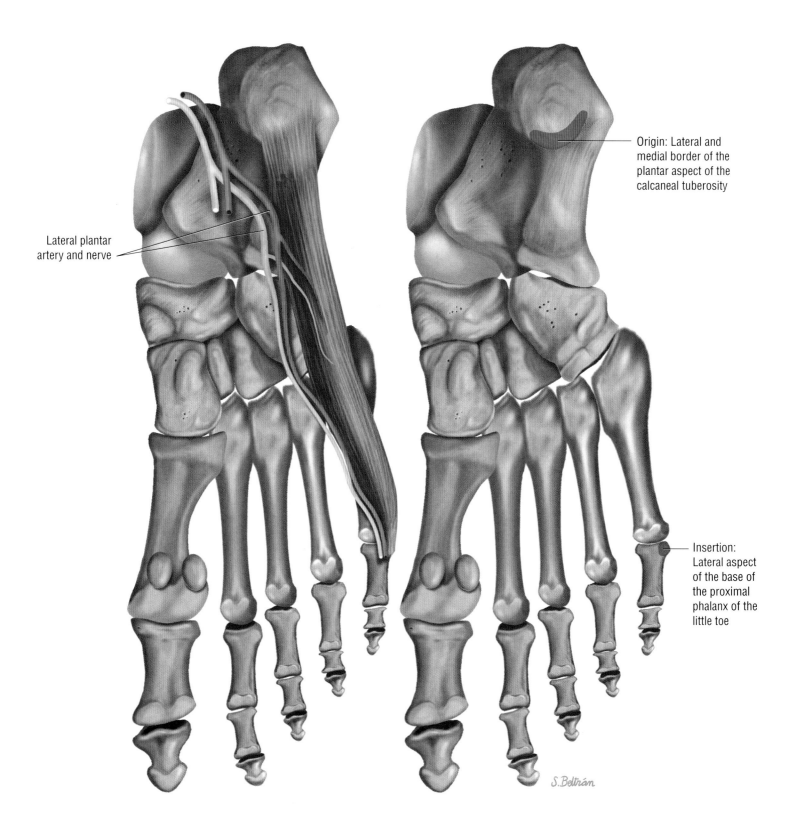

Lateral plantar
artery and nerve

Origin: Lateral and
medial border of the
plantar aspect of the
calcaneal tuberosity

Insertion:
Lateral aspect
of the base of
the proximal
phalanx of the
little toe

S. Beltrán

Figure 5.18 ▪ ABDUCTOR DIGITI MINIMI. The abductor digiti minimi inserts into
the plantar plate and the lateral plantar aspect of the proximal phalanx of the fifth
toe. The abductor digiti minimi abducts the fifth toe and assists in flexion. *(See
Related Muscles pg. 742, in Stoller's 3rd Edition.)*

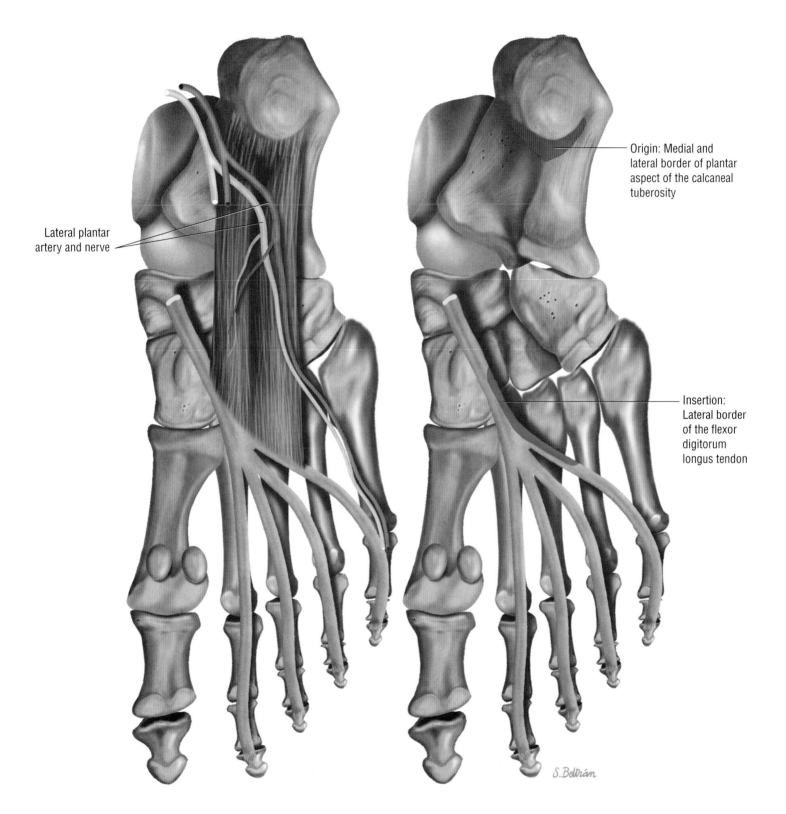

Origin: Medial and
lateral border of plantar
aspect of the calcaneal
tuberosity

Lateral plantar
artery and nerve

Insertion:
Lateral border
of the flexor
digitorum
longus tendon

S. Beltrán

Figure 5.19 ■ QUADRATUS PLANTAE. The quadratus plantae originates from two
heads from the medial and lateral aspect of the calcaneus and long plantar ligaments. The quadratus plantae flexes the terminal (distal) phalanges of the lateral four
toes. *(See Related Muscles pg. 743, in Stoller's 3rd Edition.)*

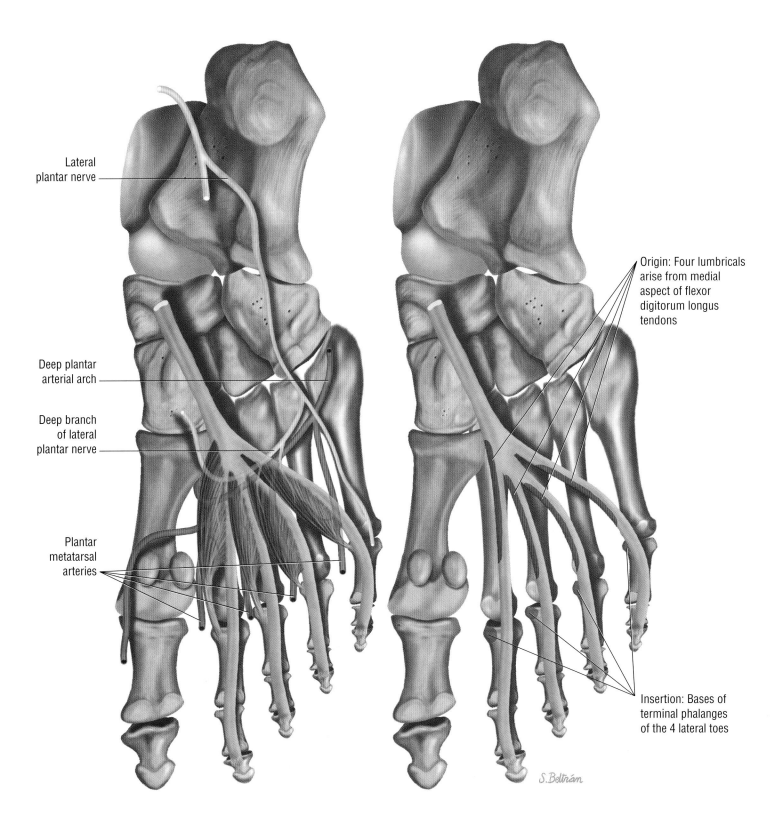

Lateral
plantar nerve

Deep plantar
arterial arch

Deep branch
of lateral
plantar nerve

Plantar
metatarsal
arteries

Origin: Four lumbricals
arise from medial
aspect of flexor
digitorum longus
tendons

Insertion: Bases of
terminal phalanges
of the 4 lateral toes

S.Beltrán

Figure 5.20 ■ **LUMBRICALS.** The lumbricals are plantar flexors of the metatarsophalangeal joint and extend the toes at the DIP and PIP joints. The lumbrical tendon inserts medially onto the extensor hood. *(See Related Muscles pg. 743, in Stoller's 3rd
Edition.)*

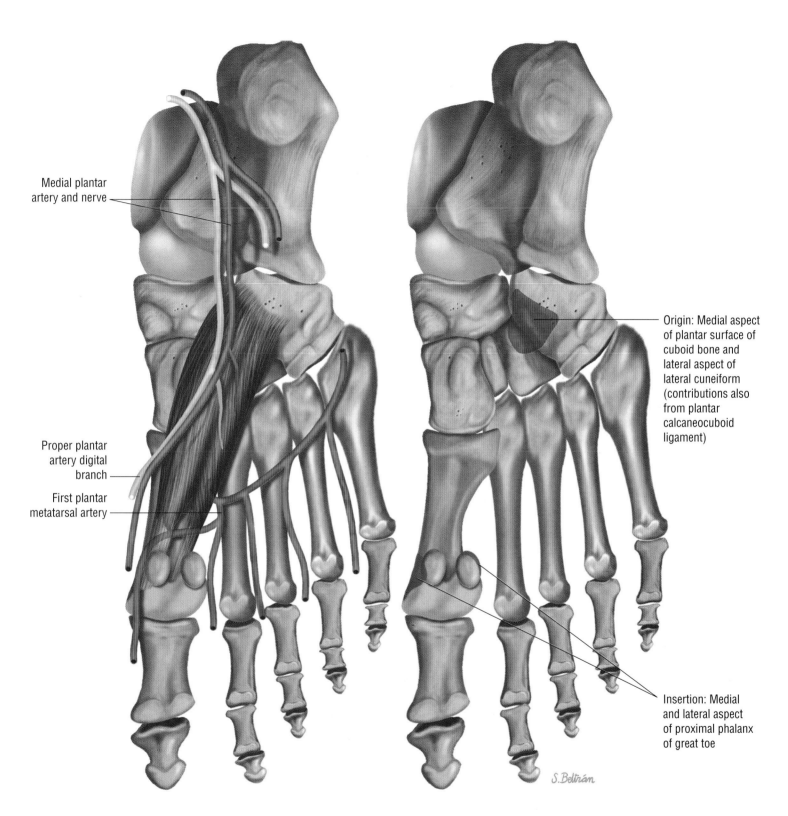

Medial plantar
artery and nerve

Proper plantar
artery digital
branch

First plantar
metatarsal artery

Origin: Medial aspect
of plantar surface of
cuboid bone and
lateral aspect of
lateral cuneiform
(contributions also
from plantar
calcaneocuboid
ligament)

Insertion: Medial
and lateral aspect
of proximal phalanx
of great toe

S.Beltrán

Figure 5.21 ■ **FLEXOR HALLUCIS BREVIS.** The flexor hallucis brevis functions in flexion of the great toe. Instability of the first metatarsophalangeal joint occurs with loss of flexor hallucis brevis function, as occurs with excision of tibial and fibula sesamoids. *(See Related Muscles pg. 744, in Stoller's 3rd Edition.)*

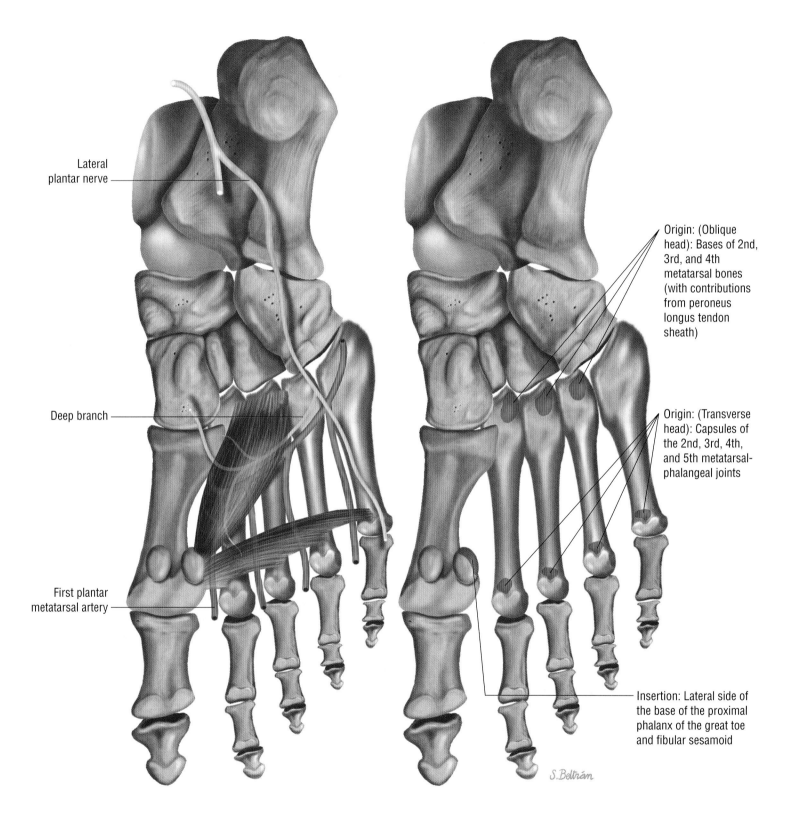

Lateral
plantar nerve

Origin: (Oblique
head): Bases of 2nd,
3rd, and 4th
metatarsal bones
(with contributions
from peroneus
longus tendon
sheath)

Deep branch

Origin: (Transverse
head): Capsules of
the 2nd, 3rd, 4th,
and 5th metatarsal-
phalangeal joints

First plantar
metatarsal artery

Insertion: Lateral side of
the base of the proximal
phalanx of the great toe
and fibular sesamoid

S.Beltrán

Figure 5.22 ■ **ADDUCTOR HALLUCIS.** The adductor hallucis has two heads and forms a conjoined tendon. The adductor hallucis adducts the great toe and assists in its flexion. *(See Related Muscles pg. 744, in Stoller's 3rd Edition.)*

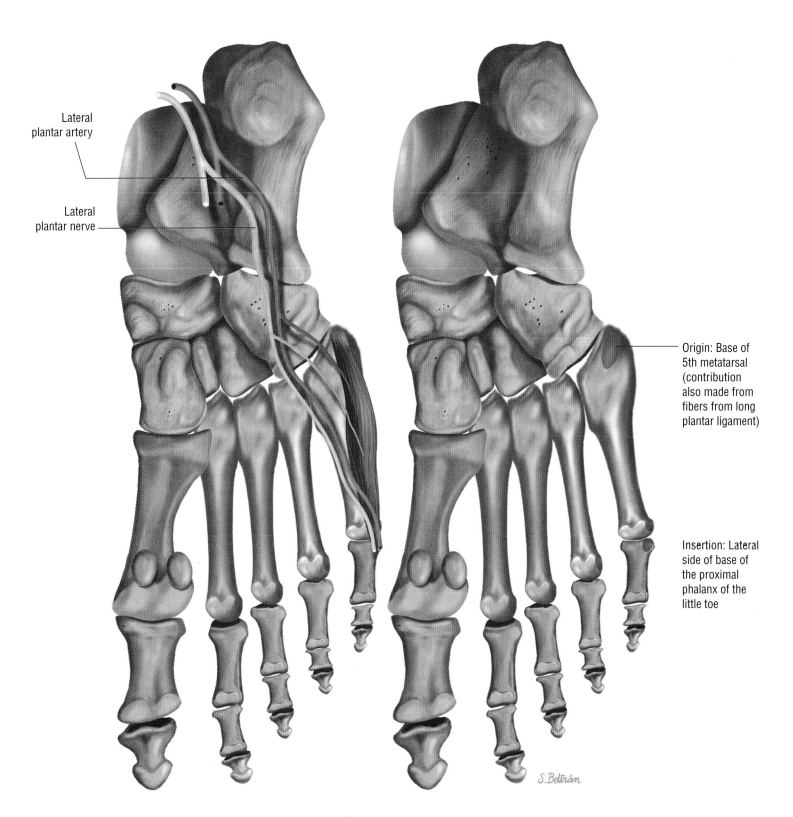

Lateral plantar artery

Lateral plantar nerve

Origin: Base of 5th metatarsal (contribution also made from fibers from long plantar ligament)

Insertion: Lateral side of base of the proximal phalanx of the little toe

S.Beltrán

Figure 5.23 ▪ **FLEXOR DIGITI MINIMI BREVIS.** The flexor digiti minimi brevis flexes the little toes. *(See Related Muscles pg. 745, in Stoller's 3rd Edition.)*

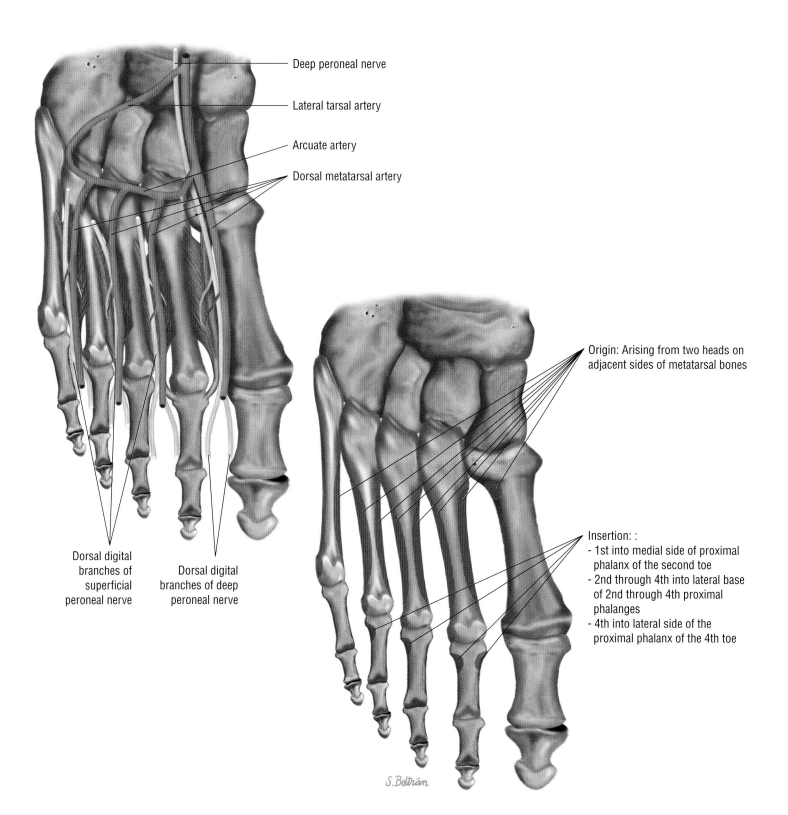

Deep peroneal nerve

Lateral tarsal artery

Arcuate artery

Dorsal metatarsal artery

Origin: Arising from two heads on
adjacent sides of metatarsal bones

Dorsal digital
branches of
superficial
peroneal nerve

Dorsal digital
branches of deep
peroneal nerve

Insertion: :
- 1st into medial side of proximal
  phalanx of the second toe
- 2nd through 4th into lateral base
  of 2nd through 4th proximal
  phalanges
- 4th into lateral side of the
  proximal phalanx of the 4th toe

S. Beltrán

Figure 5.24 ■ **DORSAL INTEROSSEI.** The four dorsal interosseous muscles stabilize
the toes and abduct the second, third, and fourth toes laterally. They also assist in the
flexion of the proximal phalanges and extension of the middle and distal phalanges.
(See Related Muscles pg. 745, in Stoller's 3rd Edition.)

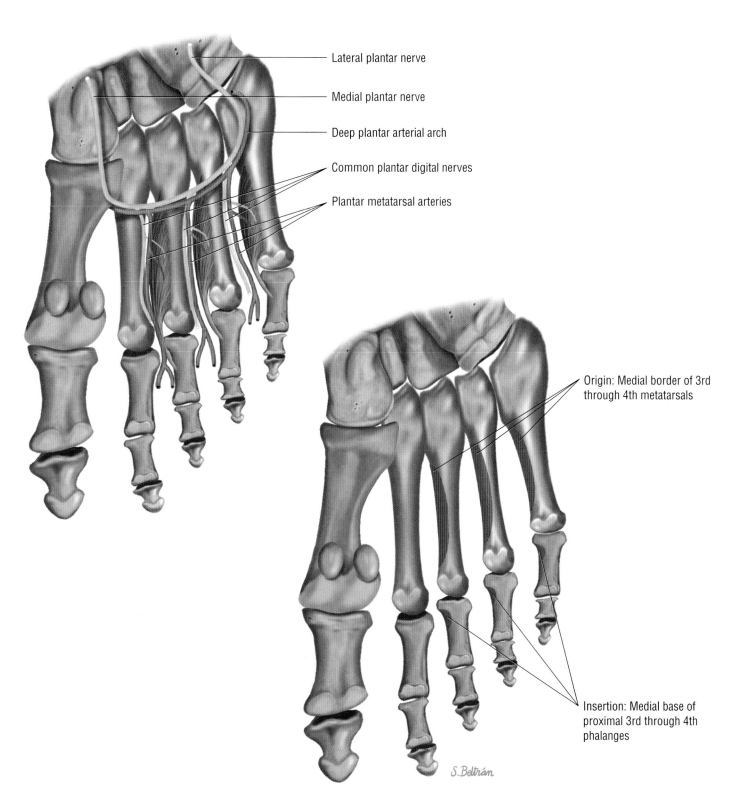

Lateral plantar nerve

Medial plantar nerve

Deep plantar arterial arch

Common plantar digital nerves

Plantar metatarsal arteries

Origin: Medial border of 3rd through 4th metatarsals

Insertion: Medial base of proximal 3rd through 4th phalanges

S. Beltrán

Figure 5.25 ■ PLANTAR INTEROSSEI. There are four dorsal and three plantar interosseous muscles. The plantar interosseous muscles function in adduction of the third, fourth, and fifth toes medially toward the axis of the second toe. They also assist in flexion of the proximal phalanges and extension of the middle and distal phalanges. *(See Related Muscles pg. 746, in Stoller's 3rd Edition.)*

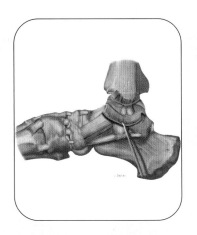

The Ankle and Foot
Anatomy and Pathology

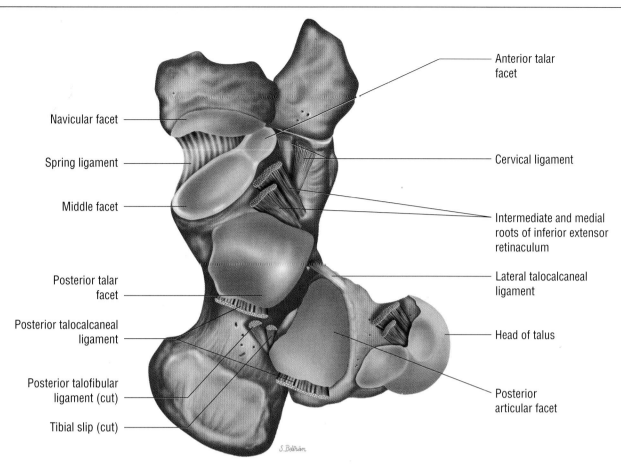

Navicular facet

Spring ligament

Middle facet

Posterior talar facet

Posterior talocalcaneal ligament

Posterior talofibular ligament (cut)

Tibial slip (cut)

Anterior talar facet

Cervical ligament

Intermediate and medial roots of inferior extensor retinaculum

Lateral talocalcaneal ligament

Head of talus

Posterior articular facet

Figure 5.26 ■ Talocalcaneal and talonavicular joints with the talus everted to demonstrate the talar and calcaneal articular surfaces. *(See Subtalar Joint pg. 797 and 798, in Stoller's 3rd Edition.)*

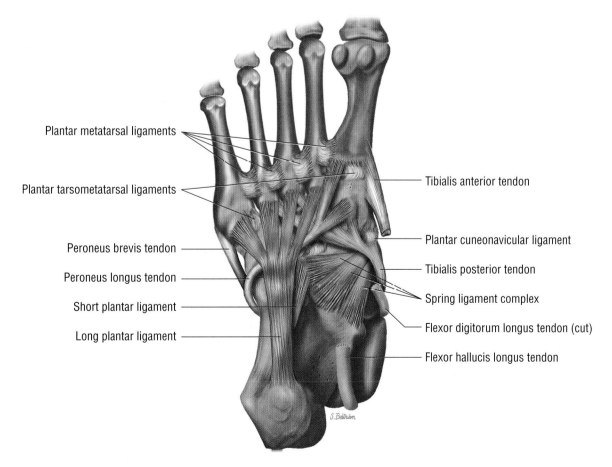

Plantar metatarsal ligaments

Plantar tarsometatarsal ligaments

Peroneus brevis tendon

Peroneus longus tendon

Short plantar ligament

Long plantar ligament

Tibialis anterior tendon

Plantar cuneonavicular ligament

Tibialis posterior tendon

Spring ligament complex

Flexor digitorum longus tendon (cut)

Flexor hallucis longus tendon

Figure 5.27 ■ Ligaments and tendons of the plantar surface of the foot (superficial layer). *(See Muscles of the Sole of the Foot pgs. 798 and 811, in Stoller's 3rd Edition.)*

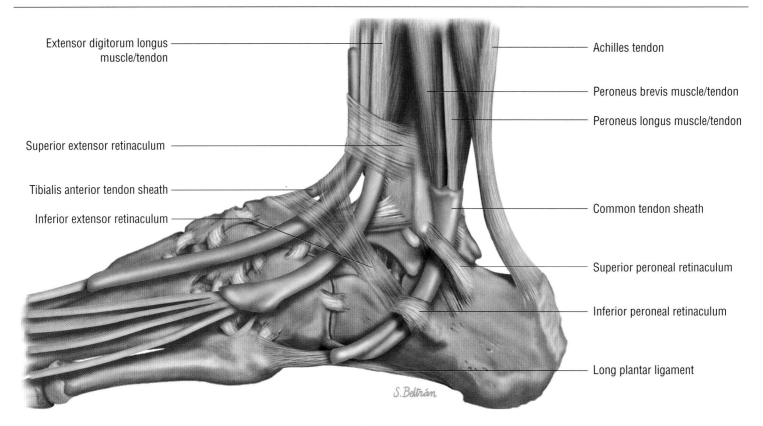

Extensor digitorum longus muscle/tendon

Superior extensor retinaculum

Tibialis anterior tendon sheath

Inferior extensor retinaculum

Achilles tendon

Peroneus brevis muscle/tendon

Peroneus longus muscle/tendon

Common tendon sheath

Superior peroneal retinaculum

Inferior peroneal retinaculum

Long plantar ligament

Figure 5.28 ■ Lateral view of the ankle tendons and tendon sheaths. *(See Regional Anatomy of the Ankle pgs. 796 and 800, in Stoller's 3rd Edition.)*

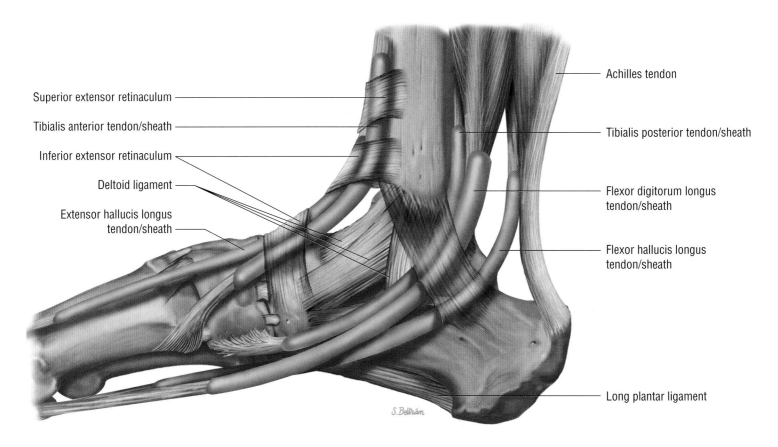

Superior extensor retinaculum

Tibialis anterior tendon/sheath

Inferior extensor retinaculum

Deltoid ligament

Extensor hallucis longus tendon/sheath

Achilles tendon

Tibialis posterior tendon/sheath

Flexor digitorum longus tendon/sheath

Flexor hallucis longus tendon/sheath

Long plantar ligament

Figure 5.29 ■ Medial view of the ankle tendons and tendon sheaths. *(See Regional Anatomy of the Ankle pgs. 796 and 801, in Stoller's 3rd Edition.)*

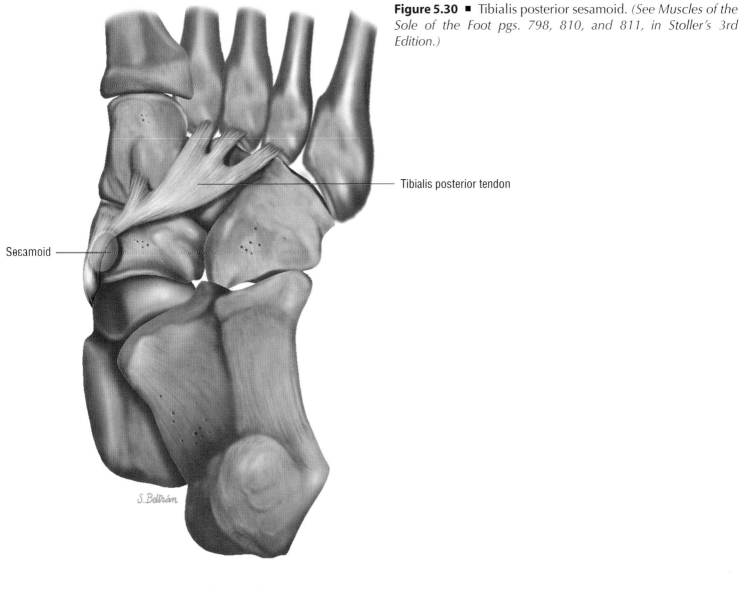

Figure 5.30 ■ Tibialis posterior sesamoid. *(See Muscles of the Sole of the Foot pgs. 798, 810, and 811, in Stoller's 3rd Edition.)*

Tibialis posterior tendon

Sesamoid

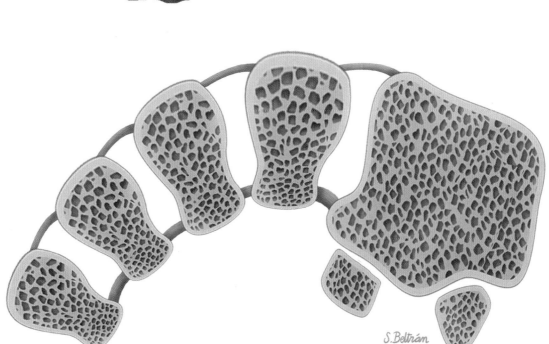

Figure 5.31 ■ The transverse arch of the foot in coronal section at the level of the first metatarsal sesamoids. *(See Arches of the Foot pg. 813, in Stoller's 3rd Edition.)*

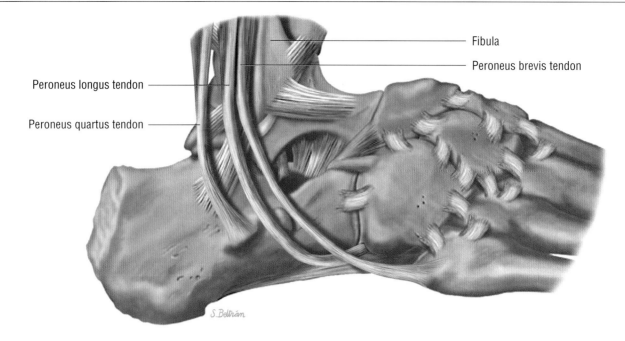

Peroneus longus tendon

Peroneus quartus tendon

Fibula

Peroneus brevis tendon

Figure 5.32 ▪ Peroneus quartus accessory muscle shown posterior to the peroneal tendons. *(See Anatomic Variants pgs. 802 and 820, in Stoller's 3rd Edition.)*

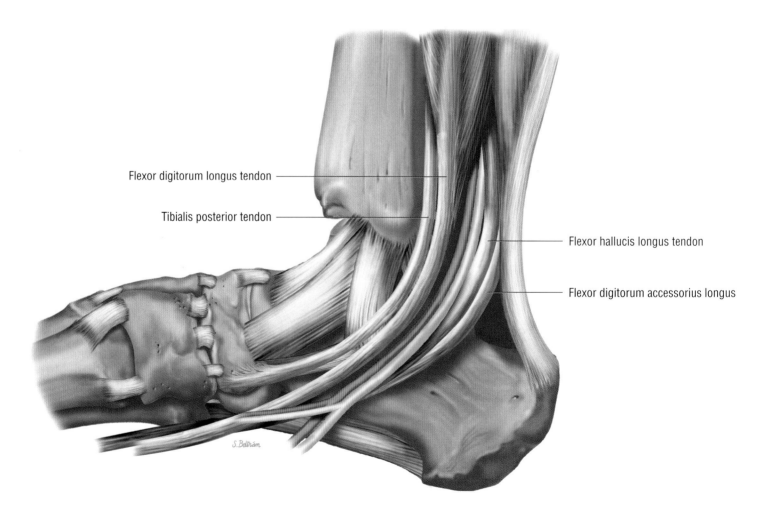

Flexor digitorum longus tendon

Tibialis posterior tendon

Flexor hallucis longus tendon

Flexor digitorum accessorius longus

Figure 5.33 ▪ Flexor digitorum accessorius longus (FDAL) demonstrated in the tarsal tunnel medial and superficial to the flexor hallucis longus (FHL) muscle.*(See Anatomic Variants pgs. 802 and 820, in Stoller's 3rd Edition.)*

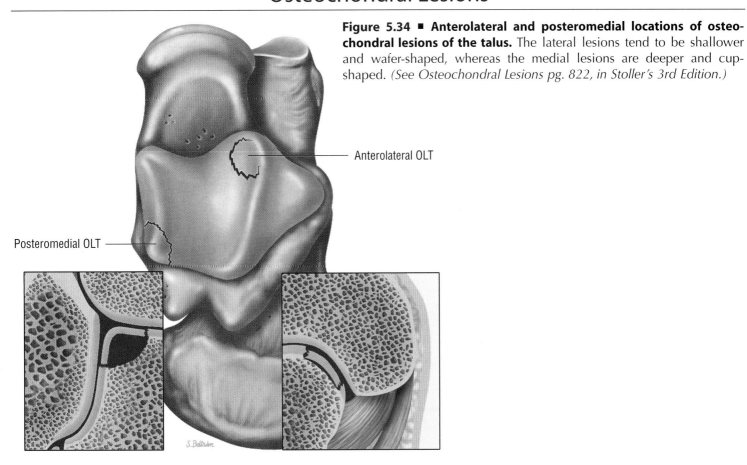

Figure 5.34 ■ Anterolateral and posteromedial locations of osteochondral lesions of the talus. The lateral lesions tend to be shallower and wafer-shaped, whereas the medial lesions are deeper and cup-shaped. *(See Osteochondral Lesions pg. 822, in Stoller's 3rd Edition.)*

Anterolateral OLT

Posteromedial OLT

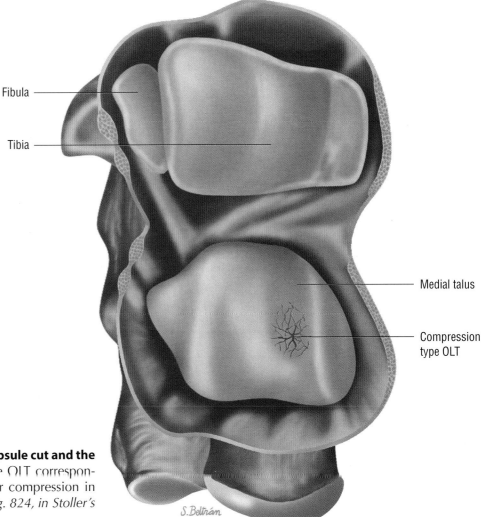

Fibula

Tibia

Medial talus

Compression type OLT

Figure 5.35 ■ Color illustration with the capsule cut and the tibia and fibula reflected. Compression-type OLT corresponding with an area of subchondral trabecular compression in stage I lesion. *(See Osteochondral Lesions pg. 824, in Stoller's 3rd Edition.)*

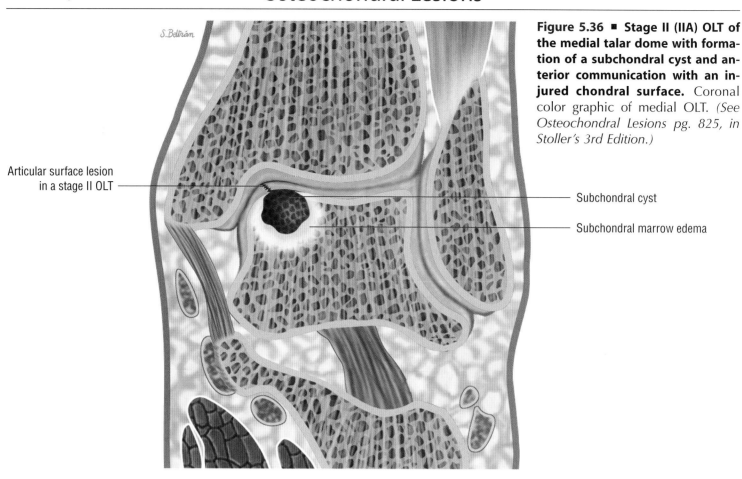

S.Beltrán

Articular surface lesion
in a stage II OLT

Subchondral cyst

Subchondral marrow edema

Figure 5.36 ■ Stage II (IIA) OLT of the medial talar dome with formation of a subchondral cyst and anterior communication with an injured chondral surface. Coronal color graphic of medial OLT. *(See Osteochondral Lesions pg. 825, in Stoller's 3rd Edition.)*

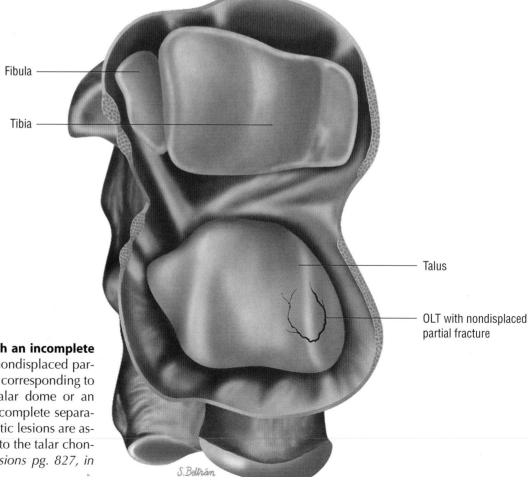

Fibula

Tibia

Talus

OLT with nondisplaced
partial fracture

S.Beltrán

Figure 5.37 ■ Stage II (IIB) OLT with an incomplete separation from the talar dome. A nondisplaced partial fracture shown in a color graphic corresponding to either a communication with the talar dome or an open articular surface lesion with incomplete separation of the fragment. Subchondral cystic lesions are associated with extension of a fracture to the talar chondral surface. *(See Osteochondral Lesions pg. 827, in Stoller's 3rd Edition.)*

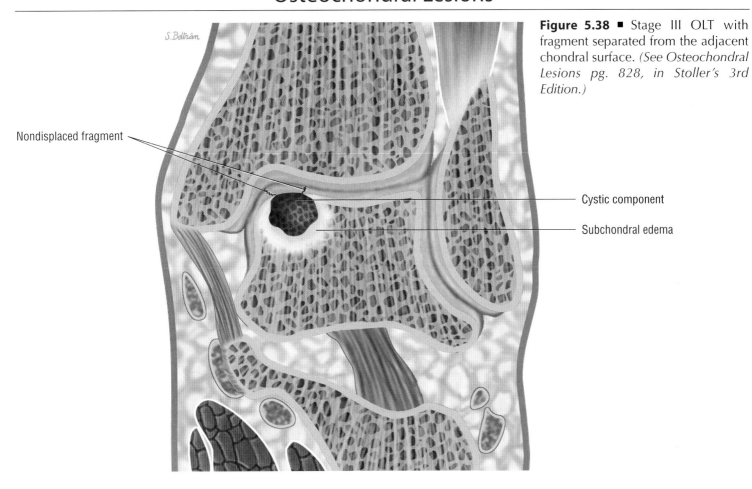

Nondisplaced fragment

Cystic component

Subchondral edema

Figure 5.38 ■ Stage III OLT with fragment separated from the adjacent chondral surface. *(See Osteochondral Lesions pg. 828, in Stoller's 3rd Edition.)*

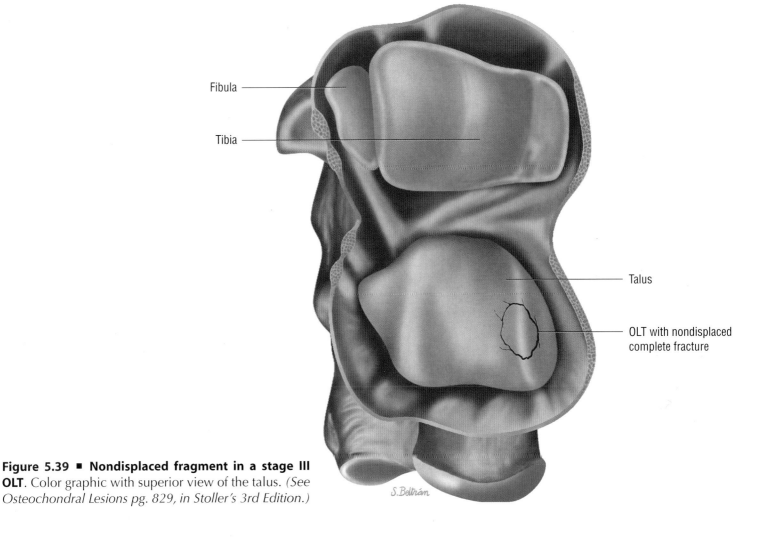

Fibula

Tibia

Talus

OLT with nondisplaced complete fracture

Figure 5.39 ■ **Nondisplaced fragment in a stage III OLT**. Color graphic with superior view of the talus. *(See Osteochondral Lesions pg. 829, in Stoller's 3rd Edition.)*

Osteochondral Lesions

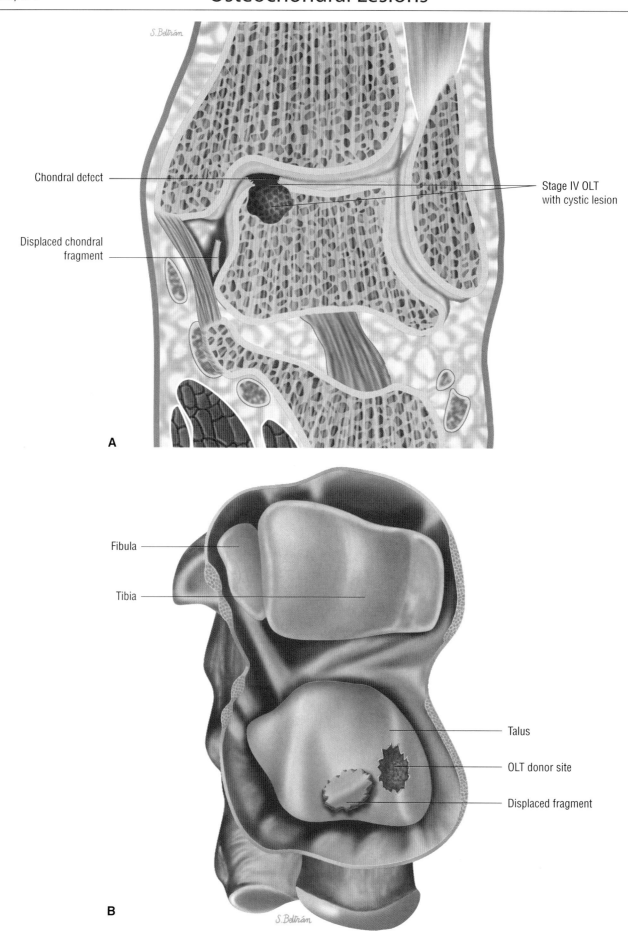

Figure 5.40 ■ **(A)** Stage IV OLT with interruption of the subchondral plate, subchondral cystic change, and medially displaced chondral fragment on a coronal section color illustration. **(B)** Displaced fragment from a medial talar dome donor site in OLT on a color graphic superior view of the talus with the tibia and fibula resected. *(See Osteochondral Lesions pg. 830, in Stoller's 3rd Edition.)*

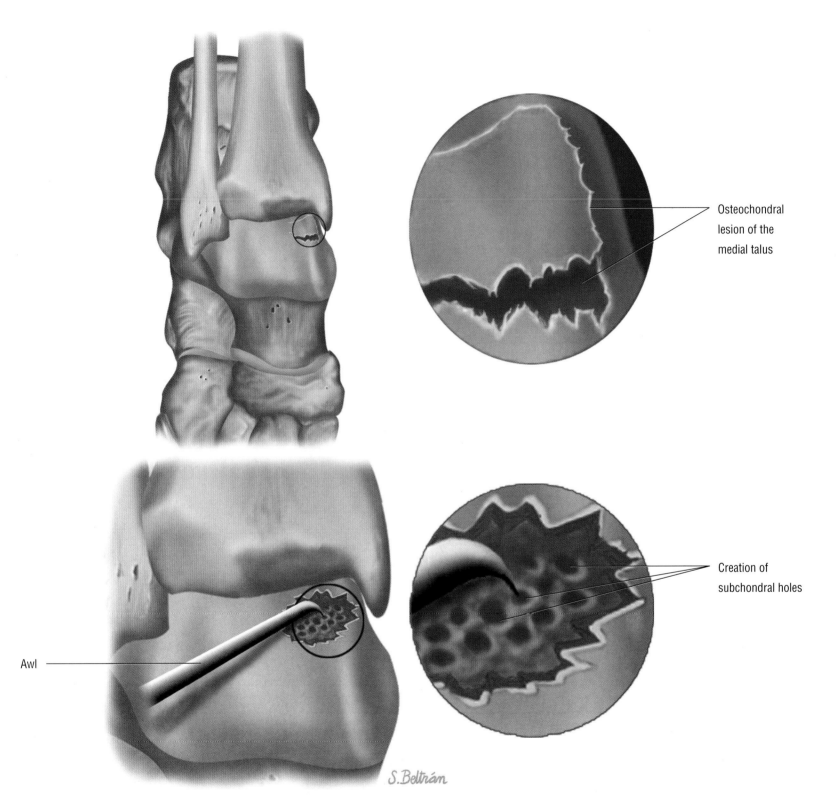

Osteochondral lesion of the medial talus

Creation of subchondral holes

Awl

Figure 5.41 ■ Microfracture treatment of a medial talar lesion. The microfracture awl is typically introduced through the contralateral arthroscopic portal. The awl is used to create subchondral holes in the bed of the lesion. *(See Osteochondral Lesions pg. 832, in Stoller's 3rd Edition.)*

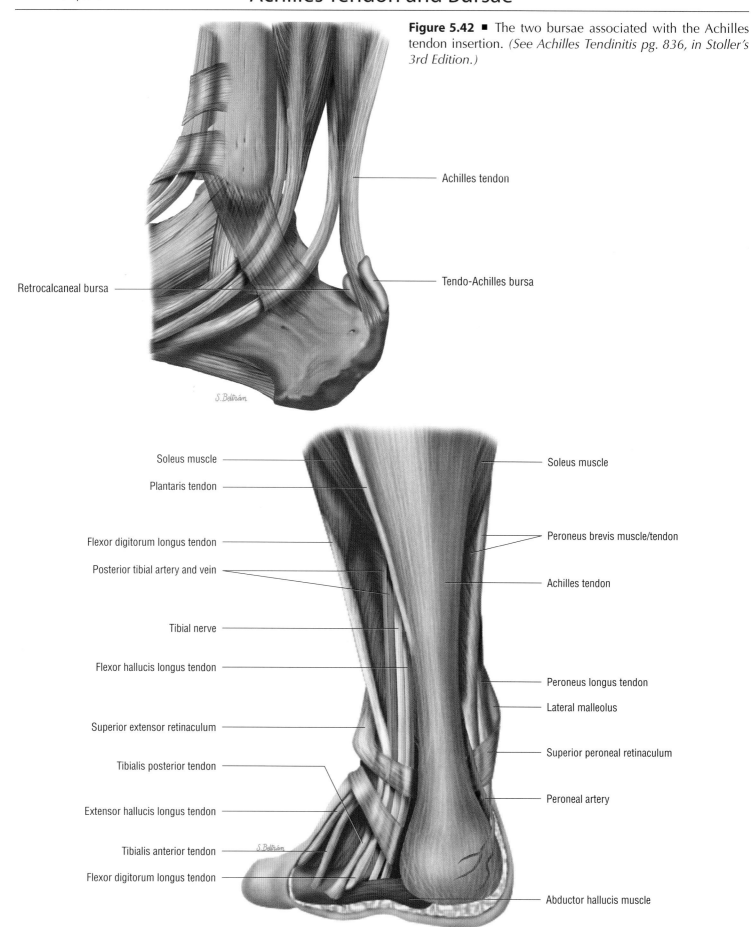

Figure 5.42 ■ The two bursae associated with the Achilles tendon insertion. *(See Achilles Tendinitis pg. 836, in Stoller's 3rd Edition.)*

Achilles tendon

Tendo-Achilles bursa

Retrocalcaneal bursa

Soleus muscle

Plantaris tendon

Flexor digitorum longus tendon

Posterior tibial artery and vein

Tibial nerve

Flexor hallucis longus tendon

Superior extensor retinaculum

Tibialis posterior tendon

Extensor hallucis longus tendon

Tibialis anterior tendon

Flexor digitorum longus tendon

Soleus muscle

Peroneus brevis muscle/tendon

Achilles tendon

Peroneus longus tendon

Lateral malleolus

Superior peroneal retinaculum

Peroneal artery

Abductor hallucis muscle

Figure 5.43 ■ **Posterior view of the hindfoot demonstrating the relation of the Achilles tendon to the posterior neurovascular bundle.** The musculotendinous junction of the triceps surae (the medial and lateral heads of the gastrocnemius and soleus muscles) marks the superior extent of the Achilles tendon. *(See Achilles Tendinitis pg. 833, in Stoller's 3rd Edition.)*

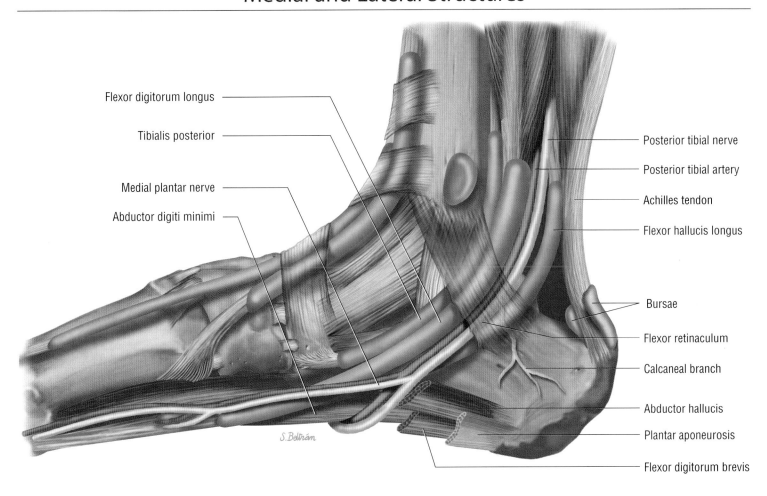

Flexor digitorum longus

Tibialis posterior

Medial plantar nerve

Abductor digiti minimi

Posterior tibial nerve

Posterior tibial artery

Achilles tendon

Flexor hallucis longus

Bursae

Flexor retinaculum

Calcaneal branch

Abductor hallucis

Plantar aponeurosis

Flexor digitorum brevis

Figure 5.44 ■ Medial soft tissue structures at the level of the calcaneus. *(See Foot pg. 801, in Stoller's 3rd Edition.)*

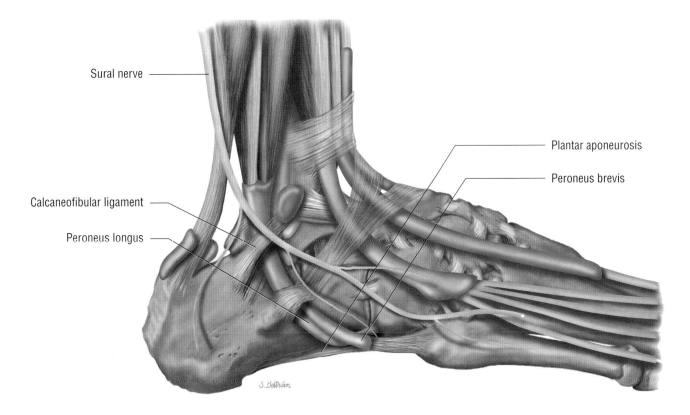

Sural nerve

Calcaneofibular ligament

Peroneus longus

Plantar aponeurosis

Peroneus brevis

Figure 5.45 ■ Lateral soft tissue structures at the level of the calcaneus. *(See Foot pg. 800, in Stoller's 3rd Edition.)*

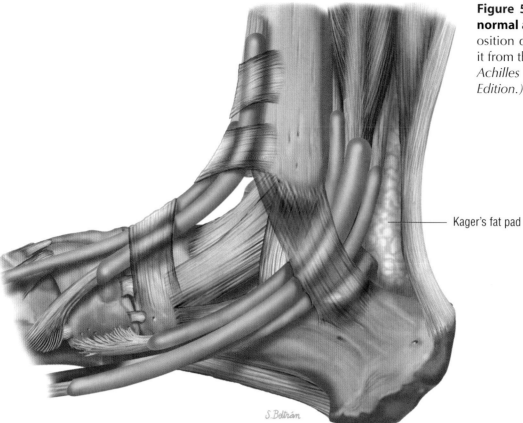

Figure 5.46 ■ Lateral color graphic of the normal anatomy of Kager's fat pad. Fat deposition deep to the Achilles tendon separates it from the deep compartment of the leg. *(See Achilles Tendinitis pg. 834, in Stoller's 3rd Edition.)*

Kager's fat pad

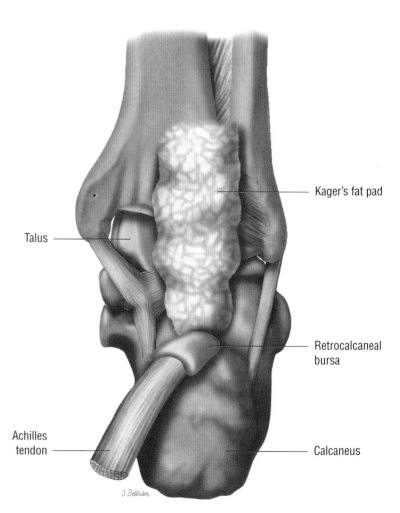

Kager's fat pad

Talus

Retrocalcaneal bursa

Achilles tendon

Calcaneus

Figure 5.47 ■ Disk-shaped retrocalcaneal bursa, posterior coronal perspective. *(See Achilles Tendinitis pg. 836, in Stoller's 3rd Edition.)*

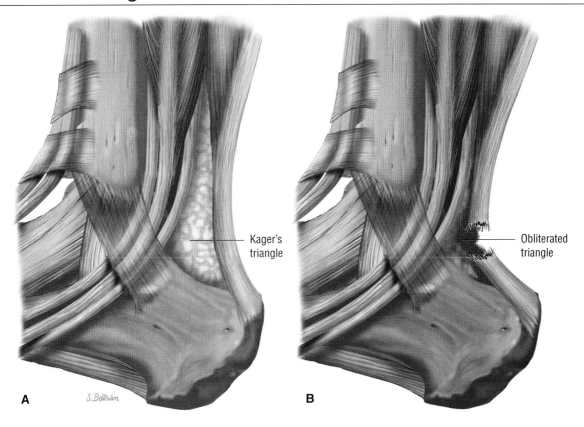

A S.Beltrán   **B**

Figure 5.48 ▪ Kager's triangle is normally formed by the anterior aspect of the Achilles tendon, posterosuperior aspect of the calcaneus, and deep flexors of the foot. (A) Normal Kager's triangle. **(B)** Distorted Kager's triangle. *(See Partial and Complete Tears of the Achilles Tendon pg. 846, in Stoller's 3rd Edition.)*

Kager's triangle

Obliterated triangle

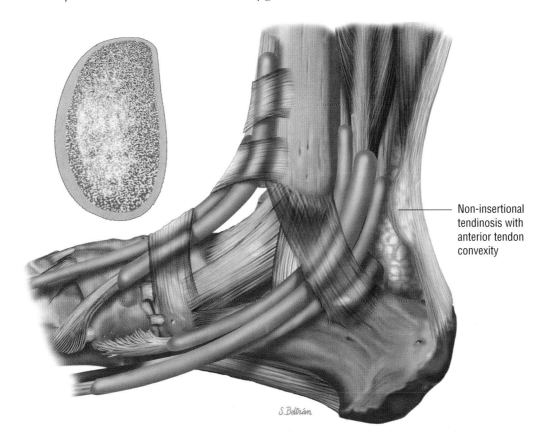

Non-insertional tendinosis with anterior tendon convexity

Figure 5.49 ▪ Non-insertional tendinosis proximal to the os calcis insertion of the Achilles tendon. Intratendinosis degeneration (yellow) is shown on the cross-section through the affected tendon segment. *(See Achilles Tendinitis pg. 838, in Stoller's 3rd Edition.)*

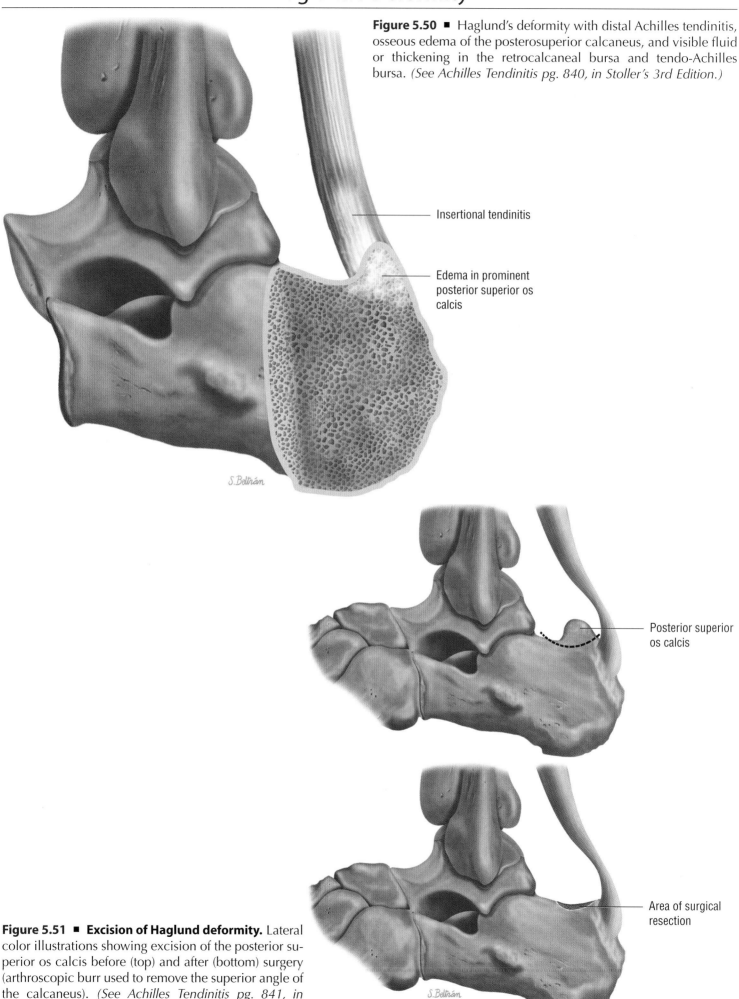

Figure 5.50 ■ Haglund's deformity with distal Achilles tendinitis, osseous edema of the posterosuperior calcaneus, and visible fluid or thickening in the retrocalcaneal bursa and tendo-Achilles bursa. *(See Achilles Tendinitis pg. 840, in Stoller's 3rd Edition.)*

Insertional tendinitis

Edema in prominent posterior superior os calcis

Posterior superior os calcis

Area of surgical resection

Figure 5.51 ■ **Excision of Haglund deformity.** Lateral color illustrations showing excision of the posterior superior os calcis before (top) and after (bottom) surgery (arthroscopic burr used to remove the superior angle of the calcaneus). *(See Achilles Tendinitis pg. 841, in Stoller's 3rd Edition.)*

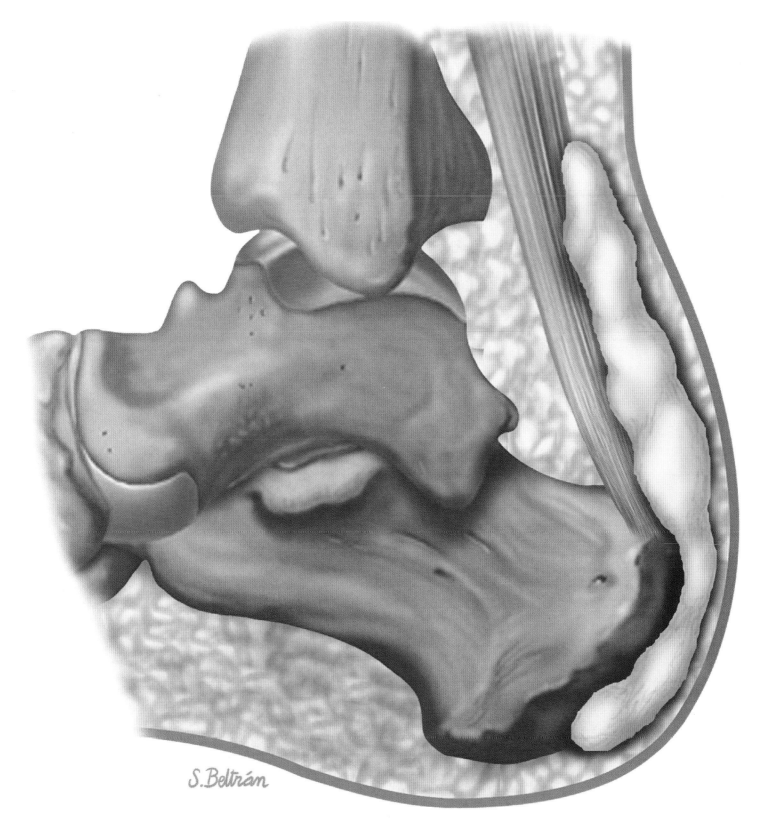

Figure 5.52 ■ Xanthomas of the Achilles tendon with a large soft-tissue component and diffuse infiltration of the Achilles tendon on a sagittal color graphic. *(See Achilles Tendinitis pg. 842, in Stoller's 3rd Edition.)*

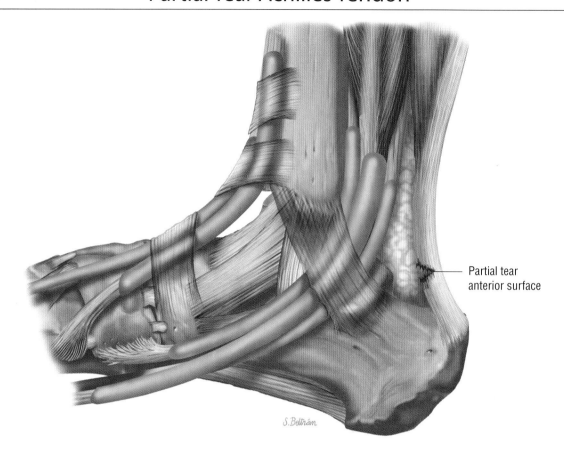

Partial tear
anterior surface

Figure 5.53 ■ Anterior surface partial tear of the Achilles tendon on a lateral color graphic. *(See Partial and Complete Tears of the Achilles Tendon pg. 843, in Stoller's 3rd Edition.)*

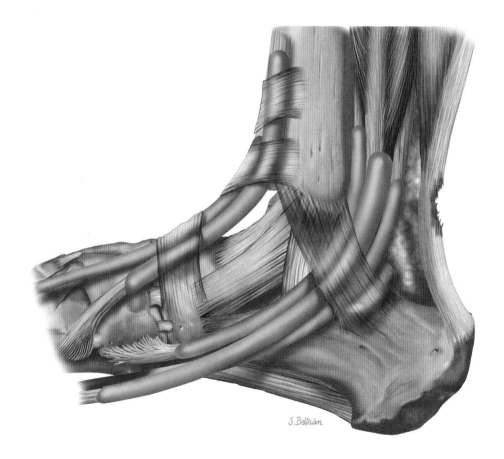

Figure 5.54 ■ Posterior surface partial tear of the Achilles tendon proximal to the os calcis. *(See Partial and Complete Tears of the Achilles Tendon pg. 843, in Stoller's 3rd Edition.)*

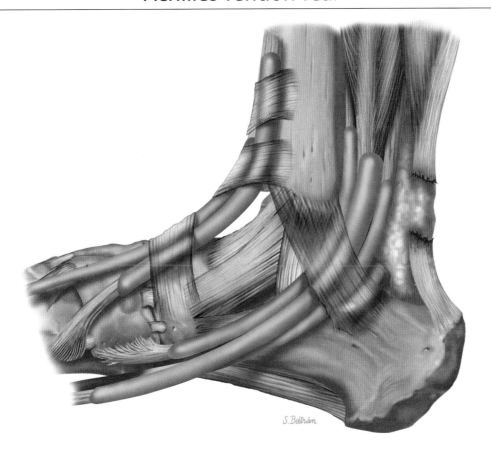

Figure 5.55 ■ Focal complete tear of the Achilles tendon with less than 3 cm of retraction. *(See Partial and Complete Tears of the Achilles Tendon pg. 845, in Stoller's 3rd Edition.)*

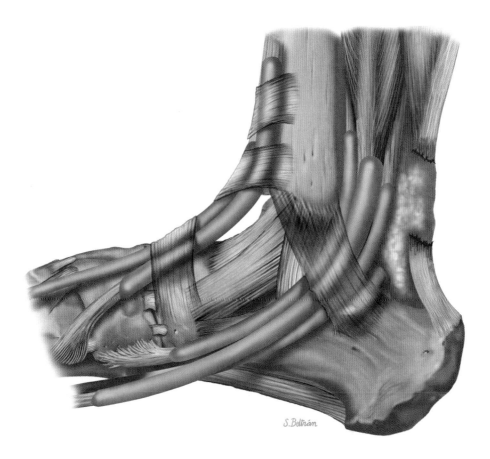

Figure 5.56 ■ Type 3 or complete rupture of the Achilles tendon with a tendinous gap of 3 to 6 cm. *(See Partial and Complete Tears of the Achilles Tendon pg. 846, in Stoller's 3rd Edition.)*

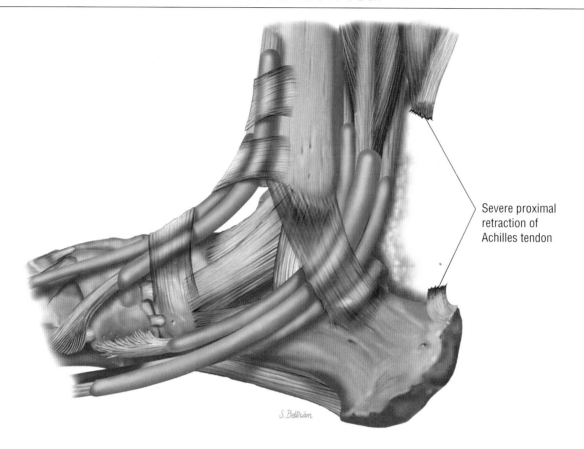

Figure 5.57 ■ **Complete Achilles rupture with greater than 6 cm of proximal tendon retraction.** Fat fills the tendinous gap site proximally. *(See Partial and Complete Tears of the Achilles Tendon pg. 847, in Stoller's 3rd Edition.)*

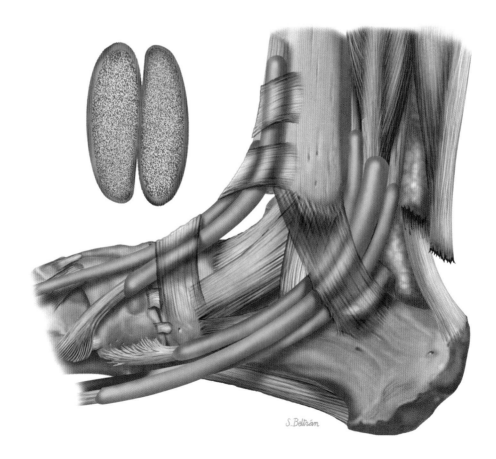

Figure 5.58 ■ Partial overlap of torn Achilles tendon ends. *(See Partial and Complete Tears of the Achilles Tendon pg. 848, in Stoller's 3rd Edition.)*

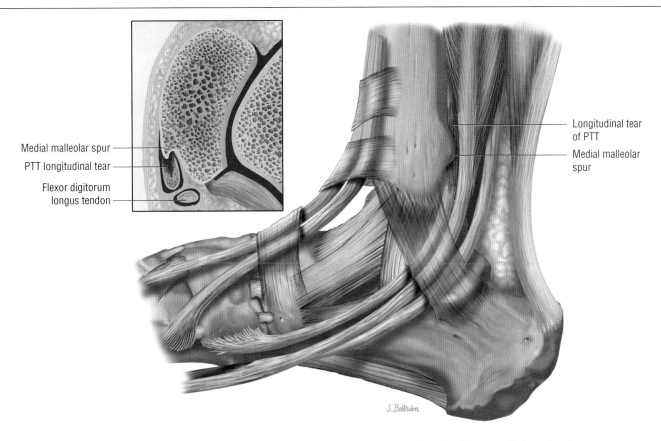

Figure 5.59 ■ **Type 1 tibialis posterior tendon tear (PTT) associated with a medial malleolus osseous spur.** The normal tibialis posterior tendon is approximately twice the cross-sectional diameter of the flexor digitorum longus. In a type 1 tear, the PTT may demonstrate increased thickening, with a cross-sectional diameter up to 5 to 10 times larger than the adjacent flexor digitorum longus tendon. Lateral graphic with an axial insert. *(See Tibialis Posterior Injuries pg. 851, in Stoller's 3rd Edition.)*

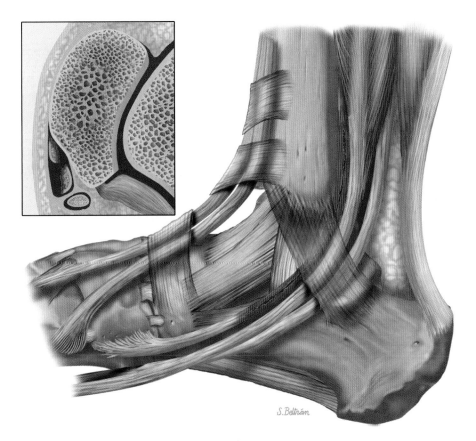

Figure 5.60 ■ **Type 2 tibialis posterior tear with the generation of two subtendons.** Lateral color graphic with axial inset. *(See Tibialis Posterior Injuries pg. 853, in Stoller's 3rd Edition.)*

Tibialis Posterior Tendon Tear

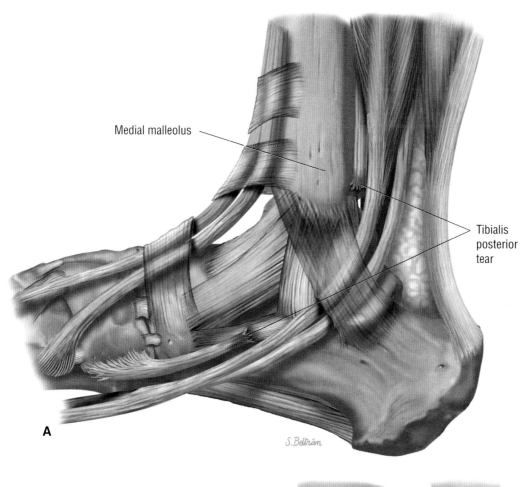

Medial malleolus

Tibialis posterior tear

A

S.Beltrán

Figure 5.61 ■ (A) Type 3 tibialis posterior tendon tear with complete tendinous gap. (B) Normal arch (top) compared to pes planus (bottom). The loss of the medial longitudinal arch and hindfoot valgus is associated with tibialis posterior tendon rupture. *Based on Ferkel RD. Arthroscopic Surgery: the foot and Ankle. Philadelphia: Lippincott-Raven, 1996. (See Tibialis Posterior Injuries pg. 855, in Stoller's 3rd Edition.)*

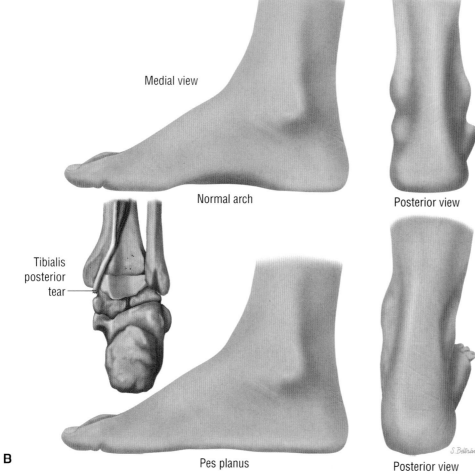

Medial view

Normal arch

Posterior view

Tibialis posterior tear

Pes planus

Posterior view

B

S.Beltrán

Figure 5.62 ■ **Plantar view color illustration of the distal insertions of the tibialis posterior tendon to the tuberosity of the navicular plantar surface of all the cuneiform bones, the sustentaculum tali, and the cuboid (not shown).** The posterior component of the tibialis posterior inserts of the anterior aspect of the spring ligament. *(See Tibialis Posterior Injuries pg. 857, in Stoller's 3rd Edition.)*

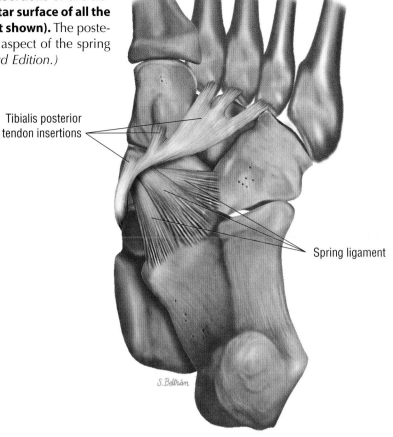

Tibialis posterior tendon insertions

Spring ligament

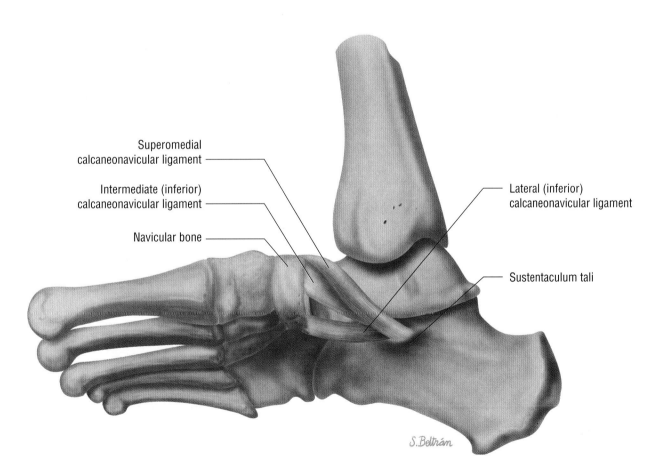

Superomedial calcaneonavicular ligament

Intermediate (inferior) calcaneonavicular ligament

Navicular bone

Lateral (inferior) calcaneonavicular ligament

Sustentaculum tali

Figure 5.63 ■ **Spring ligament complex anatomy.** Lateral-plantar oblique view. *(See Spring Ligament Complex and Pathology pg. 858, in Stoller's 3rd Edition.)*

Spring Ligament

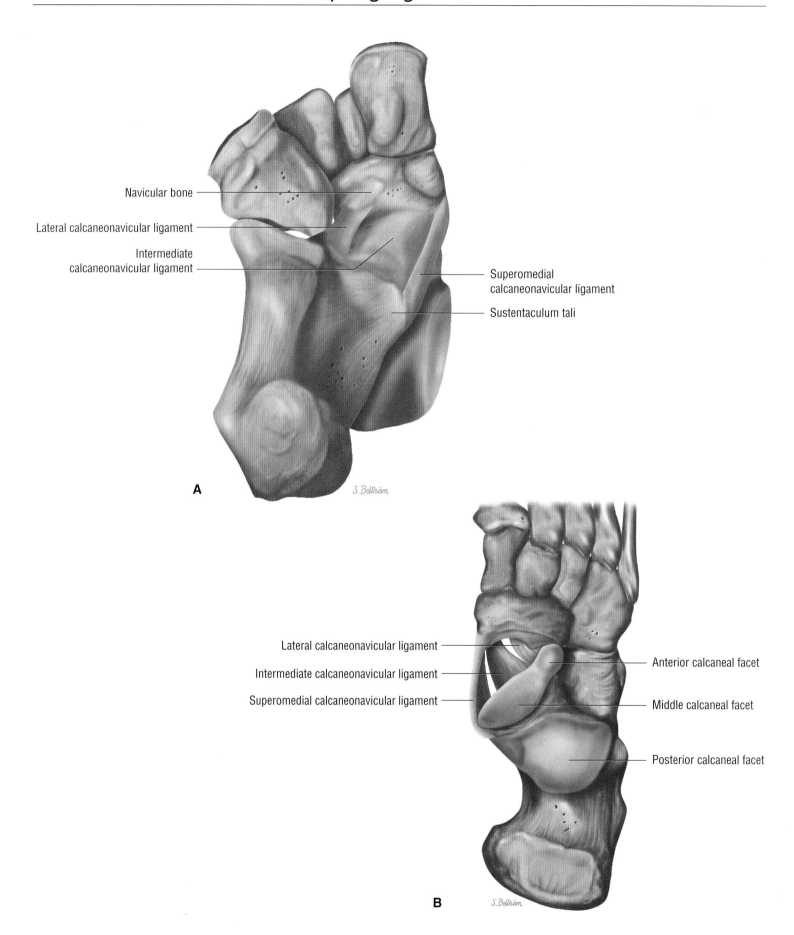

A

B

Figure 5.64 ■ Spring ligament complex anatomy. Plantar **(A)** and superior **(B)** views. *(See Spring Ligament Complex and Pathology pg. 858, in Stoller's 3rd Edition.)*

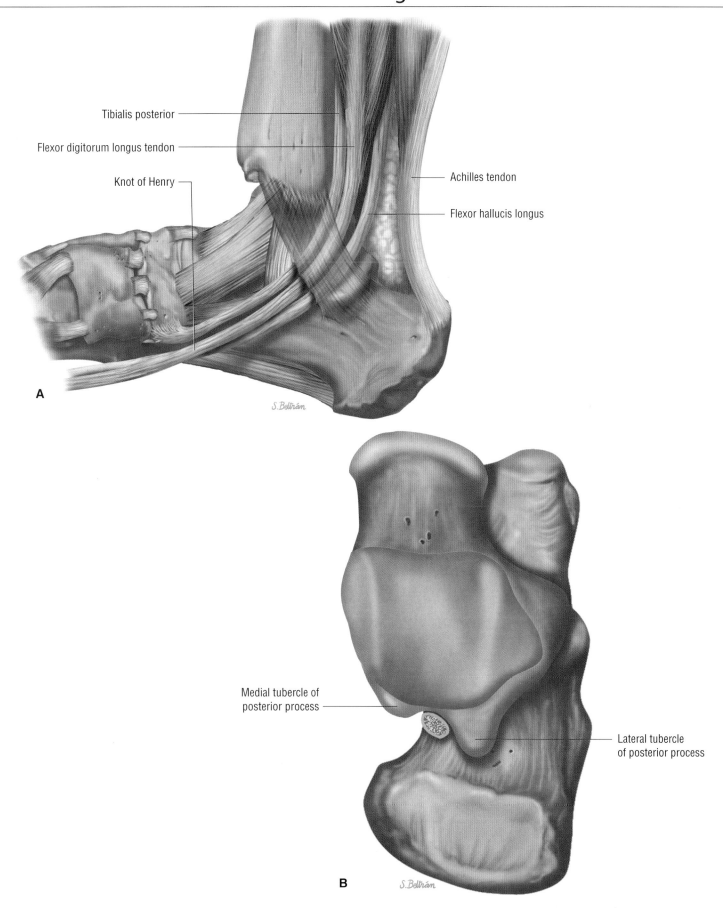

Tibialis posterior

Flexor digitorum longus tendon

Knot of Henry

Achilles tendon

Flexor hallucis longus

A

S.Beltrán

Medial tubercle of
posterior process

Lateral tubercle
of posterior process

B   S.Beltrán

Figure 5.65 ■ The flexor hallucis longus (FHL) is associated with three fibroosseous tunnels: a tunnel between the talar tubercles, a second tunnel deep to the sustentaculum tali, and a third tunnel between the hallucal sesamoids. *(A)* Lateral color illustration showing the course of the FHL and the knot of Henry where the flexor digitorum longus and flexor hallucis longus cross. The FHL is located between the medial and lateral talar tubercles on **(B)**. *(See Flexor Hallucis Longus Abnormalities pg. 863, in Stoller's 3rd Edition.)*

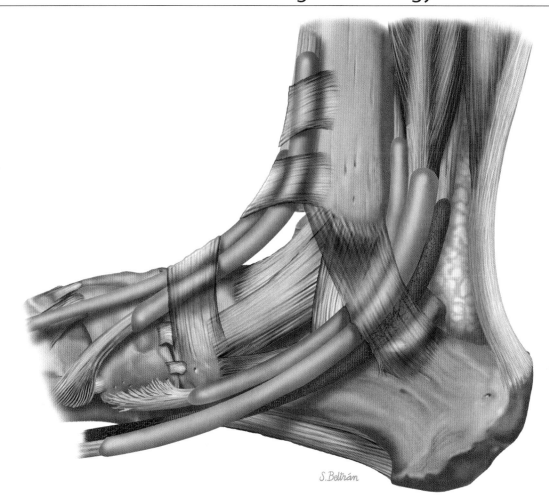

Figure 5.66 ■ Flexor hallucis longus (FHL) tenosynovitis. Tendinitis of the FHL posterior to the medial malleolus is known as dancer's tendinitis. Medial perspective lateral color illustration showing injury of the FHL as it passes through the fibroosseous tunnel from the posterior aspect of the talus to the level of the sustentaculum tali; it acts like a rope through a pulley. *(See Flexor Hallucis Longus Abnormalities pg. 864, in Stoller's 3rd Edition.)*

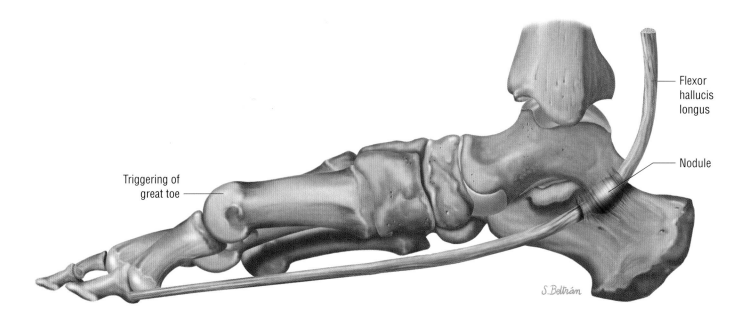

Flexor hallucis longus

Nodule

Triggering of great toe

Figure 5.67 ■ Hallux saltans may develop as the FHL binds as it passes through the fibroosseous tunnel on the medial side of the foot. A nodular partial tear of the FHL may cause triggering of the big toe. *(See Flexor Hallucis Longus Abnormalities pg. 867, in Stoller's 3rd Edition.)*

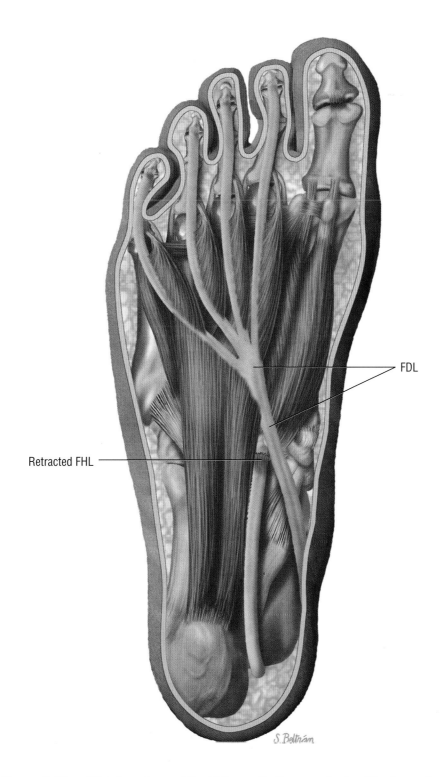

FDL

Retracted FHL

S. Beltrán

Figure 5.68 ■ Distal rupture of the FHL results from acute dorsiflexion or laceration. The fibrous slip connecting the FHL and flexor digitorum longus (FDL) at Henry's knot limits the retraction of FHL proximal to this point. FHL tears proximal to Henry's knot may be associated with tendon recoil into the calf. Plantar view color illustration of FHL distal rupture. *(See Flexor Hallucis Longus Abnormalities pg. 868, in Stoller's 3rd Edition.)*

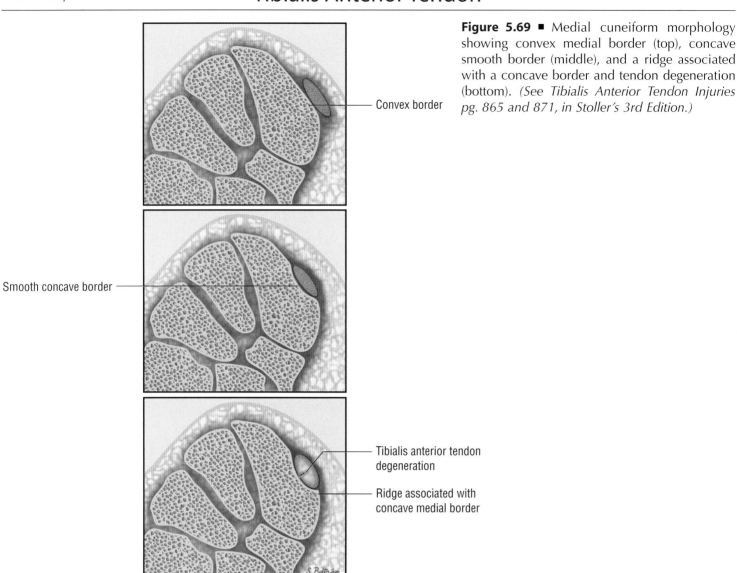

Convex border

Smooth concave border

Tibialis anterior tendon
degeneration

Ridge associated with
concave medial border

Figure 5.69 ■ Medial cuneiform morphology showing convex medial border (top), concave smooth border (middle), and a ridge associated with a concave border and tendon degeneration (bottom). *(See Tibialis Anterior Tendon Injuries pg. 865 and 871, in Stoller's 3rd Edition.)*

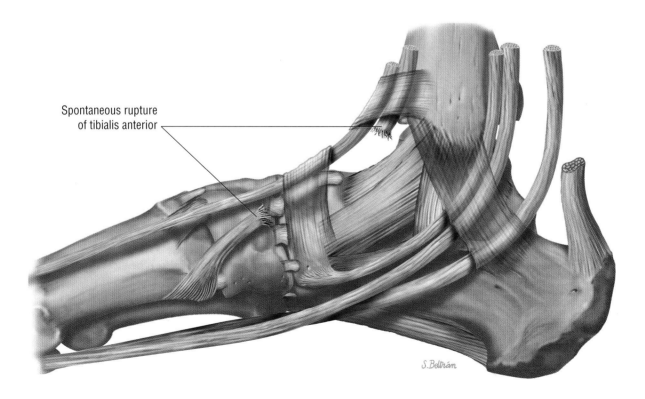

Spontaneous rupture
of tibialis anterior

Figure 5.70 ■ Spontaneous rupture of the tibialis anterior tendon in its distal course.
(See Tibialis Anterior Tendon Injuries pg. 872, in Stoller's 3rd Edition.)

Figure 5.71 ▪ **Partial tear of the tibialis anterior on a lateral color illustration.** The tibialis anterior tendon has a relatively straight course deep to the superior extensor retinaculum. There is a potential site of compression and paratenonitis as the tibialis anterior courses between the deep and superficial superior subdivisions of the superomedial band of the inferior extensor retinaculum. The distal tibialis anterior courses deep to the inferior subdivision of the superomedial band of the inferior extensor retinaculum and inferomedial band of the inferior extensor retinaculum. *(See Tibialis Anterior Tendon Injuries pg. 872, in Stoller's 3rd Edition.)*

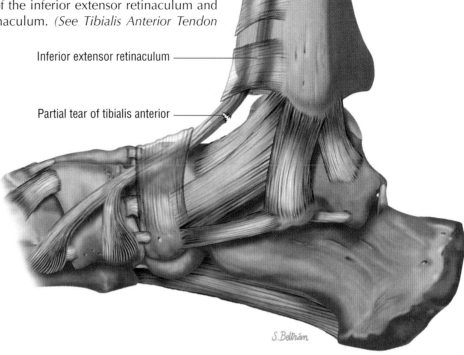

Inferior extensor retinaculum

Partial tear of tibialis anterior

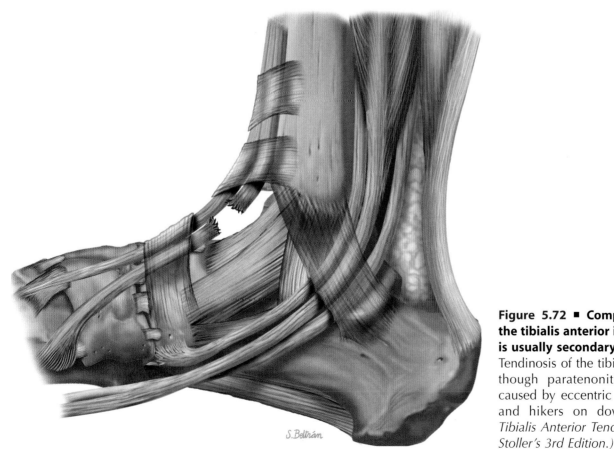

Figure 5.72 ▪ **Complete discontinuity of the tibialis anterior in younger individuals is usually secondary to tendon laceration.** Tendinosis of the tibialis anterior is rare, although paratenonitis may be indirectly caused by eccentric contraction in runners and hikers on downhill surfaces. *(See Tibialis Anterior Tendon Injuries pg. 872, in Stoller's 3rd Edition.)*

Peroneal Tendons

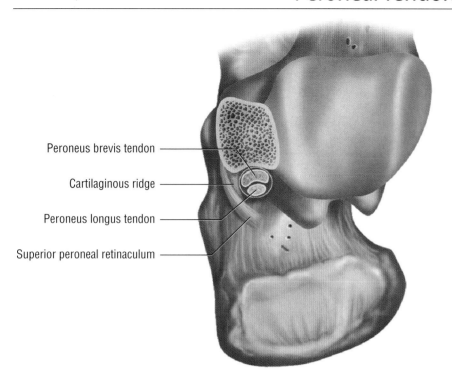

Peroneus brevis tendon

Cartilaginous ridge

Peroneus longus tendon

Superior peroneal retinaculum

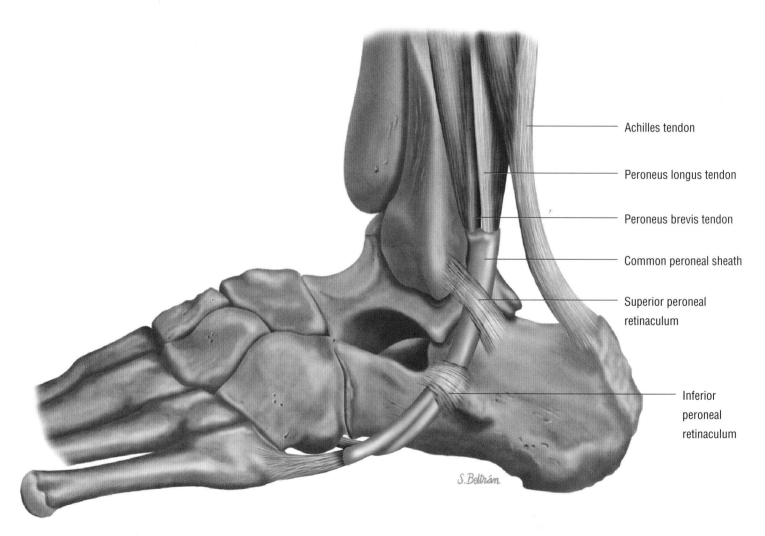

Achilles tendon

Peroneus longus tendon

Peroneus brevis tendon

Common peroneal sheath

Superior peroneal retinaculum

Inferior peroneal retinaculum

Figure 5.73 ▪ Normal relationship of the peroneal tendons to the distal fibula and common synovial sheath of the peroneal tendons posterior to the lateral malleolus. The peroneus brevis makes two turns in its course: one at the fibular groove and the other at the peroneal tubercle. The peroneus longus makes three turns; at the fibular groove, the peroneal tubercle, and the cuboid notch (os peroneum). *(See Peroneal Tendon Abnormalities pg. 873, in Stoller's 3rd Edition.)*

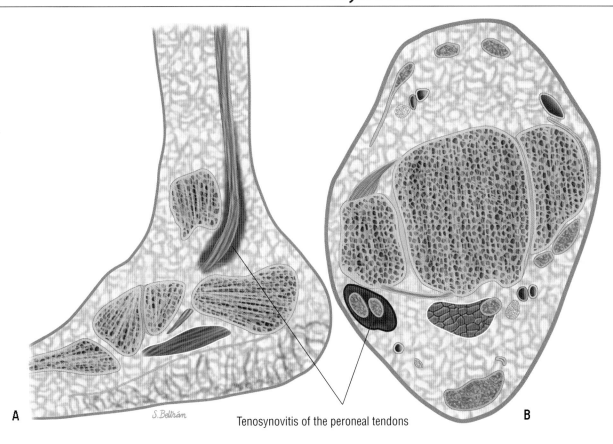

Tenosynovitis of the peroneal tendons

Figure 5.74 ▪ **Tenosynovitis of the peroneal tendons.** **(A)** Sagittal section. **(B)** Axial section. *(See Peroneus Brevis Tendon Tear pg. 875, in Stoller's 3rd Edition.)*

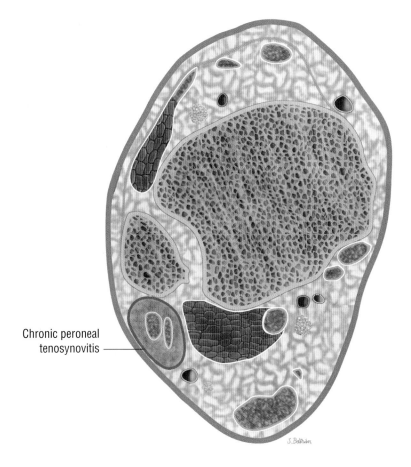

Chronic peroneal tenosynovitis

Figure 5.75 ▪ Chronic peroneal tenosynovitis with thickened synovium. *(See Peroneus Brevis Tendon Tear pg. 875, in Stoller's 3rd Edition.)*

Figure 5.76 ▪ Color illustration of a peroneus brevis partial tear. Tenosynovitis (paratenonitis) with tendinosis, including longitudinal tears and tendinosis of the peroneus brevis, usually occurs at the level of the fibular groove at the distal lateral malleolus. *(See Peroneus Brevis Tendon Tears pg. 876, in Stoller's 3rd Edition.)*

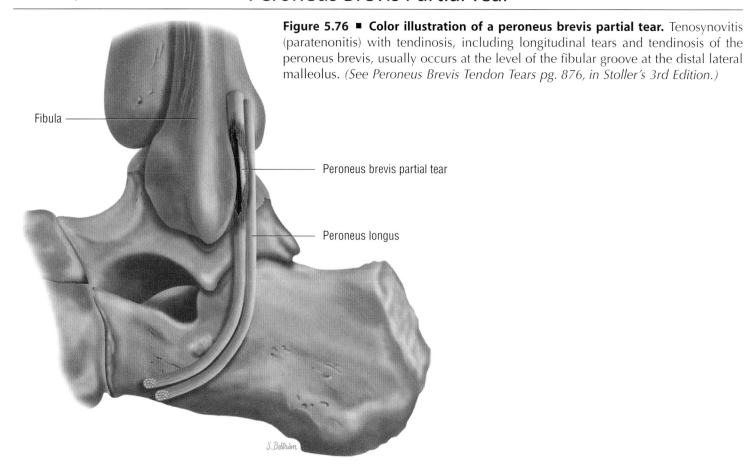

Fibula

Peroneus brevis partial tear

Peroneus longus

S.Beltrán

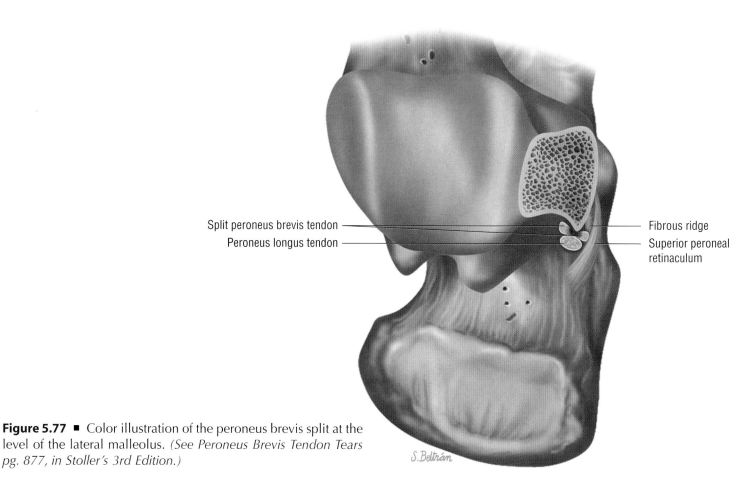

Split peroneus brevis tendon

Peroneus longus tendon

Fibrous ridge

Superior peroneal retinaculum

Figure 5.77 ▪ Color illustration of the peroneus brevis split at the level of the lateral malleolus. *(See Peroneus Brevis Tendon Tears pg. 877, in Stoller's 3rd Edition.)*

S.Beltrán

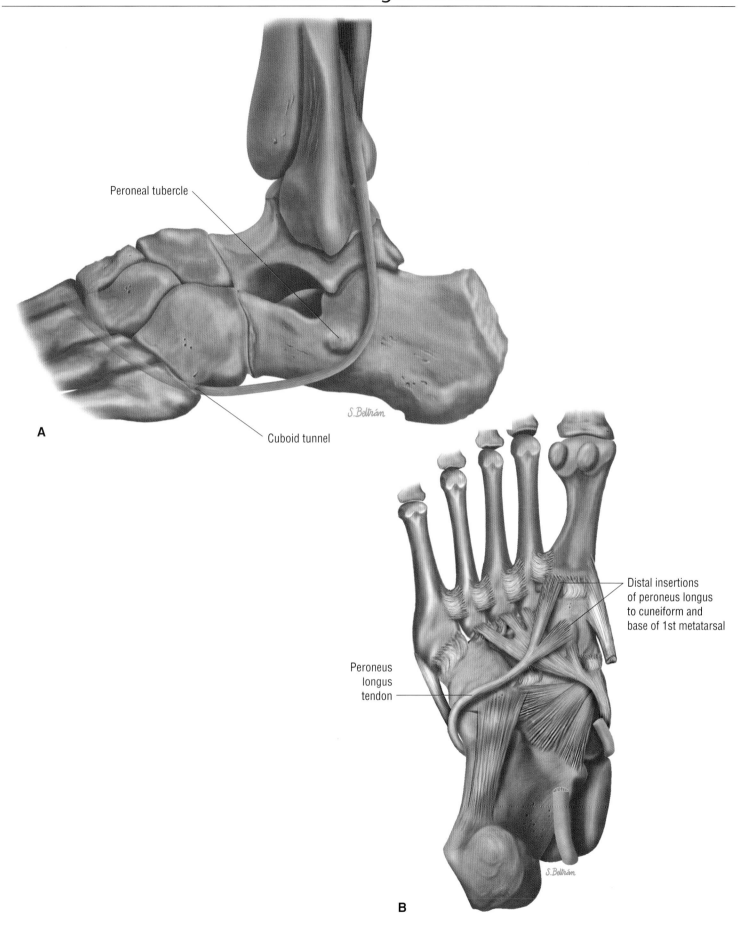

Peroneal tubercle

Cuboid tunnel

A

Distal insertions
of peroneus longus
to cuneiform and
base of 1st metatarsal

Peroneus
longus
tendon

B

Figure 5.78 ■ **(A)** Normal anatomy of the peroneus longus tendon below the peroneal tubercle and within the cuboid groove. In the plantar aspect (sole) of the foot, the peroneus longus receives a second synovial sheath from the groove of the cuboid to its insertion on the base of the first metatarsal and medial cuneiform. **(B)** Plantar course of the peroneus longus is shown on a plantar perspective color illustration. *(See Peroneus Longus Tendon Tear pg. 881, in Stoller's 3rd Edition.)*

Peroneus Brevis and Longus Tendon Split

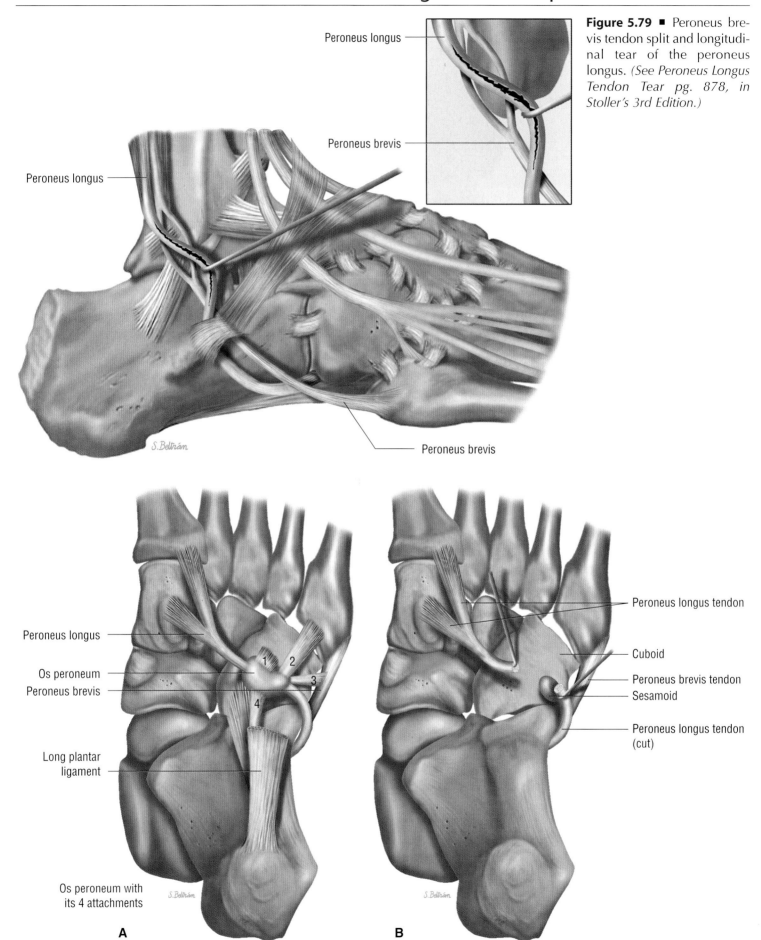

Figure 5.79 ■ Peroneus brevis tendon split and longitudinal tear of the peroneus longus. *(See Peroneus Longus Tendon Tear pg. 878, in Stoller's 3rd Edition.)*

Peroneus longus

Peroneus brevis

Peroneus longus

Peroneus brevis

Peroneus longus

Os peroneum

Peroneus brevis

Long plantar ligament

Os peroneum with its 4 attachments

Peroneus longus tendon

Cuboid

Peroneus brevis tendon

Sesamoid

Peroneus longus tendon (cut)

A

B

Figure 5.80 ■ **(A)** Soft tissue attachments of the os peroneum. **(B)** Peroneus longus tendon tear associated with proximal os peroneum displacement in the painful os peroneum syndrome (POPS). *(See Peroneus Longus Tendon Tear pgs. 878 and 883, in Stoller's 3rd Edition.)*

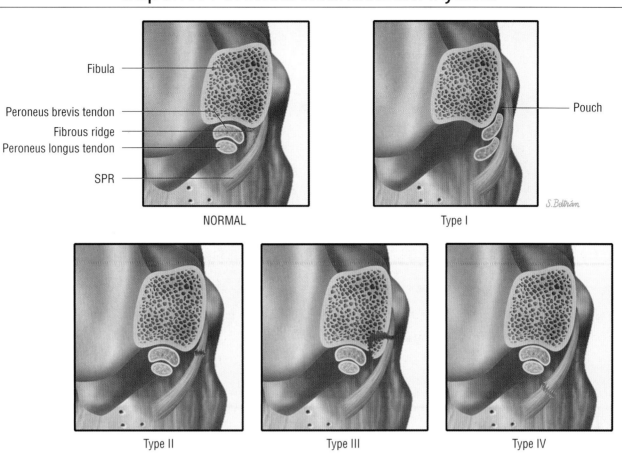

Figure 5.81 ■ Spectrum of superior peroneal retinaculum (SPR) injuries based on Oden's surgical classification. In the normal SPR, the retinaculum originates from the distal fibula, and a small fibrous ridge is identified. A type I injury represents stripping of the SPR from the distal fibula and formation of a potential pouch lateral to the distal fibula. This pouch is associated with subluxation or dislocation of the peroneal tendons. In a type II injury, the SPR is avulsed from its fibular insertion. In a type III injury, there is an osseous avulsion from the distal fibula. Type IV injuries are associated with SPR disruption at its posterior attachment. *(See Superior Peroneal Retinacular Tears pg. 884, in Stoller's 3rd Edition.)*

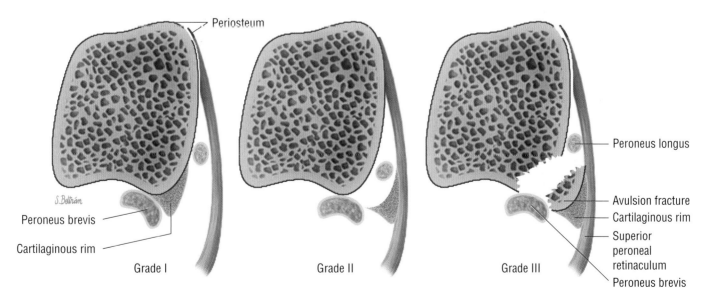

Figure 5.82 ■ Peroneal tendon grades of subluxation-dislocation. Based on *Coughlin MJ, Mann RA, Saltzman CL. Surgery of the Foot and Ankle. Philadelphia: Mosby Elsevier, 2007. (See Superior Peroneal Retinacular Tears pg. 884, in Stoller's 3rd Edition.)*

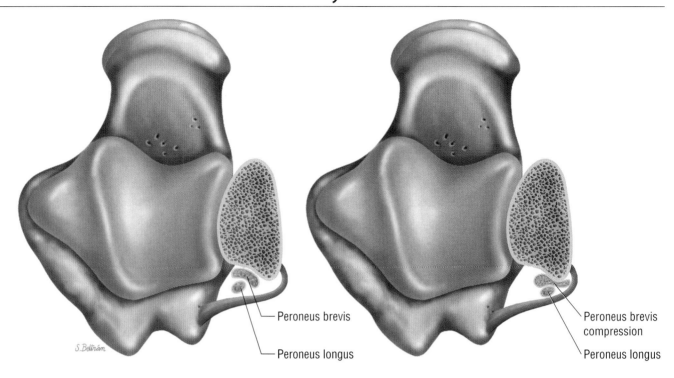

Peroneus brevis

Peroneus longus

Peroneus brevis compression

Peroneus longus

Figure 5.83 ■ Compression of peroneus brevis tendon with retinacular stripping. *(See Superior Peroneal Retinacular Tears pg. 884, in Stoller's 3rd Edition.)*

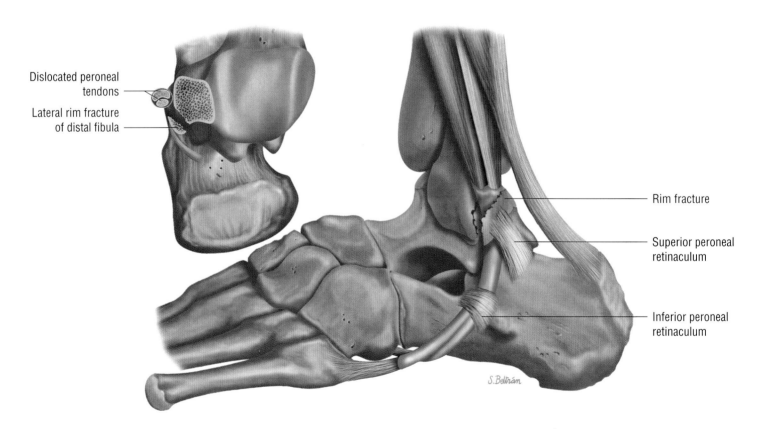

Dislocated peroneal tendons

Lateral rim fracture of distal fibula

Rim fracture

Superior peroneal retinaculum

Inferior peroneal retinaculum

Figure 5.84 ■ A rim fracture of the lateral aspect of the lateral malleolus is associated with recurrent subluxation and dislocation of the peroneal tendons, as shown on lateral and superior view illustrations. *(See Superior Peroneal Retinacular Tears pg. 886, in Stoller's 3rd Edition.)*

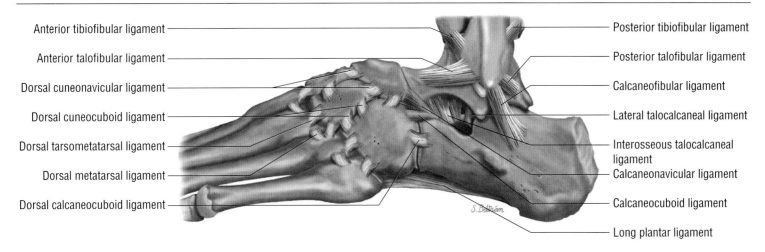

Anterior tibiofibular ligament

Anterior talofibular ligament

Dorsal cuneonavicular ligament

Dorsal cuneocuboid ligament

Dorsal tarsometatarsal ligament

Dorsal metatarsal ligament

Dorsal calcaneocuboid ligament

Posterior tibiofibular ligament

Posterior talofibular ligament

Calcaneofibular ligament

Lateral talocalcaneal ligament

Interosseous talocalcaneal ligament

Calcaneonavicular ligament

Calcaneocuboid ligament

Long plantar ligament

Figure 5.85 ■ Lateral ligaments of the ankle in a lateral view color illustration. *(See Lateral Ligament Complex Injuries pg. 888, in Stoller's 3rd Edition.)*

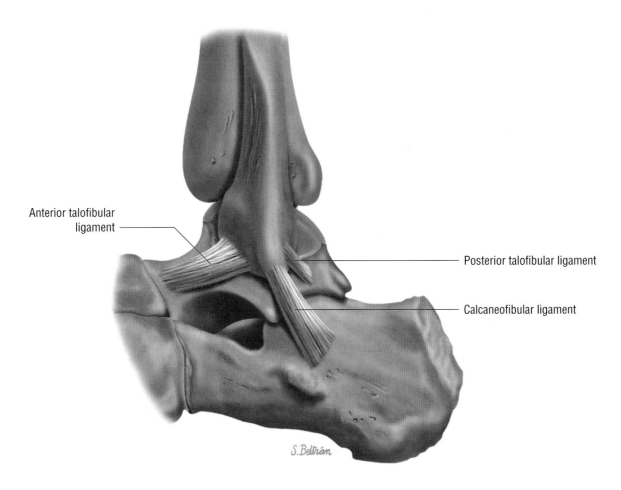

Anterior talofibular ligament

Posterior talofibular ligament

Calcaneofibular ligament

Figure 5.86 ■ The lateral ligaments along with the talus and fibular define the lateral gutter. *(See Lateral Ligament Complex Injuries pg. 889, in Stoller's 3rd Edition.)*

Ankle Ligaments and Lateral Gutter

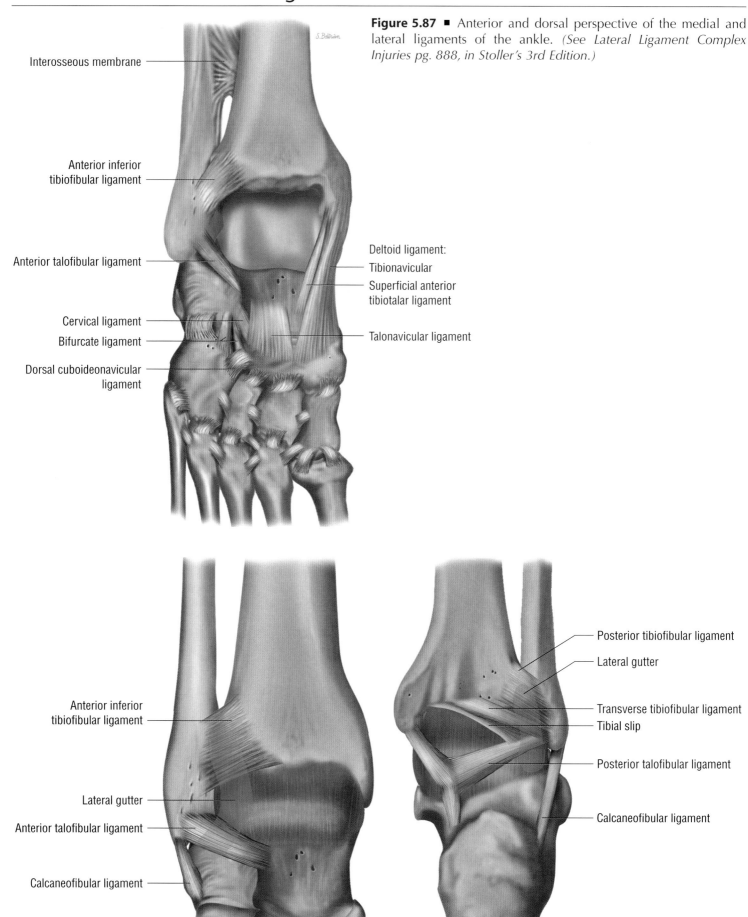

Interosseous membrane

Anterior inferior tibiofibular ligament

Anterior talofibular ligament

Cervical ligament

Bifurcate ligament

Dorsal cuboideonavicular ligament

Figure 5.87 ■ Anterior and dorsal perspective of the medial and lateral ligaments of the ankle. *(See Lateral Ligament Complex Injuries pg. 888, in Stoller's 3rd Edition.)*

Deltoid ligament:
Tibionavicular
Superficial anterior tibiotalar ligament

Talonavicular ligament

Anterior inferior tibiofibular ligament

Lateral gutter

Anterior talofibular ligament

Calcaneofibular ligament

Posterior tibiofibular ligament

Lateral gutter

Transverse tibiofibular ligament
Tibial slip

Posterior talofibular ligament

Calcaneofibular ligament

A

B

Figure 5.88 ■ **(A)** Lateral gutter, anterior perspective. **(B)** Lateral gutter, posterior perspective. *A Based on Coughlin MJ, Mann RA, Saltzman CL. Surgery of the foot and ankle. Philadelphia: Mosby Elsevier, 2007. (See Lateral Ligament Complex Injuries pg. 889, in Stoller's 3rd Edition.)*

Figure 5.89 ■ Anterior drawer test. With the tibia secured, the heel is pulled forward and internally rotated. With a double ligament tear there will be increased subluxation of the talus anteriorly on the distal tibia. *Based on Ferkel RD. Arthroscopic surgery: the foot and ankle. Philadelphia: Lippincott-Raven, 1996. (See Anterior Talofibular Ligament Tear pg. 890, in Stoller's 3rd Edition.)*

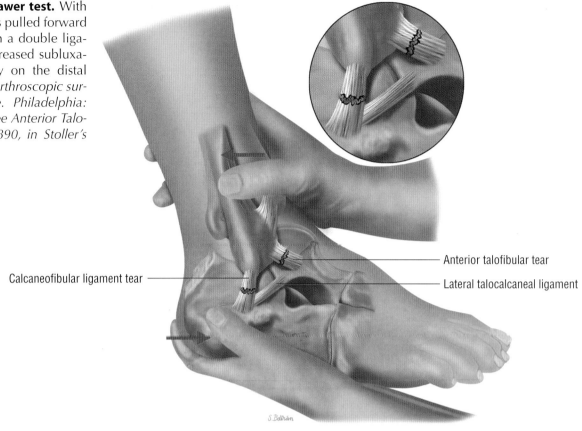

Calcaneofibular ligament tear

Anterior talofibular tear

Lateral talocalcaneal ligament

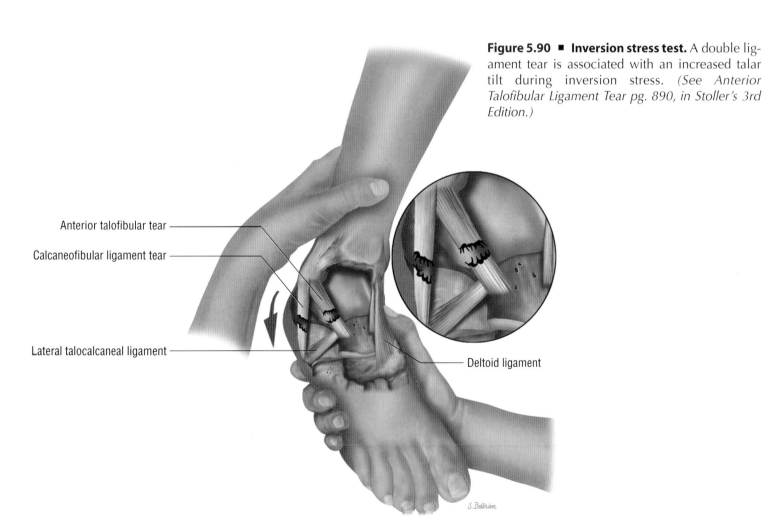

Figure 5.90 ■ Inversion stress test. A double ligament tear is associated with an increased talar tilt during inversion stress. *(See Anterior Talofibular Ligament Tear pg. 890, in Stoller's 3rd Edition.)*

Anterior talofibular tear

Calcaneofibular ligament tear

Lateral talocalcaneal ligament

Deltoid ligament

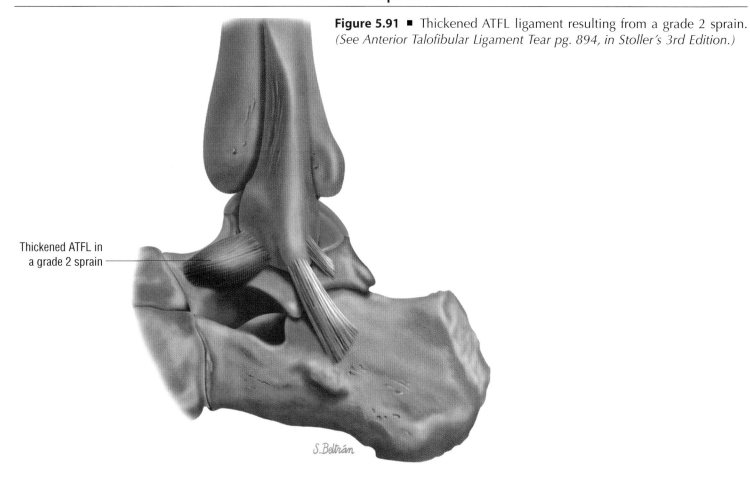

Figure 5.91 ▪ Thickened ATFL ligament resulting from a grade 2 sprain. *(See Anterior Talofibular Ligament Tear pg. 894, in Stoller's 3rd Edition.)*

Thickened ATFL in a grade 2 sprain

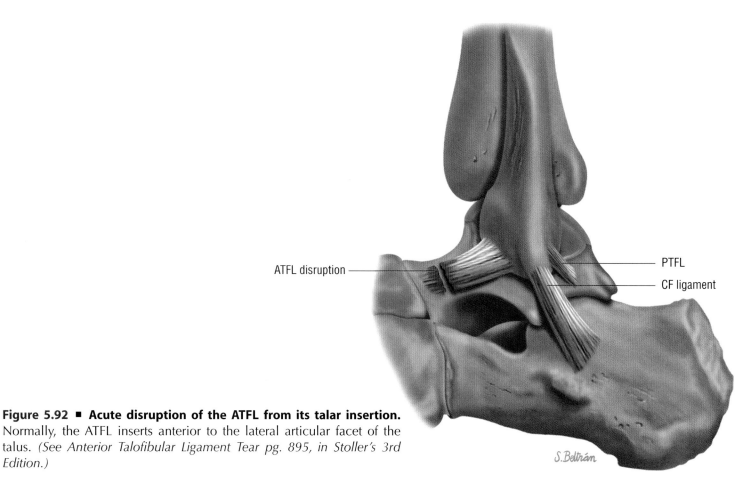

ATFL disruption

PTFL

CF ligament

Figure 5.92 ▪ Acute disruption of the ATFL from its talar insertion. Normally, the ATFL inserts anterior to the lateral articular facet of the talus. *(See Anterior Talofibular Ligament Tear pg. 895, in Stoller's 3rd Edition.)*

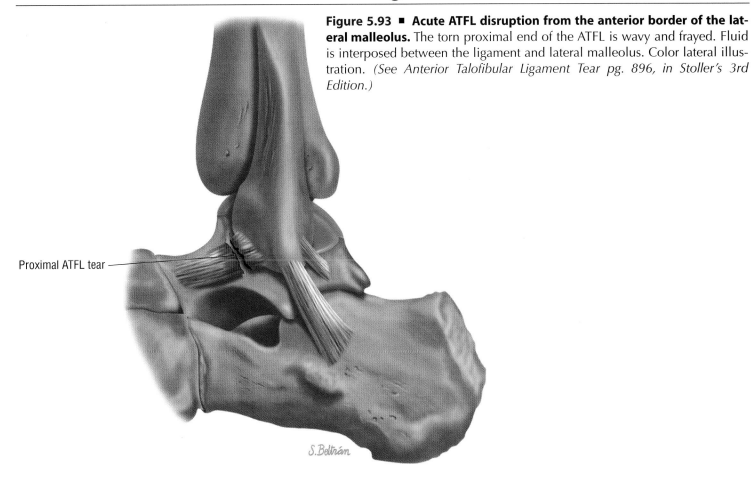

Proximal ATFL tear

Figure 5.93 ▪ **Acute ATFL disruption from the anterior border of the lateral malleolus.** The torn proximal end of the ATFL is wavy and frayed. Fluid is interposed between the ligament and lateral malleolus. Color lateral illustration. *(See Anterior Talofibular Ligament Tear pg. 896, in Stoller's 3rd Edition.)*

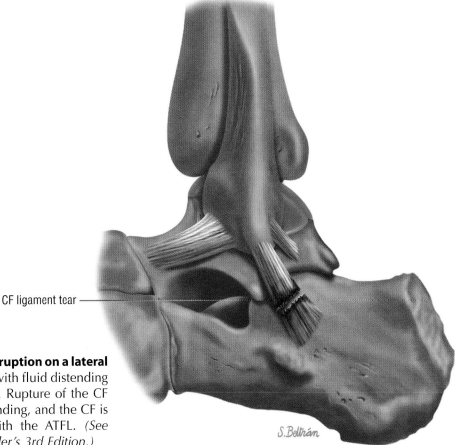

CF ligament tear

Figure 5.94 ▪ **Calcaneofibular (CF) ligament disruption on a lateral color illustration.** CF injuries may be associated with fluid distending the peroneal tendon sheath as a secondary sign. Rupture of the CF ligament does not usually occur as an isolated finding, and the CF is the second ligament injured in association with the ATFL. *(See Calcaneo-fibular Ligament Sprain pg. 899, in Stoller's 3rd Edition.)*

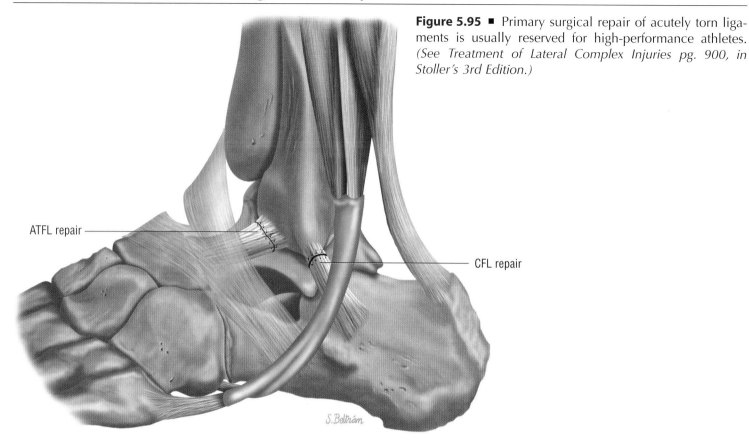

Figure 5.95 ▪ Primary surgical repair of acutely torn ligaments is usually reserved for high-performance athletes. *(See Treatment of Lateral Complex Injuries pg. 900, in Stoller's 3rd Edition.)*

ATFL repair

CFL repair

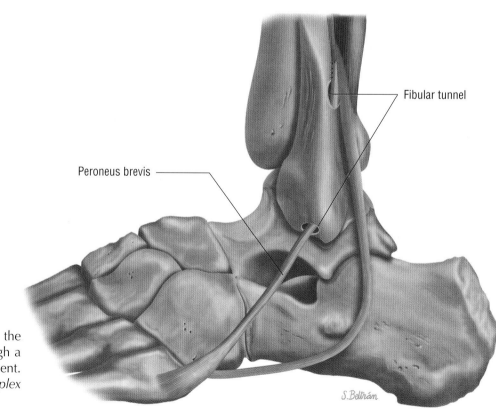

Fibular tunnel

Peroneus brevis

Figure 5.96 ▪ In the Evans procedure, the peroneus brevis tendon is rerouted through a fibular tunnel with proximal reattachment. *(See Treatment of Lateral Ligament Complex Injuries pg. 901, in Stoller's 3rd Edition.)*

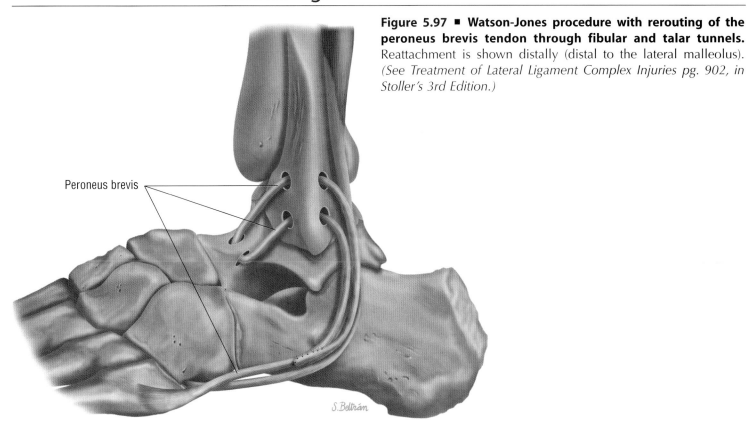

Figure 5.97 ▪ **Watson-Jones procedure with rerouting of the peroneus brevis tendon through fibular and talar tunnels.** Reattachment is shown distally (distal to the lateral malleolus). *(See Treatment of Lateral Ligament Complex Injuries pg. 902, in Stoller's 3rd Edition.)*

Peroneus brevis

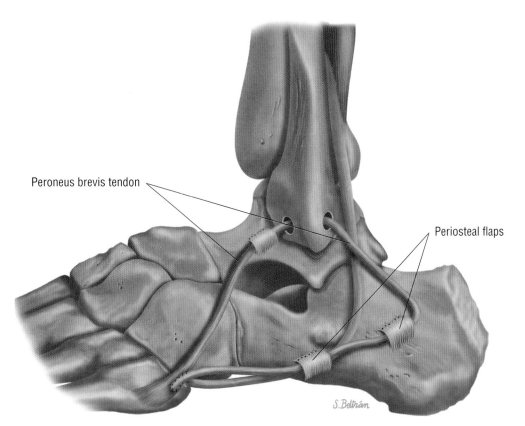

Peroneus brevis tendon

Periosteal flaps

Figure 5.98 ▪ Lateral color illustration of the Chrisman-Snook procedure with the split peroneus brevis tendon coursing through a fibular tunnel and secured to the talus and calcaneus with the use of periosteal flaps. *(See Treatment of Lateral Complex Injuries pg. 902, in Stoller's 3rd Edition.)*

Superficial and Deep Deltoid Ligaments

Superficial deltoid ligament:

Superficial posterior tibiotalar

Tibionavicular

Tibioligamentous

Tibiocalcaneal

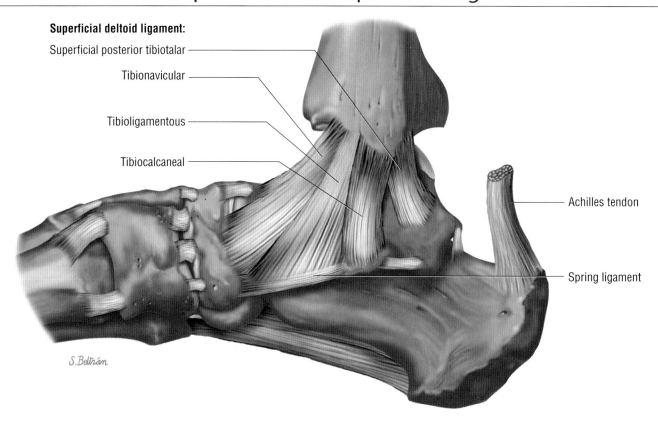

Achilles tendon

Spring ligament

S.Beltrán

Figure 5.99 ■ Superficial layer of the deltoid ligament. *(See Medial Ligament Complex Injuries/Deltoid Ligament Sprain pg. 903, in Stoller's 3rd Edition.)*

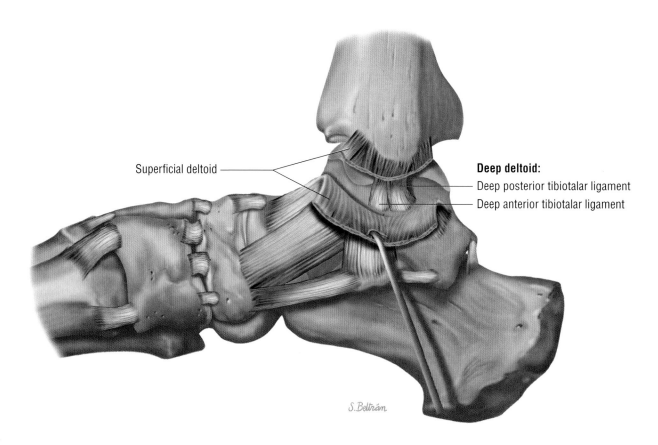

Superficial deltoid

Deep deltoid:
Deep posterior tibiotalar ligament
Deep anterior tibiotalar ligament

S.Beltrán

Figure 5.100 ■ Components of the deep deltoid ligament. *(See Medial Ligament Complex Injuries/Deltoid Ligament Sprain pg. 904, in Stoller's 3rd Edition.)*

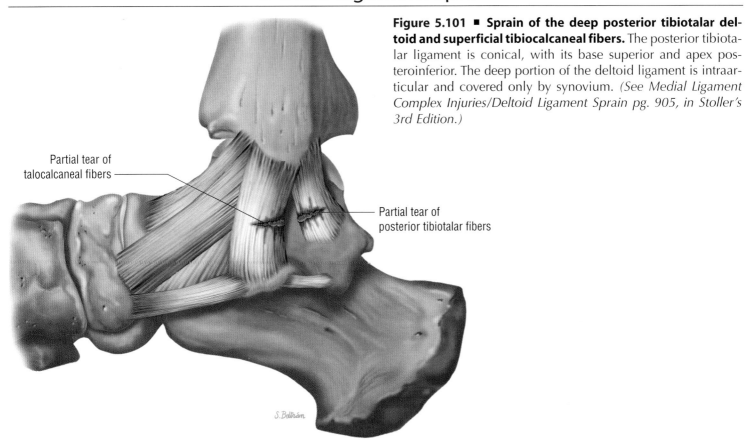

Figure 5.101 ■ **Sprain of the deep posterior tibiotalar deltoid and superficial tibiocalcaneal fibers.** The posterior tibiotalar ligament is conical, with its base superior and apex posteroinferior. The deep portion of the deltoid ligament is intraarticular and covered only by synovium. *(See Medial Ligament Complex Injuries/Deltoid Ligament Sprain pg. 905, in Stoller's 3rd Edition.)*

Partial tear of talocalcaneal fibers

Partial tear of posterior tibiotalar fibers

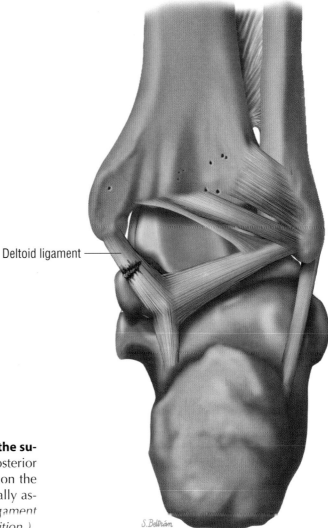

Deltoid ligament

Figure 5.102 ■ **Posterior view color illustration of a partial tear of the superficial and deep fibers of the deltoid ligament.** The deep layer posterior tibiotalar ligament runs obliquely inferiorly and posteriorly to insert on the medial surface of the talus. Posterior tibiotalar ligament sprain is usually associated with severe lateral collateral ligament sprain. *(See Medial Ligament Complex Injuries/Deltoid Ligament Sprain pg. 906, in Stoller's 3rd Edition.)*

Ligaments of the Syndesmosis

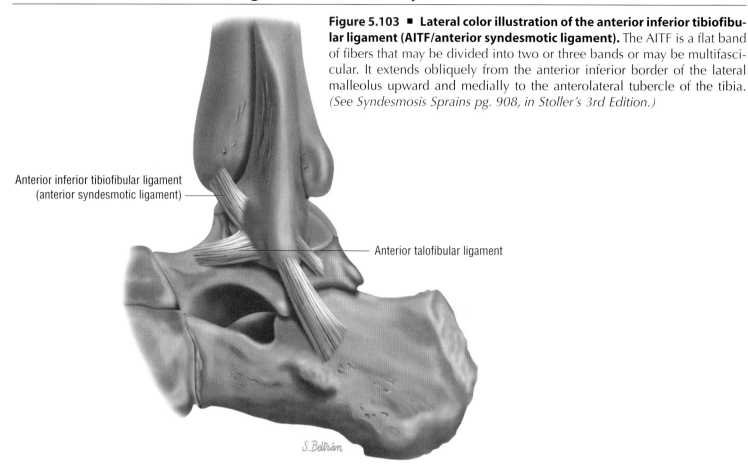

Figure 5.103 ■ **Lateral color illustration of the anterior inferior tibiofibular ligament (AITF/anterior syndesmotic ligament).** The AITF is a flat band of fibers that may be divided into two or three bands or may be multifascicular. It extends obliquely from the anterior inferior border of the lateral malleolus upward and medially to the anterolateral tubercle of the tibia. *(See Syndesmosis Sprains pg. 908, in Stoller's 3rd Edition.)*

Anterior inferior tibiofibular ligament (anterior syndesmotic ligament)

Anterior talofibular ligament

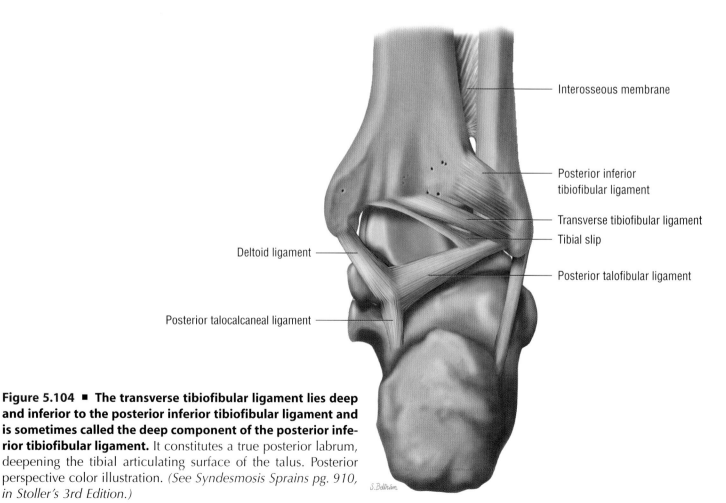

Interosseous membrane

Posterior inferior tibiofibular ligament

Transverse tibiofibular ligament

Tibial slip

Posterior talofibular ligament

Deltoid ligament

Posterior talocalcaneal ligament

Figure 5.104 ■ **The transverse tibiofibular ligament lies deep and inferior to the posterior inferior tibiofibular ligament and is sometimes called the deep component of the posterior inferior tibiofibular ligament.** It constitutes a true posterior labrum, deepening the tibial articulating surface of the talus. Posterior perspective color illustration. *(See Syndesmosis Sprains pg. 910, in Stoller's 3rd Edition.)*

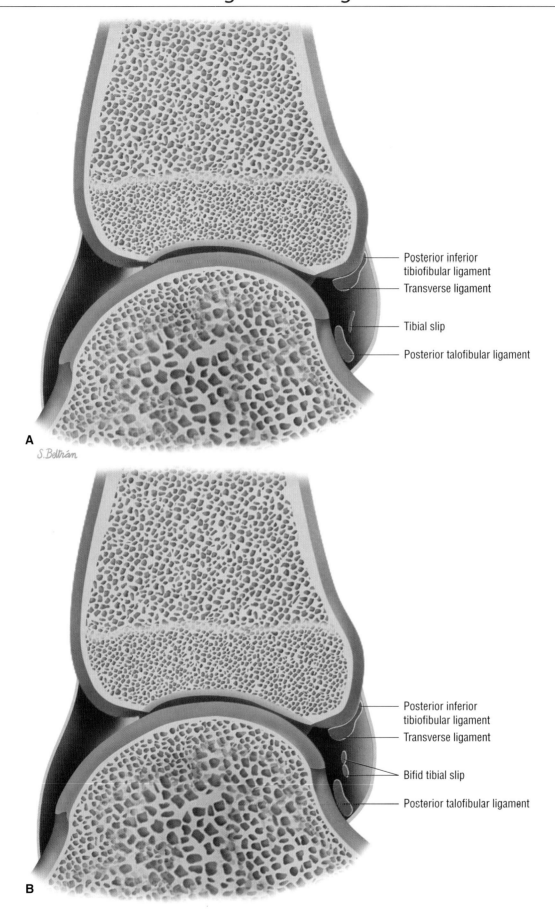

S.Beltrán

Posterior inferior
tibiofibular ligament

Transverse ligament

Tibial slip

Posterior talofibular ligament

A

Posterior inferior
tibiofibular ligament

Transverse ligament

Bifid tibial slip

Posterior talofibular ligament

B

Figure 5.105 ▪ Sagittal illustrations showing the relationship of the posterior ligaments and variation in the tibial slip anatomy. (A) Single tibial slip. (B) Bifid tibial slip. (See *Syndesmosis Sprains* pg. 912 and *Posterior Impingement* pg. 928, in *Stoller's 3rd Edition*.)

Anterior Syndesmotic Ligament Injury

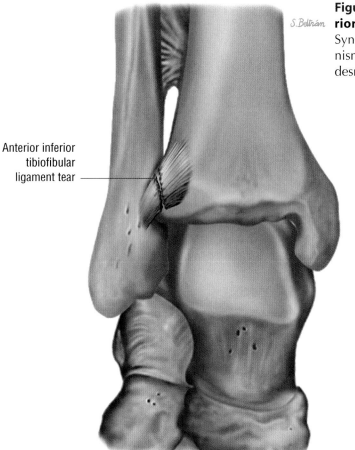

Anterior inferior
tibiofibular
ligament tear

Figure 5.106 ▪ Tear of the anterior inferior tibiofibular (AITF/anterior syndesmotic) ligament on a coronal color illustration. Syndesmosis injuries are associated with an external rotation mechanism, although hyperdorsiflexion also may lead to tears of the syndesmosis. *(See Syndesmosis Sprains pg. 914, in Stoller's 3rd Edition.)*

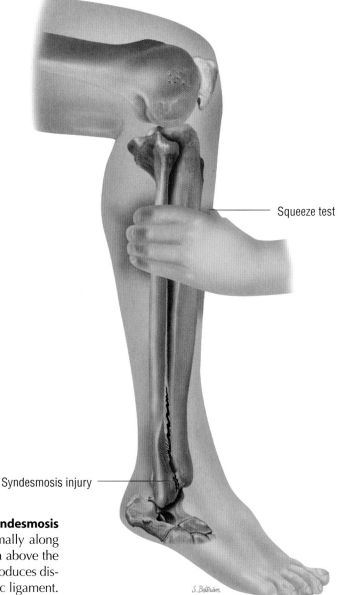

Squeeze test

Syndesmosis injury

Figure 5.107 ▪ The "squeeze test" is used clinically to diagnose syndesmosis injuries. By palpating directly over the syndesmosis and more proximally along the interosseous membrane, the fibular is compressed against the tibia above the midpoint of the calf. The test is positive when proximal compression produces distal pain in the area of the torn interosseous membrane and syndesmotic ligament. Anterolateral view illustration. *(See Syndesmosis Sprains pg. 915, in Stoller's 3rd Edition.)*

Syndesmotic Ligament Injury

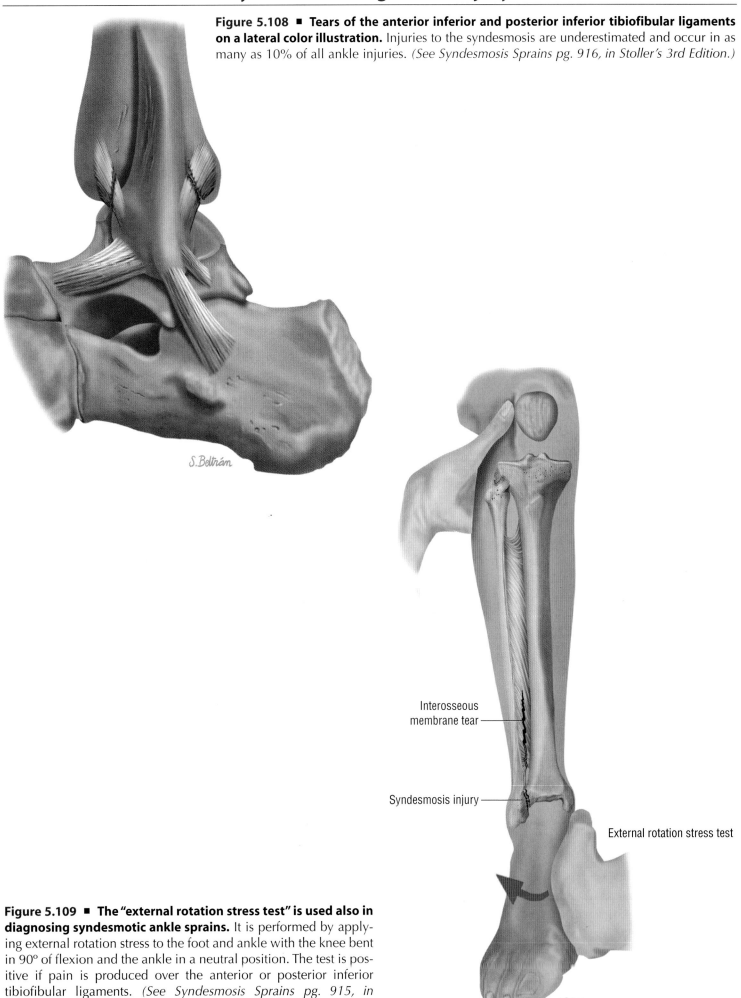

Figure 5.108 ■ **Tears of the anterior inferior and posterior inferior tibiofibular ligaments on a lateral color illustration.** Injuries to the syndesmosis are underestimated and occur in as many as 10% of all ankle injuries. *(See Syndesmosis Sprains pg. 916, in Stoller's 3rd Edition.)*

Interosseous membrane tear

Syndesmosis injury

External rotation stress test

Figure 5.109 ■ **The "external rotation stress test" is used also in diagnosing syndesmotic ankle sprains.** It is performed by applying external rotation stress to the foot and ankle with the knee bent in 90° of flexion and the ankle in a neutral position. The test is positive if pain is produced over the anterior or posterior inferior tibiofibular ligaments. *(See Syndesmosis Sprains pg. 915, in Stoller's 3rd Edition.)*

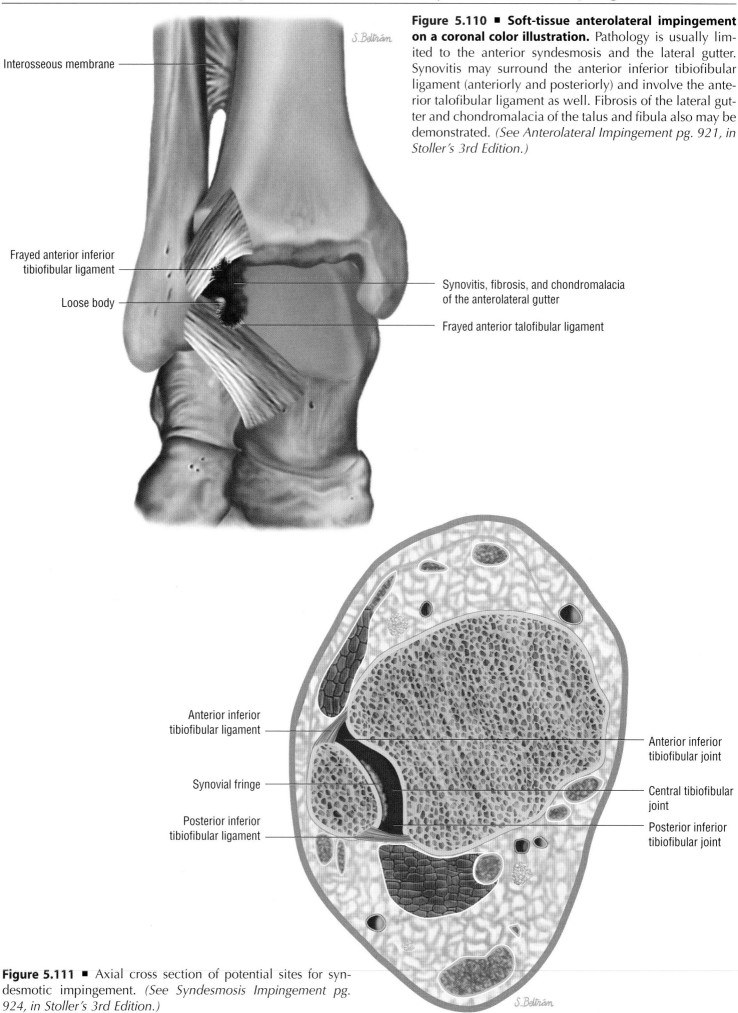

Figure 5.110 ■ **Soft-tissue anterolateral impingement on a coronal color illustration.** Pathology is usually limited to the anterior syndesmosis and the lateral gutter. Synovitis may surround the anterior inferior tibiofibular ligament (anteriorly and posteriorly) and involve the anterior talofibular ligament as well. Fibrosis of the lateral gutter and chondromalacia of the talus and fibula also may be demonstrated. *(See Anterolateral Impingement pg. 921, in Stoller's 3rd Edition.)*

Interosseous membrane

Frayed anterior inferior tibiofibular ligament

Loose body

Synovitis, fibrosis, and chondromalacia of the anterolateral gutter

Frayed anterior talofibular ligament

Anterior inferior tibiofibular ligament

Synovial fringe

Posterior inferior tibiofibular ligament

Anterior inferior tibiofibular joint

Central tibiofibular joint

Posterior inferior tibiofibular joint

Figure 5.111 ■ Axial cross section of potential sites for syndesmotic impingement. *(See Syndesmosis Impingement pg. 924, in Stoller's 3rd Edition.)*

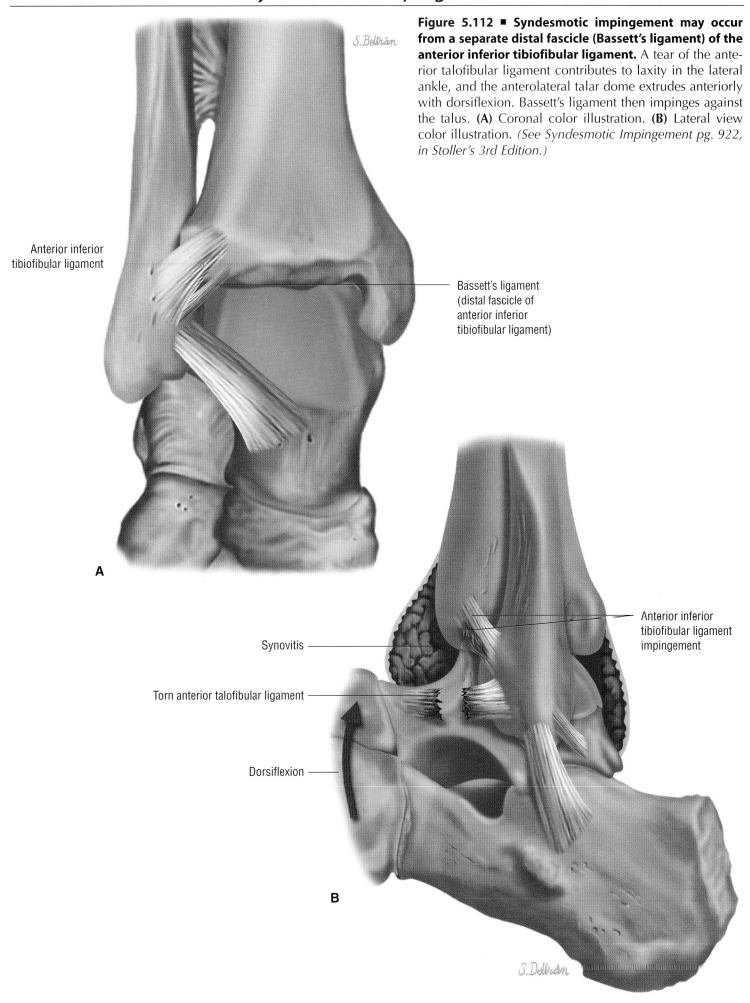

Figure 5.112 ▪ Syndesmotic impingement may occur from a separate distal fascicle (Bassett's ligament) of the anterior inferior tibiofibular ligament. A tear of the anterior talofibular ligament contributes to laxity in the lateral ankle, and the anterolateral talar dome extrudes anteriorly with dorsiflexion. Bassett's ligament then impinges against the talus. **(A)** Coronal color illustration. **(B)** Lateral view color illustration. *(See Syndesmotic Impingement pg. 922, in Stoller's 3rd Edition.)*

Anterior inferior tibiofibular ligament

Bassett's ligament (distal fascicle of anterior inferior tibiofibular ligament)

A

Synovitis

Torn anterior talofibular ligament

Dorsiflexion

Anterior inferior tibiofibular ligament impingement

B

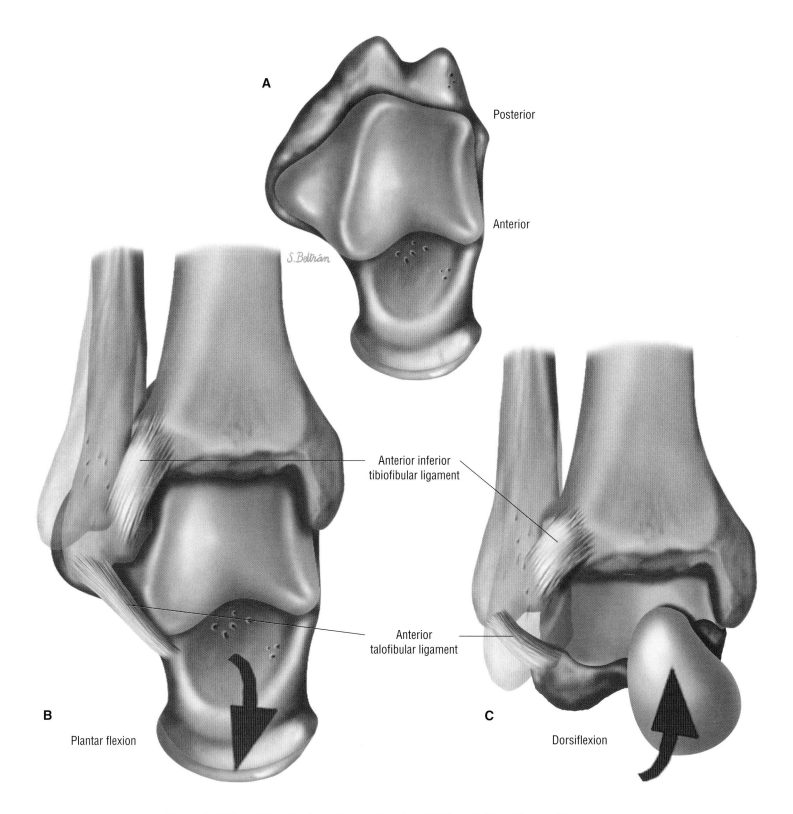

Figure 5.113 ■ Tibiofibular joint mechanics. (A) The width of the trochlear surface of the talus is smaller posteriorly than anteriorly. **(B)** During plantarflexion of the ankle, the malleoli are approximated actively as the lateral malleolus is pulled inferiorly and rotated medially. **(C)** With dorsiflexion of the ankle, the lateral malleolus moves always from the medial malleolus and is pulled slightly superiorly as the fibular is medially rotated. *Based on Ferkel RD. Arthroscopic Surgery: The foot and ankle. Philadelphia: Lippincott-Raven, 1996. (See Syndesmosis Impingement pg. 923, in Stoller's 3rd Edition.)*

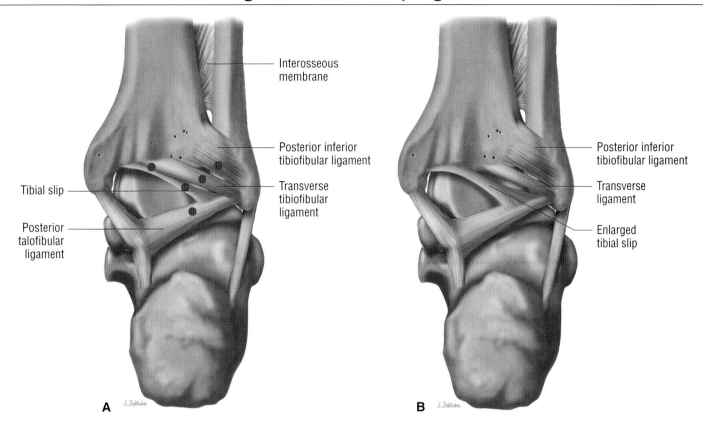

Figure 5.114 ■ **(A)** Posterior soft-tissue impingement sites. **(B)** Enlarged tibial slip and mildly attenuated transverse ligament as a variant of the posterior ligaments. *A based on Ferkel RD. Arthroscopic surgery: the foot and ankle. Philadelphia: Lippincott-Raven, 1996. (See Posterior Impingement pg. 926, in Stoller's 3rd Edition.)*

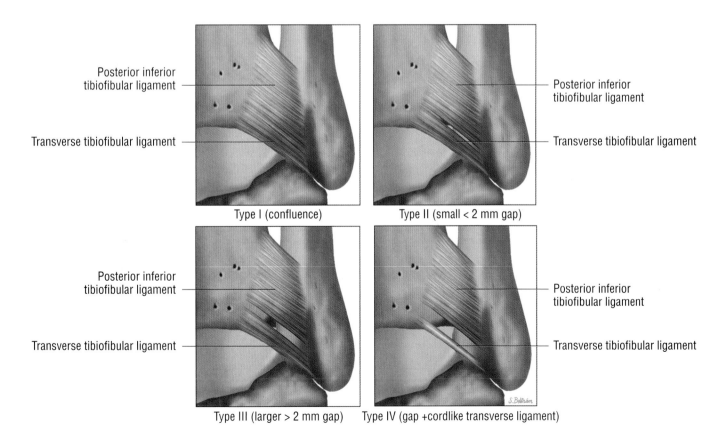

Figure 5.115 ■ Posterior inferior tibiofibular ligament (PITFL) and transverse tibiofibular ligament subtypes. *Based on Coughlin MJ, Mann RA, Saltzman CL. Surgery of the foot and ankle. Philadelphia: Mosby Elsevier, 2007. (See Posterior Impingement pgs. 926, 927, and 928, in Stoller's 3rd Edition.)*

Figure 5.116 ■ Posterior impingement with synovitis involving the posterior ligaments on color illustration with posterior perspective. *(See Posterior Impingement pg. 927, in Stoller's 3rd Edition.)*

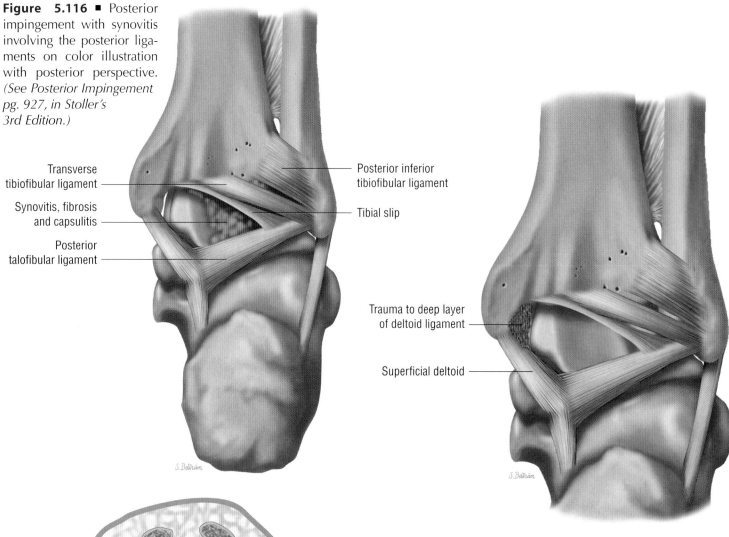

Transverse
tibiofibular ligament

Synovitis, fibrosis
and capsulitis

Posterior
talofibular ligament

Posterior inferior
tibiofibular ligament

Tibial slip

Trauma to deep layer
of deltoid ligament

Superficial deltoid

Figure 5.117 ■ Posteromedial impingement secondary to disruption of the deep fibers of the deltoid ligament (posterior talotibial component) with associated thickened synovial response deep to the tibialis posterior tendon. *(See Anteromedial and Posteromedial Impingement pg. 930, in Stoller's 3rd Edition.)*

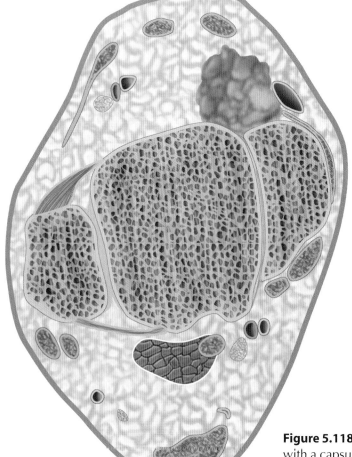

Figure 5.118 ■ Anteromedial impingement with soft-tissue thickening associated with a capsular component and a torn anterior component of the deltoid ligament. *(See Anteromedial and Posteromedial Impingement pg. 928, in Stoller's 3rd Edition.)*

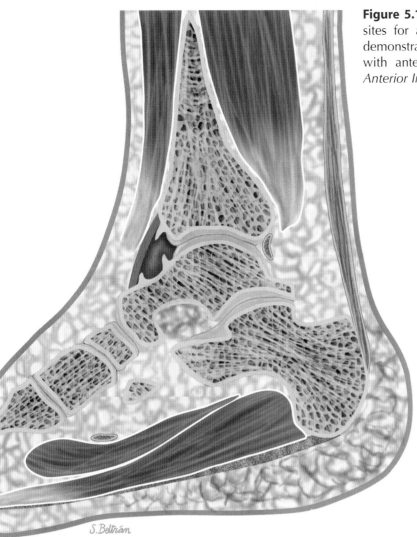

Figure 5.119 ■ **(A)** Lateral color illustration showing potential sites for anterior tibiotalar spurs. **(B)** Lateral color illustration demonstrates complications of anterior osseous impingement with anterior osteophytes, synovitis, and a loose body. *(See Anterior Impingement pg. 932, in Stoller's 3rd Edition.)*

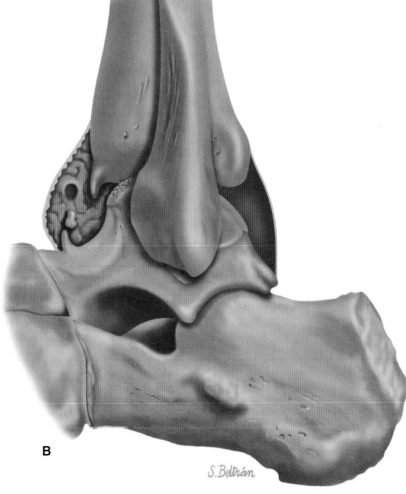

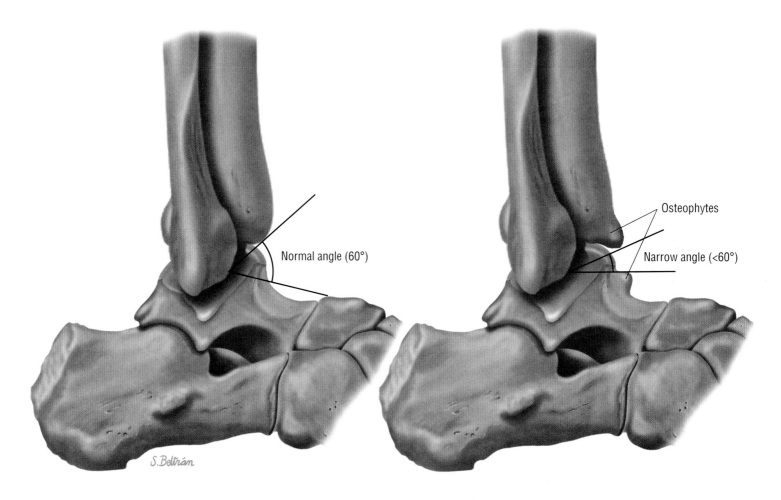

Figure 5.120 ■ **(A)** The normal angle between the distal tibia and the talar neck should be 60° or greater. **(B)** The presence of osteophytes on the distal tibia or talus can narrow the angle to less than 60°. *Based on Ferkel RD. Arthroscopic surgery: the foot and ankle. Philadelphia: Lippincott-Raven, 1996. (See Anterior Impingement pg. 933, in Stoller's 3rd Edition.)*

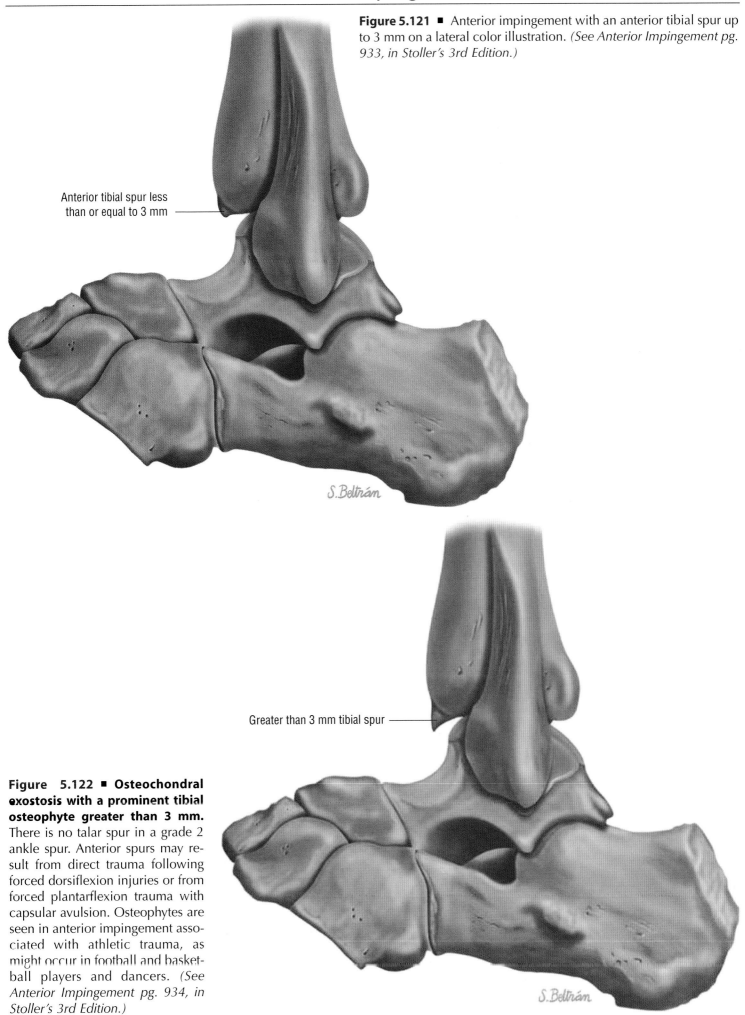

Figure 5.121 ▪ Anterior impingement with an anterior tibial spur up to 3 mm on a lateral color illustration. *(See Anterior Impingement pg. 933, in Stoller's 3rd Edition.)*

Anterior tibial spur less than or equal to 3 mm

Greater than 3 mm tibial spur

Figure 5.122 ▪ **Osteochondral exostosis with a prominent tibial osteophyte greater than 3 mm.** There is no talar spur in a grade 2 ankle spur. Anterior spurs may result from direct trauma following forced dorsiflexion injuries or from forced plantarflexion trauma with capsular avulsion. Osteophytes are seen in anterior impingement associated with athletic trauma, as might occur in football and basketball players and dancers. *(See Anterior Impingement pg. 934, in Stoller's 3rd Edition.)*

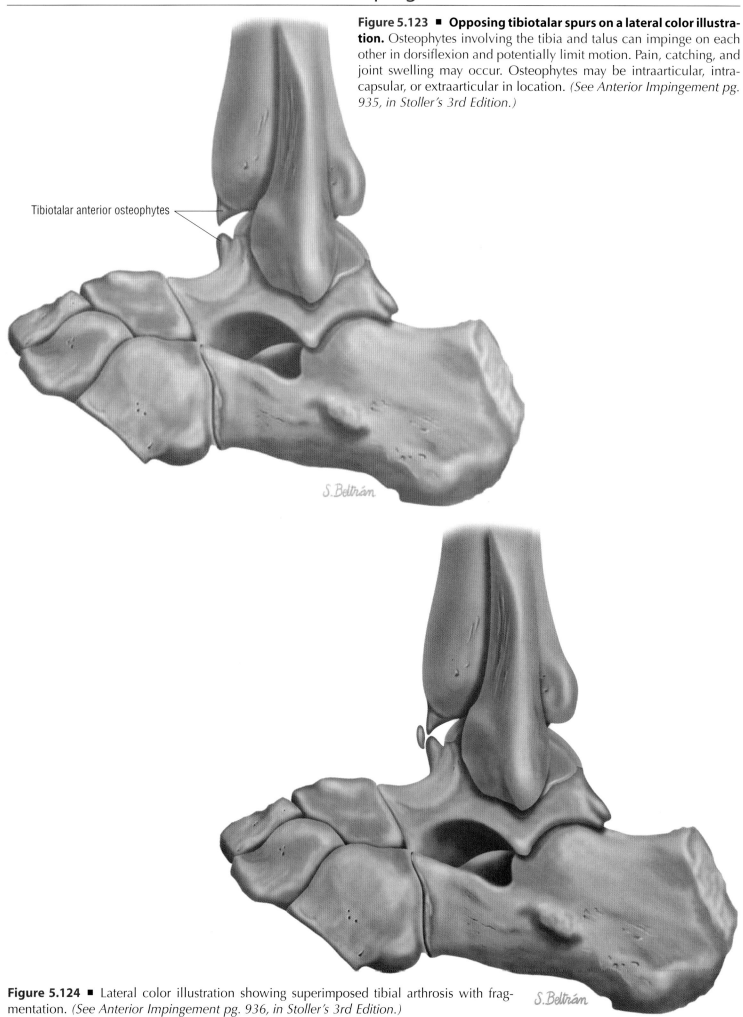

Figure 5.123 ■ **Opposing tibiotalar spurs on a lateral color illustration.** Osteophytes involving the tibia and talus can impinge on each other in dorsiflexion and potentially limit motion. Pain, catching, and joint swelling may occur. Osteophytes may be intraarticular, intracapsular, or extraarticular in location. *(See Anterior Impingement pg. 935, in Stoller's 3rd Edition.)*

Tibiotalar anterior osteophytes

Figure 5.124 ■ Lateral color illustration showing superimposed tibial arthrosis with fragmentation. *(See Anterior Impingement pg. 936, in Stoller's 3rd Edition.)*

Figure 5.125 ■ **Axial view of the tarsal canal.** Note the location of the interosseous talocalcaneal and cervical ligaments. There is a 45° angle of orientation of the long axis of the sinus tarsi to the lateral aspect of the calcaneus. *(See Sinus Tarsi Syndrome pg. 939, in Stoller's 3rd Edition.)*

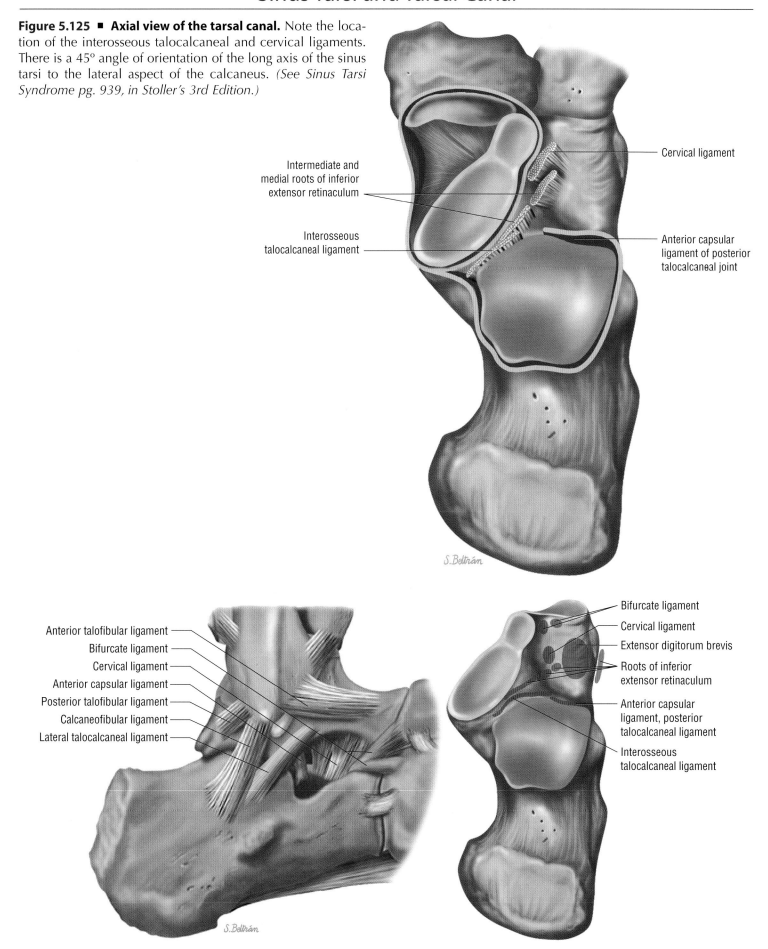

Cervical ligament

Intermediate and medial roots of inferior extensor retinaculum

Interosseous talocalcaneal ligament

Anterior capsular ligament of posterior talocalcaneal joint

S.Beltrán

Anterior talofibular ligament
Bifurcate ligament
Cervical ligament
Anterior capsular ligament
Posterior talofibular ligament
Calcaneofibular ligament
Lateral talocalcaneal ligament

Bifurcate ligament
Cervical ligament
Extensor digitorum brevis
Roots of inferior extensor retinaculum
Anterior capsular ligament, posterior talocalcaneal ligament
Interosseous talocalcaneal ligament

S.Beltrán

Figure 5.126 ■ **Ligaments of the subtalar joint. (A)** Superficial lateral view of the subtalar joint with bones and ligaments. From this position, the interosseous ligament cannot be seen. **(B)** Superior view of the insertion sites on the calcaneus with the talus removed. *(See Sinus Tarsi Syndrome pg. 937, in Stoller's 3rd Edition.)*

Sinus Tarsi and Tarsal Canal

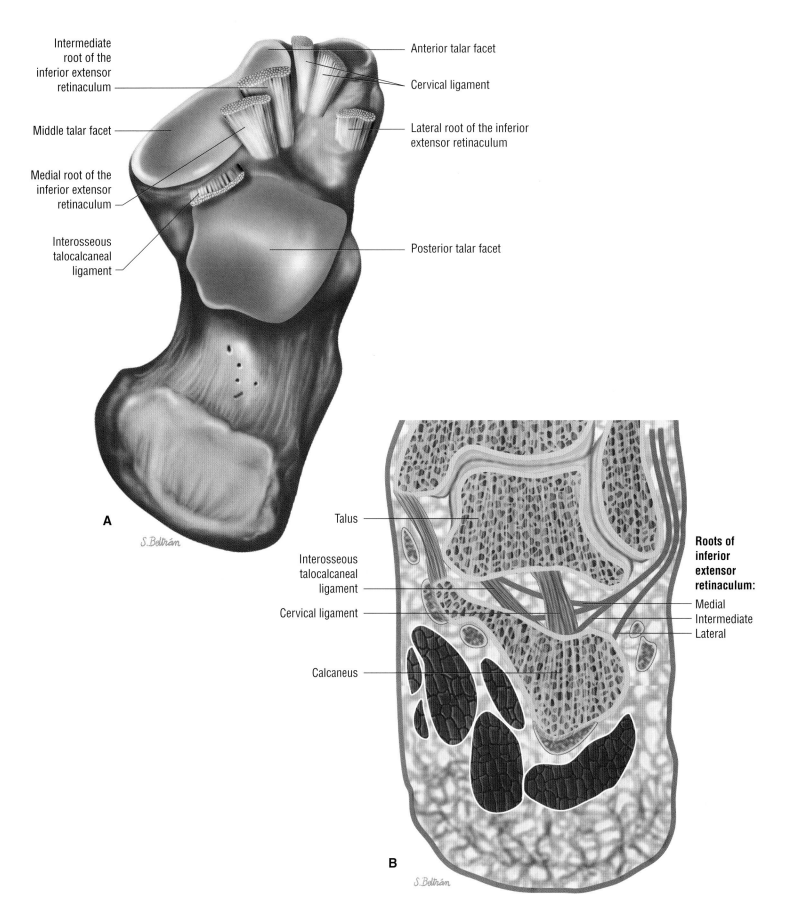

Intermediate root of the inferior extensor retinaculum

Middle talar facet

Medial root of the inferior extensor retinaculum

Interosseous talocalcaneal ligament

Anterior talar facet

Cervical ligament

Lateral root of the inferior extensor retinaculum

Posterior talar facet

A

S. Beltrán

Talus

Interosseous talocalcaneal ligament

Cervical ligament

Calcaneus

Roots of inferior extensor retinaculum:
Medial
Intermediate
Lateral

B

S. Beltrán

Figure 5.127 ■ Tarsal canal and sinus tarsi anatomy on an axial superior view color graphic **(A)**, and a color coronal section **(B)**. *(See Sinus Tarsi Syndrome pg. 938, in Stoller's 3rd Edition.)*

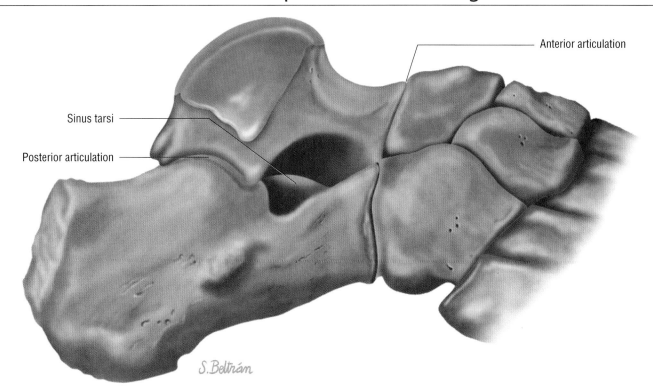

Figure 5.128 ■ **Lateral view of the sinus tarsi.** The sinus tarsi and tarsal canal separate the anterior and posterior articulations of the subtalar joint. The sagittal plane of section helps to demonstrate the anatomy more clearly. *(See Sinus Tarsi Syndrome pg. 939, in Stoller's 3rd Edition.)*

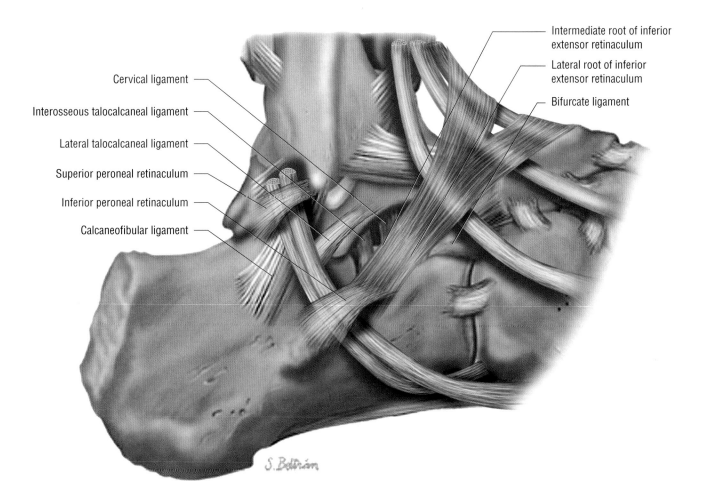

Figure 5.129 ■ Lateral view of the superficial or peripheral ligaments. *(See Sinus Tarsi Syndrome pg. 941, in Stoller's 3rd Edition.)*

Subtalar Joint Ligaments

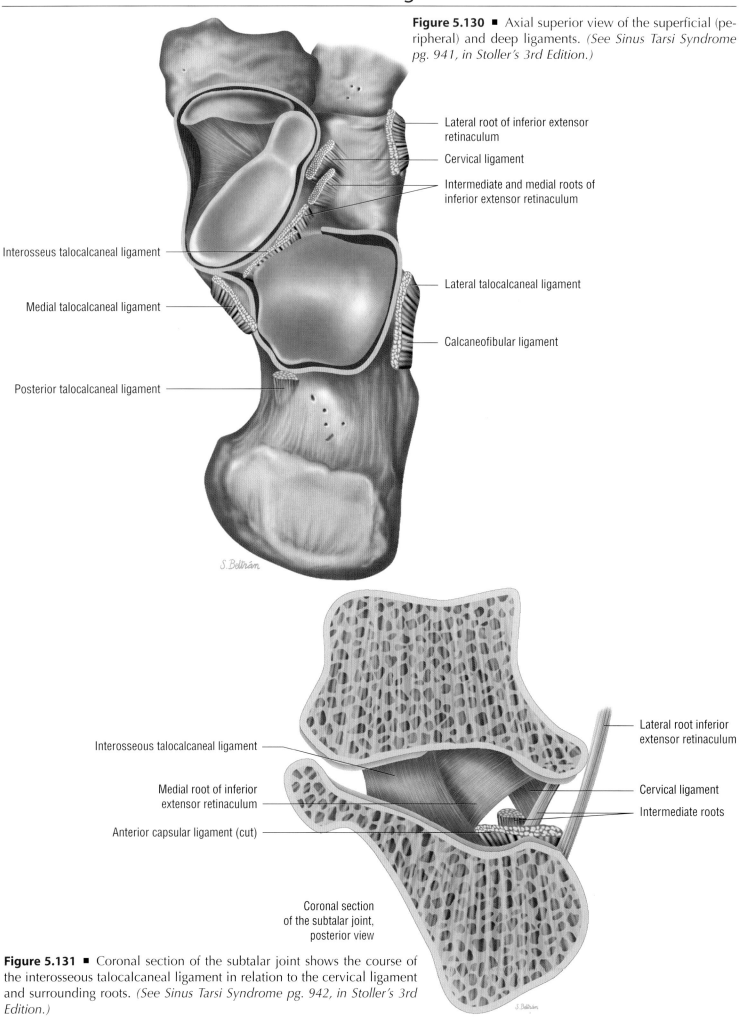

Figure 5.130 ■ Axial superior view of the superficial (peripheral) and deep ligaments. *(See Sinus Tarsi Syndrome pg. 941, in Stoller's 3rd Edition.)*

Lateral root of inferior extensor retinaculum

Cervical ligament

Intermediate and medial roots of inferior extensor retinaculum

Interosseus talocalcaneal ligament

Lateral talocalcaneal ligament

Medial talocalcaneal ligament

Calcaneofibular ligament

Posterior talocalcaneal ligament

S. Beltrán

Interosseous talocalcaneal ligament

Lateral root inferior extensor retinaculum

Medial root of inferior extensor retinaculum

Cervical ligament

Intermediate roots

Anterior capsular ligament (cut)

Coronal section of the subtalar joint, posterior view

Figure 5.131 ■ Coronal section of the subtalar joint shows the course of the interosseous talocalcaneal ligament in relation to the cervical ligament and surrounding roots. *(See Sinus Tarsi Syndrome pg. 942, in Stoller's 3rd Edition.)*

Figure 5.132 ▪ **Sinus tarsi syndrome with synovitis of the synovial recesses and inflammation of the fat contained within the sinus tarsi.** The majority of cases of sinus tarsi syndrome involve trauma, usually related to a significant inversion sprain. Scarring and degenerative changes to the soft-tissue structures of the sinus tarsi are associated with pain. *(See Sinus Tarsi Syndrome pg. 943, in Stoller's 3rd Edition.)*

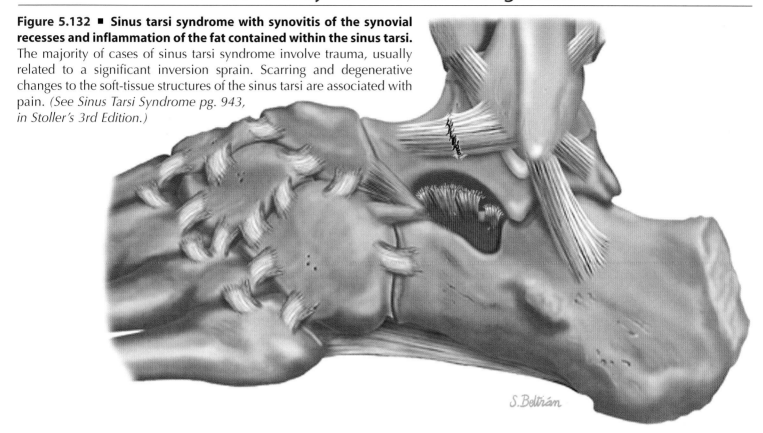

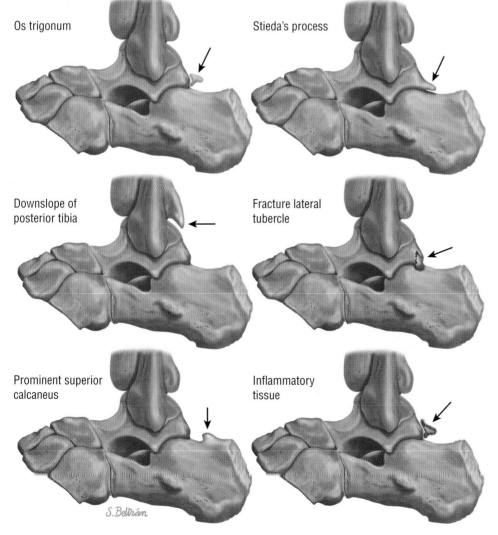

Os trigonum

Stieda's process

Downslope of posterior tibia

Fracture lateral tubercle

Prominent superior calcaneus

Inflammatory tissue

Figure 5.133 ▪ Lateral perspective color illustrations of the os trigonum and related anatomic structures in the differential diagnosis of posterior impingement. *(See Os Trigonum Syndrome pg. 945, in Stoller's 3rd Edition.)*

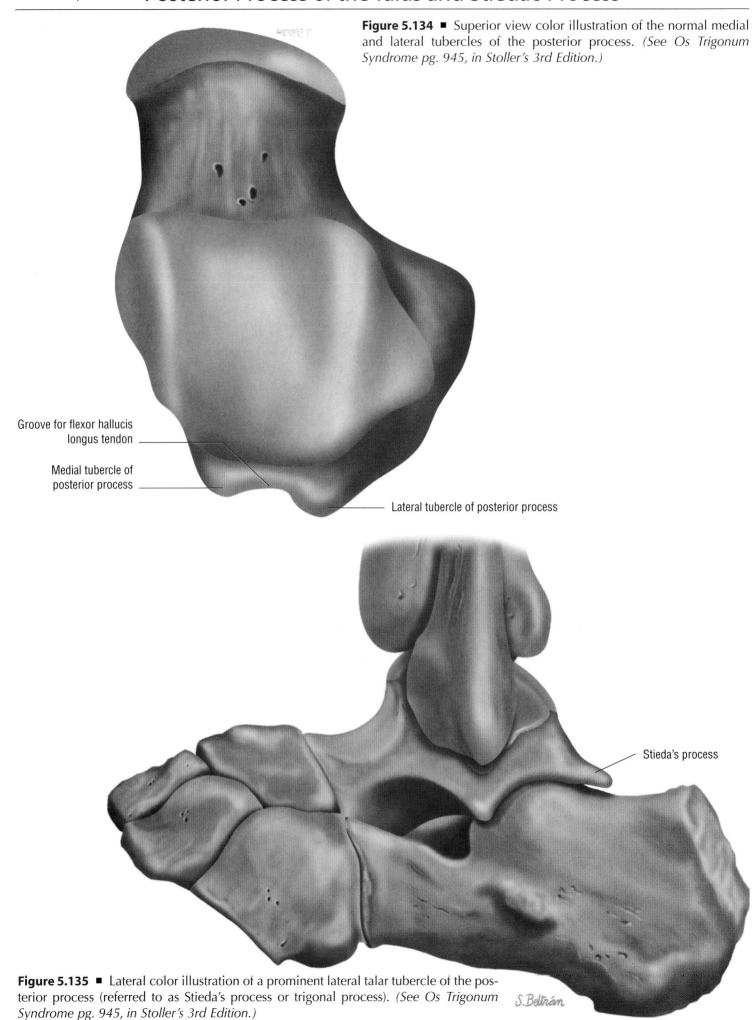

Figure 5.134 ■ Superior view color illustration of the normal medial and lateral tubercles of the posterior process. *(See Os Trigonum Syndrome pg. 945, in Stoller's 3rd Edition.)*

Groove for flexor hallucis longus tendon

Medial tubercle of posterior process

Lateral tubercle of posterior process

Stieda's process

Figure 5.135 ■ Lateral color illustration of a prominent lateral talar tubercle of the posterior process (referred to as Stieda's process or trigonal process). *(See Os Trigonum Syndrome pg. 945, in Stoller's 3rd Edition.)*

S. Beltrán

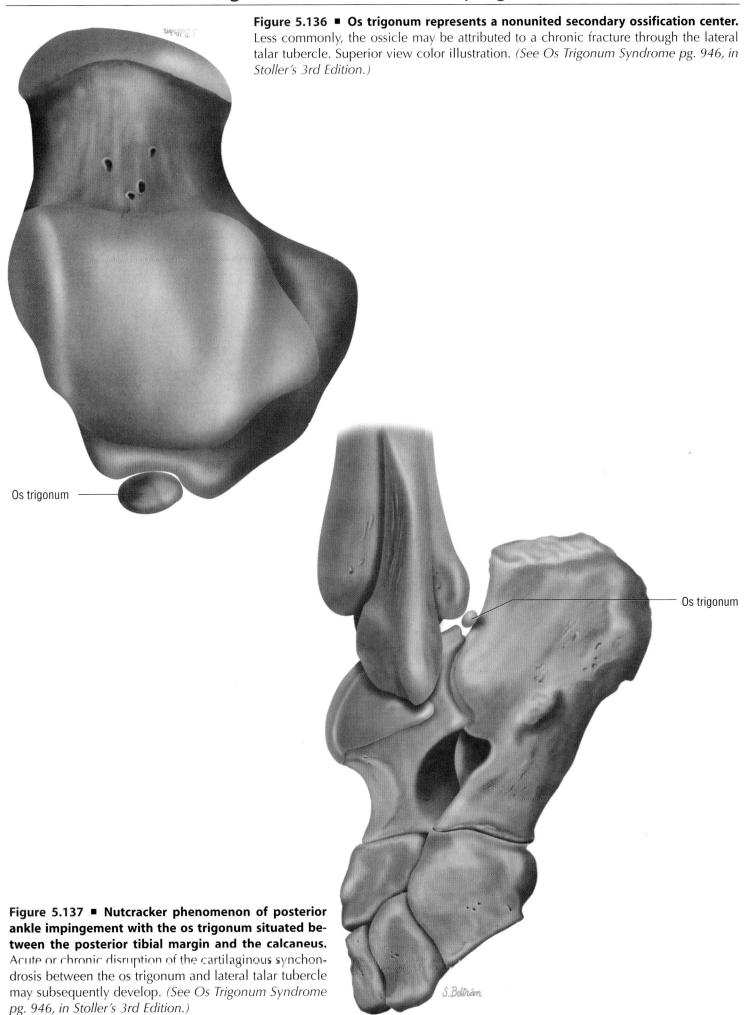

Figure 5.136 ▪ Os trigonum represents a nonunited secondary ossification center. Less commonly, the ossicle may be attributed to a chronic fracture through the lateral talar tubercle. Superior view color illustration. *(See Os Trigonum Syndrome pg. 946, in Stoller's 3rd Edition.)*

Os trigonum

Os trigonum

Figure 5.137 ▪ Nutcracker phenomenon of posterior ankle impingement with the os trigonum situated between the posterior tibial margin and the calcaneus. Acute or chronic disruption of the cartilaginous synchondrosis between the os trigonum and lateral talar tubercle may subsequently develop. *(See Os Trigonum Syndrome pg. 946, in Stoller's 3rd Edition.)*

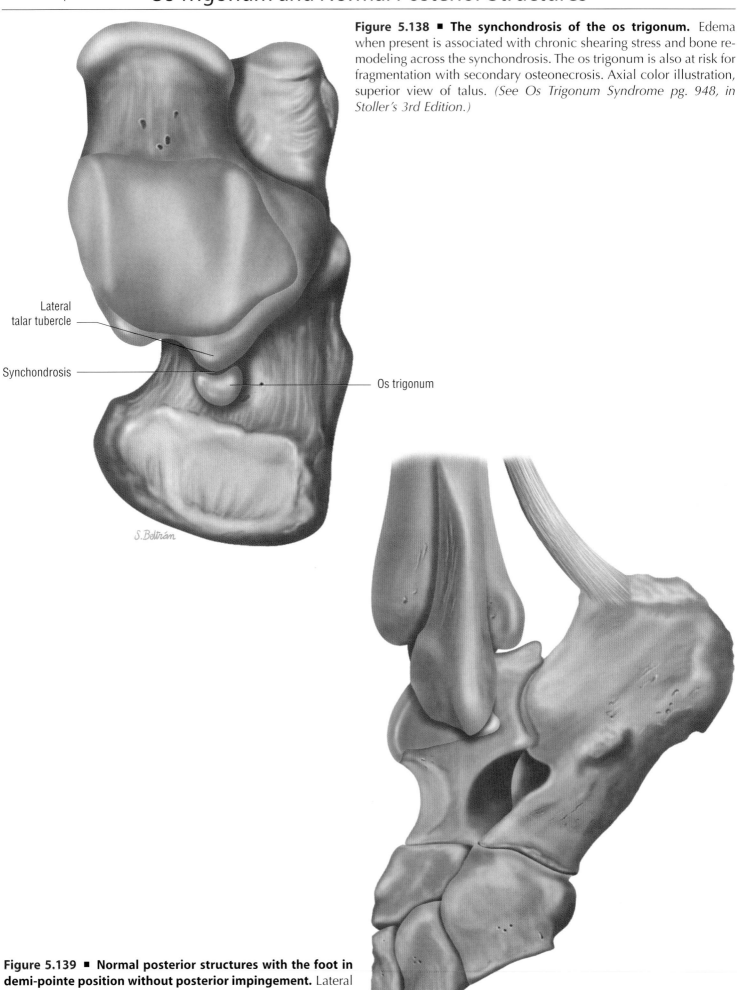

Figure 5.138 ▪ The synchondrosis of the os trigonum. Edema when present is associated with chronic shearing stress and bone remodeling across the synchondrosis. The os trigonum is also at risk for fragmentation with secondary osteonecrosis. Axial color illustration, superior view of talus. *(See Os Trigonum Syndrome pg. 948, in Stoller's 3rd Edition.)*

Lateral
talar tubercle

Synchondrosis

Os trigonum

S.Beltrán

Figure 5.139 ▪ Normal posterior structures with the foot in demi-pointe position without posterior impingement. Lateral color illustration. *(See Os Trigonum Syndrome pg. 950, in Stoller's 3rd Edition.)*

S.Beltrán

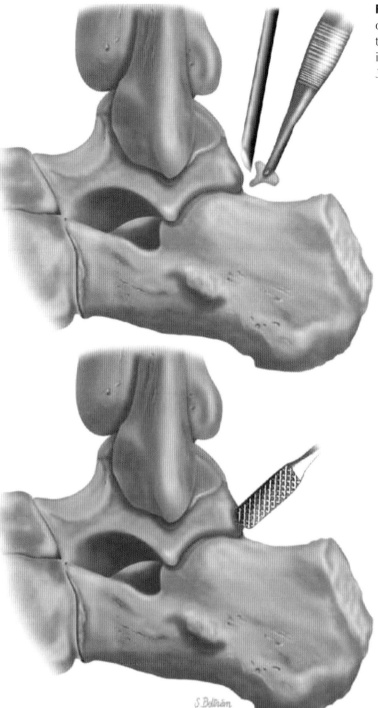

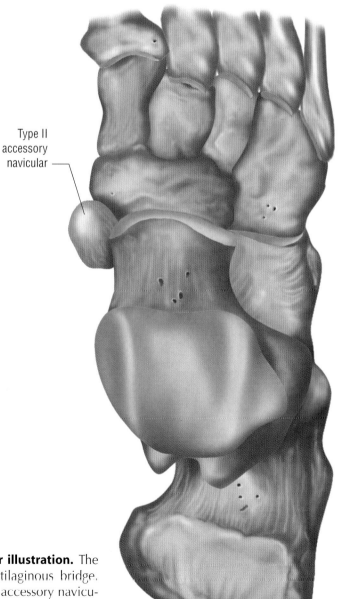

Figure 5.140 ▪ **Excision of an os trigonum.** A nonunion of the os trigonum shows significant motion at its fibrous attachment to the talus and irregularity and chondromalacia and fibrosis at its insertion. *(See Os Trigonum Syndrome pg. 951, in Stoller's 3rd Edition.)*

Type II accessory navicular

Figure 5.141 ▪ **Type II accessory navicular on a superior view color illustration.** The connection of the accessory ossification is through a fibrous or cartilaginous bridge. Repetitive contraction of the tibialis posterior tendon insertion onto the accessory navicular can generate painful shearing forces across the synchondrosis at the level of the medial aspect of the midfoot. *(See Accessory Navicular pg. 953, in Stoller's 3rd Edition.)*

Figure 5.142 ▪ **Hallux MTP capsular-ligamentous-sesamoid complex demonstrates the relationship of the plantar plate distal to the sesamoids and between the sesamoid-phalangeal ligaments.** The plantar plate is a strong fibrous structure that has a firm attachment to the proximal phalanx and a less substantial attachment to the metatarsal neck. The medial and lateral collateral ligaments consist of an MTP and a metatarsosesamoid ligament. The medial and lateral sesamoid-phalangeal ligaments are directly adjacent to the plantar plate and also bridge and stabilize the sesamoids to the proximal phalanx. *(See Turf Toe pg. 958, in Stoller's 3rd Edition.)*

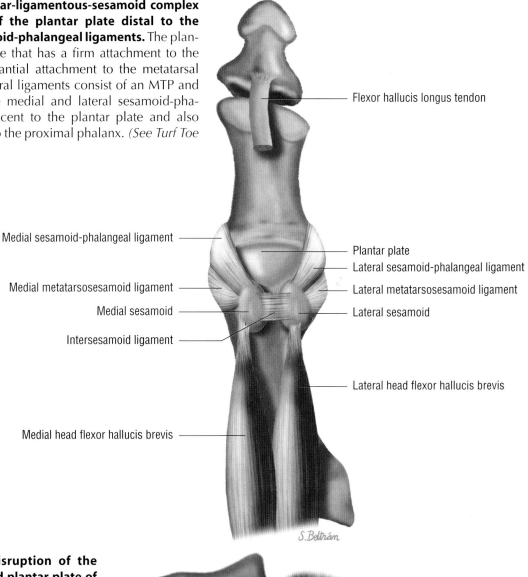

Flexor hallucis longus tendon

Medial sesamoid-phalangeal ligament

Plantar plate
Lateral sesamoid-phalangeal ligament

Medial metatarsosesamoid ligament

Lateral metatarsosesamoid ligament

Medial sesamoid

Lateral sesamoid

Intersesamoid ligament

Lateral head flexor hallucis brevis

Medial head flexor hallucis brevis

S. Beltrán

Figure 5.143 ▪ **Turf toe with disruption of the sesamoid-phalangeal ligament and plantar plate of the first (hallux) MTP joint.** Lateral color illustration of a retracted sesamoid and disruption of the plantar plate complex. *(See Turf Toe pg. 959, in Stoller's 3rd Edition.)*

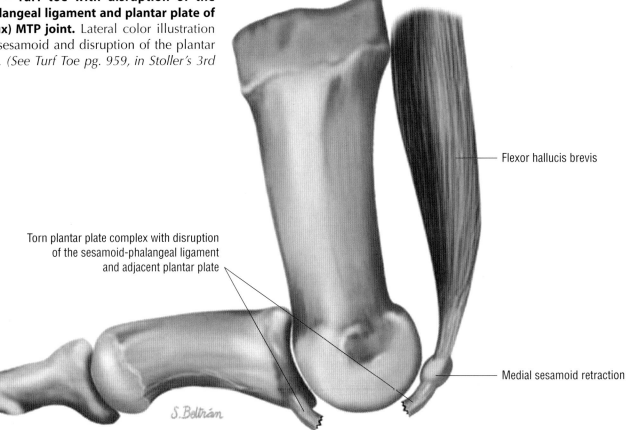

Flexor hallucis brevis

Torn plantar plate complex with disruption of the sesamoid-phalangeal ligament and adjacent plantar plate

Medial sesamoid retraction

S. Beltrán

Figure 5.144 ■ Hyperextension mechanism of injury to the first metatarsophalangeal joint in turf toe. *(See Turf Toe pg. 959, in Stoller's 3rd Edition.)*

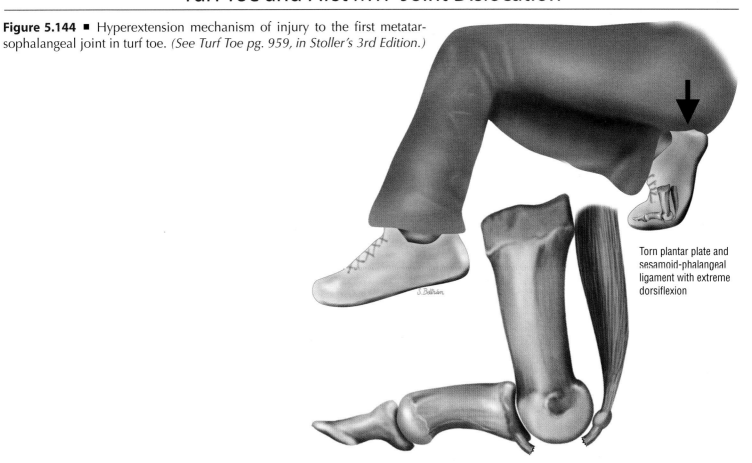

Torn plantar plate and sesamoid-phalangeal ligament with extreme dorsiflexion

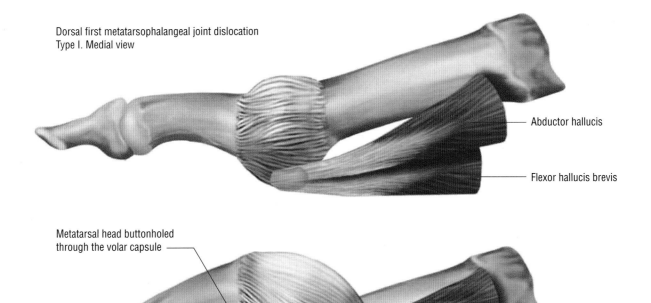

Dorsal first metatarsophalangeal joint dislocation Type I. Medial view

Abductor hallucis

Flexor hallucis brevis

Metatarsal head buttonholed through the volar capsule

Figure 5.145 ■ **Dorsal first metatarsophalangeal joint dislocation with the first metatarsal and buttonholed through the volar joint capsule.** The intact inters-esamoid ligament, plantar plate complex, and conjoint tendon attachments prevent reduction. *Based on Coughlin MJ, Mann RA, Saltzman CL. Surgery of the foot and ankle. Philadelphia: Mosby Elsevier, 2007. (See Turf Toe pgs. 952, 954, and 955–961, in Stoller's 3rd Edition.)*

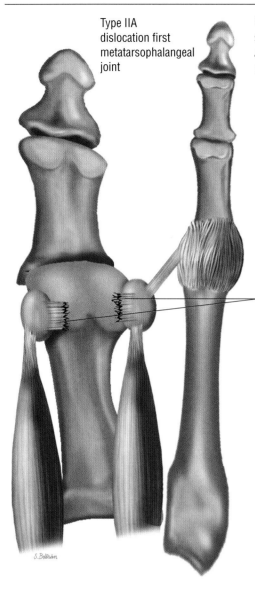

Type IIA dislocation first metatarsophalangeal joint

Intersesamoid ligament disruption

Figure 5.146 ▪ First metatarsophalangeal joint dislocation with a torn interosseous sesamoid ligament. *Based on Coughlin MJ, Mann RA, Saltzman CL. Surgery of the foot and ankle. Philadelphia: Mosby Elsevier, 2007. (See Turf Toe pgs. 952, 954, and 955–961, in Stoller's 3rd Edition.)*

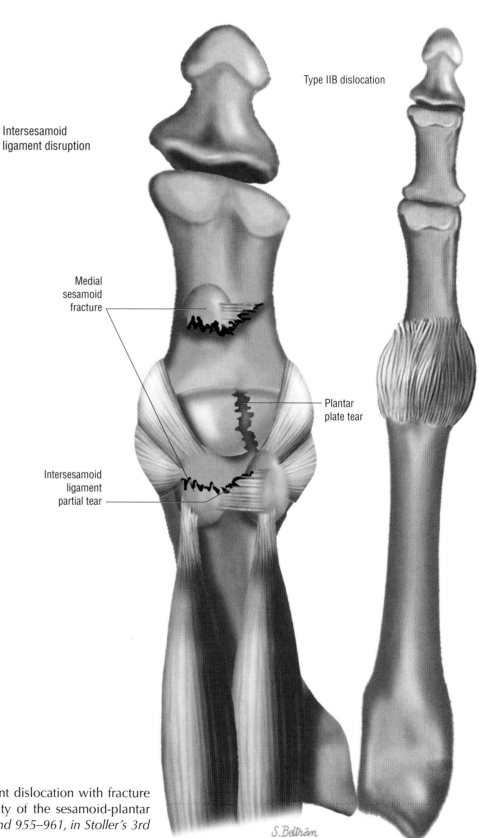

Type IIB dislocation

Medial sesamoid fracture

Plantar plate tear

Intersesamoid ligament partial tear

Figure 5.147 ▪ First metatarsophalangeal joint dislocation with fracture of the medial sesamoid and loss of continuity of the sesamoid-plantar plate complex. *(See Turf Toe pgs. 952, 954, and 955–961, in Stoller's 3rd Edition.)*

Figure 5.148 ■ Turf toe with traumatic separation of a bipartite sesamoid. The sesamoid-phalangeal ligament and plantar plate were intact. Lateral color illustration. *(See Turf Toe pg. 960, in Stoller's 3rd Edition.)*

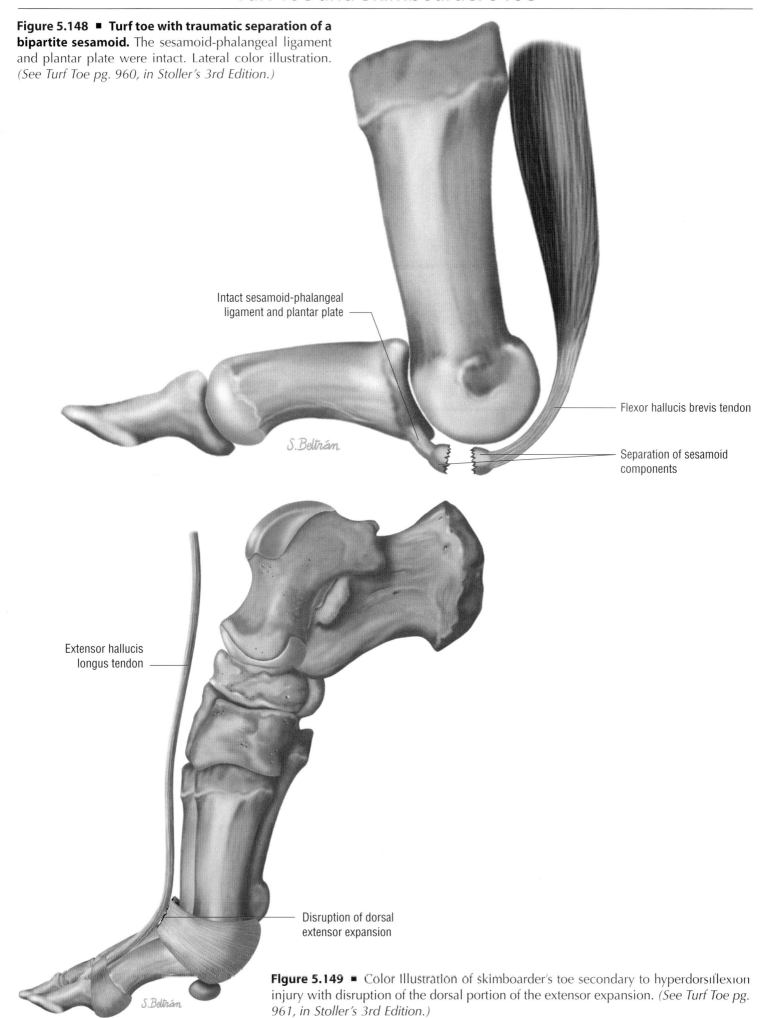

Intact sesamoid-phalangeal ligament and plantar plate

Flexor hallucis brevis tendon

Separation of sesamoid components

S.Beltrán

Extensor hallucis longus tendon

Disruption of dorsal extensor expansion

Figure 5.149 ■ Color illustration of skimboarder's toe secondary to hyperdorsiflexion injury with disruption of the dorsal portion of the extensor expansion. *(See Turf Toe pg. 961, in Stoller's 3rd Edition.)*

S.Beltrán

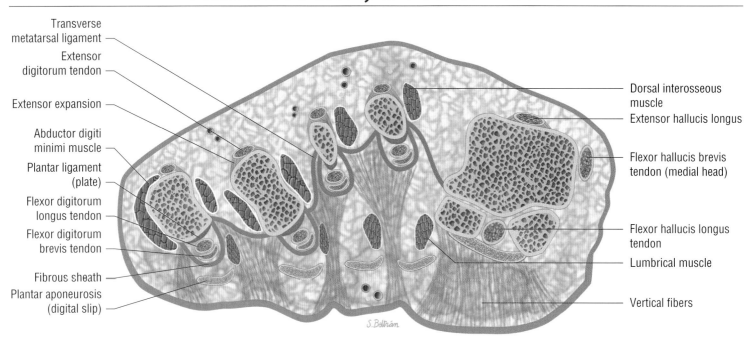

Transverse metatarsal ligament

Extensor digitorum tendon

Extensor expansion

Abductor digiti minimi muscle

Plantar ligament (plate)

Flexor digitorum longus tendon

Flexor digitorum brevis tendon

Fibrous sheath

Plantar aponeurosis (digital slip)

Dorsal interosseous muscle

Extensor hallucis longus

Flexor hallucis brevis tendon (medial head)

Flexor hallucis longus tendon

Lumbrical muscle

Vertical fibers

Figure 5.150 ■ Coronal color section through the sesamoids. The sesamoids vary in morphology from semiovoid to circular to bean-shaped. The medial sesamoid is usually larger and can be bi-, tri-, or quadripartite. *(See Sesamoid Dysfunction pg. 962, in Stoller's 3rd Edition.)*

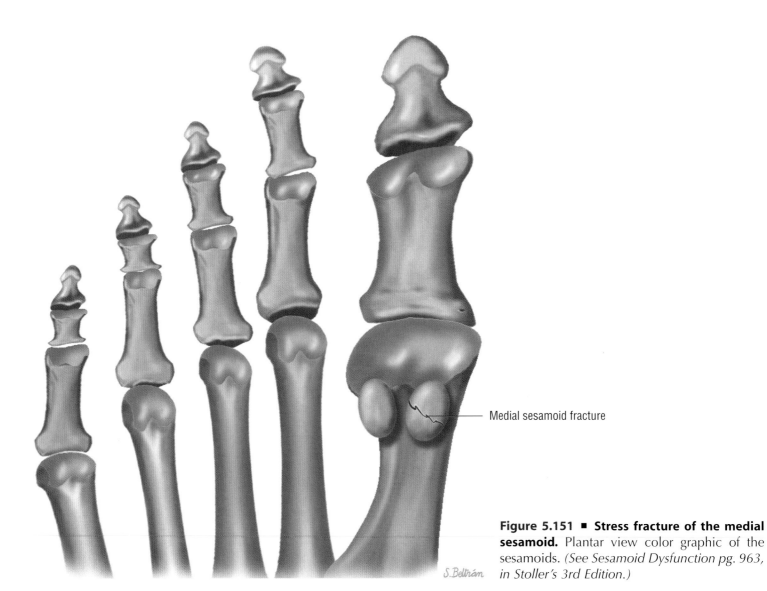

Medial sesamoid fracture

Figure 5.151 ■ Stress fracture of the medial sesamoid. Plantar view color graphic of the sesamoids. *(See Sesamoid Dysfunction pg. 963, in Stoller's 3rd Edition.)*

Figure 5.152 ▪ Hallux valgus deformity on superior view color illustration. There is subluxation of the first MTP base. With subluxation of the tibial sesamoid there is erosion of the crista of the metatarsal head. The crista normally helps maintain alignment and prevents lateral subluxation of the tibial sesamoid. The first metatarsal may deviate both medially and dorsally. Metatarsus primus varus (medial inclination of the first metatarsal) with dorsal splaying of the first and fifth metatarsal heads occurs in hallux valgus. *(See Sesamoid Dysfunction pg. 964, in Stoller's 3rd Edition.)*

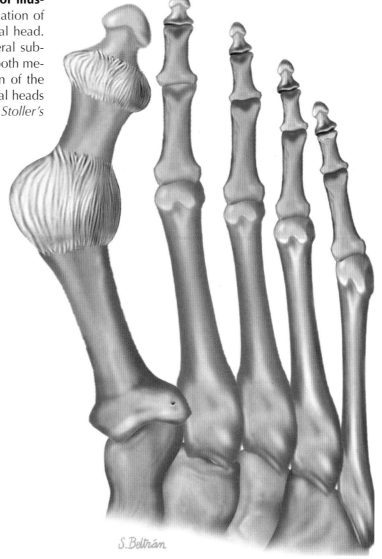

Dorsal osteophyte

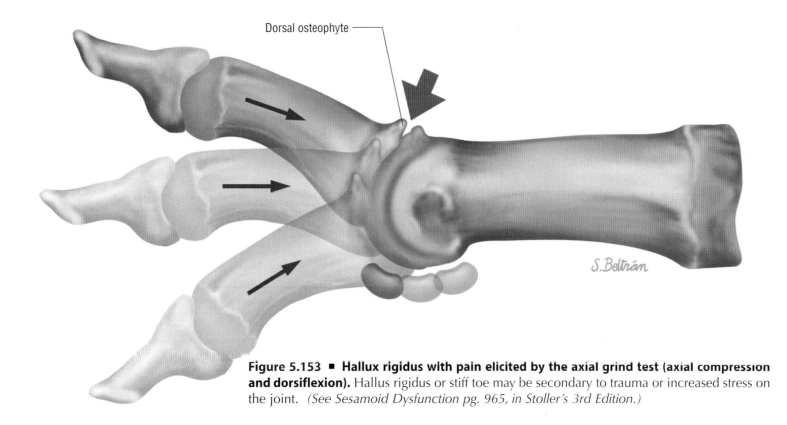

Figure 5.153 ▪ Hallux rigidus with pain elicited by the axial grind test (axial compression and dorsiflexion). Hallus rigidus or stiff toe may be secondary to trauma or increased stress on the joint. *(See Sesamoid Dysfunction pg. 965, in Stoller's 3rd Edition.)*

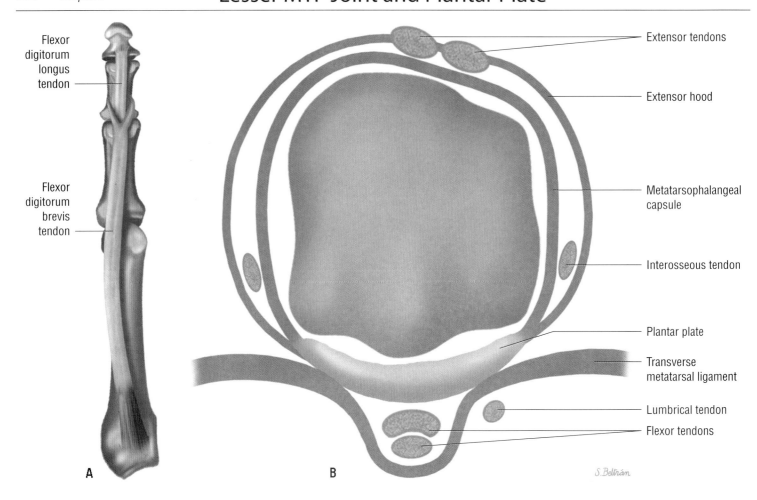

Flexor digitorum longus tendon

Flexor digitorum brevis tendon

Extensor tendons

Extensor hood

Metatarsophalangeal capsule

Interosseous tendon

Plantar plate

Transverse metatarsal ligament

Lumbrical tendon

Flexor tendons

A

B

S. Beltrán

Figure 5.154 ■ **(A)** Flexor digitorum longus and brevis insertions. **(B)** Axial section of the lesser toe metatarsal head at the level of the metatarsophalangeal joint. *Based on Coughlin MJ, Mann RA, Saltzman CL. Surgery of the foot and ankle. Philadelphia: Mosby Elsevier, 2007. (See Plantar Plate Injuries of the Lesser Metatarsophalangeal Joints pg. 965–968, in Stoller's 3rd Edition.)*

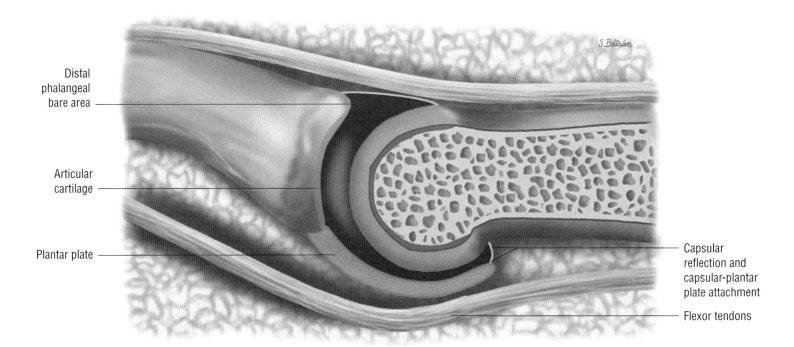

Distal phalangeal bare area

Articular cartilage

Plantar plate

Capsular reflection and capsular-plantar plate attachment

Flexor tendons

Figure 5.155 ■ **MTP joint plantar plate anatomy.** The plantar plate is directly deep to the superior border of the flexor tendons. There is normal undercutting of the plantar plate at the base of the proximal phalanx at the interface with hyaline articular cartilage. Lateral view color illustration. *(See Plantar Plate Injuries of the Lesser Metatarsophalangeal Joints pg. 967, in Stoller's 3rd Edition.)*

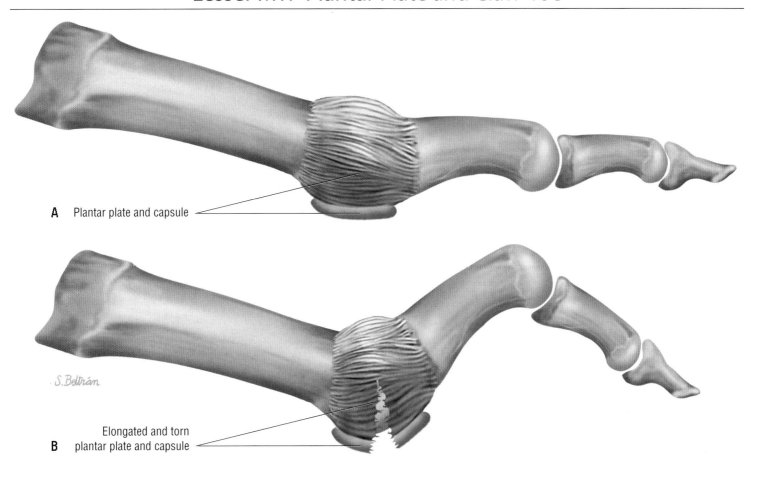

A Plantar plate and capsule

B Elongated and torn plantar plate and capsule

Figure 5.156 ■ Lesser MTP joint plantar plate and capsule intact **(A)** and disrupted **(B)**. *(See Plantar Plate Injuries of the Lesser Metatarsophalangeal Joints pg. 968, in Stoller's 3rd Edition.)*

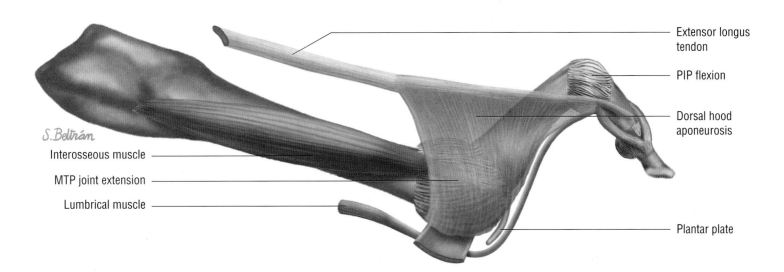

Extensor longus tendon

PIP flexion

Dorsal hood aponeurosis

Interosseous muscle

MTP joint extension

Lumbrical muscle

Plantar plate

Figure 5.157 ■ **A claw-toe deformity represents a hammertoe deformity (flexion deformity at the PIP joint with MP dorsiflexion and the DIP in neutral or hyperextension) with the addition of a hyperextension deformity at the MP joint.** Hammertoe and claw toe are examples of sagittal plane deformities. Lateral color illustration. *(See Plantar Plate Injuries of the Lesser Metatarsophalangeal Joints pg. 969, in Stoller's 3rd Edition.)*

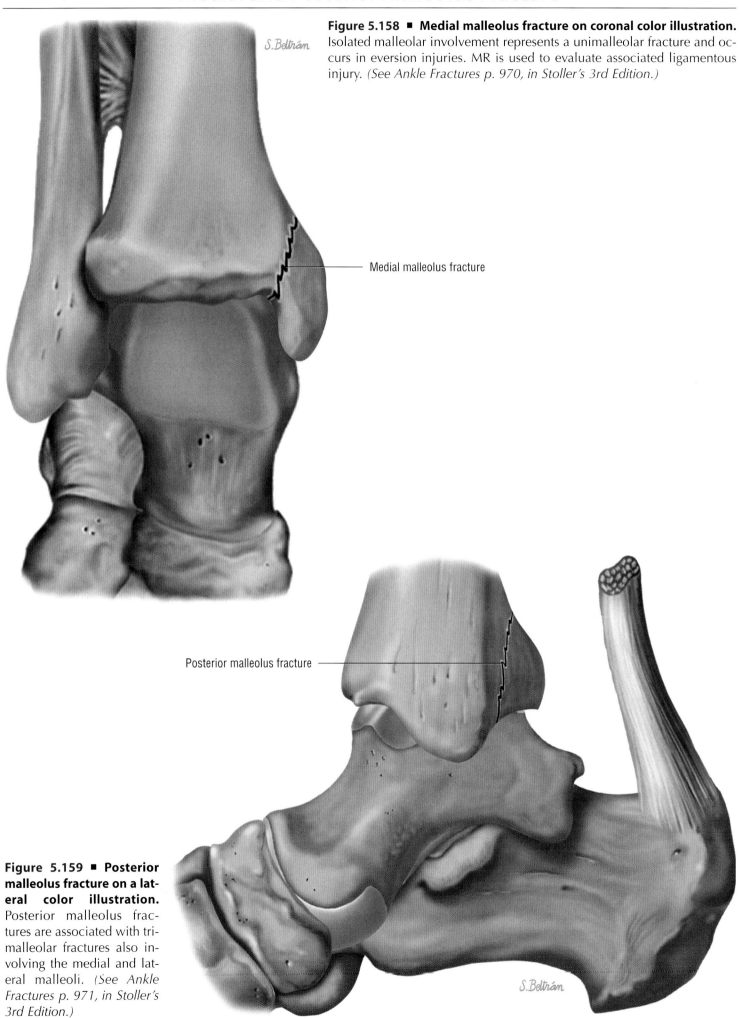

Figure 5.158 ■ Medial malleolus fracture on coronal color illustration. Isolated malleolar involvement represents a unimalleolar fracture and occurs in eversion injuries. MR is used to evaluate associated ligamentous injury. *(See Ankle Fractures p. 970, in Stoller's 3rd Edition.)*

Medial malleolus fracture

Posterior malleolus fracture

Figure 5.159 ■ Posterior malleolus fracture on a lateral color illustration. Posterior malleolus fractures are associated with trimalleolar fractures also involving the medial and lateral malleoli. *(See Ankle Fractures p. 971, in Stoller's 3rd Edition.)*

Tillaux and Triplane Fracture

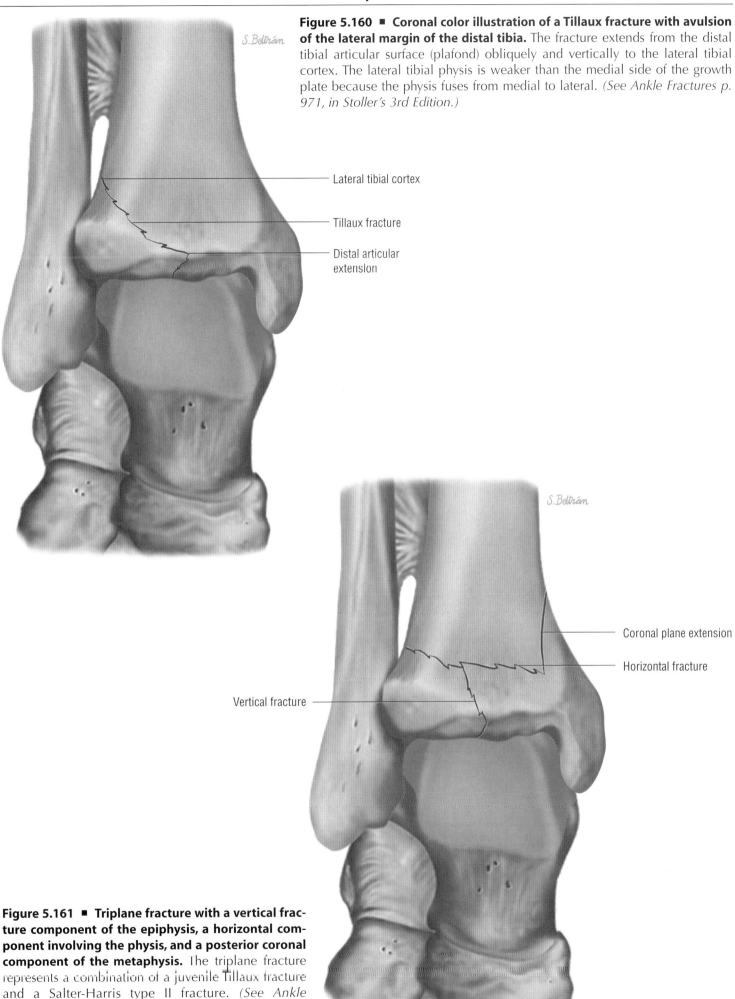

Figure 5.160 ■ **Coronal color illustration of a Tillaux fracture with avulsion of the lateral margin of the distal tibia.** The fracture extends from the distal tibial articular surface (plafond) obliquely and vertically to the lateral tibial cortex. The lateral tibial physis is weaker than the medial side of the growth plate because the physis fuses from medial to lateral. *(See Ankle Fractures p. 971, in Stoller's 3rd Edition.)*

Lateral tibial cortex

Tillaux fracture

Distal articular extension

Coronal plane extension

Horizontal fracture

Vertical fracture

Figure 5.161 ■ **Triplane fracture with a vertical fracture component of the epiphysis, a horizontal component involving the physis, and a posterior coronal component of the metaphysis.** The triplane fracture represents a combination of a juvenile Tillaux fracture and a Salter-Harris type II fracture. *(See Ankle Fractures p. 972, in Stoller's 3rd Edition.)*

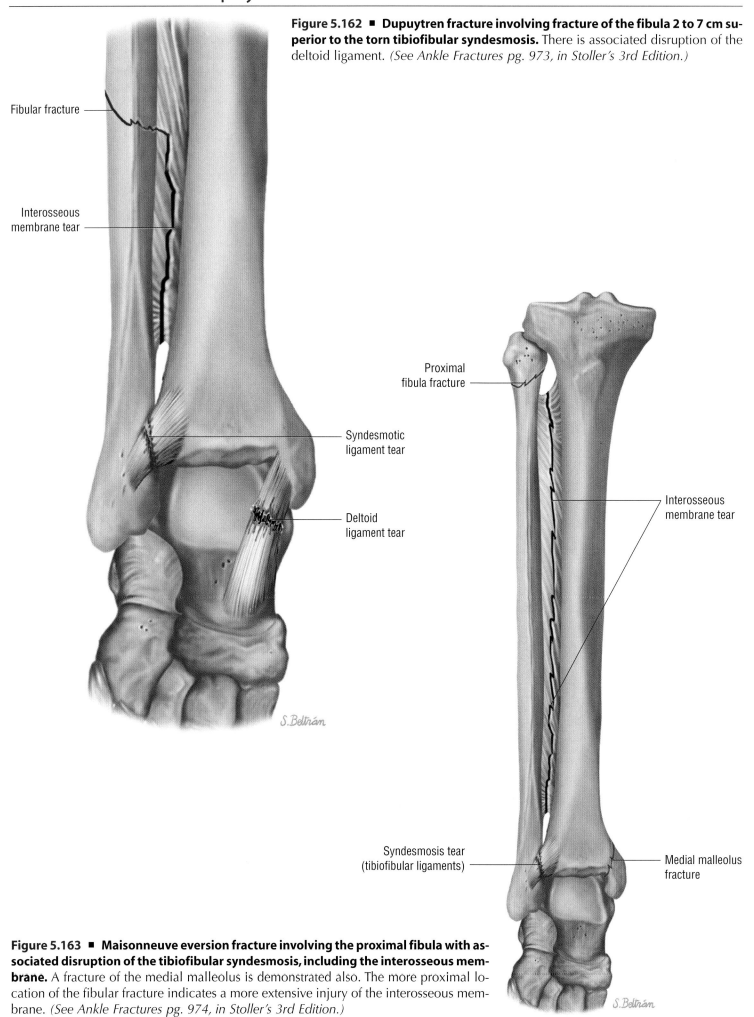

Fibular fracture

Interosseous membrane tear

Figure 5.162 ▪ Dupuytren fracture involving fracture of the fibula 2 to 7 cm superior to the torn tibiofibular syndesmosis. There is associated disruption of the deltoid ligament. *(See Ankle Fractures pg. 973, in Stoller's 3rd Edition.)*

Syndesmotic ligament tear

Deltoid ligament tear

Proximal fibula fracture

Interosseous membrane tear

Syndesmosis tear (tibiofibular ligaments)

Medial malleolus fracture

S. Beltrán

Figure 5.163 ▪ Maisonneuve eversion fracture involving the proximal fibula with associated disruption of the tibiofibular syndesmosis, including the interosseous membrane. A fracture of the medial malleolus is demonstrated also. The more proximal location of the fibular fracture indicates a more extensive injury of the interosseous membrane. *(See Ankle Fractures pg. 974, in Stoller's 3rd Edition.)*

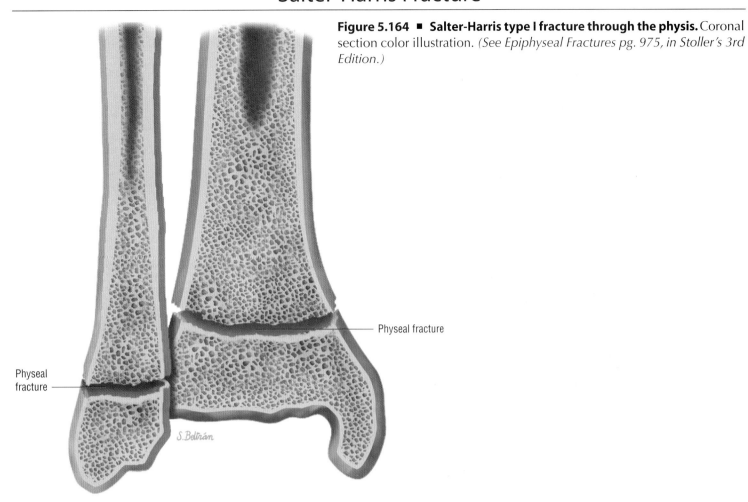

Figure 5.164 ■ **Salter-Harris type I fracture through the physis.** Coronal section color illustration. *(See Epiphyseal Fractures pg. 975, in Stoller's 3rd Edition.)*

Physeal fracture

Physeal fracture

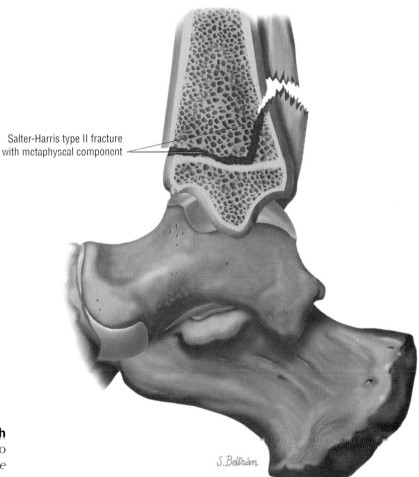

Salter-Harris type II fracture with mctaphyscal component

Figure 5.165 ■ **Salter-Harris type II fracture through the physis and metaphysis of the distal tibia.** There is no epiphyseal extension. Lateral color illustration. *(See Epiphyseal Fractures pg. 977, in Stoller's 3rd Edition.)*

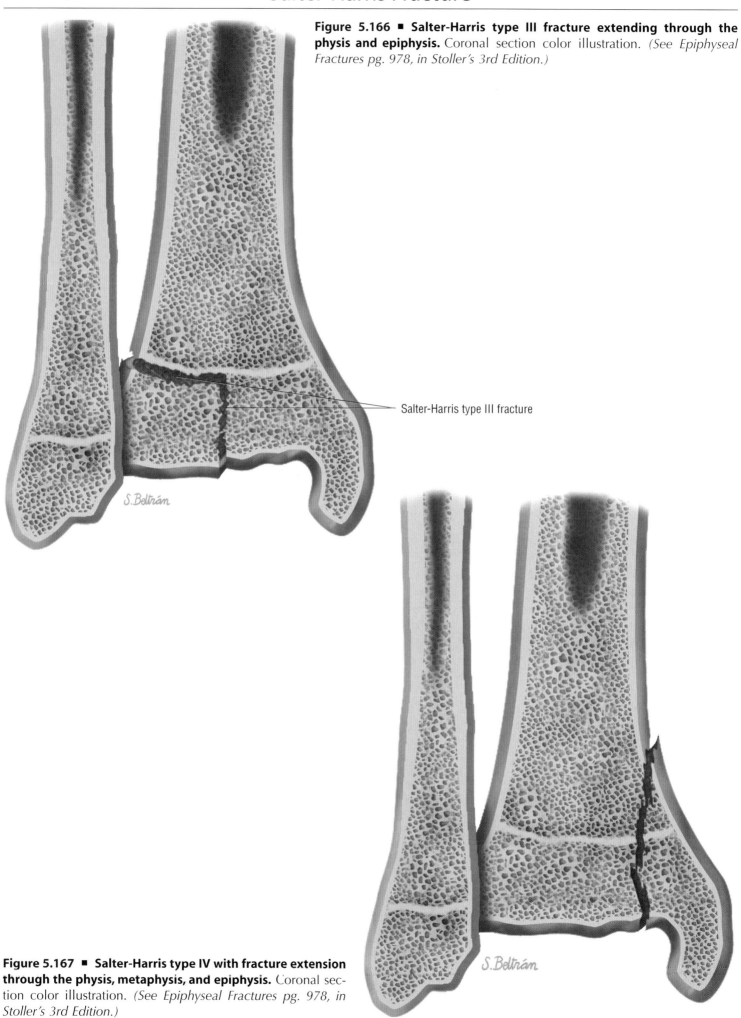

Figure 5.166 ■ Salter-Harris type III fracture extending through the physis and epiphysis. Coronal section color illustration. *(See Epiphyseal Fractures pg. 978, in Stoller's 3rd Edition.)*

Salter-Harris type III fracture

S.Beltrán

Figure 5.167 ■ Salter-Harris type IV with fracture extension through the physis, metaphysis, and epiphysis. Coronal section color illustration. *(See Epiphyseal Fractures pg. 978, in Stoller's 3rd Edition.)*

S.Beltrán

Figure 5.168 ▪ **Essex-Lopresti calcaneal fracture with central depression and subtalar extension.** Up to 75% of calcaneal fractures extend into the subtalar joint. Subtalar fracture types are subdivided further into either joint-depression or tongue-type fractures. In the Rowe classification there is subtalar joint involvement in stage IV and stage V (central depression) injuries. *(See Fractures of the Calcaneus pg. 979, in Stoller's 3rd Edition.)*

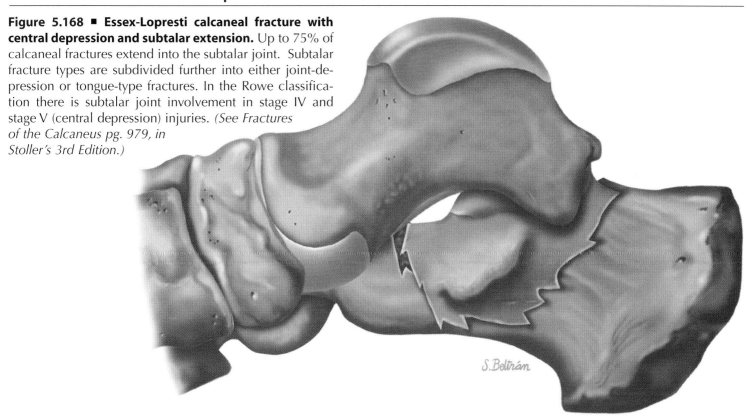

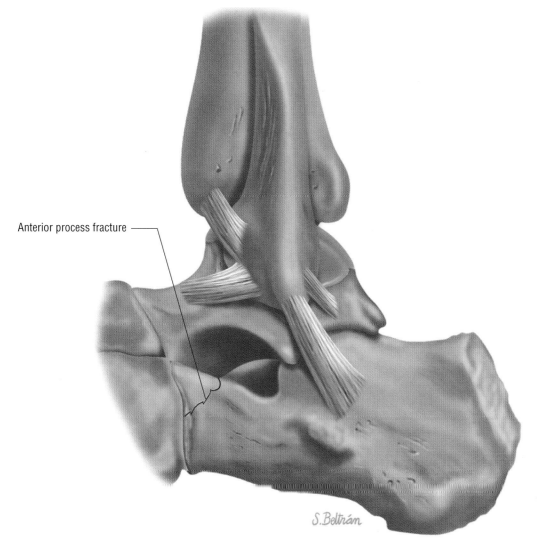

Anterior process fracture

Figure 5.169 ▪ Fracture of the anterior process of the calcaneus on a lateral perspective color illustration. *(See Fractures of the Calcaneus pg. 980, in Stoller's 3rd Edition.)*

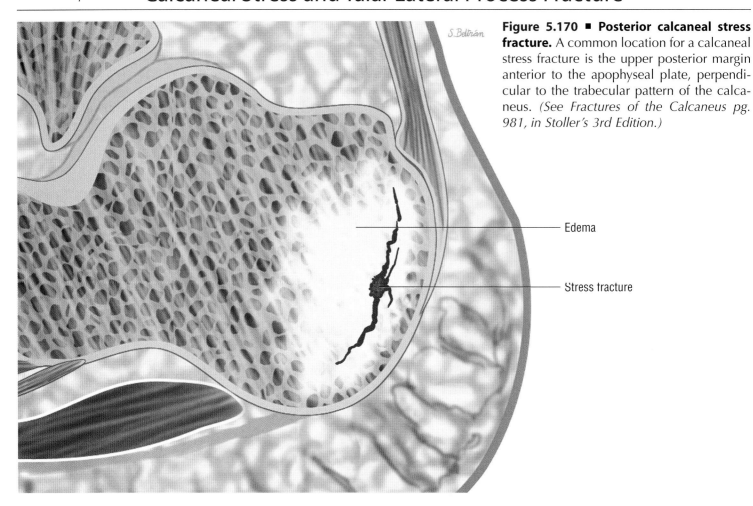

Figure 5.170 ▪ Posterior calcaneal stress fracture. A common location for a calcaneal stress fracture is the upper posterior margin anterior to the apophyseal plate, perpendicular to the trabecular pattern of the calcaneus. *(See Fractures of the Calcaneus pg. 981, in Stoller's 3rd Edition.)*

Edema

Stress fracture

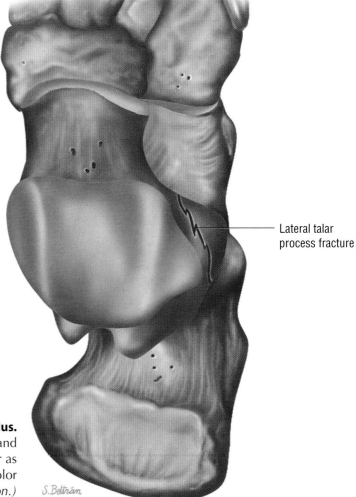

Lateral talar process fracture

Figure 5.171 ▪ Snowboarder's or lateral process fracture of the talus. The mechanism of injury is related to eversion of an axial-loaded and dorsiflexed ankle. A lateral process fracture may be classified further as a simple comminuted fracture or as a chip fracture. Superior view color illustration. *(See Fractures of the Talus pg. 982, in Stoller's 3rd Edition.)*

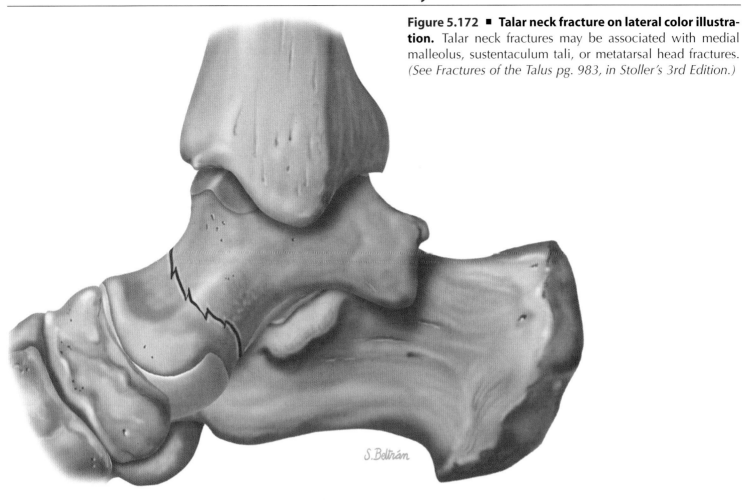

Figure 5.172 ▪ **Talar neck fracture on lateral color illustration.** Talar neck fractures may be associated with medial malleolus, sustentaculum tali, or metatarsal head fractures. *(See Fractures of the Talus pg. 983, in Stoller's 3rd Edition.)*

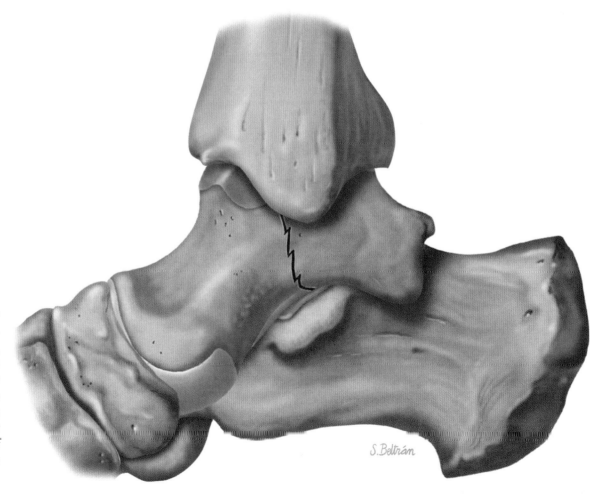

Figure 5.173 ▪ **Talar body fracture on a lateral color illustration.** The mechanism of injury is axial loading or shear force. Associated injuries include fractures of the calcaneus, tibia, or talar neck. *(See Fractures of the Talus pg. 983, in Stoller's 3rd Edition.)*

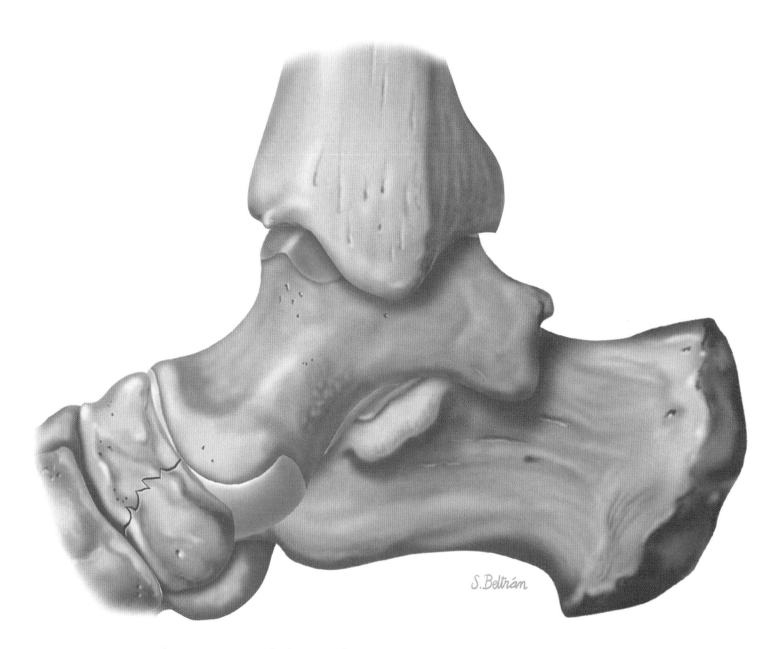

Figure 5.174 ■ **Navicular stress fracture involving the central to medial aspect of the dorsum of the navicular.** Edema is often prominent in the sagittal plane, whereas fracture morphology is visualized in the axial plane. Delayed union and nonunion are potential risks secondary to the relative avascularity and increased shear forces that occur in this region. Lateral color graphic. *(See Navicular Fractures pg. 987, in Stoller's 3rd Edition.)*

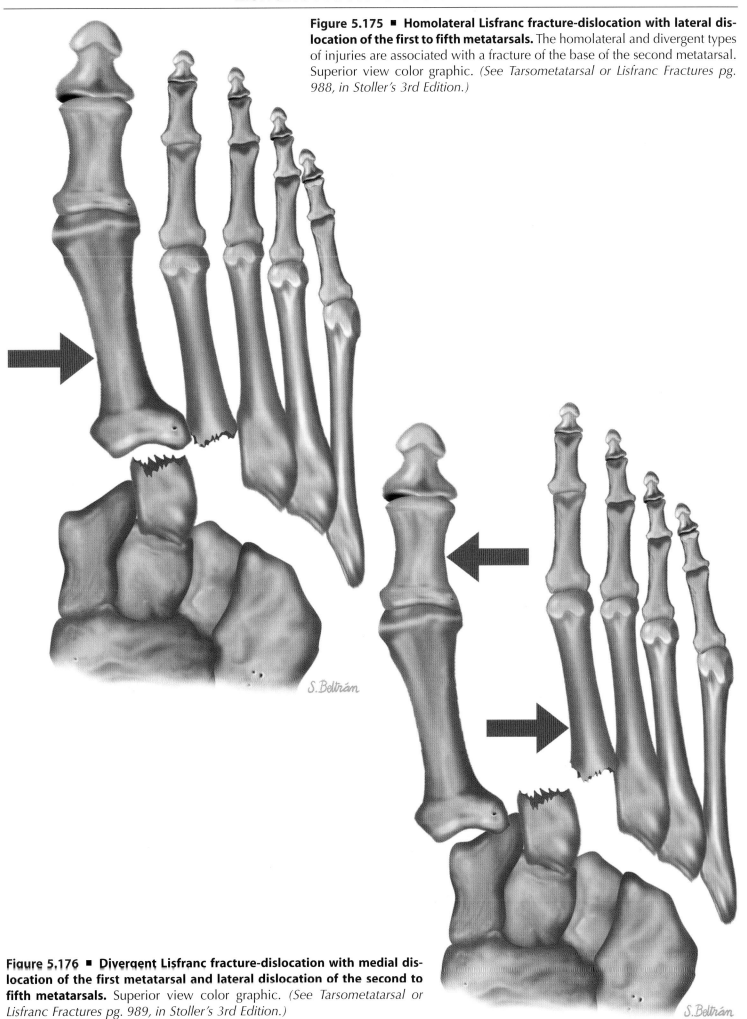

Figure 5.175 ■ **Homolateral Lisfranc fracture-dislocation with lateral dislocation of the first to fifth metatarsals.** The homolateral and divergent types of injuries are associated with a fracture of the base of the second metatarsal. Superior view color graphic. *(See Tarsometatarsal or Lisfranc Fractures pg. 988, in Stoller's 3rd Edition.)*

Figure 5.176 ■ **Divergent Lisfranc fracture-dislocation with medial dislocation of the first metatarsal and lateral dislocation of the second to fifth metatarsals.** Superior view color graphic. *(See Tarsometatarsal or Lisfranc Fractures pg. 989, in Stoller's 3rd Edition.)*

Lisfranc Fracture-Dislocation

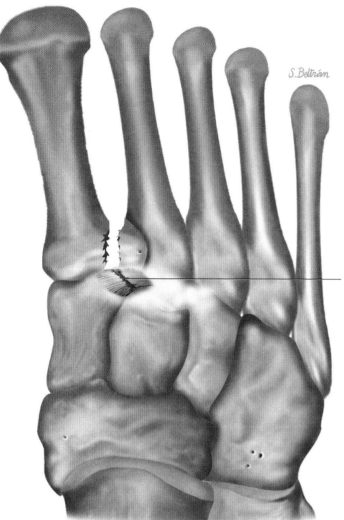

Figure 5.177 ▪ Homolateral type Lisfranc fracture-dislocation with lateral displacement. Transverse (superior view) color illustration. Associated fractures in a Lisfranc tarsometatarsal dislocation occur at the base of the second or third metatarsals, medial or intermediate cuneiforms, or the navicular bone. *(See Tarsometatarsal or Lisfranc Fractures pg. 991, in Stoller's 3rd Edition.)*

Lisfranc ligament tear

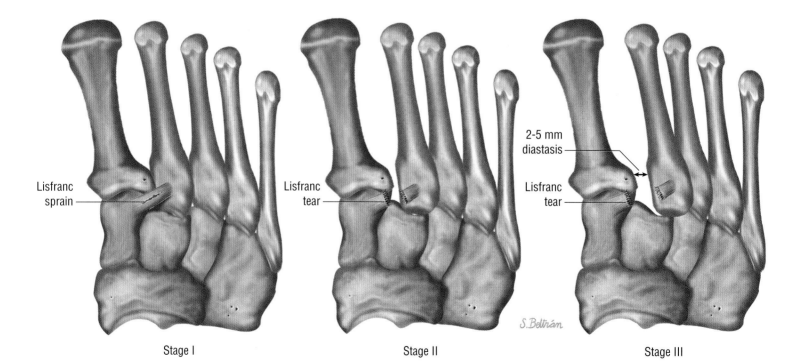

Lisfranc sprain

Lisfranc tear

Lisfranc tear

2-5 mm diastasis

Stage I

Stage II

Stage III

Figure 5.178 ▪ Classification of Lisfranc midfoot sprains. *Based on Coughlin MJ, Mann RA, Saltzman CL. Surgery of the foot and ankle. Philadelphia: Mosby Elsevier, 2007. (See Tarsometatarsal or Lisfranc Fractures pg. 988, in Stoller's 3rd Edition.)*

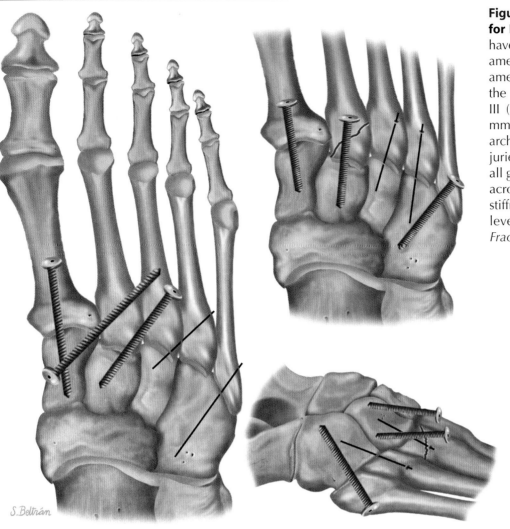

Figure 5.179 ■ Surgical fixation options for Lisfranc joint injuries. Lisfranc injuries have been classified as stage I (Lisfranc ligament sprain), stage II (ruptured Lisfranc ligament with a 2- to 5 mm diaphysis between the first and second metatarsals), and stage III (rupture of Lisfranc's ligament with >5 mm of diastasis and loss of longitudinal arch height). ORIF is used for stage III injuries. Athletes may require early ORIF for all grade 2 and 3 sprains. Screws are placed across the tarsometatarsal joint to create stiffness, support the arch, and form a rigid lever. *(See Tarsometatarsal or Lisfranc Fractures pg. 993, in Stoller's 3rd Edition.)*

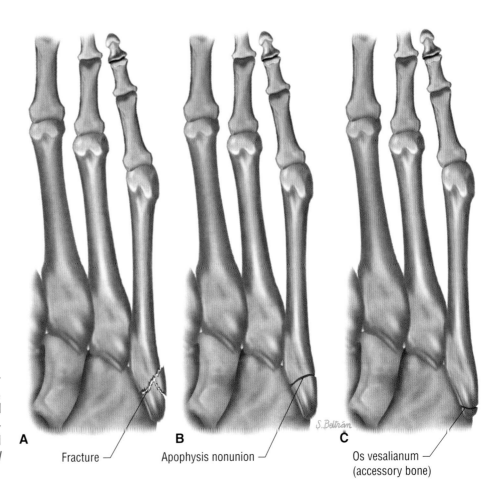

Figure 5.180 ■ Comparison of the morphology of a proximal fifth metatarsal fracture **(A)**, nonunion of the metatarsal apophysis **(B)**, and an os vesalianum **(C)**. Note the irregular margins of a fracture site and the more proximal location of the os vesalianum. *(See Metatarsal Fractures pg. 994, in Stoller's 3rd Edition.)*

A — Fracture

B — Apophysis nonunion

C — Os vesalianum (accessory bone)

Metatarsal Fractures

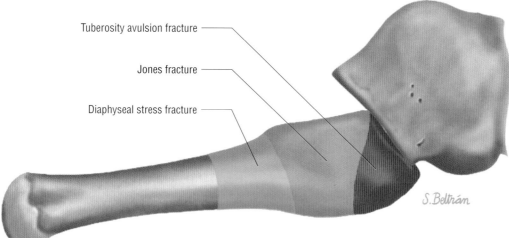

Tuberosity avulsion fracture
Jones fracture
Diaphyseal stress fracture

Figure 5.181 ▪ **Lateral color illustration of the three zones of proximal fifth metatarsal fractures:** (1) tuberosity avulsion fractures; (2) Jones fractures at the junction of the metaphysis and diaphysis; and (3) diaphyseal stress fractures. Avulsion fractures of the tuberosity are the most common type. Contraction of the peroneus brevis tendon secondary to an inversion injury may result in this fracture. The Jones fracture and more distal diaphyseal stress fractures are susceptible to nonunion. *(See Metatarsal Fractures pg. 994, in Stoller's 3rd Edition.)*

Figure 5.182 ▪ **Open reduction and internal fixation of a Jones fracture.** Displaced fractures often require open reduction and internal fixation. Screw fixation and bone grafting are also treatment options. *(See Metatarsal Fractures pg. 994, in Stoller's 3rd Edition.)*

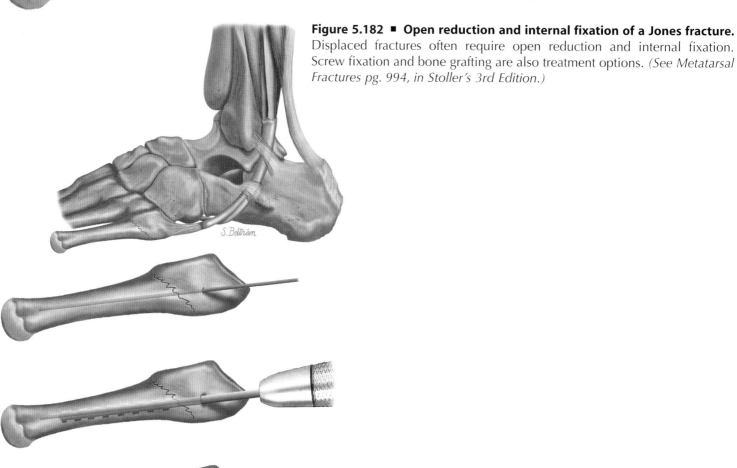

Figure 5.183 ▪ **Second metatarsal base stress fractures are frequently seen in ballet dancers.** Cessation of training for up to 6 weeks or until pain with weight-bearing subsides, is necessary for healing. MR findings may persist after clinical healing. Lateral color illustration. *(See Metatarsal Fractures pg. 997, in Stoller's 3rd Edition.)*

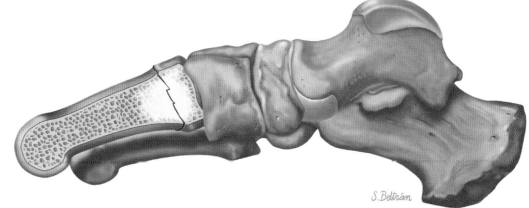

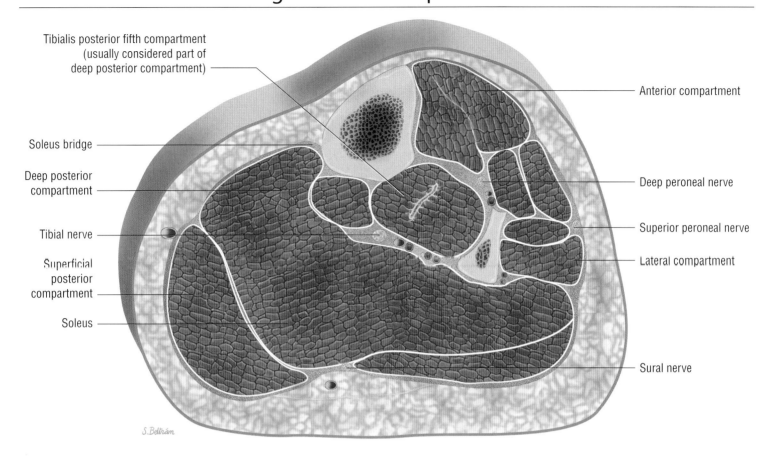

Tibialis posterior fifth compartment (usually considered part of deep posterior compartment)

Soleus bridge

Deep posterior compartment

Tibial nerve

Superficial posterior compartment

Soleus

Anterior compartment

Deep peroneal nerve

Superior peroneal nerve

Lateral compartment

Sural nerve

Figure 5.184 ■ Compartments of the leg. The soleus bridge consists of the tough superficial investing fascia of the soleus and inserts along the posteromedial border of the tibia. *(See Compartment Syndrome pgs. 996–1000, in Stoller's 3rd Edition.)*

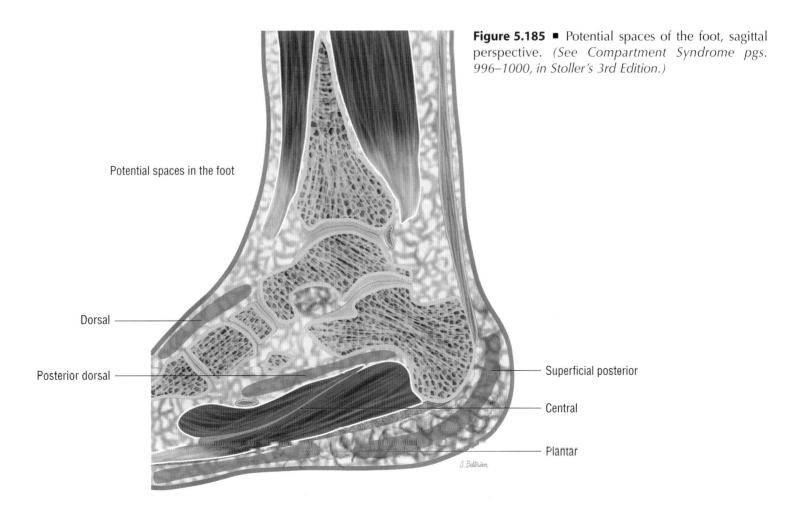

Figure 5.185 ■ Potential spaces of the foot, sagittal perspective. *(See Compartment Syndrome pgs. 996–1000, in Stoller's 3rd Edition.)*

Potential spaces in the foot

Dorsal

Posterior dorsal

Superficial posterior

Central

Plantar

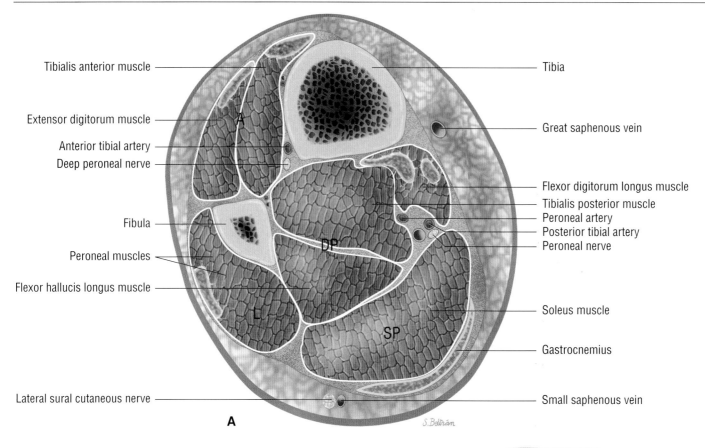

Tibialis anterior muscle

Extensor digitorum muscle

Anterior tibial artery

Deep peroneal nerve

Fibula

Peroneal muscles

Flexor hallucis longus muscle

Lateral sural cutaneous nerve

Tibia

Great saphenous vein

Flexor digitorum longus muscle

Tibialis posterior muscle

Peroneal artery

Posterior tibial artery

Peroneal nerve

Soleus muscle

Gastrocnemius

Small saphenous vein

A

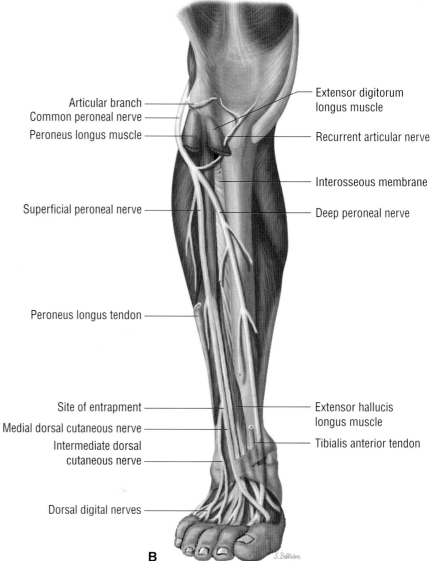

Articular branch

Common peroneal nerve

Peroneus longus muscle

Superficial peroneal nerve

Peroneus longus tendon

Site of entrapment

Medial dorsal cutaneous nerve

Intermediate dorsal
cutaneous nerve

Dorsal digital nerves

Extensor digitorum
longus muscle

Recurrent articular nerve

Interosseous membrane

Deep peroneal nerve

Extensor hallucis
longus muscle

Tibialis anterior tendon

B

Figure 5.186 ■ **(A)** The lower leg contains four major compartments (A, L, SP, DP): the anterior compartment, the lateral compartment, the superficial posterior compartment, and the deep posterior compartment. The tibialis posterior is sometimes classified as its own separate compartment and not grouped with the deep posterior compartment. **(B)** Anterior color illustration showing the relationship of the deep peroneal nerve to the anterior compartment. Weakness of dorsiflexion or toe extension, paresthesias of the dorsum of the foot, first web space numbness, and foot drop may be seen in anterior compartment syndrome. The superficial peroneal nerve is contained within the lateral compartment. The sural nerve is within the superficial posterior compartment. The posterior tibial nerve is contained within the deep posterior compartment. (See *Compartment Syndrome pg. 998, in Stoller's 3rd Edition.*)

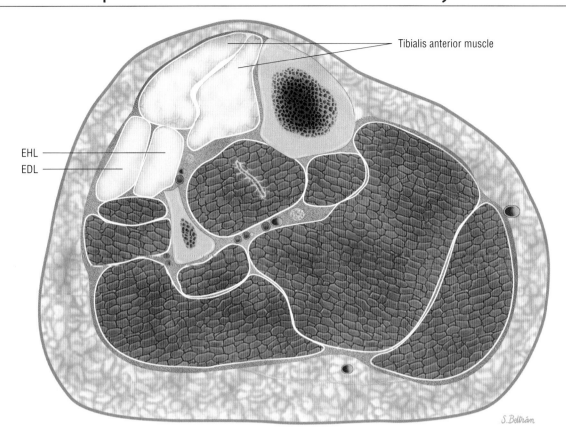

EHL
EDL

Tibialis anterior muscle

S.Beltrán

Figure 5.187 ▪ **Anterior compartment syndrome involving the tibialis anterior, extensor digitorum longus (EDL), and extensor hallucis longus (EHL) muscles.** The inelastic fascial sheath and increased volume of the involved muscles are associated with edema and relative muscle hypertrophy. Myofiber damage and an increase in osmotic pressure contribute to decreased blood flow. The anterior compartment is the most common of the four compartments involved, followed by the deep posterior compartment, the lateral compartment, and the superficial posterior compartment. Axial color illustration. *(See Compartment Syndrome pg. 1000, in Stoller's 3rd Edition.)*

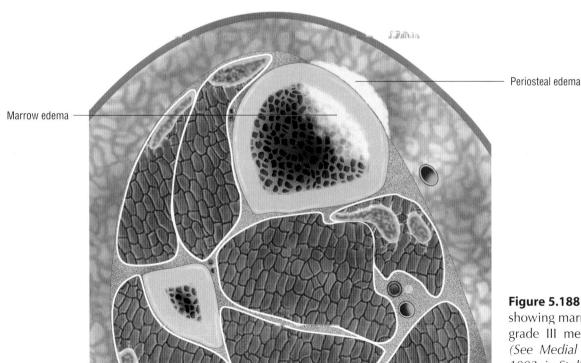

Marrow edema

Periosteal edema

S.Beltrán

Figure 5.188 ▪ Axial color cross section showing marrow and periosteal edema in grade III medial tibial stress syndrome. *(See Medial Tibial Stress Syndrome pg. 1002, in Stoller's 3rd Edition.)*

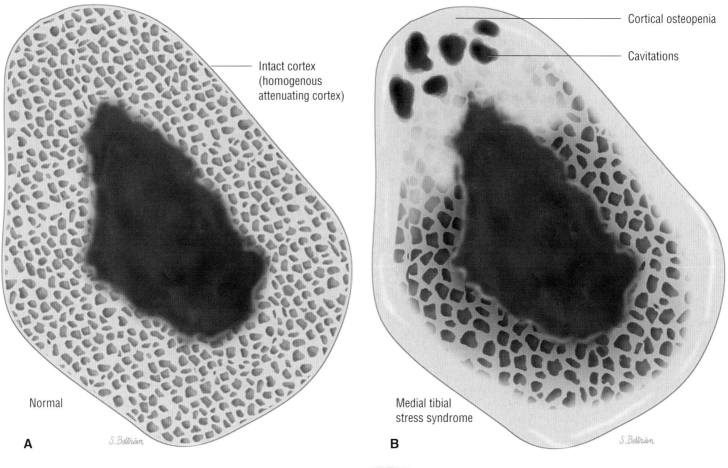

Intact cortex
(homogenous
attenuating cortex)

Normal

S.Beltrán

A

Cortical osteopenia

Cavitations

Medial tibial
stress syndrome

S.Beltrán

B

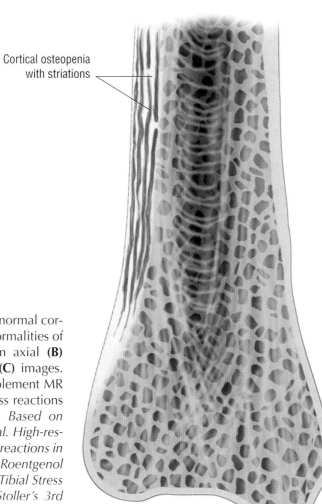

Cortical osteopenia
with striations

Medial tibial
stress syndrome

S.Beltrán

C

Figure 5.189 ■ CT findings of a normal cortex pattern **(A)** compared to abnormalities of medial tibial stress syndrome in axial **(B)** and multiplanar reconstruction **(C)** images. CT studies may be used to complement MR findings in exercise-induced stress reactions (medial tibial stress syndrome). *Based on Gaeta M, Minutoli F, Vinci S, et al. High-resolution CT grading of tibial stress reactions in distance runners. AJR; Am J Roentgenol 2006;187: 789–93. (See Medial Tibial Stress Syndrome pgs. 1000–1003, in Stoller's 3rd Edition.)*

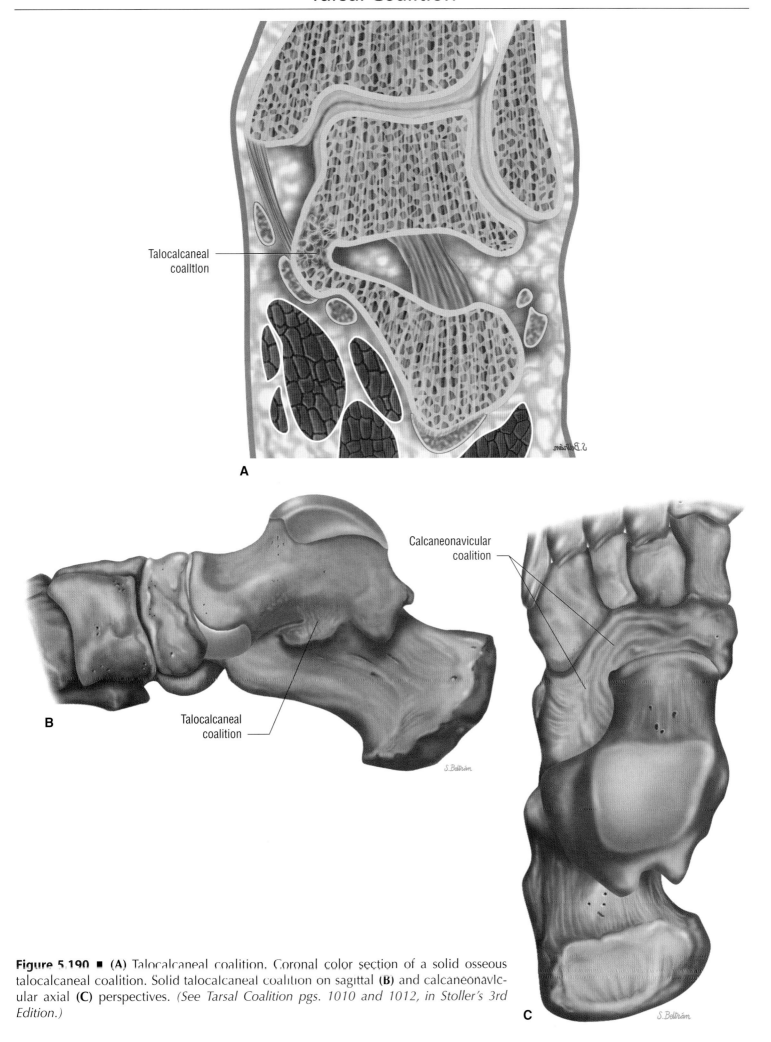

A

Talocalcaneal
coalition

B

Talocalcaneal
coalition

Calcaneonavicular
coalition

C

Figure 5.190 ■ (A) Talocalcaneal coalition. Coronal color section of a solid osseous talocalcaneal coalition. Solid talocalcaneal coalition on sagittal (B) and calcaneonavicular axial (C) perspectives. *(See Tarsal Coalition pgs. 1010 and 1012, in Stoller's 3rd Edition.)*

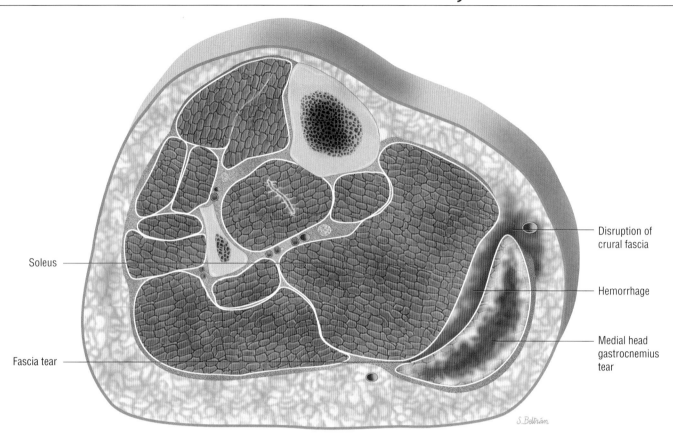

Soleus

Disruption of
crural fascia

Hemorrhage

Medial head
gastrocnemius
tear

Fascia tear

S. Beltrán

Figure 5.191 ■ Grade 2 strain of the medial head of the gastrocnemius with disruption of the fascial layer between the soleus and gastrocnemius and discontinuity of the crural fascia medially. *(See Gastrocnemius-Soleus Strain pgs. 1003 and 1007, in Stoller's 3rd Edition.)*

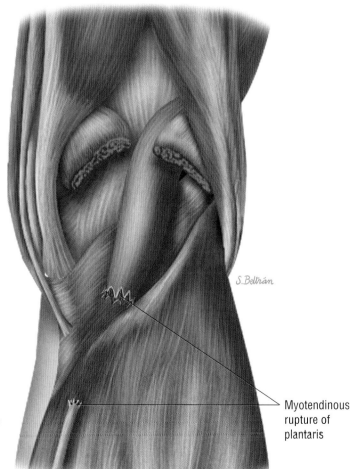

S. Beltrán

Myotendinous
rupture of
plantaris

Figure 5.192 ■ **Plantaris myotendinous rupture with the path of hemorrhage corresponding to the course of the retracted plantaris tendon.** Posterior view coronal color graphic. *(See Plantaris Rupture pg. 1008, in Stoller's 3rd Edition.)*

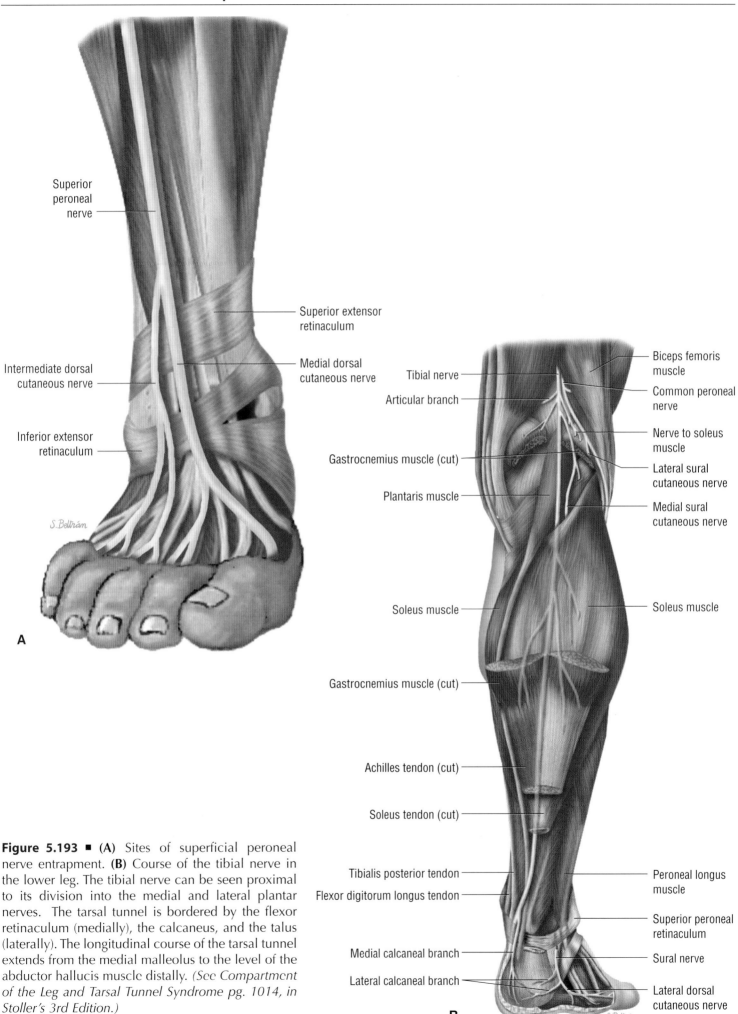

Superior peroneal nerve

Superior extensor retinaculum

Medial dorsal cutaneous nerve

Intermediate dorsal cutaneous nerve

Inferior extensor retinaculum

S. Beltrán

A

Tibial nerve

Articular branch

Gastrocnemius muscle (cut)

Plantaris muscle

Soleus muscle

Gastrocnemius muscle (cut)

Achilles tendon (cut)

Soleus tendon (cut)

Tibialis posterior tendon

Flexor digitorum longus tendon

Medial calcaneal branch

Lateral calcaneal branch

Biceps femoris muscle

Common peroneal nerve

Nerve to soleus muscle

Lateral sural cutaneous nerve

Medial sural cutaneous nerve

Soleus muscle

Peroneal longus muscle

Superior peroneal retinaculum

Sural nerve

Lateral dorsal cutaneous nerve

B

Figure 5.193 ■ **(A)** Sites of superficial peroneal nerve entrapment. **(B)** Course of the tibial nerve in the lower leg. The tibial nerve can be seen proximal to its division into the medial and lateral plantar nerves. The tarsal tunnel is bordered by the flexor retinaculum (medially), the calcaneus, and the talus (laterally). The longitudinal course of the tarsal tunnel extends from the medial malleolus to the level of the abductor hallucis muscle distally. *(See Compartment of the Leg and Tarsal Tunnel Syndrome pg. 1014, in Stoller's 3rd Edition.)*

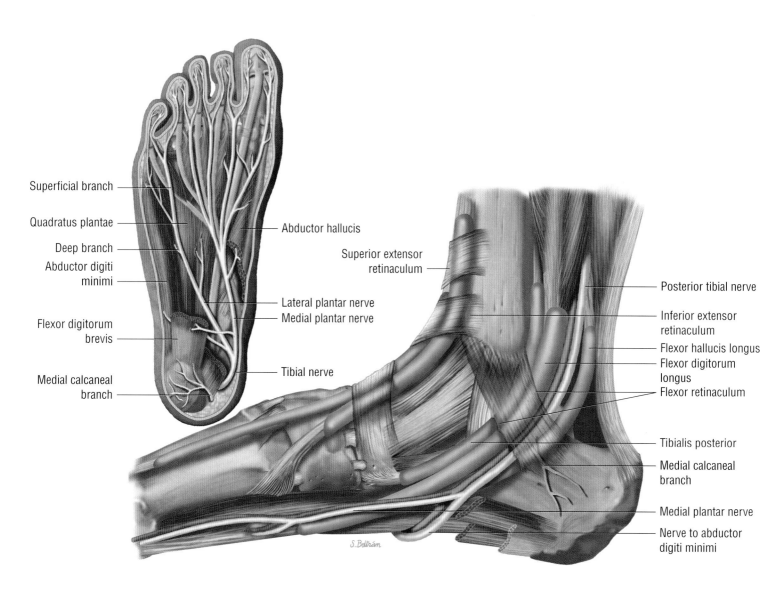

Superficial branch

Quadratus plantae

Deep branch

Abductor digiti minimi

Flexor digitorum brevis

Medial calcaneal branch

Abductor hallucis

Superior extensor retinaculum

Lateral plantar nerve

Medial plantar nerve

Tibial nerve

Posterior tibial nerve

Inferior extensor retinaculum

Flexor hallucis longus

Flexor digitorum longus

Flexor retinaculum

Tibialis posterior

Medial calcaneal branch

Medial plantar nerve

Nerve to abductor digiti minimi

S. Beltrán

Figure 5.194 ■ The posterior tibial nerve is located between the flexor digitorum longus and the flexor hallucis longus divides into the medial and lateral plantar nerves and gives off calcaneal branches. *(See Tarsal Tunnel Syndrome pgs. 1014 and 1015, in Stoller's 3rd Edition.)*

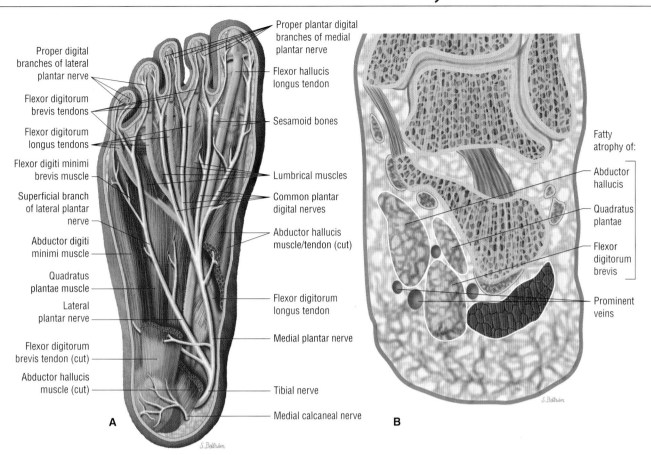

Figure 5.195 ■ **(A) Axial plantar view of plantar nerves.** The tibial nerve divides into its two terminal branches (the lateral and medial plantar nerves) as it passes through the tarsal tunnel. These terminal branches supply the muscles on the plantar aspect of the foot. **(B)** Prominent veins in association with denervation hyperintensity of the abductor hallucis, quadratus plantae, and flexor digitorum brevis. *(See Tarsal Tunnel Syndrome pgs. 1015 and 1016, in Stoller's 3rd Edition.)*

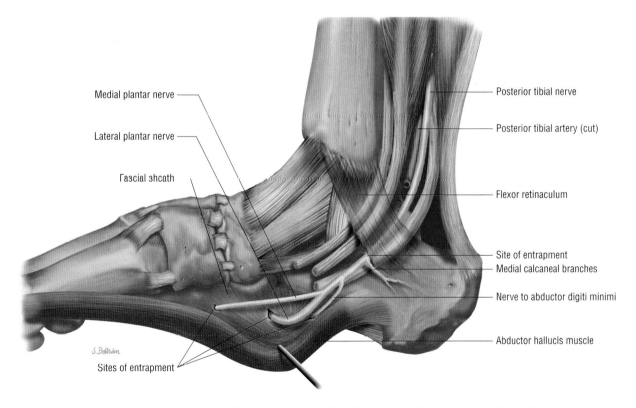

Figure 5.196 ■ **Potential sites of entrapment of the tibial nerve.** Compression of the tibial nerve or its lateral and medial plantar nerve branches may result in tarsal tunnel syndrome. Pain or sensory disturbances of the sole of the foot and palsies of the intrinsic foot muscles may result. *(See Tarsal Tunnel Syndrome pg. 1015, in Stoller's 3rd Edition.)*

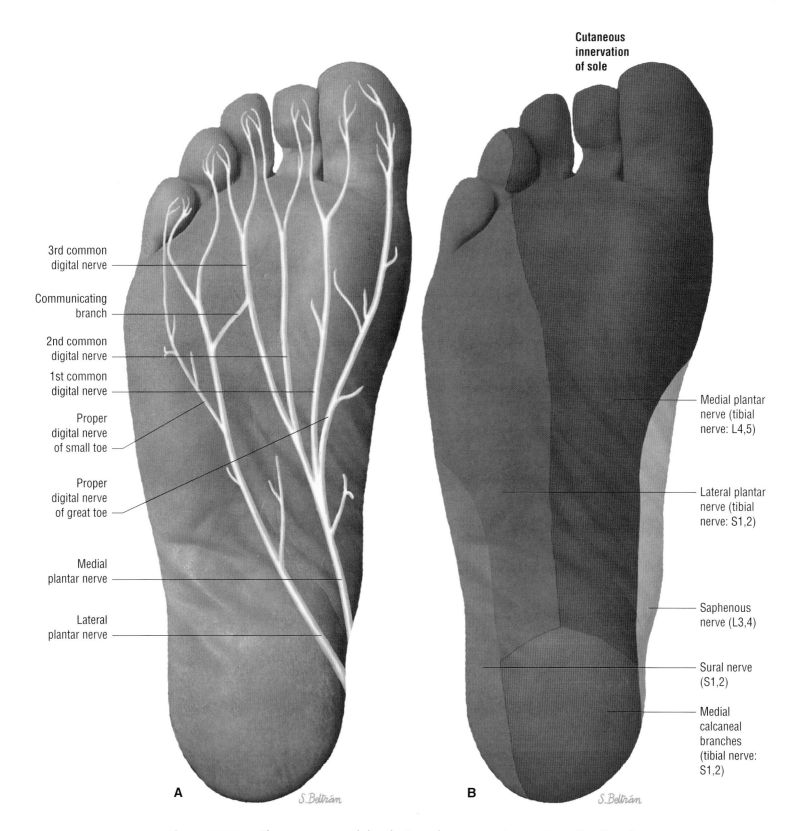

Cutaneous innervation of sole

3rd common digital nerve

Communicating branch

2nd common digital nerve

1st common digital nerve

Proper digital nerve of small toe

Proper digital nerve of great toe

Medial plantar nerve

Lateral plantar nerve

Medial plantar nerve (tibial nerve: L4,5)

Lateral plantar nerve (tibial nerve: S1,2)

Saphenous nerve (L3,4)

Sural nerve (S1,2)

Medial calcaneal branches (tibial nerve: S1,2)

A

B

S. Beltrán

S. Beltrán

Figure 5.197 ■ Plantar nerves and distribution of cutaneous innervation. *(See Tarsal Tunnel Syndrome pg. 1016, in Stoller's 3rd Edition.)*

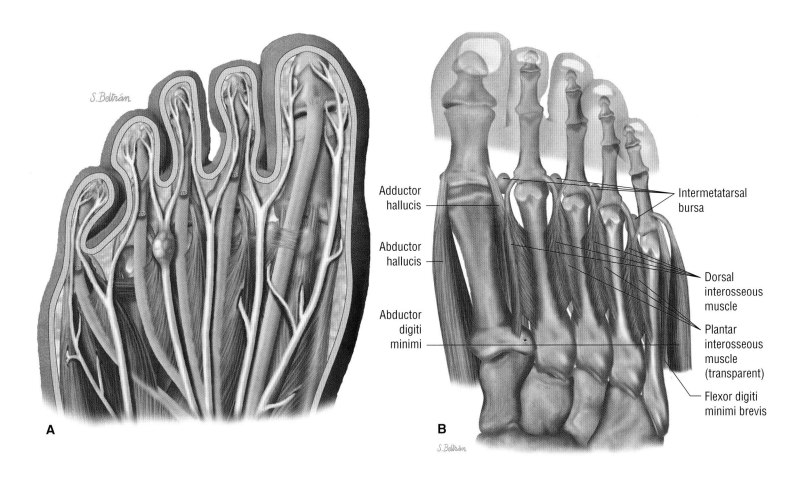

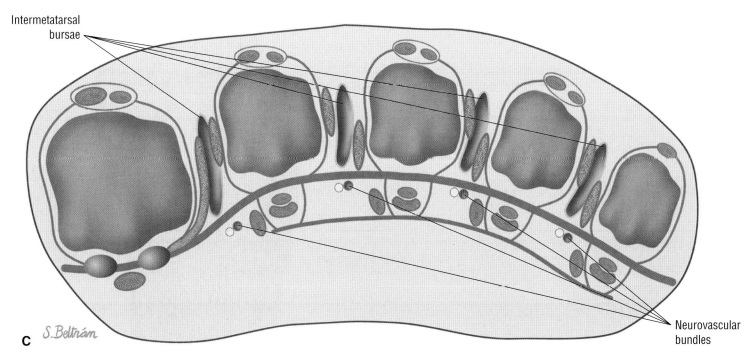

Figure 5.198 ■ **(A)** Morton's neuroma with localized fusiform enlargement of the common digital nerve between the third and fourth metatarsal heads. **(B)** and **(C)** Intermetatarsal bursa sites for potential inflammation in association with Morton's neuroma. *(See Morton's Neuroma pgs. 1018 and 1020, in Stoller's 3rd Edition.)*

Plantar Fibromatosis and Plantar Fascia

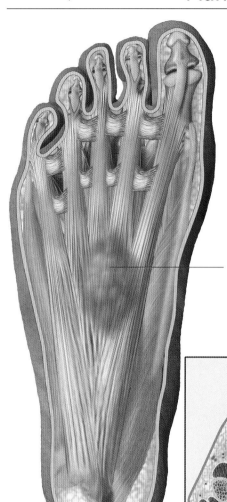

Figure 5.199 ▪ Large lesion of plantar fibromatosis with capsular margins. The long axis is parallel to the plantar aponeurosis in the sagittal plane. Axial plantar view color illustration. *(See Plantar Fibromatosis pg. 1023, in Stoller's 3rd Edition.)*

Multiple lesions of plantar fibromatosis in central and medial plantar fascia

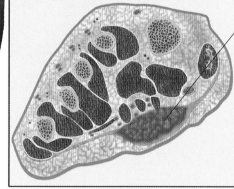

Plantar subcutaneous tissue extension of plantar fibromatosis

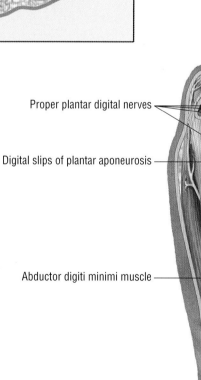

Proper plantar digital nerves

Digital slips of plantar aponeurosis

Abductor digiti minimi muscle

Flexor hallucis longus tendon

Superficial transverse metatarsal ligaments

Transverse fasciculi

Superficial branch of medial plantar artery

Abductor hallucis muscle/tendon

Plantar aponeurosis

Medial calcaneal branches of tibial nerve

Figure 5.200 ▪ The plantar fascia consists of a central aponeurosis and medial and lateral components. Plantar view axial plane color illustration. *(See Plantar Fasciitis pg. 1025, in Stoller's 3rd Edition.)*

Plantar Fasciitis and Heel Pain

Figure 5.201 ■ Palpation of the plantar fascia at the medial calcaneal tuberosity frequently elicits pain. *(See Plantar Fasciitis pg. 1026, in Stoller's 3rd Edition.)*

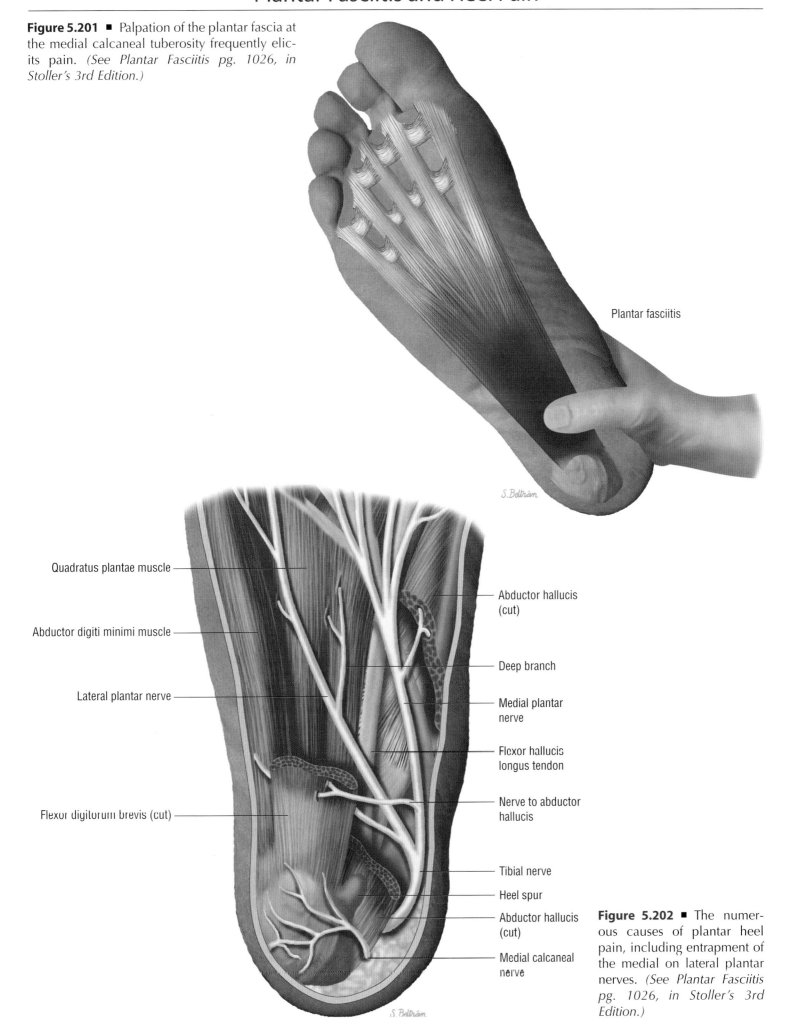

Plantar fasciitis

S. Beltrán

Quadratus plantae muscle

Abductor digiti minimi muscle

Lateral plantar nerve

Flexor digitorum brevis (cut)

Abductor hallucis (cut)

Deep branch

Medial plantar nerve

Flexor hallucis longus tendon

Nerve to abductor hallucis

Tibial nerve

Heel spur

Abductor hallucis (cut)

Medial calcaneal nerve

S. Beltrán

Figure 5.202 ■ The numerous causes of plantar heel pain, including entrapment of the medial on lateral plantar nerves. *(See Plantar Fasciitis pg. 1026, in Stoller's 3rd Edition.)*

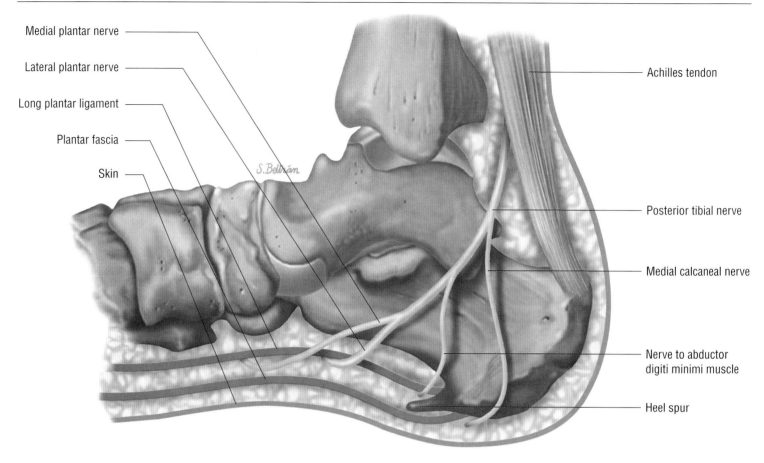

Medial plantar nerve

Lateral plantar nerve

Long plantar ligament

Plantar fascia

Skin

Achilles tendon

Posterior tibial nerve

Medial calcaneal nerve

Nerve to abductor
digiti minimi muscle

Heel spur

Figure 5.203 ■ Structures associated with the presence of heel pain. Lateral color
illustration. *(See Plantar Fasciitis pg. 1027, in Stoller's 3rd Edition.)*

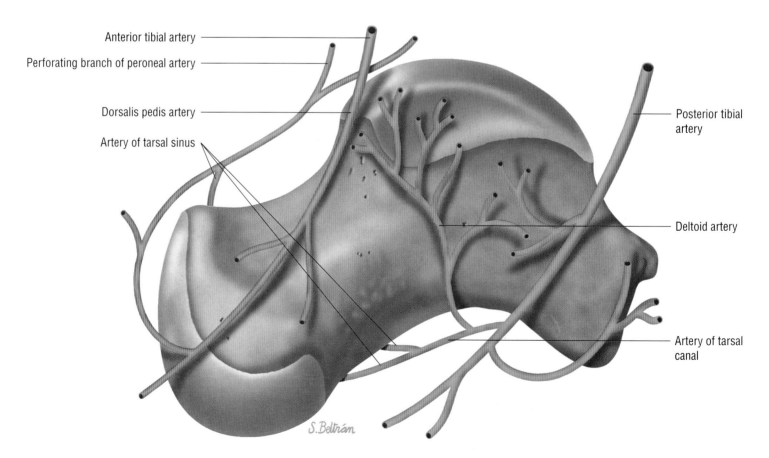

Anterior tibial artery

Perforating branch of peroneal artery

Dorsalis pedis artery

Artery of tarsal sinus

Posterior tibial
artery

Deltoid artery

Artery of tarsal
canal

Figure 5.204 ■ Talar arterial blood supply. The main artery to the body of the talus
is supplied by the artery of the tarsal canal. Lateral color graphic. *(See Avascular
necrosis of the Talus pg. 1030, in Stoller's 3rd Edition.)*

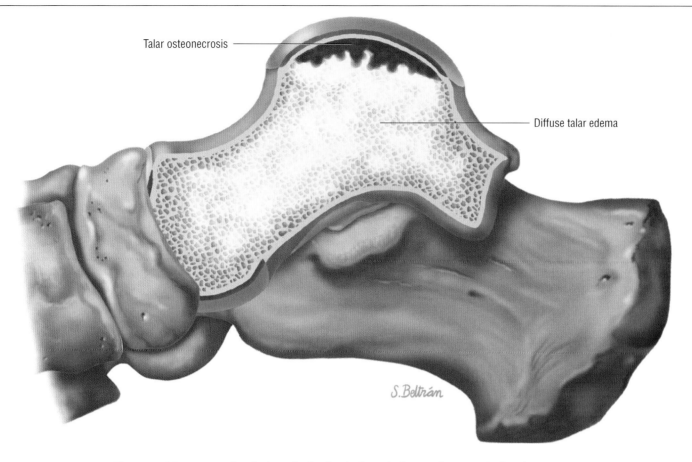

Talar osteonecrosis

Diffuse talar edema

Figure 5.205 ■ **Focal subchondral talar ischemic focus characteristic of AVN (osteonecrosis) of the talus.** The ischemic zone is well demarcated. The associated talar edema may extend diffusely in the acute stages of ischemia. Lateral color illustration. *(See Avascular Necrosis pg. 1031, in Stoller's 3rd Edition.)*

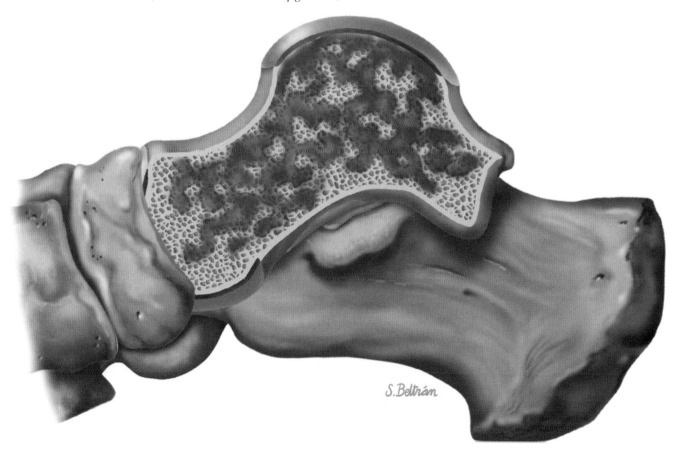

Figure 5.206 ■ Diffuse form of talar ischemia with an infarction pattern involving the entire talar body. *(See Avascular Necrosis pg. 1032, in Stoller's 3rd Edition.)*

AVN of the Talus

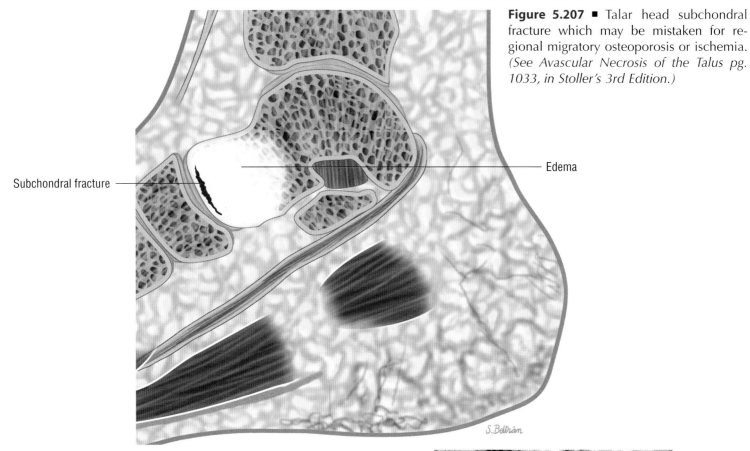

Subchondral fracture

Edema

Figure 5.207 ■ Talar head subchondral fracture which may be mistaken for regional migratory osteoporosis or ischemia. *(See Avascular Necrosis of the Talus pg. 1033, in Stoller's 3rd Edition.)*

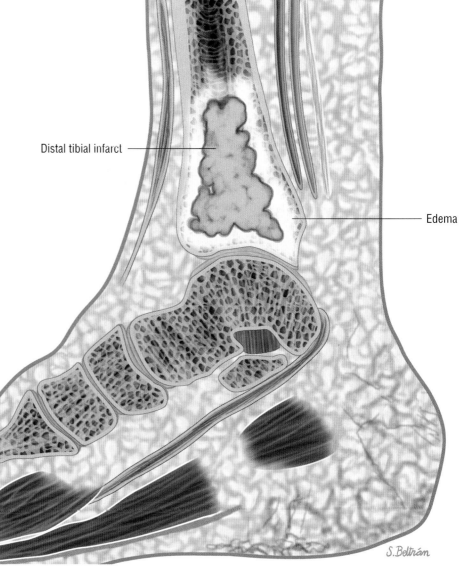

Distal tibial infarct

Edema

Figure 5.208 ■ Serpiginous distal tibial infarct pattern. *(See Avascular Necrosis of the Talus pg. 1033, in Stoller's 3rd Edition.)*

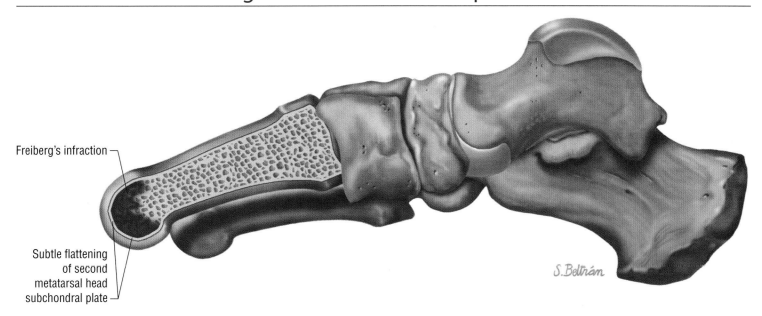

Freiberg's infraction

Subtle flattening
of second
metatarsal head
subchondral plate

Figure 5.209 ■ Lateral color illustration of Freiberg's infraction, which represents an osteochondrosis most commonly, involving the second metatarsal head. *(See Freiberg's Infractions pg. 1034, in Stoller's 3rd Edition.)*

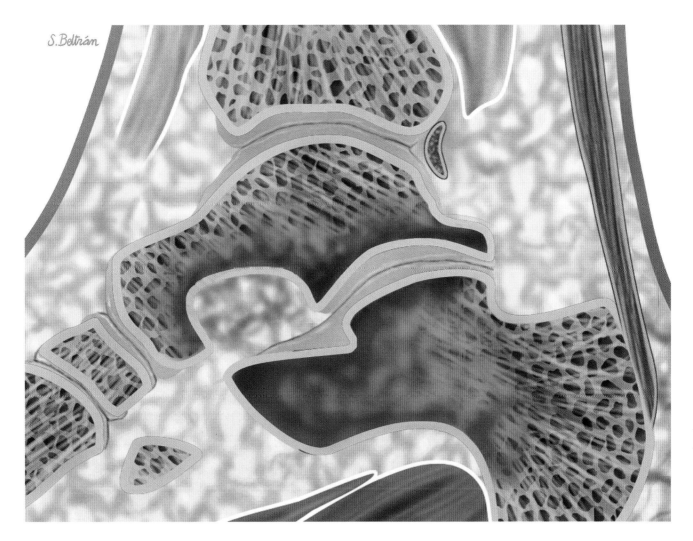

Figure 5.210 ■ **Acute neuropathic osteoarthropathy with edema of multiple regional joints without contiguous soft-tissue signal intensity changes.** Lateral color illustration. *(See Neuropathic Foot in Diabetes Mellitus pg. 1037, in Stoller's 3rd Edition.)*

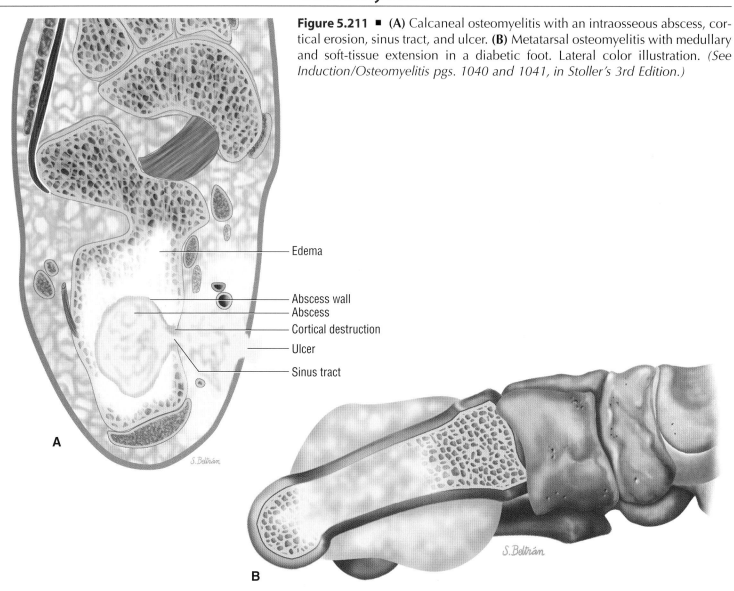

Figure 5.211 ■ **(A)** Calcaneal osteomyelitis with an intraosseous abscess, cortical erosion, sinus tract, and ulcer. **(B)** Metatarsal osteomyelitis with medullary and soft-tissue extension in a diabetic foot. Lateral color illustration. *(See Induction/Osteomyelitis pgs. 1040 and 1041, in Stoller's 3rd Edition.)*

Edema

Abscess wall
Abscess
Cortical destruction

Ulcer

Sinus tract

A

B

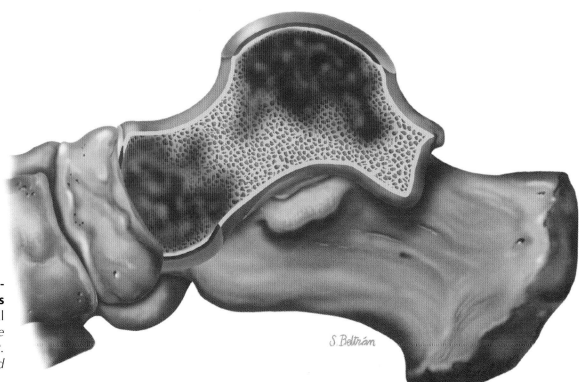

Figure 5.212 ■ **Osteomyelitis with hematogenous spread to the talus.** Lateral color illustration. *(See Infection/Osteomyelitis pg. 1042, in Stoller's 3rd Edition.)*

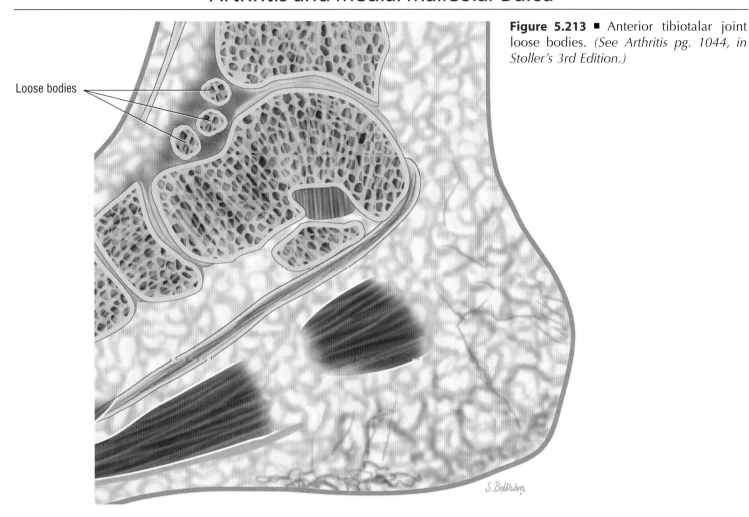

Loose bodies

Figure 5.213 ■ Anterior tibiotalar joint loose bodies. *(See Arthritis pg. 1044, in Stoller's 3rd Edition.)*

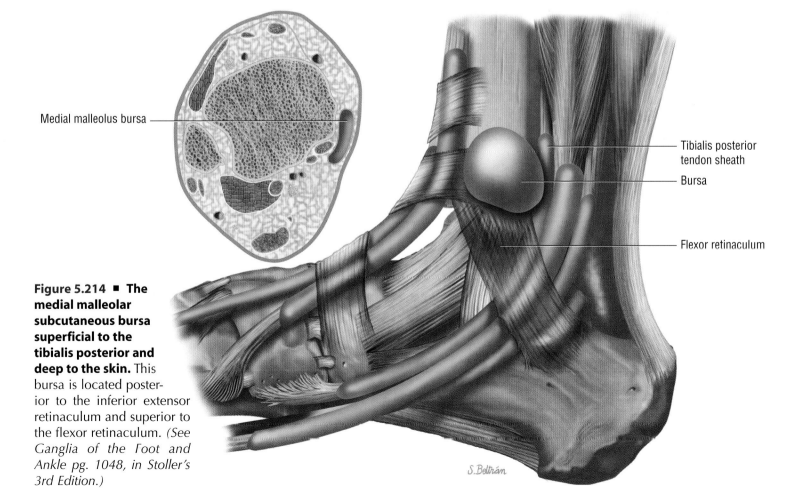

Medial malleolus bursa

Tibialis posterior tendon sheath

Bursa

Flexor retinaculum

Figure 5.214 ■ **The medial malleolar subcutaneous bursa superficial to the tibialis posterior and deep to the skin.** This bursa is located posterior to the inferior extensor retinaculum and superior to the flexor retinaculum. *(See Ganglia of the Foot and Ankle pg. 1048, in Stoller's 3rd Edition.)*

Chapter

6

Entrapment Neuropathies of the Lower Extremity

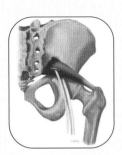

Pearls and Pitfalls & Color Illustrations

Pearls and Pitfalls

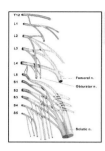

PATHOMECHANISMS

- The etiology of neuropathy may be related to mechanical or dynamic causes.
- Nerve entrapment may result in motor, sensory, and autonomic deficits.
- Nerve injury is classified in order of severity from neurapraxia, to axonotmesis, to neurotmesis.

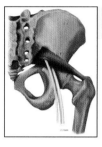

MR IMAGING TECHNIQUES

- Nerve visualization requires imaging in all three orthogonal planes using high-resolution T1-weighted images and fluid-sensitive fat-suppressed images (e.g., FS PD FSE or STIR).
- MR intravenous contrast is used to assess mass lesions associated with nerve compression.
- Normal nerves do not enhance with intravenous contrast administration.
- MR T2 neurography selectively emphasizes fluid signal from nerves.
- Chronic nerve damage is associated with fatty infiltration and decreased muscle bulk.
- Partially reversible nerve damage displays increased signal on T1- and T2-weighted images.
- In the double crush syndrome, a proximally compromised nerve is more susceptible to entrapment distally.
- Distal entrapment affects the proximal nerve in the Valleix phenomenon.

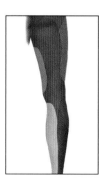

NORMAL ANATOMY

- Peripheral nerves display intermediate signal intensity on T1- and PD-weighted images with a mild increase on fluid-sensitive sequences (signal intensity usually within the intermediate range on FS PD FSE images).
- The fascicular anatomy of larger nerves demonstrates honeycomb morphology on axial images.

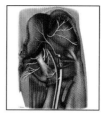

NERVE PATHOLOGY

- Nerve swelling and hyperintensity may represent an advanced process of nerve damage with fascicular and endoneurial edema.
- Muscle denervation is associated with motor nerve entrapment.
- On fluid-sensitive images, hyperintense muscle signal represents subacute denervation (denervation edema).

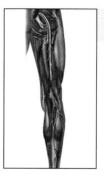

SCIATIC NERVE
(see Figures 6.2–6.5)

- Sciatic neuropathy is associated with total hip replacements, especially revisions.
- Sciatic neuropathy more commonly affects the peroneal nerve division.
- The piriformis syndrome is related to spasticity, irritability, or inflammation of the piriformis muscle.

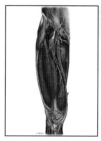

FEMORAL NERVE
(See Figures 6.6–6.7)

- The saphenous nerve is the largest branch of the femoral nerve.
- Femoral nerve compression frequently occurs underneath the inguinal ligament.
- Anterior compartment (thigh) muscle atrophy is associated with femoral nerve entrapment.
- Saphenous nerve entrapment occurs in the adductor canal.

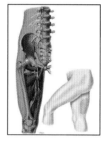

OBTURATOR NERVE
(See Figure 6.8)

- Entrapment neuropathy is usually associated with trauma and postsurgical injury to the inguinal area and pelvis.
- Pelvic tumors, including metastatic extension, may cause obturator neuropathy.
- Groin pain in athletes is associated with involvement of the anterior branch of the obturator nerve distal to the obturator tunnel.

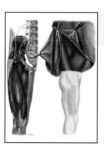

LATERAL FEMORAL CUTANEOUS NERVE
(see Figure 6.9)

- Entrapment neuropathy occurs under the inguinal ligament or as the nerve perforates the fascia lata.
- The term *meralgia paresthetica* is also used to refer to neuropathy of the lateral femoral cutaneous nerve.

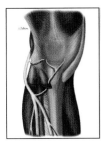

COMMON PERONEAL NERVE
(See Figure 6.10)

- The common peroneal nerve trifurcates into the recurrent articular branch to the knee capsule and the superficial peroneal and deep peroneal nerves.
- Common peroneal neuropathy usually occurs as the nerve crosses the fibular neck or as it pierces the peroneus longus muscle.

- Extrinsic compression may be associated with intraneural and extraneural ganglia originating from the proximal tibiofibular joint. Tracking proximally along the articular branch of the common peroneal nerve occurs with intra-neural ganglia.

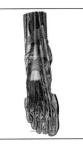

DEEP PERONEAL NERVE
(See Figure 6.11)

- The deep peroneal nerve provides motor supply to the extensor muscles of the foot and toes and carries sensation from the dorsal first web space.
- Potential sites of entrapment include the superior extensor retinaculum and, in the anterior tarsal syndrome, the inferior extensor retinaculum or talonavicular joint.

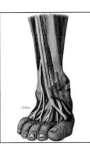

SUPERFICIAL PERONEAL NERVE
(See Figure 6.12)

- The superficial peroneal nerve provides motor innervation to the peroneus longus and brevis muscles.
- Entrapment occurs as the nerve pierces the deep fascia of the leg.

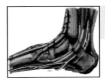

TIBIAL NERVE
(See Figures 6.13–6.17)

- The tibial nerve is the largest division of the sciatic nerve.
- **Tibial neuropathies include:**
  - ☐ Proximal tibial neuropathy
  - ☐ Tarsal tunnel syndrome
  - ☐ Medial plantar neuropathy
  - ☐ Lateral plantar neuropathy
  - ☐ Morton's neuroma (interdigital neuropathy)
  - ☐ Joplin's neuroma (medial plantar proper digital neuropathy)
- The tarsal tunnel syndrome is caused by trauma, space-occupying lesions, or foot deformities.
- **Distal foot entrapment neuropathies include:**
  - ☐ Medial calcaneal neuropathy
  - ☐ Medial plantar neuropathy
  - ☐ Lateral plantar nerve entrapment and entrapment of the nerve to the abductor digiti minimi
- Morton's neuroma is the result of damage to the interdigital nerve by entrapment or ischemia and represents a degenerative process.
- Joplin's neuroma is an entrapment neuropathy of the plantar proper digital nerve.

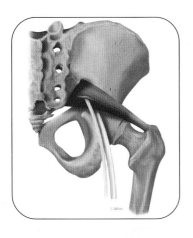

Entrapment Neuropathies of the Lower Extremity

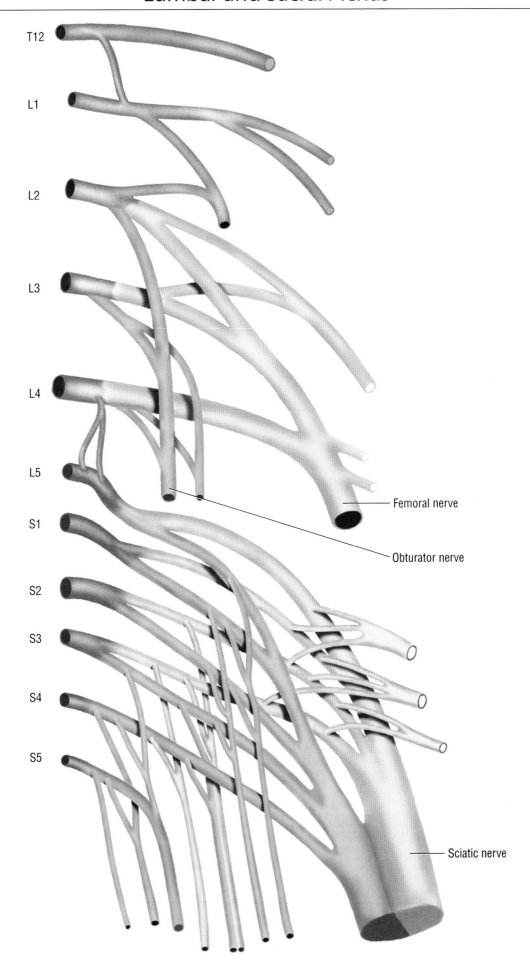

Figure 6.1 ■ The origins of the three major nerves supplying the lower extremity: the sciatic nerve, the femoral nerve, and the obturator nerve. (Green: Anterior division; Yellow: Posterior division.) *(See Entrapment Neuropathies of the Lower Extremity pg. 1052, in Stoller's 3rd Edition.)*

Sciatic Nerve

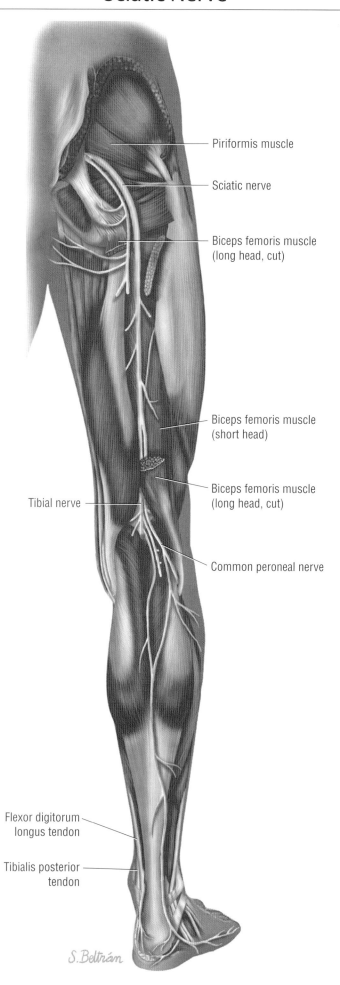

Piriformis muscle

Sciatic nerve

Biceps femoris muscle
(long head, cut)

Biceps femoris muscle
(short head)

Biceps femoris muscle
(long head, cut)

Tibial nerve

Common peroneal nerve

Flexor digitorum
longus tendon

Tibialis posterior
tendon

S. Beltrán

Figure 6.2 ■ A posterior view of the right lower extremity demonstrating the sciatic nerve and its tibial and peroneal divisions. *(See Sciatic Nerve pg. 1057, in Stoller's 3rd Edition.)*

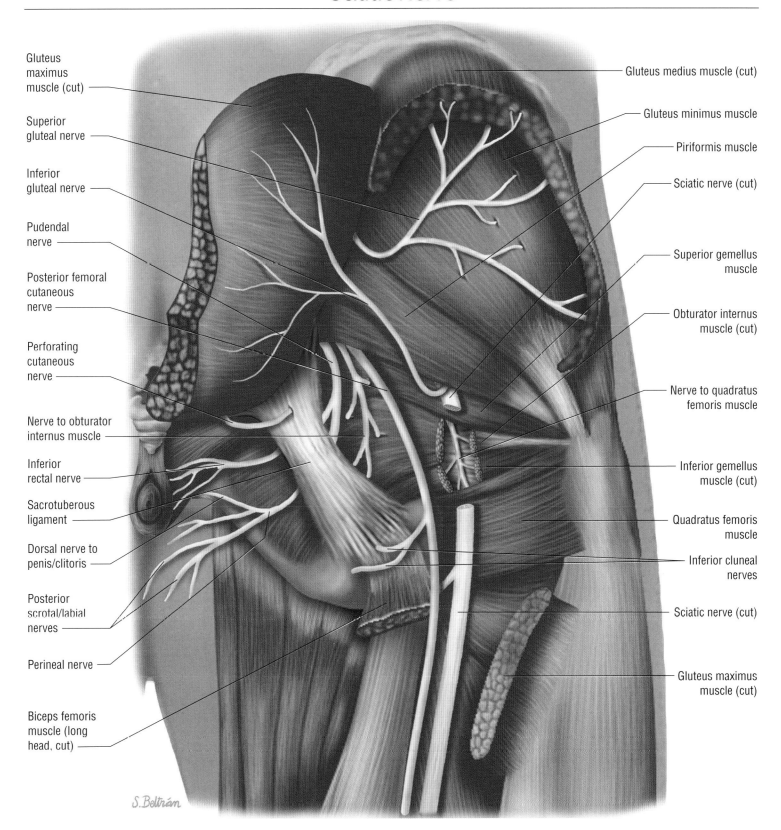

Gluteus maximus muscle (cut)

Superior gluteal nerve

Inferior gluteal nerve

Pudendal nerve

Posterior femoral cutaneous nerve

Perforating cutaneous nerve

Nerve to obturator internus muscle

Inferior rectal nerve

Sacrotuberous ligament

Dorsal nerve to penis/clitoris

Posterior scrotal/labial nerves

Perineal nerve

Biceps femoris muscle (long head, cut)

Gluteus medius muscle (cut)

Gluteus minimus muscle

Piriformis muscle

Sciatic nerve (cut)

Superior gemellus muscle

Obturator internus muscle (cut)

Nerve to quadratus femoris muscle

Inferior gemellus muscle (cut)

Quadratus femoris muscle

Inferior cluneal nerves

Sciatic nerve (cut)

Gluteus maximus muscle (cut)

S. Beltrán

Figure 6.3 ■ A posterior view of the sciatic nerve in the greater sciatic foramen.
The nerve descends anterior to the piriformis muscle and successively posterior to the superior gemellus, obturator internus, inferior gemellus, and quadratus femoris muscles. *(See Sciatic Nerve pg. 1058, in Stoller's 3rd Edition.)*

Sensory Innervation of the Lower Extremity

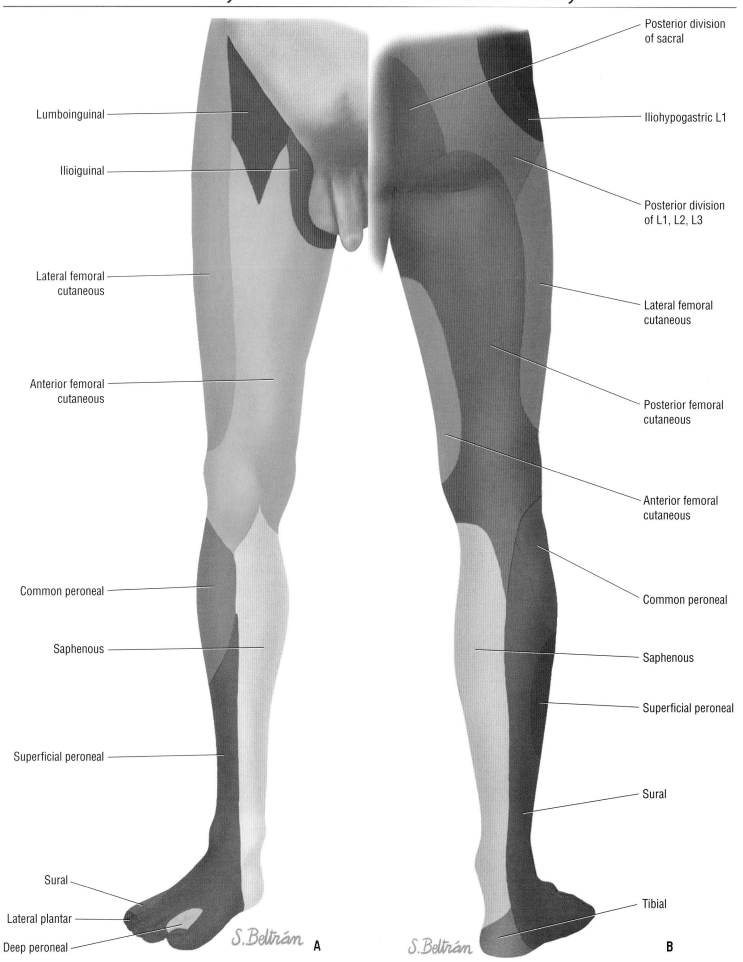

Lumboinguinal

Ilioiguinal

Lateral femoral
cutaneous

Anterior femoral
cutaneous

Common peroneal

Saphenous

Superficial peroneal

Sural

Lateral plantar

Deep peroneal

Posterior division
of sacral

Iliohypogastric L1

Posterior division
of L1, L2, L3

Lateral femoral
cutaneous

Posterior femoral
cutaneous

Anterior femoral
cutaneous

Common peroneal

Saphenous

Superficial peroneal

Sural

Tibial

S. Beltrán A

S. Beltrán B

Figure 6.4 ■ Anterior **(A)** and posterior **(B)** views of the sensory innervation of the lower extremity. *(See Sciatic Nerve pg. 1059, in Stoller's 3rd Edition.)*

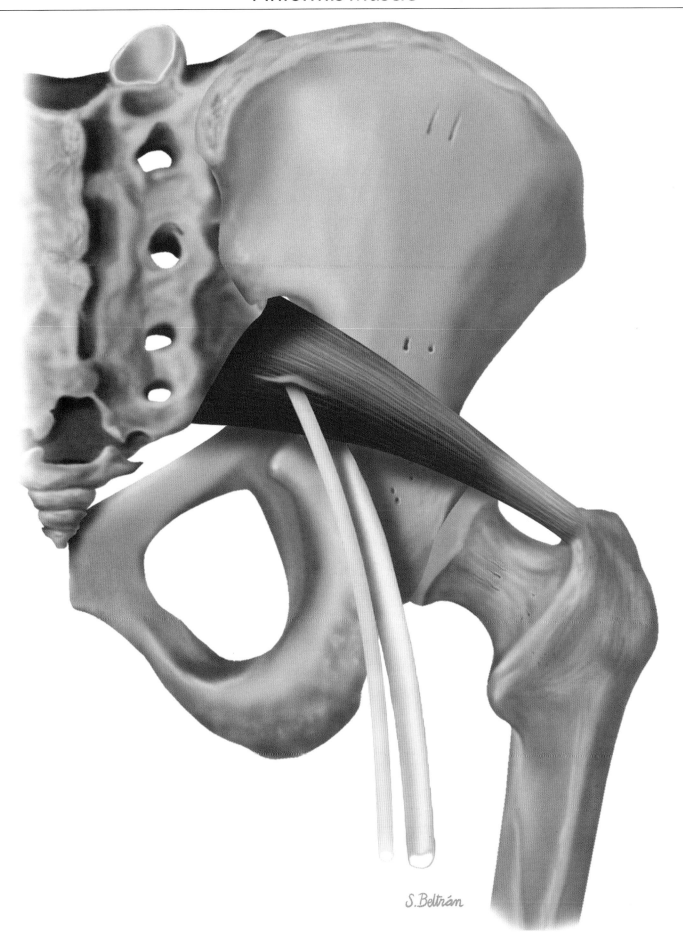

Figure 6.5 ▪ The piriformis muscle pierced by the peroneal division of the sciatic nerve (anatomic variation). *(See Piriformis Muscle Syndrome pg. 1061, in Stoller's 3rd Edition.)*

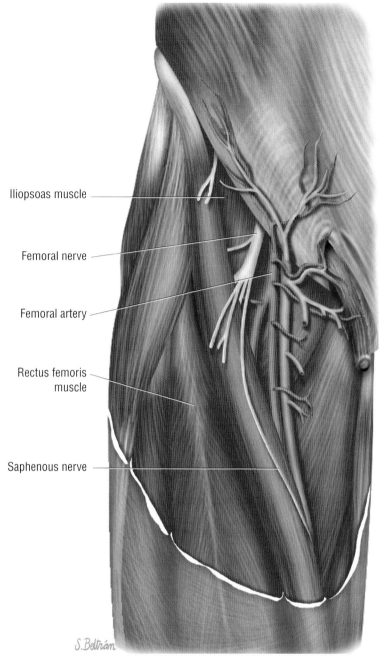

Iliopsoas muscle

Femoral nerve

Femoral artery

Rectus femoris
muscle

Saphenous nerve

S.Beltrán

Figure 6.6 ■ The femoral nerve and its branches. *(See Femoral Nerve pgs. 1065–1067, in Stoller's 3rd Edition.)*

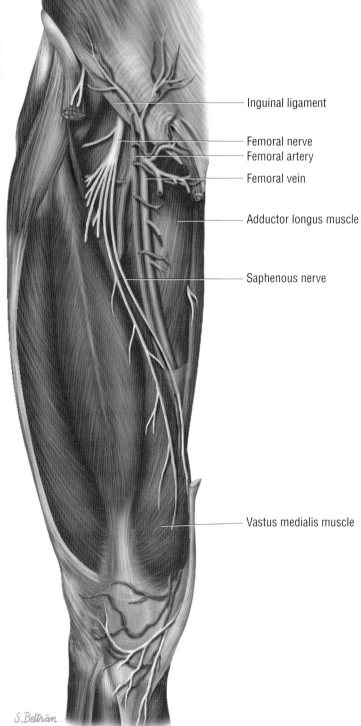

Inguinal ligament

Femoral nerve
Femoral artery

Femoral vein

Adductor longus muscle

Saphenous nerve

Vastus medialis muscle

S.Beltrán

Figure 6.7 ■ The saphenous nerve as it descends down the thigh to enter the adductor canal. *(See Femoral Nerve pgs. 1065–1067, in Stoller's 3rd Edition.)*

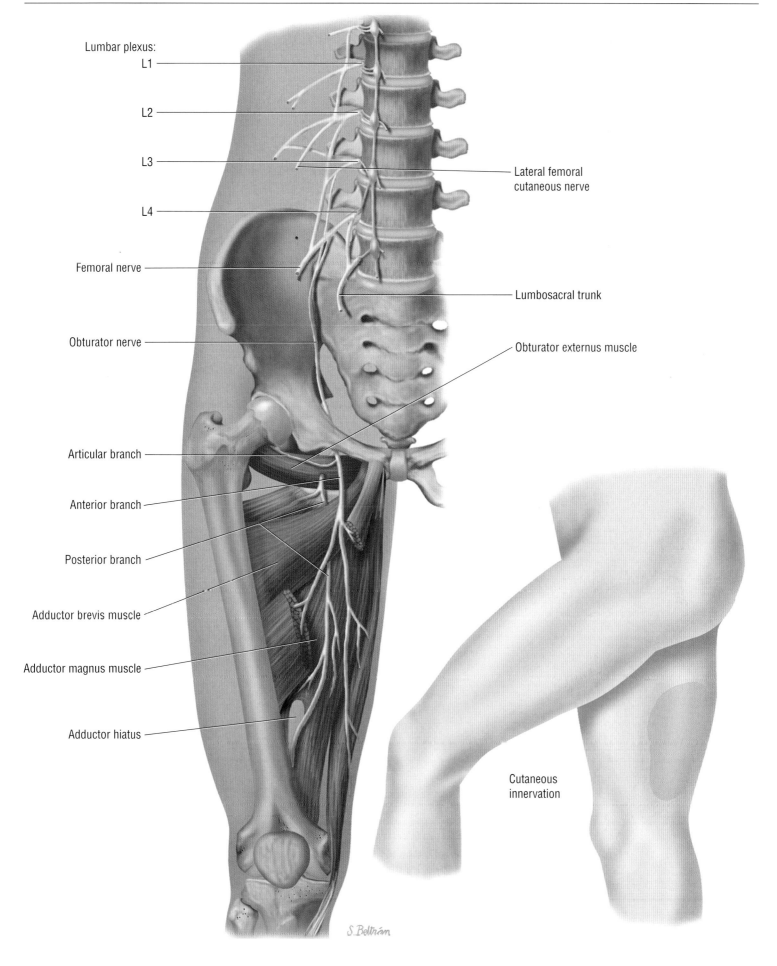

Lumbar plexus:
L1
L2
L3
L4

Femoral nerve

Obturator nerve

Articular branch

Anterior branch

Posterior branch

Adductor brevis muscle

Adductor magnus muscle

Adductor hiatus

Lateral femoral cutaneous nerve

Lumbosacral trunk

Obturator externus muscle

Cutaneous innervation

S. Beltrán

Figure 6.8 ■ The normal obturator nerve. The insert shows the sensory distribution of the nerve along the medial thigh. *(See Obturator Nerve pg. 1069, in Stoller's 3rd Edition.)*

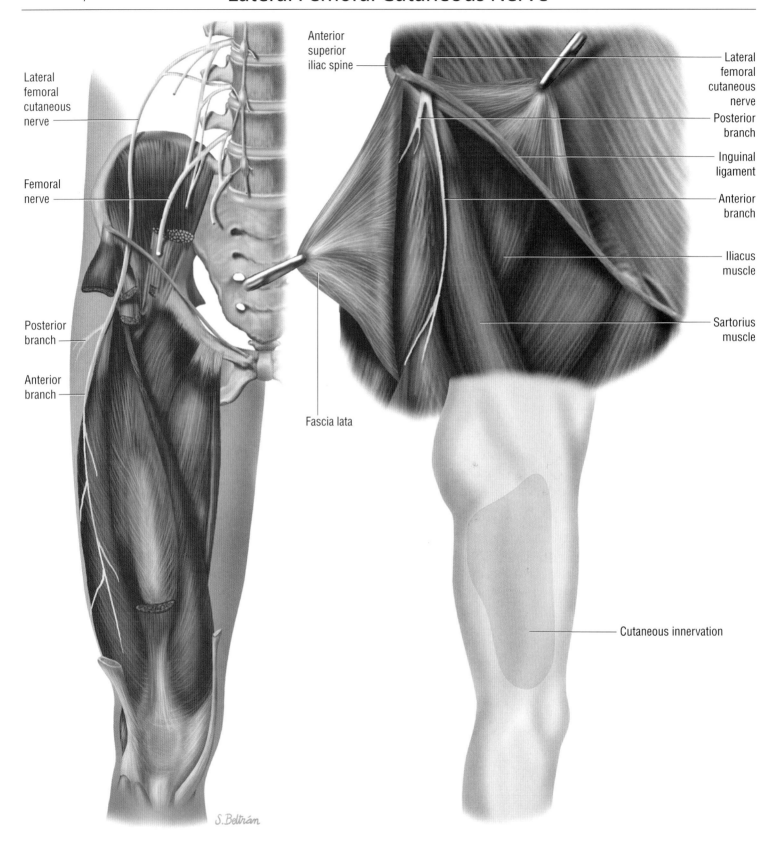

Figure 6.9 ▪ The lateral femoral cutaneous nerve as it dives under the inguinal ligament close to the anterior superior iliac spine. The insert shows the sensory distribution of the nerve along the lateral thigh. *(See Lateral Femoral Cutaneous Nerve pg. 1071, in Stoller's 3rd Edition.)*

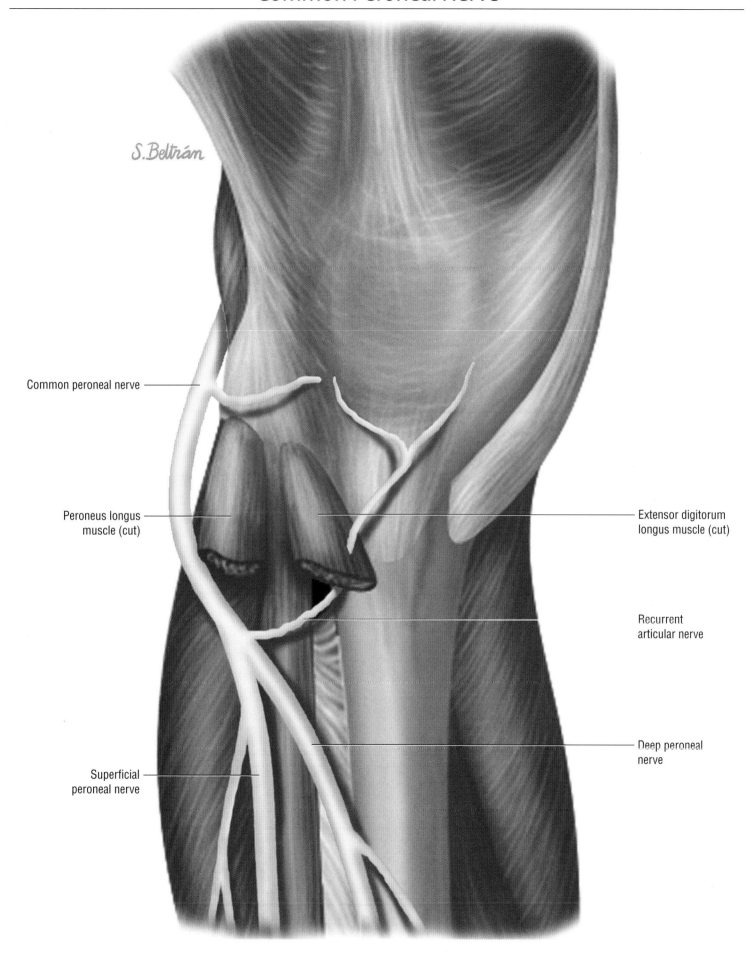

Common peroneal nerve

Peroneus longus
muscle (cut)

Extensor digitorum
longus muscle (cut)

Recurrent
articular nerve

Deep peroneal
nerve

Superficial
peroneal nerve

S. Beltrán

Figure 6.10 ▪ Anterior view of the knee depicting the common peroneal nerve and its branches winding around the fibular neck, deep to the peroneus longus muscle. *(See Common Peroneal Nerve pg. 1073, in Stoller's 3rd Edition.)*

Figure 6.11 ▪ Anterior view of the foot demonstrating the three most common locations for deep peroneal nerve entrapment. *(See Deep Peroneal Nerve pg. 1076, in Stoller's 3rd Edition.)*

Superior extensor retinaculum

Inferior extensor retinaculum

Deep peroneal nerve

S.Beltrán

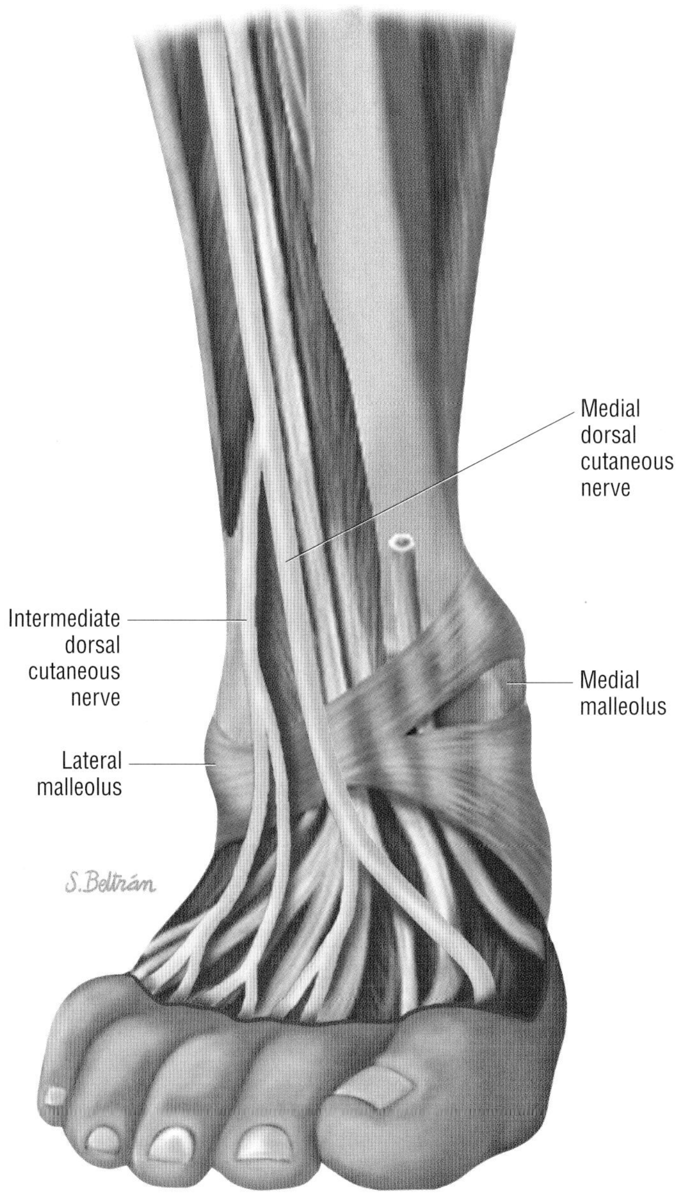

Medial dorsal cutaneous nerve

Intermediate dorsal cutaneous nerve

Lateral malleolus

Medial malleolus

S.Beltrán

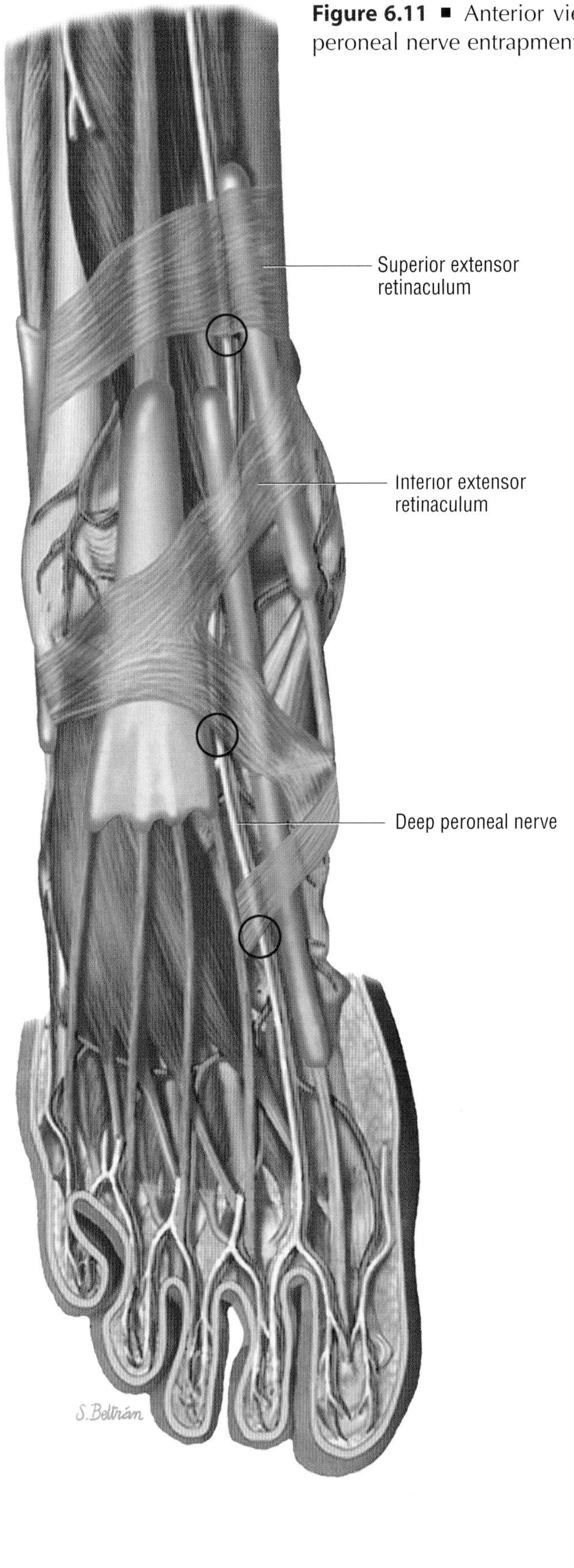

Figure 6.12 ▪ **The superficial peroneal nerve as it pierces the deep fascia of the lateral compartment.** Inversion injury can cause stretching of the nerve against the fascia. *(See Superficial Peroneal Nerve pg. 1079, in Stoller's 3rd Edition.)*

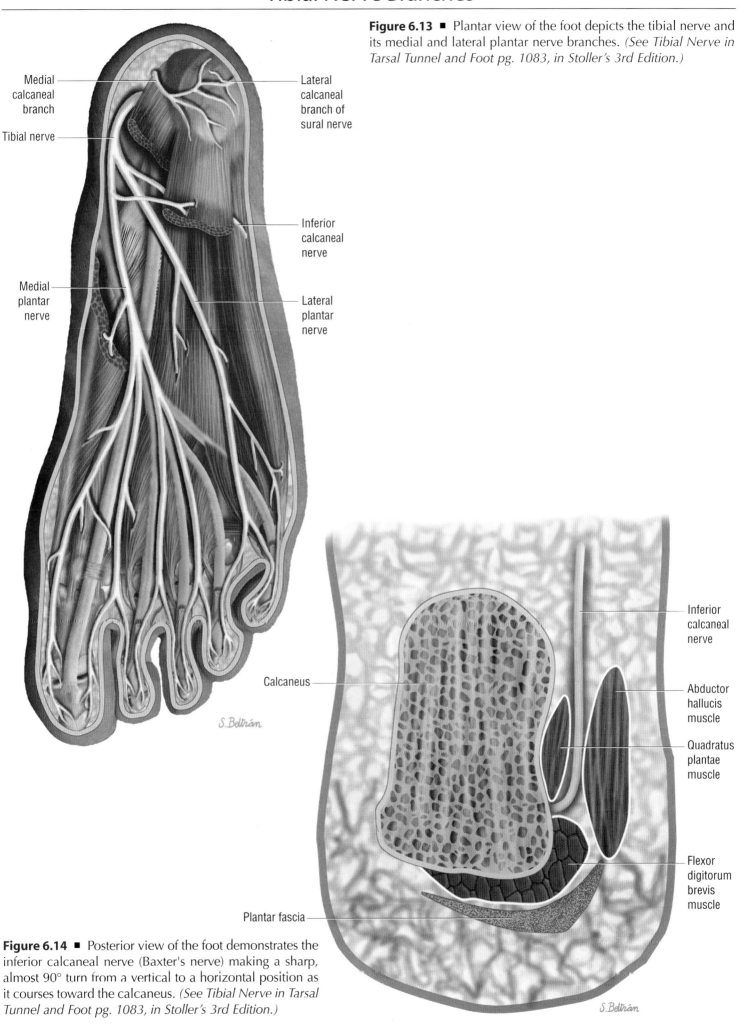

Figure 6.13 ■ Plantar view of the foot depicts the tibial nerve and its medial and lateral plantar nerve branches. *(See Tibial Nerve in Tarsal Tunnel and Foot pg. 1083, in Stoller's 3rd Edition.)*

Medial calcaneal branch

Tibial nerve

Medial plantar nerve

Lateral calcaneal branch of sural nerve

Inferior calcaneal nerve

Lateral plantar nerve

S.Beltrán

Calcaneus

Plantar fascia

Inferior calcaneal nerve

Abductor hallucis muscle

Quadratus plantae muscle

Flexor digitorum brevis muscle

S.Beltrán

Figure 6.14 ■ Posterior view of the foot demonstrates the inferior calcaneal nerve (Baxter's nerve) making a sharp, almost 90° turn from a vertical to a horizontal position as it courses toward the calcaneus. *(See Tibial Nerve in Tarsal Tunnel and Foot pg. 1083, in Stoller's 3rd Edition.)*

Figure 6.15 ■ **The tarsal tunnel.** The tibial nerve and its branches descend, deep to the flexor retinaculum, along with the flexor tendons and vascular structures. *(See Tibial Nerve in Tarsal Tunnel and Foot pg. 1082, in Stoller's 3rd Edition.)*

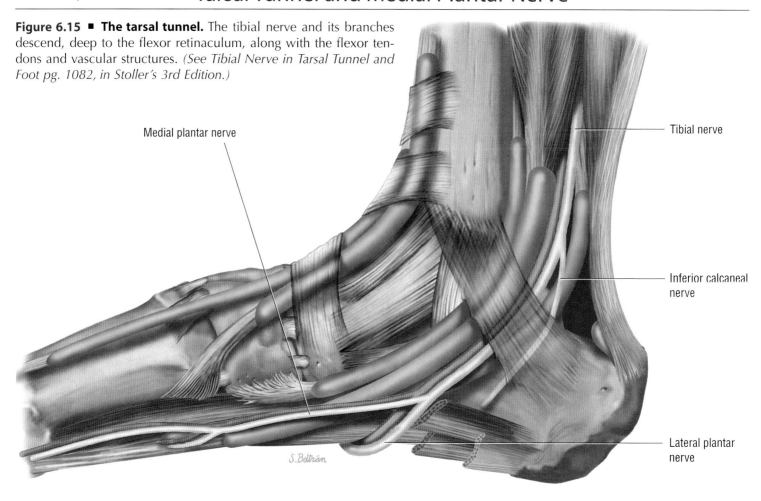

Medial plantar nerve

Tibial nerve

Inferior calcaneal nerve

Lateral plantar nerve

S.Beltrán

Figure 6.16 ■ Compression of the medial plantar nerve at the knot of Henry. *(See Medial Plantar Nerve Entrapment pg. 1088, in Stoller's 3rd Edition.)*

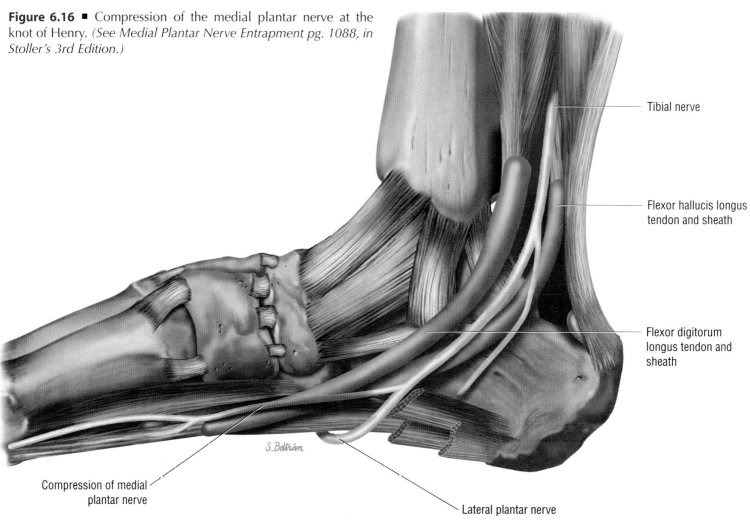

Tibial nerve

Flexor hallucis longus tendon and sheath

Flexor digitorum longus tendon and sheath

Compression of medial plantar nerve

Lateral plantar nerve

S.Beltrán

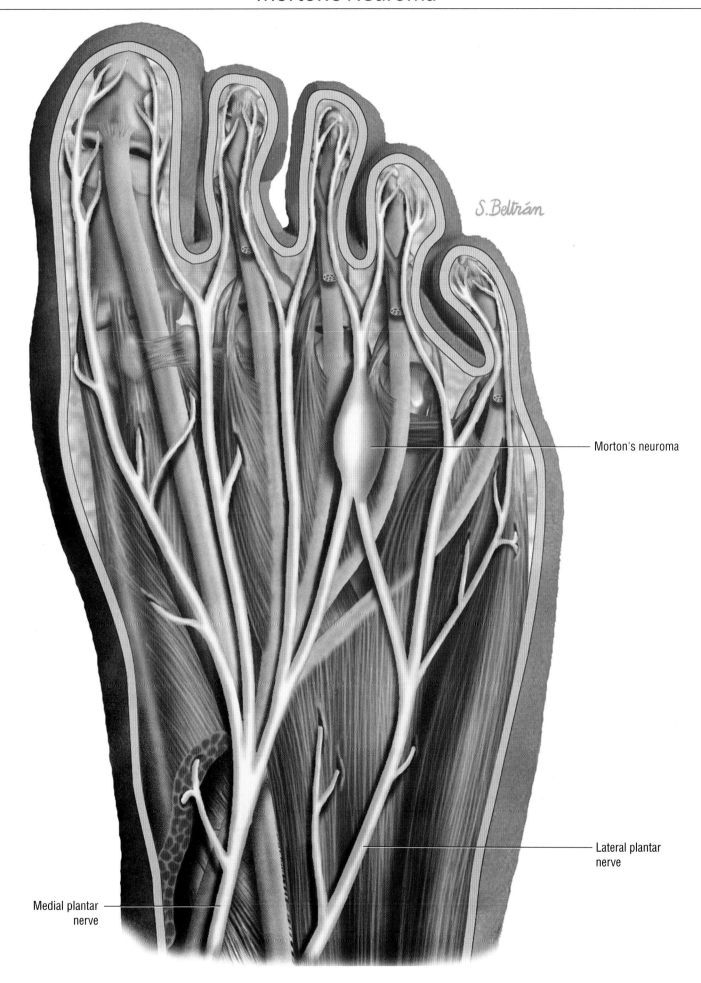

S.Beltrán

Morton's neuroma

Lateral plantar
nerve

Medial plantar
nerve

Figure 6.17 ■ A third interdigital Morton's neuroma at the confluence of the terminal branches of the medial and lateral plantar nerves. *(See Morton's Neuroma pg. 1092, in Stoller's 3rd Edition.)*

Figure 6.18 ■ The posterior leg, showing the formation of the sural nerve from the tibial and peroneal contributions. *(See Sural Nerve pg. 1095, in Stoller's 3rd Edition.)*

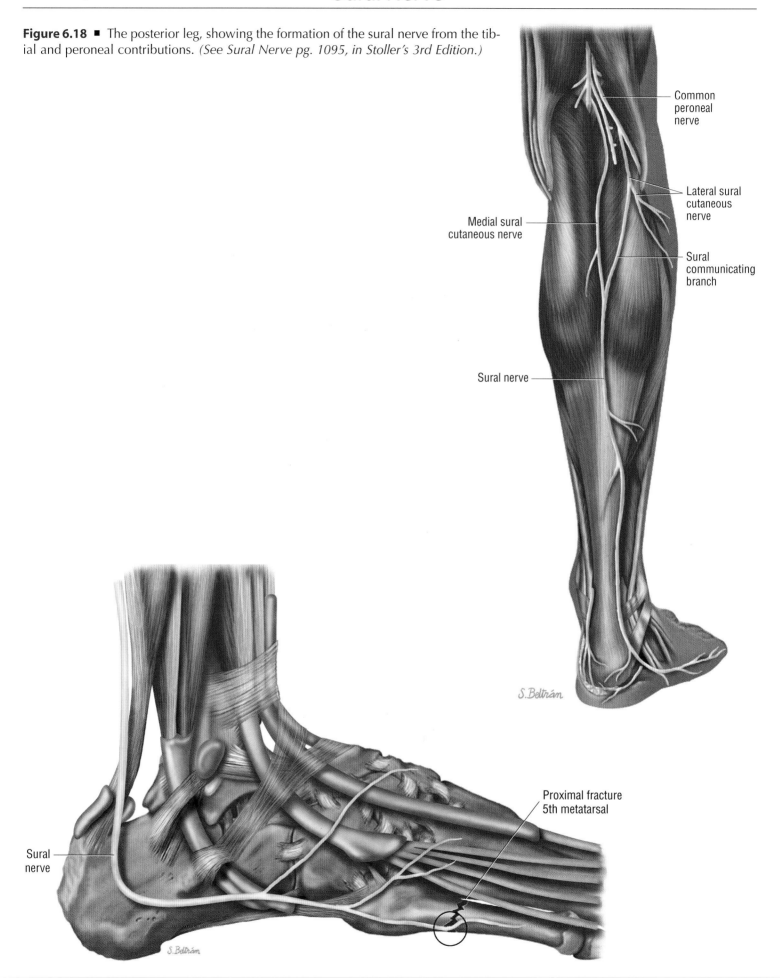

Figure 6.19 ■ Sural nerve entrapment secondary to a fracture of the base of the fifth metatarsal. *(See Sural Nerve pg. 1096, in Stoller's 3rd Edition.)*

Chapter

7

Articular Cartilage

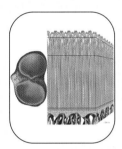

Pearls and Pitfalls & Color Illustrations

Pearls and Pitfalls

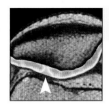

MATRIX ASSESSMENT USING MRI
(see Figures 7.1–7.6)

Proteoglycan assessment: Assess relative fixed charge density (FCD) of negatively charged glycosaminoglycans.

■ Sodium MR imaging
- ☐ No contrast required
- ☐ Standard for newer FCD techniques
- ☐ Requires multinuclear spectroscopy and special coils
- ☐ Limited by longer scan times to obtain adequate signal-to-noise ratio

■ Delayed gadolinium-enhanced MRI of cartilage (dGEMRIC)
- ☐ Indirect T1 following Gd-DTPA penetration → index of $[Gd]_{cartilage}$ proportional to the $[GAG]_{tissue}$
- ☐ Requires intravenous injection of gadolinium, followed by exercise and delay before scanning

■ T1 rho (T1ρ) imaging
- ☐ No contrast required
- ☐ Spin-locking pulse requires more RF power (specific absorption rate may limit number of slices)
- ☐ Less susceptible to regional field inhomogeneities

Collagen assessment: Assess collagen orientation throughout cartilage thickness.

■ T2 mapping
- ☐ No contrast required
- ☐ Subject to magic angle and chemical shift effects in vivo

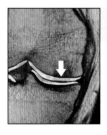

MICROFRACTURE
(see Figures 7.7–7.9)

Principles
- ■ Formation of reparative cartilage by recruitment of multipotential stem cells released from subchondral bone.
- ■ Does not preclude other subsequent forms of cartilage repair.

Procedure
- ■ Performed using arthroscopic approach.
- ■ Very small holes are created, to a depth of 4 mm, through the subchondral plate.

Imaging findings
■ Early postoperative period
- ☐ Reparative cartilage is hyperintense to native cartilage
- ☐ Subchondral bone marrow edema pattern

■ Late postoperative period
- ☐ Signal intensity of reparative cartilage decreases as it matures
- ☐ Subchondral bone marrow edema pattern diminishes
- ☐ Overgrowth of subchondral bone may be present

Diagnostic checklist
- ■ Degree of filling of defect by reparative tissue.
- ■ Morphology of reparative tissue.
- ■ Presence or absence of delamination.
- ■ Peripheral integration (fissures at repair–native tissue interface).
- ■ Assessment of host cartilage.

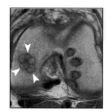

OSTEOCHONDRAL AUTOGRAFTS
(see Figures 7.7, 7.10)

Principles
- ■ Restoration of articular cartilage surface by osteochondral plugs harvested from a different region of the knee in the same individual.
- ■ Plugs are typically harvested from the far anterior margin of the condyle or the side of the intercondylar notch.
- ■ Technique is suitable for a large defect (several plugs are typically used).

Procedure
- ■ One-stage procedure is performed using arthroscopic or open-joint approach.
- ■ Osteochondral plugs are harvested from relatively non–weight-bearing areas of the knee and transplanted to the site of articular defect in the same individual.
- ■ Multiple plugs can be transferred.

Imaging findings
■ Early postoperative period
- ☐ Subchondral bone marrow edema pattern

■ Late postoperative period
- ☐ Subchondral bone marrow edema pattern diminishes

Diagnostic checklist
- ■ Degree of filling of defect by transplanted osteochondral plugs.
- ■ Restoration of radius of curvature of joint surface.
- ■ Presence or absence of displacement.
- ■ Peripheral integration of repair cartilage and osseous components.
- ■ Morphology of autologous bone.
- ■ Assessment of host cartilage.

Pitfalls
- ■ Do not mistake low-signal condensation of trabeculae at the periphery of the plug using the "press fit" technique for lack of osseous integration.

Advantages
- ■ Repair can be performed for a large defect.

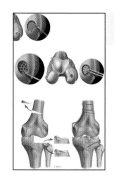

OSTEOCHONDRAL ALLOGRAFT (OCA)
(see Figure 7.7)

Principles

- Articular cartilage resurfacing with one or more osteochondral plugs harvested from a human cadaver.
- Repair is suitable for large defects (several plugs may be used).
- No donor-site morbidity.

Procedure

- Fresh or cryopreserved cadaveric plug(s) are harvested aseptically and transplanted.
- Osteochondral allograft plugs may be pressed to fit in position or fixed by biodegradable or metallic pins if deemed mechanically unstable at the time of surgery.

Imaging findings

- **Early postoperative period (0–3 months)**
  - Graft bone marrow edema pattern
- **Late postoperative period (3–6 months)**
  - Graft bone marrow edema pattern diminishes
- **Features of rejection**
  - Graft bone marrow edema pattern persists after 6 to 12 months
  - Graft collapse
  - Fluid signal intensity at graft–host interface

Diagnostic checklist

- Degree of filling of defect by transplanted osteochondral plugs.
- Restoration of radius of curvature of joint surface.
- Morphology of repair.
- Presence or absence of displacement.
- Peripheral integration of repair cartilage.
- Incorporation of allograft bone.
- Assessment of host cartilage.

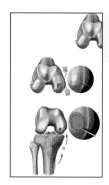

AUTOLOGOUS CHONDROCYTE IMPLANTATION (ACI)
(see Figure 7.7)

Principles

- Articular cartilage resurfacing technique using tissue-cultured autologous articular cartilage cells.

Procedure

- Two-stage procedure:
  1. Healthy articular cartilage is harvested using arthroscopy, and chondrocytes are extracted and grown in tissue culture for 3 to 5 weeks.
  2. Periosteum is harvested via arthrotomy and sewn over the cartilage defect with the cambium layer facing toward the defect. The edges of periosteum are secured with fibrin glue or suture. The cultured chondrocyte suspension is then injected under the periosteum.

Imaging findings

- **Early postoperative period**
  - Reparative cartilage is hyperintense to native cartilage and periosteal cover
  - Subchondral bone marrow edema pattern
  - ± Hypertrophy of periosteal cover
- **Late postoperative period**
  - Signal intensity of reparative cartilage decreases as it matures, approaching that of adjacent cartilage
  - Subchondral bone marrow edema pattern diminishes

Diagnostic checklist

- Degree of filling of defect.
- Morphology of repair.
- Presence or absence of displacement.
- Peripheral integration with adjacent native cartilage and underlying bone.
- Assessment of host cartilage.

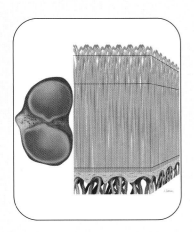

Articular Cartilage

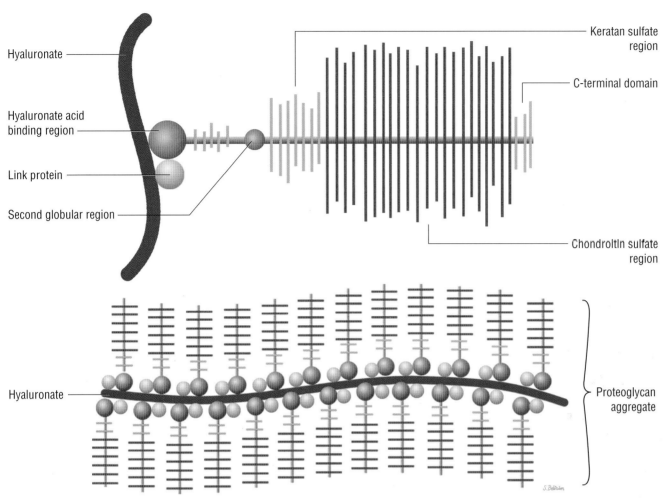

Hyaluronate

Hyaluronate acid binding region

Link protein

Second globular region

Keratan sulfate region

C-terminal domain

Chondroitin sulfate region

Figure 7.1 ■ Structure and composition of articular cartilage. The hydrophilic proteoglycans bind and link to both small and large diameter collagen fibers. The glycosaminoglycans of the proteoglycan aggregate include both chondroitin and keratin sulfate. *(See Introduction to Cartilage Structure pgs. 1100 and 1101, in Stoller's 3rd Edition.)*

Hyaluronate

Proteoglycan aggregate

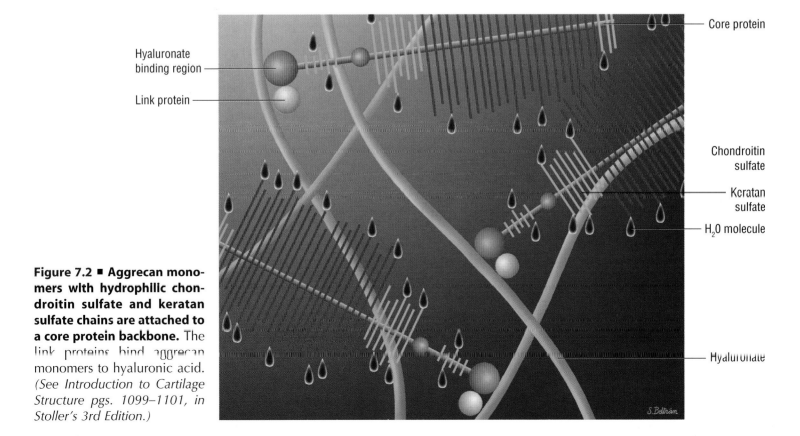

Hyaluronate binding region

Link protein

Core protein

Chondroitin sulfate

Keratan sulfate

H_2O molecule

Hyaluronate

Figure 7.2 ■ Aggrecan monomers with hydrophilic chondroitin sulfate and keratan sulfate chains are attached to a core protein backbone. The link proteins bind aggrecan monomers to hyaluronic acid. *(See Introduction to Cartilage Structure pgs. 1099–1101, in Stoller's 3rd Edition.)*

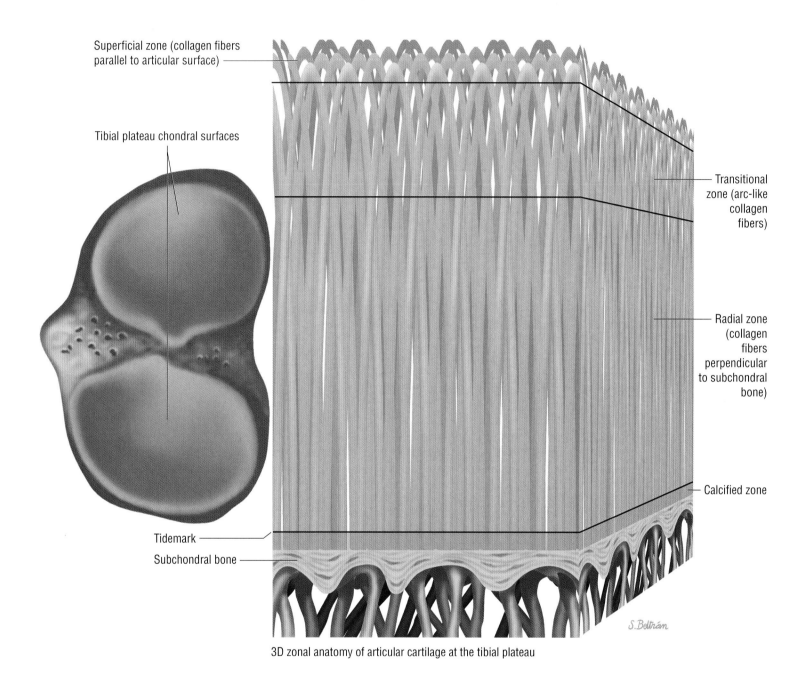

Superficial zone (collagen fibers parallel to articular surface)

Tibial plateau chondral surfaces

Transitional zone (arc-like collagen fibers)

Radial zone (collagen fibers perpendicular to subchondral bone)

Calcified zone

Tidemark

Subchondral bone

S. Beltrán

3D zonal anatomy of articular cartilage at the tibial plateau

Figure 7.3 ■ **Zonal anatomy of the articular cartilage demonstrating the superficial, transitional, radial, and calcified zones.** Tibial plateau chondral surfaces are shown as representative chondral surfaces. *(See Introduction to Cartilage Structure pgs. 1099–1101, in Stoller's 3rd Edition.)*

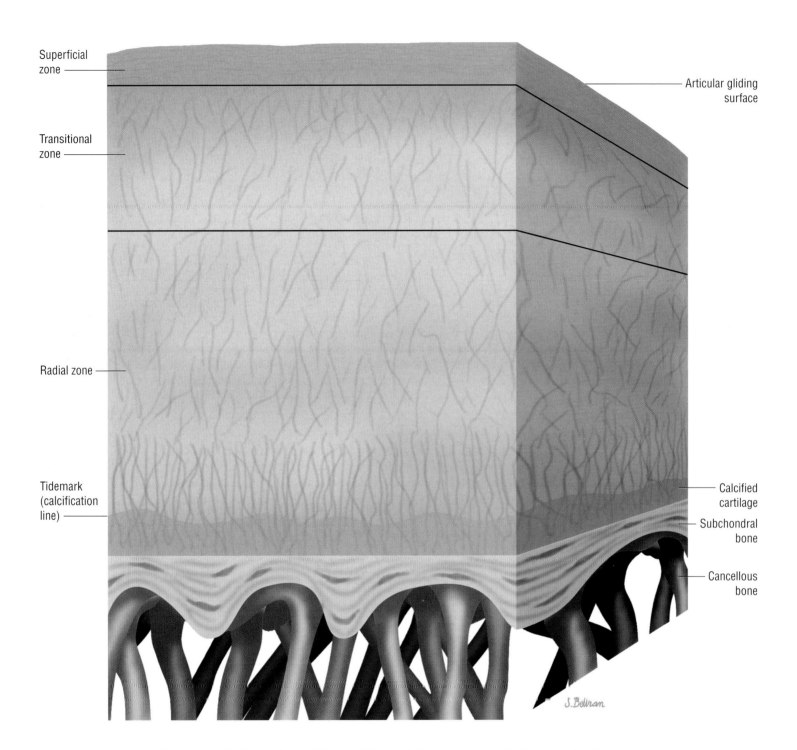

Superficial zone

Transitional zone

Radial zone

Tidemark (calcification line)

Articular gliding surface

Calcified cartilage

Subchondral bone

Cancellous bone

J. Beltran

Figure 7.4 ■ The collagen fibers of the radial zone are oriented perpendicular to the subchondral plate and anchor articular cartilage to bone. Collagen fibers form arcades in the transitional zone and are directed parallel to the surface in the superficial zone. *(See Introduction to Cartilage Structure pgs. 1099–1101, in Stoller's 3rd Edition.)*

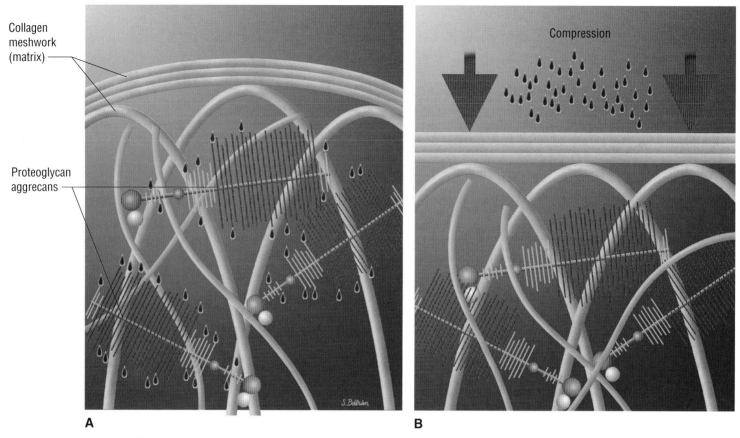

Collagen
meshwork
(matrix)

Proteoglycan
aggrecans

A

Compression

B

Figure 7.5 ■ **(A)** Matrix volume is maintained by negatively charged glycosamino-glycan side chains which repel each other and attract water. Osmotic swelling is limited by the tensile strength of the collagen network. **(B)** The effect of matrix compression pushes glycosamino side chains together, releasing water and decreasing matrix volume. Further compression of articular cartilage is limited by the osmotic pressure and the repulsive force generated by the increased negative charge density relative to the externally applied compressive force. *(See Introduction to Cartilage Structure pgs. 1099–1100, in Stoller's 3rd Edition.)*

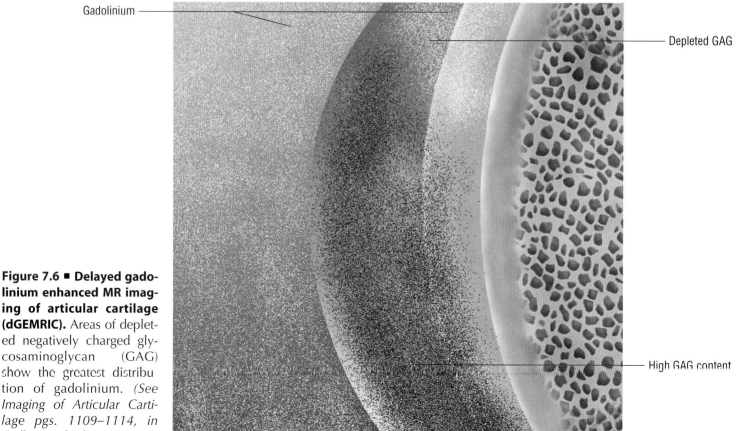

Gadolinium

Depleted GAG

High GAG content

Figure 7.6 ■ **Delayed gadolinium enhanced MR imaging of articular cartilage (dGEMRIC).** Areas of depleted negatively charged glycosaminoglycan (GAG) show the greatest distribution of gadolinium. *(See Imaging of Articular Cartilage pgs. 1109–1114, in Stoller's 3rd Edition.)*

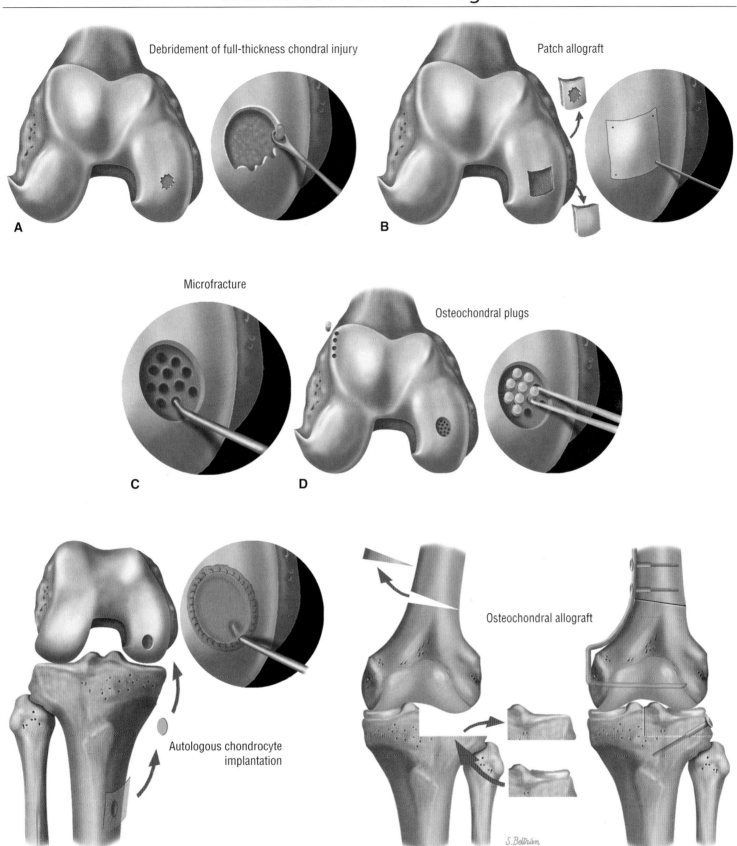

Figure 7.7 ■ Cartilage resurfacing procedures. (A) Abrasion chondroplasty with debridement of a full-thickness chondral defect. **(B)** Patch or shell allograft using a matched osteochondral graft. **(C)** Microfracture using surgical awls to penetrate the subchondral bone up to 4 mm. **(D)** Osteochondral plugs harvested and transferred as a mosaicplasty. **(E)** Autologous chondrocyte implantation (ACI) performed with cultured chondrocytes, which are injected into the chondral defect. The periosteum is sewn and sealed with fibrin glue. The subchondral plate is intact. **(F)** Osteochondral allograft is transferred into an area of excised bone and cartilage. A concomitant osteotomy restores mechanical alignment. *(Based on Miller MD, Howard RF, Plancher KD. Surgical Atlas of Sports Medicine. Philadelphia: Saunders, Elsevier.) (See Cartilage Imaging in Repair pgs. 1119–1130, in Stoller's 3rd Edition.)*

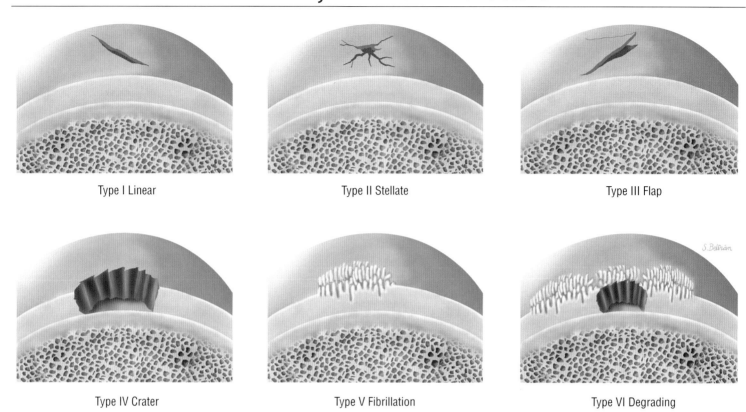

Type I Linear   Type II Stellate   Type III Flap

Type IV Crater   Type V Fibrillation   Type VI Degrading

Figure 7.8 ▪ Classification of articular cartilage injury as developed by Baurer and Jackson *(Based on Baurer M, Jackson RW. Chondral lesions of the femoral condyles: A system of arthroscopic classifications. Arthroscopy 1988; 4: 97–102.) (See Cartilage Imaging pg. 1106, in Stoller's 3rd Edition.)*

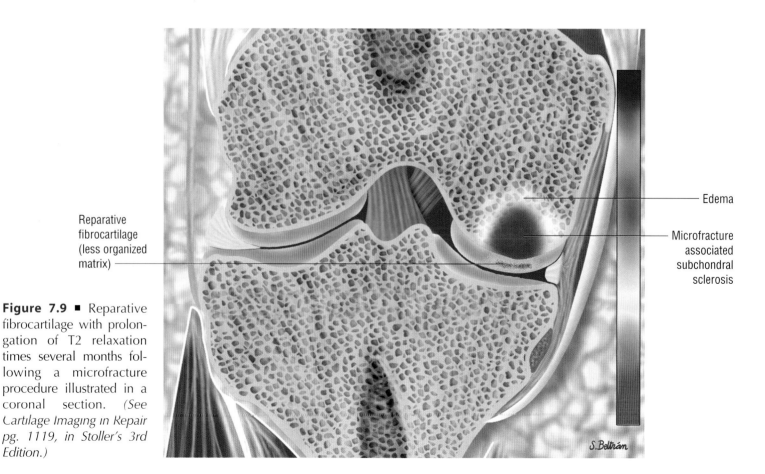

Reparative fibrocartilage (less organized matrix)

Edema

Microfracture associated subchondral sclerosis

Figure 7.9 ▪ Reparative fibrocartilage with prolongation of T2 relaxation times several months following a microfracture procedure illustrated in a coronal section. *(See Cartilage Imaging in Repair pg. 1119, in Stoller's 3rd Edition.)*

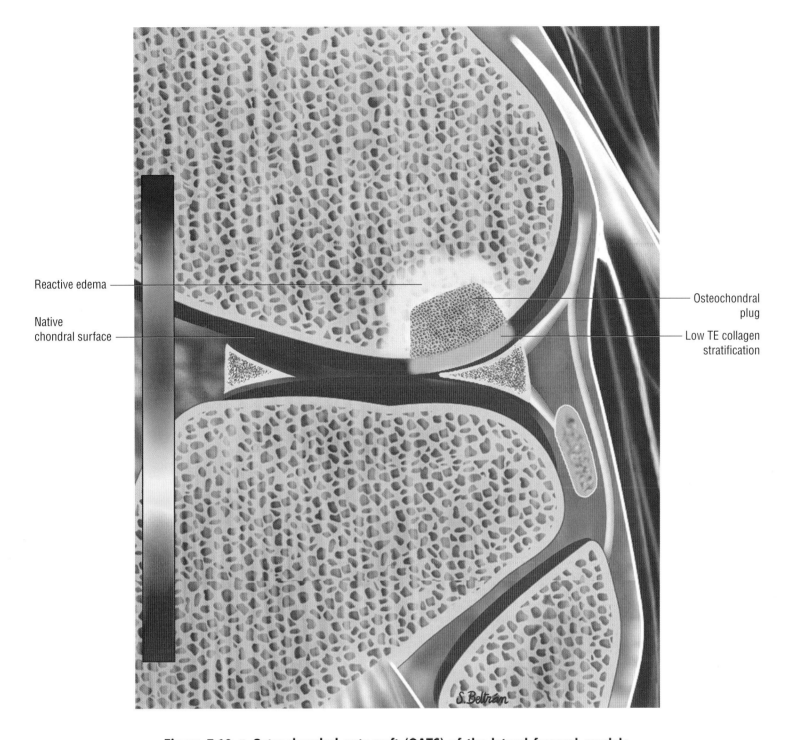

Reactive edema

Native
chondral surface

Osteochondral
plug

Low TE collagen
stratification

S. Beltran

**Figure 7.10 ■ Osteochondral autograft (OATS) of the lateral femoral condyle
with low TE value stratification of the chondral surface illustrated in a sagittal section.** The subchondral osseous component of the osteochondral plug is not proud
and effectively restores the curvature of the overlying chondral surface. *(See
Cartilage Imaging in Repair pg. 1122, in Stoller's 3rd Edition.)*

8

The Shoulder

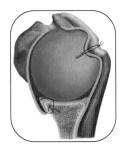

Pearls and Pitfalls & Color Illustrations

Pearls and Pitfalls

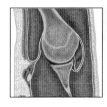

ROUTINE PROTOCOLS
(See Figure 8.22)

- Position arm in partial external rotation.
- Coronal oblique images are performed parallel to the course of the supraspinatus tendon.

- FS PD FSE coronal oblique images are sensitive to rotator cuff degeneration and fluid signal, and T2 FSE coronal images are required to distinguish between tendinosis and tear.
- Axial FS PD FSE images are sensitive for the detection of small paralabral cysts as markers for labral tears.
- Rotator cuff tears should be measured in the coronal and sagittal planes.
- The glenoid fossa is evaluated in the sagittal plane for patterns of glenoid rim and fossa sclerosis associated with instability and osteoarthritis.
- ABER (abduction external rotation) images in conjunction with MR arthrography are helpful in evaluating the postoperative labrum and nondisplaced (e.g., Perthes) labral tears.

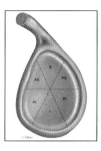

GLENOHUMERAL JOINT AND CAPSULE
(See Figures 8.23–8.38)

- The BLC is classified as type 1, 2, or 3.
- Type 1 BLC has the superior labrum firmly attached to the superior pole of the glenoid.
- The superior labral sulcus in BLC types 2 and 3 should not be mistaken for the more anterior (anterosuperior quadrant) sublabral foramen (also known as the sublabral hole).

- The IGHL contributes to the anterior labrum through its anterior band. The anterior band may be prominent and overlay a small or even absent anterosuperior labrum as a normal variation.
- The MGHL may be cord-like, absent, thin, or redundant on MR.
- The superior glenohumeral and coracohumeral ligaments stabilize the long head of the biceps tendon by forming the biceps pulley or sling in the rotator cuff interval.

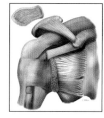

SHOULDER IMPINGEMENT
(See Figures 8.47–8.59)

- Impingement syndrome, a clinical diagnosis, is characterized by a range of MR findings from tendinosis to rotator cuff tears.
- Intrinsic impingement is associated with shoulder instability.

- Primary extrinsic impingement is associated with abrasion of the rotator cuff against the inferior surface of the acromion.
- Subacromial keel spurs are located on the anteroinferior lateral portion of the acromion.
- Acromial thickness is important in planning subacromial decompression procedures.
- The AC joint may hypertrophy, but it is not responsible for true impingement.
- The imaging reference to hypertrophy of the coracoacromial ligament correlates with fraying or fragmentation of the ligament in association with impingement.
- A symptomatic os acromiale is associated with marrow edema on either side of the synchondrosis.
- Degenerative tendinopathy or intrinsic tendon degeneration associated with eccentric tensile overload may be the primary pathology in impingement.
- Rotator cuff tendinosis is most conspicuous on FS PD FSE images. It does not demonstrate hyperintensity on T2 FSE images. Partial- and full-thickness tears are hyperintense on both FS PD FSE and T2 FSE sequences, unless associated with chronic scarring or granulation tissue.

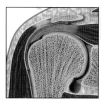

ROTATOR CUFF TEARS
(See Figures 8.60–8.86)

- Partial-thickness rotator cuff tears are articular, bursal, or interstitial (intrasubstance).
- The PASTA lesion is a partial articular-sided supraspinatus tendon avulsion and corresponds to the articular surface delamination tears visualized on MR.

- The bursal puddle sign of localized hyperintense fluid signal on coronal oblique MR images correlates with a bursal-side rotator cuff tear.
- Intramuscular rotator cuff cysts communicate with partial- or full-thickness cuff tears.
- Coronal images identify an intact stump of cuff tendon attaching to the greater tuberosity in cuff tears proximal to the tendinous footprint.
- A wavy contour ("cuff wave sign") of the retracted cuff tendon is associated with an easier cuff reattachment as the tissue is more compliant and less scarred.
- Sagittal images are used to evaluate far anterior supraspinatus tendon tears.
- Retracted rotator cuff tears are associated with an increase in cross-sectional diameter on sagittal images.

- The normal (without atrophy) supraspinatus muscle nearly occupies the suprascapular fossa as assessed on sagittal images.
- The biceps tendon may be medially subluxed or dislocated anteriorly, deep or within the substance of a torn distal subscapularis tendon.
- Rotator cuff tendon retears may be associated with partial or complete tendon retraction and/or granulation tissue at the tear site stimulating apparent cuff continuity.

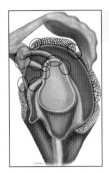

MICROINSTABILITY
(See Figure 8.87)

- The structures involved in microinstability include the biceps, the biceps pulley, the biceps root attachment, the rotator cuff, and the rotator cuff interval.
- Microinstability does not refer to anteroinferior instability, but instead denotes pathologic conditions in the superior half of the shoulder.

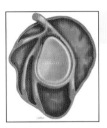

SLAC LESIONS
(See Figure 8.88)

- The SLAC lesion is associated with an articular-side partial-thickness anterior supraspinatus tendon lesion.
- The SLAC lesion is combined with the anterior component of a SLAP 2 tear.

- The SLAC lesion is a type of instability and not an impingement lesion.

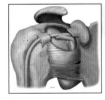

ROTATOR CUFF INTERVAL
(See Figures 8.89–8.90)

- The rotator interval is contained between the supraspinatus and subscapularis tendons.
- The CHL is a bursal structure and the SGHL is an articular structure.

- The confluence of the medial CHL and SGHL is an articular structure.
- The confluence of the medial CHL and SGHL forms the biceps pulley within the rotator cuff interval.
- Failure of the biceps pulley or sling is associated with medial subluxations and dislocations of the biceps tendon.

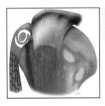

BICEPS PULLEY LESIONS
(See Figures 8.91–8.98)

- Biceps pulley lesions are associated with tearing of the deep fibers of the distal subscapularis and articular surface of the distal supraspinatus tendon.

- The medially dislocated biceps tendon is displaced either intra-articularly, between the coracohumeral ligament and the subscapularis tendon, or extra-articularly.
- Intra-articular dislocation is associated with disruption of the lesser tuberosity attachment of the subscapularis tendon and the SGHL–CHL complex.

- Extra-articular subluxation is associated with an anterolateral supraspinatus tendon tear with extension into the lateral coracohumeral ligament.

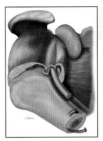

ANTEROSUPERIOR IMPINGEMENT
(See Figures 8.99–8.100)

- Anterosuperior impingement is associated with a tear of the biceps pulley and involvement of the deep subscapularis tendon. A partial articular-side supraspinatus tear may coexist.
- Anterosuperior labral tearing exists with decentralization of the humeral head occurring with adduction and internal rotation.

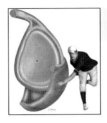

THROWING SHOULDER
(See Figures 8.101–8.111)

- A SLAP 2 or posterior SLAP 2 lesion causes the dead arm.
- Repetitive tensile loading during follow-through results in a tight posterior band of the IGHL.

- The tight posterior band bowstrings the humeral head in the late cocking phase, resulting in a posterosuperior shift of the glenohumeral contact point.
- Glenohumeral internal rotation deficit (GIRD) is an acquired loss of internal rotation resulting from the tight posterior band of the IGL.
- Peel-back posterior SLAP 2 lesions and posterior articular surface tears of the supraspinatus represent the net effect of the shift of the glenohumeral rotation contact point with a loss of internal rotation and gain of external rotation.
- Pseudolaxity of the anterior IGHL results from a reduced cam effect of the proximal humerus, which allows for an even greater degree of external rotation.
- On sagittal MR images, eccentric posterior glenoid rim sclerosis may precede the development of the peel-back labral lesion.

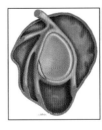

ANTERIOR INSTABILITY
(See Figures 8.112–8.129)

- The IGHL can fail at its attachment to the inferior pole of the glenoid (Bankart), mid-ligament, or at the attachment to the anatomic neck of the humerus (HAGL).
- Bankart, Perthes, ALPSA, and HAGL lesions may produce anterior instability.

- The Bankart lesion may be osseous or primarily soft tissue.
- Atraumatic anterior instability is a component of multidirectional instability (MDI).

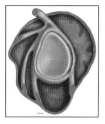

POSTERIOR INSTABILITY
(See Figures 8.130–8.133)

- The reverse Hill-Sachs and the reverse Bankart lesions are associated with posterior instability.
- The reverse HAGL lesion is characterized by tearing of the posterior capsule at the humeral attachment.

- Posterosuperior labral tears may occur as part of posterior SLAP 2 or posterior peel-back lesions.
- The Bennett lesion occurs in the throwing athlete and is visualized as an extra-articular posterior ossification.

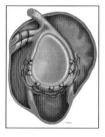

MULTIDIRECTIONAL INSTABILITY
(See Figure 8.134)

- Referred to as either MDI (multidirectional instability) or AMBRI (atraumatic multidirectional instability, bilateral treated with rehabilitation or inferior capsular shift).
- MDI must include a component of inferior instability (anteroinferior or posteroinferior).

- MR findings in MDI may include subtle anterior and posterior glenoid rim sclerosis or static humeral head subluxation in the axial plane.
- A pancapsular plication is used to selectively tighten lax ligaments.

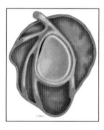

NORMAL VARIATIONS
(See Figures 8.135–8.141)

- The sublabral foramen is located in the anterosuperior quadrant of the glenoid fossa. The biceps labral sulcus is identified at the level of the superior pole of the glenoid in the 12-o'clock position.

- The MGL may be cord-like, thin, or absent.
- When cord-like, the MGL presents as an isolated variation or in conjunction with a prominent anterior band of the IGL or as part of the Buford complex.
- Because there is no anterosuperior labrum in the Buford complex, a sublabral foramen cannot exist. In the presence of a prominent anterior band of the IGHL and a Buford complex, the anterior band may form an apparent or pseudo-sublabral foramen above the equator.

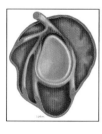

SLAP TEARS
(See Figures 8.142–8.155)

- A biceps labral sulcus greater than 5 mm is abnormal.
- Superior paralabral cysts that often extend into the spinoglenoid notch communicate with SLAP 2 or posterior SLAP 2 (peel-back) lesions.

- Inferior displacement of the superior labrum (relative to the biceps labral junction) is associated with bucket-handle SLAP morphology.

- SLAP tears are grouped into 10 subtypes. Four primary types were initially described and six further types were subsequently characterized.
- The SLAP 2 or classic SLAP lesion is subdivided further into anterior SLAP 2 in the SLAC lesion and posterior SLAP 2 in the posterior peel-back lesion.
- A SLAP fracture is a posterosuperior medial humeral head chondral fracture in association with a SLAP lesion.

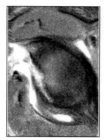

MR OF LABRAL TEARS

- The coronal oblique plane is used to assess both the superior labrum at the superior pole of the glenoid and the IGLLC at the inferior pole of the glenoid.
- The sagittal oblique plane is useful in identifying normal variations in the MGHL and the anterior band of the IGHL relative to the corresponding morphology of the anterior labrum in the axial plane. The sagittal oblique plane demonstrates bucket-handle SLAP tear patterns.
- The labrum usually tears in an entire quadrant on more than one image location.

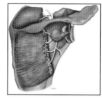

PARALABRAL CYSTS
(See Figures 8.156–8.158)

- Paralabral cysts frequently communicate with a SLAP 2 or posterior-type SLAP 2 lesion.
- A paralabral cyst usually coexists with a labral tear but may be associated with degenerative arthritis.

- Suprascapular notch cysts are associated with edema or atrophy of the supraspinatus and infraspinatus.
- Spinoglenoid notch cysts are associated with edema or atrophy of the infraspinatus.
- Inferior paralabral cysts are associated with isolated denervation of the teres minor muscle.

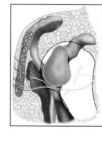

QUADRILATERAL SPACE SYNDROME
(See Figures 8.156–8.161)

- The posterior branch of the axillary nerve courses adjacent to the inferior pole of the glenoid and inferior joint capsule and then divides into a branch to the teres minor muscle and a superolateral brachial cutaneous nerve branch.

- The quadrilateral space syndrome is more commonly associated with denervation edema or atrophy restricted to the teres minor muscle, although the teres minor and deltoid are supplied by the axillary nerve.

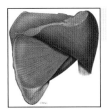

PARSONAGE-TURNER SYNDROME
(See Figures 8.162–8.163)

- Parsonage-Turner syndrome is characterized by acute painful brachial neuritis.
- Supraspinatus and infraspinatus; supraspinatus, infraspinatus, and deltoid; and infraspinatus and teres minor are potential patterns of affected muscle groups.
- FS PD FSE images show all hyperintense muscles involved in the sagittal plane.

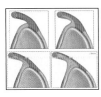

BICEPS TENDON
(See Figures 8.164–8.166)

- The biceps tendon origin includes the posterosuperior labrum and supraglenoid tubercle medial to the BLC.
- The CHL-SGHL complex and not the transverse humeral ligament provides the stability of the biceps tendon in the intertubercular sulcus (groove).
- Intra-articular biceps tendinosis may be overestimated on sagittal images secondary to the magic-angle effect.
- Biceps tenosynovitis is visualized with hyperintense fluid or intermediate to hyperintense signal in the presence of thickened synovium.
- Biceps tendon ruptures occur at the biceps anchor or within the rotator cuff interval.

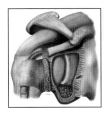

ADHESIVE CAPSULITIS
(See Figure 8.167)

- Acute adhesive capsulitis demonstrates a hyperintense and thickened IGHL on coronal FS PD FSE images. Associated synovial hypertrophy is shown as intermediate signal intensity and occupies the space created by the axillary pouch.
- Residual or chronic thickening of the axillary pouch does not demonstrate hyperintensity on coronal FS PD FSE images.
- Adhesive capsulitis may coexist with synovitis in other joint locations, including the rotator cuff interval and subscapularis recess.
- The axillary nerve is susceptible to injury during transection of the axillary pouch in arthroscopic treatment of adhesive capsulitis. Arthroscopic capsular release should be considered when conservative management or manipulation is unsuccessful.

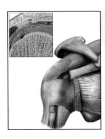

CALCIFIC TENDINITIS
(See Figures 8.168–8.169)

- Calcific tendinitis is visualized best as hypointensity on a T2* GRE sequence.
- The semiliquid state of calcium hydroxyapatite may demonstrate heterogeneous hyperintensity on FS PD FSE images, although hypointensity is still characteristic on T2* GRE images.
- The supraspinatus and infraspinatus are the most commonly affected tendons.

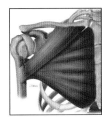

PECTORALIS MAJOR TEAR
(See Figure 8.170)

- The bilaminar pectoralis major tendon is formed from the sternocostal and clavicular heads of the pectoralis muscle.
- Partial musculotendinous pectoralis major tears with combined sternal and clavicular head involvement are the most common presentation.
- Axial MR images must include the humeral diaphyseal insertion of the lateral lip of the bicipital groove. Coronal oblique images are prescribed parallel to the course of the pectoralis muscle.

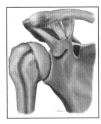

ACROMIOCLAVICULAR SEPARATIONS
(See Figures 8.171–8.172)

- AC separations range from AC ligament sprains to complete disruption of the AC joint capsule and coracoclavicular ligaments.
- Displacement between the coracoid and clavicle and the position of the distal clavicle relative to the acromial facet are assessed on sagittal and coronal images.
- Associated fractures may occur in the coracoid, acromion, or clavicle.

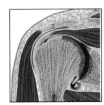

ARTHRITIS
(See Figures 8.173–8.175)

- Central and posterior glenoid wear with sclerosis and cartilage loss is typically seen in osteoarthritis.
- Loose bodies are frequently located in the subscapularis recess.
- Coronal images demonstrate the medial and inferior projection of humeral head osteophytes. Spurring also is present directed from the inferior pole of the glenoid.
- Severe glenohumeral osteoarthritis may be associated with reactive subchondral marrow edema.
- Rheumatoid-related synovial hypertrophy or pannus is intermediate in signal intensity on FS PD FSE images and will enhance with intravenous contrast.
- Rotator cuff tears are commonly seen in association with rheumatoid arthritis.
- Rice bodies are hypointense on FS PD FSE images and represent detached fibrotic synovial villi.

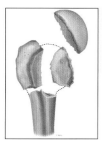

FRACTURES OF THE PROXIMAL HUMERUS AND OSTEOCHONDRAL LESIONS
(See Figures 8.176–8.179)

- Proximal humeral fractures have been grouped into involvement of the anatomic neck, greater tuberosity, lesser tuberosity, and surgical neck.

- Fracture displacement and angulation requires correlation of coronal and axial images.

- A chondral SLAP fracture involves the posteromedial superior humeral head.

- In acute fractures, T2* GRE images may be useful if hyperintense marrow edema obscures fracture site morphology or if a number of segments are involved.

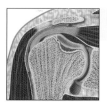

AVASCULAR NECROSIS
(See Figures 8.180–8.181)

- Although the risk of avascular necrosis (AVN) increases with three and four-part fractures, displacement is not required to cause osseous ischemia.

- MR findings of AVN may be subchondral or metaphyseal in location.

- Extended hyperintense marrow edema of the proximal humerus is often associated with the more acute stages of AVN.

- Sagittal images are helpful in assessing early subchondral collapse with a flattening in the humeral head contour.

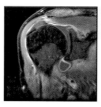

INFECTION

- T1-weighted images in at least one plane provide yellow marrow fat contrast relative to the patchy hypointensity of osseous osteomyelitis.

- T2* GRE images, although not sensitive for infection, can increase specificity in the diagnosis of osteomyelitis if areas of trabecular hyperintensity are shown. A non-marrow-sensitive sequence that demonstrates hyperintensity in association with joint sepsis is consistent with the spread or extension of osteomyelitis.

- Intravenous contrast, although not specific for osteomyelitis, is used to enhance soft tissue tracts and abscesses, which may communicate with adjacent osseous erosions.

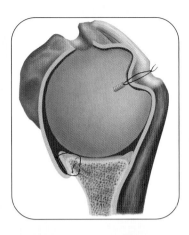

The Shoulder

Muscle

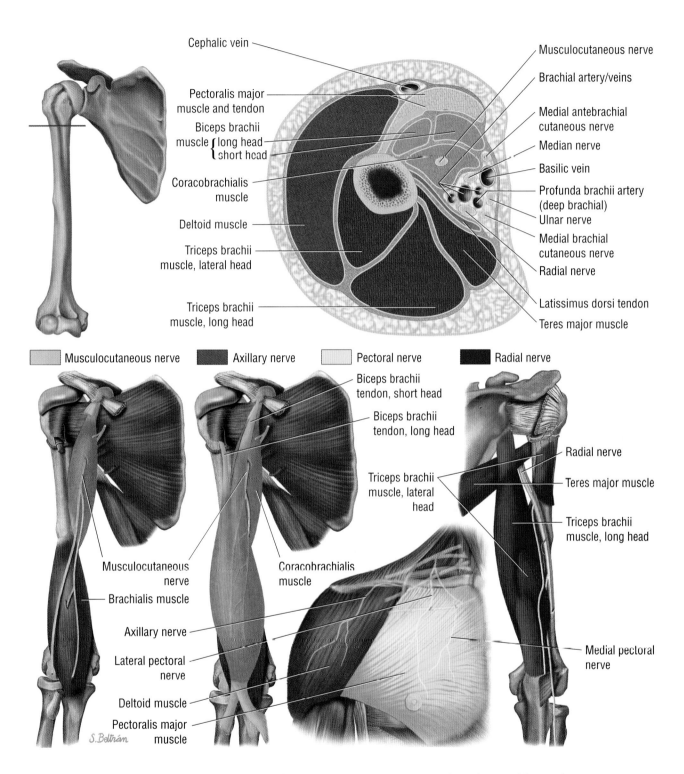

Figure 8.1 ■ Upper Arm Muscle Innervation. *Cross section based on Vahlensiech M, Genant HK, Reiter M. MRI of the Musculoskeletal System. New York/Stuttgart: Thieme, 2000. (See Related Muscles pgs. 1141–1159, in Stoller's 3rd Edition.)*

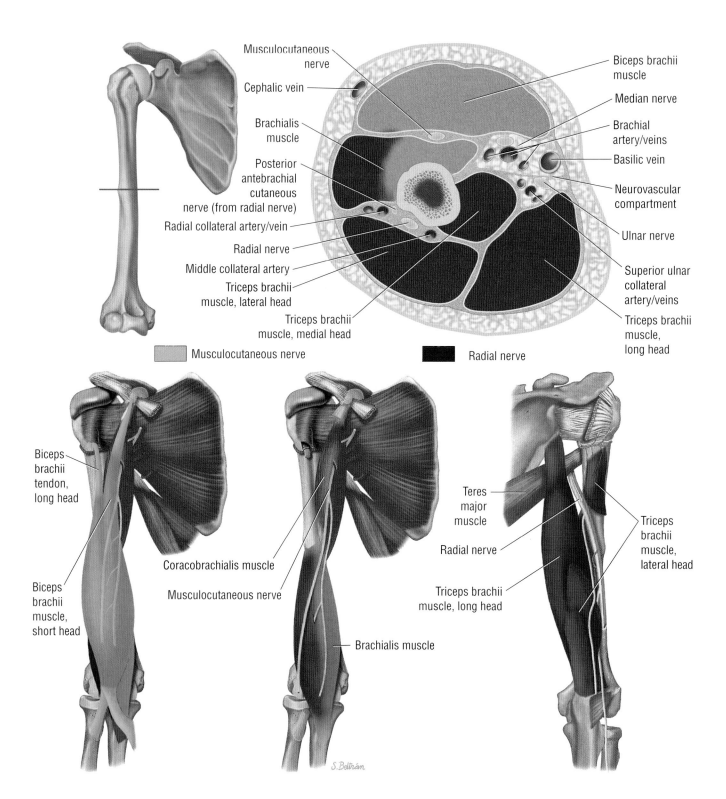

Figure 8.2 ■ Mid-Arm Muscle Innervation. *Cross section based on Vahlensiech M, Genant HK, Reiter M. MRI of the Musculoskeletal System. New York/Stuttgart: Thieme, 2000. (See Related Muscles pgs. 1141–1159, in Stoller's 3rd Edition.)*

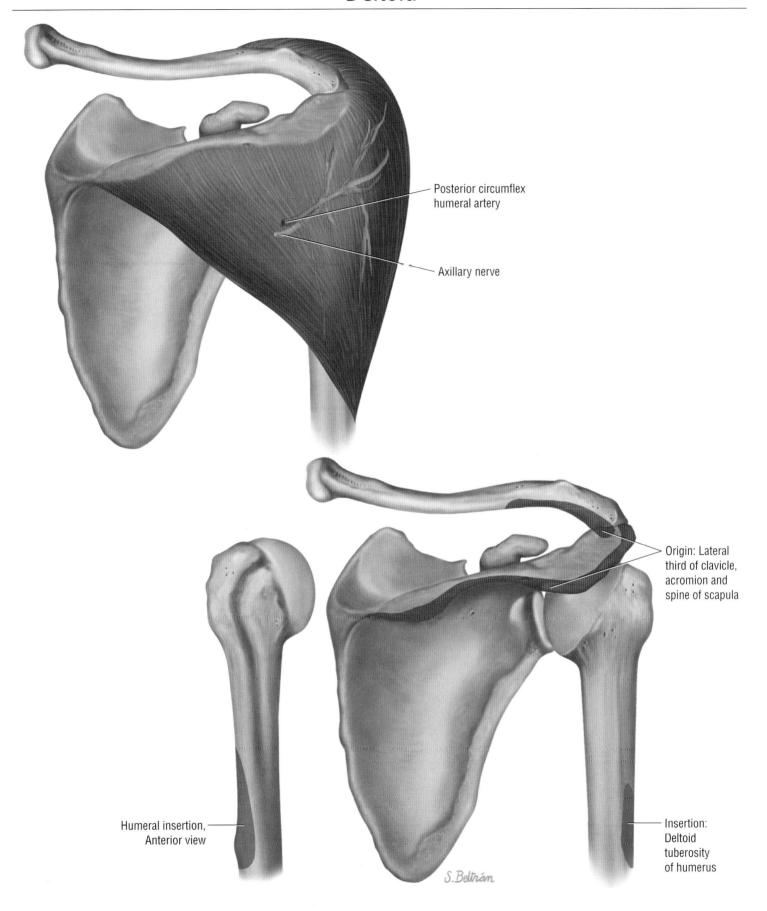

Posterior circumflex
humeral artery

Axillary nerve

Origin: Lateral
third of clavicle,
acromion and
spine of scapula

Humeral insertion,
Anterior view

Insertion:
Deltoid
tuberosity
of humerus

S. Beltrán

Figure 8.3 ■ DELTOID. The deltoid abducts the arm and represents the largest of the glenohumeral muscles. The deltoid is multipennate, with an anterolateral raphe, and is important in any form of arm elevation. It Is active throughout the entire arc of glenohumeral abduction, even if the supraspinatus muscle Is Inactive. *(See Related Muscles pg. 1144, in Stoller's 3rd Edition.)*

Subscapularis

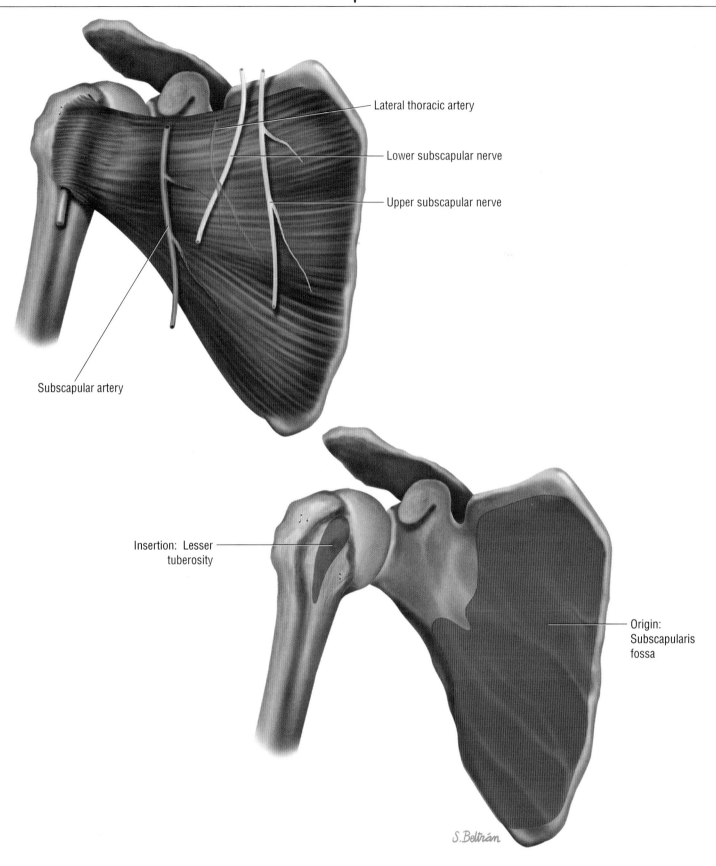

Lateral thoracic artery

Lower subscapular nerve

Upper subscapular nerve

Subscapular artery

Insertion: Lesser tuberosity

Origin: Subscapularis fossa

S.Beltrán

Figure 8.4 ▪ SUBSCAPULARIS. The subscapularis muscle represents the anterior compartment of the rotator cuff. It internally rotates and flexes the humerus. The superior two thirds of the muscle has a tendinous distribution dispersed within the muscle belly, converging into a single large tendon laterally. The inferior third of the subscapularis is muscular throughout its course. *(See Related Muscles pg. 1145, in Stoller's 3rd Edition.)*

Supraspinatus

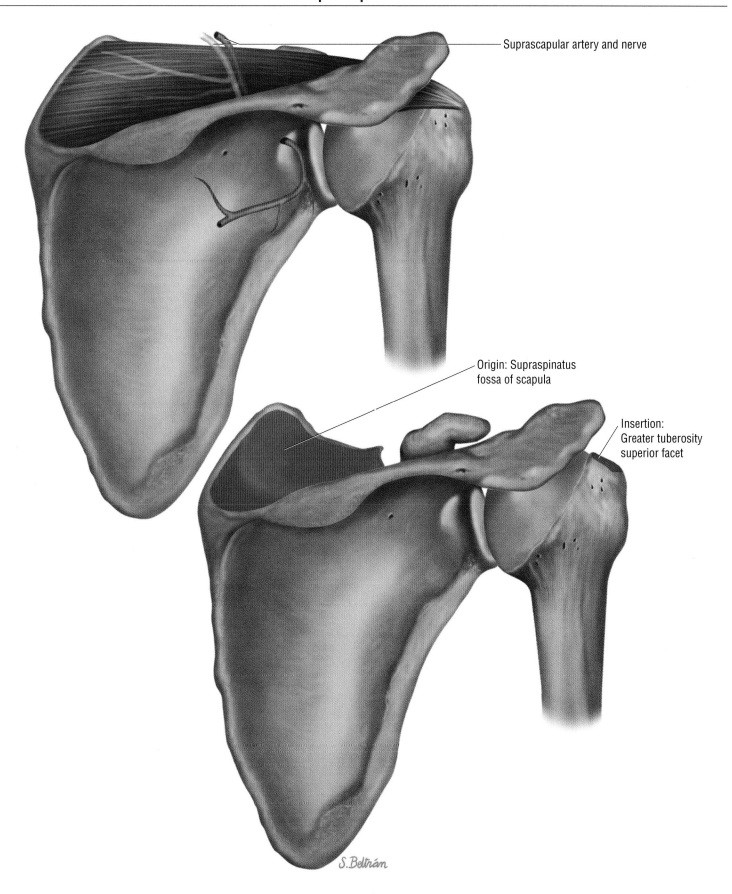

Suprascapular artery and nerve

Origin: Supraspinatus
fossa of scapula

Insertion:
Greater tuberosity
superior facet

S.Beltrán

Figure 8.5 ■ SUPRASPINATUS. The supraspinatus initiates abduction of the arm
and is active during the entire arc of scapular plane abduction. The parallel independent collagen fascicles permit differential excursion of segments of the tendon.
The supraspinatus exerts maximal effort at approximately 30° of abduction and functions with the rotator cuff as a humeral head depressor. *(See Related Muscles pg.
1146, in Stoller's 3rd Edition.)*

Infraspinatus

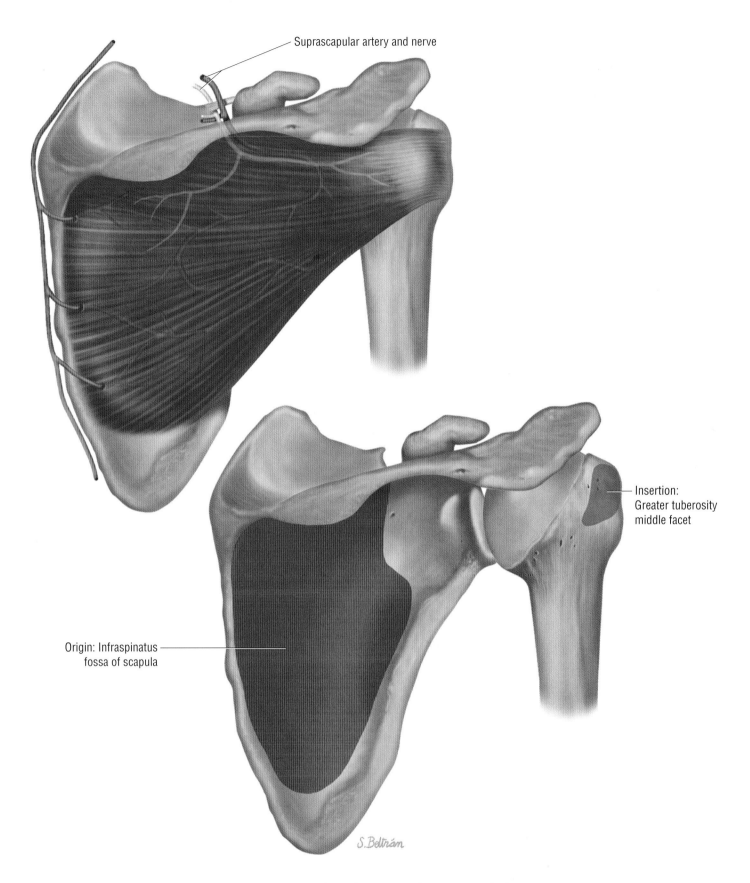

Suprascapular artery and nerve

Insertion:
Greater tuberosity
middle facet

Origin: Infraspinatus
fossa of scapula

S.Beltrán

Figure 8.6 ▪ INFRASPINATUS. The infraspinatus functions with the teres minor to externally rotate and extend the humerus. The infraspinatus is more active with the arm in the adducted position and accounts for up to 60% of external rotation force. The infraspinatus contributes to the humeral head depressor action of the rotator cuff. *(See Related Muscles pg. 1147, in Stoller's 3rd Edition.)*

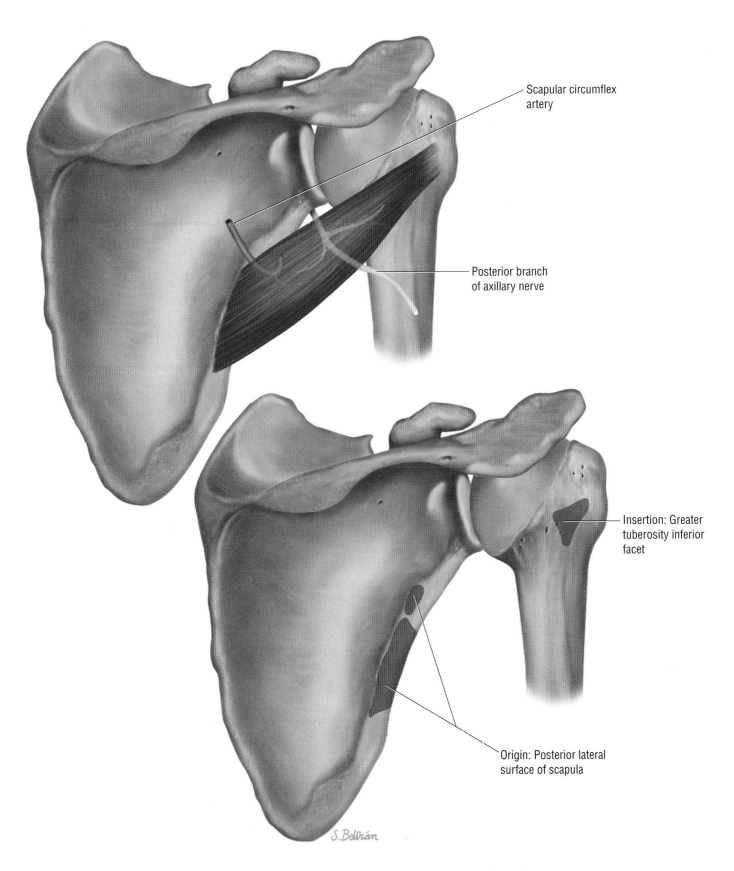

Scapular circumflex artery

Posterior branch of axillary nerve

Insertion: Greater tuberosity inferior facet

Origin: Posterior lateral surface of scapula

S.Beltrán

Figure 8.7 ▪ TERES MINOR. The teres minor functions with the infraspinatus to externally rotate and extend the humerus. The teres minor is active with the shoulder in 90° of elevation. *(See Related Muscles pg. 1148, in Stoller's 3rd Edition.)*

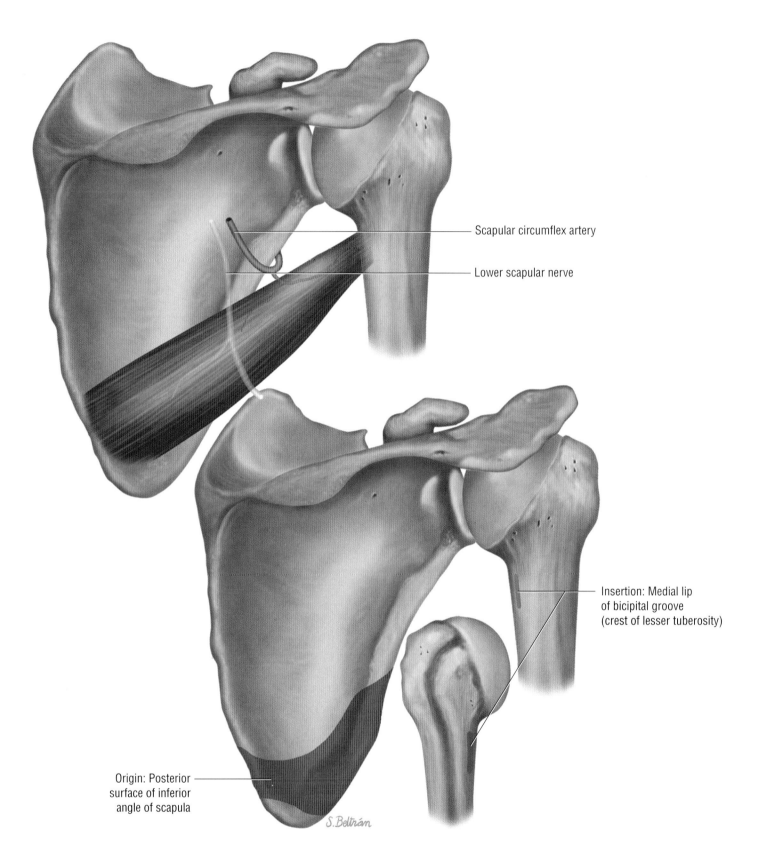

Scapular circumflex artery

Lower scapular nerve

Insertion: Medial lip
of bicipital groove
(crest of lesser tuberosity)

Origin: Posterior
surface of inferior
angle of scapula

S. Beltrán

Figure 8.8 ■ TERES MAJOR. The teres major internally rotates and adducts the arm. The axillary nerve and posterior humeral circumflex artery pass superior to the upper border of the teres major through the quadrilateral space. The quadrilateral space is bordered also by the teres minor, the triceps, and the humerus. The teres major functions with the latissimus dorsi muscle in humeral extension, internal rotation, and adduction. *(See Related Muscles pg. 1149, in Stoller's 3rd Edition.)*

Coracobrachialis

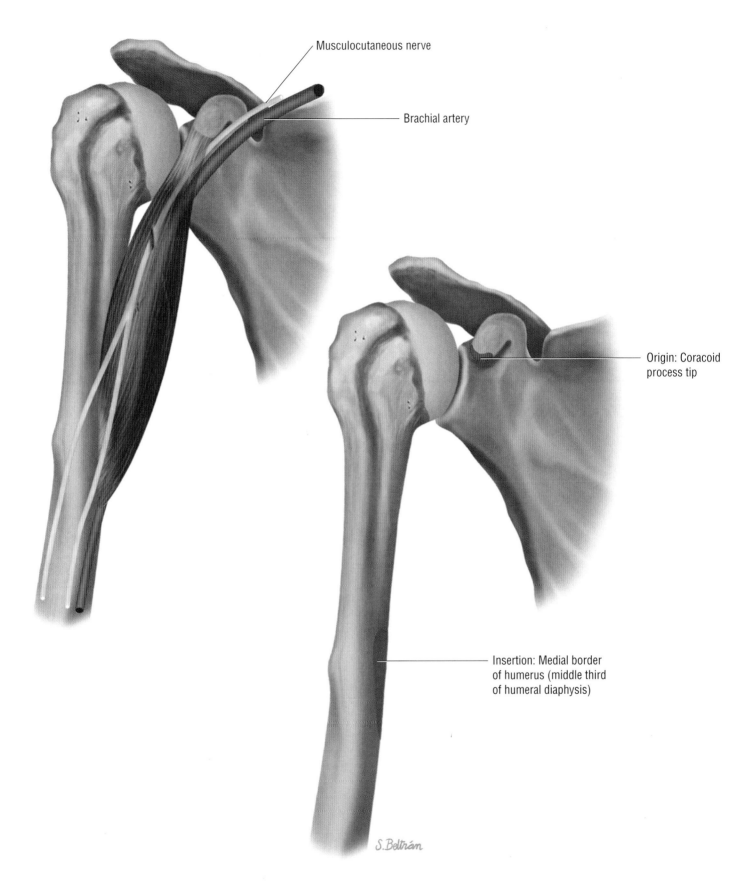

Musculocutaneous nerve

Brachial artery

Origin: Coracoid process tip

Insertion: Medial border of humerus (middle third of humeral diaphysis)

S. Beltrán

Figure 8.9 ■ CORACOBRACHIALIS. The coracobrachialis flexes and adducts the arm. The coracobrachialis and the short head of the biceps have a conjoined tendon origin at the coracoid. *(See Related Muscles pg. 1150, in Stoller's 3rd Edition.)*

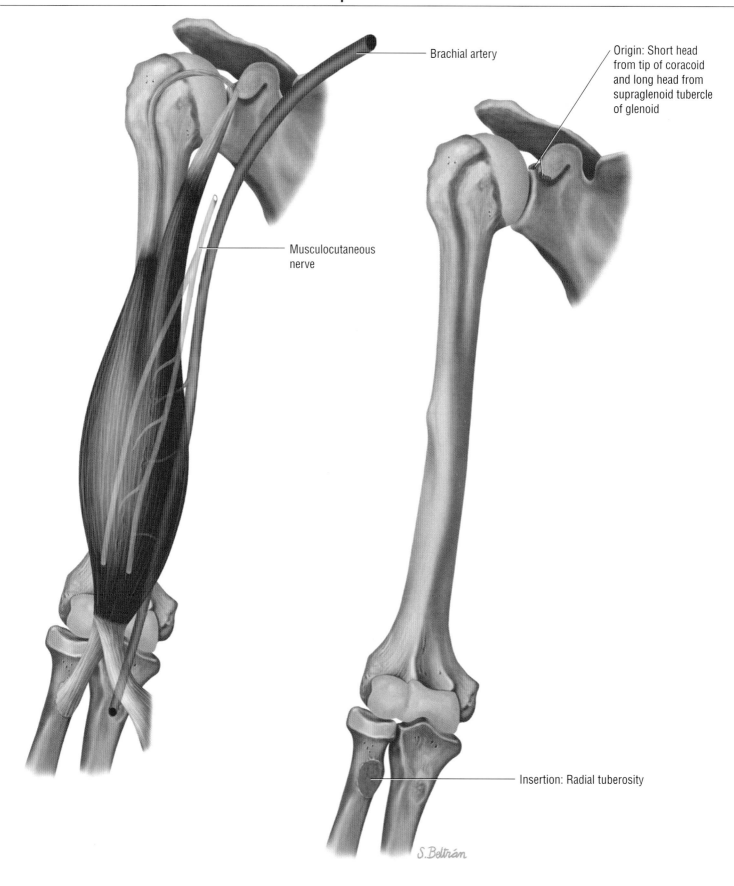

Brachial artery

Origin: Short head
from tip of coracoid
and long head from
supraglenoid tubercle
of glenoid

Musculocutaneous
nerve

Insertion: Radial tuberosity

S. Beltrán

Figure 8.10 ■ BICEPS BRACHII. The biceps brachii functions to flex and supinate
the forearm. The long head of the biceps tendon (LHBT) has origins at the superior
pole of the glenoid and the posterosuperior labrum of the biceps labral complex. The
LHBT extends within the synovial sheath of the glenohumeral joint. The long and
short head muscle bellies join at the level of the deltoid insertion on the humerus.
(See Related Muscles pg. 1151, in Stoller's 3rd Edition.)

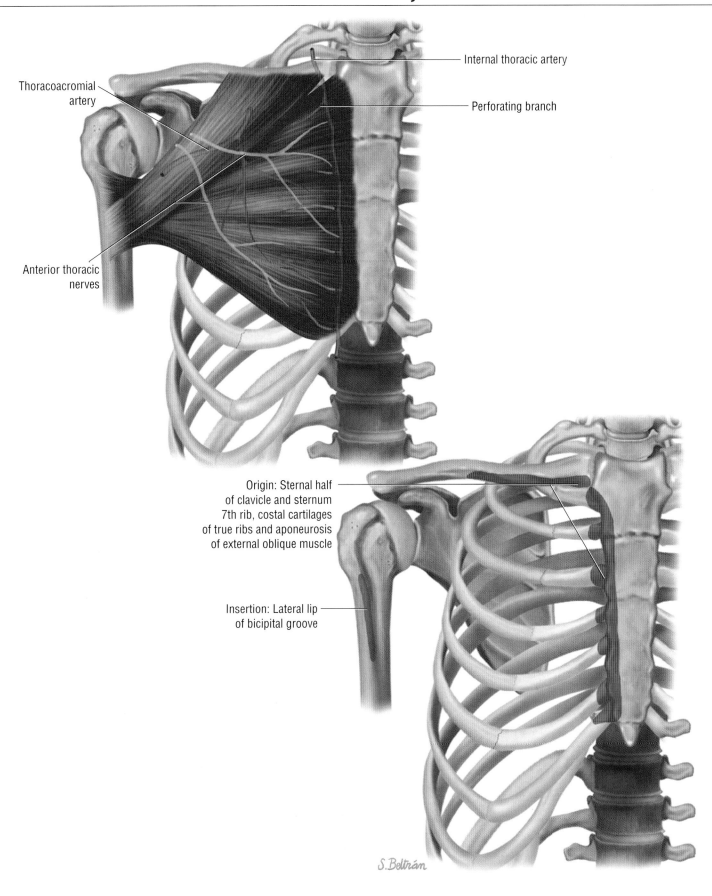

Thoracoacromial artery

Anterior thoracic nerves

Internal thoracic artery

Perforating branch

Origin: Sternal half of clavicle and sternum 7th rib, costal cartilages of true ribs and aponeurosis of external oblique muscle

Insertion: Lateral lip of bicipital groove

S. Beltrán

Figure 8.11 ▪ PECTORALIS MAJOR. The pectoralis major muscle adducts the arm and internally rotates the humerus. The pectoralis major has an upper clavicular and a lower sternocostal head. The clavicular head contributes to the anterior lamina of the broad flat tendon insertion to the humerus, whereas the more distal and deep sternocostal head fibers form the posterior lamina of the tendinous insertion. *(See Related Muscles pg. 1152, in Stoller's 3rd Edition.)*

Pectoralis Minor

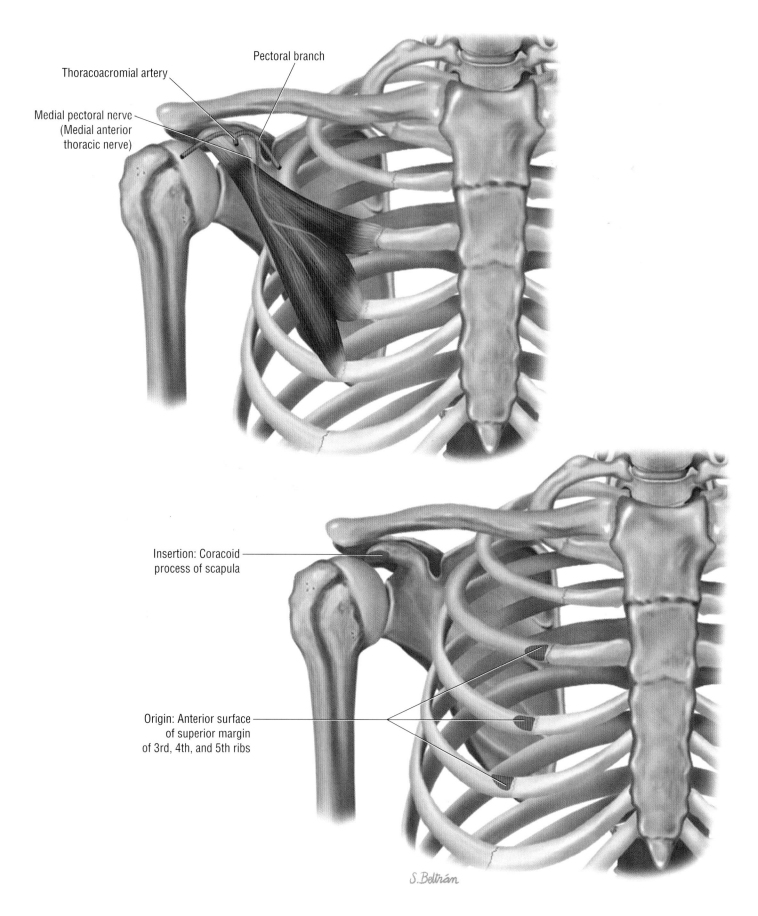

Thoracoacromial artery

Pectoral branch

Medial pectoral nerve
(Medial anterior
thoracic nerve)

Insertion: Coracoid
process of scapula

Origin: Anterior surface
of superior margin
of 3rd, 4th, and 5th ribs

S.Beltrán

Figure 8.12 ▪ PECTORALIS MINOR. The pectoralis minor and major are internal rotators and flexors of the shoulder joint. The pectoralis minor helps stabilize the scapula. *(See Related Muscles pg. 1153, in Stoller's 3rd Edition.)*

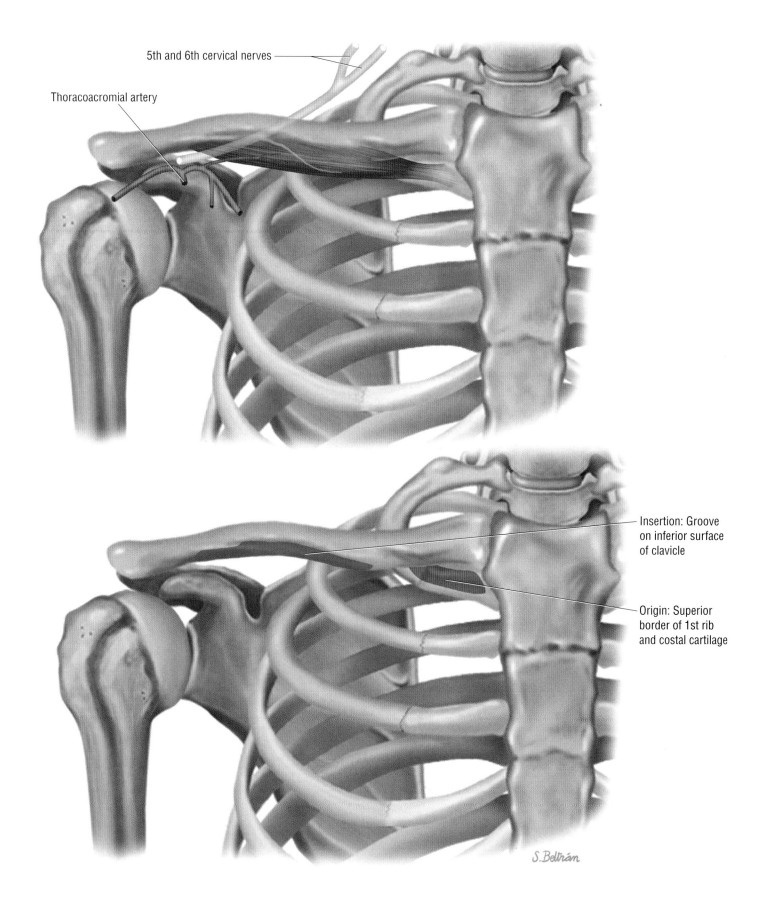

5th and 6th cervical nerves

Thoracoacromial artery

Insertion: Groove on inferior surface of clavicle

Origin: Superior border of 1st rib and costal cartilage

S. Beltrán

Figure 8.13 ■ SUBCLAVIUS. The subclavius muscle functions to depress the clavicle. *(See Related Muscles pg. 1153, in Stoller's 3rd Edition.)*

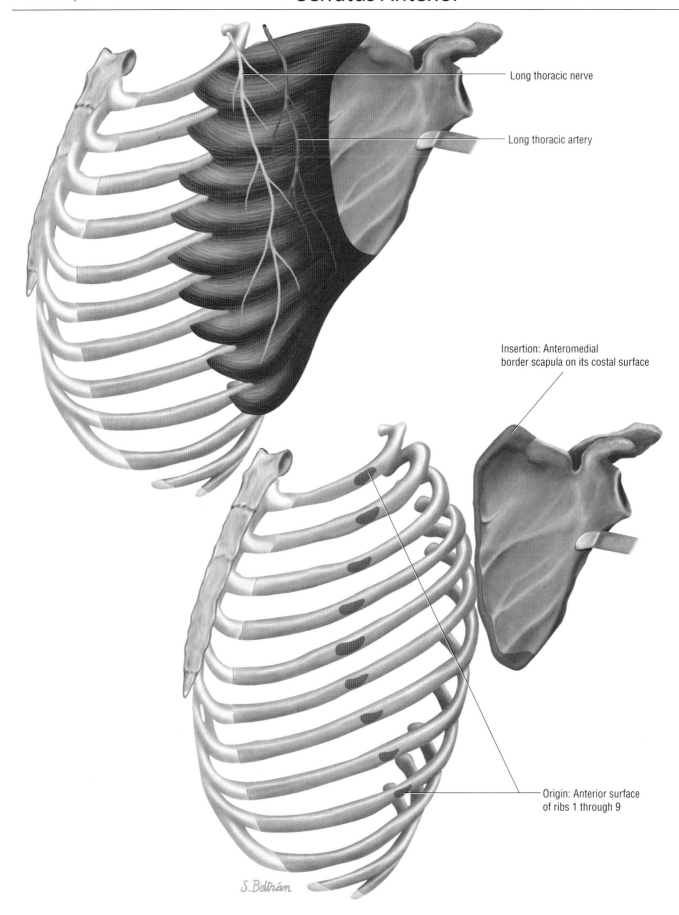

Long thoracic nerve

Long thoracic artery

Insertion: Anteromedial
border scapula on its costal surface

Origin: Anterior surface
of ribs 1 through 9

S.Beltrán

Figure 8.14 ■ SERRATUS ANTERIOR. The serratus anterior muscle holds the scapula to the chest wall, protracting and allowing for upward rotation. The serratus anterior originates from the outer surface of the first eight or nine ribs. Injury to the long thoracic nerve with absence of serratus function produces a winged scapula with forward flexion of the arm. *(See Related Muscles pg. 1154, in Stoller's 3rd Edition.)*

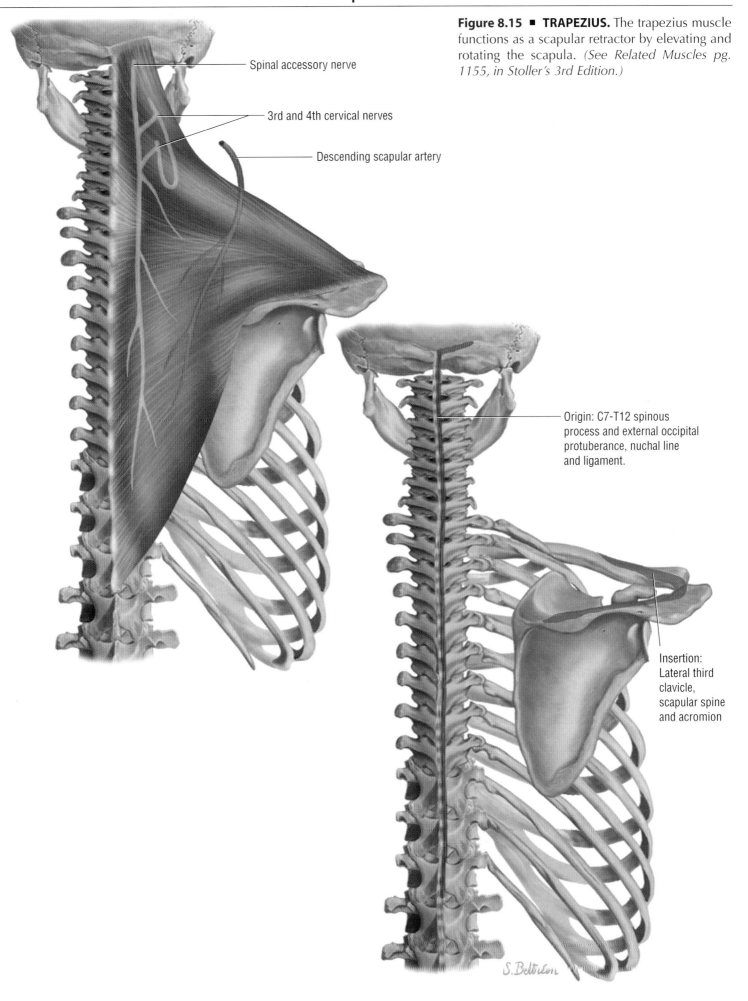

Figure 8.15 ■ TRAPEZIUS. The trapezius muscle functions as a scapular retractor by elevating and rotating the scapula. *(See Related Muscles pg. 1155, in Stoller's 3rd Edition.)*

Spinal accessory nerve

3rd and 4th cervical nerves

Descending scapular artery

Origin: C7-T12 spinous process and external occipital protuberance, nuchal line and ligament.

Insertion: Lateral third clavicle, scapular spine and acromion

S.Beltrilon

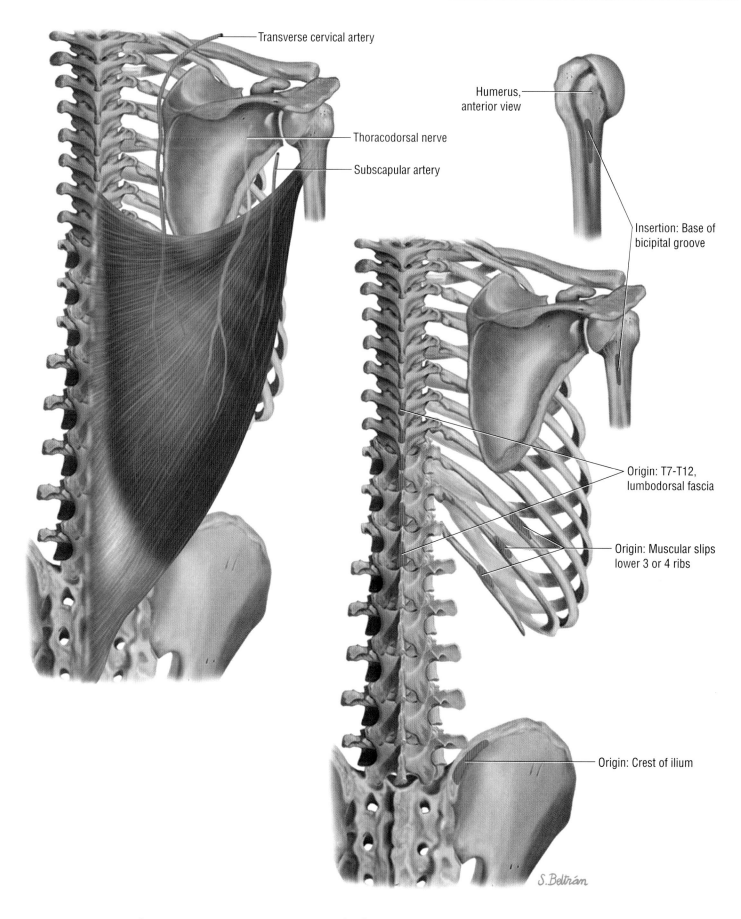

Transverse cervical artery

Humerus,
anterior view

Thoracodorsal nerve

Subscapular artery

Insertion: Base of
bicipital groove

Origin: T7-T12,
lumbodorsal fascia

Origin: Muscular slips
lower 3 or 4 ribs

Origin: Crest of ilium

S. Beltrán

Figure 8.16 ▪ LATISSIMUS DORSI. The latissimus dorsi, which adducts, extends, and internally rotates the humerus, forms the posterior axillary fold. The thoracodorsal nerve arises from the posterior cord and innervates the muscle. *(See Related Muscles pg. 1156, in Stoller's 3rd Edition.)*

Rhomboid Major

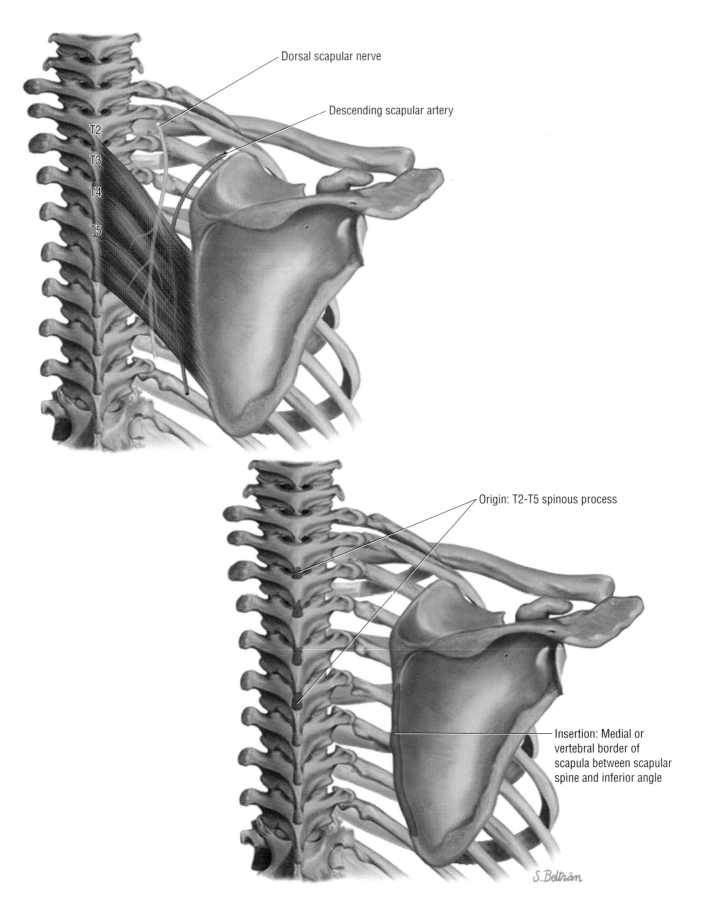

Figure 8.17 ■ RHOMBOID MAJOR. The rhomboid major muscle adducts the scapula, participating in its retraction and elevation. *(See Related Muscles pg. 1157, in Stoller's 3rd Edition.)*

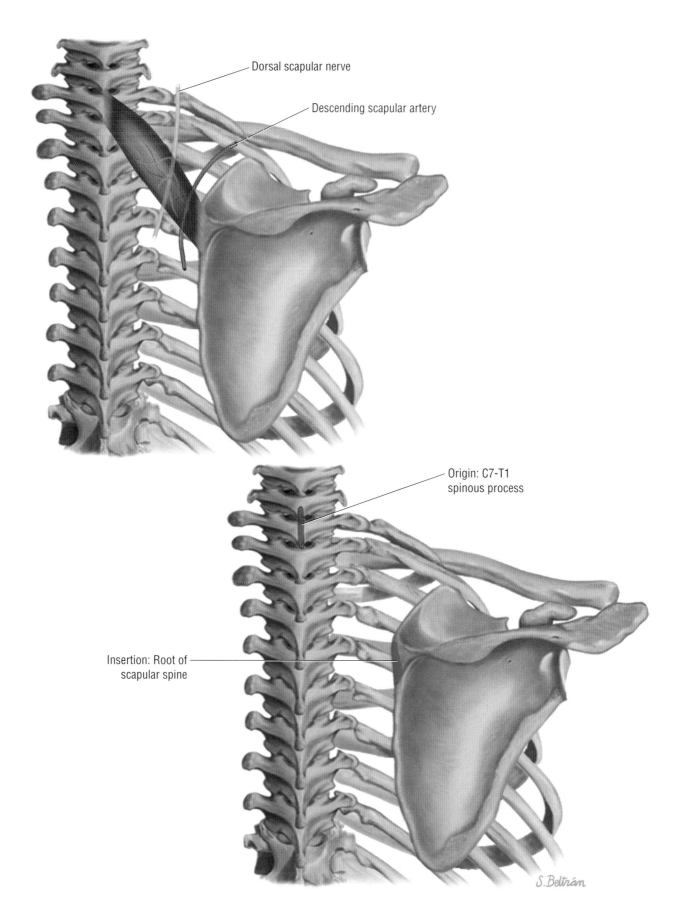

Dorsal scapular nerve

Descending scapular artery

Origin: C7-T1 spinous process

Insertion: Root of scapular spine

S. Beltrán

Figure 8.18 ■ RHOMBOID MINOR. The rhomboid minor and the rhomboid major retract the scapula and participate in elevation of the scapula. *(See Related Muscles pg. 1158, in Stoller's 3rd Edition.)*

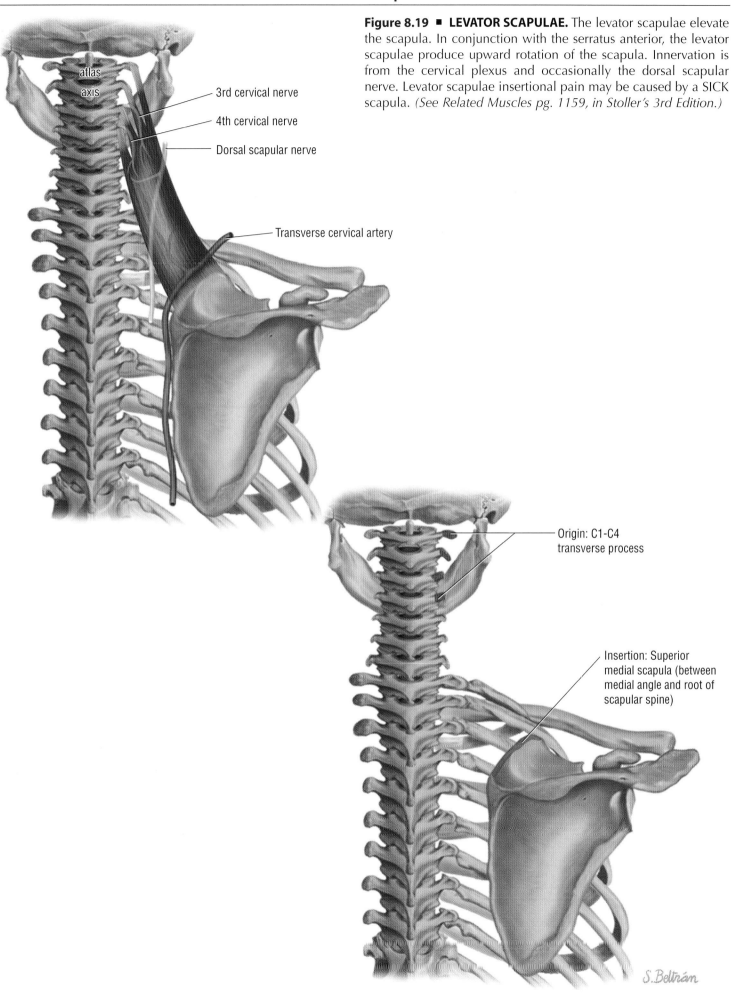

atlas
axis

3rd cervical nerve

4th cervical nerve

Dorsal scapular nerve

Transverse cervical artery

Origin: C1-C4
transverse process

Insertion: Superior
medial scapula (between
medial angle and root of
scapular spine)

Figure 8.19 ▪ LEVATOR SCAPULAE. The levator scapulae elevate the scapula. In conjunction with the serratus anterior, the levator scapulae produce upward rotation of the scapula. Innervation is from the cervical plexus and occasionally the dorsal scapular nerve. Levator scapulae insertional pain may be caused by a SICK scapula. *(See Related Muscles pg. 1159, in Stoller's 3rd Edition.)*

S. Beltrán

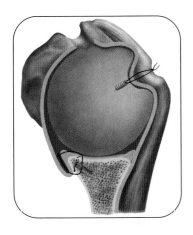

The Shoulder

Anatomy and Pathology

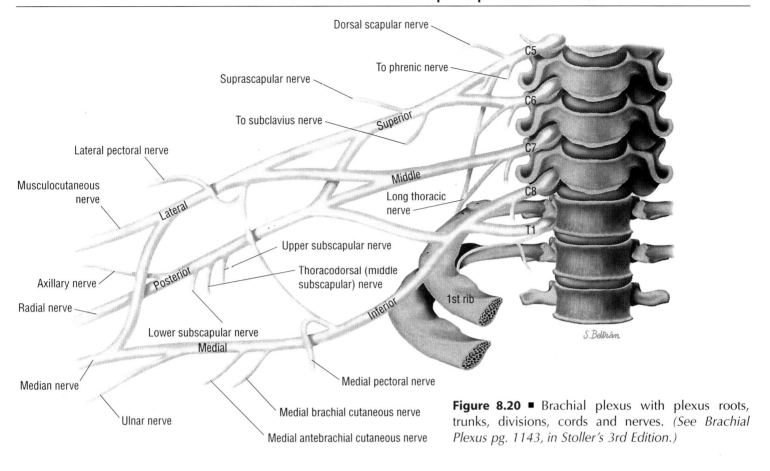

Dorsal scapular nerve

To phrenic nerve

Suprascapular nerve

To subclavius nerve

Superior

Lateral pectoral nerve

Musculocutaneous nerve

Lateral

Middle

Long thoracic nerve

Axillary nerve

Posterior

Upper subscapular nerve

Thoracodorsal (middle subscapular) nerve

Radial nerve

Inferior

1st rib

Lower subscapular nerve

Medial

Median nerve

Medial pectoral nerve

Ulnar nerve

Medial brachial cutaneous nerve

Medial antebrachial cutaneous nerve

C5
C6
C7
C8
T1

S. Beltrán

Figure 8.20 ■ Brachial plexus with plexus roots, trunks, divisions, cords and nerves. *(See Brachial Plexus pg. 1143, in Stoller's 3rd Edition.)*

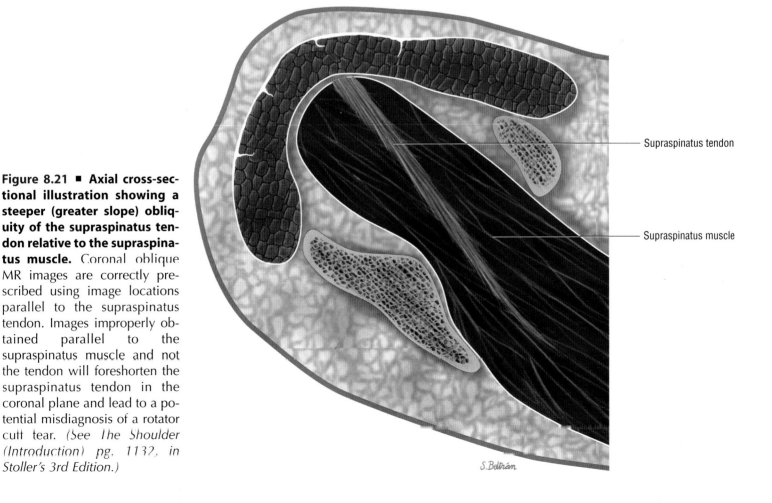

Figure 8.21 ■ **Axial cross-sectional illustration showing a steeper (greater slope) obliquity of the supraspinatus tendon relative to the supraspinatus muscle.** Coronal oblique MR images are correctly prescribed using image locations parallel to the supraspinatus tendon. Images improperly obtained parallel to the supraspinatus muscle and not the tendon will foreshorten the supraspinatus tendon in the coronal plane and lead to a potential misdiagnosis of a rotator cuff tear. *(See The Shoulder (Introduction) pg. 1132, in Stoller's 3rd Edition.)*

Supraspinatus tendon

Supraspinatus muscle

S. Beltrán

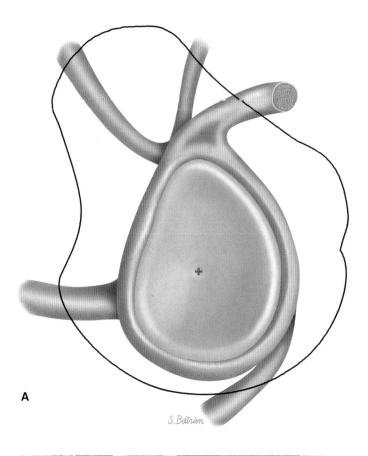

A

S. Beltrán

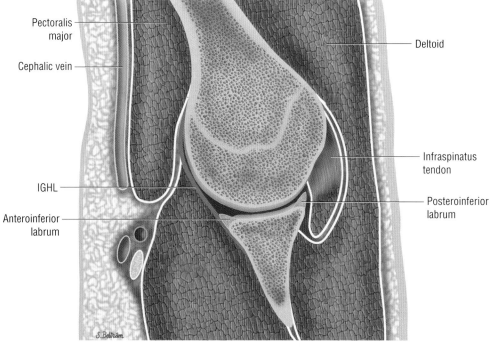

Pectoralis major

Cephalic vein

Deltoid

IGHL

Infraspinatus tendon

Anteroinferior labrum

Posteroinferior labrum

S. Beltrán

B

Figure 8.22 ■ **(A)** Normal central point (red cross) of glenohumeral rotation with arm positioned in abduction and external rotation. **(B)** Axial oblique ABER (abduction and external rotation) anatomy illustrated at the level of the IGHL labral complex. *(See ABER Technique pgs. 1138 and 1139, in Stoller's 3rd Edition.)*

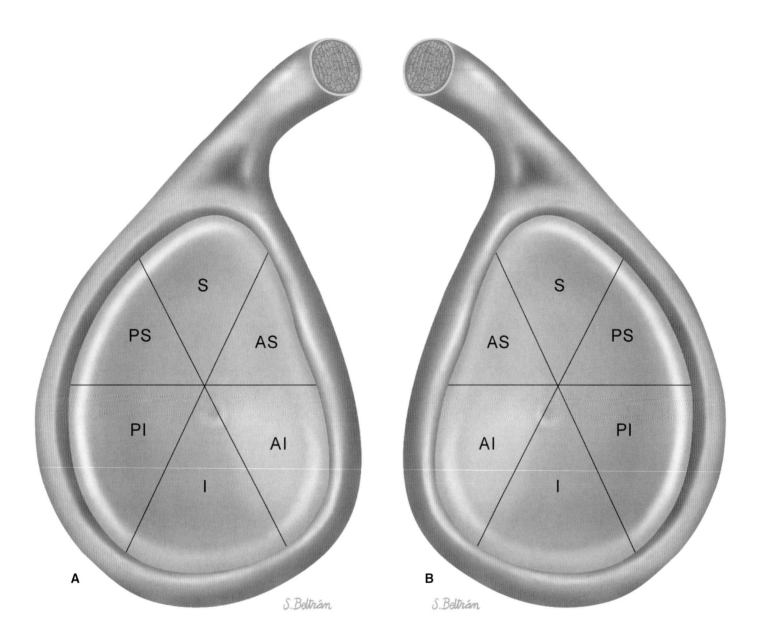

Figure 8.23 ▪ Six quadrants of the glenoid. MR units may default to a display of sagittal images of the shoulder from a left-shoulder perspective even if the right shoulder was imaged. It is accepted practice to describe a lesion by its quadrant. The description of the superior pole as 12 O'Clock and the inferior pole as 6 O'Clock is accurate for the right and left shoulders. To avoid mistaking right for left, however, use of the 3 O'Clock or 9 O'Clock positions should be avoided. **(A)** Illustration using a right-shoulder perspective. **(B)** Left-shoulder perspective. S, superior; AS, antero-posterior; AI, anteroinferior; I, inferior; PS, posterosuperior; PI, posteroinferior. *(See Glenoid Labrum pgs. 1197 and 1199, in Stoller's 3rd Edition.)*

Labral Attachments

Type A labrum

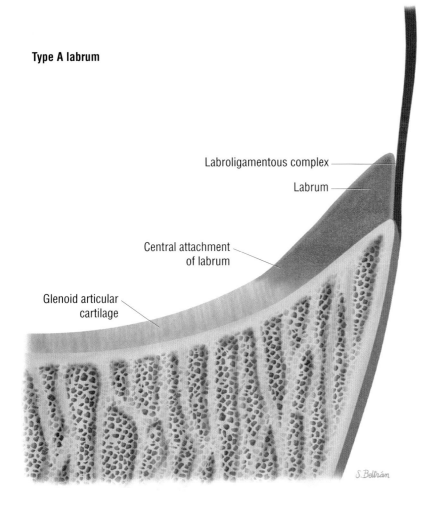

Labroligamentous complex

Labrum

Central attachment
of labrum

Glenoid articular
cartilage

Figure 8.24 ■ The superior wedge labrum is characterized by a firm attachment of the anterior, posterior, and inferior labrum to the glenoid articular surfaces, with no free central edge. The superior labrum is, however, triangular in cross-section and its central free edge is separated and overlaps the articular cartilage at the biceps labral complex. An associated anterosuperior sublabral foramen is common in this labral type. *(See Labral Types pgs. 1200 and 1201, in Stoller's 3rd Edition.)*

Type B labrum

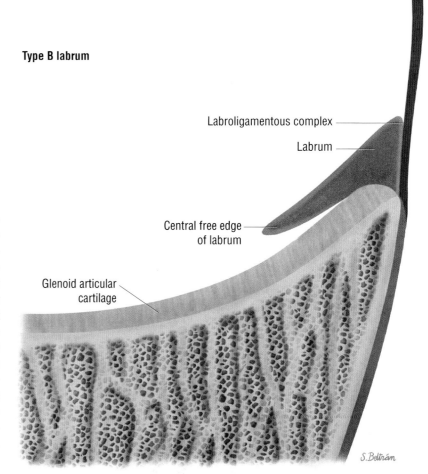

Labroligamentous complex

Labrum

Central free edge
of labrum

Glenoid articular
cartilage

Figure 8.25 ■ The posterior wedge labrum is characterized by a posterior wedged-shaped labrum attached only at its periphery. A probe can be passed between the articular cartilage and the overlapping posterior labrum. When present, a well-defined posterior band of the IGL may overlap a relatively small posterior labrum, analogous to the anterior wedge labrum that occurs with a prominent anterior band. Anteriorly, superiorly, and inferiorly the labrum is firmly attached to the glenoid so that a probe cannot be passed between the glenoid articular surface and the labrum. The superior labrum is smaller than in the superior wedge labrum and is more firmly attached to the articular cartilage of the superior glenoid, as seen in the type 1 biceps labral complex (BLC 1). *(See Labral Types pgs. 1200 and 1202, in Stoller's 3rd Edition.)*

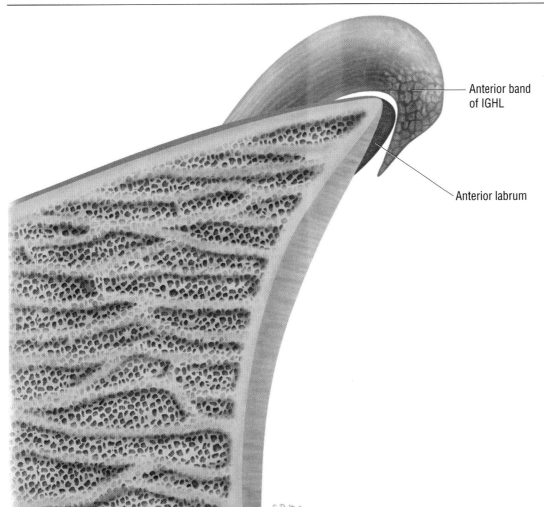

Figure 8.26 ■ **The anterior wedge labrum is firmly attached to the glenoid articular surface inferiorly, posteriorly, and superiorly.** The anterior band (AB) of the IGHL, however, is thick and prominent and covers or overlaps the anterior labrum anterior to the anterior glenoid rim. The anterior wedge labrum may be defined further into two subtypes. The first subtype has a small anterior superior labrum, as already described, whereas the second subtype has an absent anterosuperior labrum underneath or deep to the prominent anterior band. Deep to the prominent anterior band of the IGHL, the anterior rim articular cartilage may taper and become thin peripherally. *(See Labral Types pgs. 1200 and 1203, in Stoller's 3rd Edition.)*

Figure 8.27 ■ **Another labral variation is a combination of features of the superior wedge labrum and the anterior wedge labrum.** A prominent or large anterior band of the IGL overlaps and may replace a small anterosuperior labrum. Superiorly, the labrum has a free central margin and overlaps the glenoid articular cartilage, unlike the firmly attached superior labrum found in the anterior wedge labrum. There are three subtypes of this variant. In the first subtype, there is no anterosuperior labrum. The second subtype has small anterosuperior labrum firmly attached to the glenoid articular cartilage. In a third subtype, the superior labrum and the anterior band of the IGL may blend together to form a free margin. This unattached free margin extends from the posterosuperior glenoid to the anteroinferior glenoid without an associated sub labral foramen anterosuperiorly. *(See Labral Types pgs. 1200 and 1204, in Stoller's 3rd Edition.)*

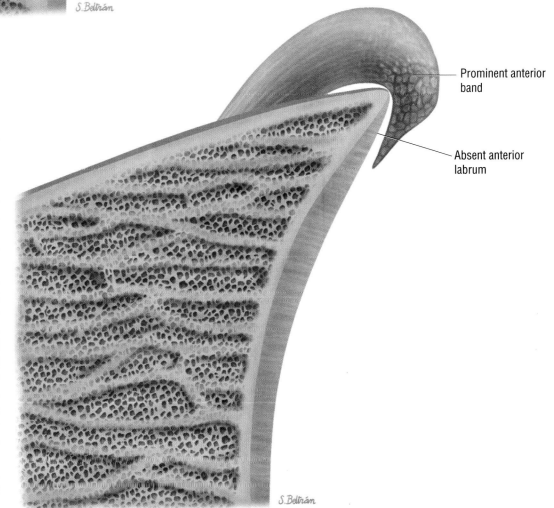

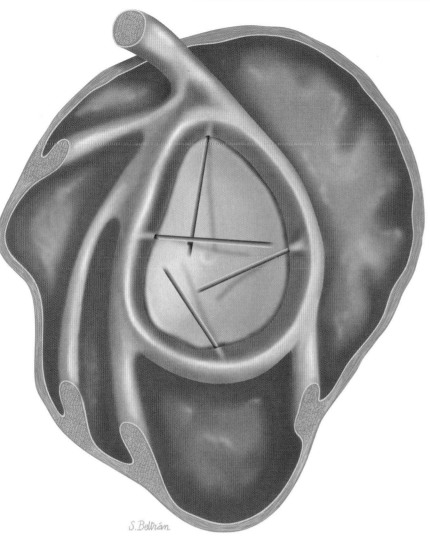

S. Beltrán.

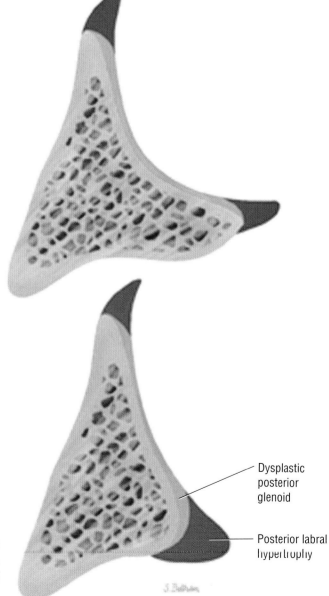

Figure 8.28 ■ **Meniscoid labrum with a circumferential free edge.** This configuration is rare, and it is
unusual to visualize an attached free margin involving the inferior labrum on MR studies. Fluid between
the inferior labrum and glenoid articular cartilage on
coronal MR images thus represents labral tearing.
Lateral color illustration with probing of the free
labral margin. *(See Labral Types pgs. 1200 and 1205,
in Stoller's 3rd Edition.)*

Dysplastic
posterior
glenoid

Posterior labral
hypertrophy

Figure 8.29 ■ Color axial section of normal posterior glenoid rim (top)
compared to severe dysplastic posterior glenoid rim (bottom) with com-
pensatory posterior labral hypertrophy. *(See Labral Types pgs. 1200 and
1206, in Stoller's 3rd Edition.)*

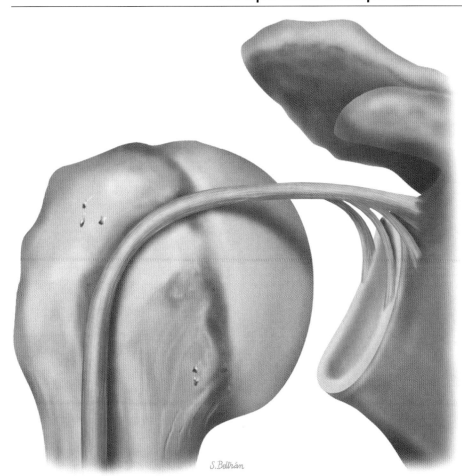

Figure 8.30 ■ Origin of the long head of the biceps with idealized attachments to the posterior labrum, supraglenoid tubercle, anterior glenoid labrum, and base of the coracoid. (Based on Detrisac DJ, Johnson LL. Biceps and subscapularis tendons. In: Detrisac DJ, Johnson LL, eds. Arthroscopic shoulder anatomy: pathologic and surgical implications. Thorofare, NJ: Slack, 1986: 21–34.) *(See Long Head of the Biceps Tendon and Biceps Labral Complex pgs. 1200 and 1207, in Stoller's 3rd Edition.)*

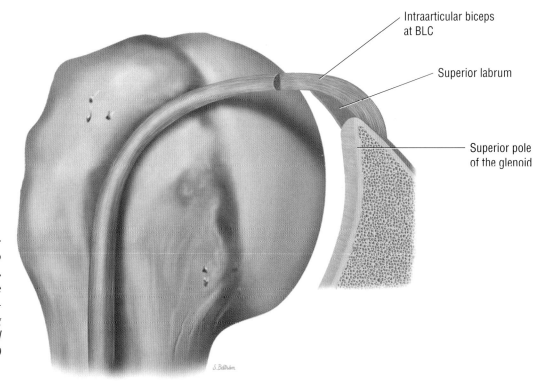

Intraarticular biceps at BLC

Superior labrum

Superior pole of the glenoid

Figure 8.31 ■ **Type 1 BLC with superior labrum firmly attached to the superior pole of the glenoid.** The type 1 BLC may be seen in the posterior wedge labrum and the anterior wedge labrum. *(See Long Head of the Biceps Tendon and Biceps Labral Complex pgs. 1200 and 1212, in Stoller's 3rd Edition.)*

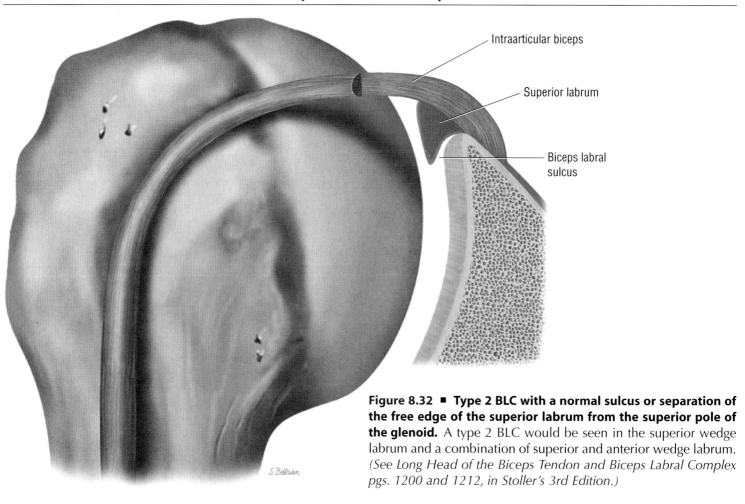

Intraarticular biceps

Superior labrum

Biceps labral
sulcus

S.Beltrán

Figure 8.32 ■ **Type 2 BLC with a normal sulcus or separation of the free edge of the superior labrum from the superior pole of the glenoid.** A type 2 BLC would be seen in the superior wedge labrum and a combination of superior and anterior wedge labrum. *(See Long Head of the Biceps Tendon and Biceps Labral Complex pgs. 1200 and 1212, in Stoller's 3rd Edition.)*

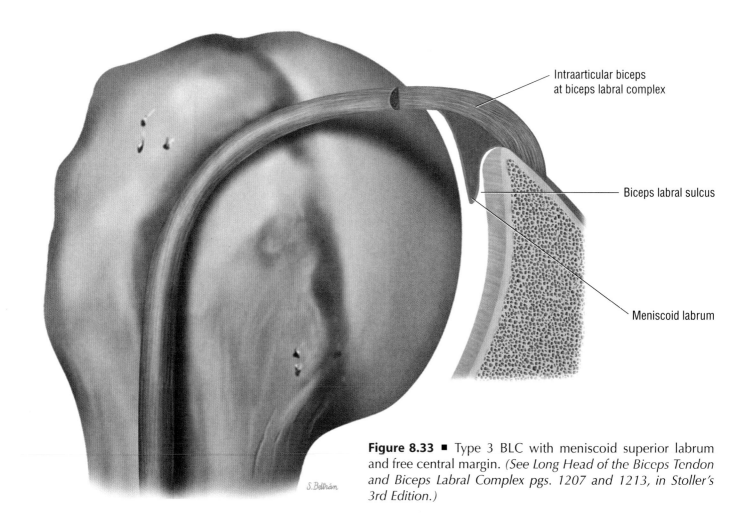

Intraarticular biceps
at biceps labral complex

Biceps labral sulcus

Meniscoid labrum

S.Beltrán

Figure 8.33 ■ Type 3 BLC with meniscoid superior labrum and free central margin. *(See Long Head of the Biceps Tendon and Biceps Labral Complex pgs. 1207 and 1213, in Stoller's 3rd Edition.)*

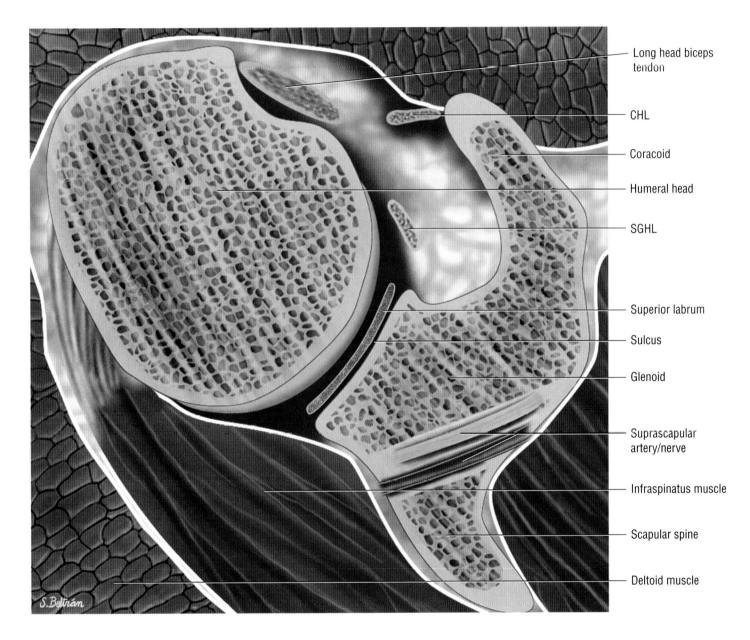

- Long head biceps tendon
- CHL
- Coracoid
- Humeral head
- SGHL
- Superior labrum
- Sulcus
- Glenoid
- Suprascapular artery/nerve
- Infraspinatus muscle
- Scapular spine
- Deltoid muscle

S.Beltrán

Figure 8.34 ■ **Type 2 BLC with normal sulcus on axial color cross-section.** This sulcus should not be mistaken for detachment of the superior labrum. *(See Long Head of the Biceps Tendon and Biceps Labral Complex pgs. 1207 and 1214, in Stoller's 3rd Edition.)*

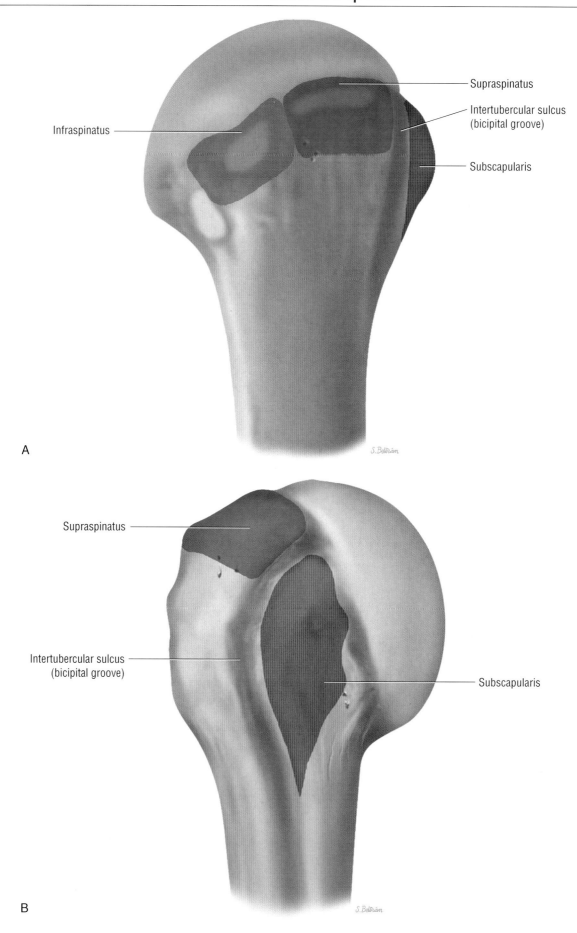

A

B

Figure 8.35 ▪ Footprints of the supraspinatus, infraspinatus, and subscapularis.
(**A**) Lateral view. (**B**) Anterior view. *(See Rotator Cuff pgs. 1227–1229, in Stoller's 3rd Edition.)*

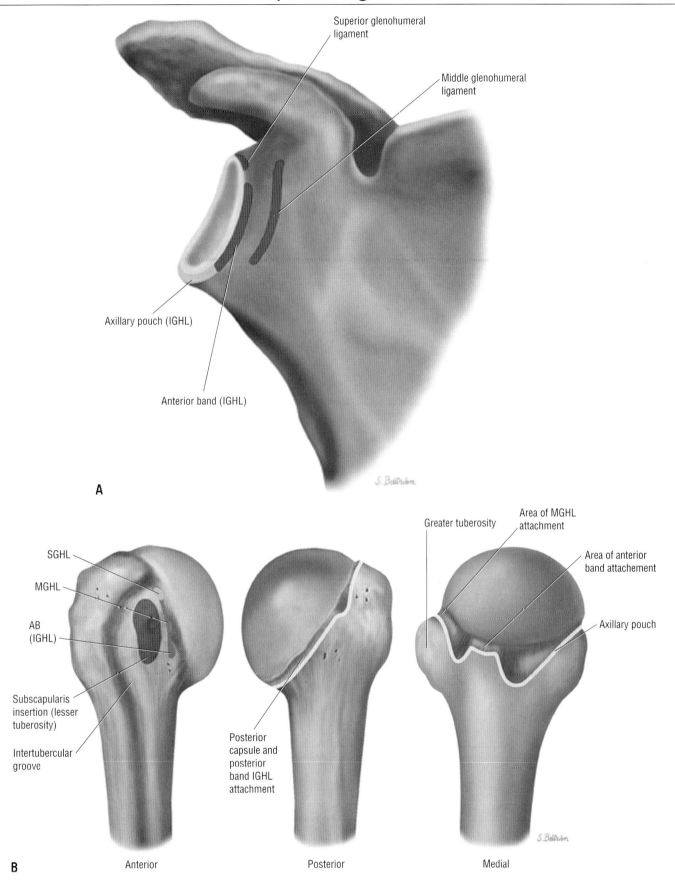

Figure 8.36 ▪ **(A)** The glenoid attachments of the anterior capsule ligaments including the superior glenohumeral ligament (SGHL or SGL), the middle glenohumeral ligament (MGHL or MGL), the anterior band of inferior glenohumeral ligament (IGHL or IGL), and the axillary pouch of IGHL. **(B)** Glenohumeral capsular and ligament attachments in anterior, posterior, and medial humeral projections. (A and B based on Detrisac DJ, Johnson LL. Biceps and subscapularis tendons. In: Detrisac DJ, Johnson LL, eds. Arthroscopic shoulder anatomy: pathologic and surgical implications. Thorofare, NJ: Slack, 1986: 21–34.) *(See Glenohumeral Ligaments pgs. 1207 and 1216, in Stoller's 3rd Edition.)*

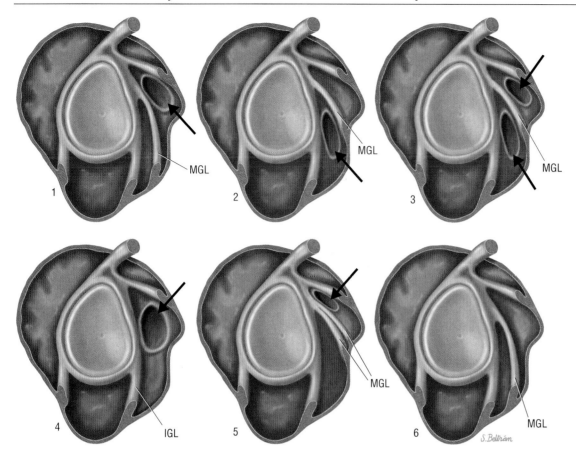

Figure 8.37 ■ **Six arrangements of synovial recesses (i.e., joint capsule variations, arrows) are described by DePalma.** Type 1: One synovial recess exists above the middle glenohumeral ligament. Type 2: One synovial recess exists below the middle glenohumeral ligament. Type 3: Two synovial recesses exist, with a superior subscapular recess above the middle glenohumeral ligament and an inferior subscapular recess below the middle glenohumeral ligament. Type 4: No middle glenohumeral ligament. Type 5: The middle glenohumeral ligament exists as two small synovial folds. Type 6: Complete absence of synovial recesses. *(See Synovial Recesses pg. 1222, in Stoller's 3rd Edition.)*

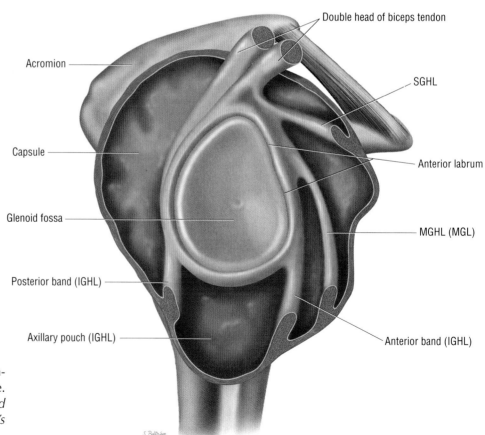

Figure 8.38 ■ Double biceps with two tendons inserting into the supraglenoid tubercle. *(See Long Head of the Biceps Tendon and Biceps Labral Complex pg. 1208, in Stoller's 3rd Edition.)*

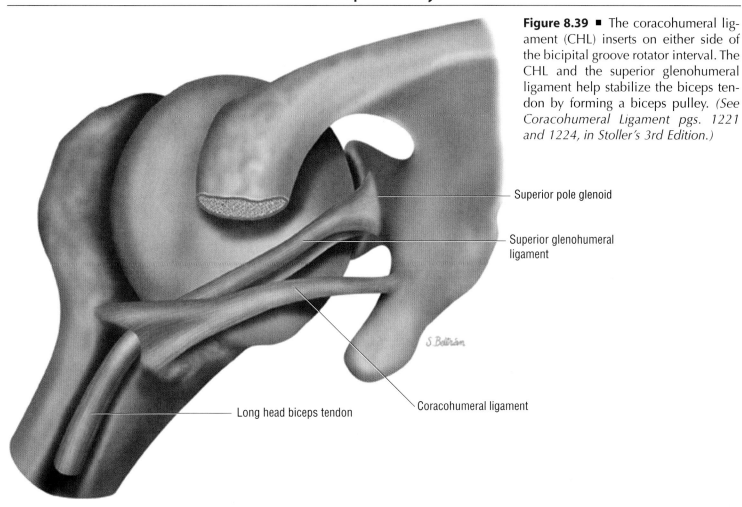

Figure 8.39 ■ The coracohumeral ligament (CHL) inserts on either side of the bicipital groove rotator interval. The CHL and the superior glenohumeral ligament help stabilize the biceps tendon by forming a biceps pulley. *(See Coracohumeral Ligament pgs. 1221 and 1224, in Stoller's 3rd Edition.)*

Superior pole glenoid

Superior glenohumeral ligament

Coracohumeral ligament

Long head biceps tendon

Figure 8.40 ■ **The biceps pulley complex is sectioned in the sagittal plane at the level of the proximal, middle, and distal rotator cuff interval.** The confluence of the CHL and SGHL occurs at the middle and distal aspects of the rotator interval. A T-shaped junction is formed between the SGHL and CHL at the mid-interval, superior to the humeral head. An anterior U-shaped sling is shown at the distal interval at the entrance to the bicipital groove. *(See Coracohumeral Ligament pgs. 1221 and 1225, in Stoller's 3rd Edition.)*

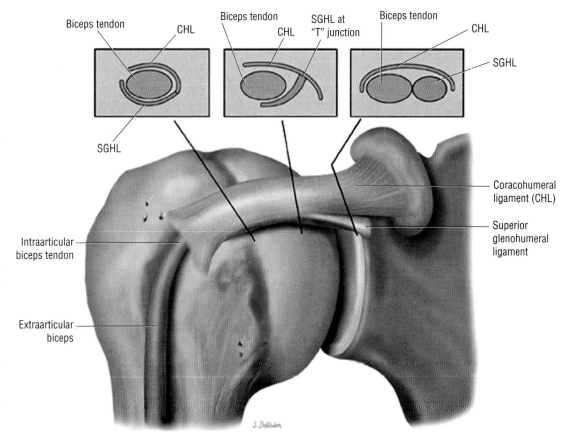

Biceps tendon
CHL
SGHL

Biceps tendon
CHL
SGHL at "T" junction

Biceps tendon
CHL
SGHL

Intraarticular biceps tendon

Extraarticular biceps

Coracohumeral ligament (CHL)

Superior glenohumeral ligament

Biceps Pulley and Rotator Cuff Cable

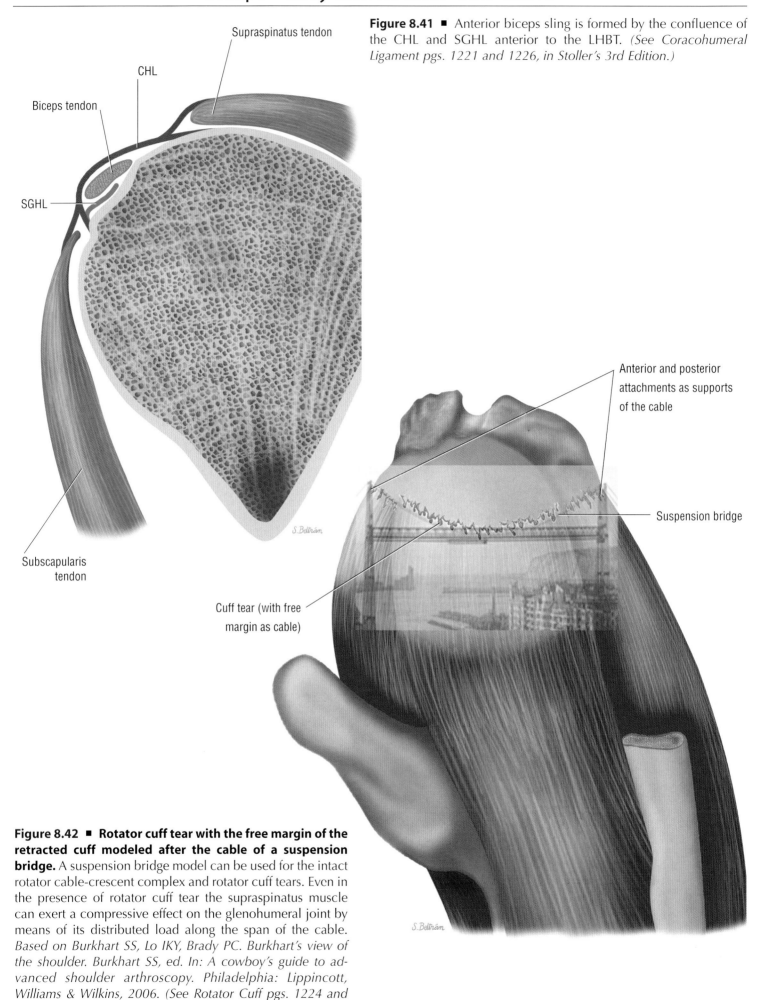

Supraspinatus tendon

CHL

Biceps tendon

SGHL

Subscapularis tendon

Figure 8.41 ■ Anterior biceps sling is formed by the confluence of the CHL and SGHL anterior to the LHBT. *(See Coracohumeral Ligament pgs. 1221 and 1226, in Stoller's 3rd Edition.)*

Anterior and posterior attachments as supports of the cable

Suspension bridge

Cuff tear (with free margin as cable)

S.Beltrán

Figure 8.42 ■ **Rotator cuff tear with the free margin of the retracted cuff modeled after the cable of a suspension bridge.** A suspension bridge model can be used for the intact rotator cable-crescent complex and rotator cuff tears. Even in the presence of rotator cuff tear the supraspinatus muscle can exert a compressive effect on the glenohumeral joint by means of its distributed load along the span of the cable. *Based on Burkhart SS, Lo IKY, Brady PC. Burkhart's view of the shoulder. Burkhart SS, ed. In: A cowboy's guide to advanced shoulder arthroscopy. Philadelphia: Lippincott, Williams & Wilkins, 2006. (See Rotator Cuff pgs. 1224 and 1230, in Stoller's 3rd Edition.)*

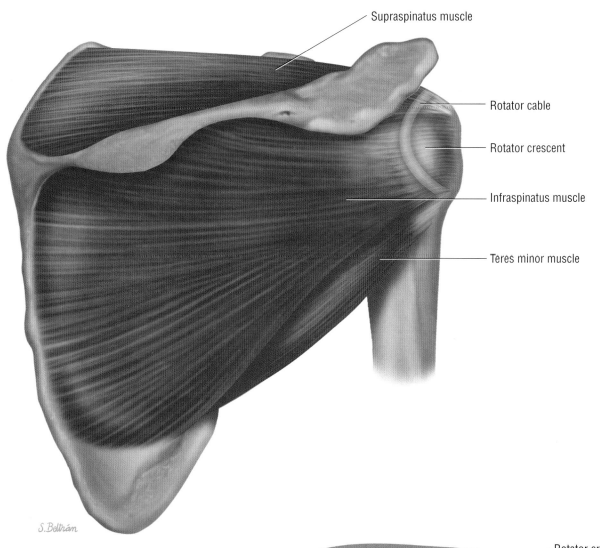

Supraspinatus muscle

Rotator cable

Rotator crescent

Infraspinatus muscle

Teres minor muscle

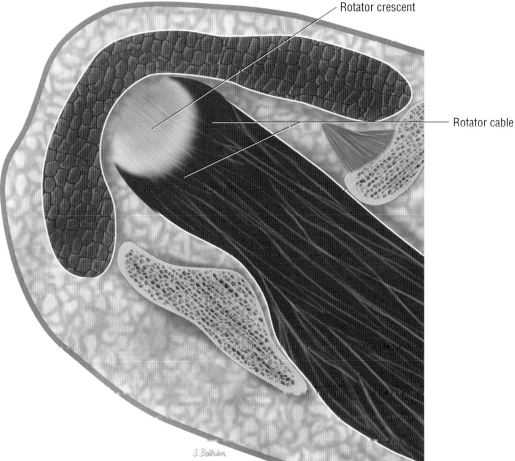

Rotator crescent

Rotator cable

Figure 8.43 ■ **(A)** The rotator cable and crescent shown from a posterior view. The cable represents thickened capsular tissue from the articular side of the cuff connecting the anterior and posterior tendon edges of the tendinous portion of the rotator cuff. An extension of the coracohumeral ligament contributes to the cable. The rotator crescent, especially the lateral portion of the supraspinatus peripheral to the cable, represents the concave portion of the cuff at risk for pathology. **(B)** A superior view of the rotator cuff ridge or cable. (See Rotator Cuff pgs. 1224 and 1230, in Stoller's 3rd Edition.)

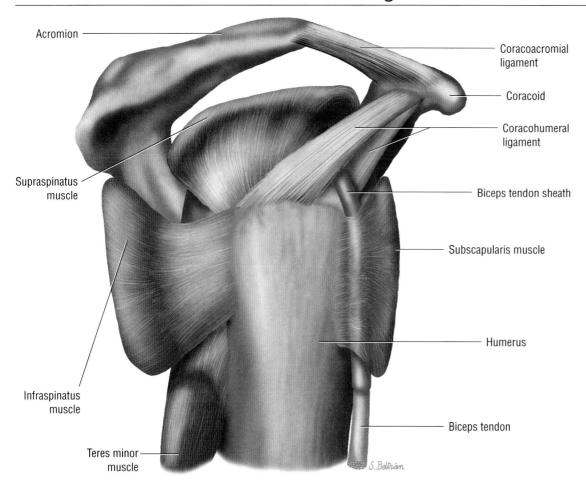

Acromion

Coracoacromial ligament

Coracoid

Coracohumeral ligament

Supraspinatus muscle

Biceps tendon sheath

Subscapularis muscle

Humerus

Infraspinatus muscle

Biceps tendon

Teres minor muscle

S. Beltrán

Figure 8.44 ▪ The coracoacromial ligament extends from the inferior surface of the acromion to the lateral aspect of the coracoid. The humeroscapular motion interface represents a relationship between the rotator cuff, the humeral head, the biceps, the coracoacromial arch, and the deltoid and the coracoid muscles. Contact and load transfer occur between the rotator cuff and coracoacromial arch. *(See Coracoacromial Ligament pgs. 1224 and 1231, in Stoller's 3rd Edition.)*

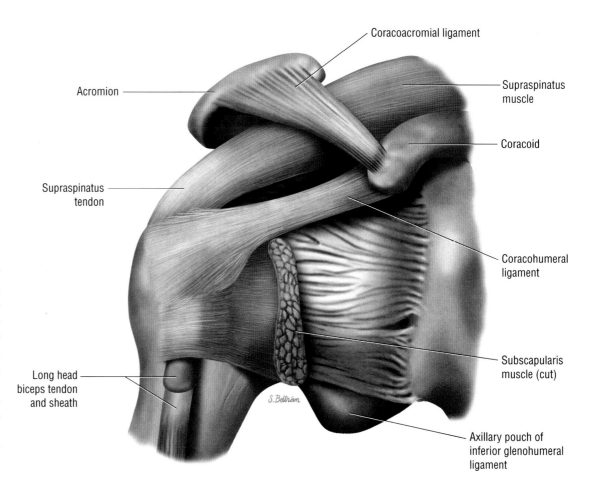

Coracoacromial ligament

Supraspinatus muscle

Acromion

Coracoid

Supraspinatus tendon

Coracohumeral ligament

Subscapularis muscle (cut)

Long head biceps tendon and sheath

S. Beltrán

Axillary pouch of inferior glenohumeral ligament

Figure 8.45 ▪ The anterior undersurface of the acromion and the coracoacromial ligament form the coracoacromial arch. The subacromial subdeltoid bursa facilitates the passage of the rotator cuff and proximal humerus under the coracoacromial arch. *(See Coracoacromial Ligament pgs. 1230 and 1232, in Stoller's 3rd Edition.)*

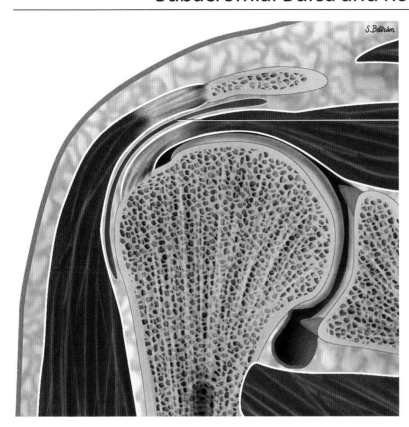

Figure 8.46 ■ **The subacromial bursa extends over the insertion of the supraspinatus superiorly and over the infraspinatus and teres minor posteriorly.** The superior surface of the bursa is in contact with the undersurface of the acromion, the coracoacromial ligament, and the origin of the mid-portion of the deltoid muscle. The superior surface of the bursa extends medially adjacent to the deep surface of the acromioclavicular joint. *(See Subacromial Bursa pgs. 1233 and 1234, in Stoller's 3rd Edition.)*

Subacromial bursa

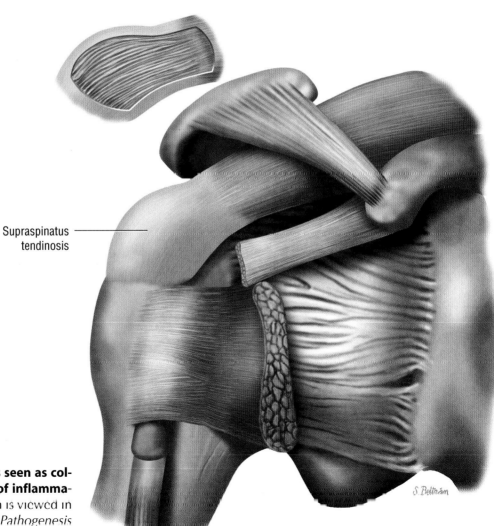

Supraspinatus tendinosis

Figure 8.47 ■ **Rotator cuff tendinosis is seen as collagen degeneration without the influx of inflammatory cells.** The thickened distal cuff tendon is viewed in an anterior coronal perspective. *(See Pathogenesis pgs. 1235 and 1236, in Stoller's 3rd Edition.)*

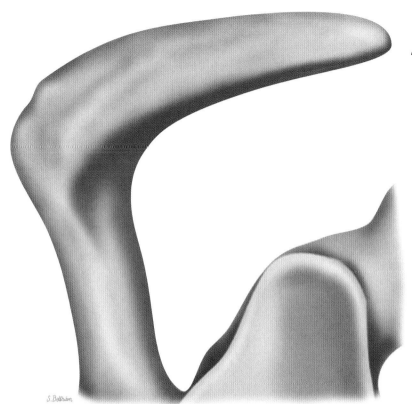

Figure 8.48 ■ Type 1 acromion with flat acromial undersurface. *(See Acromial Morphology in Impingement pgs. 1237 and 1238, in Stoller's 3rd Edition.)*

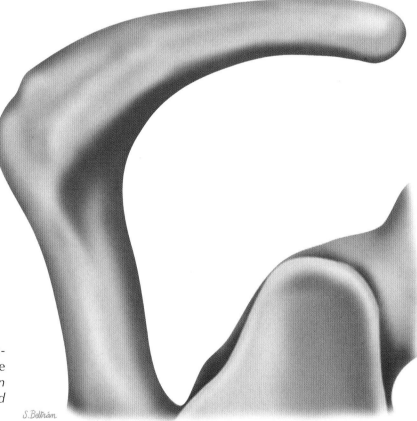

Figure 8.49 ■ Type 2 acromion with a curved convex inferior surface that parallels the contour of the humeral head. *(See Acromial Morphology in Impingement pgs. 1237 and 1238, in Stoller's 3rd Edition.)*

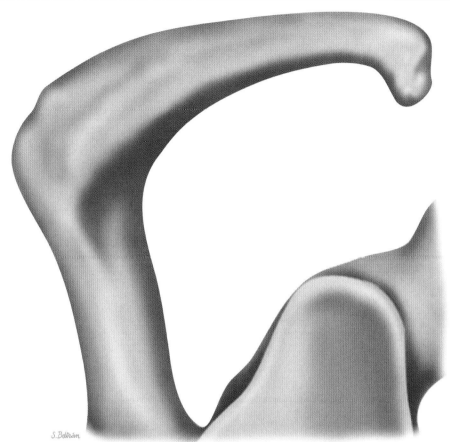

Figure 8.50 ■ Type 3 acromion with an inferiorly directed beak or hook, which contributes to narrowing of the supraspinatus outlet for the supraspinatus tendon. *(See Acromial Morphology in Impingement pgs. 1237 and 1239, in Stoller's 3rd Edition.)*

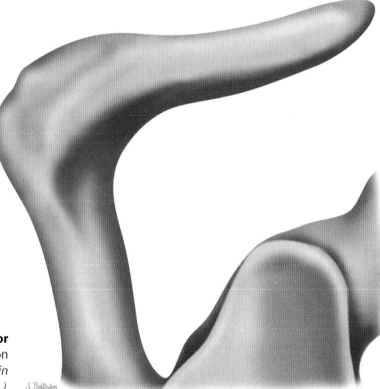

Figure 8.51 ■ **Type 4 acromion with upward or superior convexity of its inferior border.** There is no association with cuff impingement. *(See Acromial Morphology in Impingement pgs. 1237 and 1239, in Stoller's 3rd Edition.)*

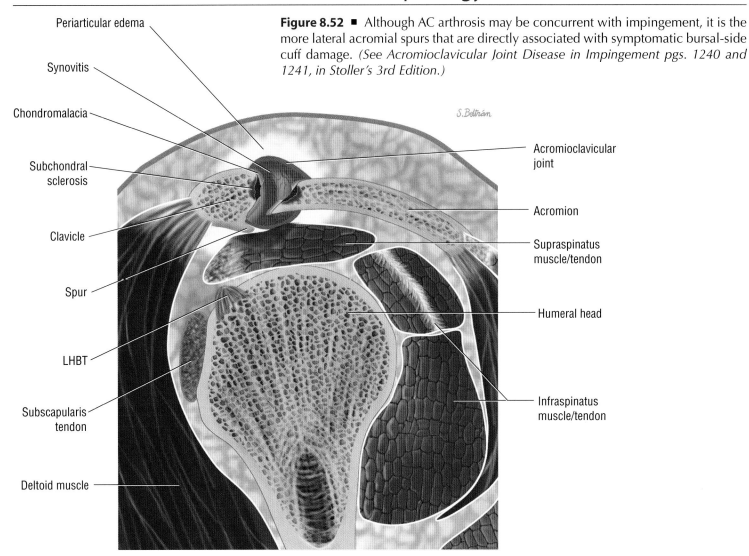

Periarticular edema

Synovitis

Chondromalacia

Subchondral sclerosis

Clavicle

Spur

LHBT

Subscapularis tendon

Deltoid muscle

Acromioclavicular joint

Acromion

Supraspinatus muscle/tendon

Humeral head

Infraspinatus muscle/tendon

Figure 8.52 ■ Although AC arthrosis may be concurrent with impingement, it is the more lateral acromial spurs that are directly associated with symptomatic bursal-side cuff damage. *(See Acromioclavicular Joint Disease in Impingement pgs. 1240 and 1241, in Stoller's 3rd Edition.)*

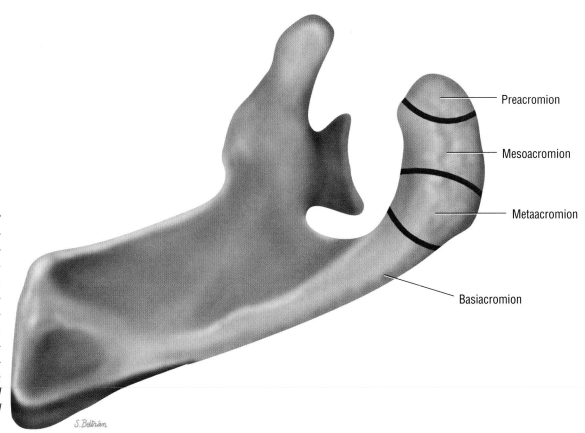

Preacromion

Mesoacromion

Metaacromion

Basiacromion

Figure 8.53 ■ **Superior view of os acromiale subtypes from distal to proximal.** These unfused ossification centers include pre-, meso-, meta-, and basiacromion based on the location of the articulation. The mesoacromion-metaacromion type is most common. *(See Os Acromiale in Impingement pgs. 1240 and 1243, in Stoller's 3rd Edition.)*

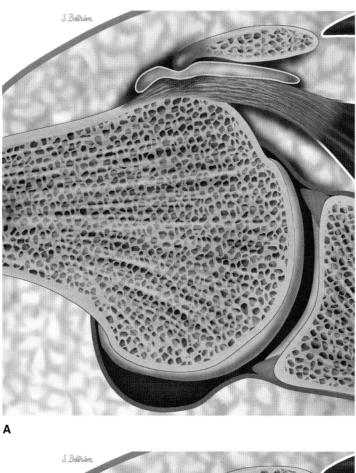

A

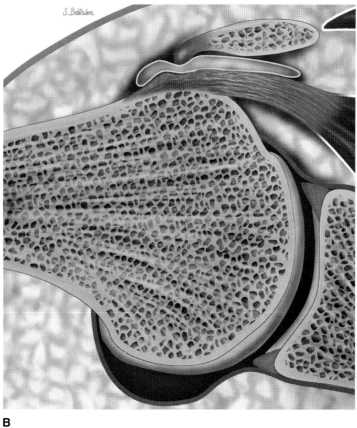

B

Figure 8.54 ■ **(A)** Subacromial impingement with subacromial bursal inflammatory changes and development of a bursal side partial tear of the rotator cuff. **(B)** Articular-side partial tear in subacromial impingement. Bursal inflammatory changes may be present with both bursal and articular side pathology. *(See Arthroscopic Classification of Impingement pg. 1249, in Stoller's 3rd Edition.)*

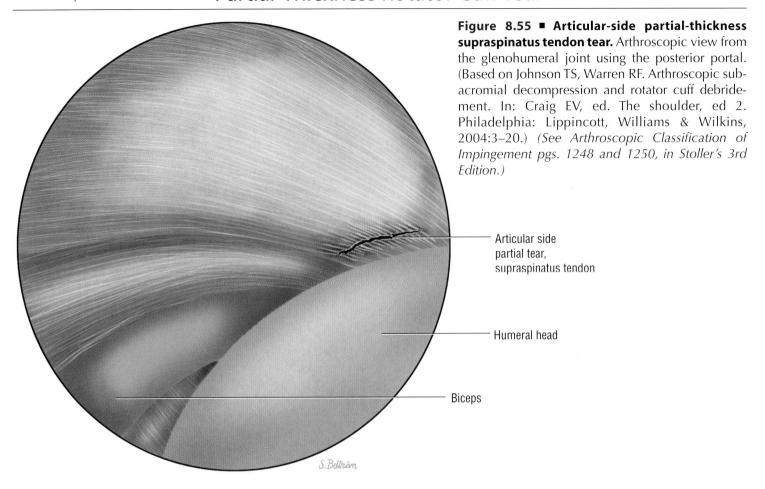

Figure 8.55 ▪ Articular-side partial-thickness supraspinatus tendon tear. Arthroscopic view from the glenohumeral joint using the posterior portal. (Based on Johnson TS, Warren RF. Arthroscopic subacromial decompression and rotator cuff debridement. In: Craig EV, ed. The shoulder, ed 2. Philadelphia: Lippincott, Williams & Wilkins, 2004:3–20.) *(See Arthroscopic Classification of Impingement pgs. 1248 and 1250, in Stoller's 3rd Edition.)*

Articular side partial tear, supraspinatus tendon

Humeral head

Biceps

S.Beltrán

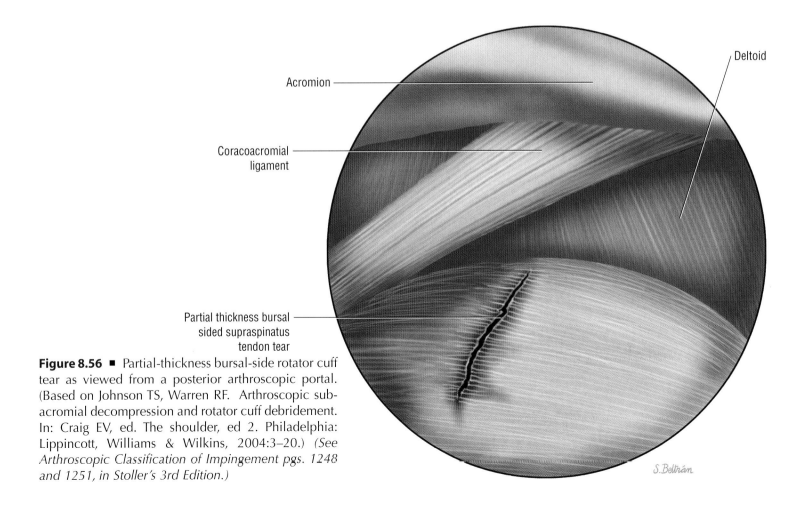

Acromion

Deltoid

Coracoacromial ligament

Partial thickness bursal sided supraspinatus tendon tear

Figure 8.56 ▪ Partial-thickness bursal-side rotator cuff tear as viewed from a posterior arthroscopic portal. (Based on Johnson TS, Warren RF. Arthroscopic subacromial decompression and rotator cuff debridement. In: Craig EV, ed. The shoulder, ed 2. Philadelphia: Lippincott, Williams & Wilkins, 2004:3–20.) *(See Arthroscopic Classification of Impingement pgs. 1248 and 1251, in Stoller's 3rd Edition.)*

S.Beltrán

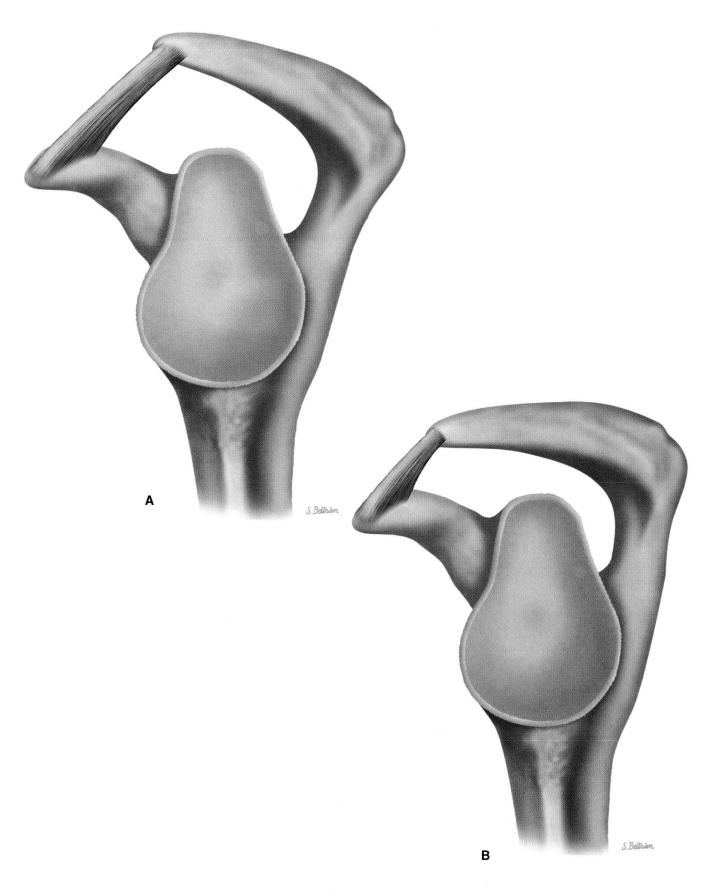

Figure 8.57 ■ **(A)** Normal upward-oriented acromial slope. **(B)** Anterior downsloping acromion with narrowed supraspinatus outlet. *(See MR Appearance of the Acromion in Impingement pgs. 1252 and 1253, in Stoller's 3rd Edition.)*

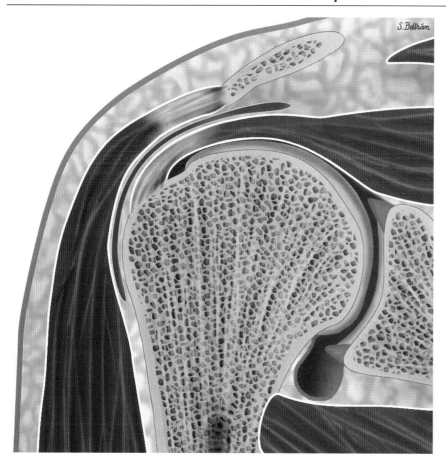

Figure 8.58 ■ Lateral downsloping acromion as viewed on coronal section. *(See MR Appearance of the Acromion in Impingement pgs. 1254 and 1255, in Stoller's 3rd Edition.)*

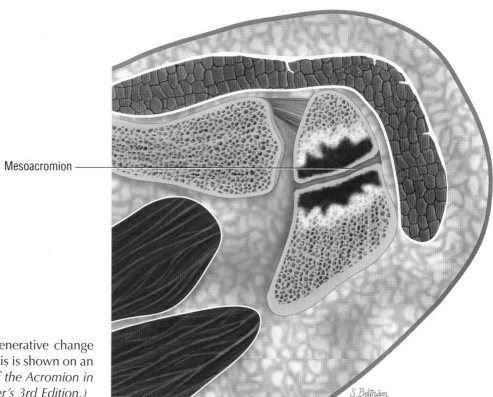

Mesoacromion

Figure 8.59 ■ A mesoacromion with degenerative change and osseous edema across the synchondrosis is shown on an axial color illustration. *(See Appearance of the Acromion in Impingement pgs. 1254 and 1257, in Stoller's 3rd Edition.)*

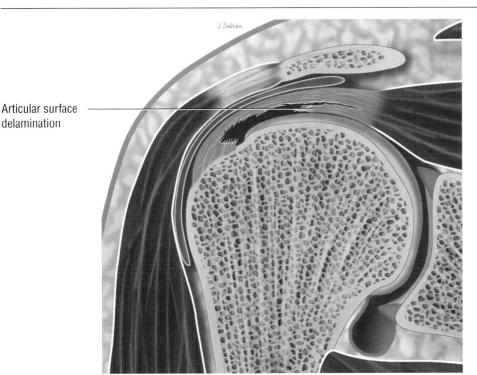

Articular surface
delamination

Figure 8.60 ■ Delamination of the articular surface of the rotator cuff that creates a substantial flap tear retracted from the remaining tendon is referred to as the PASTA (partial articular supraspinatus tendon avulsion) lesion. *(See Partial Tears pgs. 1262 and 1264, in Stoller's 3rd Edition.)*

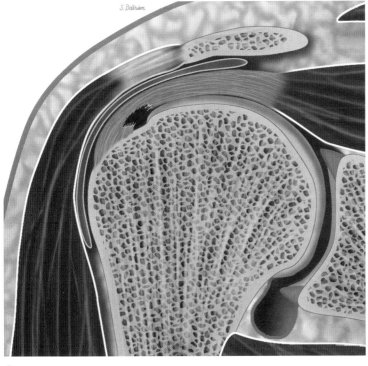

A

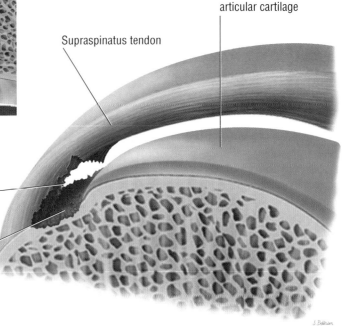

Humeral head
articular cartilage

Supraspinatus tendon

Partial cuff tear,
articular side

Greater tuberosity
erosion

B

Figure 8.61 ■ **(A)** Partial-thickness articular-side tear of the rotator cuff. **(B)** Rim-rent tear of the articular surface of the cuff with erosion of the greater tuberosity. *(See MR Appearance of Partial Tears pgs. 1262 and 1265, in Stoller's 3rd Edition.)*

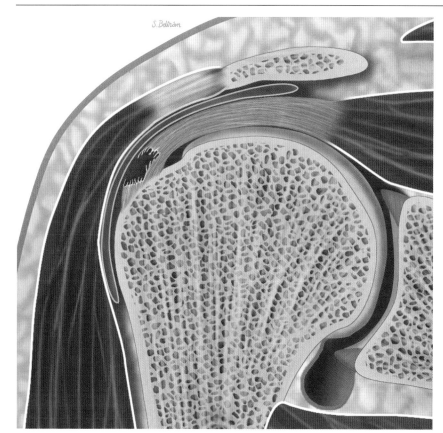

Figure 8.62 ▪ Bursal surface partial-thickness rotator cuff tear. *(See MR Appearance of Partial Tears pgs. 1262 and 1266, in Stoller's 3rd Edition.)*

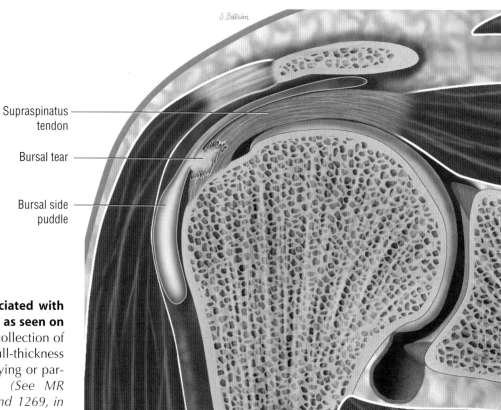

Supraspinatus tendon

Bursal tear

Bursal side puddle

Figure 8.63 ▪ **Bursal puddle sign associated with an adjacent bursal-side rotator cuff tear as seen on a color coronal section.** If this localized collection of subacromial fluid is identified without a full-thickness tear, then the diagnosis of bursal-side fraying or partial-thickness tear must be assumed. *(See MR Appearance of Partial Tears pgs. 1262 and 1269, in Stoller's 3rd Edition.)*

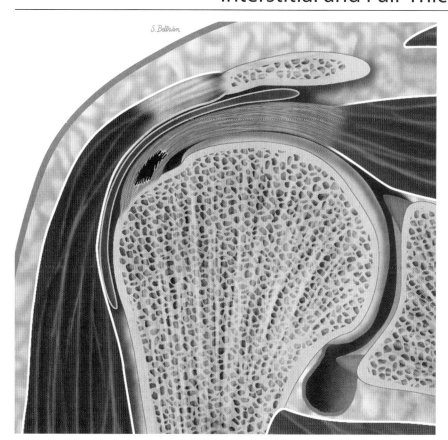

Figure 8.64 ▪ Intrasubstance or interstitial tear of the supraspinatus without bursal or articular surface extension. *(See MR Appearance of Partial Tears pgs. 1262 and 1297, in Stoller's 3rd Edition.)*

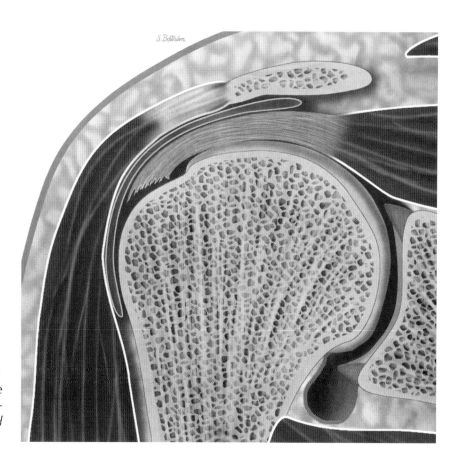

Figure 8.65 ▪ Coronal section showing a stage 1 full-thickness tear with the torn edge adjacent to the greater tuberosity. *(See MR Appearance of Full-Thickness Tears pgs. 1268 and 1273, in Stoller's 3rd Edition.)*

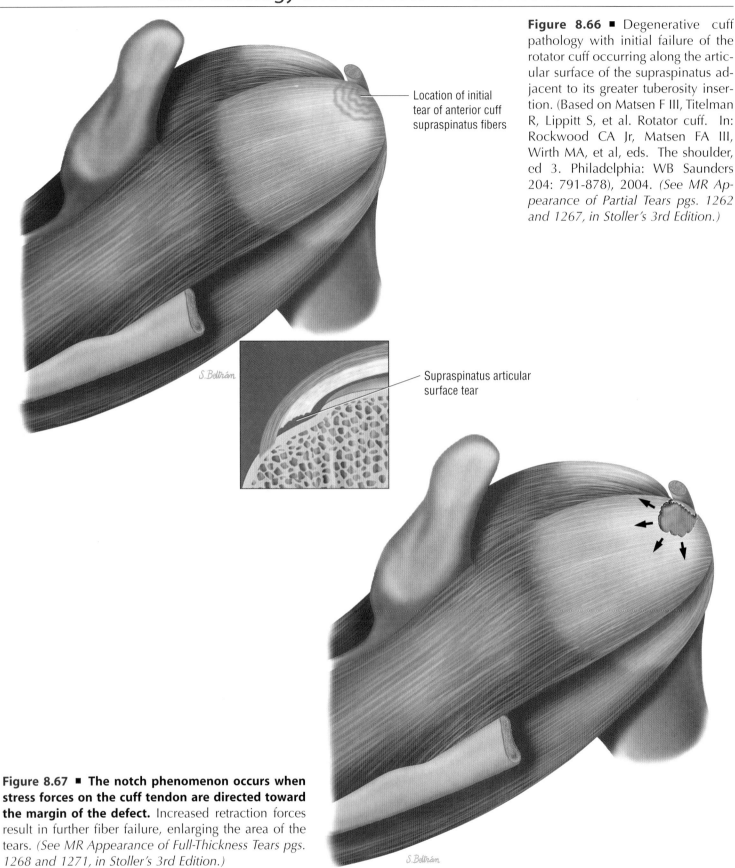

Location of initial tear of anterior cuff supraspinatus fibers

Figure 8.66 ■ Degenerative cuff pathology with initial failure of the rotator cuff occurring along the articular surface of the supraspinatus adjacent to its greater tuberosity insertion. (Based on Matsen F III, Titelman R, Lippitt S, et al. Rotator cuff. In: Rockwood CA Jr, Matsen FA III, Wirth MA, et al, eds. The shoulder, ed 3. Philadelphia: WB Saunders 204: 791-878), 2004. *(See MR Appearance of Partial Tears pgs. 1262 and 1267, in Stoller's 3rd Edition.)*

S. Beltrán

Supraspinatus articular surface tear

Figure 8.67 ■ **The notch phenomenon occurs when stress forces on the cuff tendon are directed toward the margin of the defect.** Increased retraction forces result in further fiber failure, enlarging the area of the tears. *(See MR Appearance of Full-Thickness Tears pgs. 1268 and 1271, in Stoller's 3rd Edition.)*

S. Beltrán

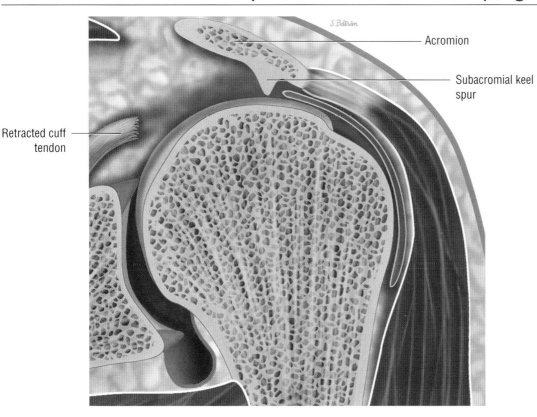

Acromion

Subacromial keel spur

Retracted cuff tendon

Figure 8.68 ■ Acromial "Keel" spur associated with a full thickness rotator cuff tear with retraction. *(See MR Appearance of the Acromion in Impingement pgs. 1251–1252, in Stoller's 3rd Edition.)*

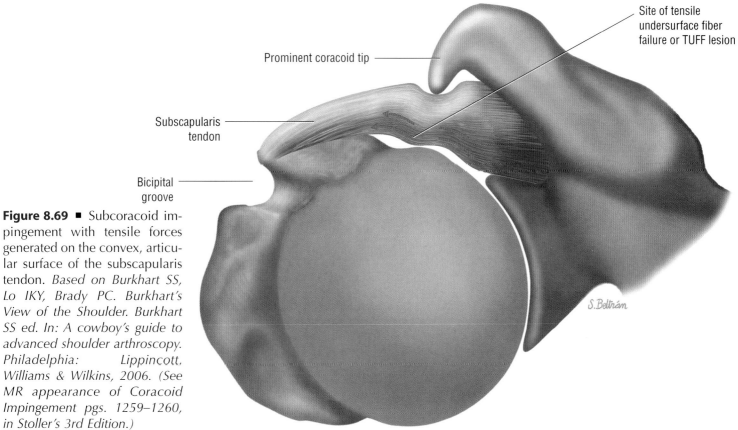

Site of tensile undersurface fiber failure or TUFF lesion

Prominent coracoid tip

Subscapularis tendon

Bicipital groove

Figure 8.69 ■ Subcoracoid impingement with tensile forces generated on the convex, articular surface of the subscapularis tendon. *Based on Burkhart SS, Lo IKY, Brady PC. Burkhart's View of the Shoulder. Burkhart SS ed. In: A cowboy's guide to advanced shoulder arthroscopy. Philadelphia: Lippincott, Williams & Wilkins, 2006. (See MR appearance of Coracoid Impingement pgs. 1259–1260, in Stoller's 3rd Edition.)*

Cuff Mobility

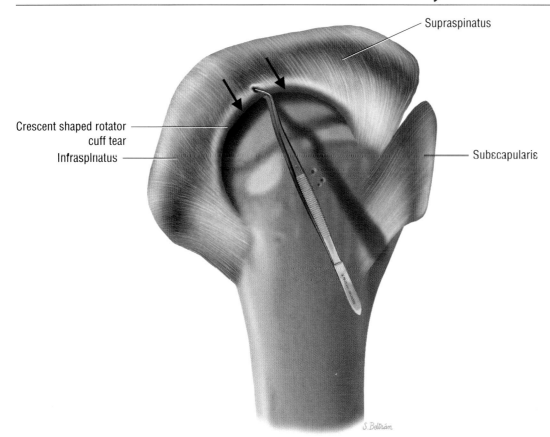

Supraspinatus

Crescent shaped rotator
cuff tear

Infraspinatus

Subscapularis

Figure 8.70 ■ Assessment of medial to lateral mobility of a rotator cuff tendon tear. *Based on Burkhart SS, Lo IKY, Brady PC. Burkhart's view of the shoulder. Burkhart SS ed. In: A cowboy's guide to advanced shoulder arthroscopy. Philadelphia: Lippincott, Williams & Wilkins, 2006. (See Full Thickness Tears pgs. 1268 and 1275–1280, in Stoller's 3rd Edition.)*

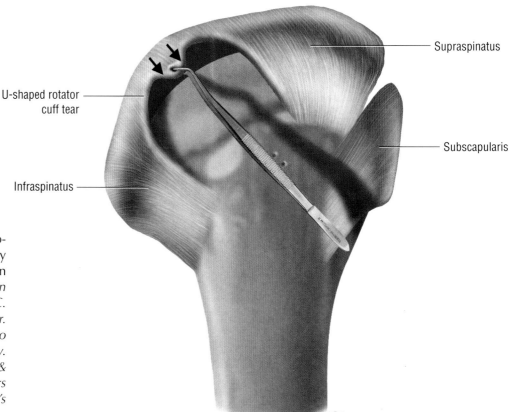

Supraspinatus

U-shaped rotator
cuff tear

Subscapularis

Infraspinatus

Figure 8.71 ■ Contracted immobile rotator cuff tear. There is limited mobility of the cuff edge with traction applied in a medial to lateral direction. *Based on Burkhart SS, Lo IKY, Brady PC. Burkhart's view of the shoulder. Burkhart SS ed. In: A cowboy's guide to advanced shoulder arthroscopy. Philadelphia: Lippincott, Williams & Wilkins, 2006. (See Full Thickness Tears pgs. 1268 and 1275–1280, in Stoller's 3rd Edition.)*

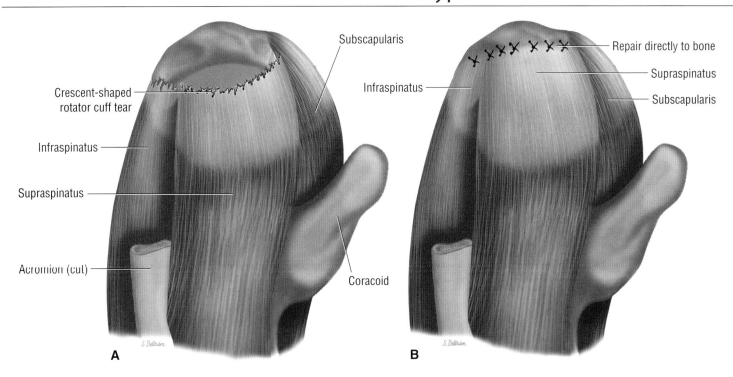

Figure 8.72 ■ Crescent-shaped rotator cuff tear **(A)** and repair directly to bone **(B)**. Rotator cuff tears can be classified as crescent-shaped tears, U-shaped tears, L-shaped and reverse L-shaped tears, and massive contracted immobile tears. *Based on Burkhart SS, Lo IKY, Brady PC. Burkhart's view of the shoulder. Burkhart SS ed. In: A cowboy's guide to advanced shoulder arthroscopy. Philadelphia: Lippincott, Williams & Wilkins, 2006. (See Full Thickness Tears pgs. 1268–1280, in Stoller's 3rd Edition.)*

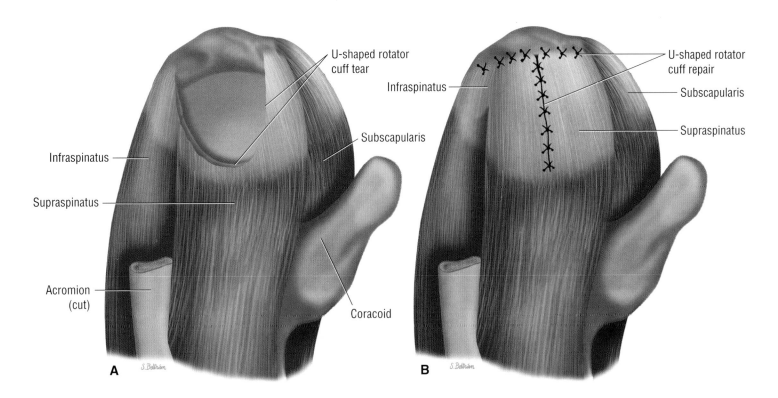

Figure 8.73 ■ **(A)** U-shaped rotator cuff tear involving the supraspinatus and infraspinatus tendons. **(B)** Repaired U-shaped tear using a side to side repair and attachment of margin to bone. *Based on Burkhart SS, Lo IKY, Brady PC. Burkhart's view of the shoulder. Burkhart SS ed. In: A cowboy's guide to advanced shoulder arthroscopy. Philadelphia: Lippincott, Williams & Wilkins, 2006. (See Full Thickness Tears pgs. 1268–1280, in Stoller's 3rd Edition.)*

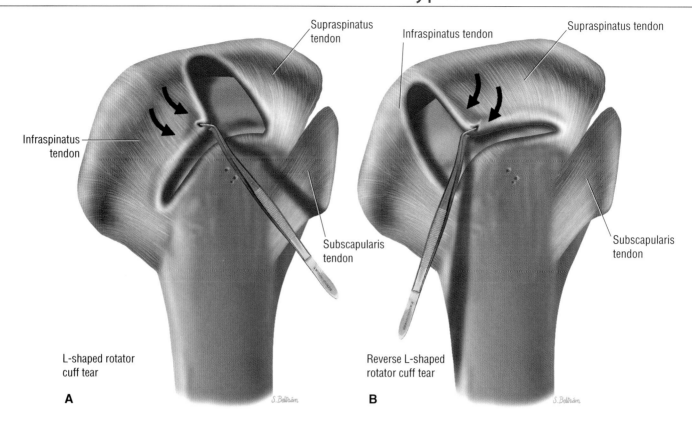

Figure 8.74 ■ L-shaped **(A)** and reverse L-shaped **(B)** rotator cuff tendon tears. *Based on Burkhart SS, Lo IKY, Brady PC. Burkhart's view of the shoulder. Burkhart SS ed. In: A cowboy's guide to advanced shoulder arthroscopy. Philadelphia: Lippincott, Williams & Wilkins, 2006. (See Full Thickness Tears pgs. 1268–1280, in Stoller's 3rd Edition.)*

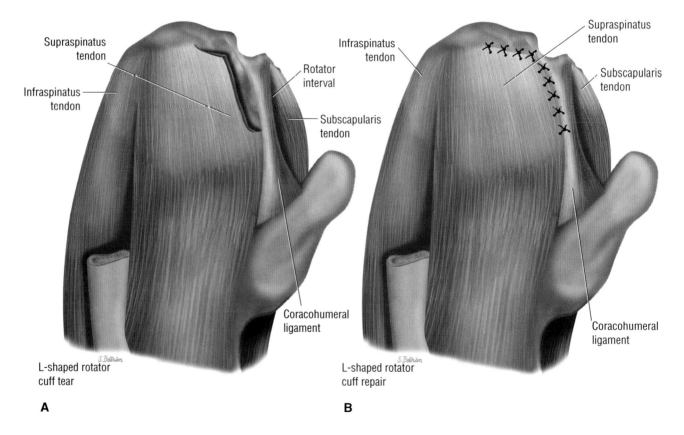

Figure 8.75 ■ **(A)** Superior view of a L-shaped rotator cuff tear. **(B)** Repair of a L-shaped tear along its longitudinal split and margin. *Based on Burkhart SS, Lo IKY, Brady PC. Burkhart's view of the shoulder. Burkhart SS ed. In: A cowboy's guide to advanced shoulder arthroscopy. Philadelphia: Lippincott, Williams & Wilkins, 2006. (See Full Thickness Tears pgs. 1268–1280, in Stoller's 3rd Edition.)*

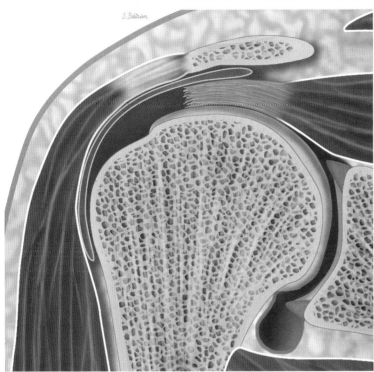

Figure 8.76 ■ Stage 2 full-thickness rotator cuff tear with supraspinatus tendon retraction superior to the humeral head. *(See Appearance of Full-Thickness Tears pgs. 1272–1273, in Stoller's 3rd Edition.)*

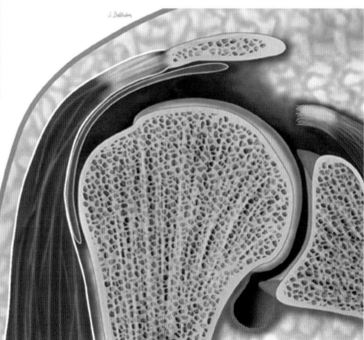

Figure 8.77 ■ Stage 3 full-thickness rotator cuff tear with tendon retraction to the level of the glenoid. *(See MR Appearance of Full-Thickness Tears pgs. 1272 and 1274, in Stoller's 3rd Edition.)*

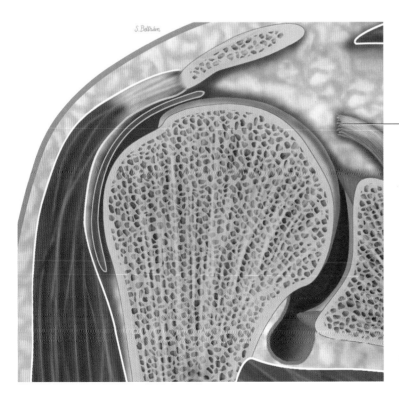

Retracted cuff with atrophy

Figure 8.78 ■ Chronic rotator cuff fatty atrophy associated with proximal retraction. *(See MR Appearance of Full-Thickness Tears pgs. 1275 and 1279, in Stoller's 3rd Edition.)*

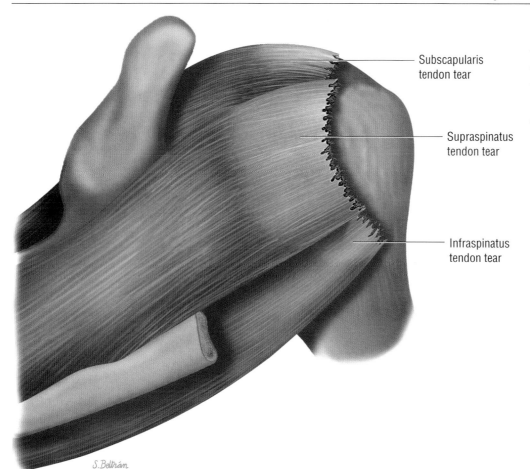

Subscapularis
tendon tear

Supraspinatus
tendon tear

Infraspinatus
tendon tear

S.Beltrán

Figure 8.79 ■ Posterosuperior view color graphic showing a massive rotator cuff tear involving the supraspinatus, infraspinatus, and suprascapularis tendon. *(See MR Appearance of Full-Thickness Tears pgs. 1275 and 1276, in Stoller's 3rd Edition.)*

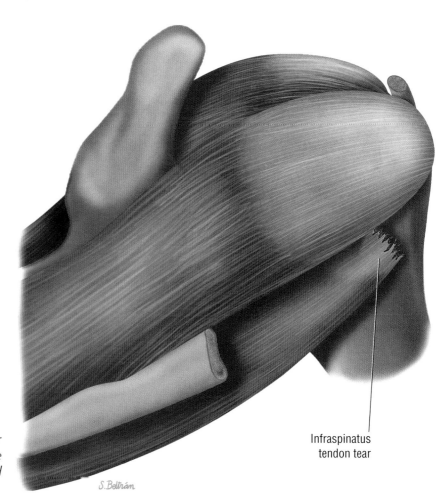

Infraspinatus
tendon tear

S.Beltrán

Figure 8.80 ■ An isolated infraspinatus tendon tear shown on a posterior superior color illustration. *(See MR Appearance of Full-Thickness Tears pgs. 1275 and 1277, in Stoller's 3rd Edition.)*

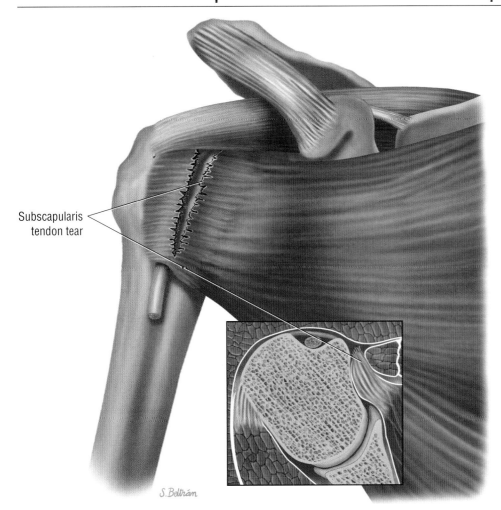

Subscapularis
tendon tear

S. Beltrán

Figure 8.81 ▪ **Isolated subscapularis tendon tear without associated biceps tendon dislocation.** Subscapularis tendon tears are associated with biceps tendon instability with laxity or disruption of the CHL-SGHL sling. SHGL tears are frequently associated with superior distal subscapularis tendon disruptions. *(See Subscapularis Tendon Tears pgs. 1280 and 1282, in Stoller's 3rd Edition.)*

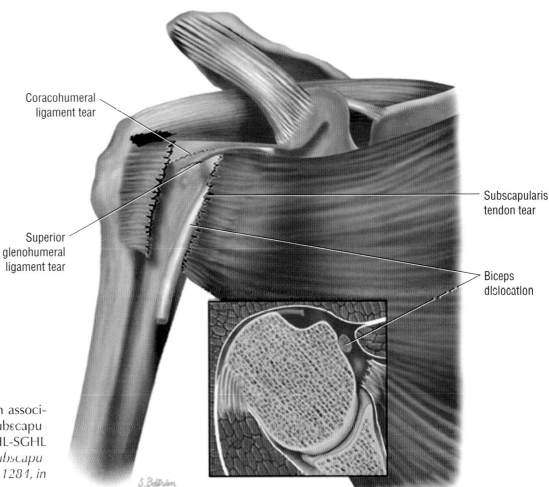

Coracohumeral
ligament tear

Superior
glenohumeral
ligament tear

Subscapularis
tendon tear

Biceps
dislocation

S. Beltrán

Figure 8.82 ▪ Biceps dislocation associated with rupture of the distal subscapularis tendon and tearing of CHL-SGHL sling. *(See MR Appearance of Subscapularis Tendon Tears pgs. 1283 and 1284, in Stoller's 3rd Edition.)*

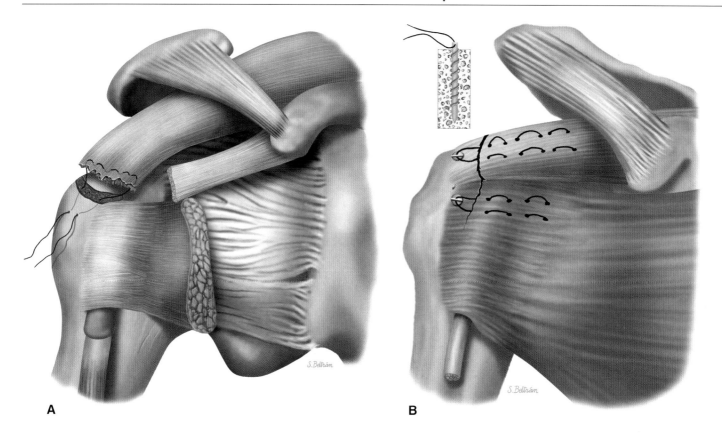

A

B

Figure 8.83 ■ **(A)** Tendon-to-bone rotator cuff repair with suturing of the edge of the distal cuff into a prepared humeral head trough. **(B)** Suture anchor repair of the supraspinatus and subscapularis tendons. Suture anchors do not preclude postoperative MR assessment. Arthroscopy spares damage to the deltoid and allows an ideal subacromial decompression. *(See Surgical Management pgs. 1288 and 1289, in Stoller's 3rd Edition.)*

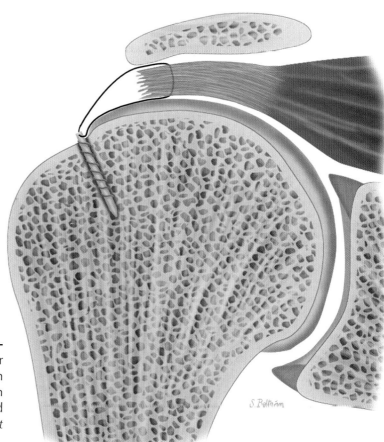

Figure 8.84 ■ **The majority of torn rotator cuffs can be repaired arthroscopically.** Suture anchor fixation of the rotator cuff tear to bone is shown. One or two sutures can be used in each suture anchor. The arthroscopic technique allows for an enhanced fixation of the cuff tendon, which can be performed with side-to-side suture anchors. *(See Surgical Management pgs. 1288 and 1289, in Stoller's 3rd Edition.)*

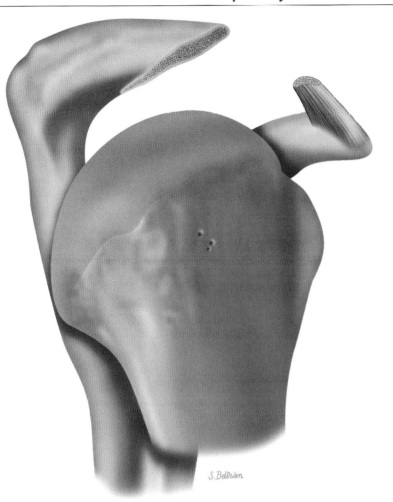

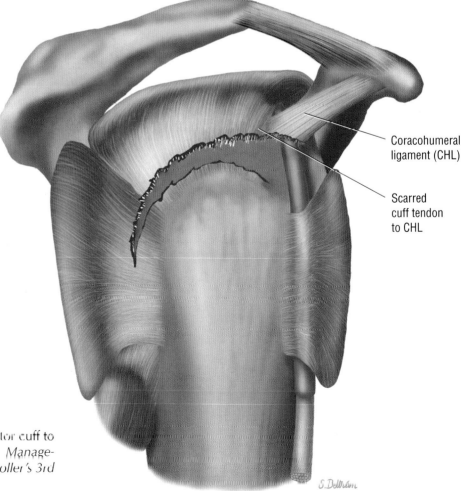

Figure 8.85 ■ Partial anterior acromioplasty. The coracoacromial ligament (CA) should be released from the acromion and not resected from under the deltoid to allow the ligament to reattach to the acromion and reconstitute the anterior arch. *(See MR Appearance of Postoperative Rotator Cuff pgs. 1286 and 1287, in Stoller's 3rd Edition.)*

Coracohumeral ligament (CHL)

Scarred cuff tendon to CHL

Figure 8.86 ■ Adherence of the retracted rotator cuff to the coracohumeral ligament. *(See Surgical Management; Complications pgs. 1290 and 1291, in Stoller's 3rd Edition.)*

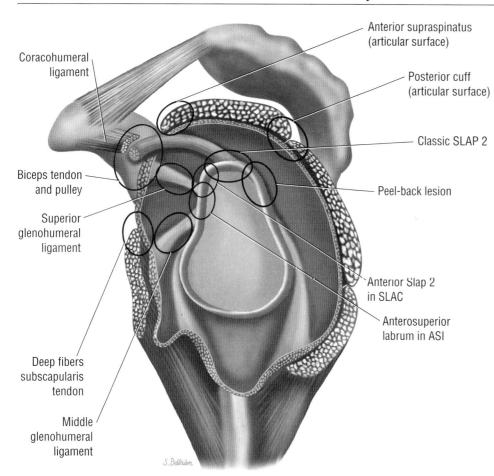

Coracohumeral ligament

Anterior supraspinatus (articular surface)

Posterior cuff (articular surface)

Classic SLAP 2

Peel-back lesion

Biceps tendon and pulley

Superior glenohumeral ligament

Anterior Slap 2 in SLAC

Anterosuperior labrum in ASI

Deep fibers subscapularis tendon

Middle glenohumeral ligament

S. Beltrán

Figure 8.87 ■ Potential sites of involvement in microinstability, including the anterior supraspinatus and anterior component of a SLAP 2 in the SLAC lesion; the posterior cuff and posterior component of a SLAP 2 in the posterior peel-back lesion; the classic anterior-to-posterior SLAP 2 lesion; anterosuperior impingement (ASI) involving the superior subscapularis, CHL-SGHL complex, the anterior supraspinatus, and anterosuperior labrum; and the middle glenohumeral ligament (MGL) in anterior laxity. *(See Microinstability pgs. 1290 and 1293, in Stoller's 3rd Edition.)*

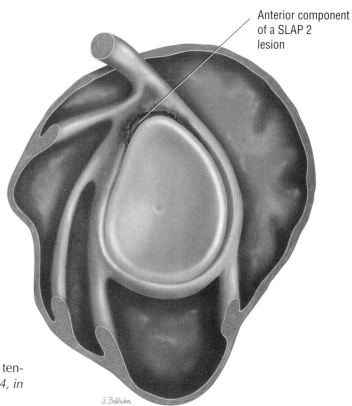

Anterior component of a SLAP 2 lesion

S. Beltrán

Figure 8.88 ■ SLAC lesion with partial articular-side supraspinatus tendon tear and anterior SLAP lesion. *(See SLAC Lesions pgs. 1292–1294, in Stoller's 3rd Edition.)*

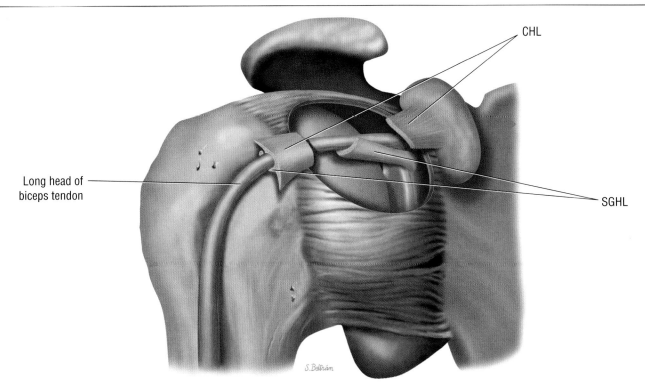

Figure 8.89 ■ **The rotator cuff interval, demonstrating the confluence of CHL and SGHL (SHL) to form the biceps pulley or sling at the entrance of the intertubercular groove.** The superior aspect of the glenohumeral joint capsule is windowed to reveal the contribution of the CHL to the roof and the SGHL to the floor of the biceps pulley. *(Based on Habermeyer P, Magosch P, Pritsch M, et al. Anterosuperior impingement of the shoulder as a result of pulley lesions: a prospective arthroscopic study. J. Shoulder Elbow Surg 2004;13(1):5). (See Rotator Cuff Interval pgs. 1293 and 1295, in Stoller's 3rd Edition.)*

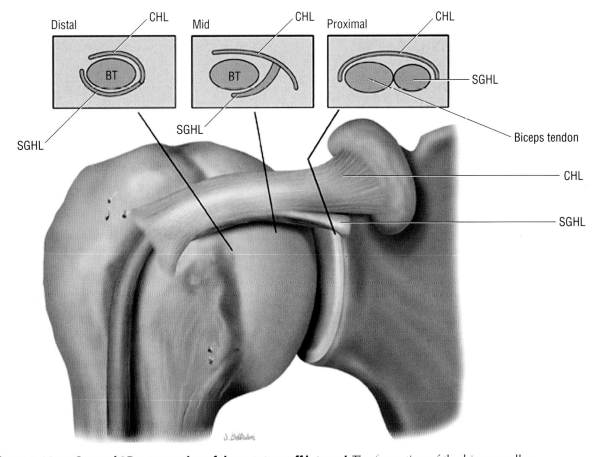

Figure 8.90 ■ **Coronal 3D perspective of the rotator cuff interval.** The formation of the biceps pulley or sling is shown from proximal, middle, and distal sections through the confluence of the CHL and SGHL. There is a T-shaped junction between the SGHL and CHL at the mid-interval, and a more U-shaped anterior sling is formed distally at the entrance of the intertubercular groove. *(See Rotator Cuff Interval pgs. 1296 and 1297, in Stoller's 3rd Edition.)*

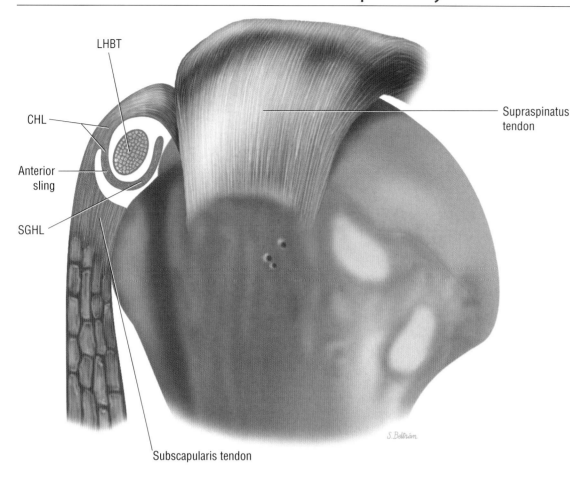

LHBT

CHL

Anterior sling

SGHL

Supraspinatus tendon

Subscapularis tendon

Figure 8.91 ▪ Biceps pulley formed by the CHL and SGHL. A 2D sagittal section of the subscapularis and a 3D perspective of the supraspinatus are shown in proximity to the pulley. Note the intimate relationship between the CHL (roof of the biceps pulley) and the anterior leading edge of the supraspinatus tendon. The medial CHL primarily contributes to the pulley, whereas the lateral CHL stabilizes the biceps (LHBT) through its attachment to the greater tuberosity. These lateral fibers are at a risk for injury with anterior and far lateral supraspinatus tears. *(See Biceps Pulley Lesions pgs. 1300 and 1301, in Stoller's 3rd Edition.)*

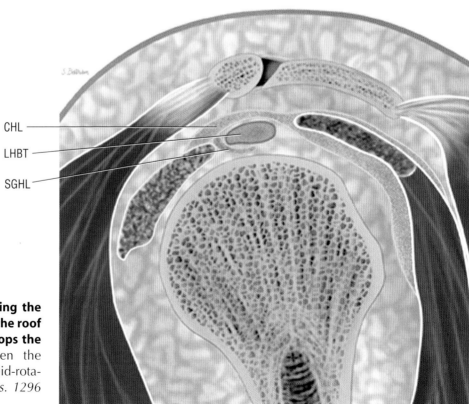

CHL

LHBT

SGHL

Figure 8.92 ▪ Sagittal color section illustrating the proximal biceps pulley with the CHL forming the roof and the SGHL forming the floor, which envelops the LHBT. Note the T-shaped junction between the CHL/roof and the SGHL/floor at the level of mid-rotator cuff interval. *(See Rotator Cuff Interval pgs. 1296 and 1298, in Stoller's 3rd Edition.)*

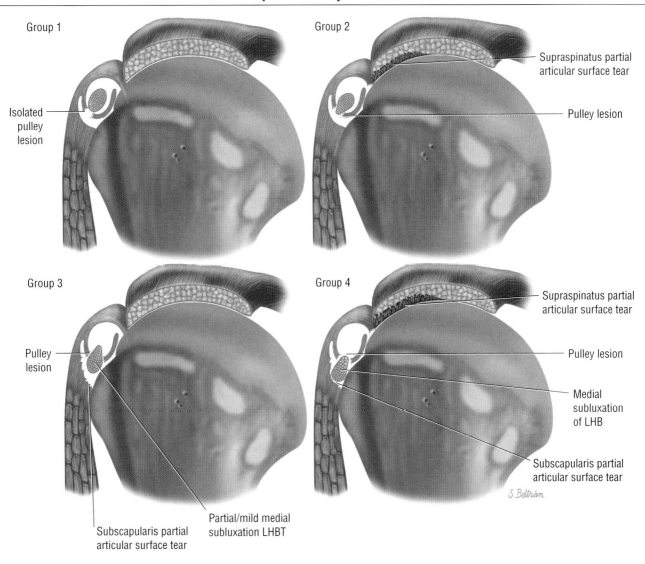

Group 1

Isolated
pulley
lesion

Group 2

Supraspinatus partial
articular surface tear

Pulley lesion

Group 3

Pulley
lesion

Subscapularis partial
articular surface tear

Partial/mild medial
subluxation LHBT

Group 4

Supraspinatus partial
articular surface tear

Pulley lesion

Medial
subluxation
of LHB

Subscapularis partial
articular surface tear

Figure 8.93 ■ **The Habermeyer classification of biceps pulley lesions groups them into four subtypes.** Type 1 lesions are isolated pulley lesions with an intact supraspinatus and subscapularis tendon. Type 2 represents a pulley lesion and a partial articular surface supraspinatus tendon tear. Type 3 is a pulley lesion with partial medial subluxation of the biceps tendon associated with a partial articular or deep surface tear of the superior distal fibers of the subscapularis tendon. Type 4 combines the pulley lesion with partial articular surface tears of both the supraspinatus and subscapularis tendons. There is frank medial subluxation of the LHBT as the contributions of the CHL (roof of the sling) and SGHL (floor of the sling) are affected. *(See Biceps Pulley Lesions pgs. 1300 and 1302, in Stoller's 3rd Edition.)*

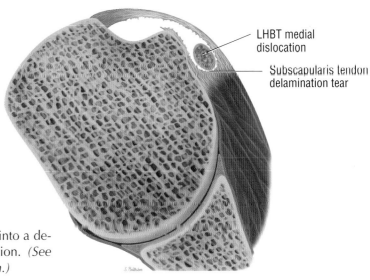

LHBT medial
dislocation

Subscapularis tendon
delamination tear

Figure 8.94 ■ Dislocation of the biceps tendon (LHBT) directly into a delamination of the subscapularis tendon on axial color illustration. *(See Biceps Pulley Lesions pgs. 1300 and 1309, in Stoller's 3rd Edition.)*

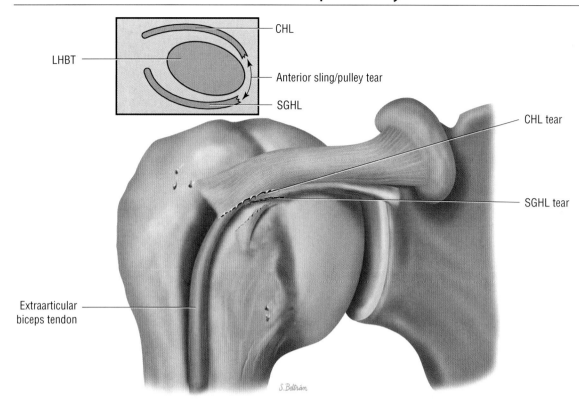

CHL

LHBT

Anterior sling/pulley tear

SGHL

CHL tear

SGHL tear

Extraarticular biceps tendon

Figure 8.95 ■ A type 1 biceps pulley lesion with a torn anterior CHL-SGHL sling. The biceps tendon (LHBT), although unstable, has not undergone subluxation. *(See Biceps Pulley Lesions pg. 1303, in Stoller's 3rd Edition.)*

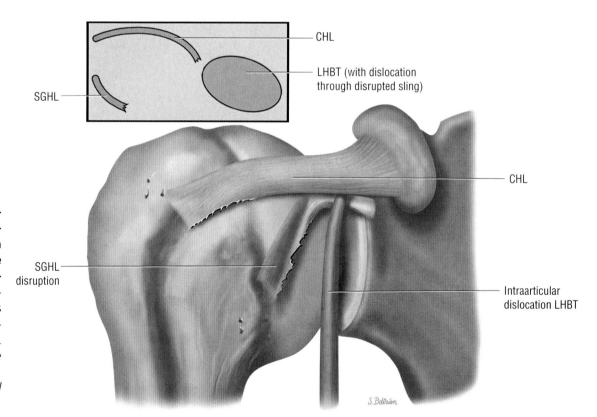

CHL

LHBT (with dislocation through disrupted sling)

SGHL

CHL

SGHL disruption

Intraarticular dislocation LHBT

Figure 8.96 ■ Intraarticular dislocation of the biceps tendon (LHBT) with complete disruption of the SGHL on a coronal color illustration. Both the insertion of the subscapularis tendon and the SGHL component of the CHL-SGHL complex are disrupted. *(See Biceps Pulley Lesions pg. 1304, in Stoller's 3rd Edition.)*

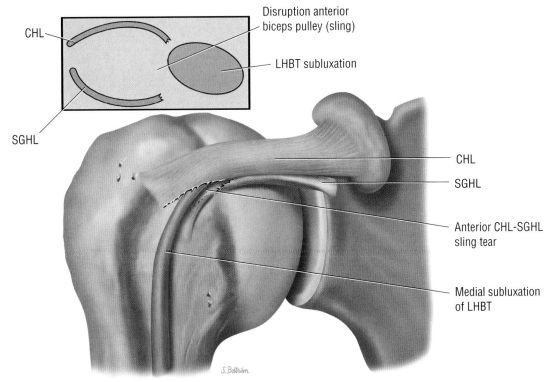

CHL

SGHL

Disruption anterior
biceps pulley (sling)

LHBT subluxation

CHL

SGHL

Anterior CHL-SGHL
sling tear

Medial subluxation
of LHBT

Figure 8.97 ■ **Coronal color illustration showing medial subluxation of the biceps tendon anterior to the subscapularis tendon and deep to the CHL.** This pathology is made possible by disruption of the anterior sling with intact lateral fibers of the CHL. The medial fibers of the CHL that directly contribute to the CHL-SGHL complex are torn in conjunction with the SGHL. *(See Biceps Pulley Lesions pgs. 1300, 1305 and 1306, in Stoller's 3rd Edition.)*

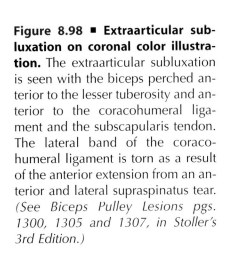

Figure 8.98 ■ **Extraarticular subluxation on coronal color illustration.** The extraarticular subluxation is seen with the biceps perched anterior to the lesser tuberosity and anterior to the coracohumeral ligament and the subscapularis tendon. The lateral band of the coracohumeral ligament is torn as a result of the anterior extension from an anterior and lateral supraspinatus tear. *(See Biceps Pulley Lesions pgs. 1300, 1305 and 1307, in Stoller's 3rd Edition.)*

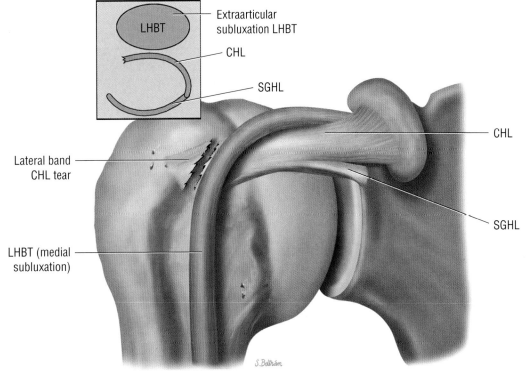

LHBT

Extraarticular
subluxation LHBT

CHL

SGHL

Lateral band
CHL tear

LHBT (medial
subluxation)

CHL

SGHL

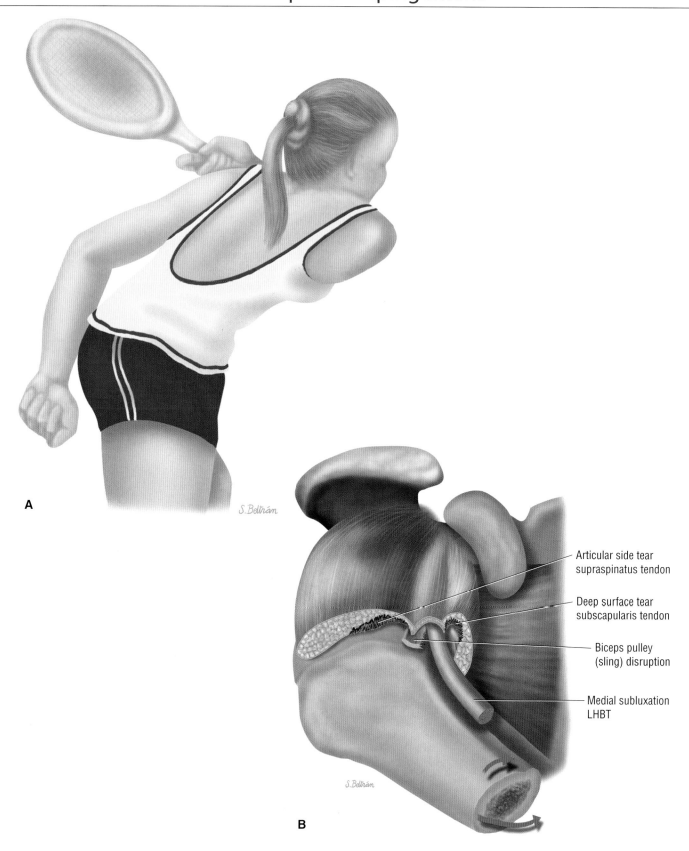

Articular side tear
supraspinatus tendon

Deep surface tear
subscapularis tendon

Biceps pulley
(sling) disruption

Medial subluxation
LHBT

A

B

Figure 8.99 ▪ Anterosuperior impingement occurring with an internal rotation and adduction mechanism. Medial subluxation of the LHBT is associated with disruption of the biceps pulley system and partial tears of the articular surface of the subscapularis and supraspinatus tendons. Medial subluxation of the LHB causes the deep or articular surface tear of the subscapularis tendon. **(A)** Color graphic of a tennis player in position of shoulder adduction and internal rotation. **(B)** Superolateral view color illustration demonstrating the association of a grade 4 biceps pulley lesion and the corresponding pathomechanics of humeral adduction and internal rotation in anterosuperior impingement. (A and B based on Habermeyer P, Magosch P, Pritsch M, et al. Anterosuperior impingement of the shoulder as a result of pulley lesions: a prospective arthroscopic study. J Shoulder Elbow Surg 2004; 13(1):5.) *(See Anterosuperior Impingement pgs. 1305, 1310 and 1311, in Stoller's 3rd Edition.)*

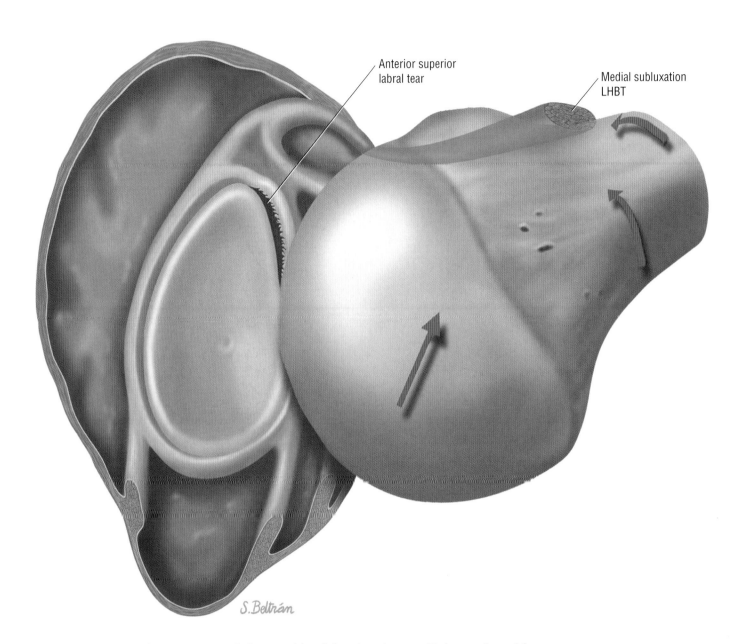

Anterior superior
labral tear

Medial subluxation
LHBT

S.Beltrán

Figure 8.100 ■ Color graphic of the glenohumeral joint as viewed from a supero-lateral exposure with the humerus adducted and internally rotated. In anterosuperior impingement (ASI), the anterosuperior labral tear occurs as the humeral head migrates into the anterosuperior quadrant against the anterior glenoid rim. The normal posterior and compressive joint retraction function of the LHB is lost in ASI secondary to the unstable medially subluxed LHB. (Based on Habermeyer P, Magosch P, Pritsch M, et al. Anterosuperior impingement of the shoulder as a result of pulley lesions: a prospective arthroscopic study. J Shoulder Elbow Surg 2004; 13(1):5.) *(See Anterosuperior Impingement pgs. 1305, 1310 and 1312, in Stoller's 3rd Edition.)*

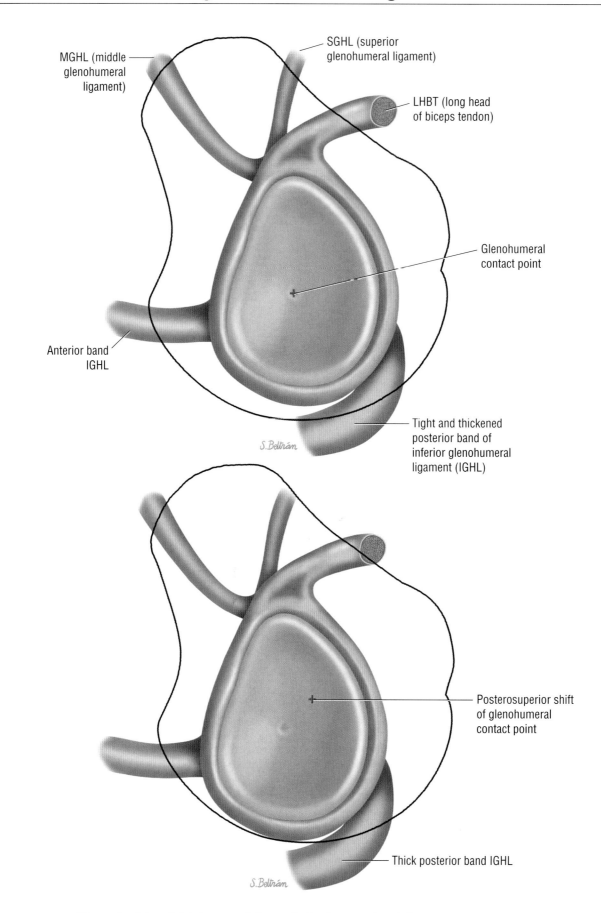

MGHL (middle glenohumeral ligament)

SGHL (superior glenohumeral ligament)

LHBT (long head of biceps tendon)

Glenohumeral contact point

Anterior band IGHL

Tight and thickened posterior band of inferior glenohumeral ligament (IGHL)

A

Posterosuperior shift of glenohumeral contact point

Thick posterior band IGHL

B

Figure 8.101 ■ **Initial steps of the pathologic cascade of changes in the throwing shoulder.** **(A)** Abduction and external rotation with a tight and thickened posterior band of the inferior glenohumeral ligament. **(B)** Posterosuperior shift of the glenohumeral contact point. *(See Throwing Shoulder pgs. 1313 and 1314, in Stoller's 3rd Edition.)*

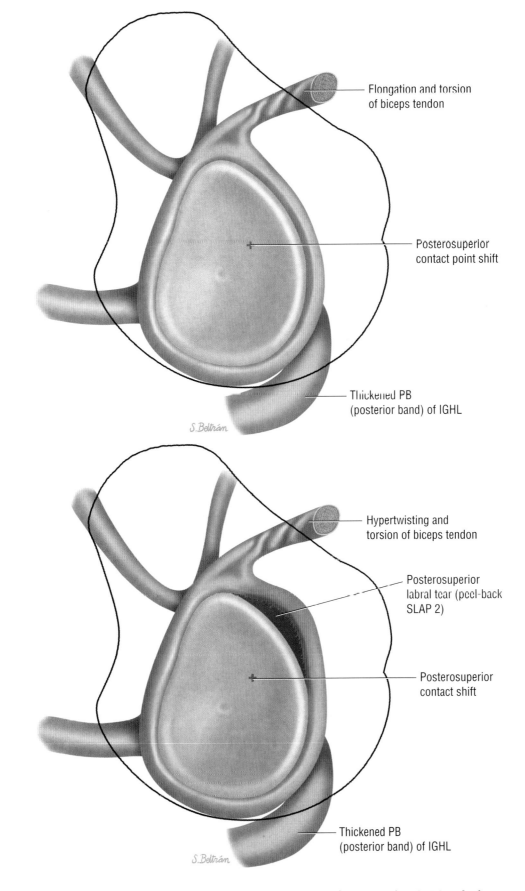

A

B

Figure 8.102 ■ Dead arm with the development of a posterior SLAP 2 lesion.
Color illustrations of glenohumeral joint from a lateral perspective. Hypertwisting
and torsion of the intraarticular biceps are shown on **(A)**, and a peel-back posterosuperior labral tear is shown on **(B)**. *(See Dead Arm pgs. 1313 and 1315, in Stoller's
3rd Edition.)*

Labels on illustration A:
- Flongation and torsion of biceps tendon
- Posterosuperior contact point shift
- Thickened PB (posterior band) of IGHL

Labels on illustration B:
- Hypertwisting and torsion of biceps tendon
- Posterosuperior labral tear (peel-back SLAP 2)
- Posterosuperior contact shift
- Thickened PB (posterior band) of IGHL

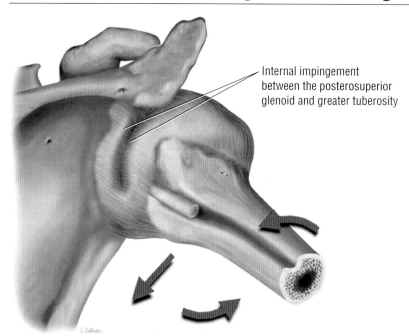

Internal impingement between the posterosuperior glenoid and greater tuberosity

Figure 8.103 ▪ **Internal impingement of the articular surface of the rotator cuff between the posterior superior glenoid and the greater tuberosity is appreciated as a normal mechanism in the position of shoulder abduction and external rotation.** Therefore, internal impingement is usually not responsible for the pathologic cascade in the throwing shoulder. *(See Dead Arm pgs. 1313 and 1316, in Stoller's 3rd Edition.)*

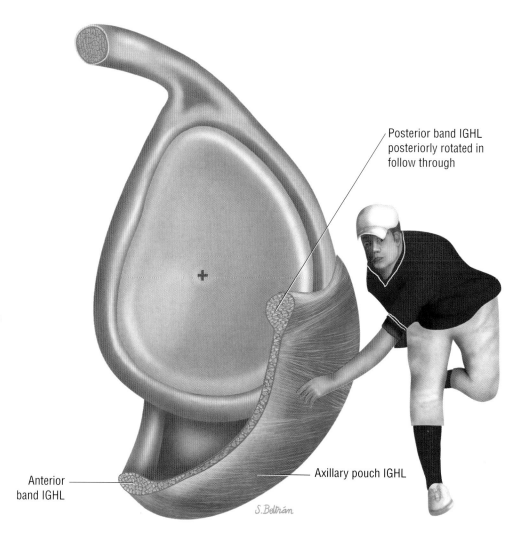

Posterior band IGHL posteriorly rotated in follow through

Figure 8.104 ▪ **Repetitive tensile loading during the follow through phase of throwing is the primary mechanism responsible for the development of the tight posteroinferior capsule.** Large distraction forces must be resisted by the posteriorly rotated IGL during follow-through. (Based on Burkhart SS, Morgan CD, Kibler WB. The disabled throwing shoulder: spectrum of pathology. Part I: Pathoanatomy and biomechanics. Arthroscopy 2003; 19(4):404.) *(See Glenohumeral Internal Rotation Deficit pgs. 1313 and 1316, in Stoller's 3rd Edition.)*

Anterior band IGHL

Axillary pouch IGHL

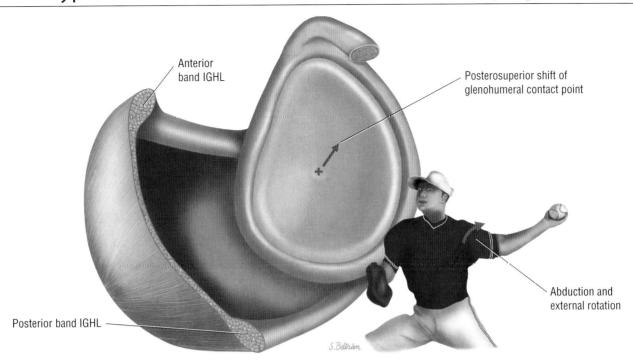

Anterior
band IGHL

Posterosuperior shift of
glenohumeral contact point

Abduction and
external rotation

Posterior band IGHL

S.Beltrán

Figure 8.105 ■ **A color graphic illustrating hyperabduction and external rotation in the late cocking phase of throwing.** In the late cocking phase of this swing, the posterior band of IGHL is bowstrung underneath the humeral head, causing a posterosuperior shift in the glenohumeral contact or rotation point. An acquired tight or contracted posterior band of the IGHL thus initiates the pathologic cascade (evident in abduction and external rotation causing GIRD). (Based on Burhart SS, Morgan CD, Kibler WB. The disabled throwing shoulder: spectrum of pathology. Part I: Pathoanatomy and biomechanics. Arthroscopy 2003; 19(4):404.) *(See Posterior Band of IGHL pgs. 1313 and 1317, in Stoller's 3rd Edition.)*

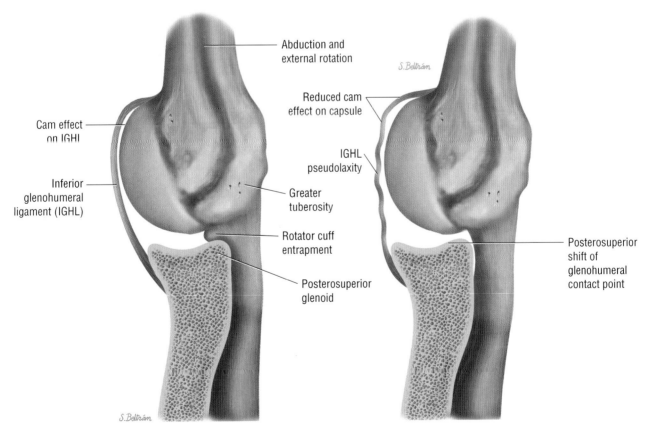

Abduction and
external rotation

S.Beltrán

Cam effect
on IGHL

Reduced cam
effect on capsule

Inferior
glenohumeral
ligament (IGHL)

IGHL
pseudolaxity

Greater
tuberosity

Rotator cuff
entrapment

Posterosuperior
glenoid

Posterosuperior
shift of
glenohumeral
contact point

S.Beltrán

Figure 8.106 ■ **(A)** Internal impingement, a normal phenomenon in all shoulders, is demonstrated with abduction and external rotation of shoulder. The greater tuberosity abuts against the posterosuperior glenoid, which entraps the rotator cuff between these two osseous structures. In throwers the posterosuperior shift of the glenohumeral contact point produces a reduction of the cam effect as the space-occupying effect of the proximal humerus on the anteroinferior capsule (IGL) is reduced. **(B)** The resultant relative laxity (shown here) or redundancy of the IGL should not be misinterpreted as anteroinferior instability. (A and B based on Burhart SS, Morgan CD, Kibler WB. The disabled throwing shoulder: spectrum of pathology. Part I: Pathoanatomy and biomechanics. Arthroscopy 2003; 19(4):404.) *(See Posterior Band of IGHL pgs. 1313 and 1318, in Stoller's 3rd Edition.)*

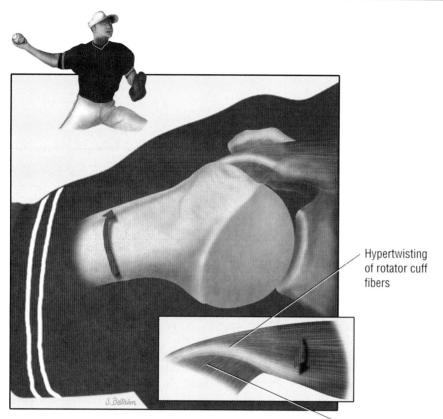

Figure 8.107 ■ Color coronal graphic of hyperexternal rotation during cocking phase of throwing, causing hypertwisting of the rotator cuff fibers. (Based on Burhart SS, Morgan CD, Kibler WB. The disabled throwing shoulder: spectrum of pathology.   Part I: Pathoanatomy and biomechanics. Arthroscopy 2003; 19(4):404.) *(See Posterior Band of IGHL pgs. 1313 and 1320, in Stoller's 3rd Edition.)*

Hypertwisting of rotator cuff fibers

Articular surface of tendon

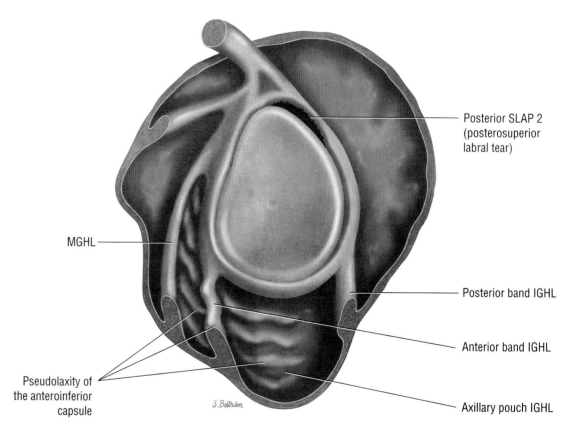

Figure 8.108 ■ Pseudolaxity of the anterior inferior capsule secondary to a break in the labral ring associated with a posterior SLAP 2 lesion is shown on a sagittal color graphic. *(See Peel-Back Lesion pgs. 1319 and 1322, in Stoller's 3rd Edition.)*

MGHL

Pseudolaxity of the anteroinferior capsule

Posterior SLAP 2 (posterosuperior labral tear)

Posterior band IGHL

Anterior band IGHL

Axillary pouch IGHL

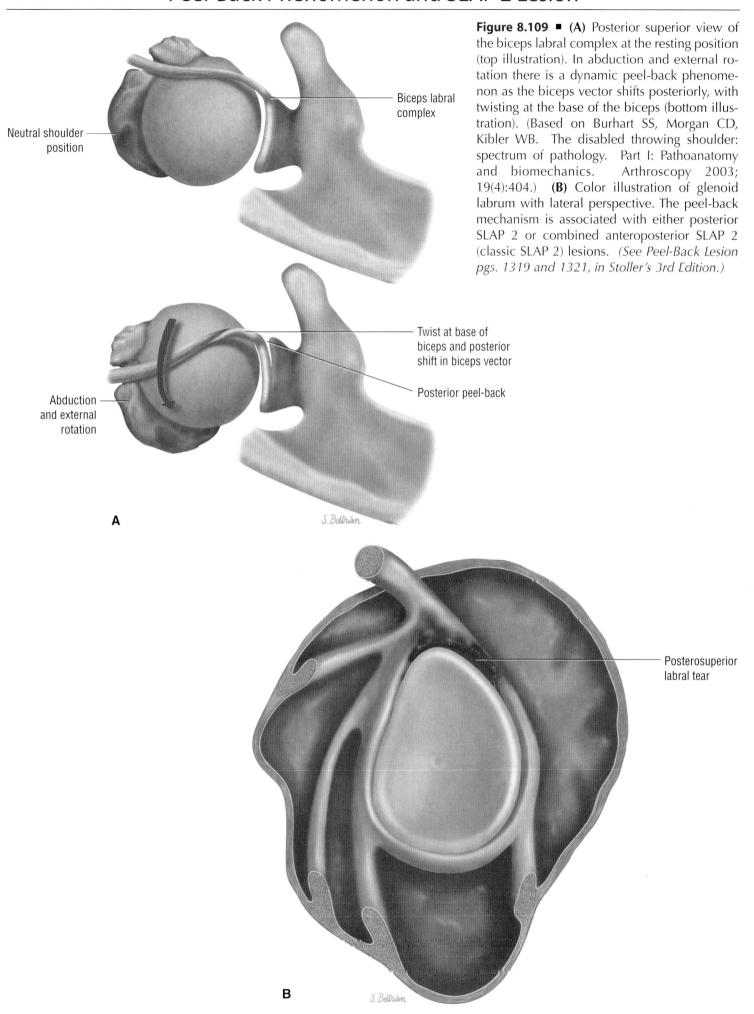

Figure 8.109 ■ **(A)** Posterior superior view of the biceps labral complex at the resting position (top illustration). In abduction and external rotation there is a dynamic peel-back phenomenon as the biceps vector shifts posteriorly, with twisting at the base of the biceps (bottom illustration). (Based on Burhart SS, Morgan CD, Kibler WB. The disabled throwing shoulder: spectrum of pathology. Part I: Pathoanatomy and biomechanics. Arthroscopy 2003; 19(4):404.) **(B)** Color illustration of glenoid labrum with lateral perspective. The peel-back mechanism is associated with either posterior SLAP 2 or combined anteroposterior SLAP 2 (classic SLAP 2) lesions. *(See Peel-Back Lesion pgs. 1319 and 1321, in Stoller's 3rd Edition.)*

Biceps labral complex

Neutral shoulder position

Twist at base of biceps and posterior shift in biceps vector

Posterior peel-back

Abduction and external rotation

A

S.Beltrán

Posterosuperior labral tear

B

S.Beltrán

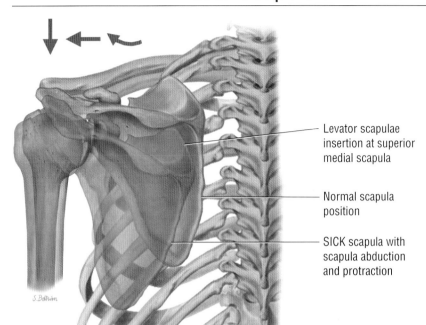

Levator scapulae
insertion at superior
medial scapula

Normal scapula
position

SICK scapula with
scapula abduction
and protraction

S. Beltrán

Figure 8.110 ■ **SICK scapula associated with scapular abduction and protraction.** Tension on the superomedial scapular insertion of the levator scapulae produces a painful tendinopathy between the medial angle and root of the scapular spine. (Based on Burkhart SS, Morgan DC, Kibler WB. The disabled throwing shoulder: spectrum of pathology. Part III: The SICK scapula, scapular dyskinesis, the kinetic chain, and rehabilitation. Arthroscopy 2003; 19(6): 641.) *(See SICK Scapula pgs. 1319 and 1323, in Stoller's 3rd Edition.)*

Figure 8.111 ■ **(A)** Proper throwing mechanics with abduction of the arm in the plane of the scapula. Note the upper arm is maintained above the horizontal plane with the elbow positioned high. **(B)** Improper mechanics with a dropped elbow position and hyperangulation of the upper arm (humerus) posterior to the plane of the scapula. (Based on Burkhart SS, Morgan DC, Kibler WB. The disabled throwing shoulder: spectrum of pathology. Part III: The SICK scapula, scapular dyskinesis, the kinetic chain, and rehabilitation. Arthroscopy 2003; 19(6): 641.) *(See Summary of the Throwing Shoulder and Dead Arm pgs. 1319 and 1323, in Stoller's 3rd Edition.)*

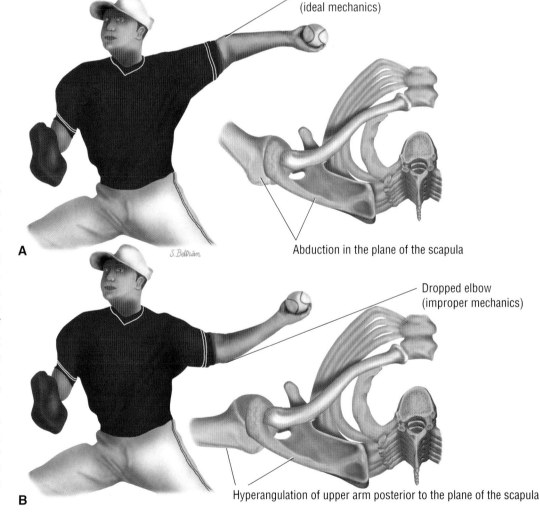

Raised elbow
(ideal mechanics)

Abduction in the plane of the scapula

S. Beltrán

A

Dropped elbow
(improper mechanics)

Hyperangulation of upper arm posterior to the plane of the scapula

B

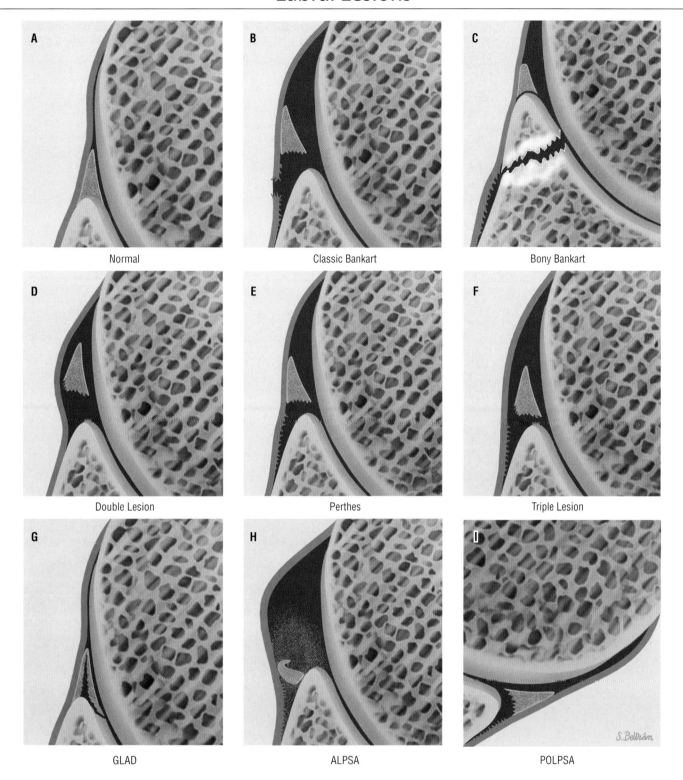

Figure 8.112 ■ **(A)** Normal anterior inferior labrum and capsule. **(B)** Classic or soft tissue Bankart with disruption of scapular periosteum. **(C)** Bony or osseous Bankart with a double labral lesion. **(D)** Double labral lesion with labral disruption from the glenoid rim and adjacent IGHL. **(E)** Perthes avulsion of the labrum and IGHL from the anterior scapular neck without periosteal disruption. **(F)** Triple labral lesion with disruption of the labrum from the glenoid rim and IGHL, with additional tearing of the IGHL from the scapular neck. **(G)** A GLAD lesion (glenoid labrum articular disruption) is known also as a GARD lesion (glenoid articular rim divot). These lesions involve a partial tear of the anterior inferior glenoid labrum with adjacent articular cartilage defect in clinically stable patients. **(H)** The ALPSA lesion is an anterior labroligamentous periosteal sleeve avulsion. **(I)** The POLPSA lesion (posterior labrocapsular periosteal sleeve avulsion). *(See Bankart Lesions pgs. 1329 and 1330, in Stoller's 3rd Edition.)*

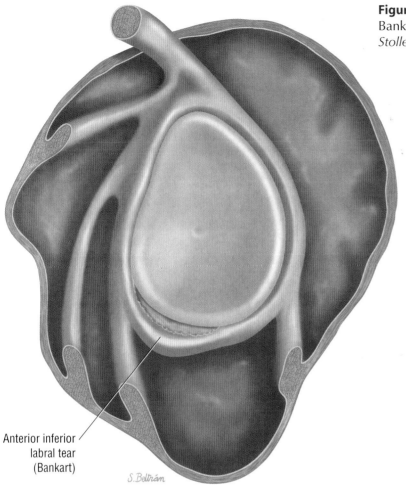

Anterior inferior
labral tear
(Bankart)

S.Beltrán

Figure 8.113 ■ Sagittal color graphic illustrating a soft tissue Bankart lesion. *(See Bankart Lesions pgs. 1329 and 1331, in Stoller's 3rd Edition.)*

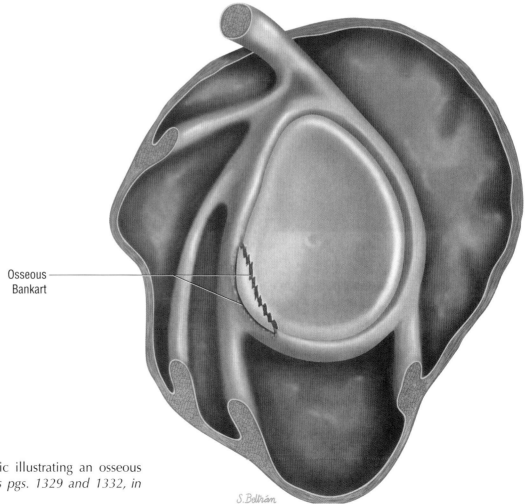

Osseous
Bankart

S.Beltrán

Figure 8.114 ■ Sagittal color graphic illustrating an osseous Bankart Lesion. *(See Bankart Lesions pgs. 1329 and 1332, in Stoller's 3rd Edition.)*

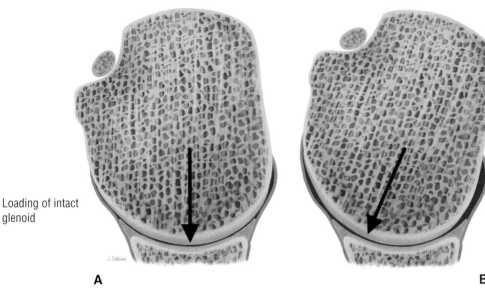

Loading of intact
glenoid

A

Figure 8.115 ■ The normal glenoid arc length resists changes in angles of humeral rotation throughout the glenoid arc length. (A) Neutral position. (B) External rotation. *Based on Burkhart SS, Lo IKY, Brady PC. Burkhart's view of the shoulder. Burkhart SS ed. In: A cowboy's guide to advanced shoulder arthroscopy. Philadelphia: Lippincott, Williams & Wilkins, 2006. (See Bankart Lesions pgs. 1335–1339, in Stoller's 3rd Edition.)*

Force vector directed
beyond the edge of the
anterior glenoid may
produce a Bankart lesion

B

Figure 8.116 ■ Osseous Bankart lesion with loss of the full glenoid arc as required to buttress against shear forces as seen in dislocation. (A) Normal glenoid fossa. (B) Bony Bankart lesion. *Based on Burkhart SS, Lo IKY, Brady PC. Burkhart's view of the shoulder. Burkhart SS ed. In: A cowboy's guide to advanced shoulder arthroscopy. Philadelphia: Lippincott, Williams & Wilkins, 2006. (See Bankart Lesions pgs. 1329 and 1333, in Stoller's 3rd Edition.)*

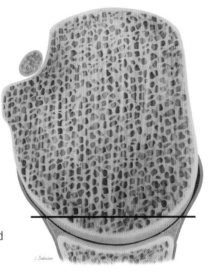

The anterior glenoid
rim deepens the
glenoid fossa

A

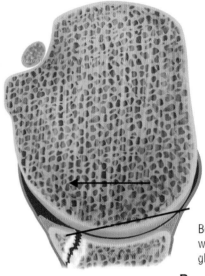

Bony Bankart
with decreased
glenoid arc

B

Figure 8.117 ■ (A) Centrally applied axial force maintains osseous glenohumeral loading in an anterior osseous-deficient glenoid. (B) The bony Bankart shortens the "safe arc" for the glenoid to overcome axial forces. A Bankart repair may fail if the axial forces are applied beyond the edge of the deficient glenoid. *Based on Burkhart SS, Lo IKY, Brady PC. Burkhart's view of the shoulder. Burkhart SS ed. In: A cowboy's guide to advanced shoulder arthroscopy. Philadelphia: Lippincott, Williams & Wilkins, 2006. (See Bankart Lesions pgs. 1329–1339, in Stoller's 3rd Edition.)*

Axial force applied
to a point beyond
the edge of a
deficient glenoid

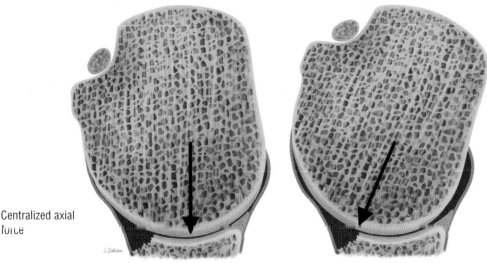

Centralized axial
force

A

B

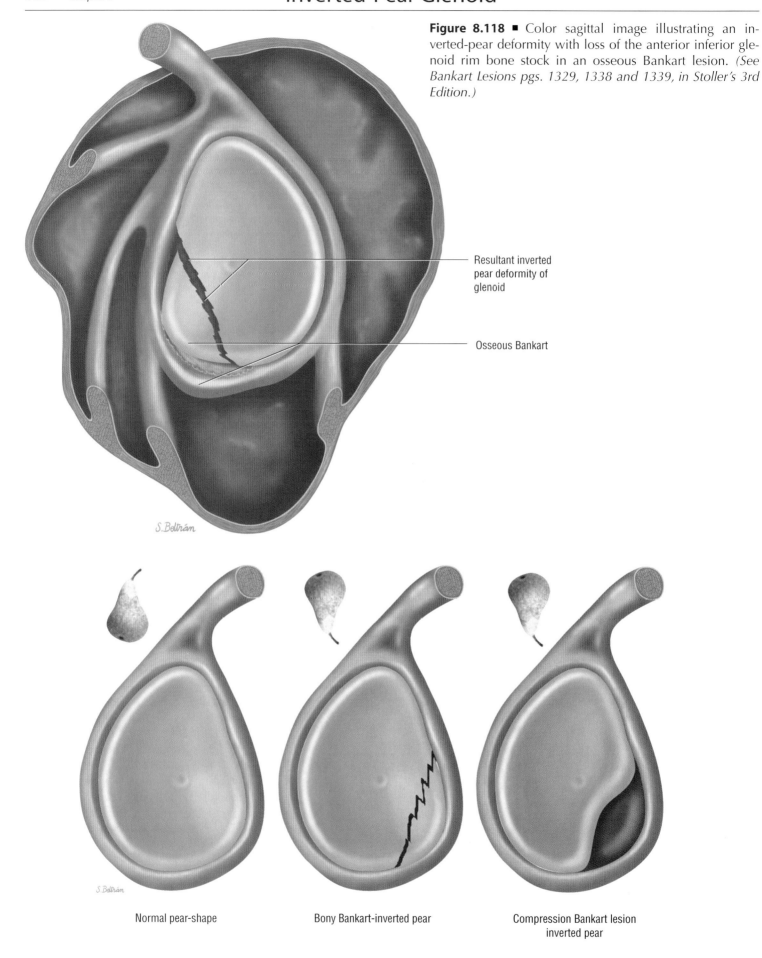

Figure 8.118 ▪ Color sagittal image illustrating an inverted-pear deformity with loss of the anterior inferior glenoid rim bone stock in an osseous Bankart lesion. *(See Bankart Lesions pgs. 1329, 1338 and 1339, in Stoller's 3rd Edition.)*

Resultant inverted pear deformity of glenoid

Osseous Bankart

Normal pear-shape

Bony Bankart-inverted pear

Compression Bankart lesion inverted pear

Figure 8.119 ▪ **(A)** Normal pear shaped glenoid with greater fossa area below the equator. **(B)** Inverted-pear morphology secondary to a bony Bankart lesion. **(C)** Compression or impaction of the anterior inferior glenoid rim, which also results in an inverted pear configuration of the glenoid fossa. *(See Bankart Lesions pgs. 1329 and 1339, in Stoller's 3rd Edition.)*

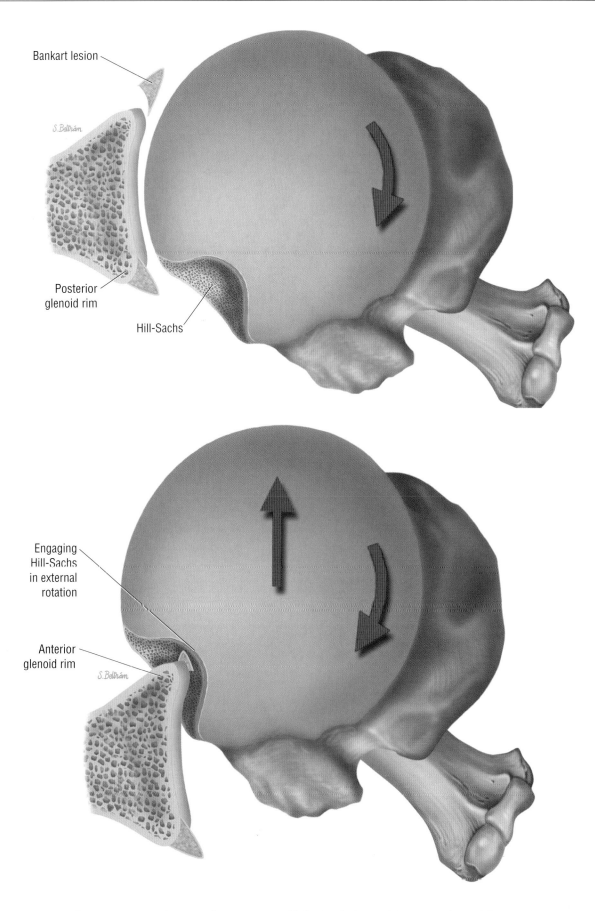

Figure 8.120 ■ Stages of engaging Hill-Sachs lesion with posterolateral humeral head defect contacting the posterior glenoid rim **(A)**, and subsequently engaging the anterior rim **(B)**. The engaging Hill-Sachs reproduces the anterior inferior instability event with humeral head displacement. *(See Bankart Repair pgs. 1335 and 1338, in Stoller's 3rd Edition.)*

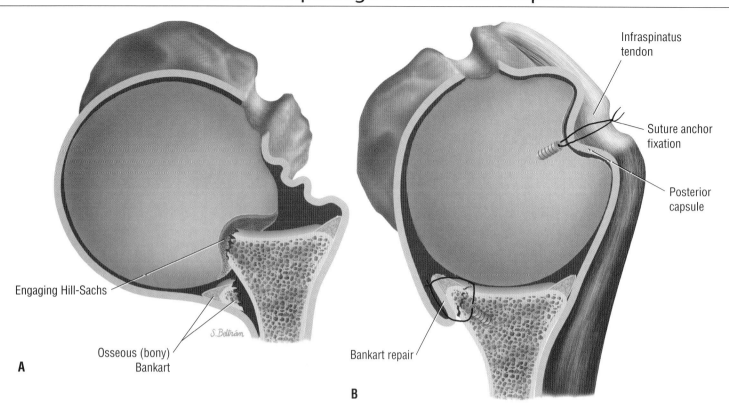

Infraspinatus
tendon

Suture anchor
fixation

Posterior
capsule

Engaging Hill-Sachs

Osseous (bony)
Bankart

A

Bankart repair

B

Figure 8.121 ■ **Hill-Sachs Remplissage arthroscopic treatment for the engaging Hill-Sachs lesion.** **(A)** Engaging Hill-Sachs lesion. **(B)** Hill-Sachs Remplissage (infraspinatus and capsular transfer) and Bankart repair. The abraded Hill-Sachs lesion is filled with the posterior capsule and by the tenodesis of the infraspinatus tendon to reduce the risk of osseous engagement. *(See Bankart Repair pgs. 1335–1339, in Stoller's 3rd Edition.)*

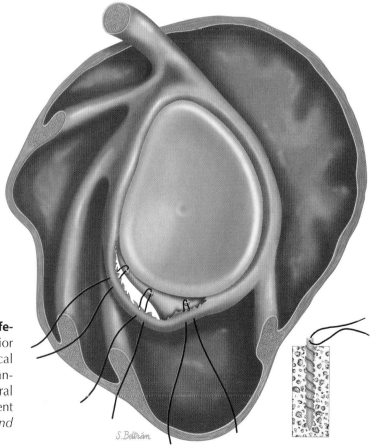

Figure 8.122 ■ **Illustration of a Bankart repair with anterior inferior suture anchors shown.** Anterior capsule and posterior-inferior capsule plication are further techniques used to improve surgical success for anterior-inferior reconstructions. The goal is to restore anterior and posterior capsular integrity and rebuild the anterior labral wedge. Associated SLAP lesions and middle glenohumeral ligament detachments are also repaired. *(See Bankart Repair pgs. 1335 and 1340, in Stoller's 3rd Edition.)*

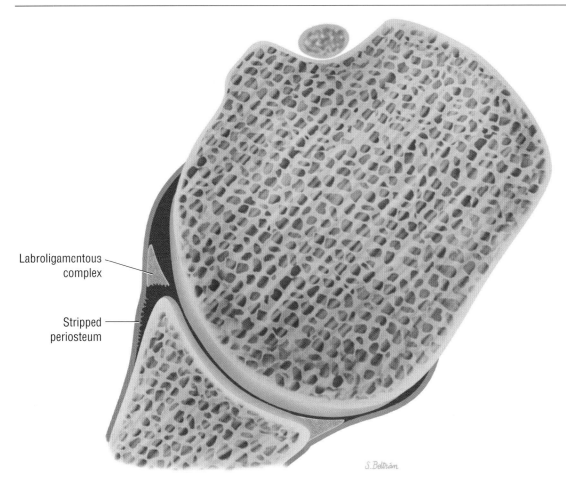

Figure 8.123 ■ Axial color graphic of Perthes lesion, a labral ligamentous avulsion with intact but medially stripped periosteum along the anterior glenoid neck. *(See Perthes Lesions pgs. 1339 and 1342, in Stoller's 3rd Edition.)*

Labroligamentous complex

Stripped periosteum

S. Beltrán

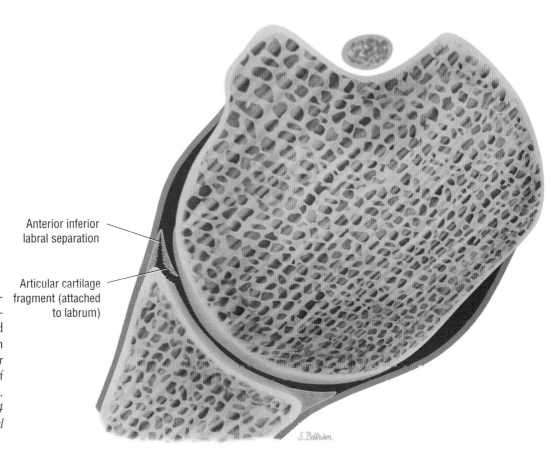

Anterior inferior labral separation

Articular cartilage fragment (attached to labrum)

Figure 8.124 ■ Axial color section of GLAD (glenolabral articular disruption) or GARD (glenoid articular rim divot) lesion with flap tear of the anterior inferior labrum and chondral defect of the adjacent articular cartilage. *(See GLAD Lesions pgs. 1344 and 1345, in Stoller's 3rd Edition.)*

S. Beltrán

ALPSA Lesion

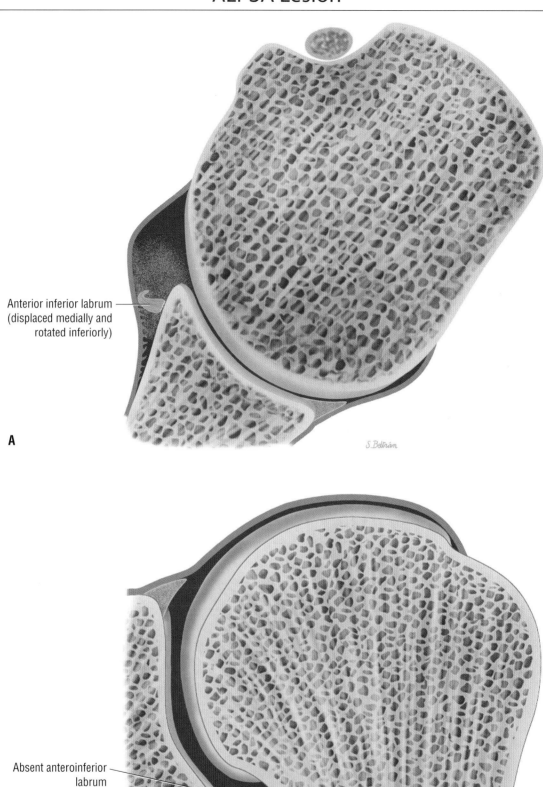

Anterior inferior labrum
(displaced medially and
rotated inferiorly)

A

Absent anteroinferior
labrum

ALPSA lesion

B

Figure 8.125 ■ **(A)** ALPSA axial (transverse plane) color illustration, and **(B)** coronal color illustration, of an ALPSA lesion (anterior labroligamentous periosteal sleeve avulsion) with medial and inferior rotation of the anteroinferior labroligamentous complex. The ALPSA is referred to also as a medialized Bankart lesion. *(See ALPSA Lesions pgs. 1339 and 1343, in Stoller's 3rd Edition.)*

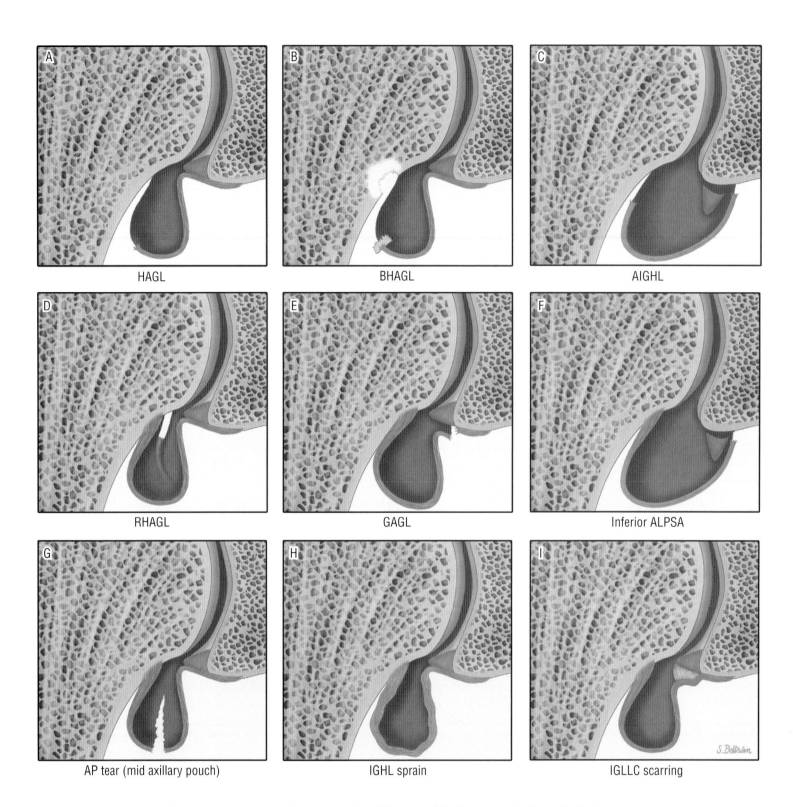

Figure 8.126 ■ Capsular IGL lesions illustrated in the coronal plane include: (A) HAGL (humeral avulsion of the glenohumeral ligament); **(B)** BHAGL (bony humeral avulsion of the glenohumeral ligament); **(C)** AIGHL (anterior inferior glenohumeral ligament); **(D)** RHAGL (reverse HAGL); **(E)** GAGL (glenohumeral avulsion of the glenohumeral ligaments); **(F)** Inferior ALPSA (anterior labroligamentous periosteal sleeve avulsion); **(G)** Mid-axillary pouch (AP) tear; **(H)** IGHL sprain; and **(I)** IGLLC (inferior glenohumeral ligament labral complex) scarring. *(See Capsular-Related Lesions pgs. 1344 and 1347, in Stoller's 3rd Edition.)*

HAGL Lesion

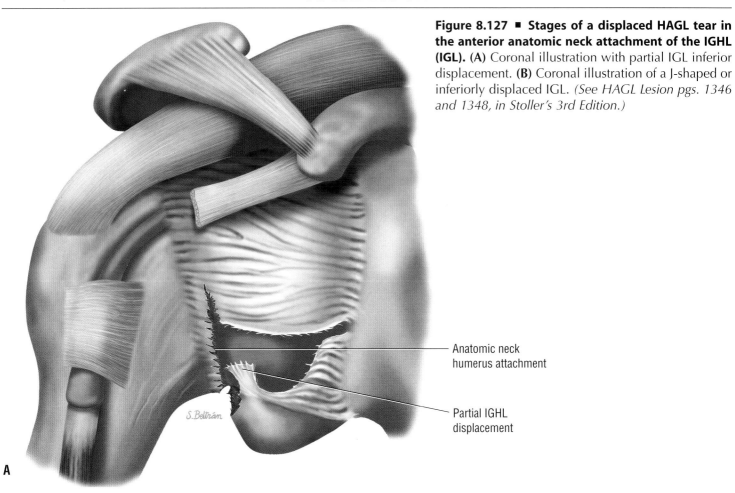

Figure 8.127 ■ **Stages of a displaced HAGL tear in the anterior anatomic neck attachment of the IGHL (IGL).** **(A)** Coronal illustration with partial IGL inferior displacement. **(B)** Coronal illustration of a J-shaped or inferiorly displaced IGL. *(See HAGL Lesion pgs. 1346 and 1348, in Stoller's 3rd Edition.)*

Anatomic neck
humerus attachment

Partial IGHL
displacement

A

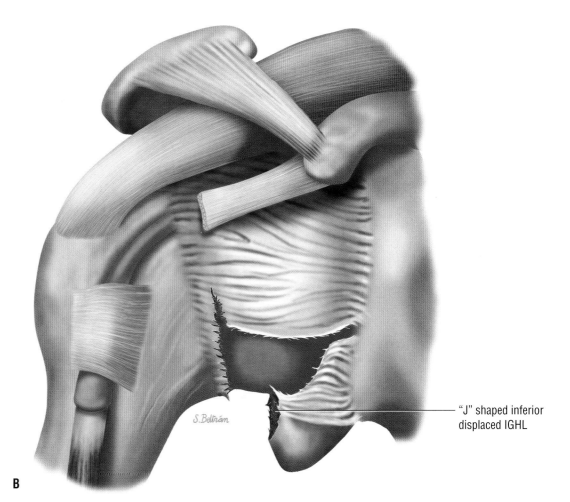

"J" shaped inferior
displaced IGHL

B

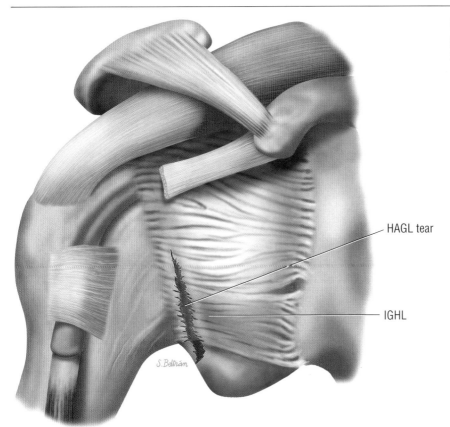

Figure 8.128 ■ HAGL lesion on coronal color graphic. *(See HAGL Lesions pgs. 1346 and 1349, in Stoller's 3rd Edition.)*

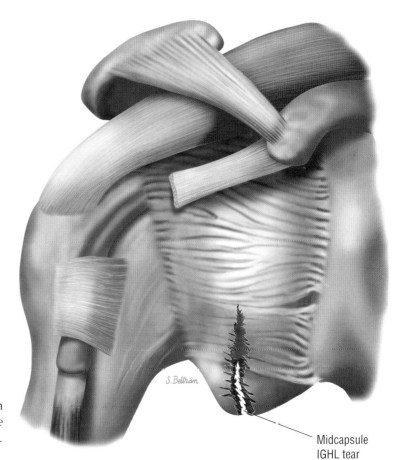

Figure 8.129 ■ Mid-axillary pouch tear of the IGHL (IGL) on a coronal color graphic centered on the axillary pouch. *(See Axillary Pouch Midligament Tears, Sprains, and Scarring pgs. 1353 and 1354, in Stoller's 3rd Edition.)*

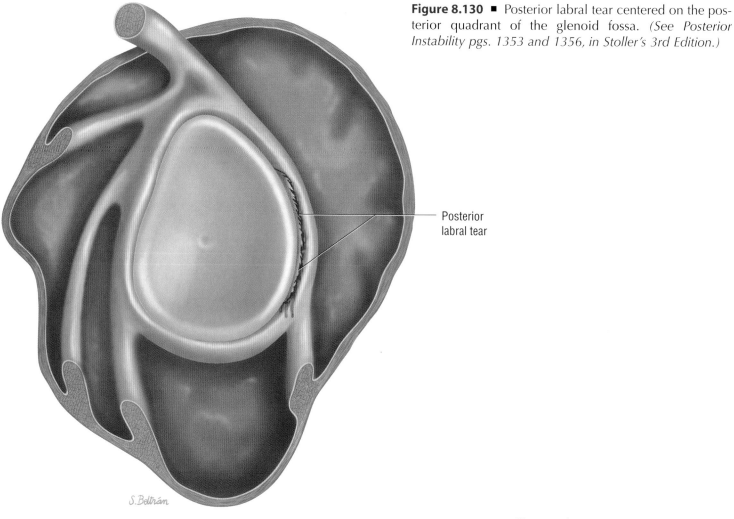

Figure 8.130 ■ Posterior labral tear centered on the posterior quadrant of the glenoid fossa. *(See Posterior Instability pgs. 1353 and 1356, in Stoller's 3rd Edition.)*

Posterior
labral tear

S. Beltrán

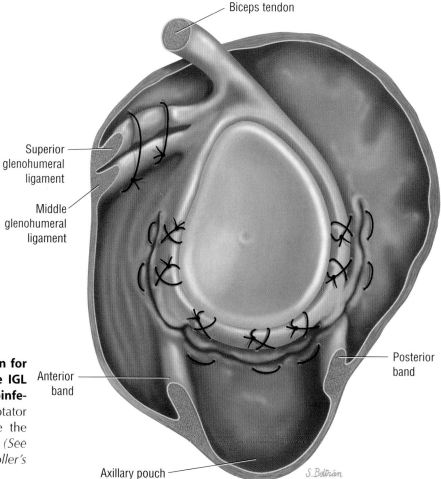

Biceps tendon

Superior
glenohumeral
ligament

Middle
glenohumeral
ligament

Posterior
band

Anterior
band

Axillary pouch

S. Beltrán

Figure 8.131 ■ **Arthroscopic pancapsular plication for treatment of multidirectional instability with the IGL and capsule folded to the labrum from the posteroinferior quadrant to the anteroinferior quadrant.** The rotator interval is closed, and the final result is to have the humeral head centralized within the glenoid fossa. *(See Multidirectional Instability pgs. 1357 and 1367, in Stoller's 3rd Edition.)*

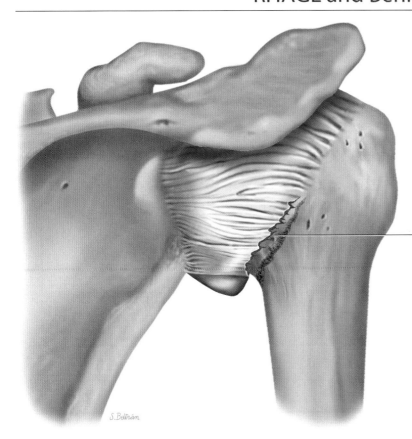

Figure 8.132 ▪ Posterior coronal color view of RHAGL with avulsion of the posterior humeral attachment of the shoulder capsule. *(See Reverse HAGL pgs. 1357 and 1362, in Stoller's 3rd Edition.)*

RHAGL posterior
capsular avulsion

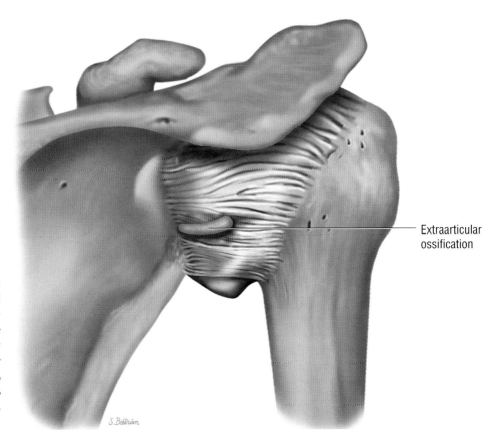

Extraarticular
ossification

Figure 8.133 ▪ **Extraarticular ossification of a Bennett lesion on posterior coronal view.** The Bennet lesion is associated with injury to the posterior superior labrum in the throwing athlete. The Bennett lesion usually occurs in the location of greatest posterior glenoid rim wear or sclerosis, and inferior to the posterosuperior peel-back lesion. *(See Bennett Lesion pgs. 1357 and 1363, in Stoller's 3rd Edition.)*

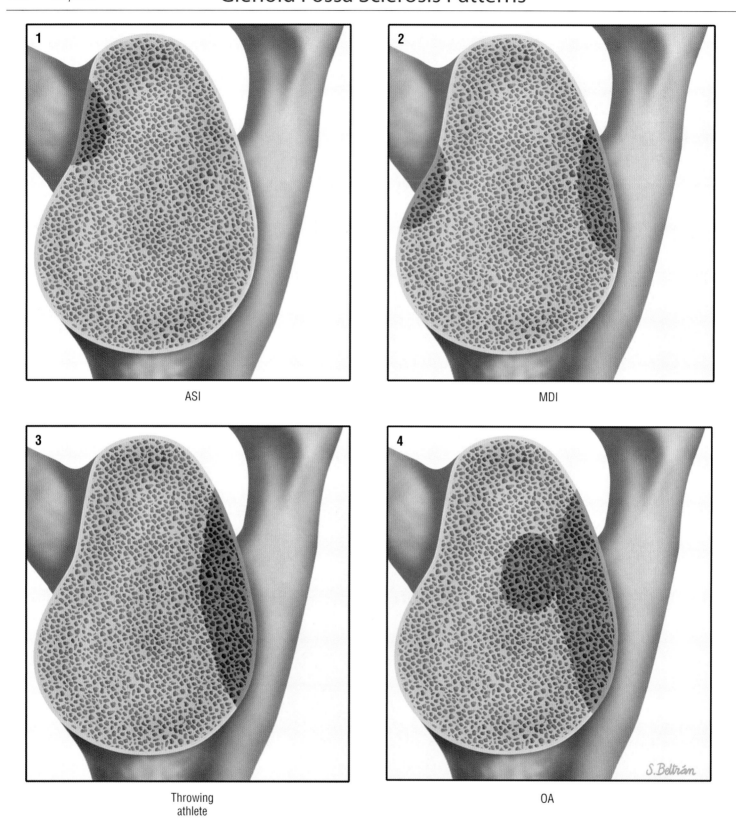

ASI

MDI

Throwing
athlete

OA

Figure 8.134 ■ Four patterns of glenoid fossa sclerosis. (1. Upper left)
Anterosuperior impingement (ASI). (2. Upper Right) Multidirectional instability
(MDI). (3. Lower left) Posterior glenoid rim wear in the throwing athlete. (4. Lower
right) Osteoarthritis pattern with central glenoid fossa and posterior glenoid wear.
(See Multidirectional Instability pgs. 1359 and 1366, in Stoller's 3rd Edition.)

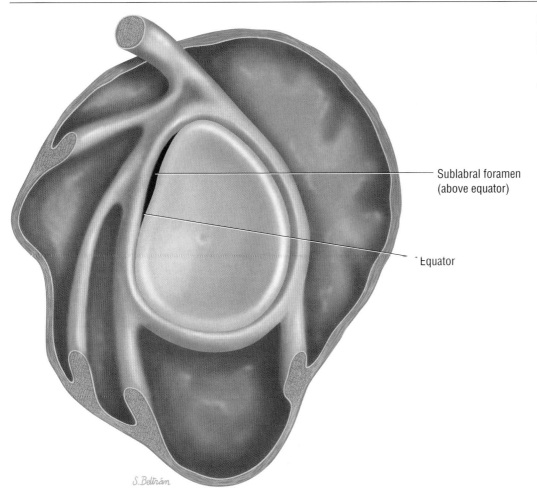

Figure 8.135 ■ Lateral view color graphic of a sublabral foramen beneath the anterior superior labrum. *(See Sublabral Foramen pgs. 1365 and 1368, in Stoller's 3rd Edition.)*

Sublabral foramen
(above equator)

Equator

S.Beltrán

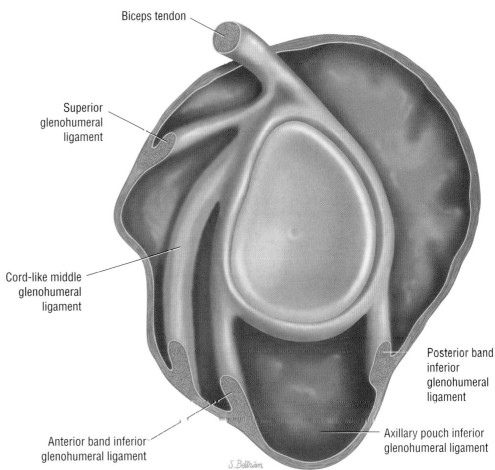

Biceps tendon

Superior
glenohumeral
ligament

Cord-like middle
glenohumeral
ligament

Anterior band inferior
glenohumeral ligament

Posterior band
inferior
glenohumeral
ligament

Axillary pouch inferior
glenohumeral ligament

S.Beltrán

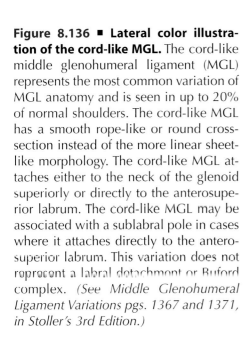

Figure 8.136 ■ **Lateral color illustration of the cord-like MGL.** The cord-like middle glenohumeral ligament (MGL) represents the most common variation of MGL anatomy and is seen in up to 20% of normal shoulders. The cord-like MGL has a smooth rope-like or round cross-section instead of the more linear sheet-like morphology. The cord-like MGL attaches either to the neck of the glenoid superiorly or directly to the anterosuperior labrum. The cord-like MGL may be associated with a sublabral pole in cases where it attaches directly to the antero-superior labrum. This variation does not represent a labral detachment or Buford complex. *(See Middle Glenohumeral Ligament Variations pgs. 1367 and 1371, in Stoller's 3rd Edition.)*

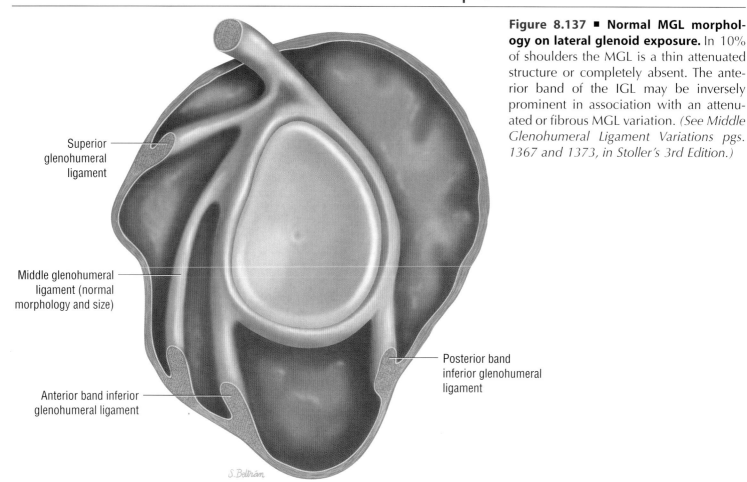

Superior
glenohumeral
ligament

Middle glenohumeral
ligament (normal
morphology and size)

Anterior band inferior
glenohumeral ligament

Posterior band
inferior glenohumeral
ligament

S.Beltrán

Figure 8.137 ■ **Normal MGL morphology on lateral glenoid exposure.** In 10% of shoulders the MGL is a thin attenuated structure or completely absent. The anterior band of the IGL may be inversely prominent in association with an attenuated or fibrous MGL variation. *(See Middle Glenohumeral Ligament Variations pgs. 1367 and 1373, in Stoller's 3rd Edition.)*

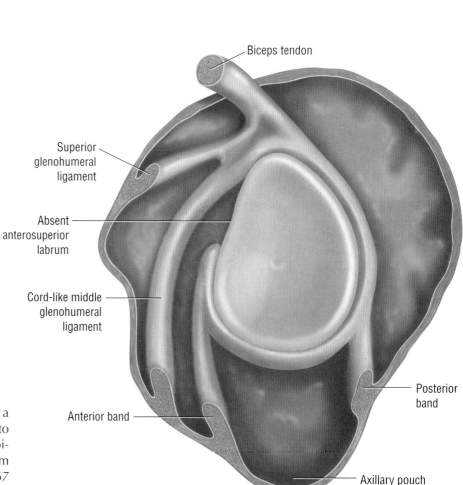

Biceps tendon

Superior
glenohumeral
ligament

Absent
anterosuperior
labrum

Cord-like middle
glenohumeral
ligament

Anterior band

Posterior
band

Axillary pouch

S.Beltrán

Figure 8.138 ■ Lateral color illustration of a Buford complex with cord-like MGL attached to superior labrum just anterior to the base of the biceps anchor, and absent anterosuperior labrum above the equator. *(See Buford Complex pgs. 1367 and 1374, in Stoller's 3rd Edition.)*

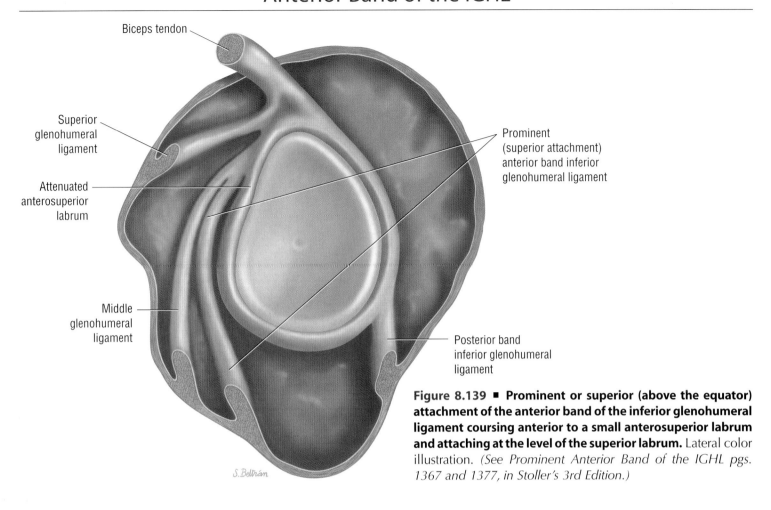

Biceps tendon

Superior glenohumeral ligament

Attenuated anterosuperior labrum

Middle glenohumeral ligament

Prominent (superior attachment) anterior band inferior glenohumeral ligament

Posterior band inferior glenohumeral ligament

S. Beltrán

Figure 8.139 ■ **Prominent or superior (above the equator) attachment of the anterior band of the inferior glenohumeral ligament coursing anterior to a small anterosuperior labrum and attaching at the level of the superior labrum.** Lateral color illustration. *(See Prominent Anterior Band of the IGHL pgs. 1367 and 1377, in Stoller's 3rd Edition.)*

Figure 8.140 ■ **Prominent anterior band of the IGHL with absent anterosuperior labrum.** This is not a Buford complex, because the MGL is not cord-like. If the anterosuperior labrum is absent, as in the case of a prominent anterior band, Buford complex, or Buford variant (cord-like MGL plus a prominent anterior band), there may be a normal sulcus between the superior labrum and superior pole of the glenoid. The high insertion of the anterior band and absent anterosuperior labrum effectively creates a sublabral foramen. *(See Prominent Anterior Band of the IGHL pgs. 1367 and 1378, in Stoller's 3rd Edition.)*

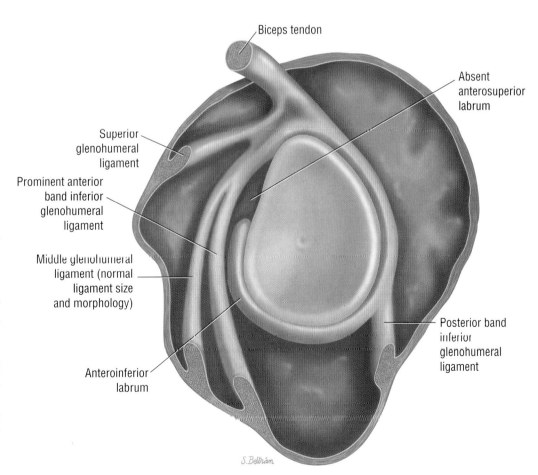

Biceps tendon

Absent anterosuperior labrum

Superior glenohumeral ligament

Prominent anterior band inferior glenohumeral ligament

Middle glenohumeral ligament (normal ligament size and morphology)

Anteroinferior labrum

Posterior band inferior glenohumeral ligament

S. Beltrán

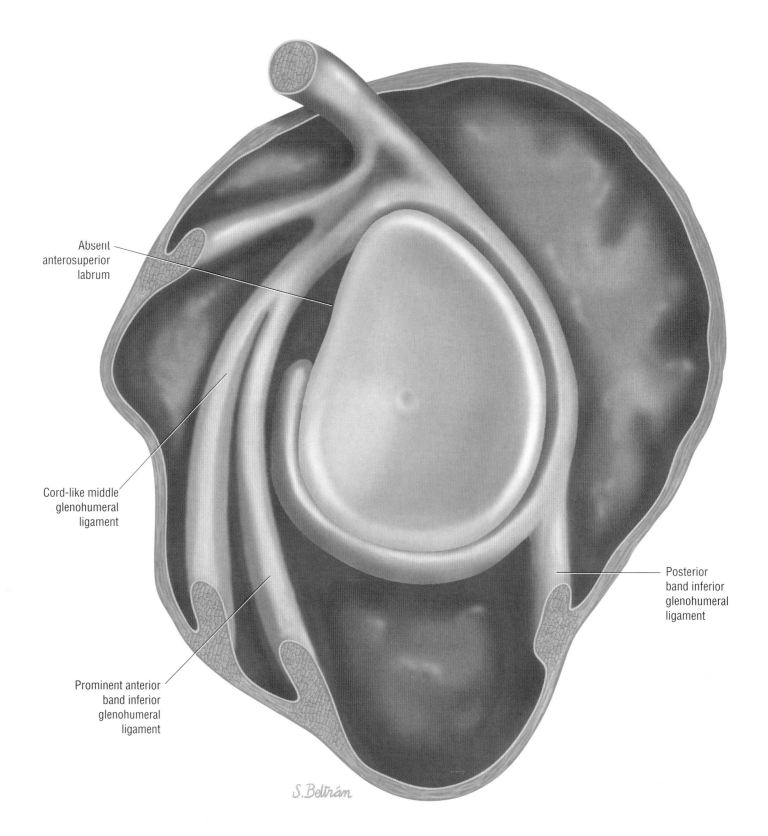

Absent
anterosuperior
labrum

Cord-like middle
glenohumeral
ligament

Prominent anterior
band inferior
glenohumeral
ligament

Posterior
band inferior
glenohumeral
ligament

S. Beltrán

Figure 8.141 ■ A prominent anterior band associated with a cord-like MGL and absent anterosuperior labrum on a lateral view color illustration. Because the MGL is cord-like, this could be considered a Buford variant. The original description of the Buford complex did not include the variant of a prominent anterior band. *(See Prominent Anterior Band of the IGHL pgs. 1367 and 1380, in Stoller's 3rd Edition.)*

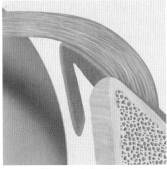

Fragmentation/loss
of labral tissue

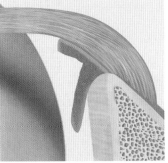

Fragmentation/loss
of labral tissue

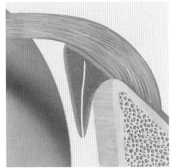

Split tear

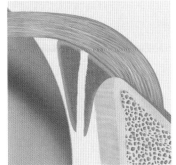

Fragmentation (displaced split)

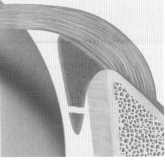

Inferior displacement/
fragmentation

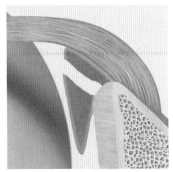

Inferior displacement/
fragmentation

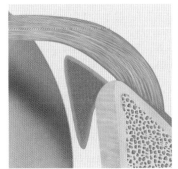

Inferior displacement

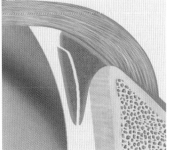

Eccentric tear

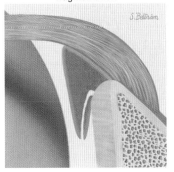

Eccentric tear

Figure 8.142 ■ Common SLAP tear variants include labral fragmentation, vertical split, inferior displacement, and eccentric tears (humeral or glenoid side). A fragmented labrum with gross displacement or absence of labral tissue is associated with bucket-handle morphology. A split of the labrum into separated triangles (double triangle sign) is associated also with a bucket-handle tear pattern. Inferior displacement of the entire superior labrum or a portion of the labrum indicates displacement of a bucket-handle tear. Linear signal without loss of labral tissue or labral displacement/fragmentation is associated with SLAP 2 lesions. There also may be complete superior labral separation from the superior pole with a widened biceps labral sulcus. *(See Classification of SLAP tears pgs. 1382 and 1385, in Stoller's 3rd Edition.)*

Figure 8.143 ■ Coronal color illustration of a SLAP fracture with a chondral divot of the superior humeral head. This type of injury is caused by impaction, often occurring in the setting of a fall onto an outstretched arm that drives the humeral head against the superior labrum and biceps anchor. These chondral fractures are more anterior and medial than the posterolateral Hill-Sachs anterior instability lesion. The SLAP fracture is frequently associated with a type 3 or 4 SLAP lesion, especially in the presence of a meniscoid-type superior labrum, which is more susceptible to injury. *(See Classification of SLAP tears pgs. 1382 and 1404, in Stoller's 3rd Edition.)*

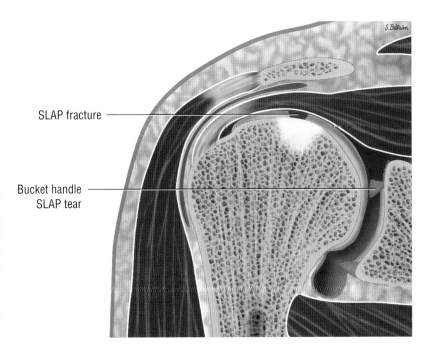

SLAP fracture

Bucket handle
SLAP tear

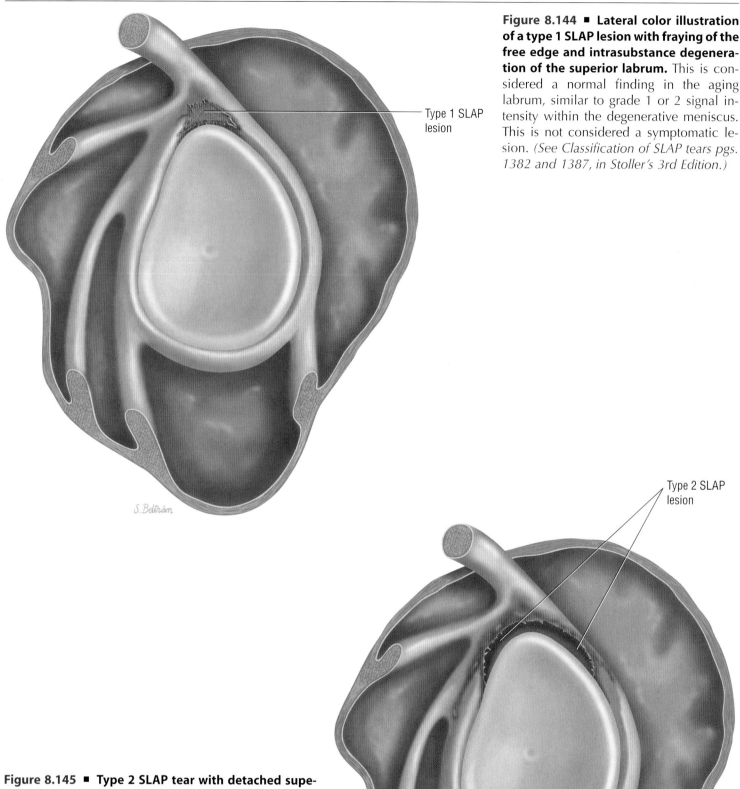

Type 1 SLAP
lesion

Figure 8.144 ■ Lateral color illustration of a type 1 SLAP lesion with fraying of the free edge and intrasubstance degeneration of the superior labrum. This is considered a normal finding in the aging labrum, similar to grade 1 or 2 signal intensity within the degenerative meniscus. This is not considered a symptomatic lesion. *(See Classification of SLAP tears pgs. 1382 and 1387, in Stoller's 3rd Edition.)*

Type 2 SLAP
lesion

Figure 8.145 ■ Type 2 SLAP tear with detached superior labrum and biceps anchor. The labral tear extends from anterior to posterior and may occur within the substance of the labrum or with complete detachment of the biceps and labrum from the superior pole of the glenoid. The term "biceps expansion" is more accurate and should be used instead of "torn biceps anchor," since the origin of the biceps tendon from the supraglenoid tubercle is not involved. The biceps tendon has a separate expansion or attachment directly to the anterior and posterior glenoid labrum. Except for the frayed appearance of the superior labrum, this SLAP lesion could be mistaken for a prominent biceps labral sulcus on coronal oblique MR images. *(See Classification of SLAP tears pgs. 1382 and 1388, in Stoller's 3rd Edition.)*

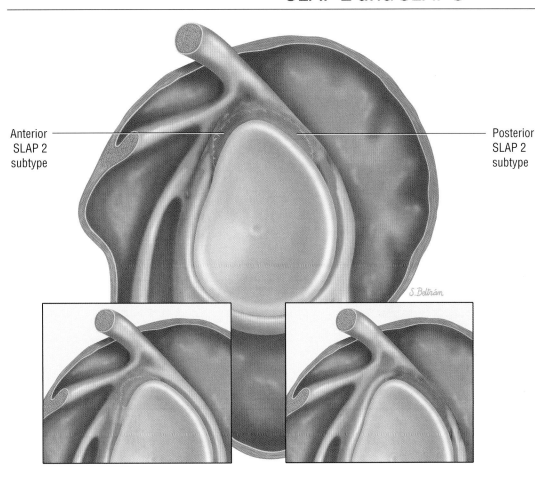

Anterior
SLAP 2
subtype

Posterior
SLAP 2
subtype

Figure 8.146 ■ **Location of anterior SLAP 2 (blue) and posterior SLAP 2 (green) subtypes.** Hemorrhage is highlighted in red. A classic type 2 SLAP lesion would involve anterior and posterior components. *(See Classification of SLAP tears pgs. 1382 and 1390, in Stoller's 3rd Edition.)*

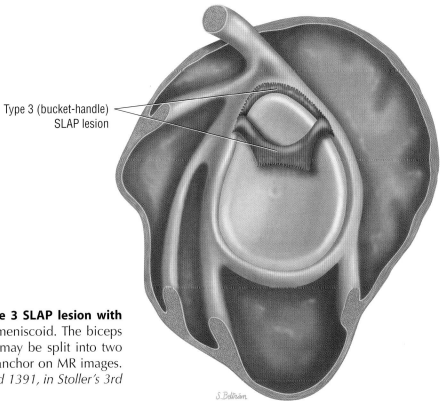

Type 3 (bucket-handle)
SLAP lesion

Figure 8.147 ■ **Lateral color illustration of a type 3 SLAP lesion with bucket-handle tear.** The superior labrum may be meniscoid. The biceps tendon attachment is intact. The bucket fragment may be split into two fragments and displaced inferiorly from the biceps anchor on MR images. *(See Classification of SLAP tears pgs. 1382, 1383 and 1391, in Stoller's 3rd Edition.)*

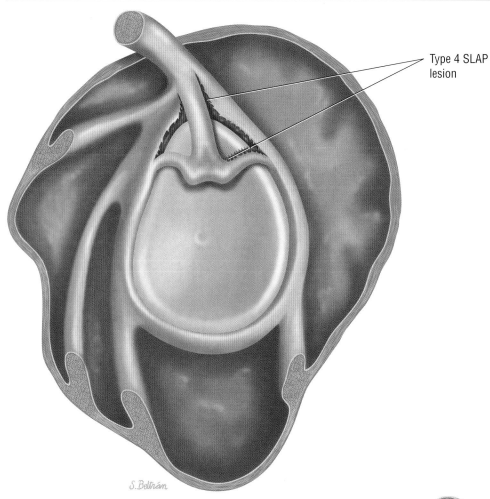

Type 4 SLAP
lesion

Figure 8.148 ■ Lateral color graphic illustrating a SLAP 4 lesion with a split or bucket-handle tear of the superior labrum that continues into the biceps tendon. *(See Classification of SLAP tears pgs. 1382, 1390 and 1394, in Stoller's 3rd Edition.)*

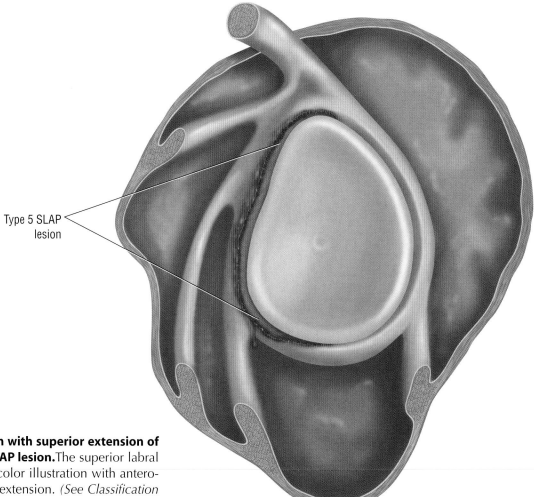

Type 5 SLAP
lesion

Figure 8.149 ■ **Type 5 SLAP lesion with superior extension of a Bankart lesion into a superior SLAP lesion.** The superior labral lesion may be type 2 or 3. Lateral color illustration with anterosuperior and anteroinferior SLAP 5 extension. *(See Classification of SLAP tears pgs. 1382, 1390 and 1396, in Stoller's 3rd Edition.)*

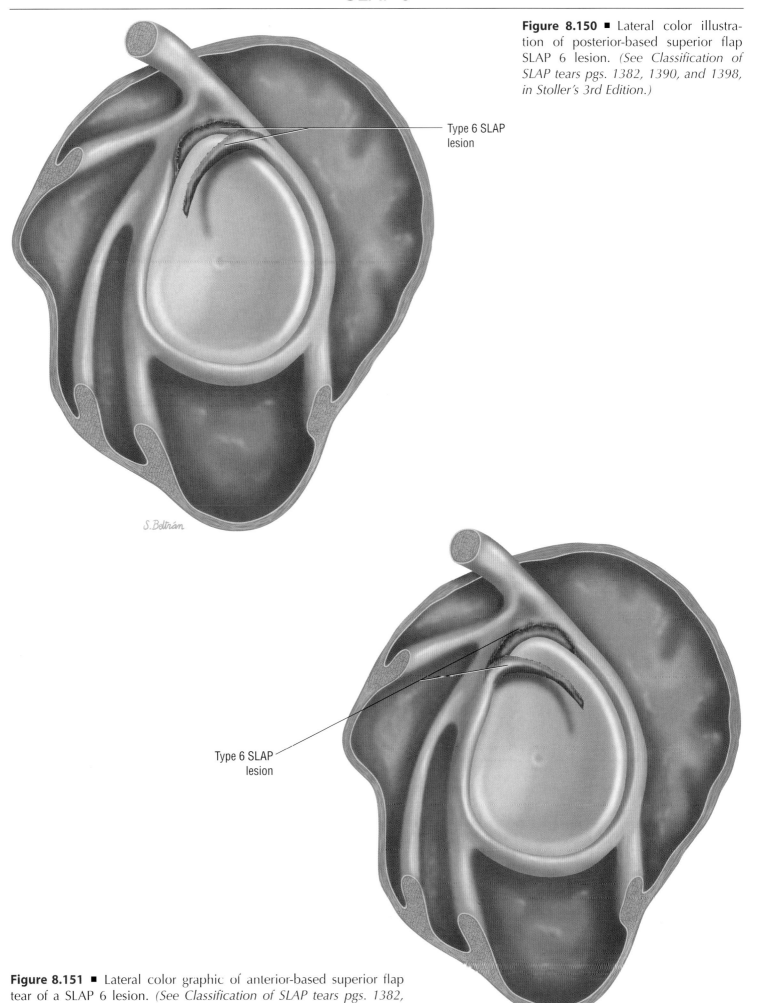

Figure 8.150 ■ Lateral color illustration of posterior-based superior flap SLAP 6 lesion. *(See Classification of SLAP tears pgs. 1382, 1390, and 1398, in Stoller's 3rd Edition.)*

Type 6 SLAP
lesion

Type 6 SLAP
lesion

S. Beltrán

S. Beltrán

Figure 8.151 ■ Lateral color graphic of anterior-based superior flap tear of a SLAP 6 lesion. *(See Classification of SLAP tears pgs. 1382, 1390, and 1399, in Stoller's 3rd Edition.)*

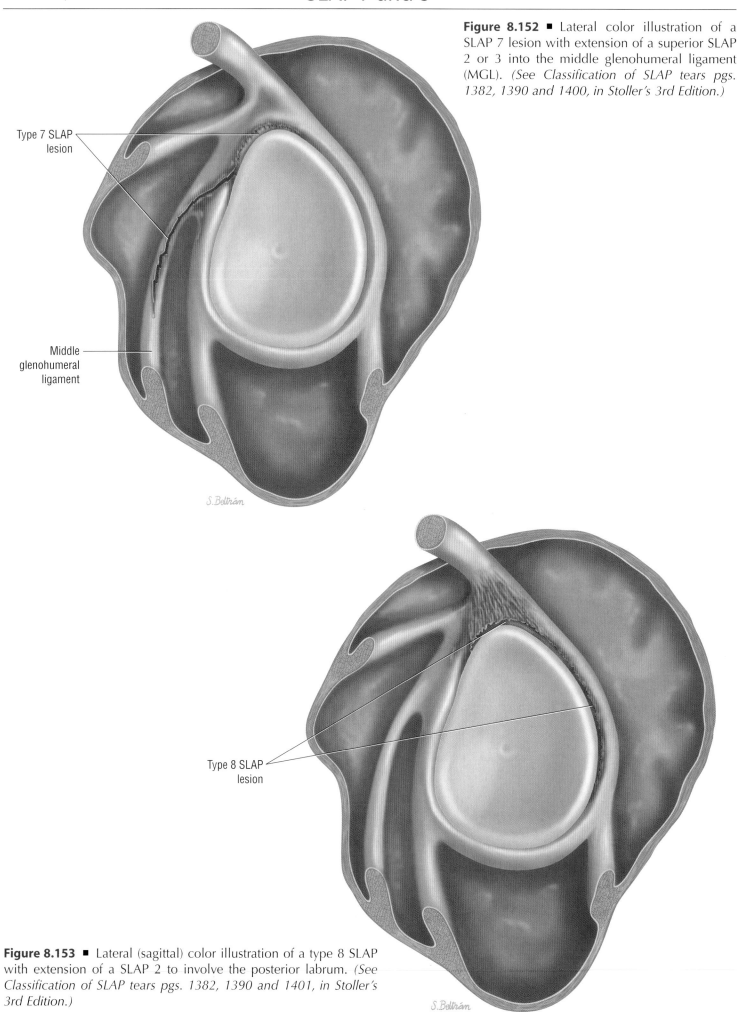

Figure 8.152 ■ Lateral color illustration of a SLAP 7 lesion with extension of a superior SLAP 2 or 3 into the middle glenohumeral ligament (MGL). *(See Classification of SLAP tears pgs. 1382, 1390 and 1400, in Stoller's 3rd Edition.)*

Type 7 SLAP lesion

Middle glenohumeral ligament

Type 8 SLAP lesion

Figure 8.153 ■ Lateral (sagittal) color illustration of a type 8 SLAP with extension of a SLAP 2 to involve the posterior labrum. *(See Classification of SLAP tears pgs. 1382, 1390 and 1401, in Stoller's 3rd Edition.)*

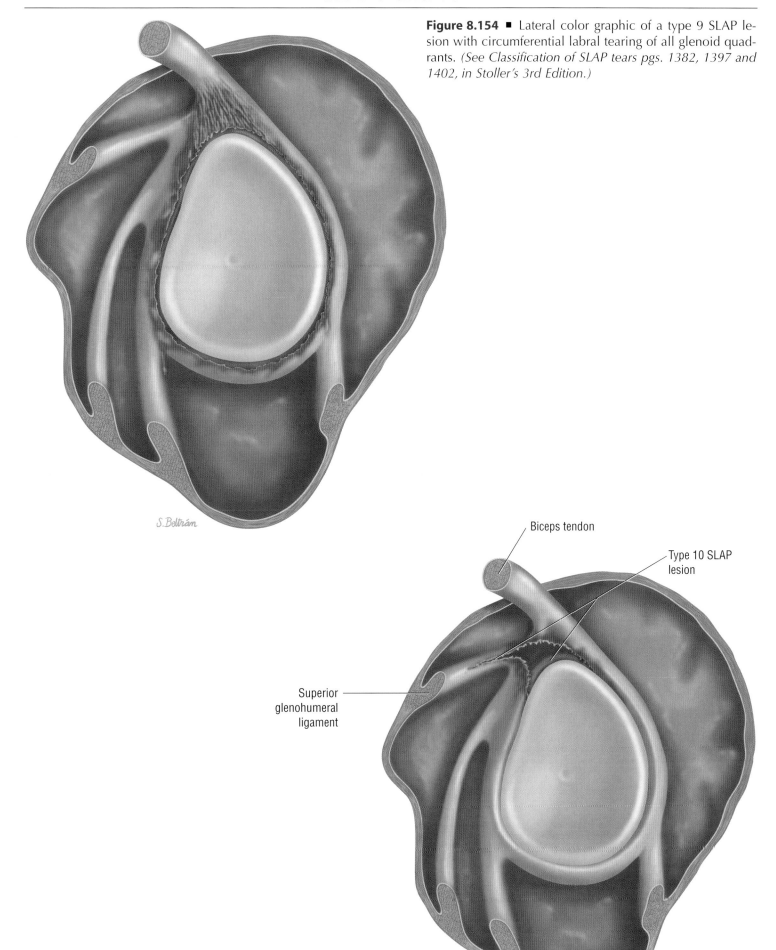

Figure 8.154 ■ Lateral color graphic of a type 9 SLAP lesion with circumferential labral tearing of all glenoid quadrants. *(See Classification of SLAP tears pgs. 1382, 1397 and 1402, in Stoller's 3rd Edition.)*

Biceps tendon

Type 10 SLAP lesion

Superior glenohumeral ligament

Figure 8.155 ■ A SLAP 10 lesion with associated rotator cuff interval involvement shown with extension in the superior glenohumeral ligament on a lateral glenoid color illustration. *(See Classification of SLAP tears pgs. 1382, 1397 and 1403, in Stoller's 3rd Edition.)*

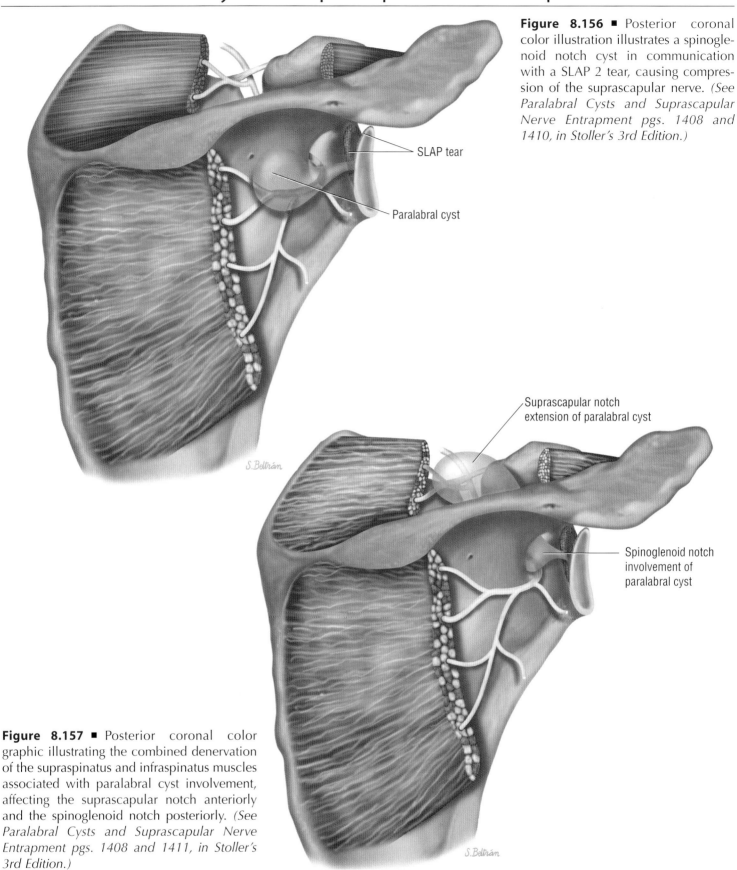

Figure 8.156 ▪ Posterior coronal color illustration illustrates a spinoglenoid notch cyst in communication with a SLAP 2 tear, causing compression of the suprascapular nerve. *(See Paralabral Cysts and Suprascapular Nerve Entrapment pgs. 1408 and 1410, in Stoller's 3rd Edition.)*

SLAP tear

Paralabral cyst

Suprascapular notch extension of paralabral cyst

Spinoglenoid notch involvement of paralabral cyst

Figure 8.157 ▪ Posterior coronal color graphic illustrating the combined denervation of the supraspinatus and infraspinatus muscles associated with paralabral cyst involvement, affecting the suprascapular notch anteriorly and the spinoglenoid notch posteriorly. *(See Paralabral Cysts and Suprascapular Nerve Entrapment pgs. 1408 and 1411, in Stoller's 3rd Edition.)*

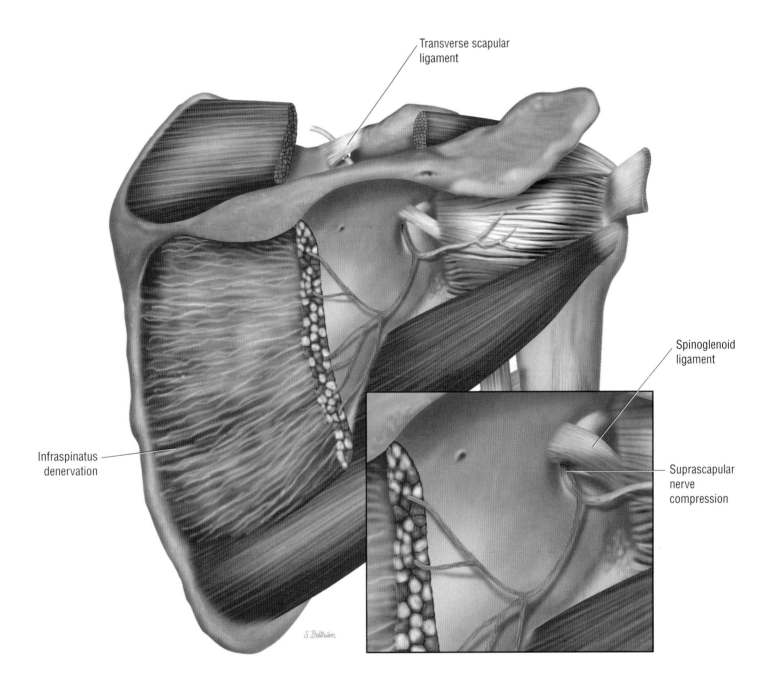

Figure 8.158 ■ **Selective or isolated infraspinatus denervation secondary to compression by a thickened spinoglenoid ligament.** The suprascapular nerve and artery enter the supraspinatus fossa through the scapular notch by passing deep to the transverse scapular ligament. The suprascapular nerve enters the infraspinatus fossa by coursing lateral to the spinoglenoid notch. The lateral margin of the spinoglenoid notch is created by the fibrous band called the spinoglenoid ligament. The suprascapular nerve is relatively immobile in this area and thus susceptible to injury or compression by paralabral cysts. In extreme abduction and external rotation (in the throwing athlete, for example), the medial tendinous margin of the supraspinatus and infraspinatus can impinge against the lateral edge of the scapula spine. This results in compression of the infraspinatus branch of the suprascapular nerve. Painless atrophy of the infraspinatus muscle in volleyball players (attributed to contraction of the infraspinatus muscle during the volleyball serving action) involves neuropathy of the inferior branch of the suprascapular nerve. *(See Paralabral Cysts and Suprascapular Nerve Entrapment pgs. 1408 and 1412, in Stoller's 3rd Edition.)*

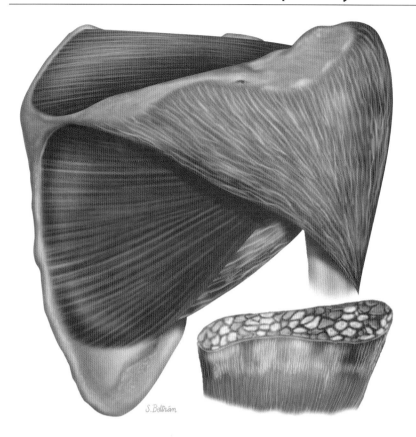

Figure 8.159 ■ **Quadrilateral space syndrome with denervation and fatty atrophy of the teres minor and deltoid.** Coronal illustration of teres minor and deltoid fatty atrophy. The axillary nerve is susceptible to entrapment by fibrous bands in the quadrilateral space when the arm is abducted and externally rotated. Selective involvement of the teres minor with posterior pain and tenderness may be present. *(See Quadrilateral Space Syndrome pgs. 1413 and 1414, in Stoller's 3rd Edition.)*

Figure 8.160 ■ The normal course of the posterior branch of the axillary nerve, which divides into the nerve to the teres minor and a superolateral brachial cutaneous nerve branch. *(See Quadrilateral Space Syndrome pgs. 1413 and 1415, in Stoller's 3rd Edition.)*

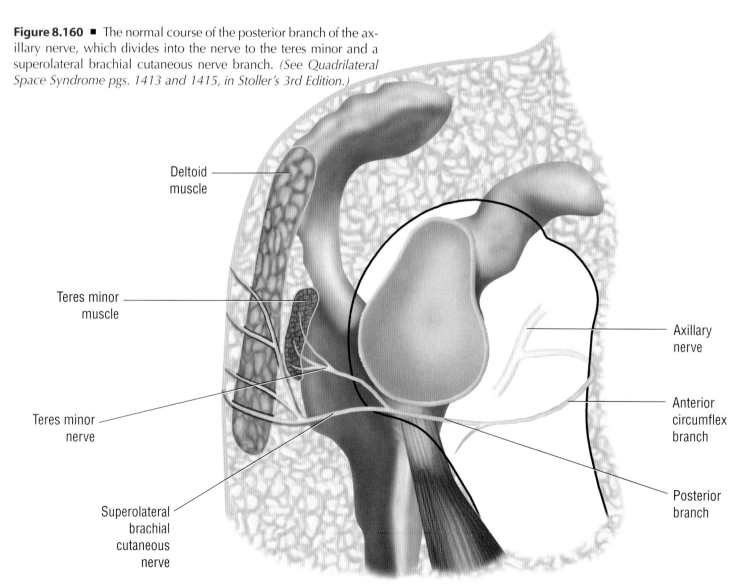

Deltoid muscle

Teres minor muscle

Teres minor nerve

Superolateral brachial cutaneous nerve

Axillary nerve

Anterior circumflex branch

Posterior branch

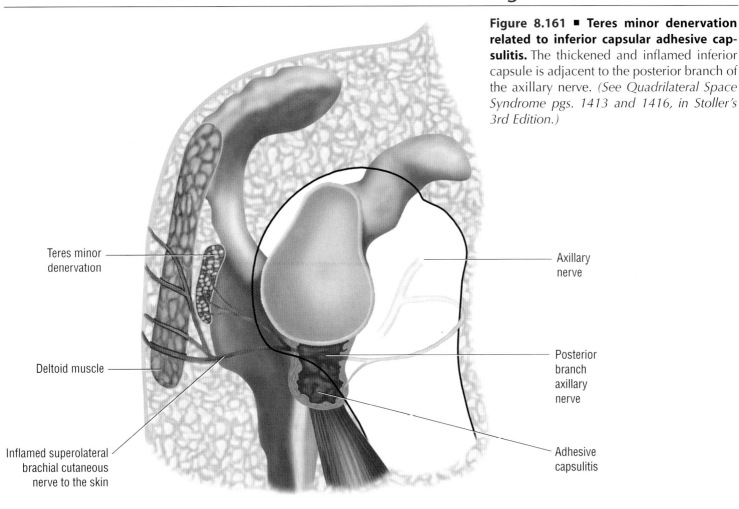

Figure 8.161 ▪ Teres minor denervation related to inferior capsular adhesive capsulitis. The thickened and inflamed inferior capsule is adjacent to the posterior branch of the axillary nerve. *(See Quadrilateral Space Syndrome pgs. 1413 and 1416, in Stoller's 3rd Edition.)*

Teres minor denervation

Deltoid muscle

Inflamed superolateral brachial cutaneous nerve to the skin

Axillary nerve

Posterior branch axillary nerve

Adhesive capsulitis

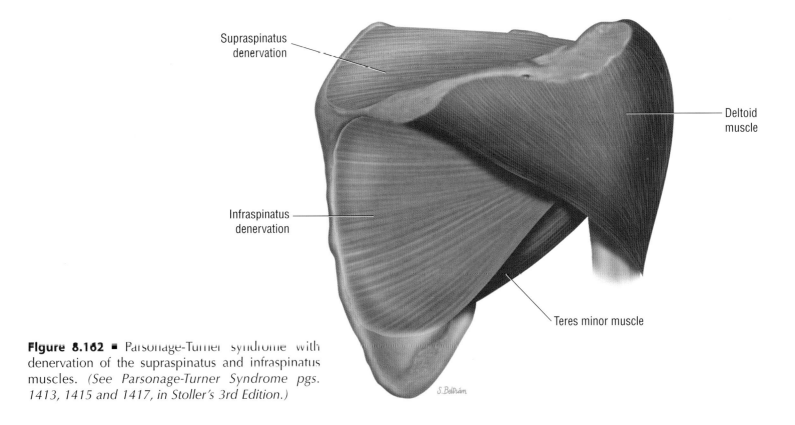

Supraspinatus denervation

Infraspinatus denervation

Deltoid muscle

Teres minor muscle

S. Beltrán

Figure 8.162 ▪ Parsonage-Turner syndrome with denervation of the supraspinatus and infraspinatus muscles. *(See Parsonage-Turner Syndrome pgs. 1413, 1415 and 1417, in Stoller's 3rd Edition.)*

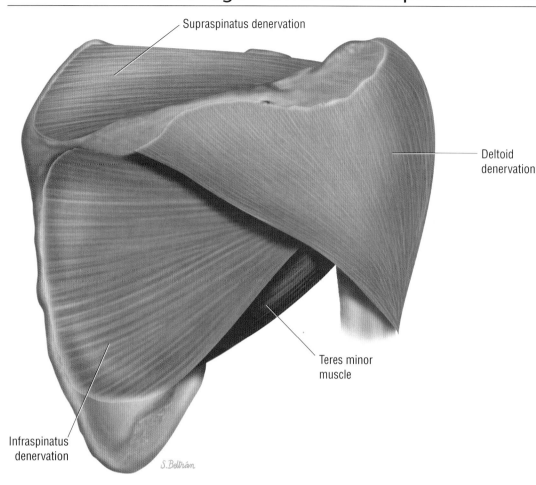

Supraspinatus denervation

Deltoid
denervation

Teres minor
muscle

Infraspinatus
denervation

S.Beltrán

Figure 8.163 ■ Color posterior coronal illustration of Parsonage-Turner variation with denervation of the supraspinatus, infraspinatus, and deltoid (suprascapular and axillary nerve innervation). *(See Parsonage-Turner Syndrome pgs. 1413, 1415 and 1418, in Stoller's 3rd Edition.)*

Figure 8.164 ■ **Variation in the biceps tendon contribution to the BLC.** These variations include: **(A)** an exclusive contribution to the posterosuperior labrum; **(B)** a primary contribution to the posterosuperior labrum and secondary involvement of the anterosuperior labrum; **(C)** equal contribution to the anterosuperior and posterosuperior labrum; and **(D)** a primary contribution to the anterosuperior labrum and secondary contribution to the posterosuperior labrum. *(See Biceps Tendon pg. 1419, in Stoller's 3rd Edition.)*

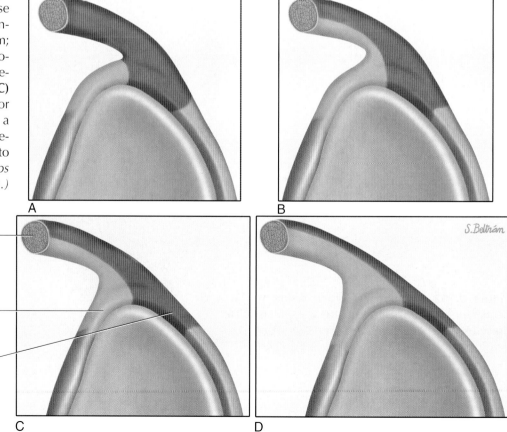

Biceps tendon

Anterosuperior
labral contribution

Posterosuperior
labral contribution

S.Beltrán

A

B

C

D

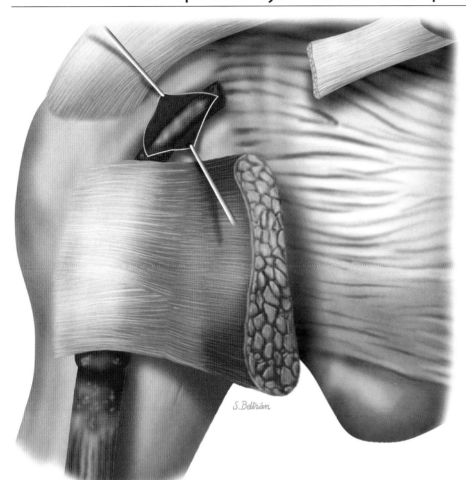

Figure 8.165 ■ **Biceps tenosynovitis with inflammation of the proximal biceps tendon sheath.** A positive Speed's test (downward force applied to the arm with the elbow extended and forearm supinated) with upper anterior arm and shoulder pain is associated with biceps tendon inflammation. *(See Biceps Tendinosis and Tenosynovitis pgs. 1421 and 1422, in Stoller's 3rd Edition.)*

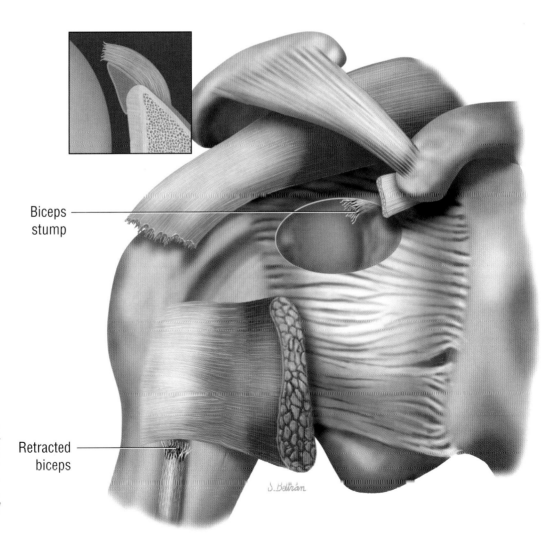

Biceps stump

Retracted biceps

Figure 8.166 ■ Coronal anterior view color illustration of rupture of the intraarticular biceps at the BLC adjacent to the biceps anchor. *(See Biceps Tendon Rupture pgs. 1423 and 1424, in Stoller's 3rd Edition.)*

Adhesive Capsulitis and Calcific Tendinitis

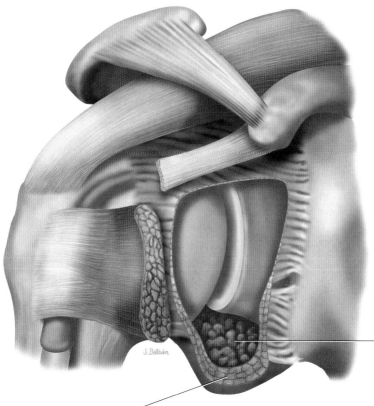

Figure 8.167 ▪ Adhesive capsulitis or frozen shoulder with thickened inflamed IGHL and synovial thickening within the axillary pouch. Idiopathic adhesive capsulitis is more common than posttraumatic or secondary adhesive capsulitis, which occurs in only 10% of cases. *(See Adhesive Capsulitis pgs. 1425 and 1426, in Stoller's 3rd Edition.)*

Synovitis

Thickened and edematous axillary pouch of inferior glenohumeral ligament

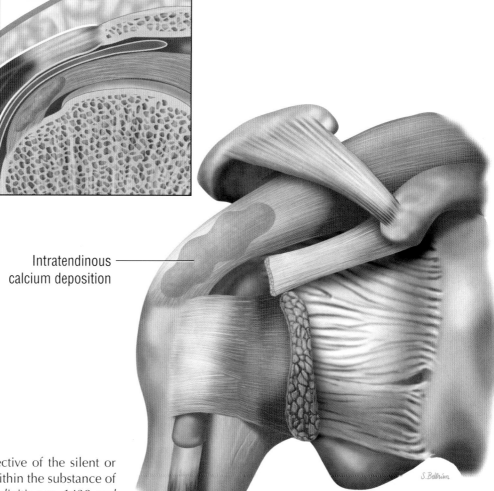

Intratendinous calcium deposition

Figure 8.168 ▪ Coronal 3D color perspective of the silent or subclinical phase of calcium deposition within the substance of the rotator cuff tendons. *(See Calcific Tendinitis pgs. 1428 and 1430, in Stoller's 3rd Edition.)*

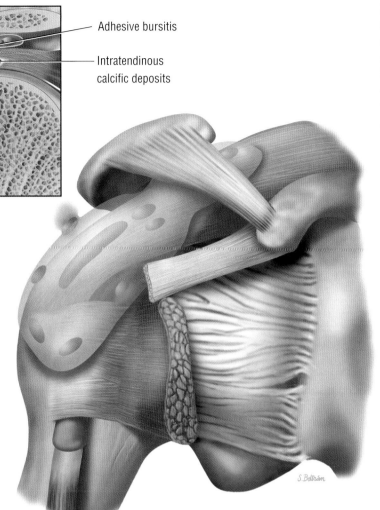

Adhesive bursitis

Intratendinous
calcific deposits

Figure 8.169 ■ **Adhesive periarthritis demonstrates intratendinous calcific deposits associated with adhesive bursitis and distension of the subacromial bursa.** Coronal 3D perspective with 2D coronal section inset in color. *(See Calcific Tendinitis pgs. 1428 and 1431, in Stoller's 3rd Edition.)*

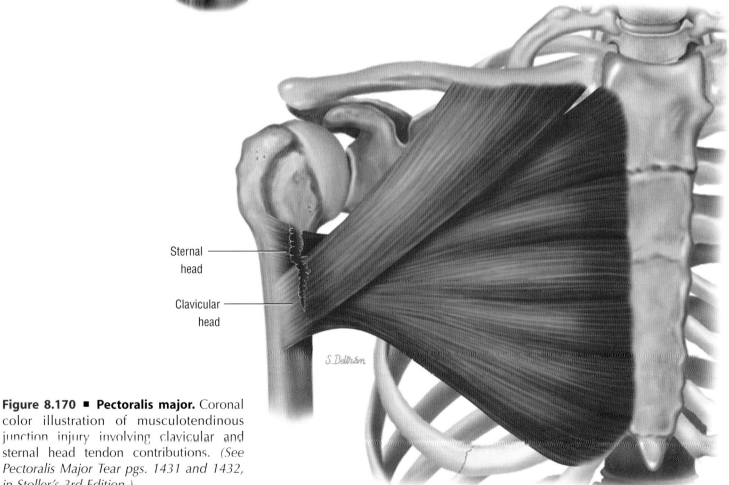

Sternal
head

Clavicular
head

Figure 8.170 ■ **Pectoralis major.** Coronal color illustration of musculotendinous junction injury involving clavicular and sternal head tendon contributions. *(See Pectoralis Major Tear pgs. 1431 and 1432, in Stoller's 3rd Edition.)*

Acromioclavicular Dislocation

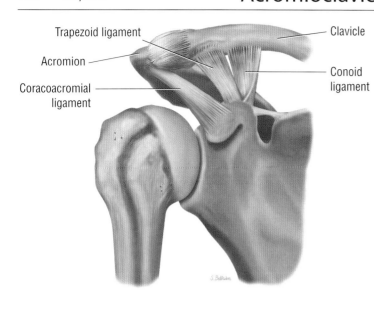

Trapezoid ligament

Acromion

Coracoacromial ligament

Clavicle

Conoid ligament

Figure 8.171 ▪ Anterior view coronal color perspective of the normal trapezoid and conoid ligaments, which function as single coracoclavicular ligament. The conoid is posterior and medial, whereas the trapezoid is anterior and lateral. *(See Acromioclavicular Separations pg. 1434, in Stoller's 3rd Edition.)*

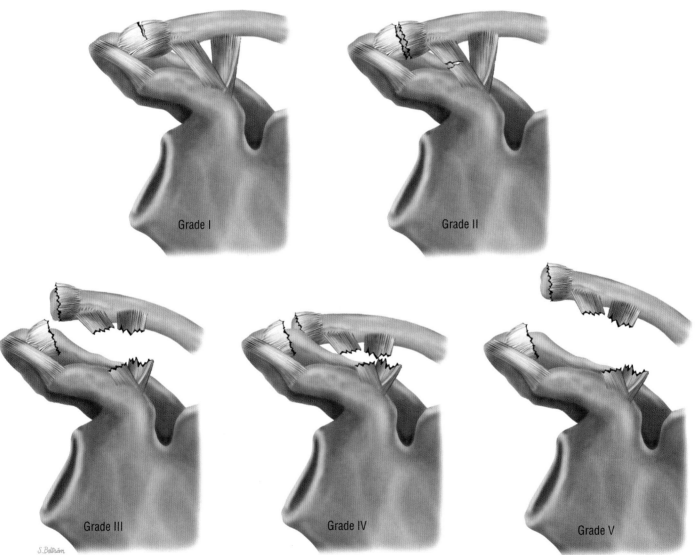

Grade I

Grade II

Grade III

Grade IV

Grade V

Figure 8.172 ▪ Grades of acromioclavicular ligamentous injuries. Type I: Intact acromioclavicular and coracoclavicular ligaments. Type II: Disruption of acromioclavicular ligaments. Type III: Disruption of acromioclavicular and coracoclavicular ligaments. Type IV: Acromioclavicular and coracoclavicular ligament disruption and posterior displacement of the clavicle into or through the trapezius muscle. Type V: Acromioclavicular and coracoclavicular ligament disruption plus injury to the deltoid and trapezius muscle attachments. There is a significant separation between the clavicle and the acromion. *(See Acromioclavicular Separations pgs. 1434 and 1435, in Stoller's 3rd Edition.)*

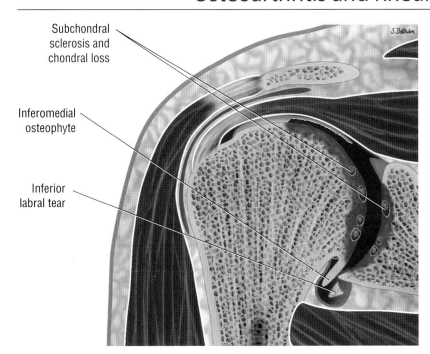

Subchondral sclerosis and chondral loss

Inferomedial osteophyte

Inferior labral tear

Figure 8.173 ▪ Advanced changes or osteoarthritis of the glenohumeral joint. Articular cartilage loss with sclerosis and subchondral cystic change is greatest in the area of the humeral head in contact with the glenoid between 60° and 100° of abduction. Characteristic large peripheral osteophytes develop inferiorly and limit rotation by effectively enlarging the diameter of the humeral head. *(See Osteoarthritis pgs. 1437 and 1439, in Stoller's 3rd Edition.)*

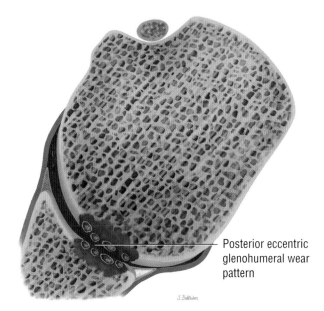

Posterior eccentric glenohumeral wear pattern

Figure 8.174 ▪ Axial color section illustrating posterior eccentric wear pattern of osteoarthritis with loss of posterior glenohumeral joint articular cartilage. *(See Osteoarthritis pgs. 1437 and 1438, in Stoller's 3rd Edition.)*

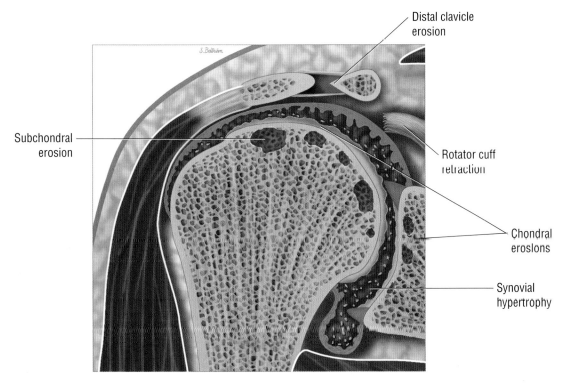

Distal clavicle erosion

Subchondral erosion

Rotator cuff retraction

Chondral erosions

Synovial hypertrophy

Figure 8.175 ▪ Rheumatoid arthritis targets the glenohumeral joint but may involve all synovial-lined joints, including the acromioclavicular and sternoclavicular joints. Marginal erosions and subchondral cysts may involve large areas of the humeral head. Glenoid destruction is associated with central or peripheral erosions. Sclerosis and osteophytosis are not common and represent the development of secondary osteoarthritis. Chondral loss, subchondral erosions, and synovial pannus are shown on this color coronal illustration. Erosion with tapering of the distal clavicle is also indicated. *(See Rheumatoid Arthritis pgs. 1437 and 1442, in Stoller's 3rd Edition.)*

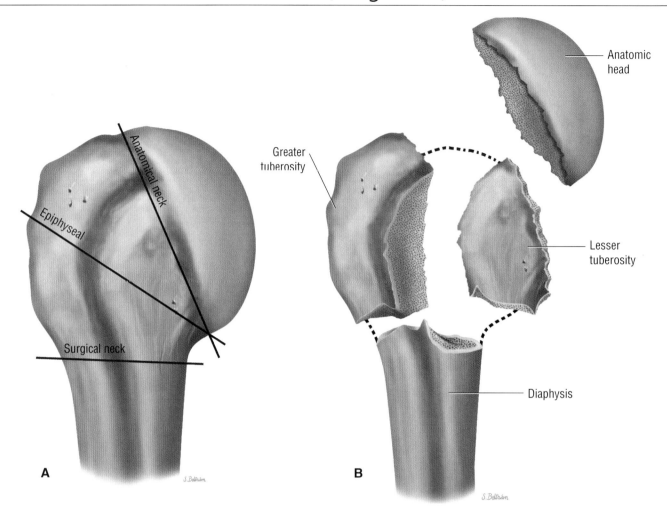

Figure 8.176 ▪ Fractures of the humeral head. (A) Original Kocher classification based on three different anatomic levels. This classification has been replaced by a description that included multiple fracture sites and differentiates between displaced and undisplaced fractures. **(B)** Division of the proximal humerus into four separate fragments based on anatomic lines of epiphyseal union. These distinct fragments are the greater tuberosity, the lesser tuberosity, the anatomic head, and the diaphysis. *(See Fractures of the Proximal Humerus and Osteochondral Lesions pgs. 1437 and 1444, in Stoller's 3rd Edition.)*

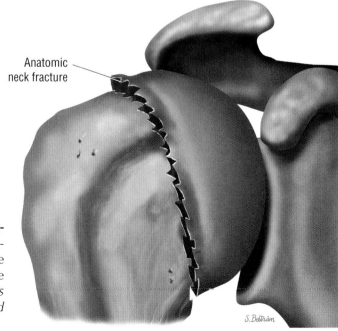

Figure 8.177 ▪ Fracture of the anatomic neck as the articular segment. A one-part fracture has no or minimal displacement or angulation. A two-part fracture has one segment displaced. A three-part fracture has two segments displaced with one tuberosity in continuity with the head. A four-part fracture has three segments displaced. *(See Fractures of the Proximal Humerus and Osteochondral Lesions pgs. 1445 and 1446, in Stoller's 3rd Edition.)*

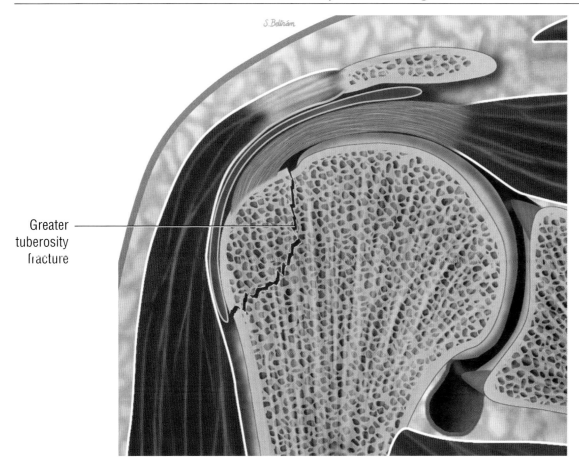

Greater
tuberosity
fracture

Figure 8.178 ▪ Nondisplaced greater tuberosity fracture. Fractures of the greater tuberosity are associated with anterior dislocations. A greater tuberosity fracture usually reduces into an acceptable anatomic position but may displace underneath the acromial process or be directed posteriorly by the pull of the rotator cuff muscles. *(See Fractures of the Proximal Humerus and Osteochondral Lesions pgs. 1437, 1445 and 1447, in Stoller's 3rd Edition.)*

Figure 8.179 ▪ Surgical neck fracture with no displacement. A fall onto the outstretched hand is the most common mechanism for a proximal humerus fracture. *(See Fractures of the Proximal Humerus and Osteochondral Lesions pgs. 1437, 1445 and 1448, in Stoller's 3rd Edition.)*

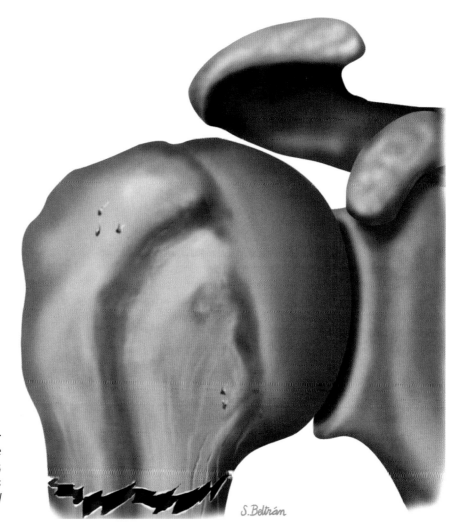

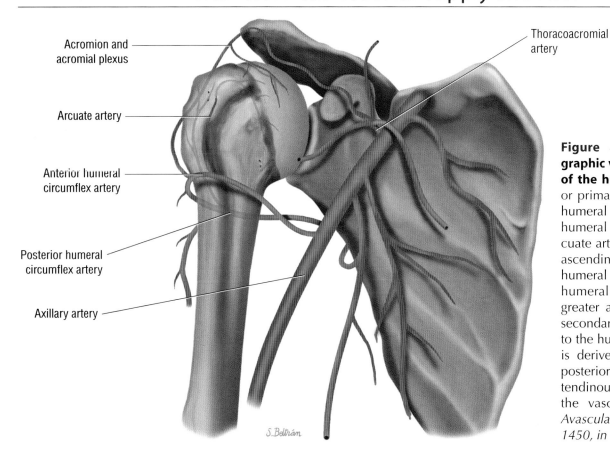

Acromion and acromial plexus

Arcuate artery

Anterior humeral circumflex artery

Posterior humeral circumflex artery

Axillary artery

Thoracoacromial artery

S.Beltrán

Figure 8.180 ▪ **Coronal color graphic view of the blood supply of the humeral head.** The major or primary vascular supply to the humeral head is from the anterior humeral circumflex artery. The arcuate artery, a continuation of the ascending branch of the anterior humeral circumflex, supplies the humeral head, including the greater and lesser tuberosities. A secondary or smaller contribution to the humeral head blood supply is derived from branches of the posterior circumflex artery and the tendinous-osseous anastomoses of the vascular rotator cuff. *(See Avascular Necrosis pgs. 1445 and 1450, in Stoller's 3rd Edition.)*

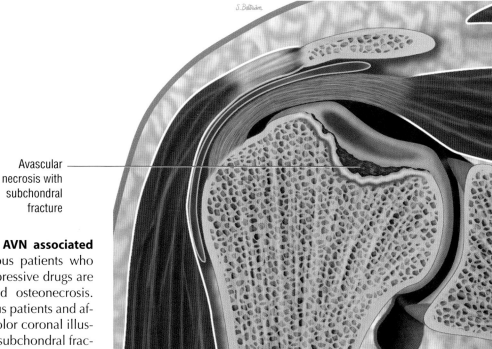

S.Beltrán

Avascular necrosis with subchondral fracture

Figure 8.181 ▪ **Localized nontraumatic AVN associated with systemic lupus erythematosus.** Lupus patients who are not on glucocorticoids or immunosuppressive drugs are at increased risk for septic arthritis and osteonecrosis. Osteonecrosis occurs in 4% to 15% of lupus patients and affects the humeral head in 80% of cases. Color coronal illustration anterior view of osteonecrosis with subchondral fractures. *(See Avascular Necrosis pgs. 1445 and 1451, in Stoller's 3rd Edition.)*

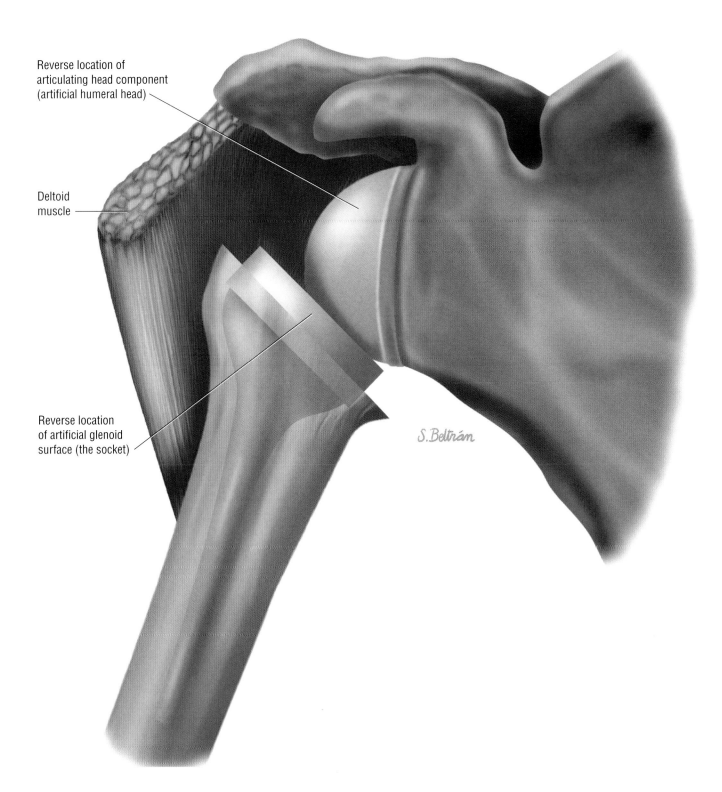

Reverse location of
articulating head component
(artificial humeral head)

Deltoid
muscle

Reverse location
of artificial glenoid
surface (the socket)

S. Beltrán

Figure 8.182 ▪ **Reverse shoulder replacement optimizes the force of the deltoid (by increasing the lever arm) and stabilizes the glenohumeral articulation by moving the center of rotation of the glenohumeral joint medially and inferiorly. This provides an increased mechanical advantage for raising the arm overhead.** Reverse prosthesis may be used to direct forces through the glenosphere, converting centrifugal or outward forces into centripetal or inward forces. *(See Shoulder Replacement pgs. 1452 and 1457, in Stoller's 3rd Edition.)*

9

The Elbow

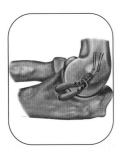

Pearls and Pitfalls & Color Illustrations

Pearls and Pitfalls

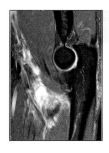

TECHNIQUES AND PROTOCOLS

- It is important to locate the joint as close to isocenter as possible, using either a prone position or an open magnet.
- Axial images must include the radial tuberosity.
- Sagittal images should have a larger field of view to evaluate a possibly retracted biceps tendon.

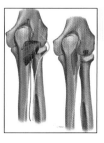

MR ANATOMY

- Axial scans are best for evaluating the neurovascular structures.
- Sagittal scans show the bony articular relationship to best advantage.
- There are normal "bare areas" at the ulnar trochlear notch and the capitellum; these should not be mistaken for pathology.
- Coronal scans are best for evaluating common tendon origins and collateral ligaments.

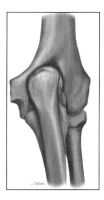

NORMAL ANATOMY OF THE ELBOW
(See Figs. 9.21–9.39)

- The elbow is a tri-arthrodial ginglymus joint.
- The medial and lateral humeral condyles are the origin of the common flexor and extensor groups of the forearm.
- The coronoid process is the key to the bony stability of the joint.
- Posterolateral stability depends on the LUCL.
- The normal but complex maturation of the elbow ossification centers can be mistaken for pathology.

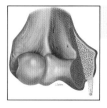

MEDIAL COLLATERAL LIGAMENT INJURY
(See Figs. 9.40–9.47)

- The anterior band of the MCL is the primary restraint to valgus stress.
- MCL rupture frequently occurs with posterior dislocation.
- The MR "T sign" is indicative of a partial tear at the sublime tubercle, which may be occult to surgical inspection.
- Strain of the flexor digitorum superficialis frequently accompanies an MCL injury.
- Lateral compartment bone bruises strongly suggest MCL disruption.

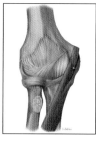

MEDIAL EPICONDYLITIS
(See Figs. 9.48–9.53)

- This is a midlife overuse injury.
- There is a frequent association with ulnar neuritis.
- Medial epicondylitis is a degenerative disorder, similar to supraspinatus and patellar tendinosis, and there is no inflammatory response.

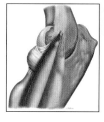

LATERAL EPICONDYLITIS
(See Figs. 9.54–9.60)

- Although common in athletes, lateral epicondylitis more frequently occurs in the general population.
- The extensor carpi radialis brevis is the tendon most often affected.
- Signal changes caused by steroid injection should not be confused with edema.
- MR is the best imaging modality for identifying high-grade lesions that are unlikely to respond to conservative therapy.

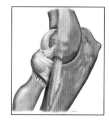

LATERAL COLLATERAL LIGAMENT INJURY
(See Fig. 9.61)

- LUCL disruption is not the only essential lesion in posterolateral rotatory instability (PLRI).
- The RCL and the LUCL play a significant role in preventing PLRI of the elbow.
- Proximal tears of the RCL and LUCL result in symptomatic PLRI.

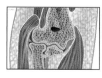

MISCELLANEOUS LATERAL ELBOW PAIN
(See Fig. 9.62)

- Consider posterior interosseous nerve impingement.
- Lateral synovial plicae may be symptomatic.

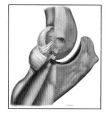

POSTERIOR DISLOCATION INJURY AND INSTABILITY
(See Figs. 9.63–9.67)

- This injury can be missed in children because of spontaneous reduction.
- Associated fractures of the coronoid, radial head, and humeral condyles may occur.
- Instability starts posterolaterally but may progress medially to involve the entire joint.
- The primary lesion of instability is no longer considered isolated insufficiency of the LUCL. The RCL and LUCL together represent the main restraint to PLRI.
- MCL tearing occurs late.
- Clinical evaluation is difficult.

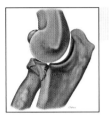

CORONOID FRACTURES
(See Figs. 9.68–9.69)

- The coronoid is the keystone of bony stability of the elbow.
- Coronoid fractures are commonly associated with elbow dislocation.

■ Fractures are graded I to III. Grade III has a poor prognosis.

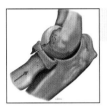

RADIAL HEAD FRACTURES
(See Figs. 9.70–9.71)

- Fractures of the radial head are the most common elbow fracture in adults.
- The typical location is the anterolateral margin of the head.

■ In association with distal radioulnar joint dislocation, the injury is called the Essex-Lopresti fracture.

■ If radial head excision is planned, it is essential to check MCL integrity.

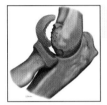

CAPITELLAR FRACTURES
(See Fig. 9.72)

- Fracture of the capitellum is rare.
- It is important to differentiate a subtle fracture from a capitellar pseudodefect.

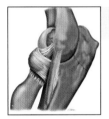

OLECRANON FRACTURES
(See Fig. 9.73)

- Olecranon fractures are frequently high-energy injuries, so a diligent check for collateral damage should be made.
- Injuries in adolescence may result in an os supratrochleare dorsale.

■ The relationship to the ulnar trochlear notch determines fracture stability.

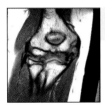

MEDIAL CONDYLAR FRACTURES

- In children the medial epicondyle may be displaced into the joint.
- The trochlear ossification center should not be mistaken for a displaced medial epicondyle.

■ If the medial epicondyle is displaced, the status and position of the ulnar nerve should be assessed carefully.

■ Involvement of the trochlear ridge determines the stability of the fracture.

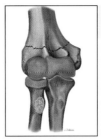

SUPRACONDYLAR FRACTURES
(See Fig. 9.74)

- This is the most common pediatric elbow injury.
- The median nerve and brachial artery are at risk.

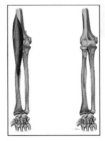

LATERAL CONDYLAR FRACTURES

- This is the most common physeal injury and is usually a Salter-Harris type IV.
- May be invisible on radiographs or CT.
- A missed fracture may result in significant loss of function or deformity.

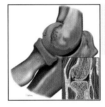

CAPITELLAR OSTEOCHONDRITIS DISSECANS
(See Fig. 9.75)

- Osteochondritis dissecans frequently leads to arthrosis.
- The lesion typically occurs anteriorly and should not be confused with capitellar pseudodefect, which occurs posteriorly.

■ Contrast-enhanced sagittal images are used to characterize and stage the lesion.

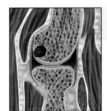

PANNER'S DISEASE
(See Figs. 9.76–9.77)

- Panner's disease occurs in childhood as opposed to osteochondritis dissecans, which typically occurs in adolescence.
- The condition is similar to Legg-Calvé-Perthes disease of the hip in that patients may recover with little or no deformity.

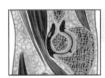

LOOSE BODIES
(See Fig. 9.80)

- The elbow is a common site for loose bodies.

■ Air bubbles may simulate loose bodies but are identified by susceptibility artifact on GRE sequences.

■ Loose bodies most commonly are found anteriorly or lodged in the trochlear notch.

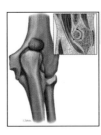

OS SUPRATROCHLEARE DORSALE
(See Fig. 9.82)

- Thought to be an accessory bone.
- May enlarge and cause symptoms.
- MR shows a deep olecranon fossa, which can help differentiate it from loose bodies.

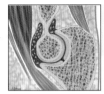

IDIOPATHIC SYNOVIAL OSTEOCHONDROMATOSIS
(See Fig. 9.81)

- The elbow is a common location of idiopathic synovial osteochondromatosis.

- It is typically a condition of middle-aged men.

- Nerve entrapment may be associated with this lesion.

- Early-stage disease may demonstrate normal articular cartilage.

- Nonossified nodules may mimic fluid on MR. A careful inspection for "septations" must be made.

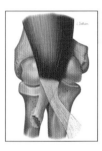

BICEPS TENDON INJURY
(See Figs. 9.83–9.88)

- This disorder is becoming increasingly common, especially in middle-aged men.

- Retraction occurs only if the lacertus fibrosus is torn.

- Pre-tear tendinosis may be accompanied by significant biceps bursal effusion.

- FS PD FSE axial and sagittal scans are the most useful sequences.

- There should be sagittal coverage to 10 cm proximal to the joint line to look for a retracted tendon.

- Consider use of the FABS position.

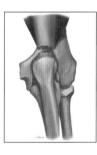

TRICEPS TENDON INJURY
(See Figs. 9.89–9.90)

- A very rare injury.

- Partial tears involve the central third of the tendon.

- Injury is frequently associated with olecranon bursitis.

- A missed triceps tear may result in severe functional disability.

- Associated Salter-Harris type II fracture of olecranon should be sought in adolescents.

- With MR it is possible to differentiate partial- from full-thickness tears.

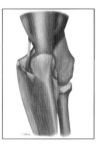

ULNAR NEUROPATHY (CUBITAL TUNNEL SYNDROME)
(See Figs. 9.91–9.99)

- The flexor carpi ulnaris aponeurosis tenses during flexion and reduces the volume of the cubital tunnel.

- The cubital tunnel retinaculum (Osborne ligament) may be anomalous or thickened and compress the nerve.

- An anomalous muscle, the anconeus epitrochlearis, may cause a mass effect.

- MCL and medial epicondylar pathology are frequent causes of cubital tunnel syndrome.

- Pre-joint compression may occur at the arcade of Struthers.

- Increased size and signal of the nerve on axial FS PD FSE scans indicate ulnar neuropathy, but engorged veins must be ruled out.

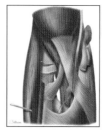

MEDIAN NERVE ENTRAPMENT
(See Figs. 9.100–9.101)

- May result from anatomic variations or enlargement of the bicipital bursa.

- Anterior interosseous nerve involvement results in weakness of the thumb and index finger.

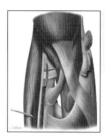

RADIAL NERVE ENTRAPMENT (POSTERIOR INTEROSSEOUS NERVE SYNDROME)
(See Figs. 9.102–9.103)

- Precubital compression produces combined wrist weakness and sensory loss.

- Cubital compression produces pain only.

- Postcubital compression results in digital weakness.

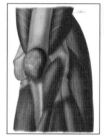

OLECRANON BURSITIS
(See Figs. 9.104–9.105)

- Most common site of bursitis in the body.

- Associated triceps tendinopathy is common.

- Systemic causes are important in older patients.

- There is associated infection in 20% of cases. Infection is best detected with contrast-enhanced imaging.

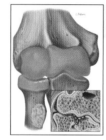

OSTEOARTHRITIS
(See Figs. 9.78–9.79, 9.106–9.107)

- Typically seen in male manual laborers.

- The coronoid and olecranon processes are usually involved.

- Overuse associated with athletics affects the ulnohumeral joint.

- Age-related changes affect the radiohumeral joint.

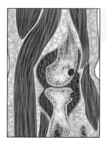

RHEUMATOID ARTHRITIS
(See Fig. 9.108)

- The elbow is affected in 20% to 50% of patients.

- Synovial hypertrophy may cause neural entrapment.

- Bone cysts occur away from load-bearing areas.

- Gadolinium enhancement shows the extent of synovial hypertrophy and can be used to monitor treatment.

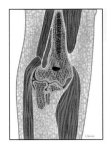

PIGMENTED VILLONODULAR SYNOVITIS

- Characterized by low-signal synovial hypertrophy.
- Usually monarticular and erodes the joint surface.
- Conditions mimicking pigmented villonodular synovitis include rheumatoid, hemophiliac, and amyloid arthropathies.

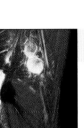

CAT SCRATCH DISEASE

- May cause epitrochlear adenopathy, which needs to be differentiated from hematoma or sarcoma.
- MR characteristics include identification of the fatty hilum of an enlarged node or visualization of a chain of nodes.

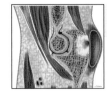

OSTEOMYELITIS
(see Figs. 9.109–9.110)

- The olecranon is the most common site of bone infection in the elbow.
- MR may provide an early diagnosis in children.

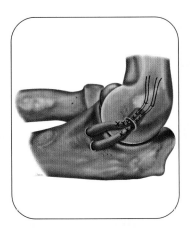

The Elbow
Muscle

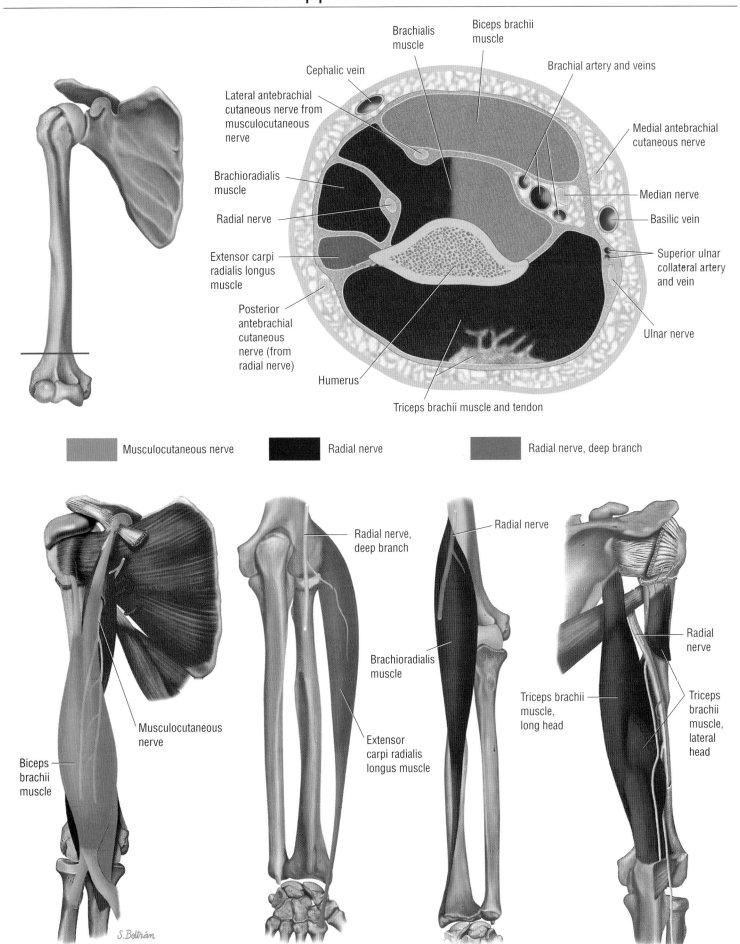

Figure 9.1 ■ Distal upper arm innervation with cross section and 3-D renderings. *Cross section based on Vahlensiech M, Genant HK, Reiter M. MRI of the musculoskeletal system. New York/Stuttgart: Thieme, 2000. (See Related Muscles pgs. 1466–1475, in Stoller's 3rd Edition.)*

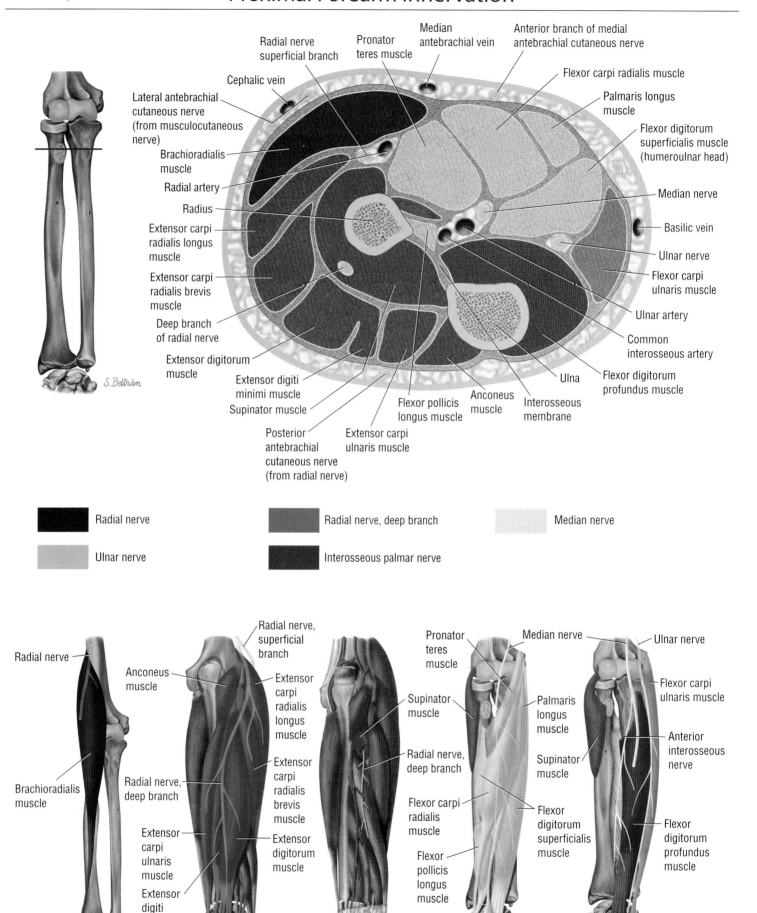

Figure 9.2 ▪ Proximal forearm innervation with cross section and 3-D renderings. *Cross section based on Vahlensiech M, Genant HK, Reiter M. MRI of the musculoskeletal system. New York/Stuttgart: Thieme, 2000. (See Related Muscles pgs. 1466–1475, in Stoller's 3rd Edition.)*

Biceps Brachii

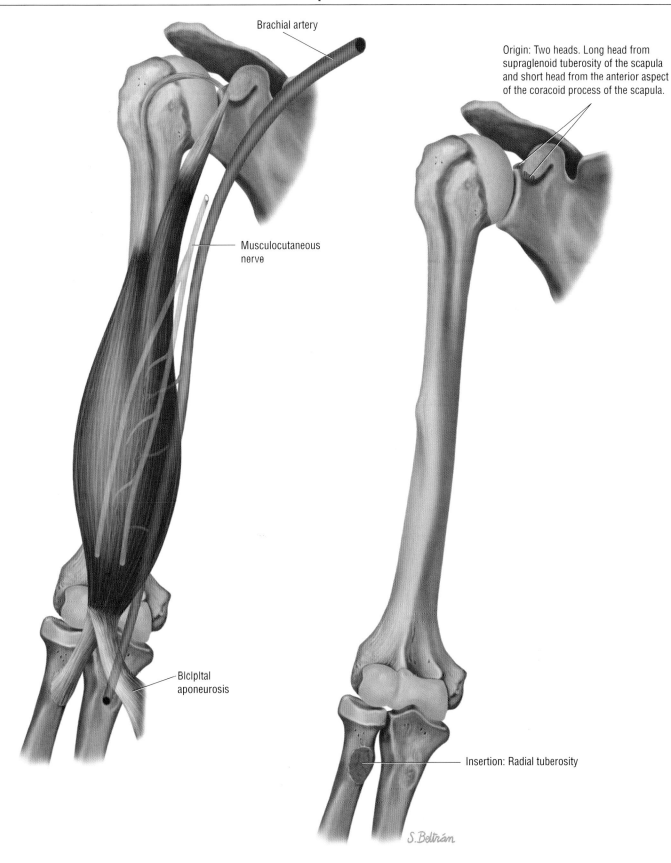

Brachial artery

Origin: Two heads. Long head from supraglenoid tuberosity of the scapula and short head from the anterior aspect of the coracoid process of the scapula.

Musculocutaneous nerve

Bicipital aponeurosis

Insertion: Radial tuberosity

S. Beltrán

Figure 9.3 ■ BICEPS BRACHII. The biceps brachii is composed of two heads and is biarticulate, spanning the shoulder and elbow joints. The distal biceps brachii tendon inserts on the radial tuberosity, with superficial fibers contributing to the bicipital aponeurosis that blends with the antebrachial fascia. Most biceps brachii tears occur proximally involving the long head; distal avulsions, however, are not uncommonly seen and are secondary to sudden or prolonged flexion against a heavy load. The biceps brachii acts as a flexor of the shoulder and elbow joints. When the elbow is flexed, the biceps brachii also acts as a powerful supinator because of its slightly medial insertion on the rotating proximal radius. *(See Related Muscles pg. 1466, in Stoller's 3rd Edition.)*

Brachialis

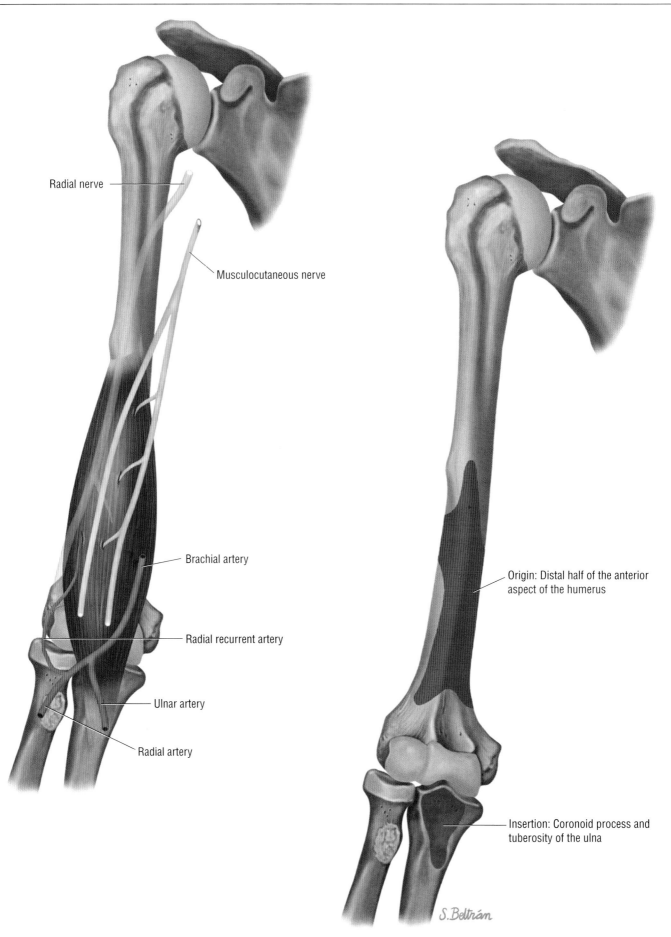

Radial nerve

Musculocutaneous nerve

Brachial artery

Radial recurrent artery

Ulnar artery

Radial artery

Origin: Distal half of the anterior aspect of the humerus

Insertion: Coronoid process and tuberosity of the ulna

S. Beltrán

Figure 9.4 ■ **BRACHIALIS.** The brachialis contributes more during isometric elbow flexion, whereas the biceps brachii is more active during dynamic elbow flexion. Isolated rupture of the brachialis muscle is a rare injury. Strains typically occur at the musculocutaneous junction. *(See Related Muscles pg. 1467, in Stoller's 3rd Edition.)*

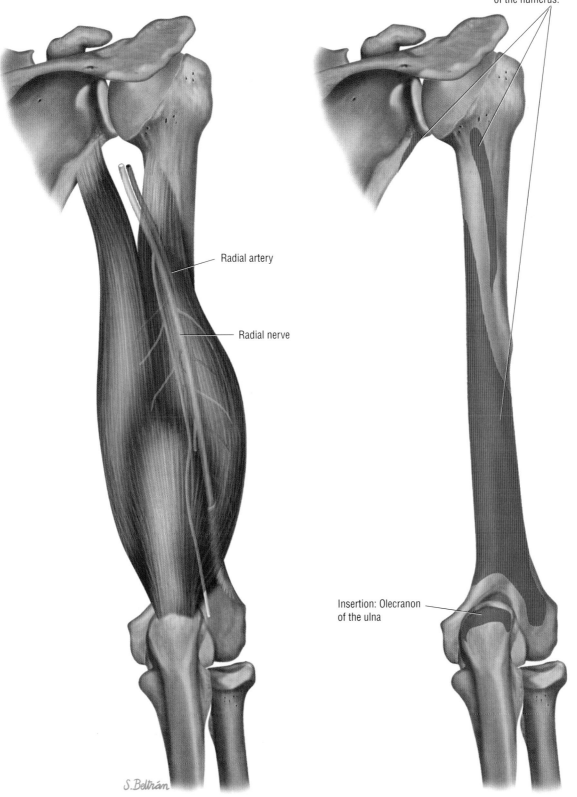

Origin: Three heads. Long head from the infraglenoid tubercle of the scapula, lateral head from the posterolateral surface of the humerus, and medial head from the mid to distal posterior aspect of the humerus.

Radial artery

Radial nerve

Insertion: Olecranon of the ulna

S. Beltrán

Figure 9.5 ■ TRICEPS BRACHII. The triceps brachii is composed of three heads. The long head of the triceps brachii is biarticulate, spanning the shoulder and elbow joints. In addition to adduction of the shoulder, the triceps brachii acts to extend the shoulder and elbow joints. The distal triceps tendon inserts on the olecranon, where avulsions can occur, typically following a fall on the outstretched upper extremity resulting in deceleration stress on an already contracted triceps. Midsubstance tendon and musculocutaneous injuries of the triceps brachii are less common. *(See Related Muscles pg. 1467, in Stoller's 3rd Edition.)*

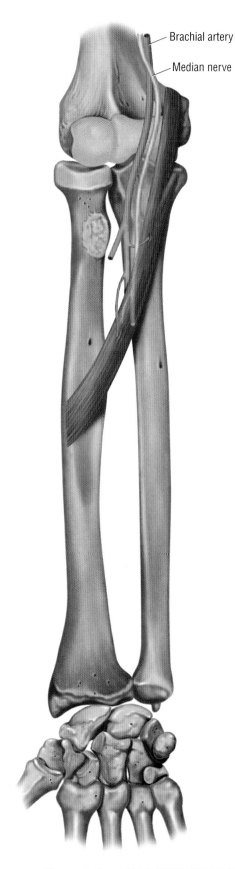

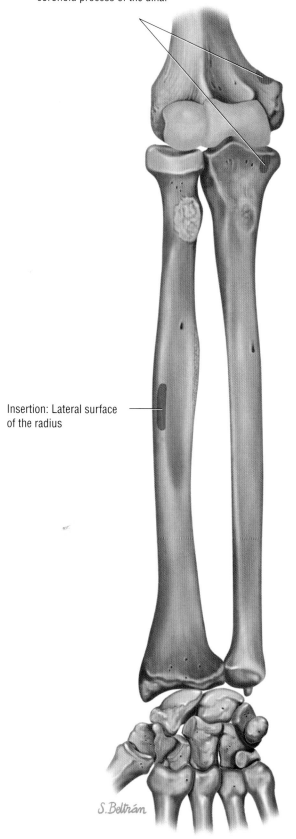

Brachial artery

Median nerve

Origin: Two heads. Humeral head originates off the medial epicondyle. Ulnar head originates from the coronoid process of the ulna.

Insertion: Lateral surface of the radius

S. Beltrán

Figure 9.6 ■ PRONATOR TERES. The pronator teres acts synergistically with the pronator quadratus to pronate the forearm. The median nerve has variable anatomy with respect to the pronator teres. Most commonly the median nerve runs between the humeral and ulnar heads of the pronator teres, but it also can travel deep to both heads as well as perforate the humeral head. Pronator syndrome results from compression of the median nerve as it courses through the pronator teres and is manifested clinically by pain in the wrist and forearm and weakness of the thenar muscles. *(See Related Muscles pg. 1468, in Stoller's 3rd Edition.)*

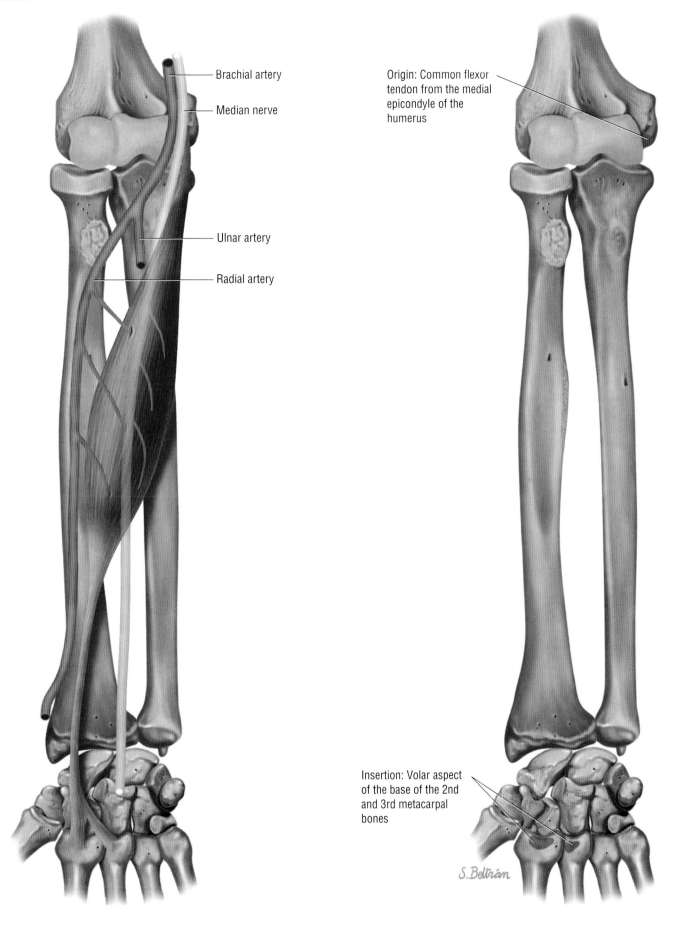

Brachial artery

Median nerve

Ulnar artery

Radial artery

Origin: Common flexor tendon from the medial epicondyle of the humerus

Insertion: Volar aspect of the base of the 2nd and 3rd metacarpal bones

S. Beltrán

Figure 9.7 ■ FLEXOR CARPI RADIALIS. The flexor carpi radialis lies radial to the palmaris longus and ulnar to the pronator teres throughout its course. It contributes to flexion and abduction of the wrist. Along with the pronator teres it is the most common tendon involved in medial epicondylitis. Distal flexor carpi radialis tendon rupture, usually occurring after a fall on the outstretched hand, can clinically mimic scaphoid fractures. *(See Related Muscles pg. 1468, in Stoller's 3rd Edition.)*

Palmaris Longus

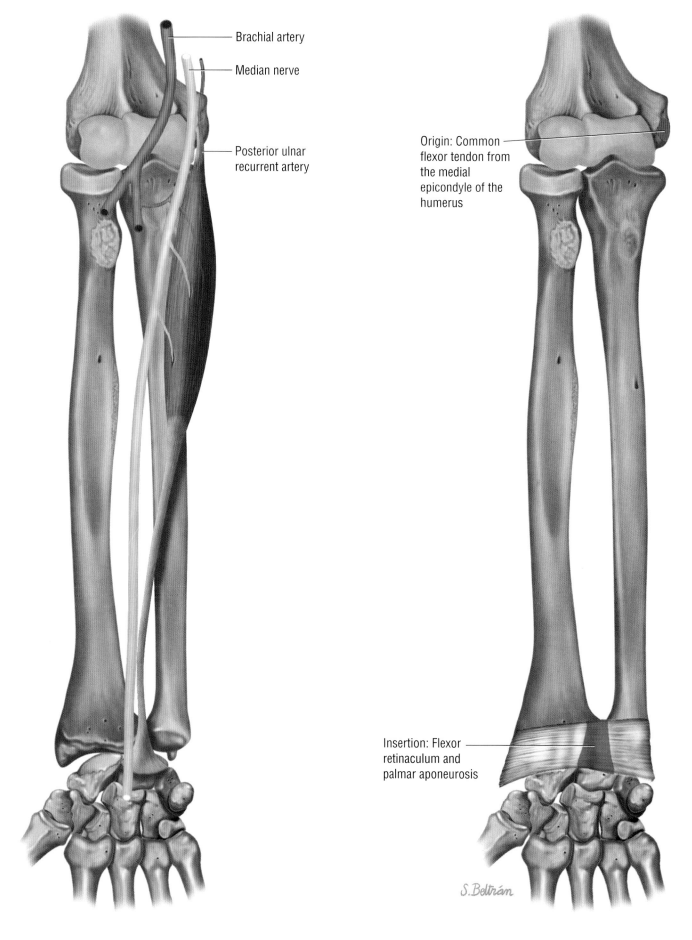

Brachial artery

Median nerve

Posterior ulnar recurrent artery

Origin: Common flexor tendon from the medial epicondyle of the humerus

Insertion: Flexor retinaculum and palmar aponeurosis

S. Beltrán

Figure 9.8 ▪ PALMARIS LONGUS. The palmaris longus is present in approximately 85% of the population and functions to flex the wrist and tighten the palmar aponeurosis. It does not have a tendon sheath but has a paratenon. It is the most commonly used tendon graft of the hand, often used for repair of the elbow MCL in throwing athletes. *(See Related Muscles pg. 1469, in Stoller's 3rd Edition.)*

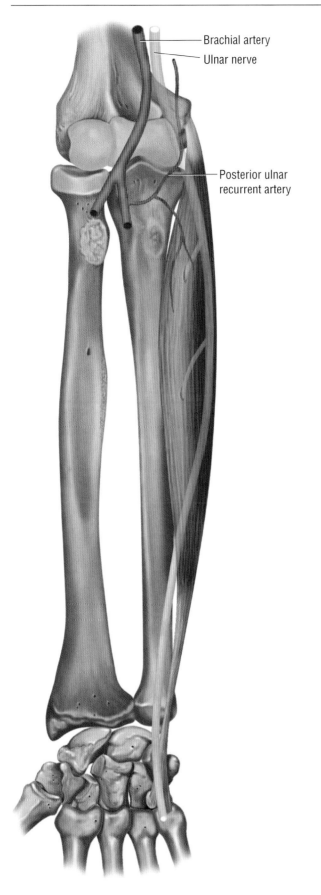

- Brachial artery
- Ulnar nerve
- Posterior ulnar recurrent artery

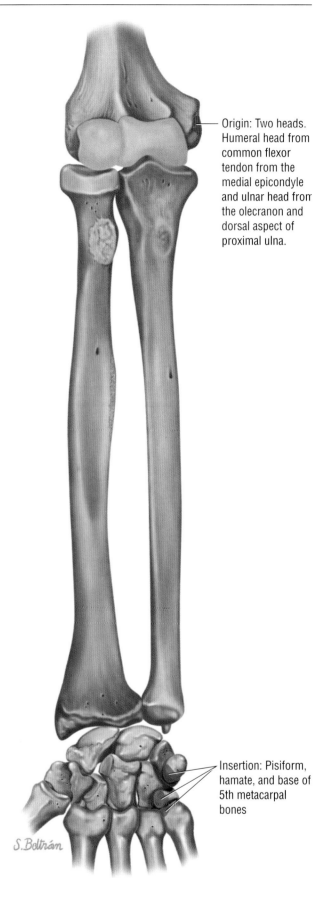

Origin: Two heads. Humeral head from common flexor tendon from the medial epicondyle and ulnar head from the olecranon and dorsal aspect of proximal ulna.

Insertion: Pisiform, hamate, and base of 5th metacarpal bones

S. Beltrán

Figure 9.9 ■ FLEXOR CARPI ULNARIS. The flexor carpi ulnaris flexes and adducts the hand. It is an important dynamic stabilizer of the pisotriquetral joint and contributes superficial fibers to the pisohamate ligament. As it is superficial and just medial to the ulnar nerve, it serves as a marker when ulnar nerve block is performed. *(See Related Muscles pg. 1469, in Stoller's 3rd Edition.)*

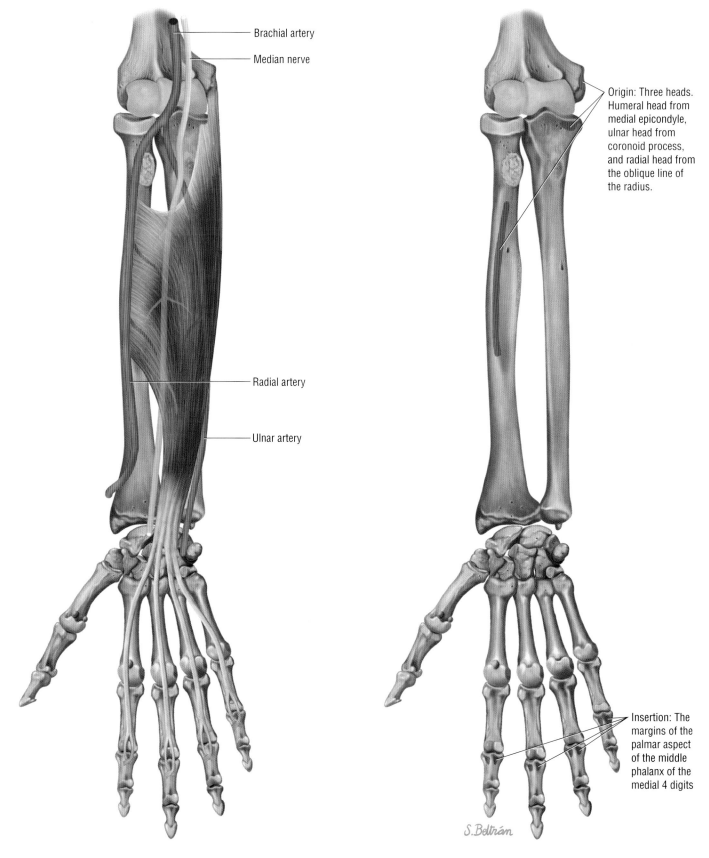

Brachial artery

Median nerve

Origin: Three heads.
Humeral head from
medial epicondyle,
ulnar head from
coronoid process,
and radial head from
the oblique line of
the radius.

Radial artery

Ulnar artery

Insertion: The
margins of the
palmar aspect
of the middle
phalanx of the
medial 4 digits

S. Beltrán

Figure 9.10 ▪ FLEXOR DIGITORUM SUPERFICIALIS. The flexor digitorum superficialis tendons
flex the middle phalanges of each finger and, using the pulley system as a fulcrum, contribute to
flexion of the fingers at the metacarpophalangeal joint. The deep fibers of the flexor digitorum superficialis origin are closely apposed with the anterior bundle of the medial collateral ligament at
the elbow, which is why edema and hemorrhage in the flexor digitorum superficialis are commonly seen in the setting of MCL tears. In the forearm, the median nerve lies just deep to the arch
of the flexor digitorum superficialis muscle, and this is an area of potential nerve compression. The
flexor digitorum superficialis divides into four musculotendinous units in the distal forearm, and
the tendons travel though the carpal tunnel before dividing again at the level of the proximal phalanges. *(See Related Muscles pg. 1470, in Stoller's 3rd Edition.)*

Flexor Digitorum Profundus

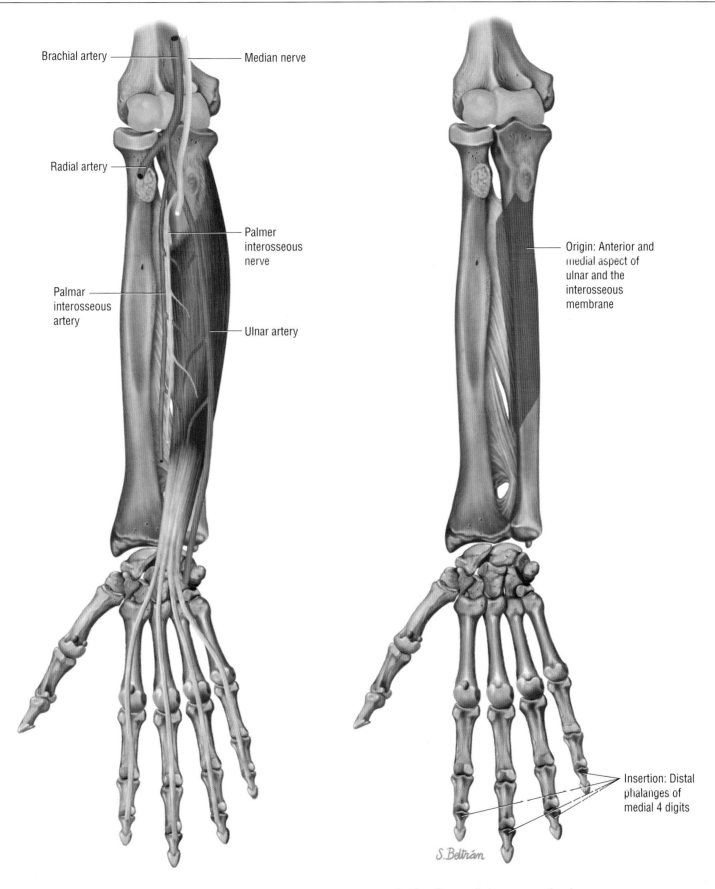

Brachial artery — —— Median nerve

Radial artery —

Palmer interosseous nerve

Palmar interosseous artery

Ulnar artery

Origin: Anterior and medial aspect of ulnar and the interosseous membrane

Insertion: Distal phalanges of medial 4 digits

S.Beltrán

Figure 9.11 ■ **FLEXOR DIGITORUM PROFUNDUS.** The flexor digitorum profundus tendons flex the distal phalanges at the distal interphalangeal joints and assist in flexion of the wrist and proximal phalanges. The flexor digitorum profundus divides into four musculotendinous units in the distal forearm, and the tendons travel though the carpal tunnel deep to the flexor digitorum superficialis tendons. Distal avulsions of a flexor digitorum profundus tendon, or "jersey finger," can occur when an athlete gets a finger caught in an opposing player's jersey. *(See Related Muscles pg. 1470, in Stoller's 3rd Edition.)*

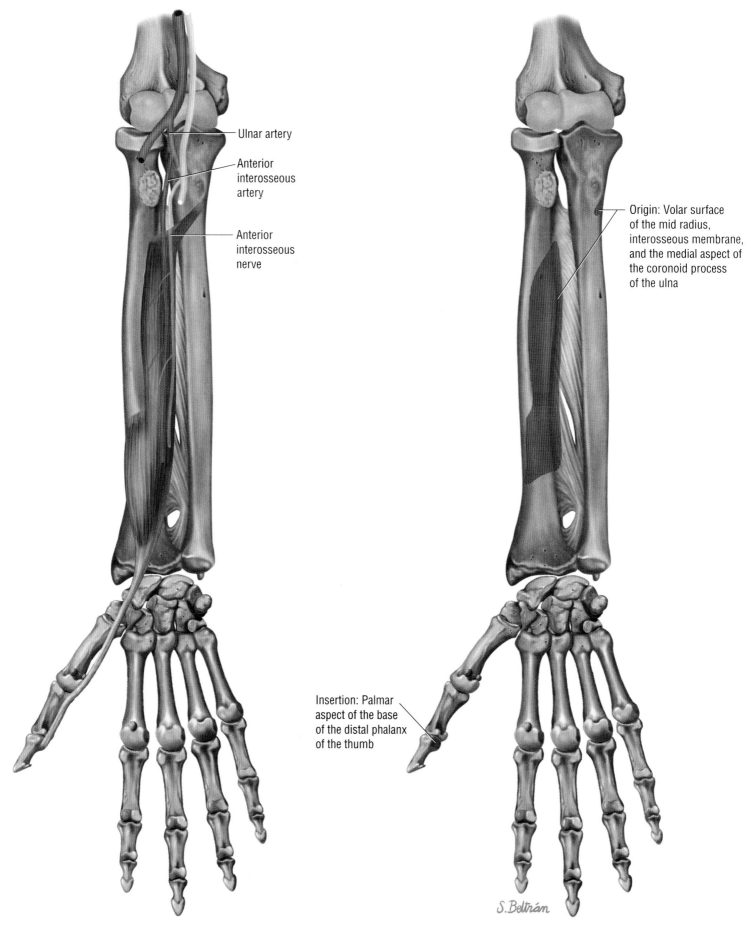

Ulnar artery

Anterior
interosseous
artery

Anterior
interosseous
nerve

Origin: Volar surface
of the mid radius,
interosseous membrane,
and the medial aspect of
the coronoid process
of the ulna

Insertion: Palmar
aspect of the base
of the distal phalanx
of the thumb

S. Beltrán

Figure 9.12 ■ FLEXOR POLLICIS LONGUS. The flexor pollicis longus flexes the thumb. Compression of the anterior interosseous nerve can lead to denervation of the flexor pollicis longus muscle, which may be isolated or concomitant with flexor digitorum profundus and pronator quadratus denervation. *(See Related Muscles pg. 1471, in Stoller's 3rd Edition.)*

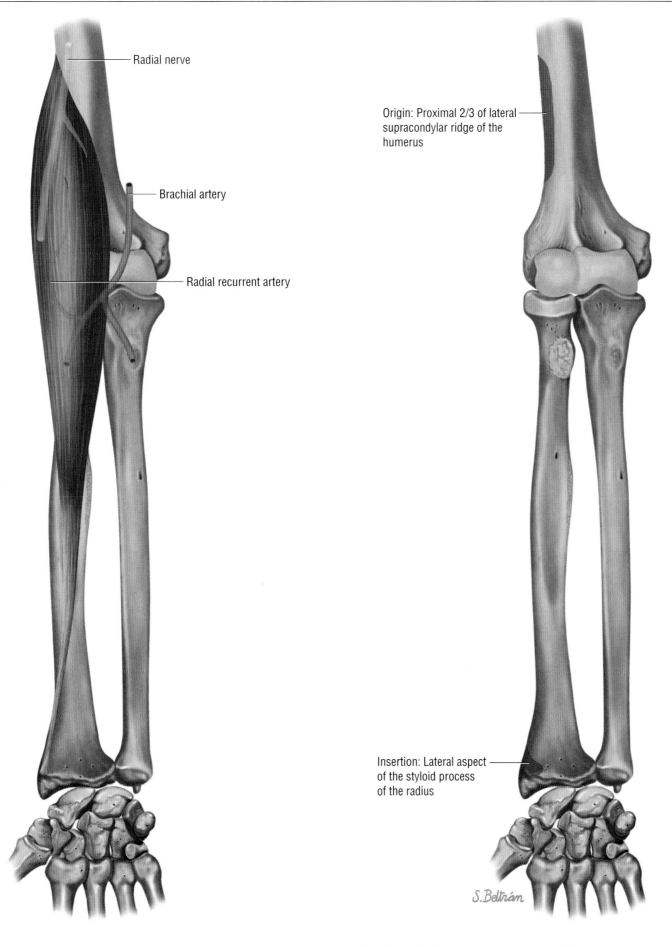

Radial nerve

Brachial artery

Radial recurrent artery

Origin: Proximal 2/3 of lateral supracondylar ridge of the humerus

Insertion: Lateral aspect of the styloid process of the radius

S. Beltrán

Figure 9.13 ■ BRACHIORADIALIS. The brachioradialis is a strong elbow flexor when the forearm is in a neutral position between supination and pronation. In forearm pronation, the brachioradialis tends to supinate as it flexes. In forearm supination, the brachioradialis tends to pronate as it flexes. *(See Related Muscles pg. 1471, in Stoller's 3rd Edition.)*

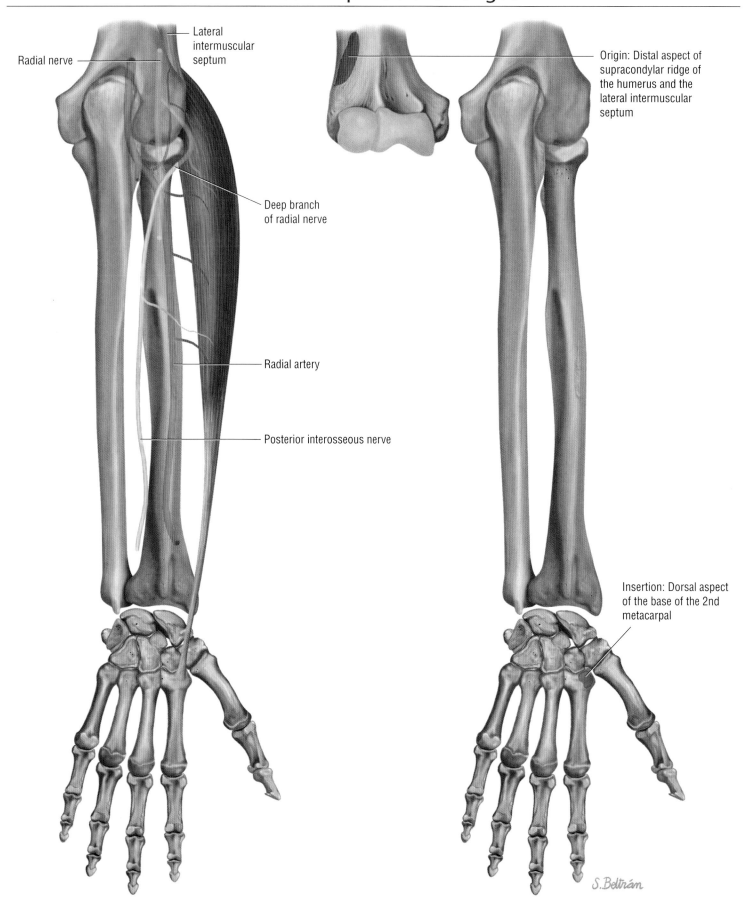

Radial nerve

Lateral
intermuscular
septum

Deep branch
of radial nerve

Radial artery

Posterior interosseous nerve

Origin: Distal aspect of
supracondylar ridge of
the humerus and the
lateral intermuscular
septum

Insertion: Dorsal aspect
of the base of the 2nd
metacarpal

S.Beltrán

Figure 9.14 ▪ EXTENSOR CARPI RADIALIS LONGUS. The extensor carpi radialis longus extends and abducts the wrist. If extensor carpi ulnaris function is lost because of posterior interosseous nerve palsy, the extensor carpi radialis causes radial deviation because normally the attachment of the extensor carpi ulnaris to the ulnar aspect of the fifth metacarpal functions to neutralize the abduction movement applied by the extensor carpi radialis longus. *(See Related Muscles pg. 1472, in Stoller's 3rd Edition.)*

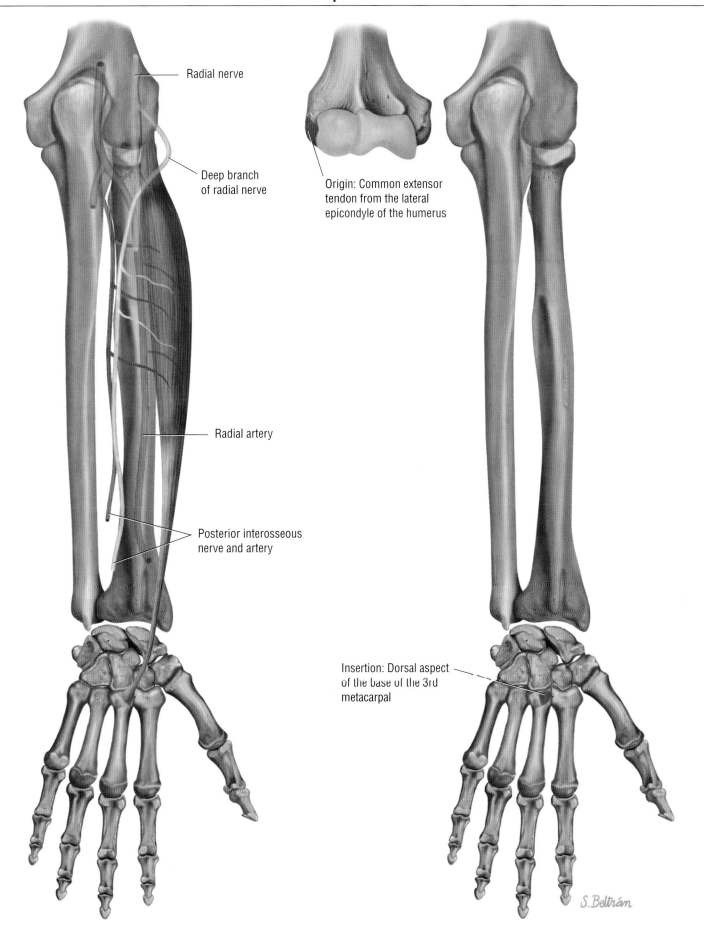

Radial nerve

Deep branch
of radial nerve

Origin: Common extensor
tendon from the lateral
epicondyle of the humerus

Radial artery

Posterior interosseous
nerve and artery

Insertion: Dorsal aspect
of the base of the 3rd
metacarpal

S. Beltrán

Figure 9.15 ▪ EXTENSOR CARPI RADIALIS BREVIS. The extensor carpi radialis brevis, which provides neutral extension of the wrist, is the most common tendon involved in lateral epicondylitis. Distal ruptures of the extensor carpi radialis brevis significantly affect wrist extension. *(See Related Muscles pg. 1472, in Stoller's 3rd Edition.)*

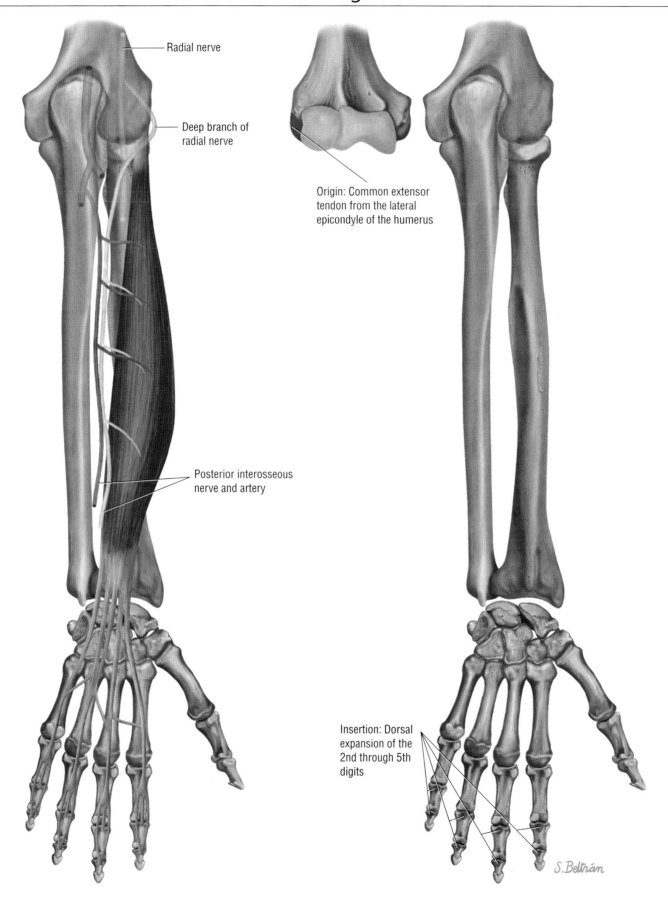

Radial nerve

Deep branch of radial nerve

Origin: Common extensor tendon from the lateral epicondyle of the humerus

Posterior interosseous nerve and artery

Insertion: Dorsal expansion of the 2nd through 5th digits

S. Beltrán

Figure 9.16 ■ EXTENSOR DIGITORUM. The extensor digitorum extends the medial four digits at the metacarpophalangeal joints and contributes to wrist extension. The proximal tendon, as part of the common extensor origin, is often involved in lateral epicondylitis. The extensor digitorum tendons are connected at the level of the metacarpal bones by fibrous bands called juncturae tendinum. Boutonnière deformity results from disruption of the central slip component of the extensor tendon at its insertion into the middle phalanx. *(See Related Muscles pg. 1473, in Stoller's 3rd Edition.)*

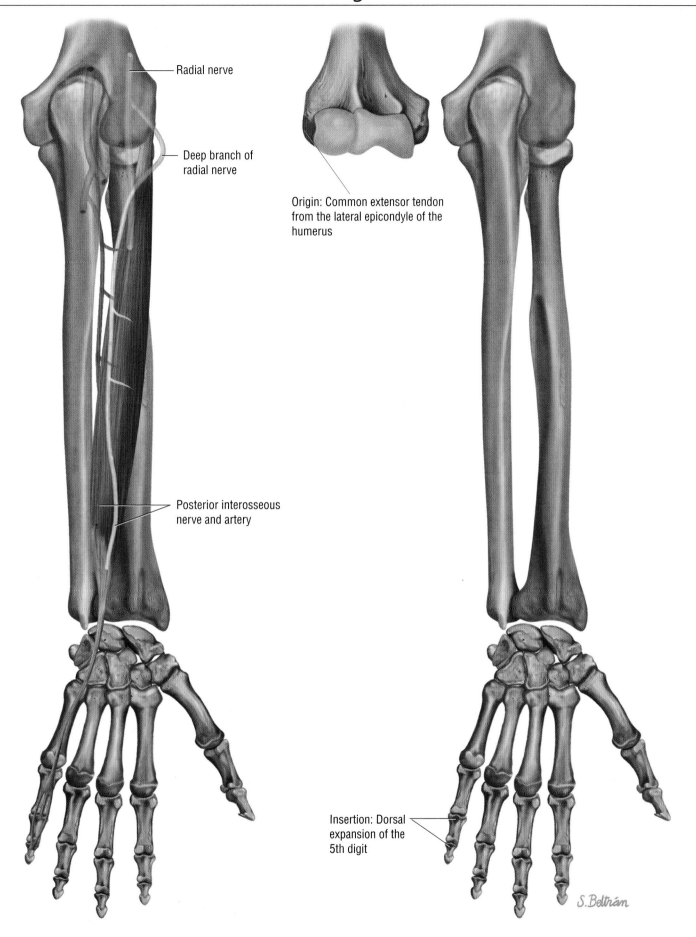

Radial nerve

Deep branch of
radial nerve

Origin: Common extensor tendon
from the lateral epicondyle of the
humerus

Posterior interosseous
nerve and artery

Insertion: Dorsal
expansion of the
5th digit

S.Beltrán

Figure 9.17 ■ EXTENSOR DIGITI MINIMI. The extensor digiti minimi extends the proximal phalanx of the little finger at the metacarpophalangeal joint and contributes to wrist extension.
Because the extensor digiti minimi tendon lies just superficial to the radioulnar articulation, it is
often the first tendon to be involved in rheumatoid arthritis. *(See Related Muscles pg. 1473, in
Stoller's 3rd Edition.)*

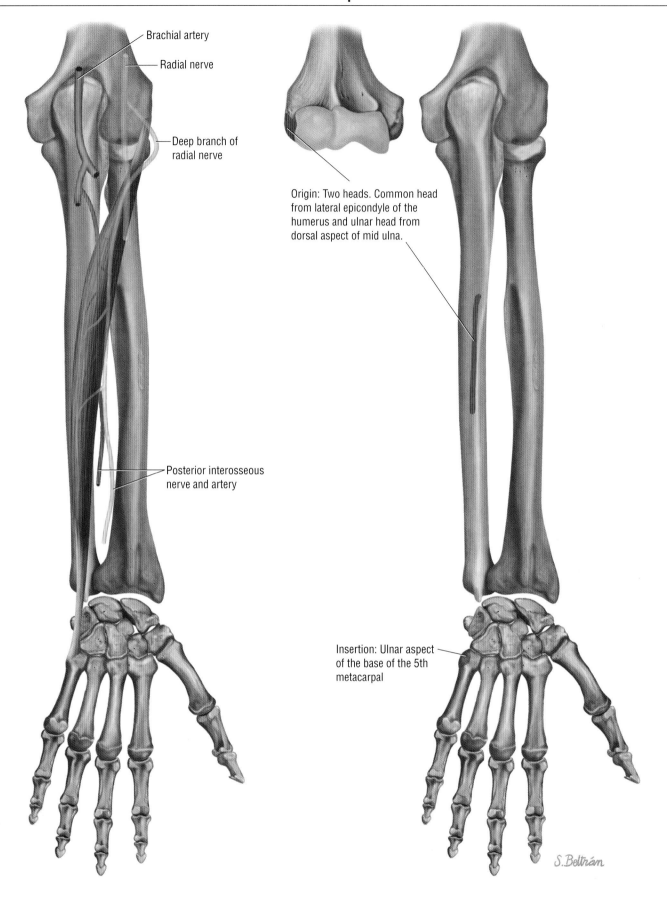

Brachial artery

Radial nerve

Deep branch of
radial nerve

Origin: Two heads. Common head
from lateral epicondyle of the
humerus and ulnar head from
dorsal aspect of mid ulna.

Posterior interosseous
nerve and artery

Insertion: Ulnar aspect
of the base of the 5th
metacarpal

S. Beltrán

Figure 9.18 ■ EXTENSOR CARPI ULNARIS. The extensor carpi ulnaris tendon extends and adducts the wrist. It is commonly affected in tendinosis and tenosynovitis as it passes through the groove on the distal ulna. Subluxation of the extensor carpi ulnaris also can occur at this location related to disruption or insufficiency of the ligament that covers the tendon in this groove. The extensor carpi ulnaris tendon subsheath is a component of the triangular fibrocartilage complex. *(See Related Muscles pg. 1474, in Stoller's 3rd Edition.)*

Anconeus

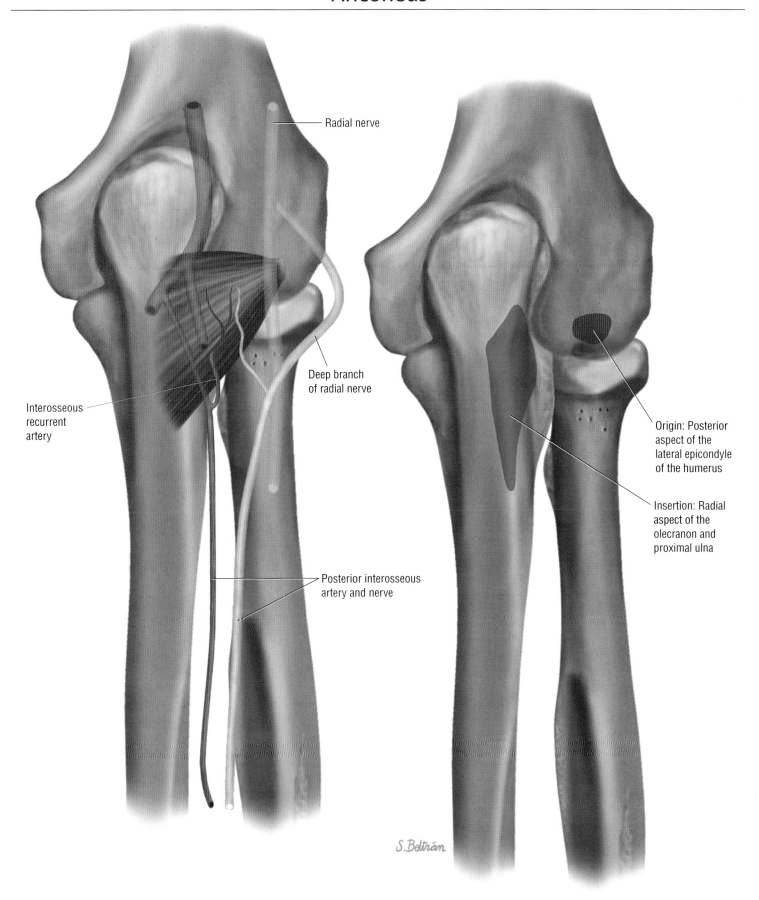

Radial nerve

Deep branch
of radial nerve

Interosseous
recurrent
artery

Posterior interosseous
artery and nerve

Origin: Posterior
aspect of the
lateral epicondyle
of the humerus

Insertion: Radial
aspect of the
olecranon and
proximal ulna

S.Beltrán

Figure 9.19 ■ ANCONEUS. The anconeus is located posterolateral to the elbow, functions to tighten the joint capsule, and is a weak extensor of the elbow. In about 10% of the population an anomalous muscle, the anconeus epitrochlearis, arises from the medial border of the olecranon and the adjacent triceps inserting into the medial epicondyle. The anconeus epitrochlearis thus is located posteromedial to the elbow and can cause compression of the ulnar nerve in the cubital tunnel. *(See Related Muscles pg. 1474, in Stoller's 3rd Edition.)*

Supinator

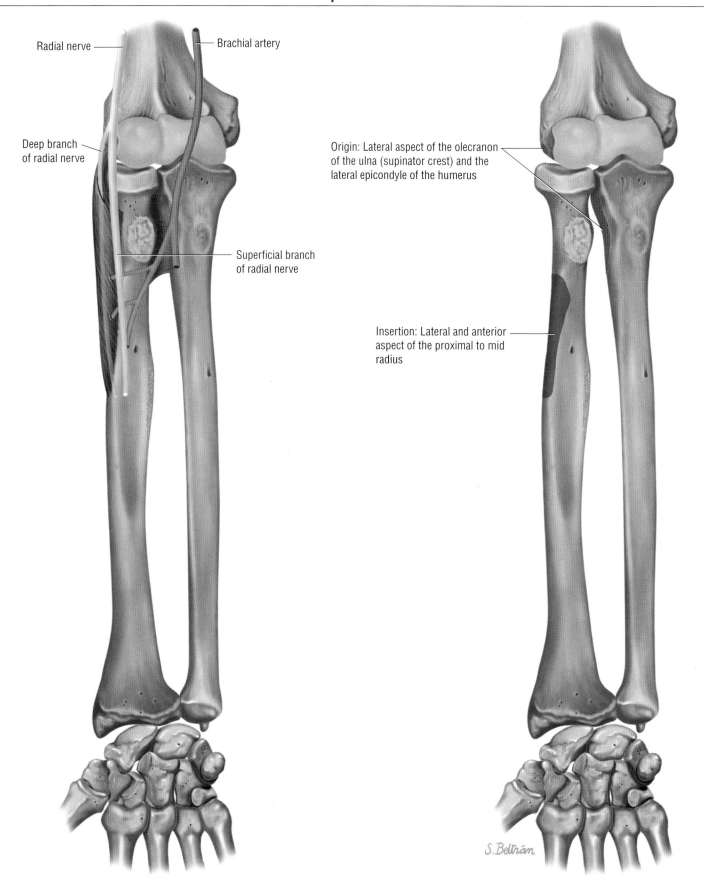

Radial nerve

Brachial artery

Deep branch
of radial nerve

Superficial branch
of radial nerve

Origin: Lateral aspect of the olecranon
of the ulna (supinator crest) and the
lateral epicondyle of the humerus

Insertion: Lateral and anterior
aspect of the proximal to mid
radius

S. Beltrán

Figure 9.20 ■ SUPINATOR. The supinator is the primary supinator of the forearm when the elbow is extended. When the elbow is flexed, the supinator and the biceps brachii work synergistically to supinate the forearm. The deep branch of the radial nerve (i.e., the posterior interosseous nerve) travels between the humeral and ulnar origins of the supinator as it courses down the forearm, posterolateral to the proximal radius. The supinator is a potential site of entrapment of this nerve. *(See Related Muscles pg. 1475, in Stoller's 3rd Edition.)*

The Elbow
Anatomy and Pathology

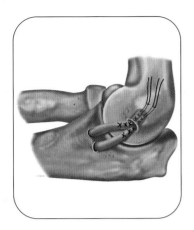

758

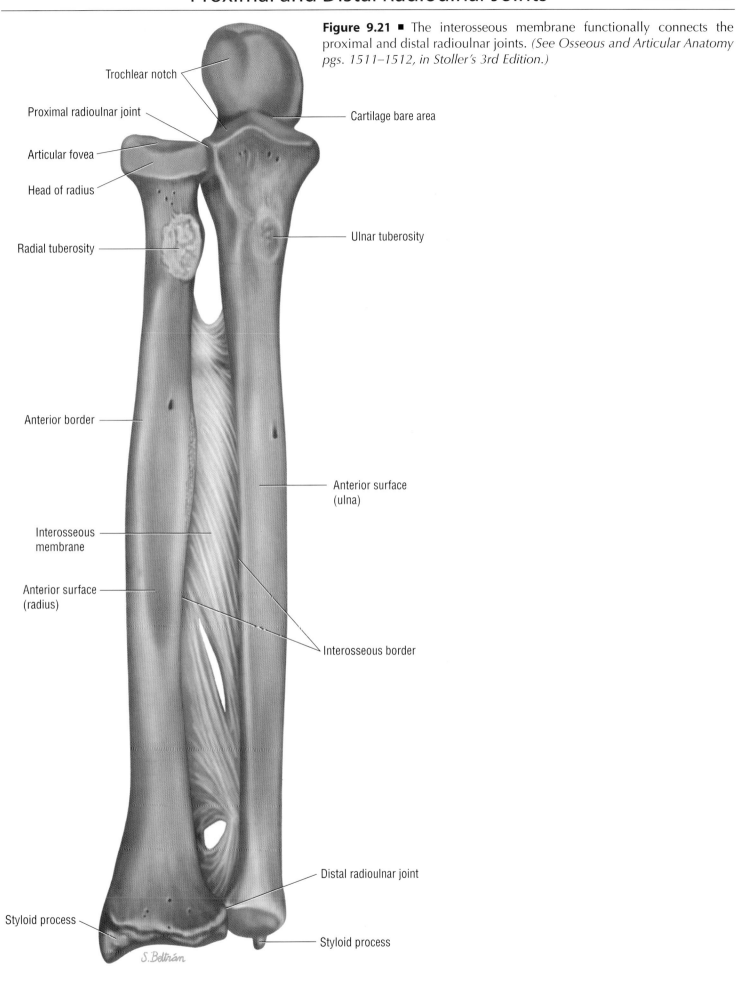

Figure 9.21 ■ The interosseous membrane functionally connects the proximal and distal radioulnar joints. *(See Osseous and Articular Anatomy pgs. 1511–1512, in Stoller's 3rd Edition.)*

Trochlear notch

Proximal radioulnar joint

Articular fovea

Head of radius

Radial tuberosity

Anterior border

Interosseous membrane

Anterior surface (radius)

Styloid process

Cartilage bare area

Ulnar tuberosity

Anterior surface (ulna)

Interosseous border

Distal radioulnar joint

Styloid process

S.Beltrán

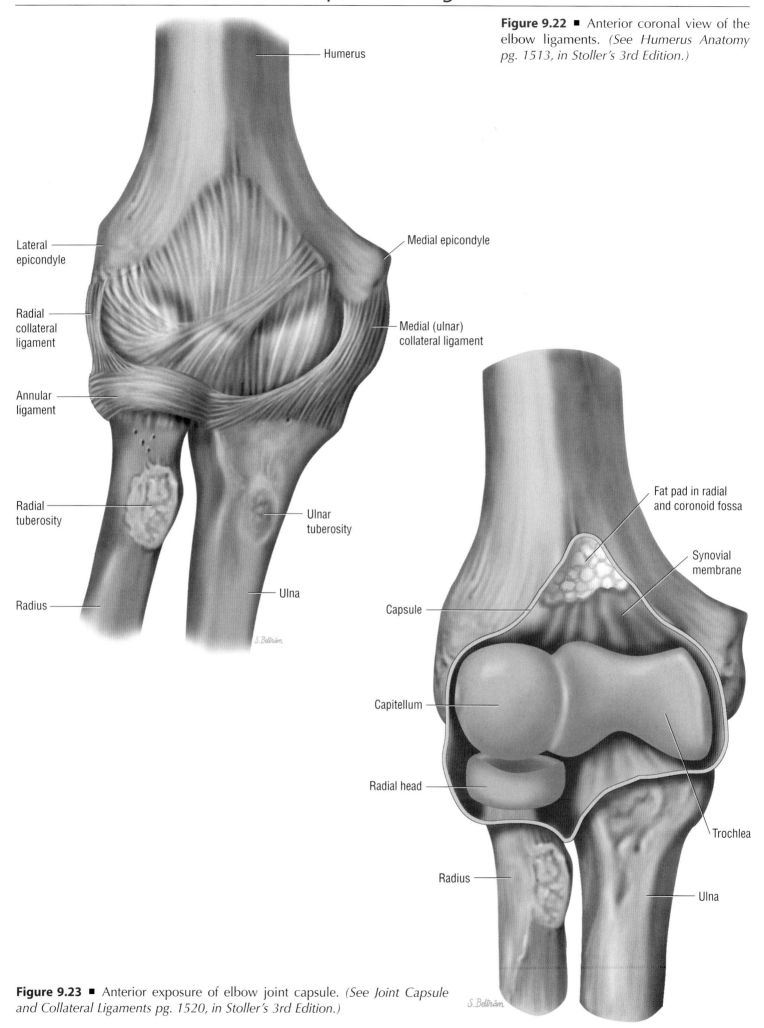

Figure 9.22 ■ Anterior coronal view of the elbow ligaments. *(See Humerus Anatomy pg. 1513, in Stoller's 3rd Edition.)*

Humerus

Lateral epicondyle

Medial epicondyle

Radial collateral ligament

Medial (ulnar) collateral ligament

Annular ligament

Radial tuberosity

Ulnar tuberosity

Radius

Ulna

Fat pad in radial and coronoid fossa

Synovial membrane

Capsule

Capitellum

Radial head

Trochlea

Radius

Ulna

Figure 9.23 ■ Anterior exposure of elbow joint capsule. *(See Joint Capsule and Collateral Ligaments pg. 1520, in Stoller's 3rd Edition.)*

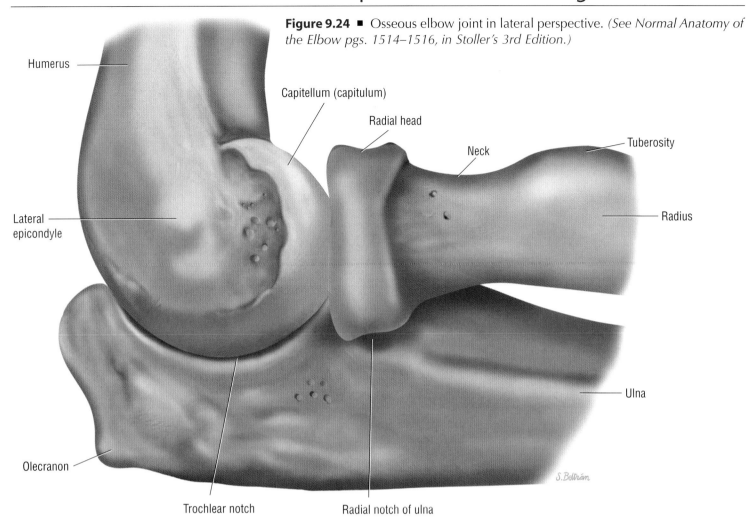

Figure 9.24 ■ Osseous elbow joint in lateral perspective. *(See Normal Anatomy of the Elbow pgs. 1514–1516, in Stoller's 3rd Edition.)*

Humerus

Capitellum (capitulum)

Radial head

Neck

Tuberosity

Lateral epicondyle

Radius

Ulna

Olecranon

Trochlear notch

Radial notch of ulna

S.Beltrán

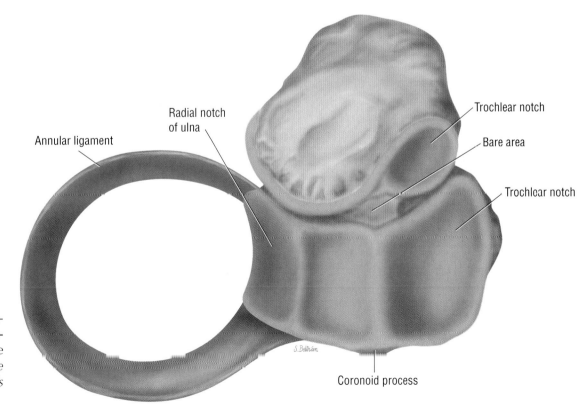

Figure 9.25 ■ Annular ligament extends from the anterior to posterior border of the radial notch of the ulna. *(See Ulna pg. 1514, in Stoller's 3rd Edition.)*

Radial notch of ulna

Annular ligament

Trochlear notch

Bare area

Trochlear notch

Coronoid process

S.Beltrán

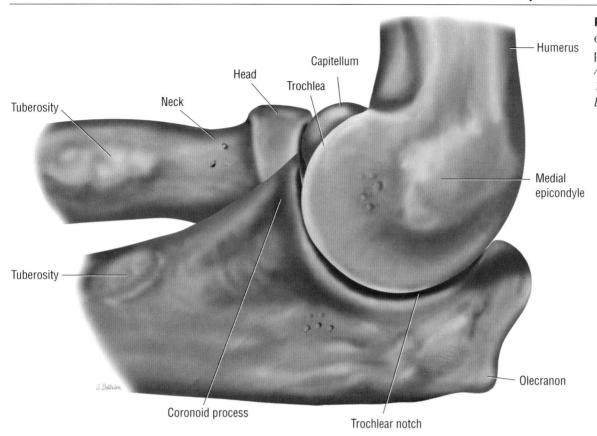

Figure 9.26 ■ Osseous elbow joint in medial perspective. *(See Normal Anatomy of the Elbow pgs. 1514–1516, in Stoller's 3rd Edition.)*

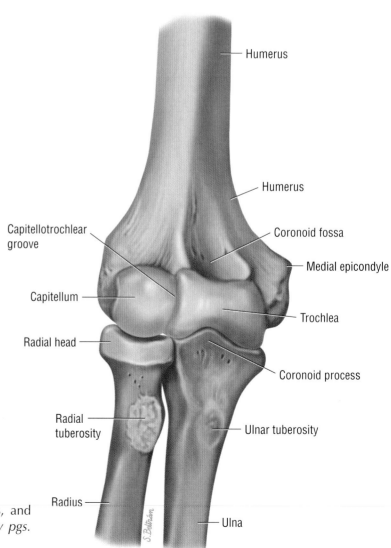

Figure 9.27 ■ Anterior view demonstrating humerus, radius, and ulna at the elbow joint. *(See Normal Anatomy of the Elbow pgs. 1512–1513, in Stoller's 3rd Edition.)*

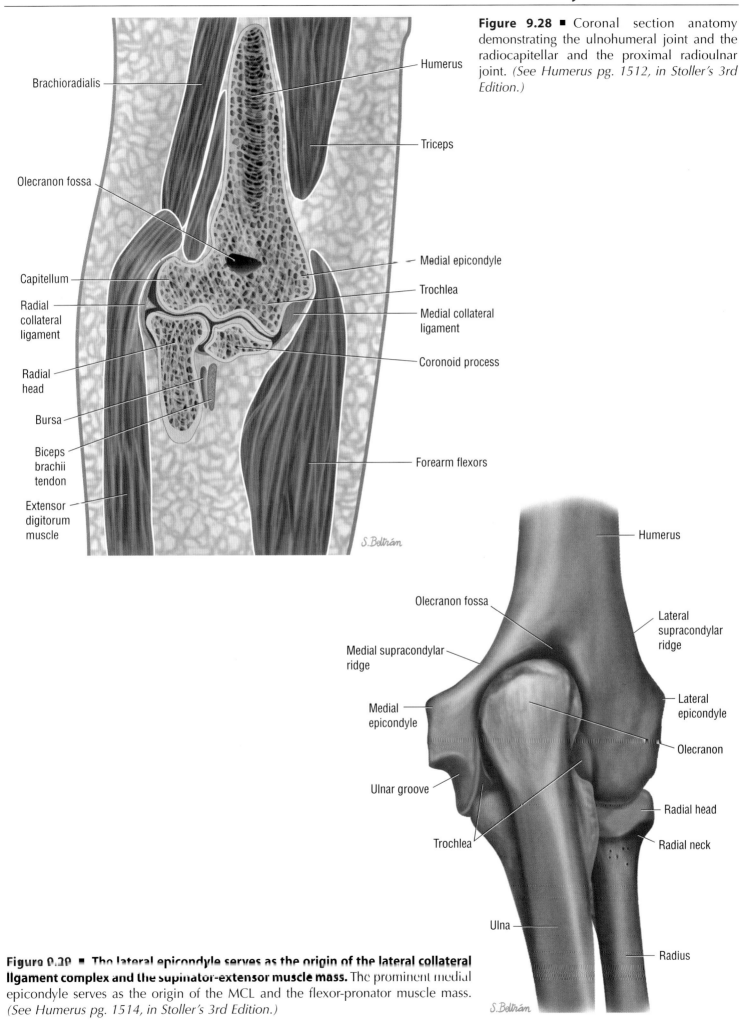

Figure 9.28 ■ Coronal section anatomy demonstrating the ulnohumeral joint and the radiocapitellar and the proximal radioulnar joint. *(See Humerus pg. 1512, in Stoller's 3rd Edition.)*

Brachioradialis

Humerus

Triceps

Olecranon fossa

Capitellum

Radial collateral ligament

Medial epicondyle

Trochlea

Medial collateral ligament

Radial head

Coronoid process

Bursa

Biceps brachii tendon

Forearm flexors

Extensor digitorum muscle

S.Beltrán

Olecranon fossa

Humerus

Medial supracondylar ridge

Lateral supracondylar ridge

Medial epicondyle

Lateral epicondyle

Ulnar groove

Olecranon

Radial head

Radial neck

Trochlea

Ulna

Radius

S.Beltrán

Figure 9.29 ■ **The lateral epicondyle serves as the origin of the lateral collateral ligament complex and the supinator-extensor muscle mass.** The prominent medial epicondyle serves as the origin of the MCL and the flexor-pronator muscle mass. *(See Humerus pg. 1514, in Stoller's 3rd Edition.)*

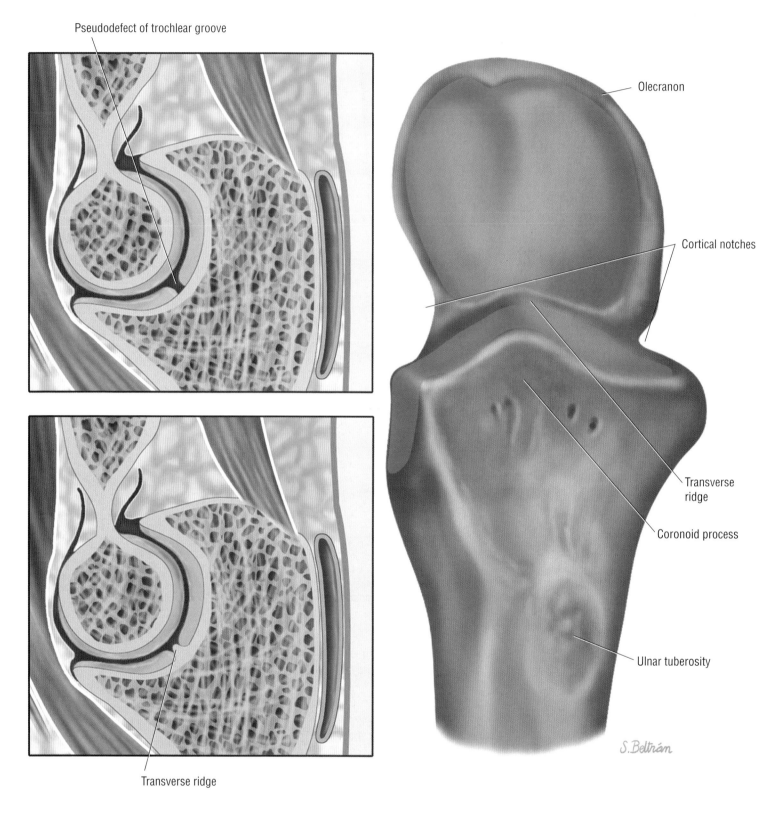

Pseudodefect of trochlear groove

Transverse ridge

Olecranon

Cortical notches

Transverse ridge

Coronoid process

Ulnar tuberosity

S. Beltrán

Figure 9.30 ■ **The cortical notches create pseudodefects of the trochlear groove on sagittal MR images.** These pseudodefects correspond to the medial and lateral edges of the waist of the trochlear groove. The transverse trochlear ridge is nonarticular and may be visualized as focal convexity along the concave trochlear groove as viewed in the sagittal plane. *(See Ulna pgs. 1515 and 1516, in Stoller's 3rd Edition.)*

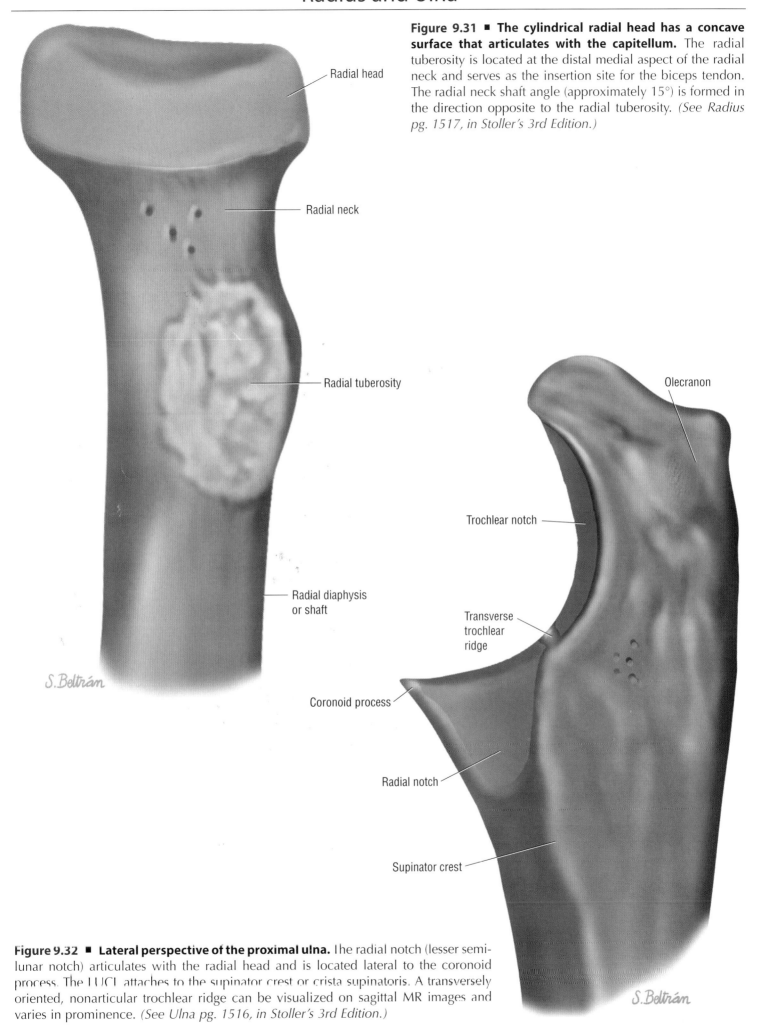

Figure 9.31 ■ The cylindrical radial head has a concave surface that articulates with the capitellum. The radial tuberosity is located at the distal medial aspect of the radial neck and serves as the insertion site for the biceps tendon. The radial neck shaft angle (approximately 15°) is formed in the direction opposite to the radial tuberosity. *(See Radius pg. 1517, in Stoller's 3rd Edition.)*

Radial head

Radial neck

Radial tuberosity

Radial diaphysis or shaft

S. Beltrán

Olecranon

Trochlear notch

Transverse trochlear ridge

Coronoid process

Radial notch

Supinator crest

S. Beltrán

Figure 9.32 ■ Lateral perspective of the proximal ulna. The radial notch (lesser semilunar notch) articulates with the radial head and is located lateral to the coronoid process. The LUCL attaches to the supinator crest or crista supinatoris. A transversely oriented, nonarticular trochlear ridge can be visualized on sagittal MR images and varies in prominence. *(See Ulna pg. 1516, in Stoller's 3rd Edition.)*

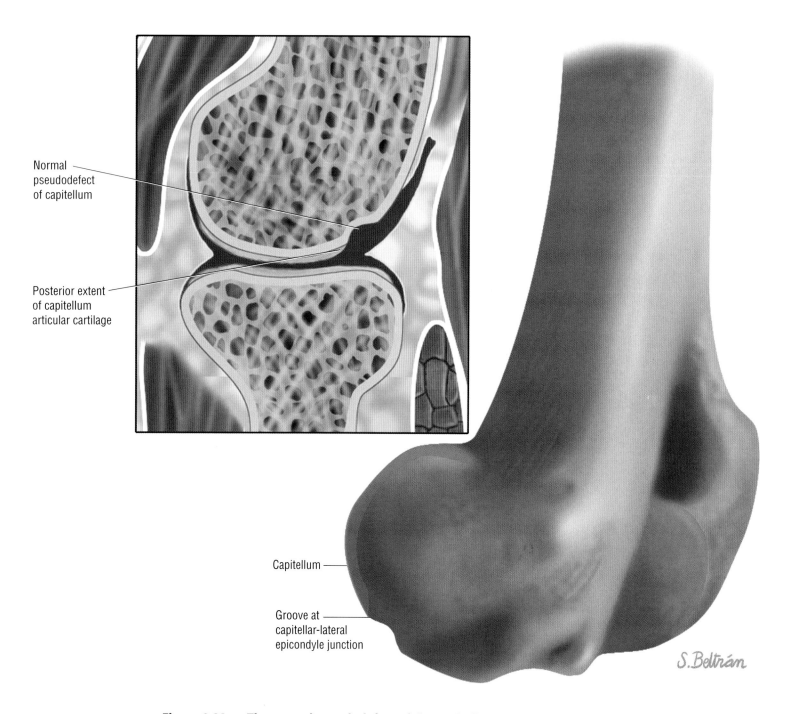

Normal
pseudodefect
of capitellum

Posterior extent
of capitellum
articular cartilage

Capitellum

Groove at
capitellar-lateral
epicondyle junction

S.Beltrán

Figure 9.33 ■ **The normal pseudodefect of the capitellum is seen at the level of the radial head capitellar joint.** Posterior to the lateral capitellar articular margin is normal groove at the junction of the capitellum and the distal humerus (lateral epicondyle). *(See Radius pgs. 1517 and 1518, in Stoller's 3rd Edition.)*

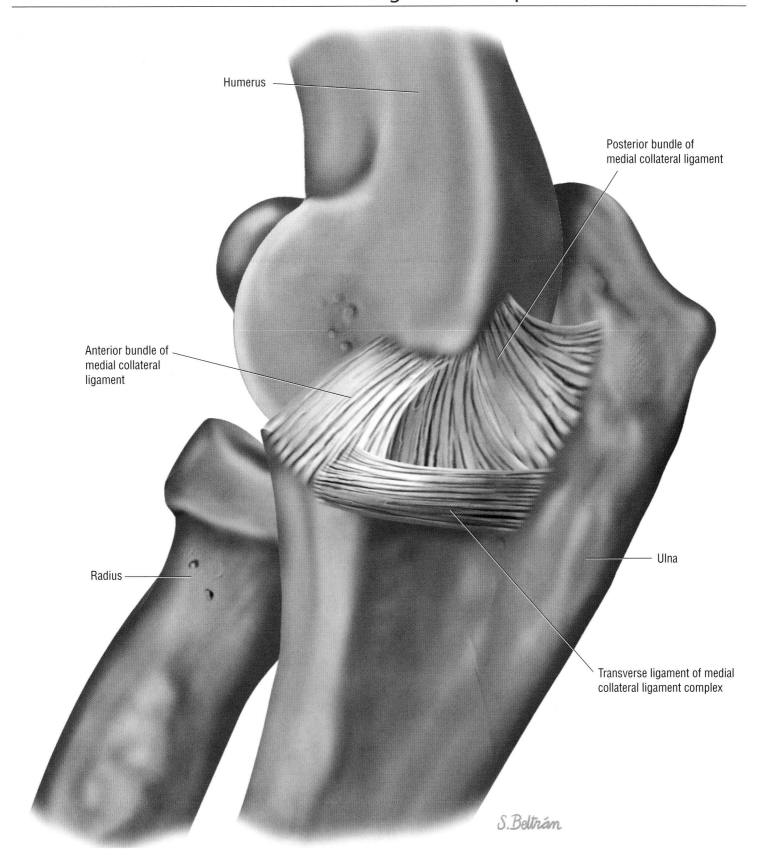

Humerus

Posterior bundle of
medial collateral ligament

Anterior bundle of
medial collateral
ligament

Ulna

Radius

Transverse ligament of medial
collateral ligament complex

S. Beltrán

Figure 9.34 ■ **The medial collateral ligament complex includes the anterior and posterior bundles and the transverse ligament (oblique band).** The posterior bundle and the transverse ligament lie at the deep margin of the ulnar nerve and make up the floor of the cubital tunnel. The functionally important anterior bundle extends from the inferior aspect of the medial epicondyle to the medial aspect of the coronoid process. The anterior, posterior, and transverse bundles of the medial collateral ligament are shown. Sagittal color illustration. *(See Medial Collateral Ligament Complex pgs. 1519 and 1521, in Stoller's 3rd Edition.)*

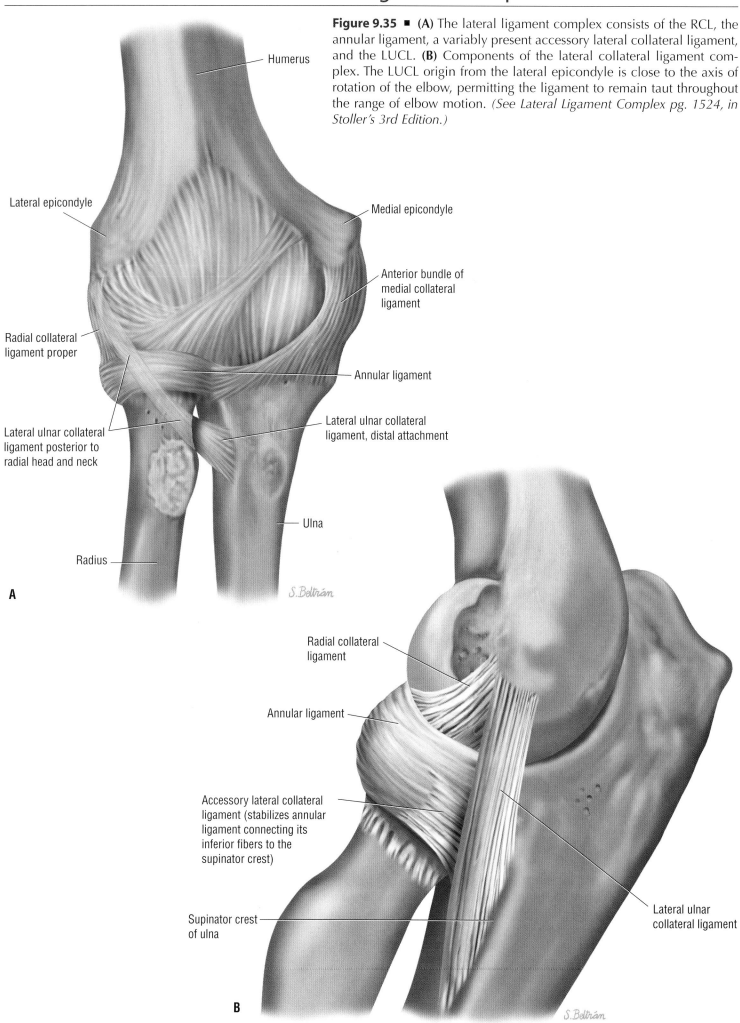

Figure 9.35 ■ (A) The lateral ligament complex consists of the RCL, the annular ligament, a variably present accessory lateral collateral ligament, and the LUCL. **(B)** Components of the lateral collateral ligament complex. The LUCL origin from the lateral epicondyle is close to the axis of rotation of the elbow, permitting the ligament to remain taut throughout the range of elbow motion. *(See Lateral Ligament Complex pg. 1524, in Stoller's 3rd Edition.)*

Humerus

Lateral epicondyle

Medial epicondyle

Anterior bundle of medial collateral ligament

Radial collateral ligament proper

Annular ligament

Lateral ulnar collateral ligament, distal attachment

Lateral ulnar collateral ligament posterior to radial head and neck

Ulna

Radius

A

Radial collateral ligament

Annular ligament

Accessory lateral collateral ligament (stabilizes annular ligament connecting its inferior fibers to the supinator crest)

Lateral ulnar collateral ligament

Supinator crest of ulna

B

Figure 9.36 ■ The LUCL, which originates more posteriorly than the RCL proper, courses superficial to the annular ligament and attaches onto the supinator crest of the ulna. *(See Lateral Ligament Complex pg. 1527, in Stoller's 3rd Edition.)*

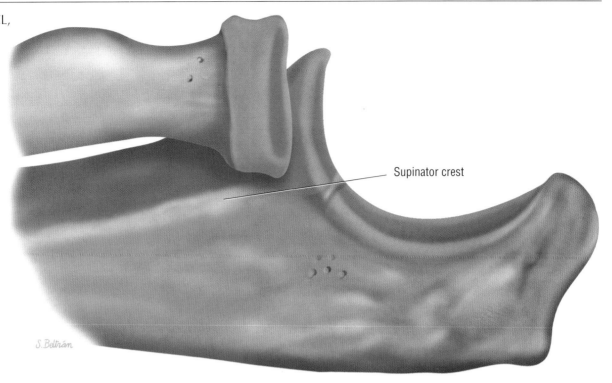

Supinator crest

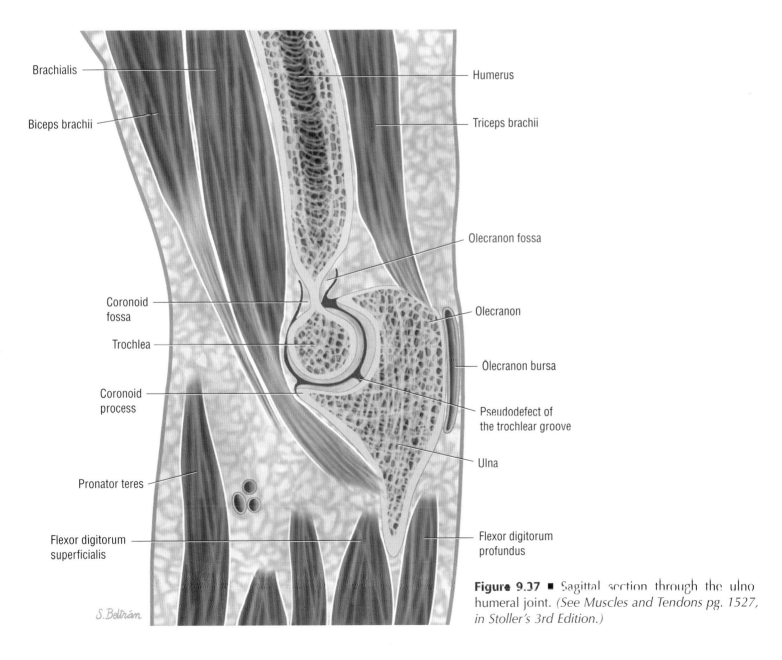

Brachialis

Biceps brachii

Humerus

Triceps brachii

Olecranon fossa

Coronoid fossa

Trochlea

Olecranon

Coronoid process

Olecranon bursa

Pseudodefect of the trochlear groove

Pronator teres

Ulna

Flexor digitorum superficialis

Flexor digitorum profundus

Figure 9.37 ■ Sagittal section through the ulnohumeral joint. *(See Muscles and Tendons pg. 1527, in Stoller's 3rd Edition.)*

Radiocapitellar Joint and Brachial Artery

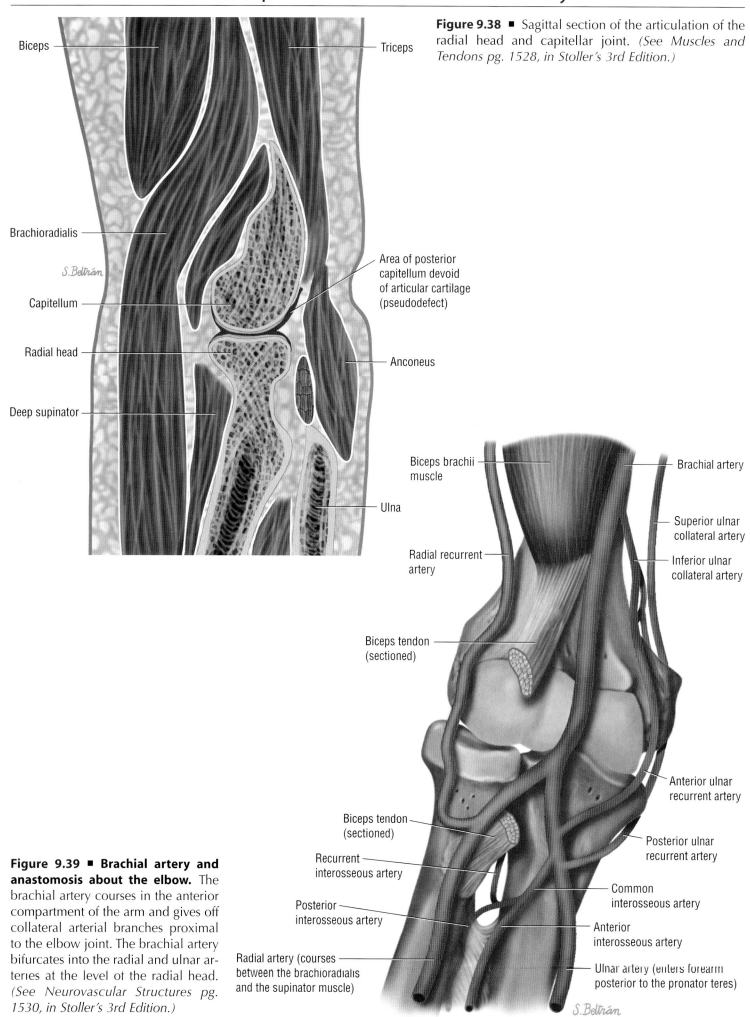

Biceps

Triceps

Brachioradialis

S.Beltrán

Capitellum

Area of posterior
capitellum devoid
of articular cartilage
(pseudodefect)

Radial head

Anconeus

Deep supinator

Ulna

Figure 9.38 ■ Sagittal section of the articulation of the radial head and capitellar joint. *(See Muscles and Tendons pg. 1528, in Stoller's 3rd Edition.)*

Biceps brachii
muscle

Brachial artery

Radial recurrent
artery

Superior ulnar
collateral artery

Inferior ulnar
collateral artery

Biceps tendon
(sectioned)

Biceps tendon
(sectioned)

Anterior ulnar
recurrent artery

Recurrent
interosseous artery

Posterior ulnar
recurrent artery

Posterior
interosseous artery

Common
interosseous artery

Anterior
interosseous artery

Radial artery (courses
between the brachioradialis
and the supinator muscle)

Ulnar artery (enters forearm
posterior to the pronator teres)

S.Beltrán

Figure 9.39 ■ **Brachial artery and anastomosis about the elbow.** The brachial artery courses in the anterior compartment of the arm and gives off collateral arterial branches proximal to the elbow joint. The brachial artery bifurcates into the radial and ulnar arteries at the level of the radial head. *(See Neurovascular Structures pg. 1530, in Stoller's 3rd Edition.)*

Figure 9.40 ▪ The anterior bundle of the MCL is the primary restraint to valgus stress. The anterior bundle can be subdivided into an anterior and posterior band, not to be confused with the posterior bundle. The anterior portion of the anterior bundle tightens during extension and the posterior portion tightens during flexion. Medial perspective sagittal color illustration. **(B)** The anterior bundle consists of parallel collagen bundles in two layers. One layer is between two synovial layers of the joint capsule. A second layer is superficial to the joint capsule and blends with the deep surface of the flexor mass. Coronal color illustration with medial epicondyle sectioned. *(See Medial Collateral Ligament Injury pg. 1531, in Stoller's 3rd Edition.)*

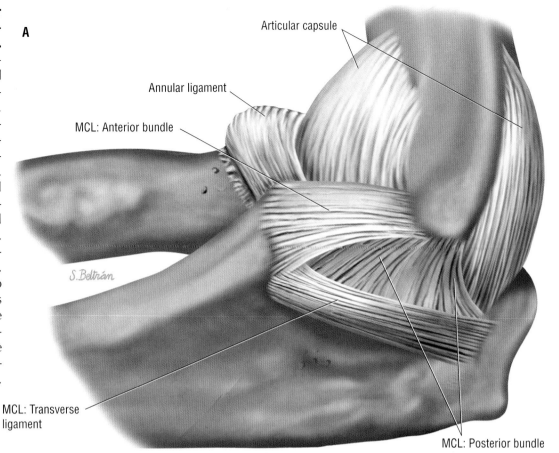

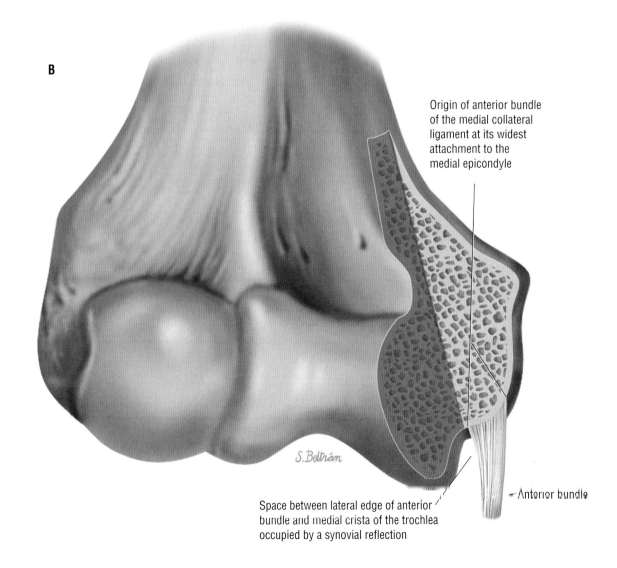

Valgus Stress in the Throwing Arm

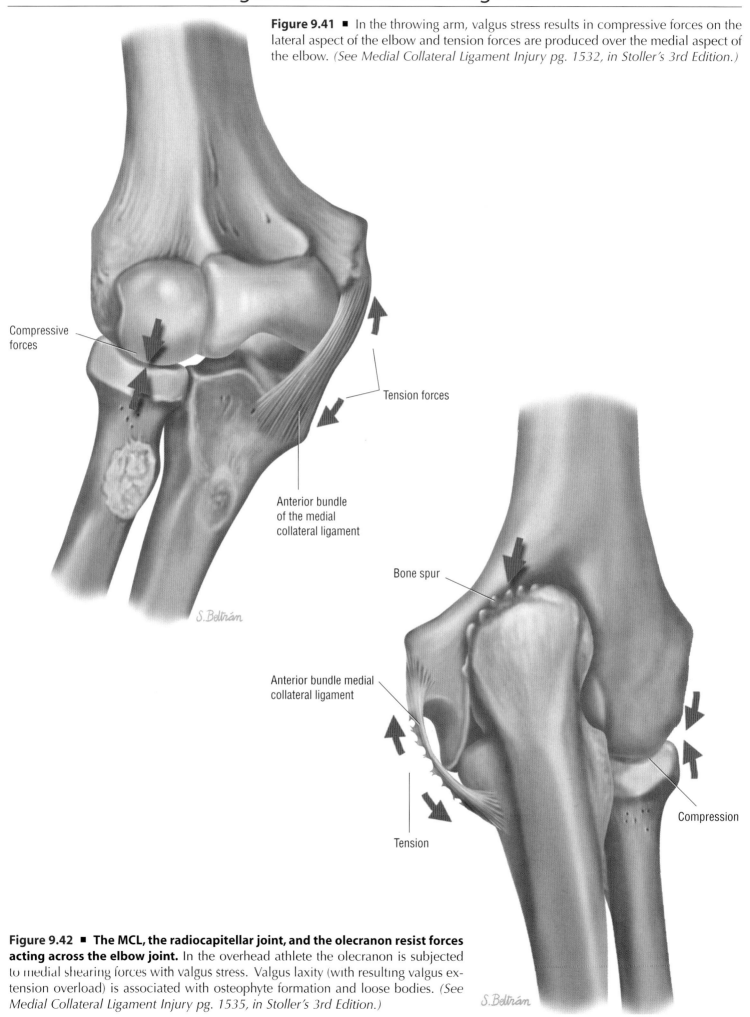

Figure 9.41 ■ In the throwing arm, valgus stress results in compressive forces on the lateral aspect of the elbow and tension forces are produced over the medial aspect of the elbow. *(See Medial Collateral Ligament Injury pg. 1532, in Stoller's 3rd Edition.)*

Compressive forces

Tension forces

Anterior bundle of the medial collateral ligament

S. Beltrán

Bone spur

Anterior bundle medial collateral ligament

Compression

Tension

Figure 9.42 ■ **The MCL, the radiocapitellar joint, and the olecranon resist forces acting across the elbow joint.** In the overhead athlete the olecranon is subjected to medial shearing forces with valgus stress. Valgus laxity (with resulting valgus extension overload) is associated with osteophyte formation and loose bodies. *(See Medial Collateral Ligament Injury pg. 1535, in Stoller's 3rd Edition.)*   *S. Beltrán*

Figure 9.43 ■ Acute rupture of the distal anterior bundle. *(See Medial Collateral Ligament Injury pg. 1536, in Stoller's 3rd Edition.)*

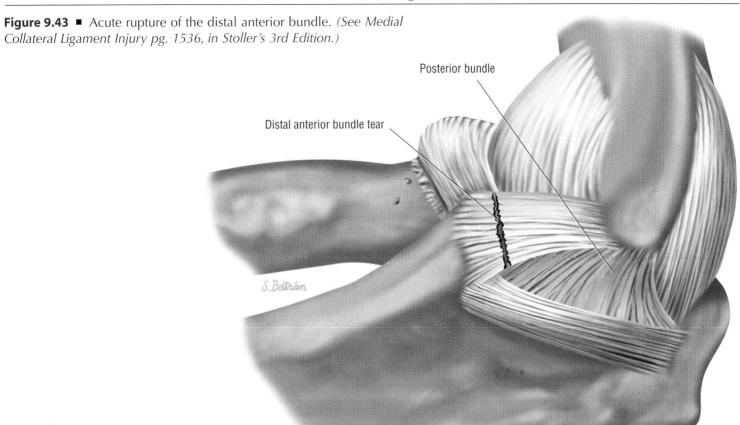

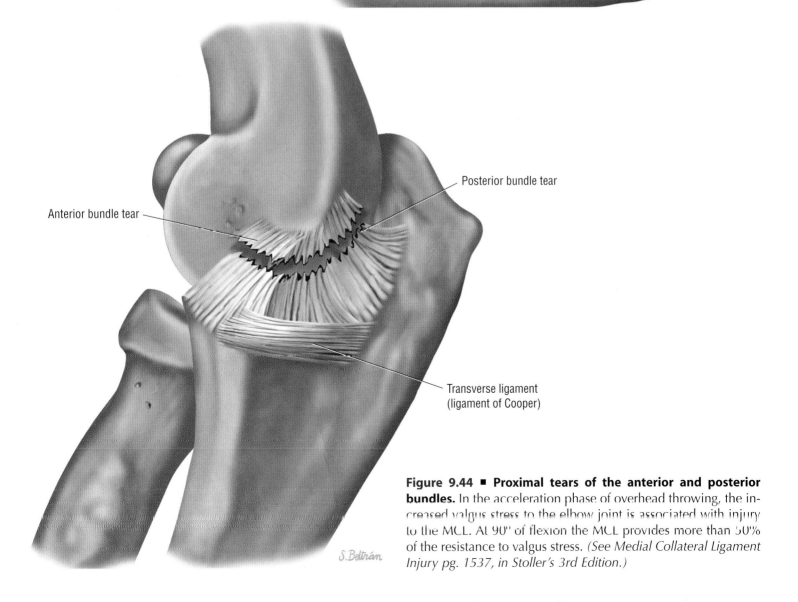

Figure 9.44 ■ Proximal tears of the anterior and posterior bundles. In the acceleration phase of overhead throwing, the increased valgus stress to the elbow joint is associated with injury to the MCL. At 90° of flexion the MCL provides more than 50% of the resistance to valgus stress. *(See Medial Collateral Ligament Injury pg. 1537, in Stoller's 3rd Edition.)*

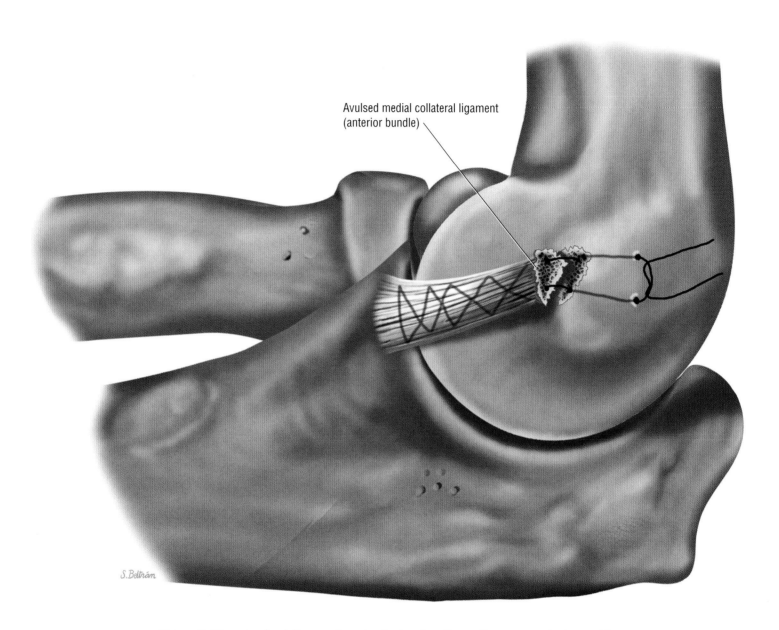

Avulsed medial collateral ligament
(anterior bundle)

S.Beltrán

Figure 9.45 ■ Avulsed ligament reattached using Bunnell suture technique. *(See Treatment pg. 1541, in Stoller's 3rd Edition.)*

Figure 9.46 ■ Medial collateral ligament (MCL or UCL) standard three-ply recon-struction. *Based on Safran MC. Elbow injuries in athletes. Clinics in Sports Medicine 2004; 23(4): xvii–xix. (See Treatment pg. 1541, in Stoller's 3rd Edition.)*

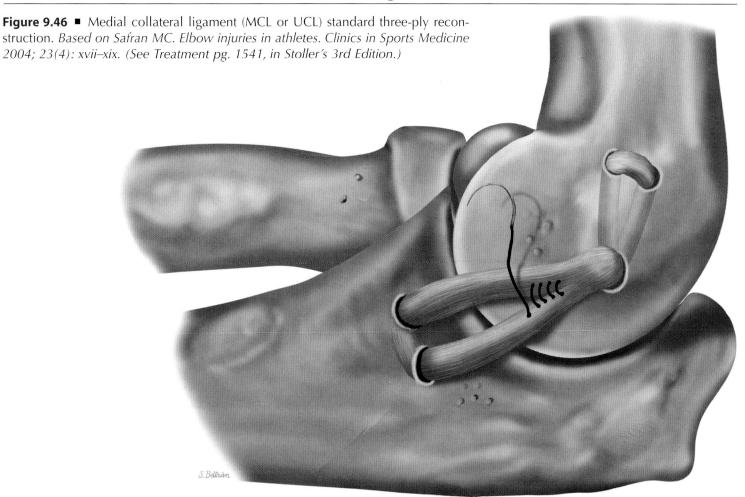

Figure 9.47 ■ The docking procedure uses a two-ply reconstruc-tion and is easier to tension the graft. *Based on Safran MC. Elbow injuries in athletes. Clinics in Sports Medicine 2004; 23(4): xvii–xix. (See Treatment pg. 1541, in Stoller's 3rd Edition.)*

Blind ended tunnels

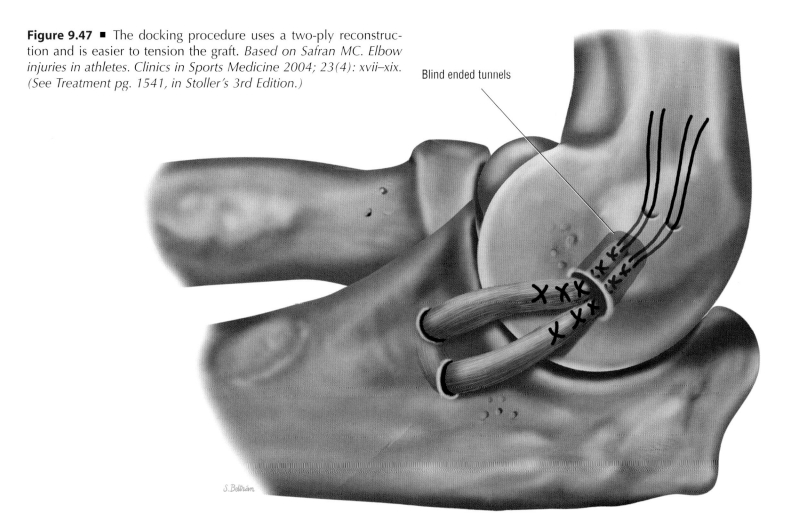

Figure 9.48 ■ **Muscle strain and partial tear of the MCL.**
Sagittal color illustration, medial perspective. In the evaluation of medial epicondylitis, especially in the throwing
athlete, the MCL should be assessed for instability secondary to excessive valgus forces. *(See Medial Epicondylitis
pg. 1542, in Stoller's 3rd Edition.)*

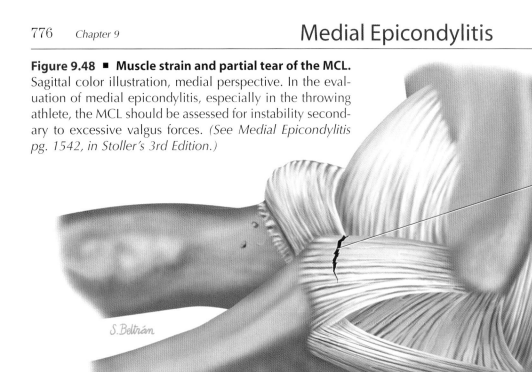

Partial tear anterior bundle
medial collateral ligament

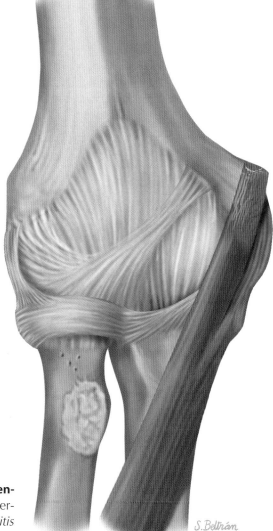

Figure 9.49 ■ **Microtear of the humeral head origin of the pronator teres with tendon degeneration and associated inflammatory synovitis.** Angiofibroblastic hyperplasia is characterized by gray and friable pathologic tissue. *(See Medial Epicondylitis
pg. 1543, in Stoller's 3rd Edition.)*

Figure 9.50 ▪ **Medial epicondylitis findings include macroscopic partial or complete tearing of the flexor-pronator origin and tears of the MCL.** Overuse tendinopathy of the flexor-pronator group is caused by chronic valgus stress and therefore often is associated with throwing sports. *(See Medial Epicondylitis pg. 1544, in Stoller's 3rd Edition.)*

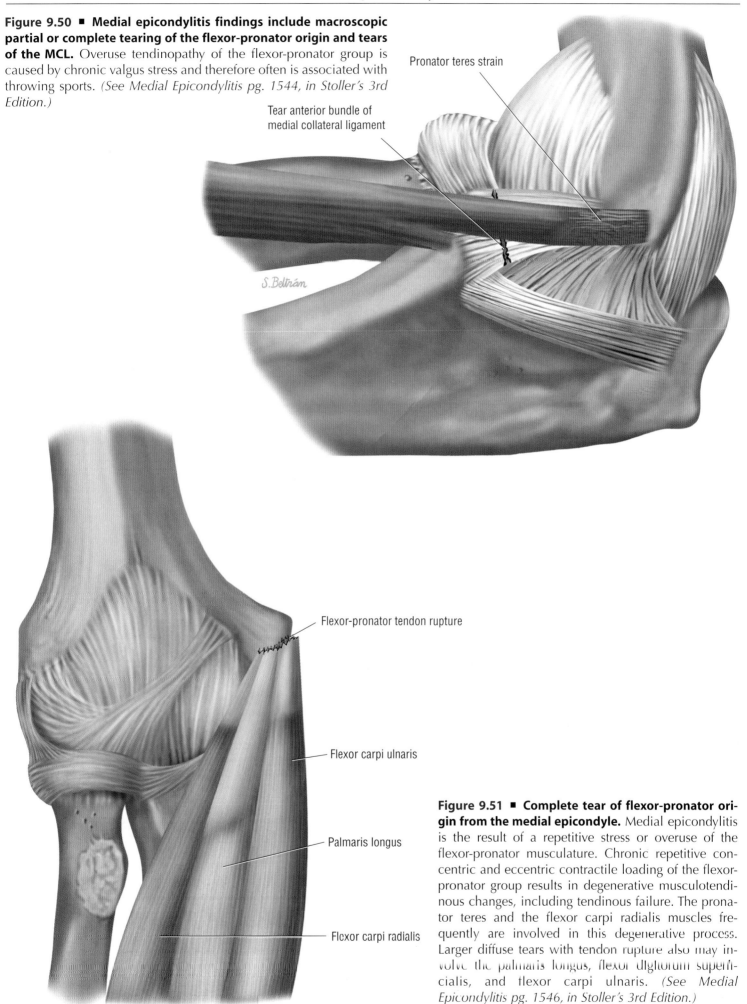

Pronator teres strain

Tear anterior bundle of medial collateral ligament

S. Beltrán

Flexor-pronator tendon rupture

Flexor carpi ulnaris

Palmaris longus

Flexor carpi radialis

Figure 9.51 ▪ **Complete tear of flexor-pronator origin from the medial epicondyle.** Medial epicondylitis is the result of a repetitive stress or overuse of the flexor-pronator musculature. Chronic repetitive concentric and eccentric contractile loading of the flexor-pronator group results in degenerative musculotendinous changes, including tendinous failure. The pronator teres and the flexor carpi radialis muscles frequently are involved in this degenerative process. Larger diffuse tears with tendon rupture also may involve the palmaris longus, flexor digitorum superficialis, and flexor carpi ulnaris. *(See Medial Epicondylitis pg. 1546, in Stoller's 3rd Edition.)*

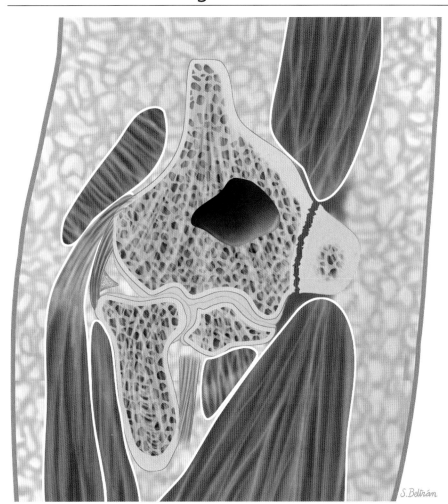

Figure 9.52 ■ Little Leaguer's elbow is an extension overload injury (valgus stress) with medial epicondylar avulsion. The childhood injury pattern is microtrauma to the apophysis and ossification center of the medial epicondyle. The adolescent pattern is an avulsion of the medial epicondyle and possible nonunion injury. *(See Little Leaguer's Elbow pg. 1547, in Stoller's 3rd Edition.)*

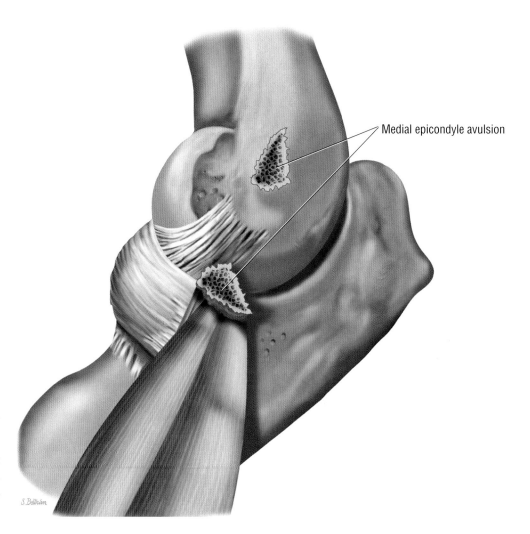

Medial epicondyle avulsion

Figure 9.53 ■ Avulsion fracture secondary to throwing stresses. There is a displaced fracture of the medial epicondyle with attached anterior bundle of the medial collateral ligament and flexor muscle mass. *(See Little Leaguer's Elbow pg. 1547, in Stoller's 3rd Edition.)*

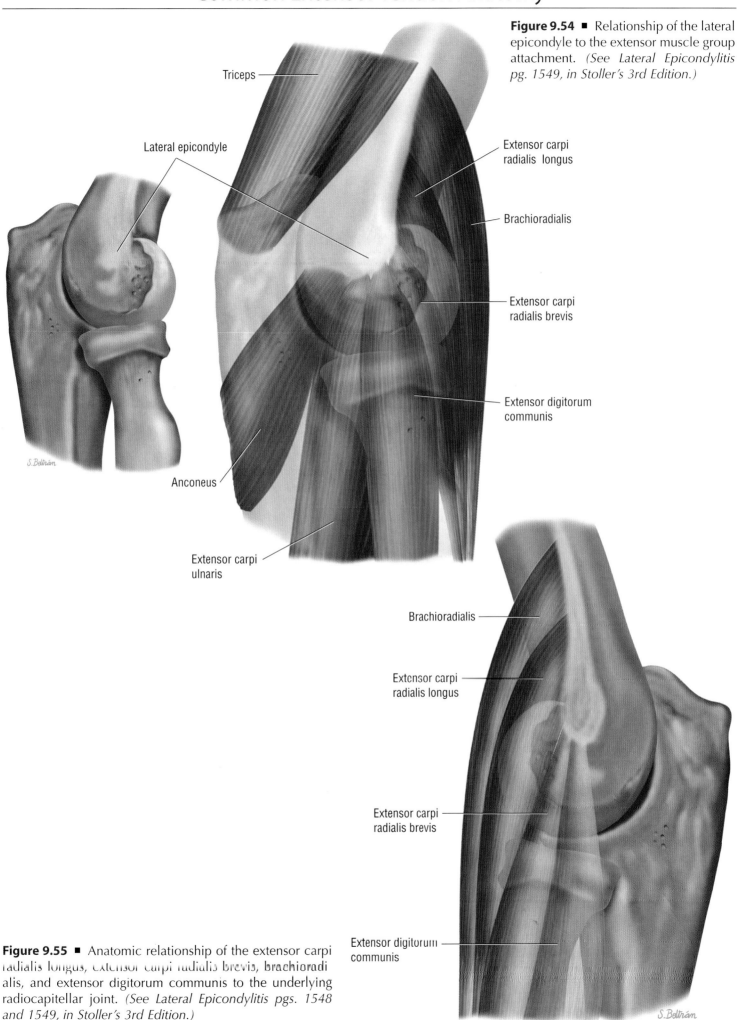

Figure 9.54 ■ Relationship of the lateral epicondyle to the extensor muscle group attachment. *(See Lateral Epicondylitis pg. 1549, in Stoller's 3rd Edition.)*

Triceps

Lateral epicondyle

Anconeus

Extensor carpi ulnaris

Extensor carpi radialis longus

Brachioradialis

Extensor carpi radialis brevis

Extensor digitorum communis

Brachioradialis

Extensor carpi radialis longus

Extensor carpi radialis brevis

Extensor digitorum communis

Figure 9.55 ■ Anatomic relationship of the extensor carpi radialis longus, extensor carpi radialis brevis, brachioradialis, and extensor digitorum communis to the underlying radiocapitellar joint. *(See Lateral Epicondylitis pgs. 1548 and 1549, in Stoller's 3rd Edition.)*

Angiofibroblastic Tendinosis

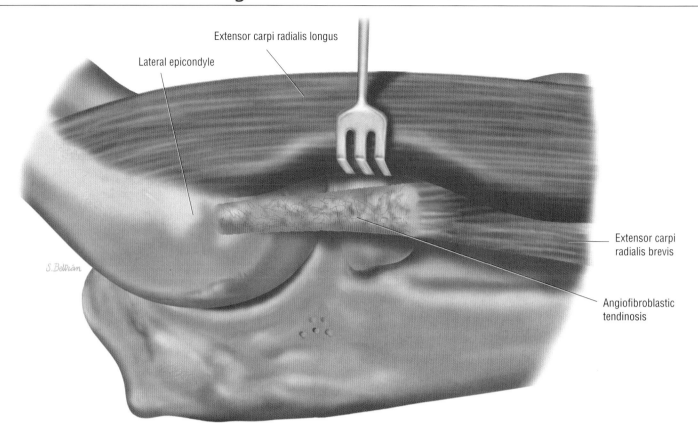

Lateral epicondyle

Extensor carpi radialis longus

Extensor carpi radialis brevis

Angiofibroblastic tendinosis

S.Beltrán

Figure 9.56 ■ Degeneration of the origin of the extensor carpi radialis brevis. *Based on Morrey BF, Thompson RCJr. The elbow; master techniques in orthopaedic surgery. New York: Raven Press, 1994. (See Lateral Epicondylitis pgs. 1550 and 1552, in Stoller's 3rd Edition.)*

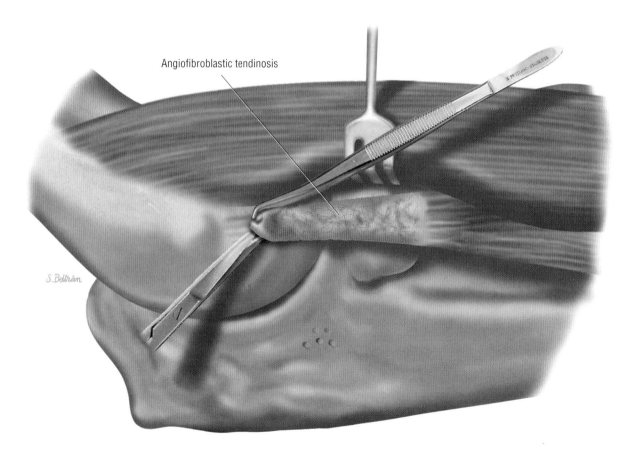

Angiofibroblastic tendinosis

S.Beltrán

Figure 9.57 ■ **Resection of degenerative and partial torn pathologic section of the extensor carpi radialis brevis origin.** The extensor aponeurosis, however, is never totally released from the epicondyle. *Based on Morrey, BF, Thompson RC Jr. The elbow; master techniques in orthopaedic surgery. New York: Raven Press, 1994. (See Lateral Epicondytitis pgs. 1550 and 1552, in Stoller's 3rd Edition.)*

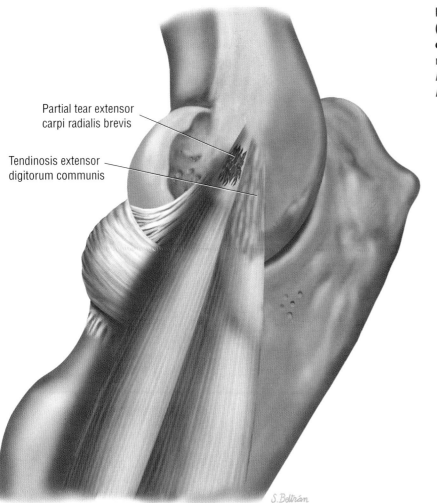

Partial tear extensor carpi radialis brevis

Tendinosis extensor digitorum communis

Figure 9.58 ▪ Partial tear with granulation tissue (angiofibroblastic tendinosis) at the origin of the extensor carpi radialis brevis. There is also tendinosis of the extensor digitorum communis. *(See Lateral Epicondylitis pg. 1550, in Stoller's 3rd Edition.)*

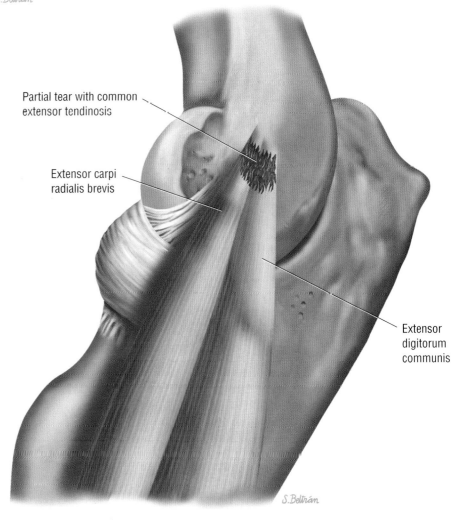

Partial tear with common extensor tendinosis

Extensor carpi radialis brevis

Extensor digitorum communis

Figure 9.59 ▪ In lateral epicondylitis, angiofibroblastic tendinosis (disorganized, immature collagen formation with immature fibroblastic and vascular elements) is secondary to eccentric or concentric overloading of the extensor muscle mass. The extensor digitorum communis also may be involved in addition to the preferentially affected extensor carpi radialis brevis. *(See Lateral Epicondylitis pg. 1552, in Stoller's 3rd Edition.)*

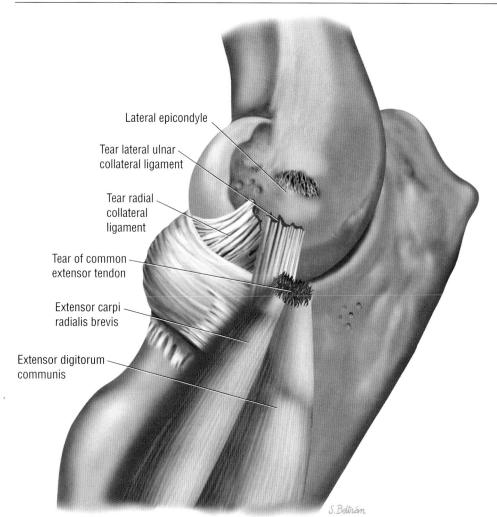

Lateral epicondyle

Tear lateral ulnar collateral ligament

Tear radial collateral ligament

Tear of common extensor tendon

Extensor carpi radialis brevis

Extensor digitorum communis

Figure 9.60 ■ **A complete massive tear of the common extensor tendon and lateral collateral ligament complex except for the annular ligament.** Lateral epicondylitis is a degenerative tendinopathy. The term "epicondylitis" is misleading, as inflammation is present only in the initial stages of the disease. Angiofibroblastic tendinosis is present with partial to complete tearing of the extensor carpi radialis brevis tendon. Lateral color illustration. *(See Lateral Collateral Ligament Injury pg. 1553, in Stoller's 3rd Edition.)*

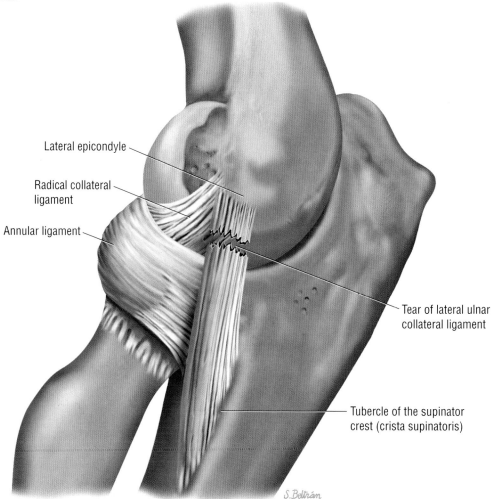

Lateral epicondyle

Radical collateral ligament

Annular ligament

Tear of lateral ulnar collateral ligament

Tubercle of the supinator crest (crista supinatoris)

Figure 9.61 ■ **Tear of the LUCL of the lateral collateral ligament complex of the elbow.** The other components of the lateral collateral ligament complex include the radial collateral ligament, the annular ligament, and the accessory lateral collateral ligament. Lateral instability of the elbow ranges from mild laxity to recurrent dislocation. *(See Lateral Collateral Ligament Injury pg. 1557, in Stoller's 3rd Edition.)*

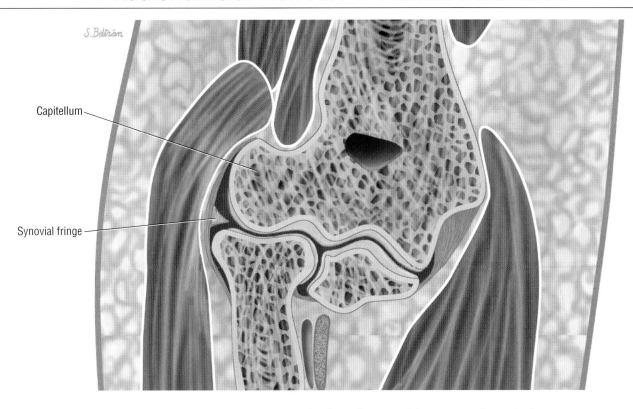

Figure 9.62 ■ **Radiohumeral meniscus.** The lateral synovial fringe or radiocapitellar meniscus is not a true fibrocartilaginous meniscus. Located posterolaterally, the synovial fringe may become inflamed or thickened. Symptoms of thickening and inflammation may mimic tennis elbow. *(See Other Causes of Lateral Elbow Pain pgs. 1555 and1559, in Stoller's 3rd Edition.)*

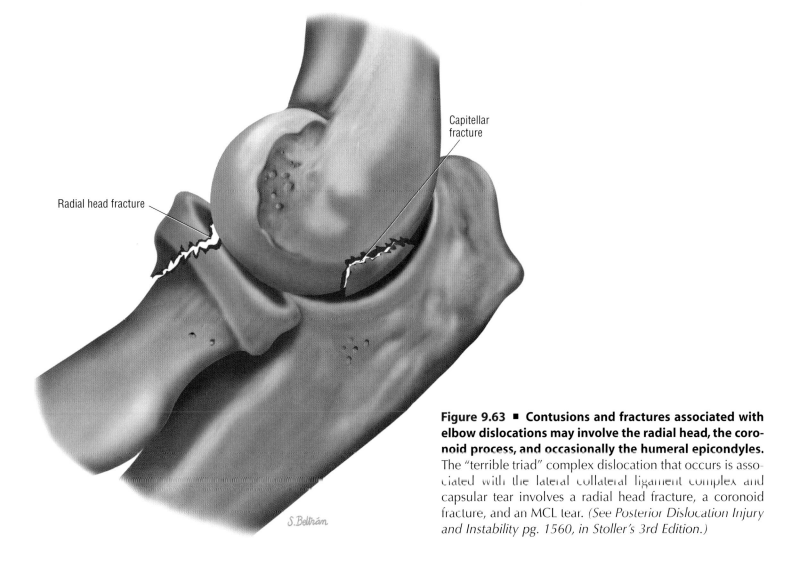

Figure 9.63 ■ **Contusions and fractures associated with elbow dislocations may involve the radial head, the coronoid process, and occasionally the humeral epicondyles.** The "terrible triad" complex dislocation that occurs is associated with the lateral collateral ligament complex and capsular tear involves a radial head fracture, a coronoid fracture, and an MCL tear. *(See Posterior Dislocation Injury and Instability pg. 1560, in Stoller's 3rd Edition.)*

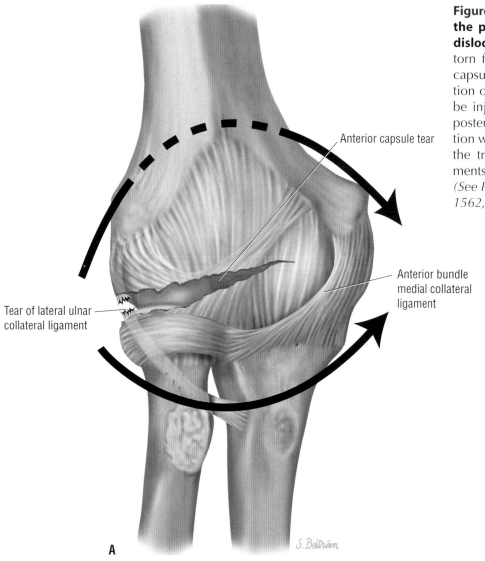

A

Figure 9.64 ■ **The circle of Horii representing the progression of structures injured in elbow dislocation.** The lateral ligamentous complex is torn first, followed by the anterior and posterior capsule, with the dislocation completed by disruption of the MCL. The MCL is the final structure to be injured and may be intact in the presence of posterolateral instability. **(A)** Coronal color illustration with anterior perspective. **(B)** Superior view of the trochlear notch, radial head, collateral ligaments, and capsule with the humerus removed. *(See Posterior Dislocation Injury and Instability pg. 1562, in Stoller's 3rd Edition.)*

Anterior capsule tear

Anterior bundle medial collateral ligament

Tear of lateral ulnar collateral ligament

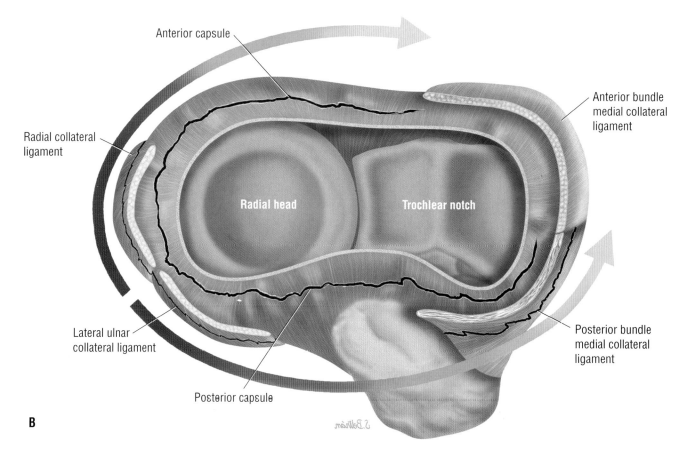

B

Anterior capsule

Radial collateral ligament

Lateral ulnar collateral ligament

Posterior capsule

Radial head

Trochlear notch

Anterior bundle medial collateral ligament

Posterior bundle medial collateral ligament

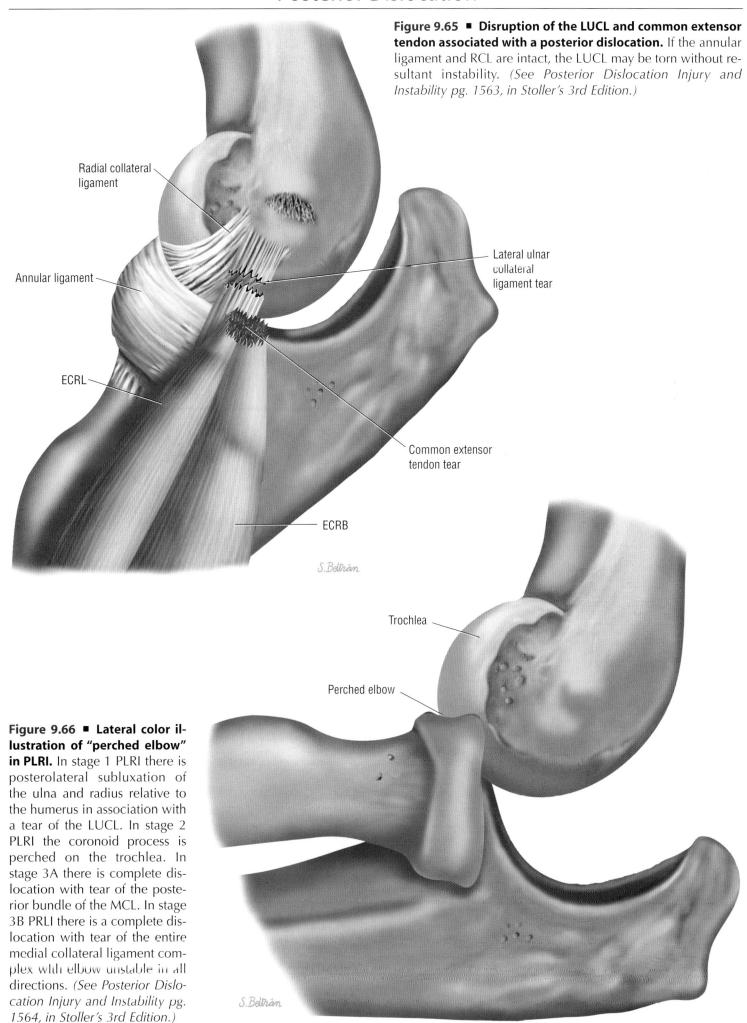

Figure 9.65 ▪ Disruption of the LUCL and common extensor tendon associated with a posterior dislocation. If the annular ligament and RCL are intact, the LUCL may be torn without resultant instability. *(See Posterior Dislocation Injury and Instability pg. 1563, in Stoller's 3rd Edition.)*

Radial collateral ligament

Annular ligament

ECRL

ECRB

Lateral ulnar collateral ligament tear

Common extensor tendon tear

Trochlea

Perched elbow

Figure 9.66 ▪ Lateral color illustration of "perched elbow" in PLRI. In stage 1 PLRI there is posterolateral subluxation of the ulna and radius relative to the humerus in association with a tear of the LUCL. In stage 2 PLRI the coronoid process is perched on the trochlea. In stage 3A there is complete dislocation with tear of the posterior bundle of the MCL. In stage 3B PRLI there is a complete dislocation with tear of the entire medial collateral ligament complex with elbow unstable in all directions. *(See Posterior Dislocation Injury and Instability pg. 1564, in Stoller's 3rd Edition.)*

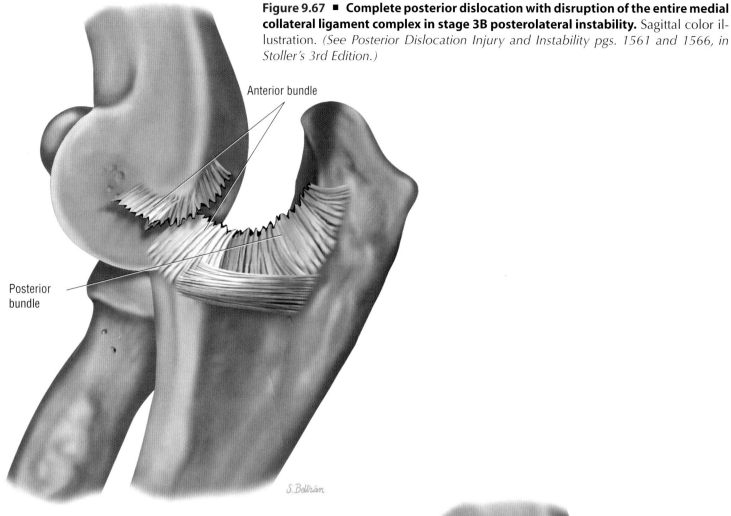

Figure 9.67 ■ **Complete posterior dislocation with disruption of the entire medial collateral ligament complex in stage 3B posterolateral instability.** Sagittal color illustration. *(See Posterior Dislocation Injury and Instability pgs. 1561 and 1566, in Stoller's 3rd Edition.)*

Anterior bundle

Posterior bundle

S.Beltrán

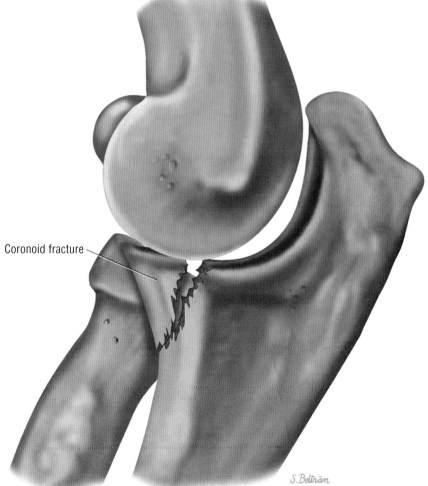

Coronoid fracture

Figure 9.68 ■ **Lateral color illustration of a coronoid process fracture.** A coronoid (Regan/Morrey) fracture is a distraction injury caused by bony avulsion of the brachialis insertion by posterior dislocation of the ulna. The etiology is related to a fall on an outstretched hand and hyperextension of the elbow. *(See Posterior Dislocation Injury and Instability pg. 1568, in Stoller's 3rd Edition.)*

S.Beltrán

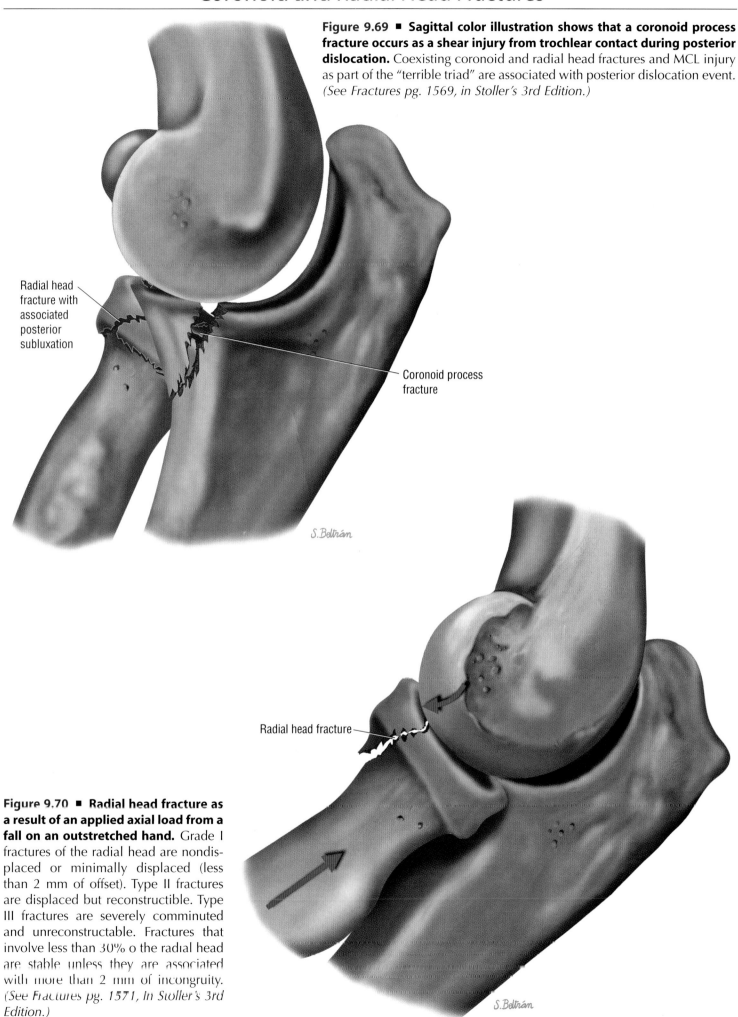

Figure 9.69 ▪ **Sagittal color illustration shows that a coronoid process fracture occurs as a shear injury from trochlear contact during posterior dislocation.** Coexisting coronoid and radial head fractures and MCL injury as part of the "terrible triad" are associated with posterior dislocation event. *(See Fractures pg. 1569, in Stoller's 3rd Edition.)*

Radial head fracture with associated posterior subluxation

Coronoid process fracture

S.Beltrán

Radial head fracture

Figure 9.70 ▪ **Radial head fracture as a result of an applied axial load from a fall on an outstretched hand.** Grade I fractures of the radial head are nondisplaced or minimally displaced (less than 2 mm of offset). Type II fractures are displaced but reconstructible. Type III fractures are severely comminuted and unreconstructable. Fractures that involve less than 30% o the radial head are stable unless they are associated with more than 2 mm of incongruity. *(See Fractures pg. 1571, In Stoller's 3rd Edition.)*

S.Beltrán

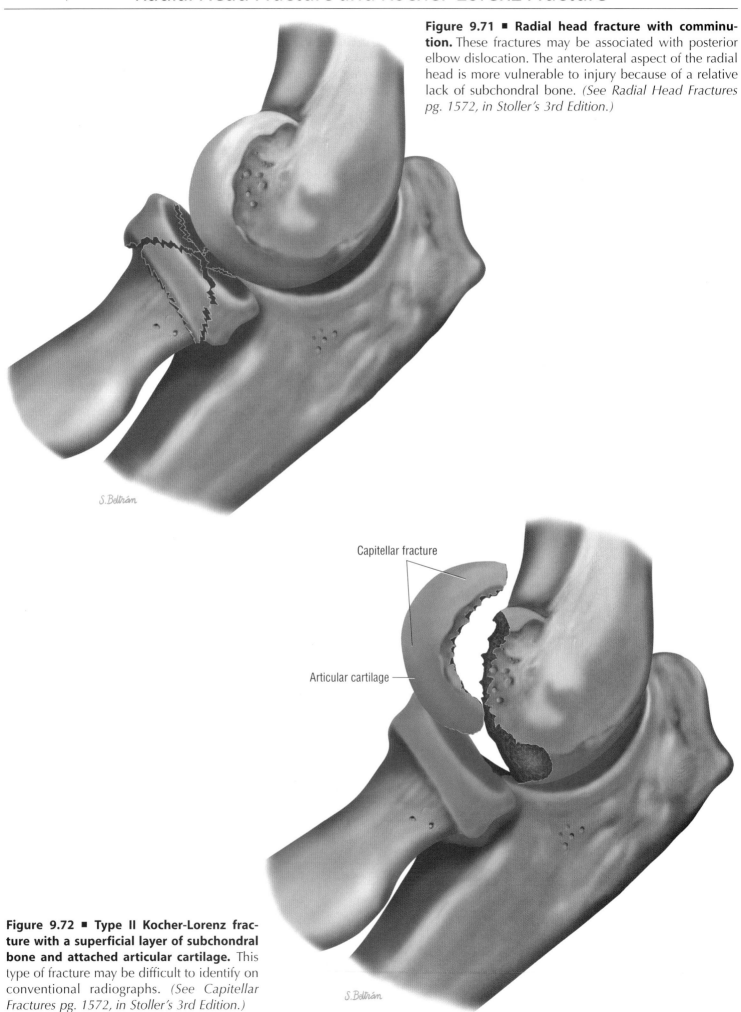

Figure 9.71 ▪ Radial head fracture with comminution. These fractures may be associated with posterior elbow dislocation. The anterolateral aspect of the radial head is more vulnerable to injury because of a relative lack of subchondral bone. *(See Radial Head Fractures pg. 1572, in Stoller's 3rd Edition.)*

Capitellar fracture

Articular cartilage

Figure 9.72 ▪ Type II Kocher-Lorenz fracture with a superficial layer of subchondral bone and attached articular cartilage. This type of fracture may be difficult to identify on conventional radiographs. *(See Capitellar Fractures pg. 1572, in Stoller's 3rd Edition.)*

S.Beltrán

S.Beltrán

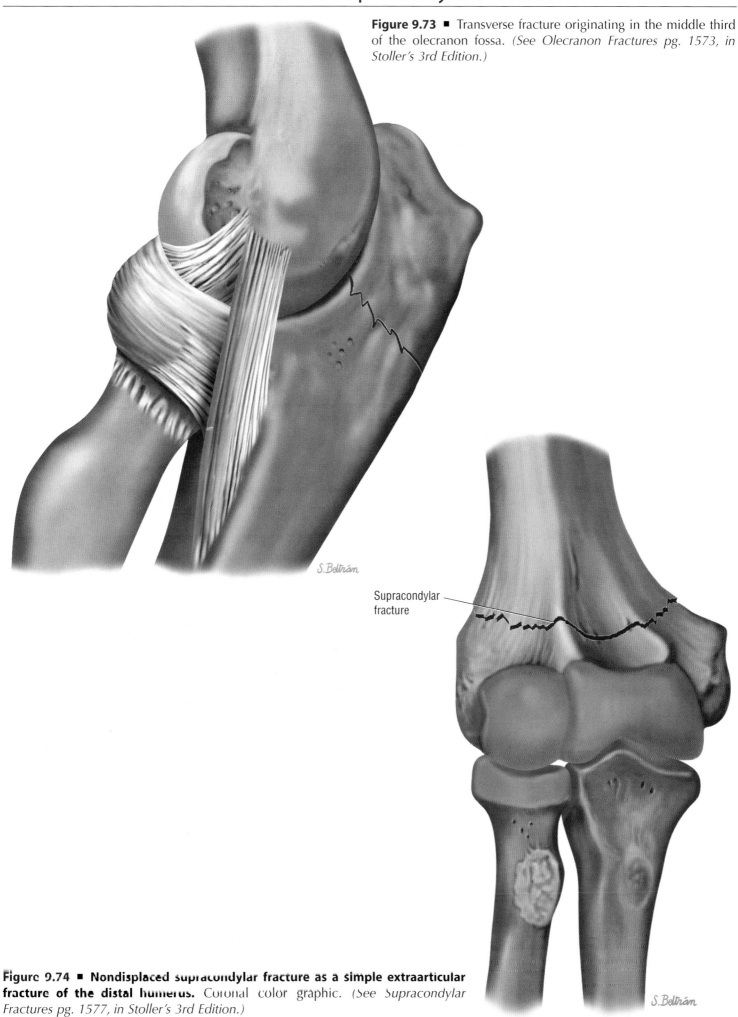

Figure 9.73 ■ Transverse fracture originating in the middle third of the olecranon fossa. *(See Olecranon Fractures pg. 1573, in Stoller's 3rd Edition.)*

S.Beltrán

Supracondylar fracture

Figure 9.74 ■ **Nondisplaced supracondylar fracture as a simple extraarticular fracture of the distal humerus.** Coronal color graphic. *(See Supracondylar Fractures pg. 1577, in Stoller's 3rd Edition.)*

S.Beltrán

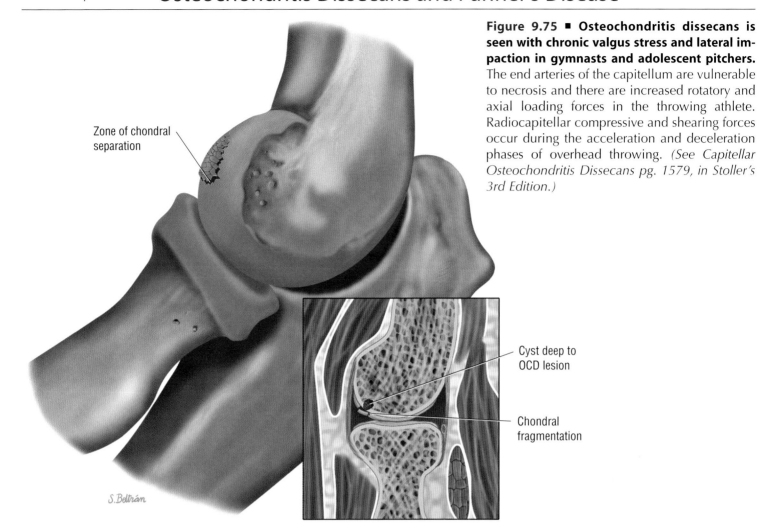

Zone of chondral separation

Cyst deep to OCD lesion

Chondral fragmentation

Figure 9.75 ▪ Osteochondritis dissecans is seen with chronic valgus stress and lateral impaction in gymnasts and adolescent pitchers. The end arteries of the capitellum are vulnerable to necrosis and there are increased rotatory and axial loading forces in the throwing athlete. Radiocapitellar compressive and shearing forces occur during the acceleration and deceleration phases of overhead throwing. *(See Capitellar Osteochondritis Dissecans pg. 1579, in Stoller's 3rd Edition.)*

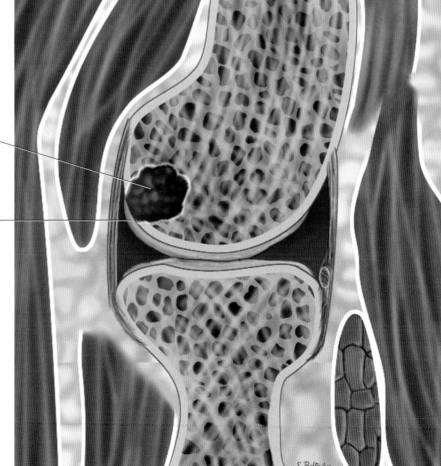

Subchondral cystic change within ischemic zone

Intact articular cartilage

Figure 9.76 ▪ Panner's disease is seen in a younger patient population (5- to 11-year-old patients) compared to osteochondritis dissecans. Loose body formation and residual deformity usually are not seen in Panner's disease. Panner's disease is associated with avascular necrosis secondary to trauma. *(See Panner's Disease pg. 1583, in Stoller's 3rd Edition.)*

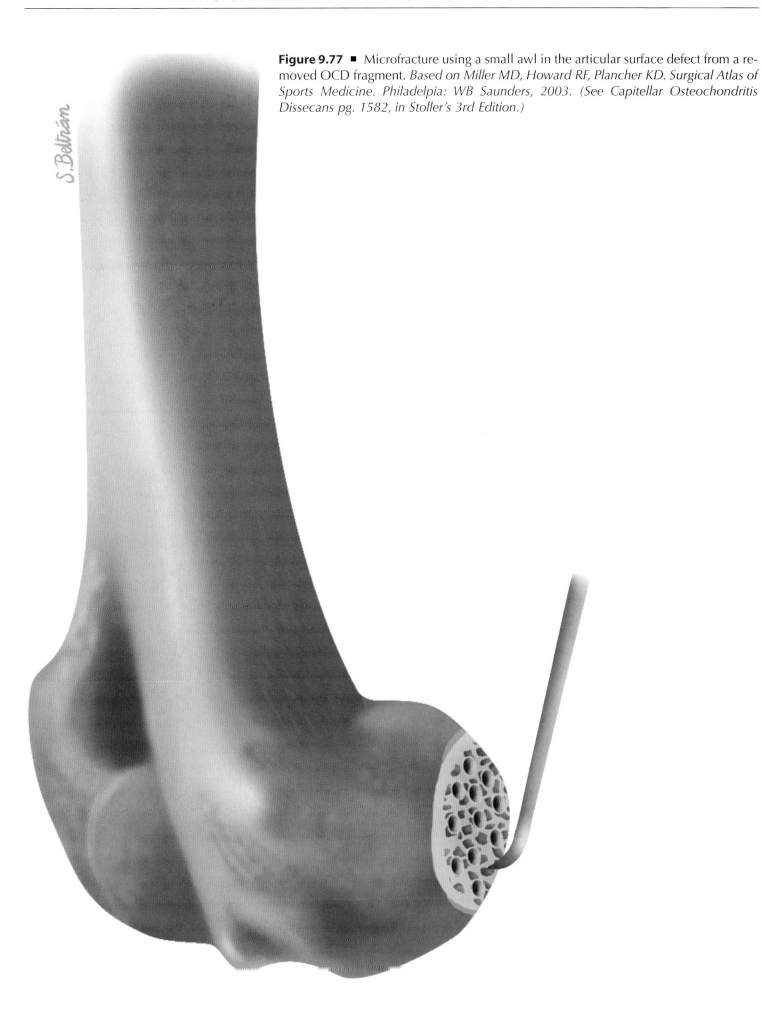

Figure 9.77 ■ Microfracture using a small awl in the articular surface defect from a removed OCD fragment. *Based on Miller MD, Howard RF, Plancher KD. Surgical Atlas of Sports Medicine. Philadelpia: WB Saunders, 2003. (See Capitellar Osteochondritis Dissecans pg. 1582, in Stoller's 3rd Edition.)*

Osteophytes

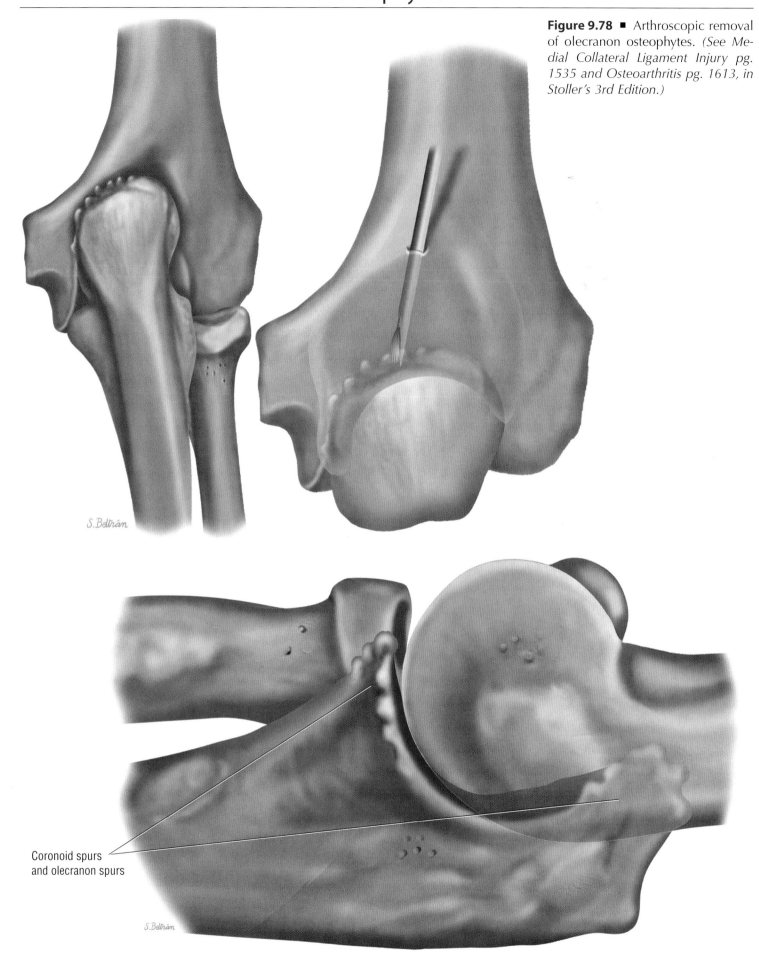

Figure 9.78 ■ Arthroscopic removal of olecranon osteophytes. *(See Medial Collateral Ligament Injury pg. 1535 and Osteoarthritis pg. 1613, in Stoller's 3rd Edition.)*

S.Beltrán

Coronoid spurs
and olecranon spurs

S.Beltrán

Figure 9.79 ■ Coronoid and olecranon osteophytes resulting from stress occurring during the follow-through phase of throwing. *(See Medial Collateral Ligament Injury pg. 1535 and Osteoarthritis pg. 1613, in Stoller's 3rd Edition.)*

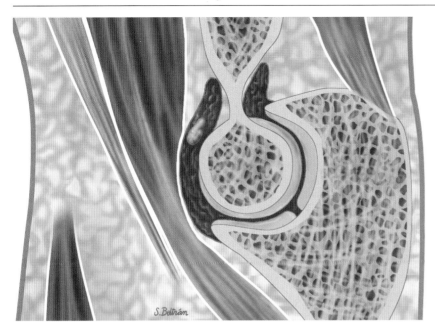

Figure 9.80 ▪ **Loose bodies form from a nidus of cartilage or an osteochondral fragment.** The loose body may be unattached or pedunculated with a tether of synovium. *(See Loose Bodies pg. 1586, in Stoller's 3rd Edition.)*

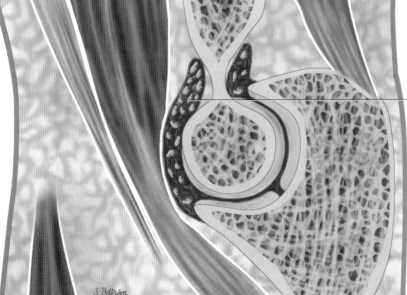

Figure 9.81 ▪ Synovial osteochondromatosis on a sagittal color section. *(See Idiopathic Synovial Osteochondromatosis pg. 1591, in Stoller's 3rd Edition.)*

Synovial osteochondromatosis with synovial proliferation

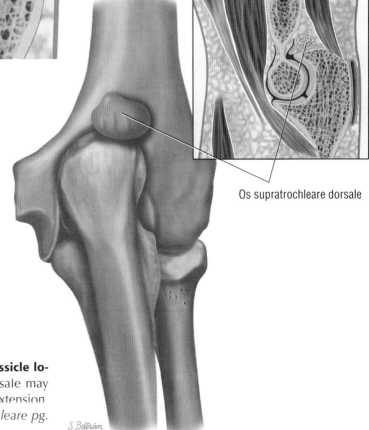

Os supratrochleare dorsale

Figure 9.82 ▪ **Os supratrochleare dorsale is an accessory ossicle located within the olecranon fossa.** The os supratrochleare dorsale may be symptomatic and associated with pain and loss of elbow extension. It is typically between 1 and 2 cm in size. *(See Os Supratrochleare pg. 1589, in Stoller's 3rd Edition.)*

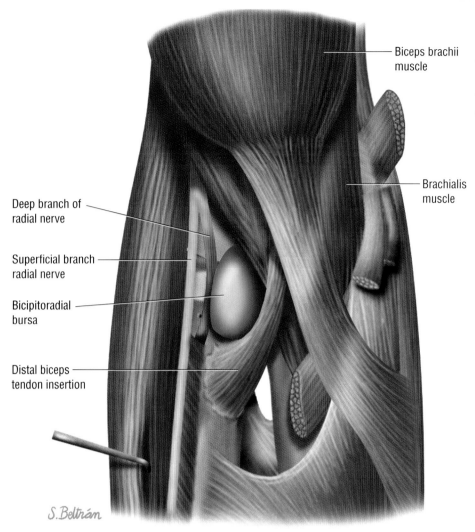

Biceps brachii
muscle

Deep branch of
radial nerve

Superficial branch
radial nerve

Bicipitoradial
bursa

Distal biceps
tendon insertion

Brachialis
muscle

S. Beltrán

Figure 9.83 ■ **Bicipitoradial bursitis may present as an antecubital mass or as pain associated with supination.** Associated abnormalities include biceps tendinopathy tears and radial tuberosity hypertrophy. Coronal color illustration. *(See Biceps Tendon Injury pgs. 1594 and 1596, in Stoller's 3rd Edition.)*

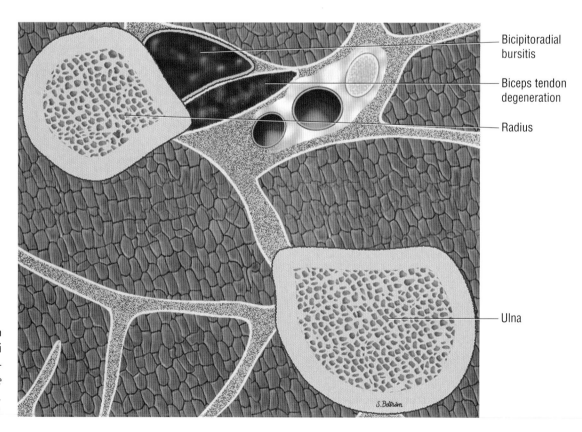

Bicipitoradial
bursitis

Biceps tendon
degeneration

Radius

Ulna

S. Beltrán

Figure 9.84 ■ Degeneration of the distal biceps brachii tendon associated with bicipitoradial (cubital) bursitis. *(See Biceps Tendon Injury pg. 1596, in Stoller's 3rd Edition.)*

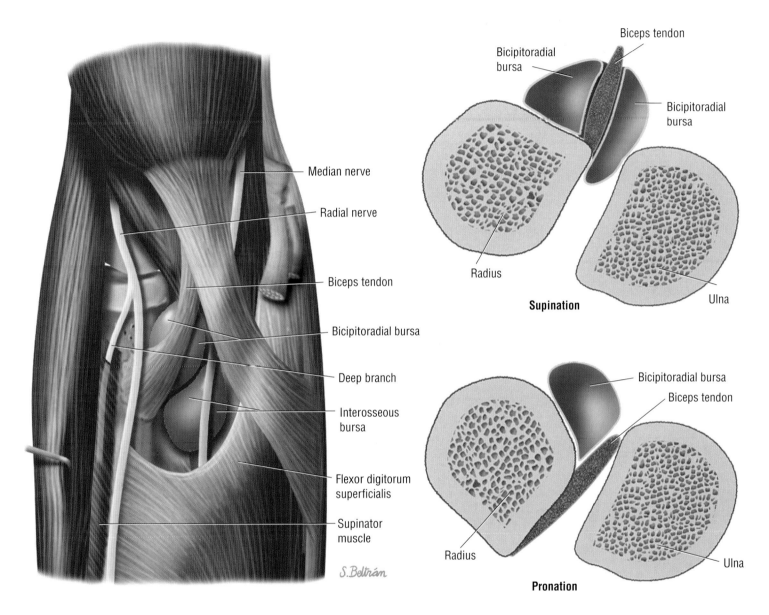

Median nerve

Radial nerve

Biceps tendon

Bicipitoradial bursa

Deep branch

Interosseous bursa

Flexor digitorum superficialis

Supinator muscle

S.Beltrán

Biceps tendon

Bicipitoradial bursa

Bicipitoradial bursa

Radius

Ulna

Supination

Bicipitoradial bursa

Biceps tendon

Radius

Ulna

Pronation

Figure 9.85 ■ In pronation, the rotation of the radial tuberosity compresses the bicipitoradial bursa between the biceps tendon and radial cortex. *Based on Skaf AY, Boutin RD, Dantas RWM, et al. Bicipitoradial bursitis: MR imaging findings in eight patients and anatomic data from contrast material opacification of bursae followed by routine radiography and MR imaging in cadavers. Radiology 1999; 212:111. (See Biceps Tendon Injury pg. 1596, in Stoller's 3rd Edition.)*

Biceps Tendon Rupture

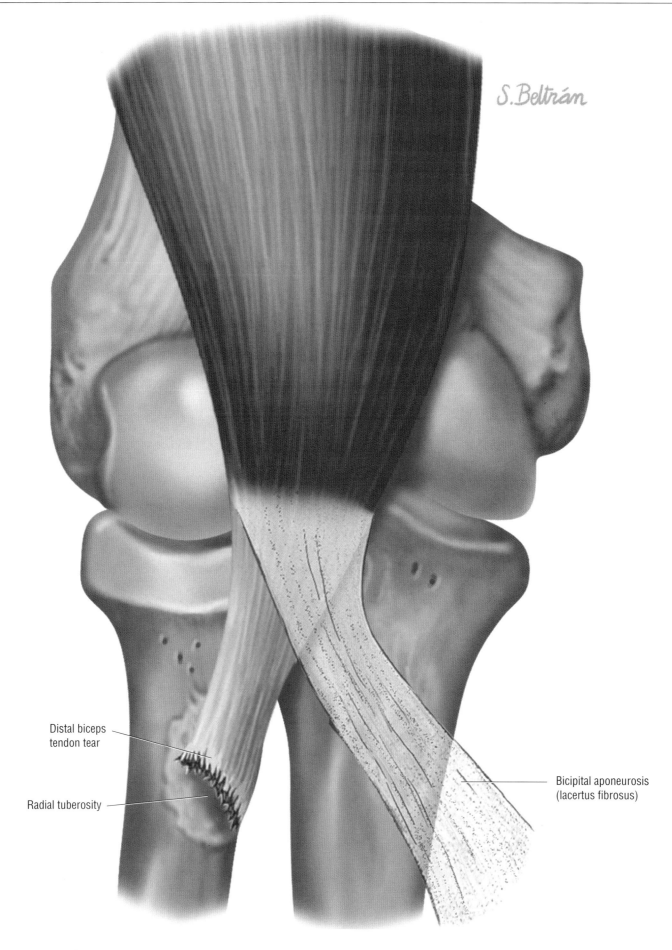

S.Beltrán

Distal biceps
tendon tear

Radial tuberosity

Bicipital aponeurosis
(lacertus fibrosus)

**Figure 9.86 ■ Coronal color illustration of distal biceps tendon rupture from the radial tuberos-
ity.** The intact lacertus fibrosus limits proximal retraction of the tendon. The lacertus fibrosus originates from the medial aspect of the biceps muscle belly and inserts onto the dorsal aspect of the
ulna. *(See Biceps Tendon Injury pgs. 1593 and 1594, in Stoller's 3rd Edition.)*

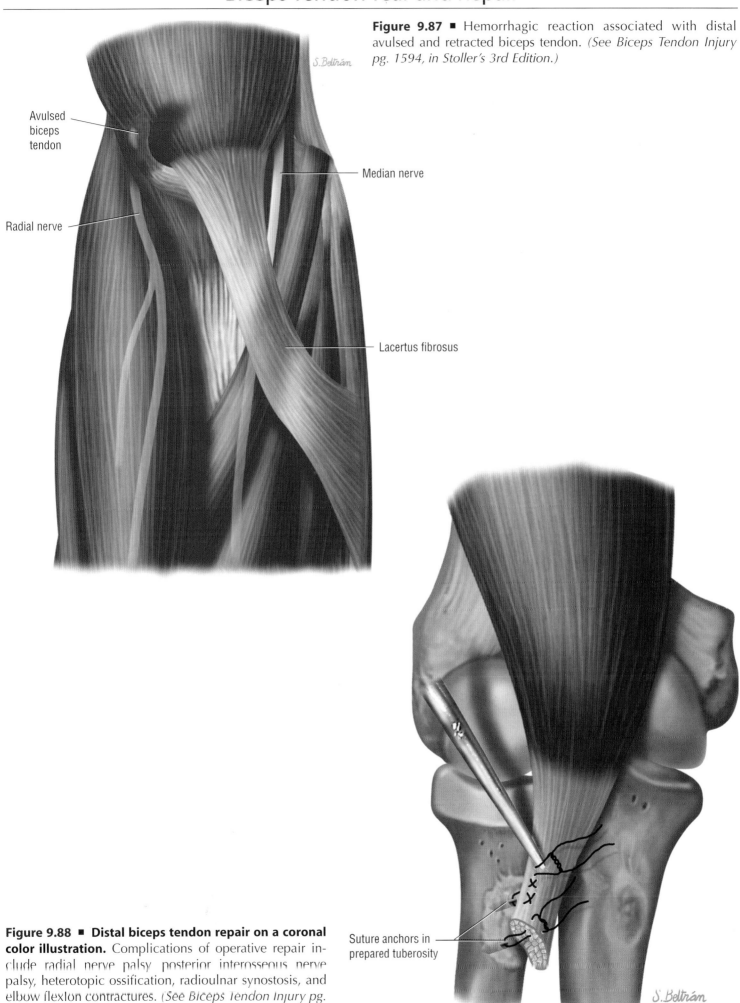

Figure 9.87 ■ Hemorrhagic reaction associated with distal avulsed and retracted biceps tendon. *(See Biceps Tendon Injury pg. 1594, in Stoller's 3rd Edition.)*

Avulsed biceps tendon

Radial nerve

Median nerve

Lacertus fibrosus

Suture anchors in prepared tuberosity

Figure 9.88 ■ **Distal biceps tendon repair on a coronal color illustration.** Complications of operative repair include radial nerve palsy, posterior interosseous nerve palsy, heterotopic ossification, radioulnar synostosis, and elbow flexion contractures. *(See Biceps Tendon Injury pg. 1598, in Stoller's 3rd Edition.)*

Triceps Tendon Rupture and Tendinosis

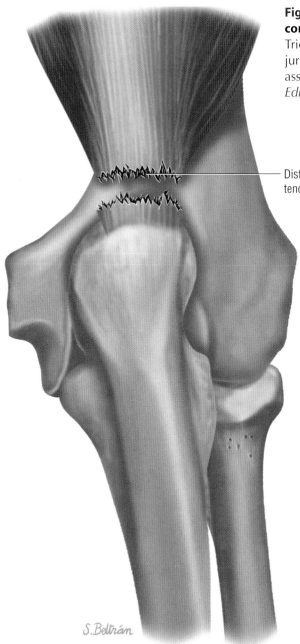

Figure 9.89 ■ **Triceps tendon rupture occurs with deceleration stress on a contracted triceps muscle or eccentric contraction against resistance.** Triceps tears occur in motorcycle accidents and football, soccer, and rugby injuries. Systemic disease, including hyperparathyroidism, and steroid use are associated etiologies. *(See Triceps Tendon Injury pg. 1600, in Stoller's 3rd Edition.)*

Distal triceps
tendon rupture

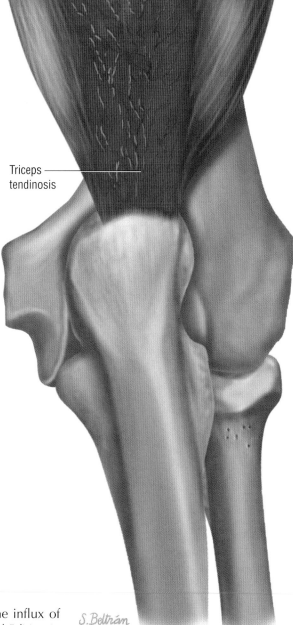

Triceps
tendinosis

Figure 9.90 ■ Tendinosis represents collagen degeneration without the influx of inflammatory cells. *(See Triceps Tendon Injury pg. 1601, in Stoller's 3rd Edition.)*

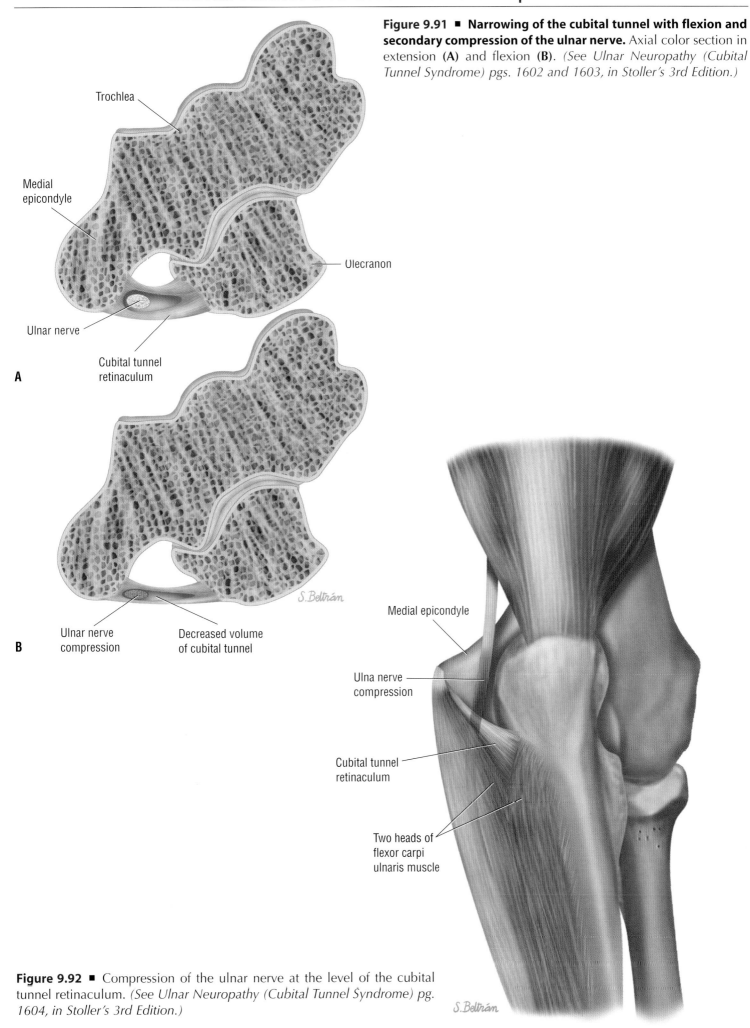

Figure 9.91 ■ **Narrowing of the cubital tunnel with flexion and secondary compression of the ulnar nerve.** Axial color section in extension **(A)** and flexion **(B)**. *(See Ulnar Neuropathy (Cubital Tunnel Syndrome) pgs. 1602 and 1603, in Stoller's 3rd Edition.)*

Trochlea

Medial epicondyle

Ulecranon

Ulnar nerve

Cubital tunnel retinaculum

A

Ulnar nerve compression

Decreased volume of cubital tunnel

B

S. Beltrán

Medial epicondyle

Ulna nerve compression

Cubital tunnel retinaculum

Two heads of flexor carpi ulnaris muscle

S. Beltrán

Figure 9.92 ■ Compression of the ulnar nerve at the level of the cubital tunnel retinaculum. *(See Ulnar Neuropathy (Cubital Tunnel Syndrome) pg. 1604, in Stoller's 3rd Edition.)*

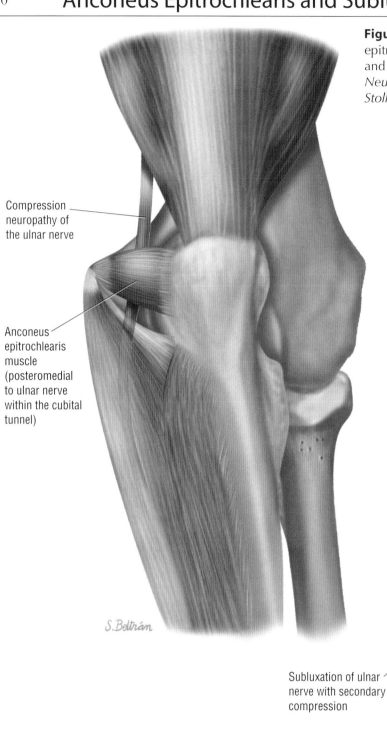

Compression neuropathy of the ulnar nerve

Anconeus epitrochlearis muscle (posteromedial to ulnar nerve within the cubital tunnel)

Figure 9.93 ■ The accessory or anomalous anconeus epitrochlearis muscle replaces the cubital tunnel retinaculum and may cause compression ulnar neuropathy. *(See Ulnar Neuropathy (Cubital Tunnel Syndrome) pgs. 1604 and 1606, in Stoller's 3rd Edition.)*

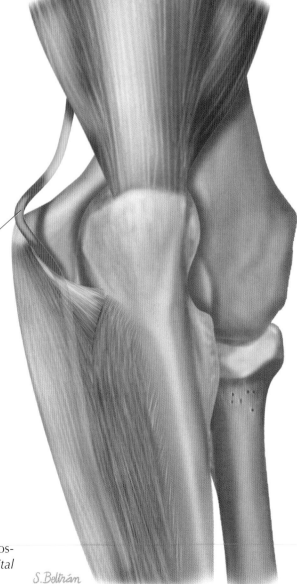

Subluxation of ulnar nerve with secondary compression

Figure 9.94 ■ Subluxation of the ulnar nerve with friction neuritis on a posterior perspective color coronal illustration. *(See Ulnar Neuropathy (Cubital Tunnel Syndrome) pg. 1607, in Stoller's 3rd Edition.)*

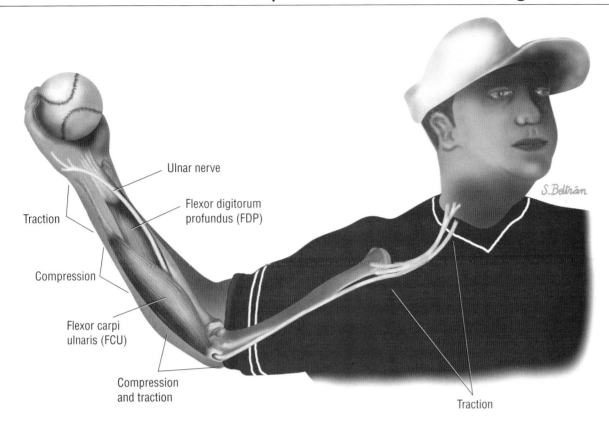

Traction

Ulnar nerve

Flexor digitorum
profundus (FDP)

Compression

Flexor carpi
ulnaris (FCU)

Compression
and traction

Traction

Figure 9.95 ■ **Traction on the ulnar nerve at the shoulder and wrist and compression of the ulnar nerve at the elbow and forearm in the throwing arm.** In the cocking position the flexor carpi ulnaris generates compressive force, increasing pressure in the cubital tunnel up to six times greater than the resting pressure. *(See Ulnar Neuropathy (Cubital Tunnel Syndrome) pg. 1608, in Stoller's 3rd Edition.)*

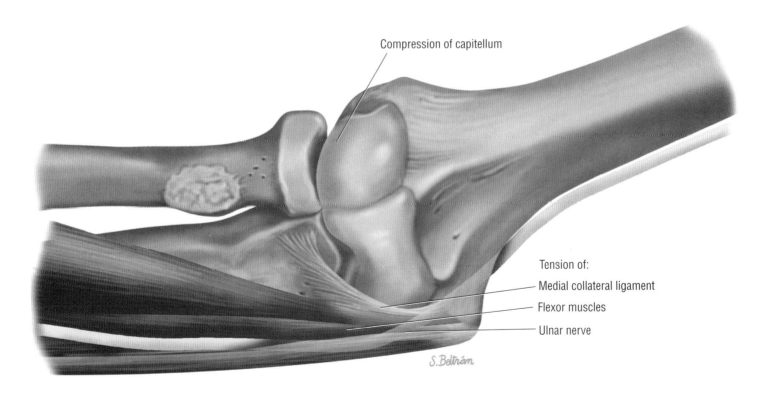

Compression of capitellum

Tension of:
Medial collateral ligament
Flexor muscles
Ulnar nerve

Figure 9.96 ■ **Injury of the elbow during throwing (early and late cocking).** There is compression of the capitellum against the radial head. Tension is generated on the medial collateral ligament, flexor muscles, and ulnar nerve. *(See Ulna Neuropathy (Cubital Tunnel Syndrome) pg. 1608, in Stoller's 3rd Edition.)*

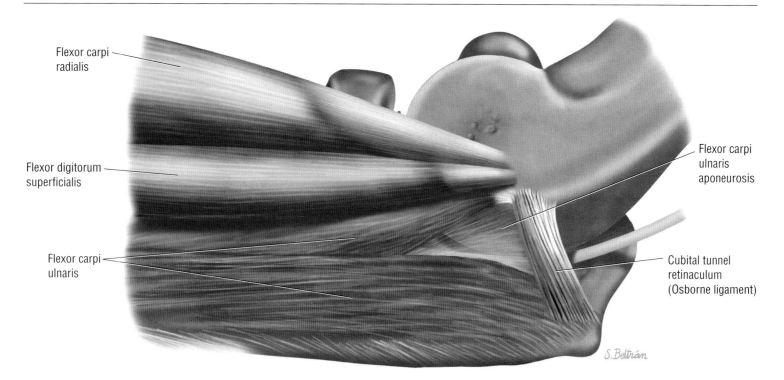

Flexor carpi radialis

Flexor digitorum superficialis

Flexor carpi ulnaris

Flexor carpi ulnaris aponeurosis

Cubital tunnel retinaculum (Osborne ligament)

S.Beltrán

Figure 9.97 ■ **The course of the ulnar nerve at the medial epicondylar groove.** Ulnar nerve compression usually occurs distal to the medial epicondyle by compression of the cubital tunnel retinaculum. *(See Ulnar Neuropathy (Cubital Tunnel syndrome) pgs. 1602–1604, in Stoller's 3rd Edition.)*

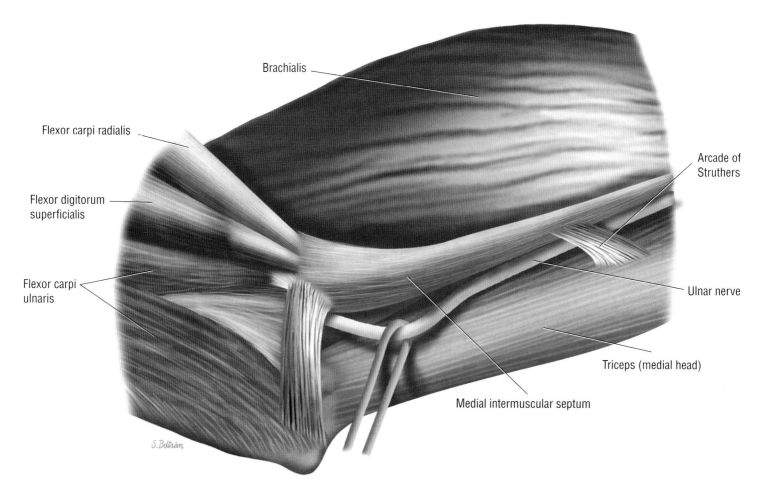

Brachialis

Flexor carpi radialis

Flexor digitorum superficialis

Flexor carpi ulnaris

Arcade of Struthers

Ulnar nerve

Triceps (medial head)

Medial intermuscular septum

S.Beltrán

Figure 9.98 ■ **The arcade of Struthers arises 8 cm proximal to the medial epicondyle.** Note the association of muscular fibers of the medial head of the triceps with the arcade. *Based on Morrey BF, Thompson RCJr. The elbow; master techniques in orthopaedic surgery. New York: Raven Press, 1994. (See Ulnar Neuropathy (Cubital Tunnel Syndrome) pgs. 1602-1604, in Stoller's 3rd Edition.)*

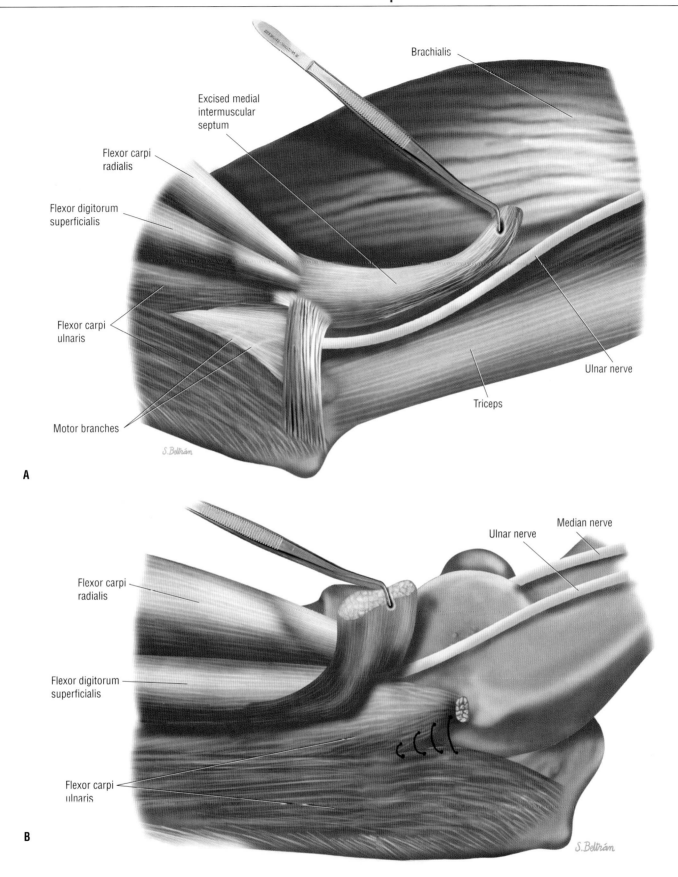

Figure 9.99 ■ **(A)** Submuscular transposition of the ulnar nerve. The proximal mobilization of the nerve extends proximally to the arcade of Struthers. **(B)** Elevation of the flexor-pronator mass allows the ulnar nerve to course in a straight path to the proximal one third of the flexor carpi ulnaris. The ulnar nerve is transposed deep to the FCU. The flexor pronator mass then is approximated. Based on Miller MD, Howard RF, Plancher KD, *Surgical Atlas of Sports Medicine.* *Philadelphia: WB Saunders, 2003. (See Ulnar Neuropathy (Cubital Tunnel Syndrome) pgs. 1602–1604, in Stoller's 3rd Edition.)*

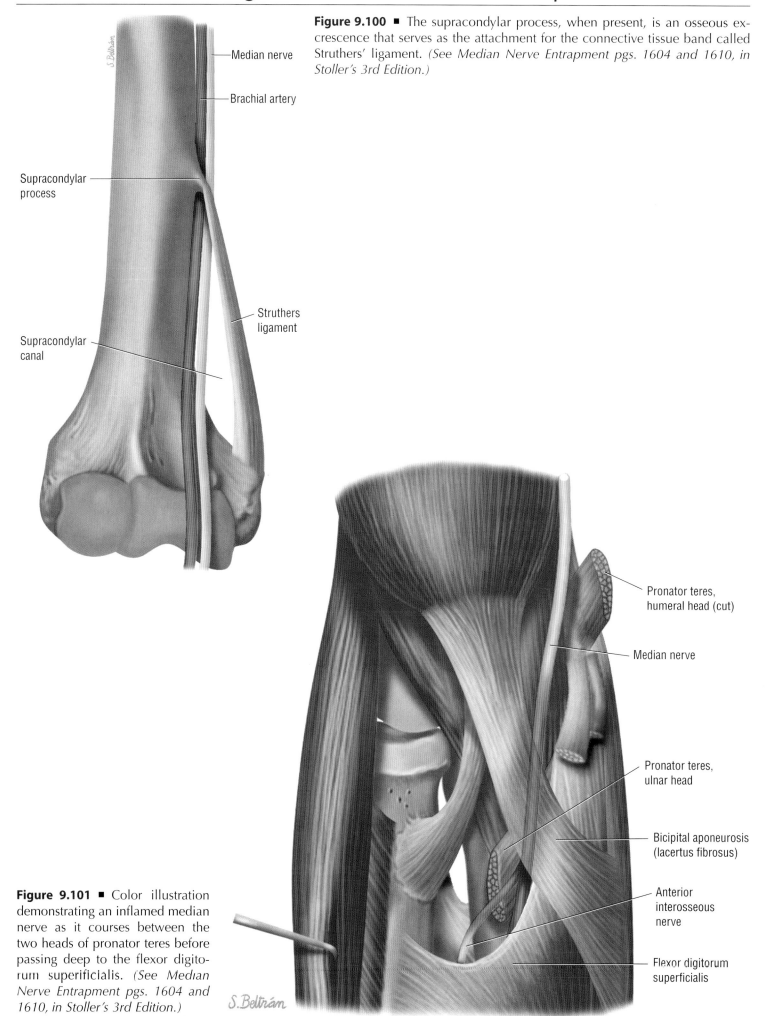

Figure 9.100 ■ The supracondylar process, when present, is an osseous excrescence that serves as the attachment for the connective tissue band called Struthers' ligament. *(See Median Nerve Entrapment pgs. 1604 and 1610, in Stoller's 3rd Edition.)*

Median nerve

Brachial artery

Supracondylar process

Supracondylar canal

Struthers ligament

Pronator teres, humeral head (cut)

Median nerve

Pronator teres, ulnar head

Bicipital aponeurosis (lacertus fibrosus)

Anterior interosseous nerve

Flexor digitorum superficialis

Figure 9.101 ■ Color illustration demonstrating an inflamed median nerve as it courses between the two heads of pronator teres before passing deep to the flexor digitorum superficialis. *(See Median Nerve Entrapment pgs. 1604 and 1610, in Stoller's 3rd Edition.)*

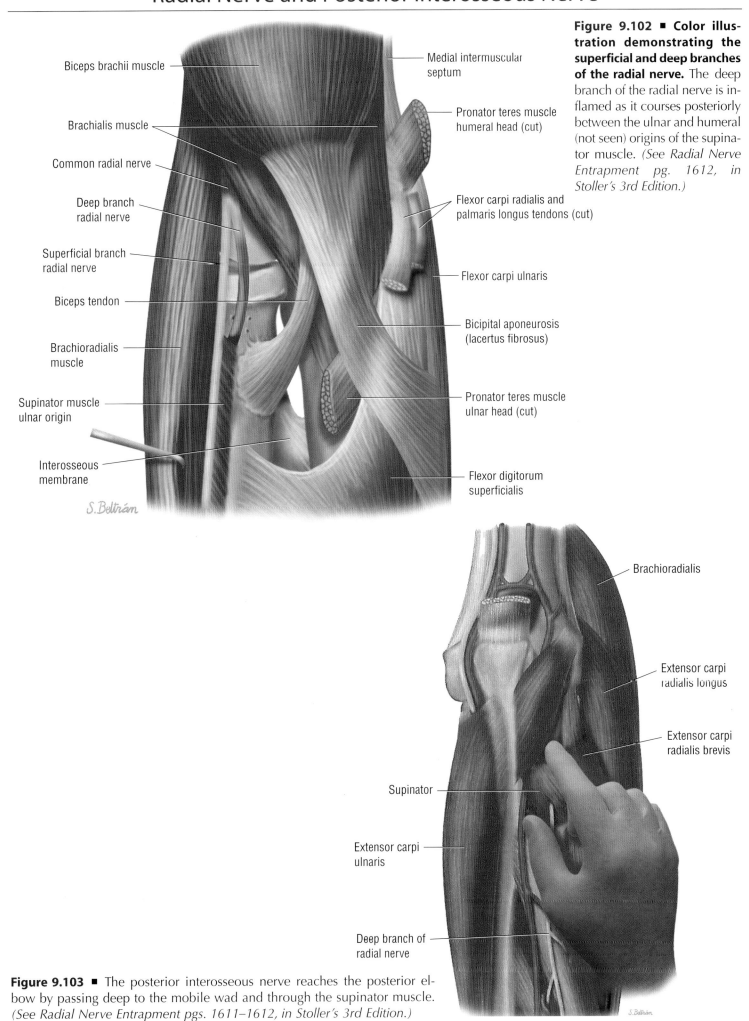

Biceps brachii muscle

Brachialis muscle

Common radial nerve

Deep branch
radial nerve

Superficial branch
radial nerve

Biceps tendon

Brachioradialis
muscle

Supinator muscle
ulnar origin

Interosseous
membrane

S. Beltrán

Medial intermuscular
septum

Pronator teres muscle
humeral head (cut)

Flexor carpi radialis and
palmaris longus tendons (cut)

Flexor carpi ulnaris

Bicipital aponeurosis
(lacertus fibrosus)

Pronator teres muscle
ulnar head (cut)

Flexor digitorum
superficialis

Figure 9.102 ■ Color illustration demonstrating the superficial and deep branches of the radial nerve. The deep branch of the radial nerve is inflamed as it courses posteriorly between the ulnar and humeral (not seen) origins of the supinator muscle. *(See Radial Nerve Entrapment pg. 1612, in Stoller's 3rd Edition.)*

Brachioradialis

Extensor carpi
radialis longus

Extensor carpi
radialis brevis

Supinator

Extensor carpi
ulnaris

Deep branch of
radial nerve

S. Beltrán

Figure 9.103 ■ The posterior interosseous nerve reaches the posterior elbow by passing deep to the mobile wad and through the supinator muscle. *(See Radial Nerve Entrapment pgs. 1611–1612, in Stoller's 3rd Edition.)*

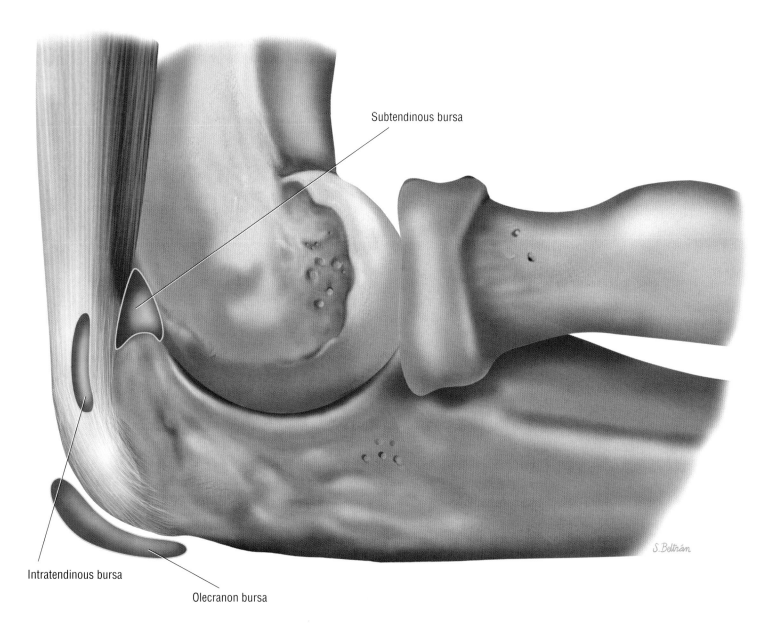

Subtendinous bursa

Intratendinous bursa

Olecranon bursa

Figure 9.104 ■ Relationship of the superficial olecranon bursa, the intratendinous bursa, and the subtendinous bursa. The subtendinous bursa is located between the olecranon tip and the triceps tendon. *(See Olecranon Bursitis pgs. 1611 and 1614, in Stoller's 3rd Edition.)*

Figure 9.105 ■ Olecranon bursitis is associated with triceps tendinopathy and tears. Inflammation of the bursa may be secondary to acute or repetitive trauma or systemic disease. Traumatic bursitis not uncommonly occurs with football injuries associated with playing on artificial turf. *(See Olecranon Bursitis pg. 1614, in Stoller's 3rd Edition.)*

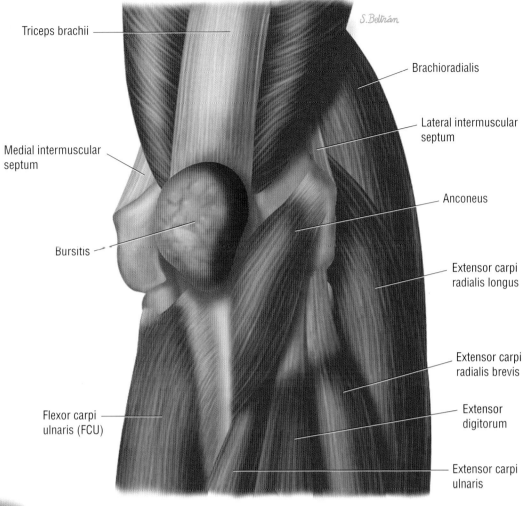

- Triceps brachii
- Brachioradialis
- Lateral intermuscular septum
- Medial intermuscular septum
- Anconeus
- Bursitis
- Extensor carpi radialis longus
- Extensor carpi radialis brevis
- Flexor carpi ulnaris (FCU)
- Extensor digitorum
- Extensor carpi ulnaris

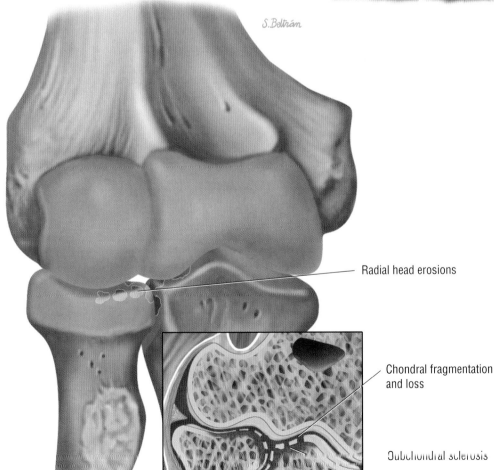

- Radial head erosions
- Chondral fragmentation and loss
- Subchondral sclerosis

Figure 9.106 ■ Arthrosis with radial head and ulnar chondral fragmentation and subchondral sclerosis in early osteoarthritis. *(See Osteoarthritis pg. 1615, in Stoller's 3rd Edition.)*

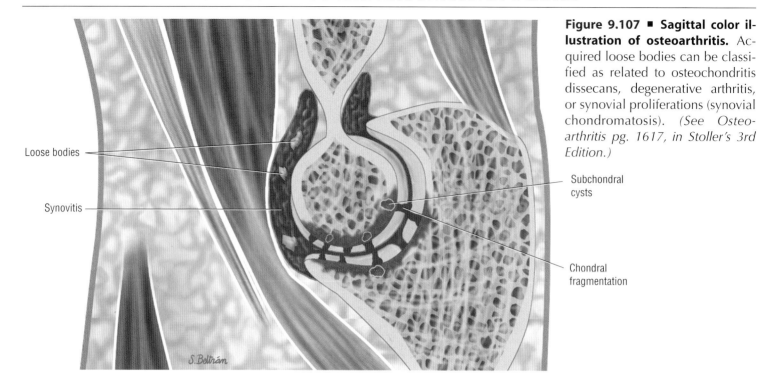

Loose bodies

Synovitis

Subchondral cysts

Chondral fragmentation

Figure 9.107 ■ Sagittal color illustration of osteoarthritis. Acquired loose bodies can be classified as related to osteochondritis dissecans, degenerative arthritis, or synovial proliferations (synovial chondromatosis). *(See Osteoarthritis pg. 1617, in Stoller's 3rd Edition.)*

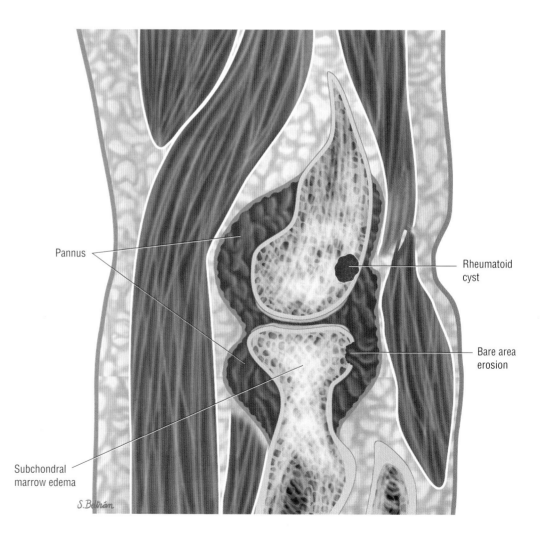

Pannus

Rheumatoid cyst

Bare area erosion

Subchondral marrow edema

Figure 9.108 ■ Rheumatoid involvement of the elbow with enhancement of inflamed synovium (pannus), cyst formation, and a bare area of ulnar erosion adjacent to the chondral surface. Subchondral marrow edema is indicated. *(See Rheumatoid Arthritis pg. 1618, in Stoller's 3rd Edition.)*

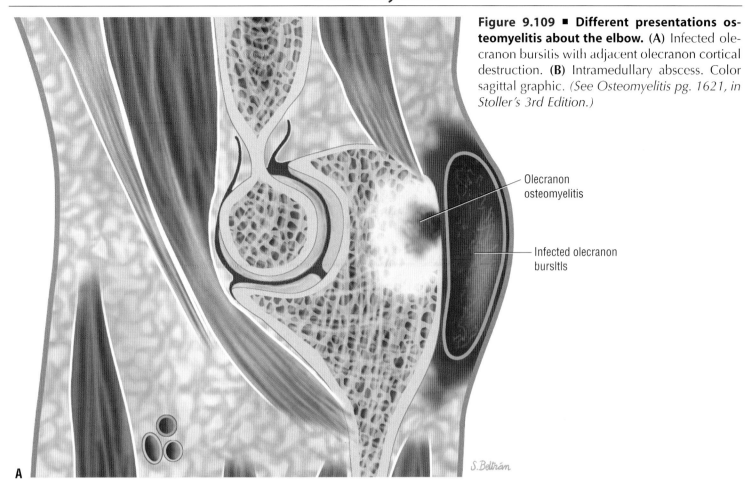

Figure 9.109 ■ **Different presentations osteomyelitis about the elbow.** (A) Infected olecranon bursitis with adjacent olecranon cortical destruction. (B) Intramedullary abscess. Color sagittal graphic. *(See Osteomyelitis pg. 1621, in Stoller's 3rd Edition.)*

Olecranon osteomyelitis

Infected olecranon bursitis

A

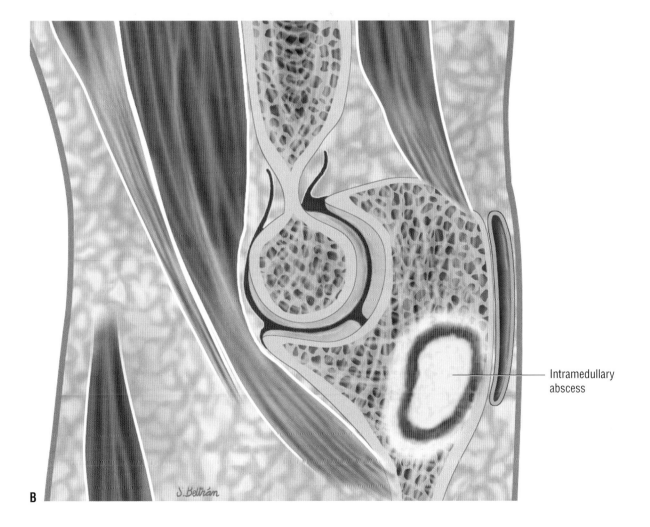

Intramedullary abscess

B

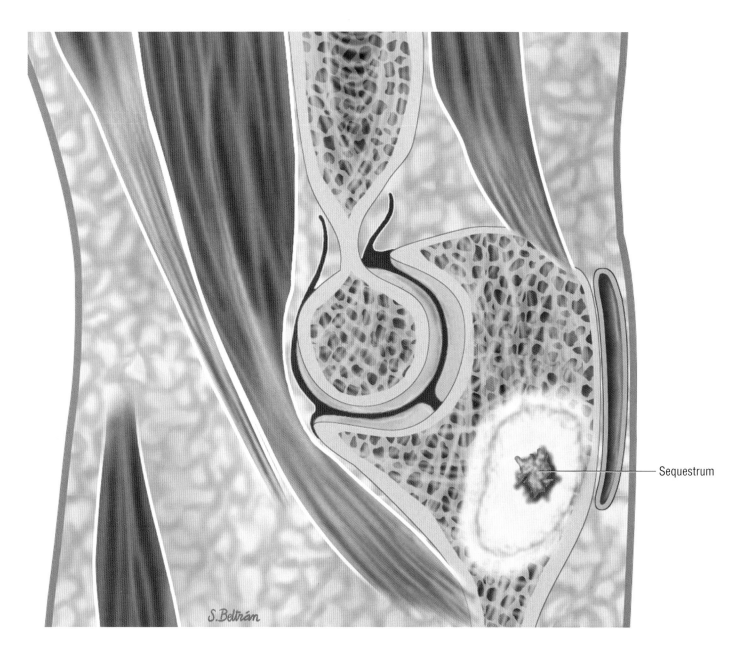

Figure 9.110 ■ Sequestrum or necrotic fragment in chronic osteomyelitis. Color sagittal graphic. *(See Osteomyelitis pg. 1621, in Stoller's 3rd Edition.)*

Chapter

10

The Wrist and Hand

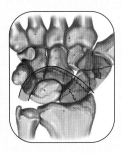

Pearls and Pitfalls & Color Illustrations

Pearls and Pitfalls

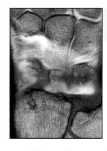

IMAGING PROTOCOLS

- MR or MR arthrography has replaced conventional single- or three-compartment arthrograms.
- Dedicated four- or eight-channel phased-array coils are required for wrist and finger imaging.

- Although TFC degeneration is best demonstrated on T2* gradient-echo images, FS PD FSE sequences are more frequently used in routine examinations to provide improved contrast between hypointense intrinsic ligaments and hyperintense fluid.

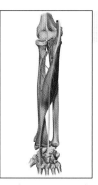

ANATOMY OF THE WRIST
(See Figures 10.29–10.37)

- The carpal bones absorb stress from the palm to the radius, change geometric shape in response to motion, and form a proximal row intercalary segment.
- The extrinsic ligaments, which connect the radius or ulna to the carpal bones or the metacarpal to the carpal bones, provide gross stability.

- The intrinsic ligaments include the intercarpal ligaments, which provide intermediate stability, and the interosseous ligaments, which provide for "fine-tune" stability.

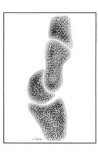

CARPAL INSTABILITIES
(See Figure 10.38)

- Carpal instabilities can be grouped as perilunar, midcarpal, or proximal.
- Perilunar instabilities include lesser arc injuries (primarily ligamentous [e.g., scapholunate or lunotriquetral injuries]) and greater arc injuries (primary osseous [e.g., scaphoid fracture]).

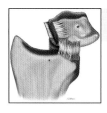

SCAPHOLUNATE LIGAMENT TEAR
(See Figures 10.39–10.42)

- All three components of the scapholunate ligament should be evaluated on coronal and axial images.
- Dorsal component scapholunate ligament tears are more likely to be symptomatic.

- Scapholunate ligament failure represents stage I perilunar instability.

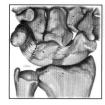

LUNOTRIQUETRAL LIGAMENT TEAR
(See Figure 10.45)

- Lunotriquetral tears may be associated with ulnocarpal impaction syndrome.
- The carpal arc offset between the triquetrum and lunate should be assessed.

- Lunotriquetral ligament injury occurs as part of stage III PLI, which includes triquetral dislocation and radiotriquetral ligament failure.

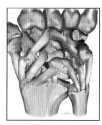

MIDCARPAL INSTABILITIES
(See Figures 10.46 and 10.47)

- Clinical signs and symptoms, including the characteristic carpal clunk, must be considered in combination with MR findings.
- Clunking of the carpus may be present in asymptomatic wrists.

- Associated capitolunate sclerosis or VISI deformity may be demonstrated on sagittal images.
- Injury with laxity of the ulnar arm of the arcuate ligament and the dorsal radiolunotriquetral ligament is seen in palmar midcarpal instability.

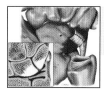

ULNOCARPAL (ULNOLUNATE) ABUTMENT SYNDROME
(See Figures 10.48–10.49)

- Eccentric lunate sclerosis (ulnar-sided) is associated with ulnocarpal abutment.

- Positive ulnar variance is not required.
- Ulnocarpal abutment represents the spectrum of findings in Palmer class 2 degenerative lesions of the TFC complex.

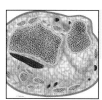

INSTABILITY OF DISTAL RADIOULNAR JOINT
(See Figures 10.50–10.52)

- Axial images in full pronation and supination are used to identify the location of the ulna relative to the sigmoid notch.

- The dorsal and volar radioulnar ligaments of the TFC are evaluated on coronal, axial, and sagittal images.
- Ulnar dorsal dislocation in hyperpronation is associated with disruption of the volar distal radioulnar ligament.
- Ulnopalmar (ulnovolar) dislocation in hypersupination occurs with disruption of the dorsal distal radioulnar ligament.

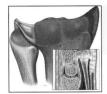

TRIANGULAR FIBROCARTILAGE COMPLEX INJURIES
(See Figures 10.53–10.56)

- Coronal T1- and PD-weighted or T2* gradient-echo images are used to improve the conspicuity of TFC intrasubstance degeneration. FS PD FSE sequences are used to evaluate contour irregularities, including partial and complete tears.

- The distal radioulnar ligaments (volar and dorsal margins of the TFC) are evaluated on coronal and sagittal images.

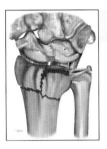

DISTAL RADIUS FRACTURES
(See Figures 10.57–10.62)

- Associated radial styloid and ulnar styloid fractures should be identified.

- Lunate fossa involvement in distal radius fractures is divided into dorsal and palmar (volar) medial components, characterized on sagittal images.

- The Melone classification divides intra-articular fractures into four components: the radial shaft, the radial styloid, dorsal medial, and volar medial segments.

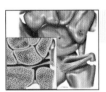

ULNAR STYLOID FRACTURES
(See Figures 10.63–10.64)

- In addition to identification of base or distal ulnar styloid fractures, TFC complex attachments should be evaluated.

- Ulnar styloid fractures are associated with distal radial fractures.

- Type 2 ulnar styloid fractures are associated with nonunion and an unstable distal radioulnar joint.

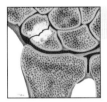

SCAPHOID FRACTURES
(See Figures 10.65–10.67)

- A trabecular fracture line may persist with intact radial and ulnar cortices in the healing phase.

- The wrist should be assessed for associated scaphoid flexion deformity and dorsiflexion instability of the lunate.

- Displaced scaphoid fractures are usually the result of an incomplete or spontaneously reduced perilunate dislocation.

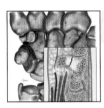

HAMATE FRACTURES
(See Figure 10.72)

- A bipartite hook or os hamuli proprium (incomplete fusion of ossification center of hook) may mimic a fracture.

- Both axial and sagittal images should be obtained before excluding a fracture.

- Other causes of ulnar-sided pain should be evaluated, including the lunotriquetral ligament in cases of chronic or healing hamate fractures.

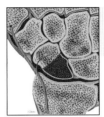

AVASCULAR NECROSIS AND NONUNION OF THE SCAPHOID
(Figure 10.73)

- Associated marrow edema is best seen on coronal FS PD FSE or STIR images.

- There may be displacement at the fracture site or DISI deformity.

- The triquetrum, lunate, and proximal scaphoid fragments slide volarly into extension in stage I perilunar instability.

- SLAC plus scaphoid nonunion presents as a scaphoid nonunion advanced collapse, or SNAC lesion.

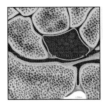

KIENBÖCK'S DISEASE
(See Figures 10.74–10.77)

- Lunate sclerosis or marrow edema is centrally located and not ulnar-sided or eccentric.

- Kienböck's disease frequently presents without a defined transverse fracture in the initial stages.

- FS PD FSE or STIR sequences should be routinely performed to identify marrow edema.

- Anteroposterior elongation of the lunate is evaluated in the sagittal plane in stage III Kienböck's disease.

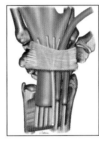

CARPAL TUNNEL SYNDROME
(See Figures 10.78–10.83)

- Thenar muscle hyperintensity (atrophy or denervation) is seen in association with positive median nerve findings.

- There may be partial to complete involvement of median nerve fascicles.

- Triscaphe volar ganglions may compress the deep surface of the carpal tunnel.

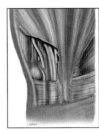

GUYON'S CANAL/ULNAR TUNNEL SYNDROME
(See Figures 10.84–10.89)

- Compression of the ulnar nerve may occur at the entrance to the ulnar tunnel, affecting the superficial branch (sensory) or the deep branch (motor).

- The deep ulnar nerve supplies motor innervation to the hypothenar, interosseous, third and fourth lumbricals, and adductor pollicis muscles.

- The superficial ulnar nerve provides sensory innervation to the skin of the hypothenar eminence and the fourth and fifth digits, and motor innervation to the palmaris brevis.

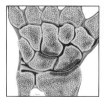

ARTHRITIS
(See Figures 10.91–10.93)

- SLAC wrist, the most common pattern of degenerative arthritis of the wrist, develops in response to scaphoid rotation.
- Initial changes of SLAC arthritis occur with degeneration of the proximal scaphoradial articulation, with subsequent development of capitolunate articular destruction.

- Advanced SLAC represents complete destruction of the scaphoradial, capitolunate, and scaphocapitate joints. There is capitate impingement on the distal radius and narrowing of the hamate–lunate joint space. The radiolunate joint is not affected because it maintains smooth articular contact.
- Triscaphe arthritis is the second most common form of degenerative arthritis of the carpus.
- A combination of SLAC and triscaphe arthritis represents the third most common form of degenerative arthritis.
- Less common degenerative disorders include ulnolunate and lunotriquetral arthritis.

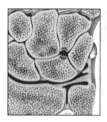

HAMATO-LUNATE IMPINGEMENT
(See Figure 10.94)

- The type II lunate has an extra facet on its ulnar aspect, which is at risk for arthrosis at its articulation with the proximal pole of the hamate.
- Coronal FS PD FSE images are used to identify early chondral erosions.

- T1-weighted images are sensitive to hamato-lunate subchondral sclerosis.

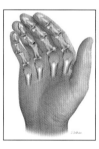

RHEUMATOID ARTHRITIS
(See Figures 10.95–10.97)

- FS PD FSE or intravenous contrast is used to identify pannus tissue.
- Chronic synovitis and inflammation are associated with capsulitis and ligamentous laxity and TFC complex tears.
- Findings in the caput ulnar syndrome include dorsal subluxation.

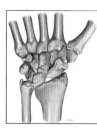

MADELUNG'S DEFORMITY
(See Figure 10.99)

- The distal radial epiphysis is triangular and medially tilted.
- Subtypes include Madelung's, reverse Madelung's, and chevron carpus.

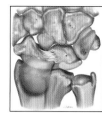

GANGLION CYSTS
(See Figure 10.100–10.101)

- The typical origin of a ganglion is dorsal to the scapholunate joint.
- Intravenous contrast is required for diagnosis when there is inhomogeneity of the ganglion signal intensity on FS PD FSE or STIR images.

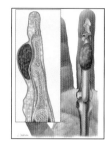

GIANT CELL TUMORS OF THE TENDON SHEATH
(See Figure 10.102)

- True osseous invasion is not typical and is suggestive of a more aggressive process.
- Reactive soft-tissue edema is atypical.
- T2* gradient-echo images are useful to document hemosiderin content.

- Enhancement with contrast is typical.

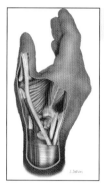

DE QUERVAIN'S TENOSYNOVITIS
(See Figures 10.103–10.105)

- Tendinosis and tenosynovitis of the abductor pollicis longus and extensor pollicis brevis are assessed at the level of the radial styloid on axial MR images.
- The striated appearance of the abductor pollicis longus is related to enlargement of tendinous slips. Longitudinal splitting is more common in the abductor pollicis longus.

- A longitudinal septum may divide the abductor pollicis longus and extensor pollicis brevis, creating a subcompartment for the extensor pollicis brevis.

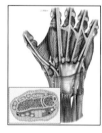

EXTENSOR CARPI ULNARIS TENDINITIS AND DYSFUNCTION
(See Figures 10.107–10.109)

- The subsheath of the extensor carpi ulnaris forms the fibro-osseous tunnel, attaches to the ulnar styloid and ulnar head, and merges with the capsule of the distal radioulnar joint and the TFC complex.

- The position of supination and ulnar deviation reproduces extensor carpi ulnaris instability. Extensor carpi ulnaris relocation occurs with pronation and radial deviation.
- Longitudinal splitting of the extensor carpi ulnaris tendon is characterized by hyperintense signal intensity and is associated with tenosynovitis.

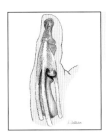

ULNAR COLLATERAL LIGAMENT TEARS OF THE THUMB
(See Figure 10.115)

- Evaluation of ulnar collateral ligament tears and Stener's lesions requires coronal images through the first metacarpophalangeal joint acquired parallel to the plane of the collateral ligaments.

- The retracted ulnar collateral ligament is seen with folded or horizontally directed fibers in Stener's lesions.

- Stener's lesion must demonstrate entrapment of the ulnar collateral ligament by adductor pollicis aponeurosis.

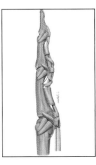

FLEXOR ANNULAR PULLEY TEARS
(See Figures 10.116–10.117)

- There are five digital annular pulleys, which are condensations of transversely oriented fibrous bands.

- The digital annular pulleys stabilize the flexor tendons during flexion and resist ulnar/radial displacement as well as palmar bowing.

- The A2 pulley (located at the proximal aspect of the proximal phalanx) and the A4 pulley (located at the midaspect of the middle phalanx) are the key stabilizing digital annular pulleys.

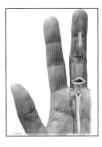

FLEXOR DIGITORUM PROFUNDUS AVULSIONS
(See Figure 10.121)

- There are three types of flexor digitorum profundus avulsion injuries: tendon retraction into the palm, retraction to the proximal interphalangeal joint, and an osseous avulsion lodged at the distal edge of the A4 pulley.

- Evaluation of the tendon course on sagittal images should be correlated with axial images. T2* gradient-echo images may be used to improve tendon contrast discrimination.

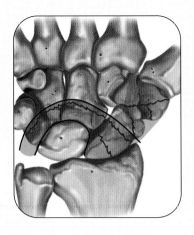

The Wrist and Hand
Muscle

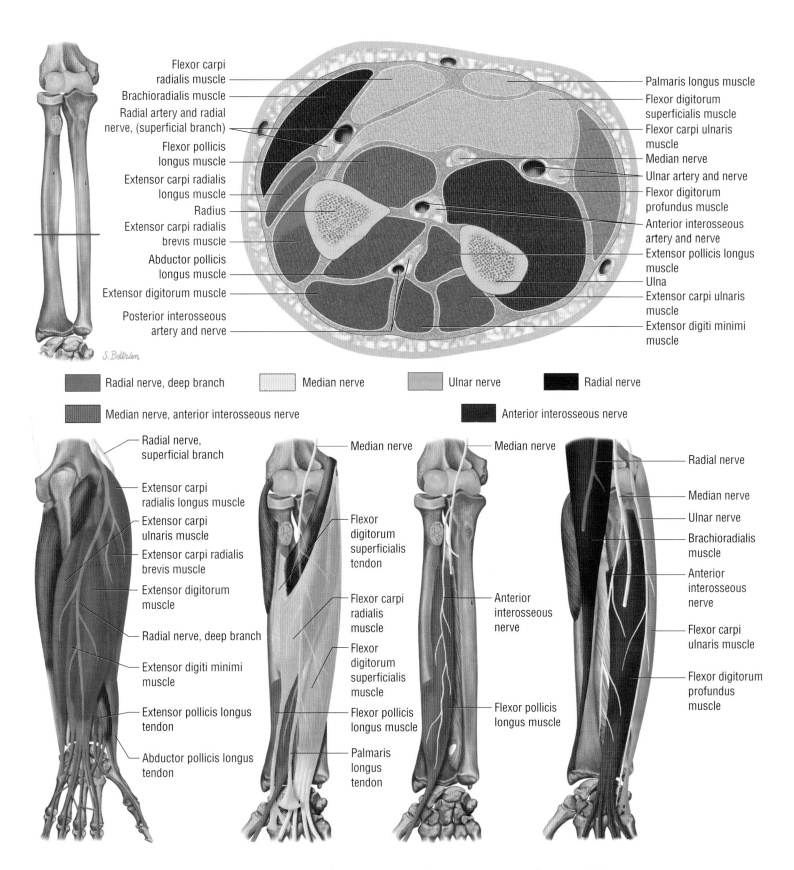

Figure 10.1 ■ Forearm muscle innervation with cross section and 3-D renderings. *Cross section based on Vahlensiech M, Genant HK, Reiter M. MRI of the musculoskeletal system. New York/Stuttgart: Thieme, 2000. (See Related Muscles of the Wrist and Hand pgs. 1631–1644, in Stoller's 3rd Edition.)*

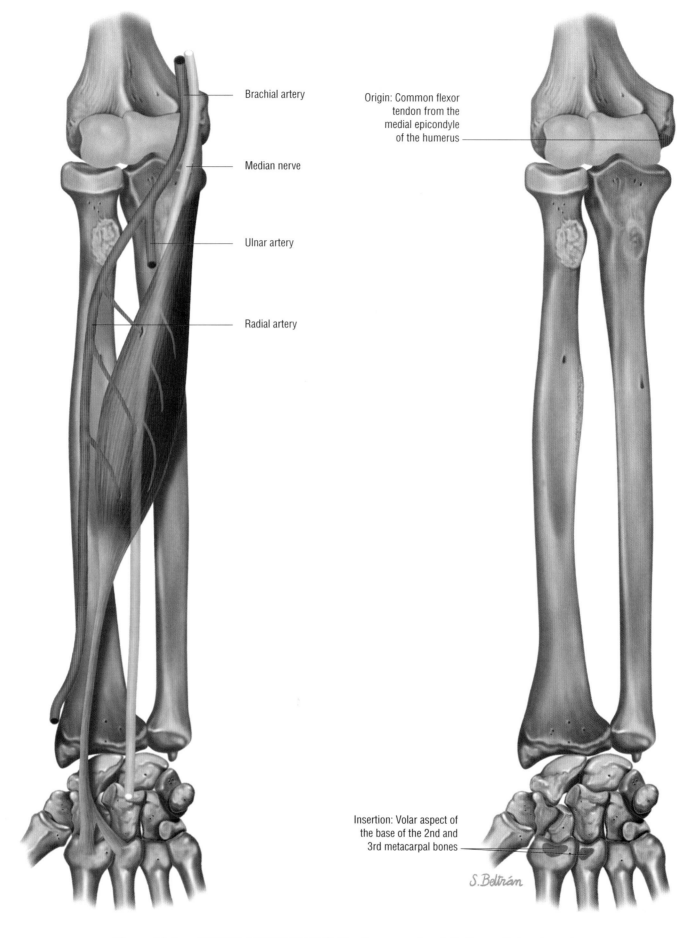

Brachial artery

Origin: Common flexor
tendon from the
medial epicondyle
of the humerus

Median nerve

Ulnar artery

Radial artery

Insertion: Volar aspect of
the base of the 2nd and
3rd metacarpal bones

S.Beltrán

Figure 10.2 ▪ FLEXOR CARPI RADIALIS. The flexor carpi radialis lies radial to the palmaris longus and ulnar to the pronator teres throughout its course. It contributes to flexion and abduction of the wrist. Distal flexor carpi radialis tendon rupture, usually occurring after a fall on the outstretched hand, can clinically mimic a scaphoid fracture. (*See Related Muscles of the Wrist and Hand pg. 1631, in Stoller's 3rd Edition.*)

Palmaris Longus

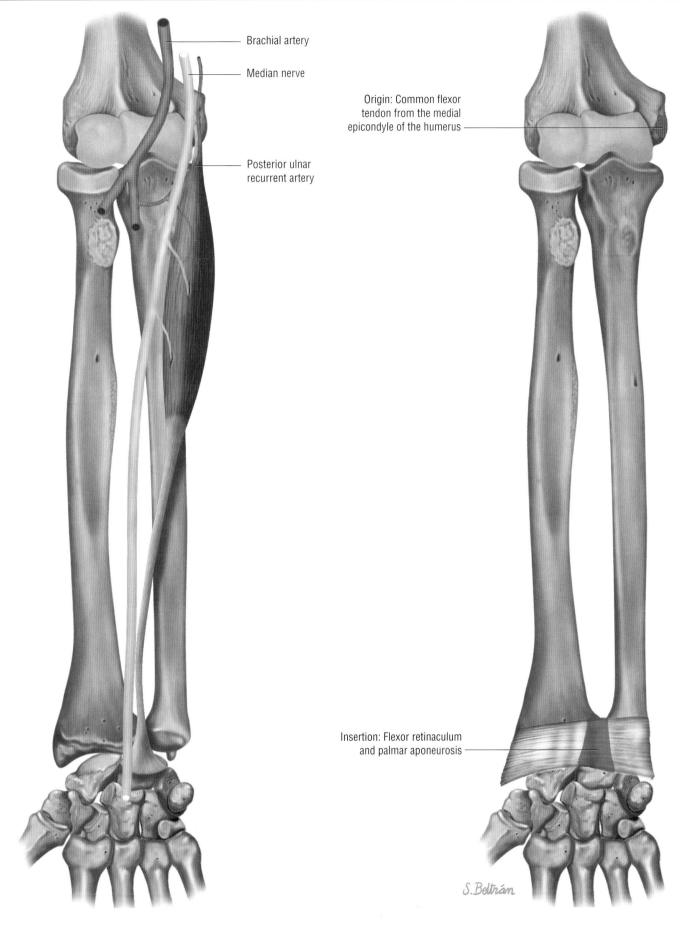

Brachial artery

Median nerve

Posterior ulnar recurrent artery

Origin: Common flexor tendon from the medial epicondyle of the humerus

Insertion: Flexor retinaculum and palmar aponeurosis

S. Beltrán

Figure 10.3 ▪ PALMARIS LONGUS. The palmaris longus is present in approximately 85% of the population and functions to flex the wrist and tighten the palmar aponeurosis. It does not have a tendon sheath but has a paratenon. *(See Related Muscles of the Wrist and Hand pg. 1632, in Stoller's 3rd Edition.)*

Flexor Carpi Ulnaris

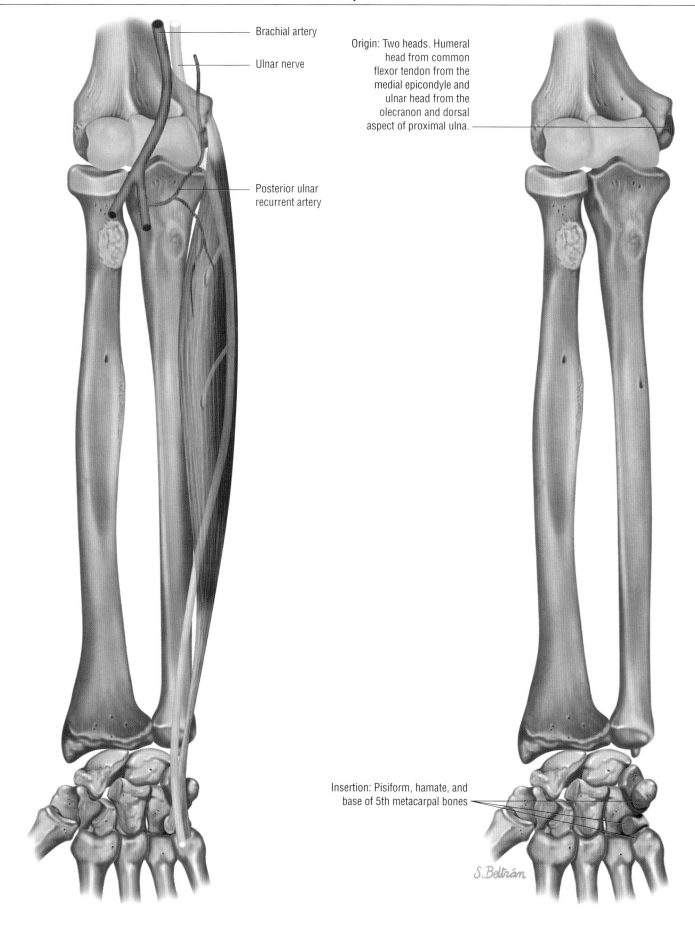

Brachial artery

Ulnar nerve

Posterior ulnar recurrent artery

Origin: Two heads. Humeral head from common flexor tendon from the medial epicondyle and ulnar head from the olecranon and dorsal aspect of proximal ulna.

Insertion: Pisiform, hamate, and base of 5th metacarpal bones

S.Beltrán

Figure 10.4 ▪ FLEXOR CARPI ULNARIS. The flexor carpi ulnaris flexes and adducts the hand. It is an important dynamic stabilizer of the pisotriquetral joint and contributes superficial fibers to the pisohamate ligament. Because it lies superficial and just medial to the ulnar nerve, it serves as a marker when ulnar nerve block is performed. *(See Related Muscles of the Wrist and Hand pg. 1632, in Stoller's 3rd Edition.)*

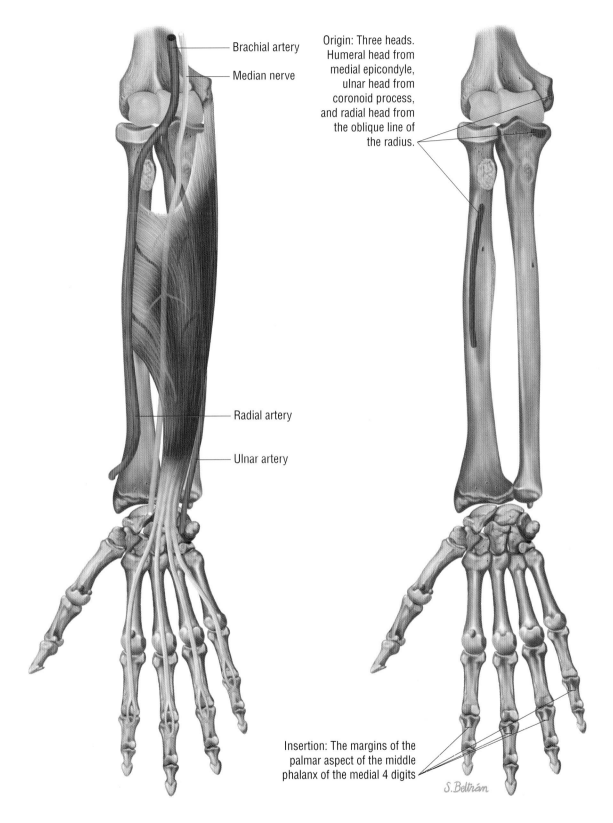

Brachial artery

Median nerve

Origin: Three heads.
Humeral head from
medial epicondyle,
ulnar head from
coronoid process,
and radial head from
the oblique line of
the radius.

Radial artery

Ulnar artery

Insertion: The margins of the
palmar aspect of the middle
phalanx of the medial 4 digits

S. Beltrán

Figure 10.5 ▪ FLEXOR DIGITORUM SUPERFICIALIS. The flexor digitorum superficialis tendons flex the middle phalanges of each finger and, using the pulley system as a fulcrum, contribute to flexion of the fingers at the metacarpophalangeal joint. In the forearm, the median nerve lies just deep to the arch of the flexor digitorum superficialis muscle, and this is an area of potential nerve compression. *(See Related Muscles of the Wrist and Hand pg. 1633, in Stoller's 3rd Edition.)*

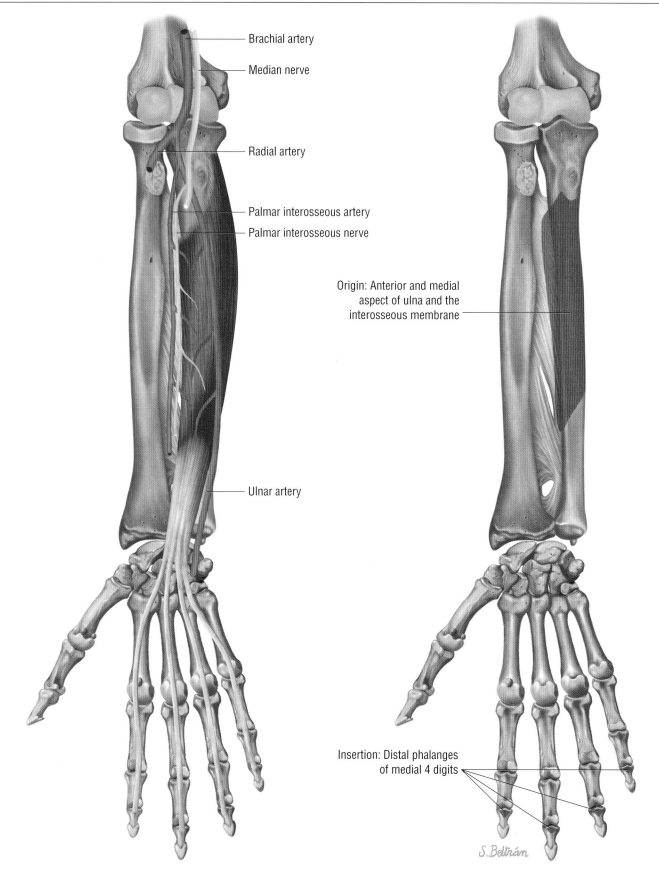

— Brachial artery

— Median nerve

— Radial artery

— Palmar interosseous artery
— Palmar interosseous nerve

Origin: Anterior and medial
aspect of ulna and the
interosseous membrane

— Ulnar artery

Insertion: Distal phalanges
of medial 4 digits

S. Beltrán

Figure 10.6 ■ FLEXOR DIGITORUM PROFUNDUS. The flexor digitorum profundus tendons flex the distal phalanges at the distal interphalangeal joints and assist in flexion of the wrist and proximal phalanges. The flexor digitorum profundus divides into four musculotendinous units in the distal forearm, and the tendons travel though the carpal tunnel deep to the flexor digitorum superficialis tendons. *(See Related Muscles of the Wrist and Hand pg. 1633, in Stoller's 3rd Edition.)*

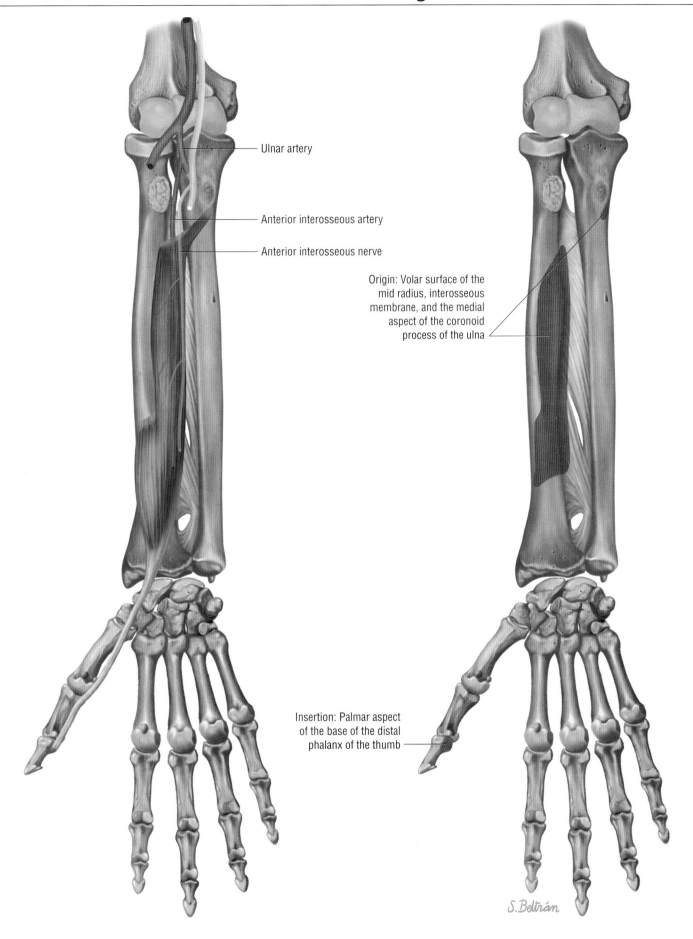

Ulnar artery

Anterior interosseous artery

Anterior interosseous nerve

Origin: Volar surface of the
mid radius, interosseous
membrane, and the medial
aspect of the coronoid
process of the ulna

Insertion: Palmar aspect
of the base of the distal
phalanx of the thumb

S. Beltrán

Figure 10.7 ■ FLEXOR POLLICIS LONGUS. The flexor pollicis longus flexes the thumb. Compression of the anterior interosseous nerve can lead to denervation of the flexor pollicis longus muscle, which may be isolated or concomitant with flexor digitorum profundus and pronator quadratus denervation. *(See Related Muscles of the Wrist and Hand pg. 1634, in Stoller's 3rd Edition.)*

Pronator Quadratus

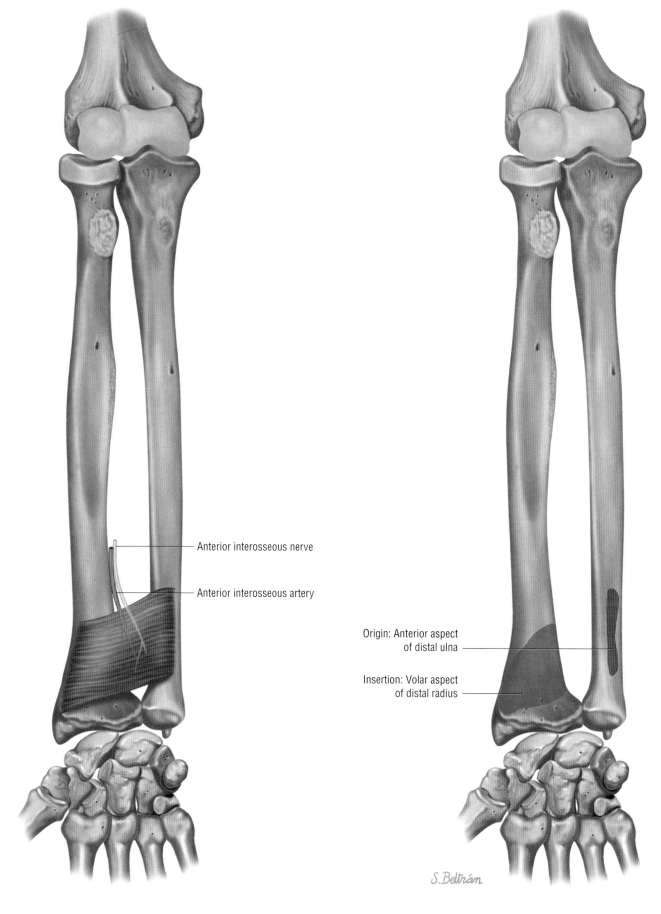

Anterior interosseous nerve

Anterior interosseous artery

Origin: Anterior aspect of distal ulna

Insertion: Volar aspect of distal radius

S.Beltrán

Figure 10.8 ▪ PRONATOR QUADRATUS. The pronator quadratus acts synergistically with the pronator teres to pronate the forearm. Denervation changes can be seen with anterior interosseous nerve compression. *(See Related Muscles of the Wrist and Hand pgs. 1631 and 1634, in Stoller's 3rd Edition.)*

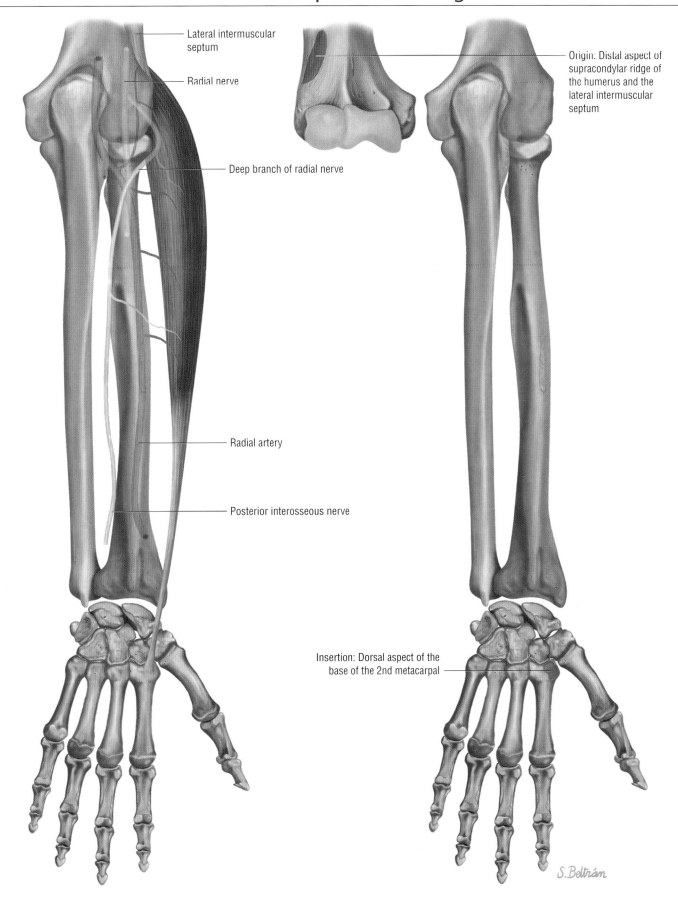

Lateral intermuscular septum

Radial nerve

Origin: Distal aspect of supracondylar ridge of the humerus and the lateral intermuscular septum

Deep branch of radial nerve

Radial artery

Posterior interosseous nerve

Insertion: Dorsal aspect of the base of the 2nd metacarpal

S. Beltrán

Figure 10.9 ■ EXTENSOR CARPI RADIALIS LONGUS. The extensor carpi radialis longus extends and abducts the wrist. If extensor carpi ulnaris function is lost because of posterior interosseus nerve palsy, the extensor carpi radialis causes radial deviation because normally the attachment of the extensor carpi ulnaris to the ulnar aspect of the fifth metacarpal functions to neutralize the abduction movement applied by the extensor carpi radialis longus. *(See Related Muscles of the Wrist and Hand pg. 1635, in Stoller's 3rd Edition.)*

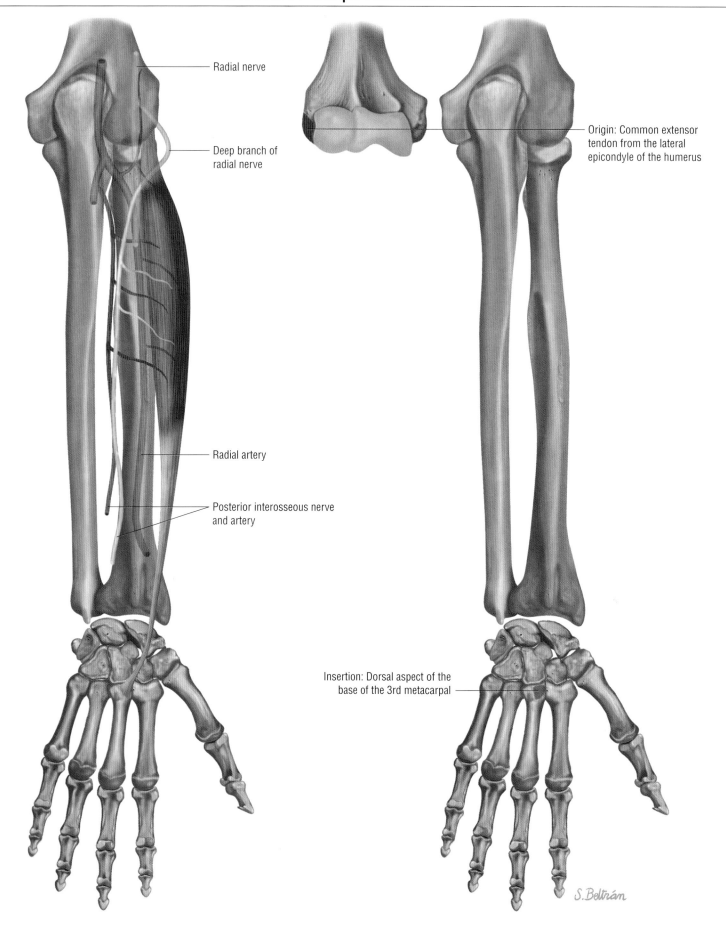

Radial nerve

Deep branch of
radial nerve

Origin: Common extensor
tendon from the lateral
epicondyle of the humerus

Radial artery

Posterior interosseous nerve
and artery

Insertion: Dorsal aspect of the
base of the 3rd metacarpal

S.Beltrán

Figure 10.10 ▪ EXTENSOR CARPI RADIALIS BREVIS. The extensor carpi radialis
brevis provides neutral extension of the wrist. Distal ruptures of the extensor carpi
radialis brevis significantly affect wrist extension. *(See Related Muscles of the Wrist
and Hand pg. 1635, in Stoller's 3rd Edition.)*

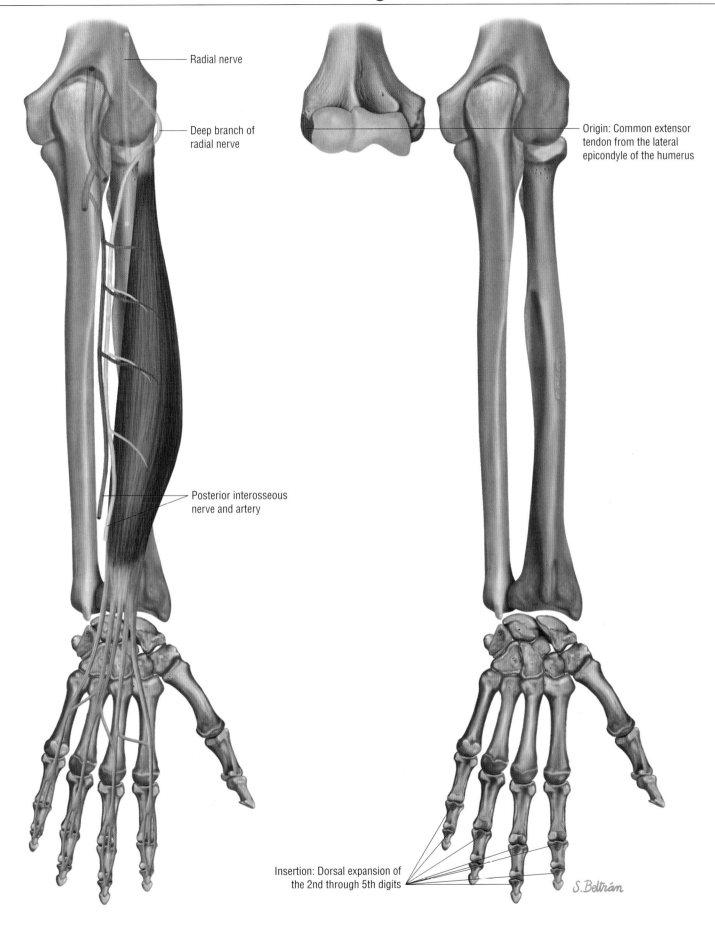

Radial nerve

Deep branch of radial nerve

Posterior interosseous nerve and artery

Origin: Common extensor tendon from the lateral epicondyle of the humerus

Insertion: Dorsal expansion of the 2nd through 5th digits

S. Beltrán

Figure 10.11 ■ EXTENSOR DIGITORUM. The extensor digitorum extends the medial four digits at the metacarpophalangeal joints and contributes to wrist extension. The extensor digitorum tendons are connected at the level of the metacarpal bones by fibrous bands called juncturae tendinum. Boutonnière deformity results from disruption of the central slip component of the extensor tendon at its insertion into the middle phalanx. *(See Related Muscles of the Wrist and Hand pgs. 1631 and 1636, in Stoller's 3rd Edition.)*

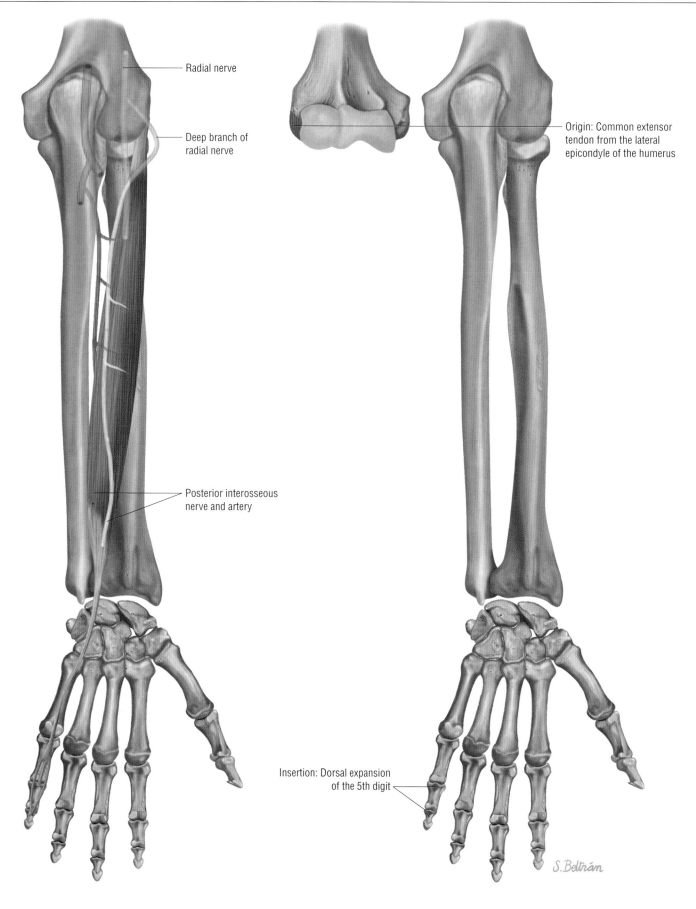

Radial nerve

Deep branch of
radial nerve

Origin: Common extensor
tendon from the lateral
epicondyle of the humerus

Posterior interosseous
nerve and artery

Insertion: Dorsal expansion
of the 5th digit

S.Beltrán

Figure 10.12 ▪ EXTENSOR DIGITI MINIMI. The extensor digiti minimi extends the
proximal phalanx of the little finger at the metacarpophalangeal joint and contributes to wrist extension. Because the extensor digiti minimi tendon lies just superficial to the radioulnar articulation, it is often the first tendon to be involved in
rheumatoid arthritis. *(See Related Muscles of the Wrist and Hand pg. 1636, in
Stoller's 3rd Edition.)*

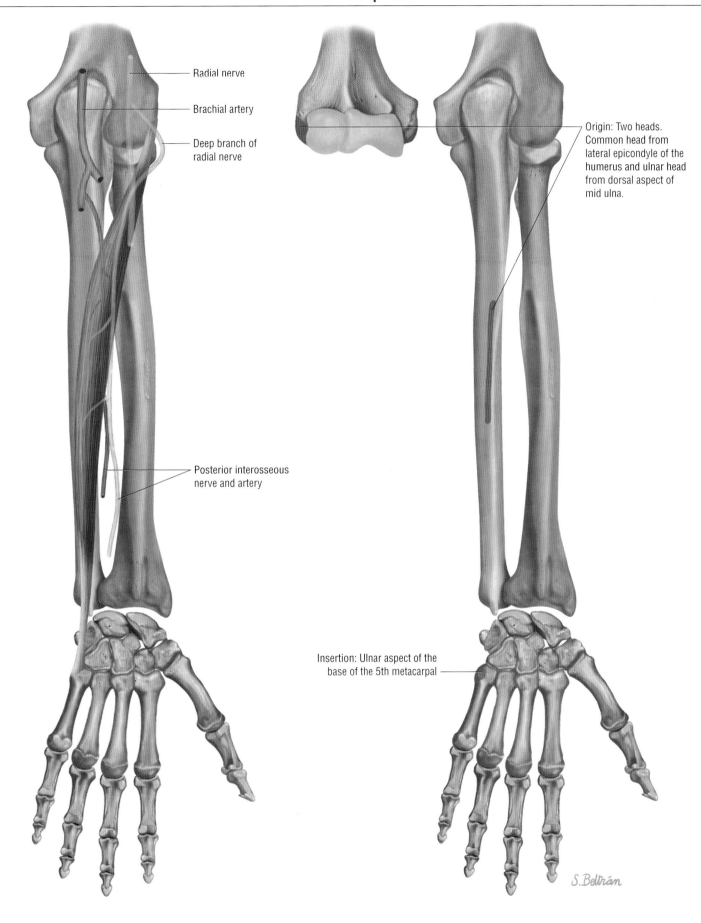

Radial nerve

Brachial artery

Deep branch of radial nerve

Origin: Two heads. Common head from lateral epicondyle of the humerus and ulnar head from dorsal aspect of mid ulna.

Posterior interosseous nerve and artery

Insertion: Ulnar aspect of the base of the 5th metacarpal

S. Beltrán

Figure 10.13 ■ **EXTENSOR CARPI ULNARIS.** The extensor carpi ulnaris tendon extends and adducts the wrist. It is commonly affected in tendinosis and tenosynovitis as it passes through the groove on the distal ulna. Subluxation of the extensor carpi ulnaris also can occur at this location related to disruption or insufficiency of the ligament that covers the tendon in this groove. The extensor carpi ulnaris tendon subsheath is a component of the triangular fibrocartilage complex. *(See Related Muscles of the Wrist and Hand pg. 1637, in Stoller's 3rd Edition.)*

Abductor Pollicis Longus

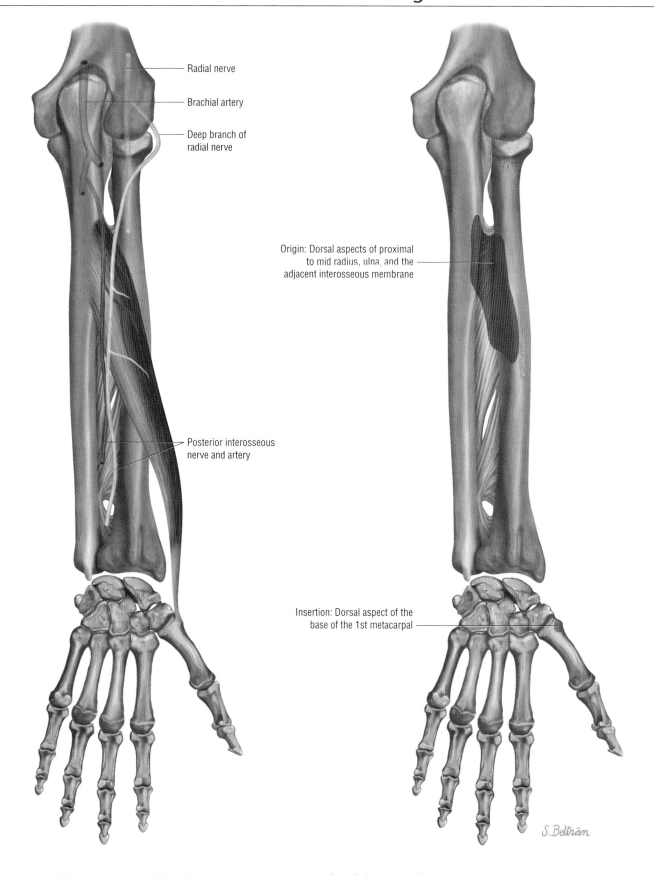

Radial nerve

Brachial artery

Deep branch of
radial nerve

Origin: Dorsal aspects of proximal
to mid radius, ulna, and the
adjacent interosseous membrane

Posterior interosseous
nerve and artery

Insertion: Dorsal aspect of the
base of the 1st metacarpal

S. Beltrán

Figure 10.14 ■ ABDUCTOR POLLICIS LONGUS. The abductor pollicis longus abducts and extends the thumb at the carpometacarpal joint. It travels in the first extensor compartment of the wrist with the extensor pollicis brevis and may become involved with a stenosing tenosynovitis located under the extensor retinaculum at the distal radial groove. This condition, known as de Quervain's tenosynovitis, is distinguished from intersection syndrome, which is a result of friction-related repetitive trauma to the second extensor compartment tendons. *(See Related Muscles of the Wrist and Hand pg. 1637, in Stoller's 3rd Edition.)*

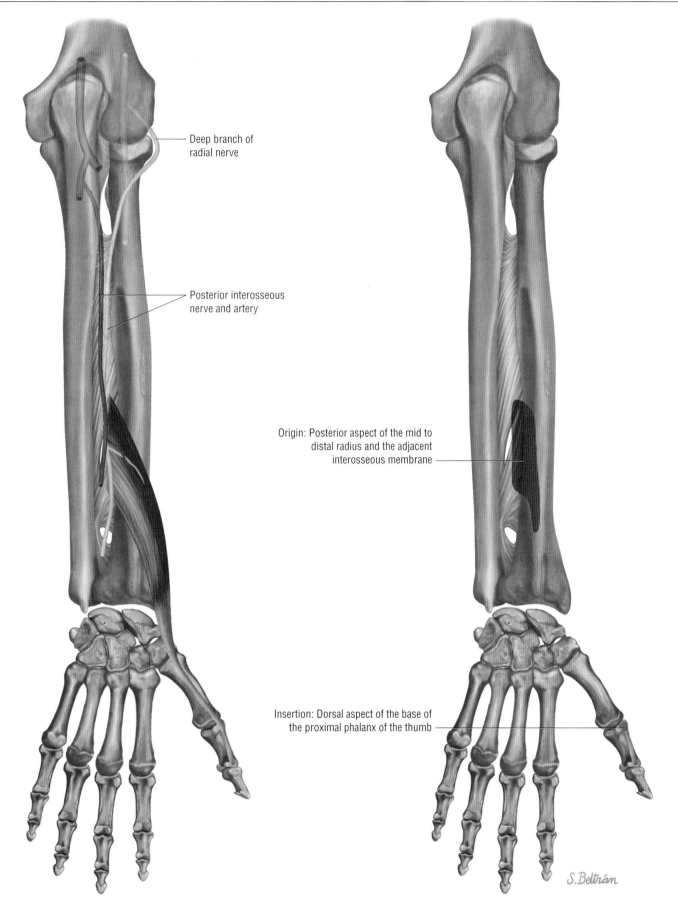

Deep branch of radial nerve

Posterior interosseous nerve and artery

Origin: Posterior aspect of the mid to distal radius and the adjacent interosseous membrane

Insertion: Dorsal aspect of the base of the proximal phalanx of the thumb

S. Beltrán

Figure 10.15 ▪ EXTENSOR POLLICIS BREVIS. The extensor pollicis brevis travels with the abductor pollicis longus in the first extensor compartment and forms the lateral margin of the anatomic snuffbox. It is usually affected concomitantly with the abductor pollicis longus in de Quervain's tenosynovitis. *(See Related Muscles of the Wrist and Hand pgs. 1631 and 1638, in Stoller's 3rd Edition.)*

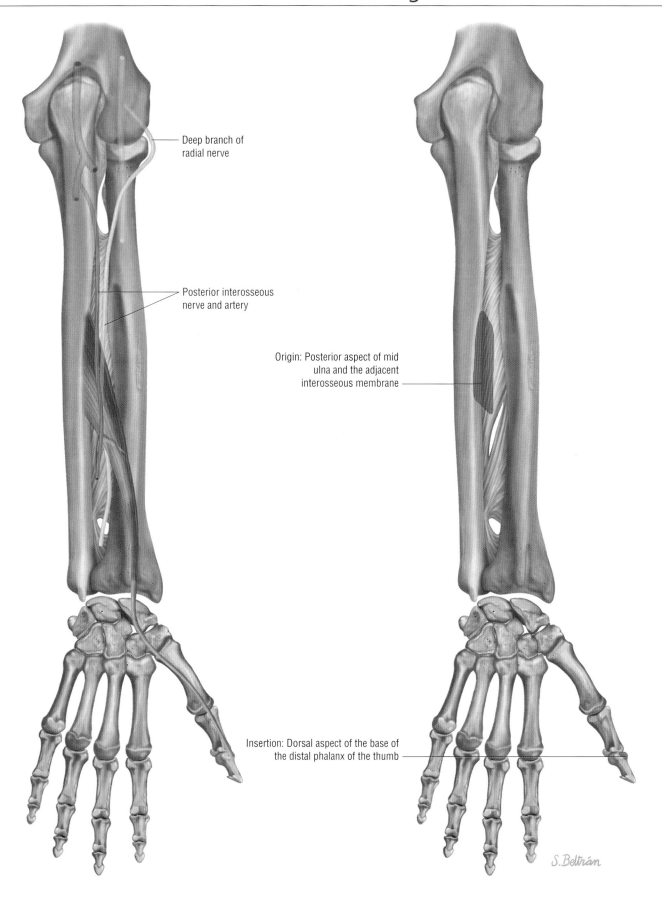

Deep branch of
radial nerve

Posterior interosseous
nerve and artery

Origin: Posterior aspect of mid
ulna and the adjacent
interosseous membrane

Insertion: Dorsal aspect of the base of
the distal phalanx of the thumb

S.Beltrán

Figure 10.16 ▪ EXTENSOR POLLICIS LONGUS. The extensor pollicis longus tendon has a separate tendon sheath throughout its course. It can be injured in Colles' fractures of the distal radius and is sometimes involved in delayed injury following conservative treatment of nondisplaced fractures. This delayed injury is thought to be related to ischemia secondary to edema or hemorrhage compromising the fibro-osseous canal. The extensor pollicis longus extends the distal phalanx of the thumb at the carpometacarpal and interphalangeal joints. *(See Related Muscles of the Wrist and Hand pgs. 1631 and 1638, in Stoller's 3rd Edition.)*

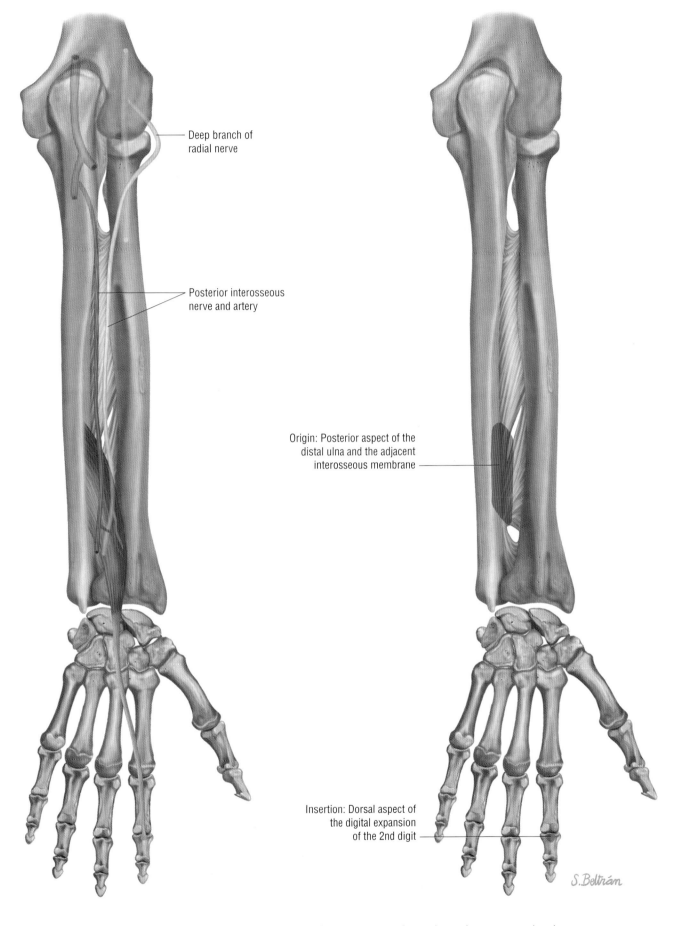

Deep branch of
radial nerve

Posterior interosseous
nerve and artery

Origin: Posterior aspect of the
distal ulna and the adjacent
interosseous membrane

Insertion: Dorsal aspect of
the digital expansion
of the 2nd digit

S. Beltrán

Figure 10.17 ■ EXTENSOR INDICIS. The extensor indicis, the only extensor that has muscle fibers that extend to or beyond the level of the radiocarpal joint, extends the second finger and contributes to wrist extension. The extensor indicis is sometimes transferred surgically to replace a torn extensor pollicis longus tendon. *(See Related Muscles of the Wrist and Hand pgs. 1631 and 1639, in Stoller's 3rd Edition.)*

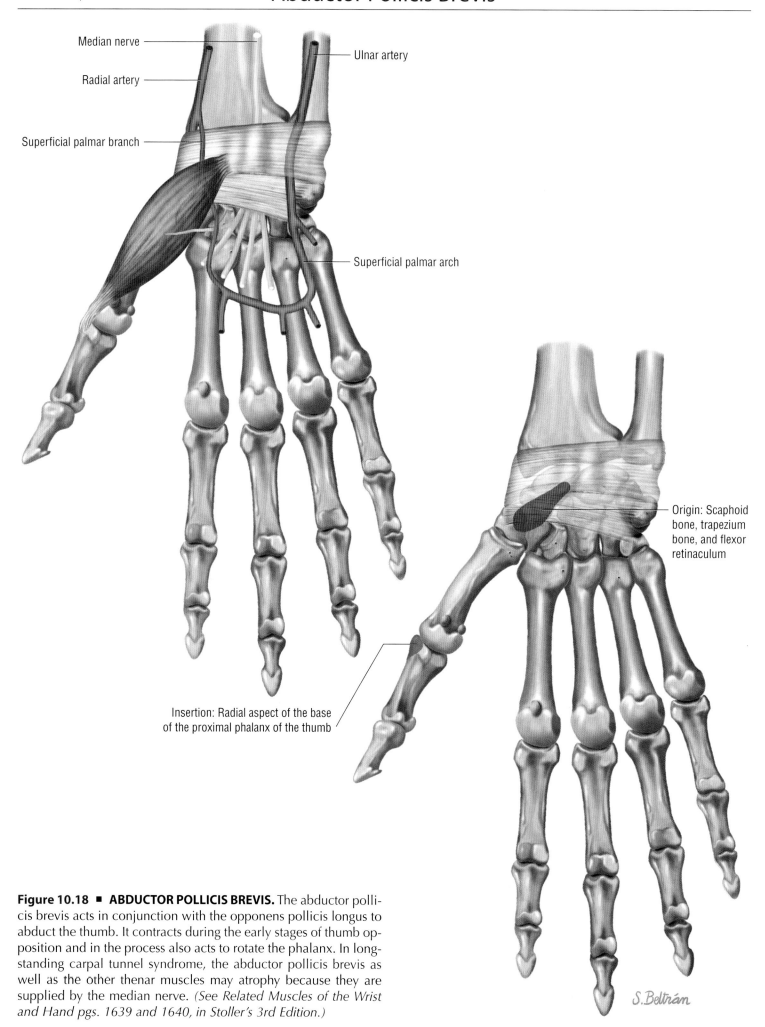

Median nerve

Ulnar artery

Radial artery

Superficial palmar branch

Superficial palmar arch

Origin: Scaphoid bone, trapezium bone, and flexor retinaculum

Insertion: Radial aspect of the base of the proximal phalanx of the thumb

S. Beltrán

Figure 10.18 ■ ABDUCTOR POLLICIS BREVIS. The abductor pollicis brevis acts in conjunction with the opponens pollicis longus to abduct the thumb. It contracts during the early stages of thumb opposition and in the process also acts to rotate the phalanx. In long-standing carpal tunnel syndrome, the abductor pollicis brevis as well as the other thenar muscles may atrophy because they are supplied by the median nerve. *(See Related Muscles of the Wrist and Hand pgs. 1639 and 1640, in Stoller's 3rd Edition.)*

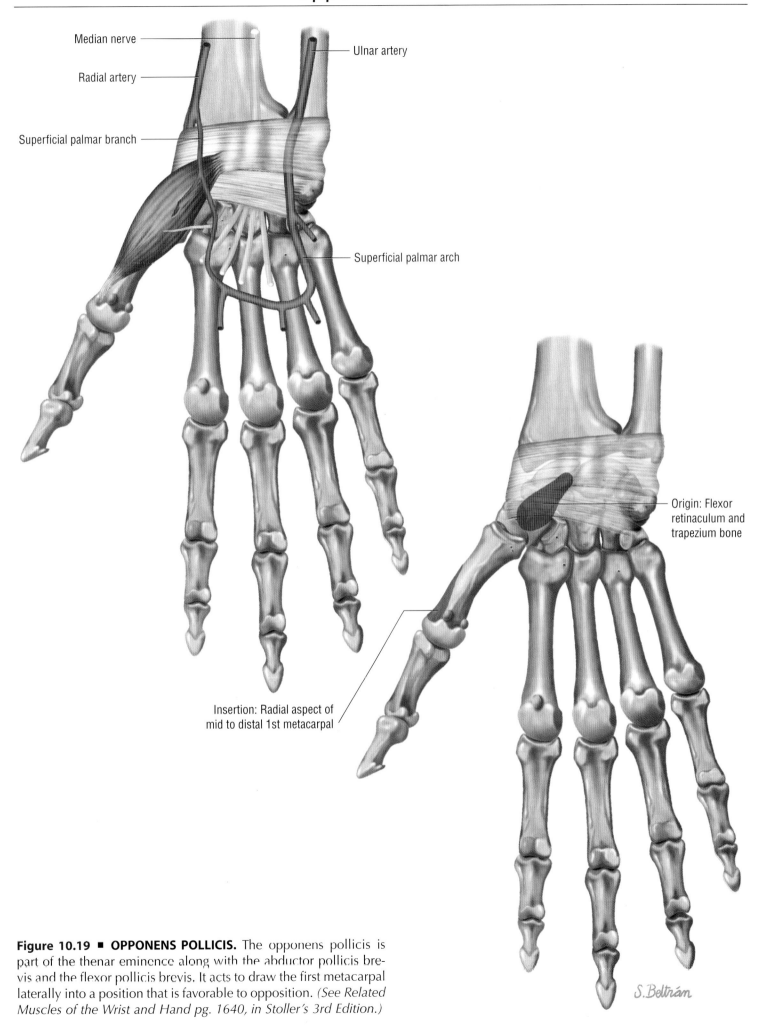

- Median nerve
- Radial artery
- Superficial palmar branch
- Ulnar artery
- Superficial palmar arch
- Origin: Flexor retinaculum and trapezium bone
- Insertion: Radial aspect of mid to distal 1st metacarpal

Figure 10.19 ■ OPPONENS POLLICIS. The opponens pollicis is part of the thenar eminence along with the abductor pollicis brevis and the flexor pollicis brevis. It acts to draw the first metacarpal laterally into a position that is favorable to opposition. *(See Related Muscles of the Wrist and Hand pg. 1640, in Stoller's 3rd Edition.)*

S. Beltrán

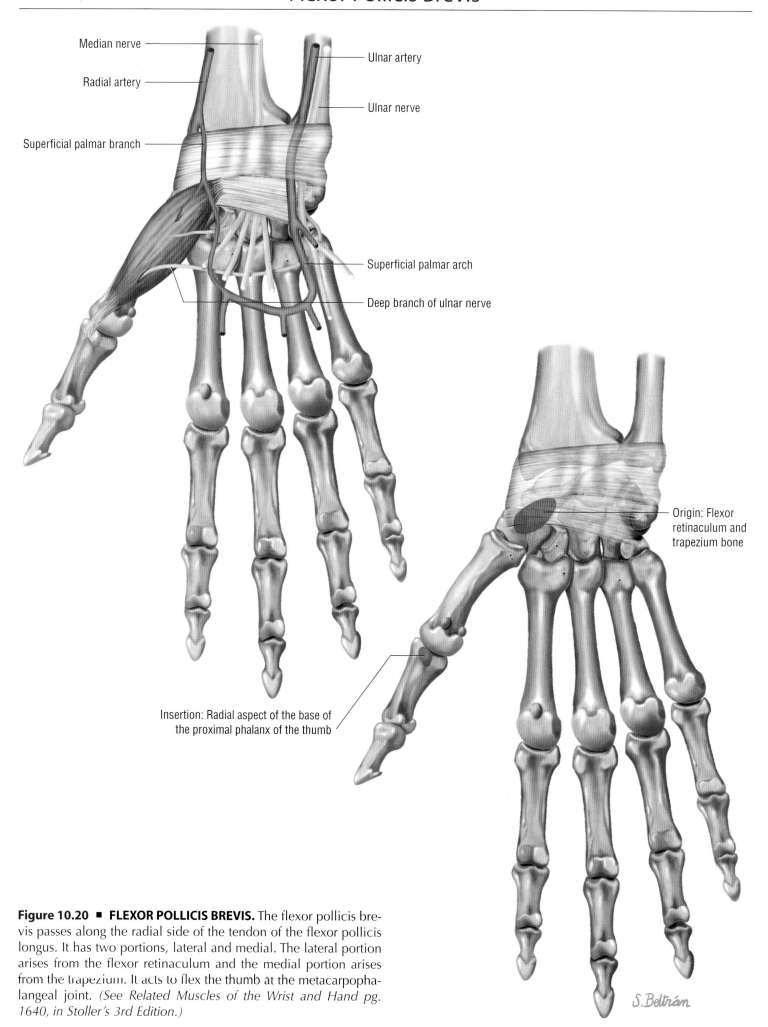

Median nerve

Radial artery

Superficial palmar branch

Ulnar artery

Ulnar nerve

Superficial palmar arch

Deep branch of ulnar nerve

Origin: Flexor retinaculum and trapezium bone

Insertion: Radial aspect of the base of the proximal phalanx of the thumb

Figure 10.20 ▪ FLEXOR POLLICIS BREVIS. The flexor pollicis brevis passes along the radial side of the tendon of the flexor pollicis longus. It has two portions, lateral and medial. The lateral portion arises from the flexor retinaculum and the medial portion arises from the trapezium. It acts to flex the thumb at the metacarpophalangeal joint. *(See Related Muscles of the Wrist and Hand pg. 1640, in Stoller's 3rd Edition.)*

S. Beltrán

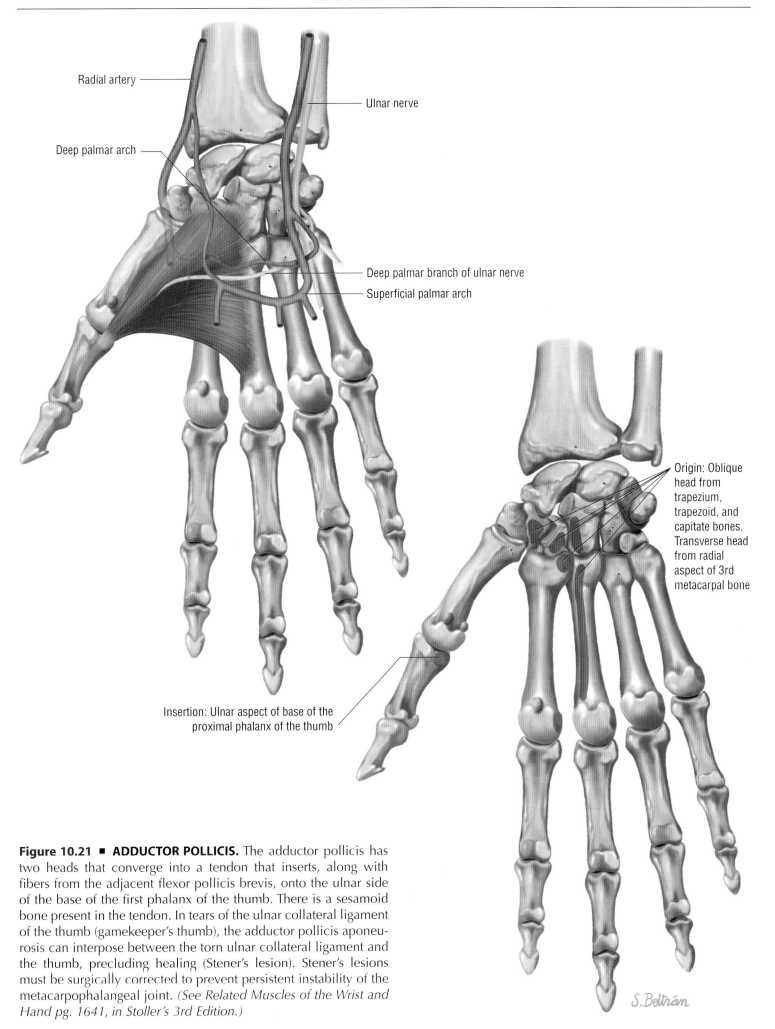

Radial artery

Ulnar nerve

Deep palmar arch

Deep palmar branch of ulnar nerve

Superficial palmar arch

Origin: Oblique head from trapezium, trapezoid, and capitate bones. Transverse head from radial aspect of 3rd metacarpal bone

Insertion: Ulnar aspect of base of the proximal phalanx of the thumb

Figure 10.21 ■ ADDUCTOR POLLICIS. The adductor pollicis has two heads that converge into a tendon that inserts, along with fibers from the adjacent flexor pollicis brevis, onto the ulnar side of the base of the first phalanx of the thumb. There is a sesamoid bone present in the tendon. In tears of the ulnar collateral ligament of the thumb (gamekeeper's thumb), the adductor pollicis aponeurosis can interpose between the torn ulnar collateral ligament and the thumb, precluding healing (Stener's lesion). Stener's lesions must be surgically corrected to prevent persistent instability of the metacarpophalangeal joint. *(See Related Muscles of the Wrist and Hand pg. 1641, in Stoller's 3rd Edition.)*

S.Beltrán

Palmaris Brevis

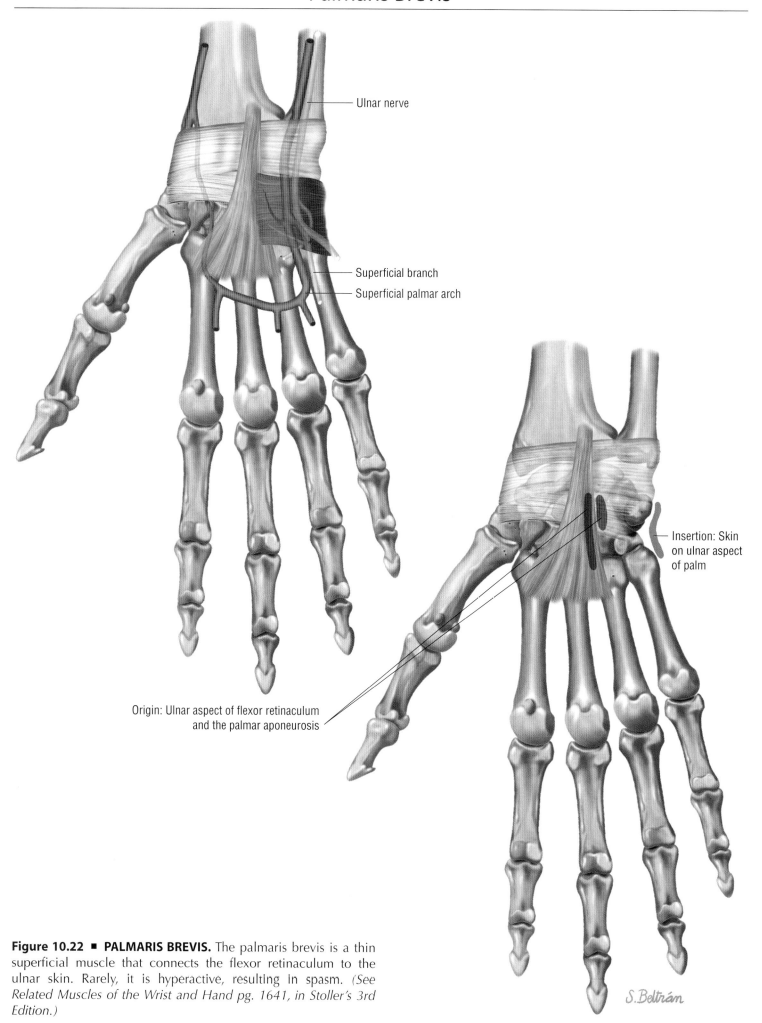

Ulnar nerve

Superficial branch

Superficial palmar arch

Insertion: Skin on ulnar aspect of palm

Origin: Ulnar aspect of flexor retinaculum and the palmar aponeurosis

Figure 10.22 ■ PALMARIS BREVIS. The palmaris brevis is a thin superficial muscle that connects the flexor retinaculum to the ulnar skin. Rarely, it is hyperactive, resulting in spasm. *(See Related Muscles of the Wrist and Hand pg. 1641, in Stoller's 3rd Edition.)*

S. Beltrán

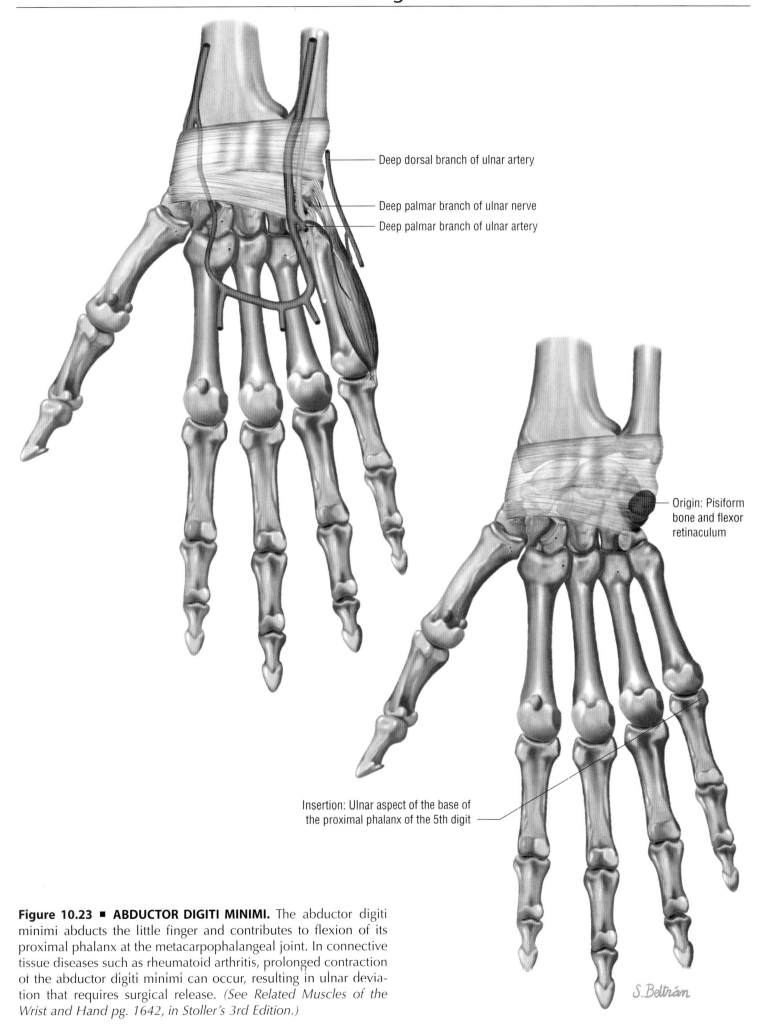

Deep dorsal branch of ulnar artery

Deep palmar branch of ulnar nerve
Deep palmar branch of ulnar artery

Origin: Pisiform bone and flexor retinaculum

Insertion: Ulnar aspect of the base of the proximal phalanx of the 5th digit

S. Beltrán

Figure 10.23 ■ ABDUCTOR DIGITI MINIMI. The abductor digiti minimi abducts the little finger and contributes to flexion of its proximal phalanx at the metacarpophalangeal joint. In connective tissue diseases such as rheumatoid arthritis, prolonged contraction of the abductor digiti minimi can occur, resulting in ulnar deviation that requires surgical release. *(See Related Muscles of the Wrist and Hand pg. 1642, in Stoller's 3rd Edition.)*

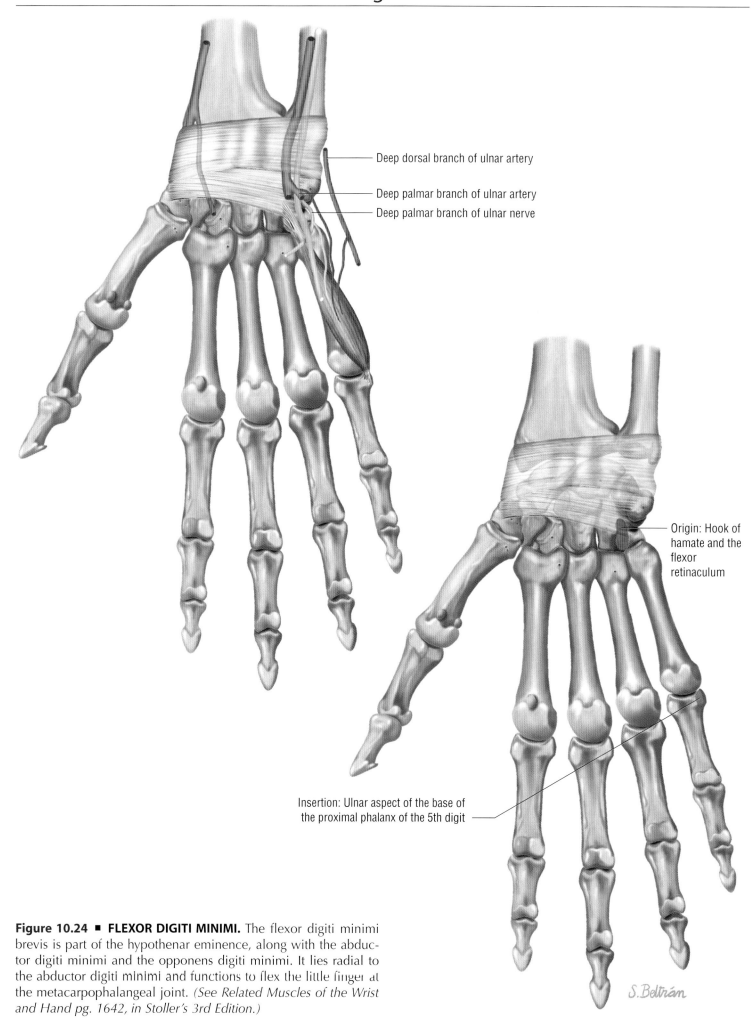

Deep dorsal branch of ulnar artery

Deep palmar branch of ulnar artery
Deep palmar branch of ulnar nerve

Origin: Hook of
hamate and the
flexor
retinaculum

Insertion: Ulnar aspect of the base of
the proximal phalanx of the 5th digit

S. Beltrán

Figure 10.24 ▪ FLEXOR DIGITI MINIMI. The flexor digiti minimi
brevis is part of the hypothenar eminence, along with the abductor digiti minimi and the opponens digiti minimi. It lies radial to
the abductor digiti minimi and functions to flex the little finger at
the metacarpophalangeal joint. *(See Related Muscles of the Wrist
and Hand pg. 1642, in Stoller's 3rd Edition.)*

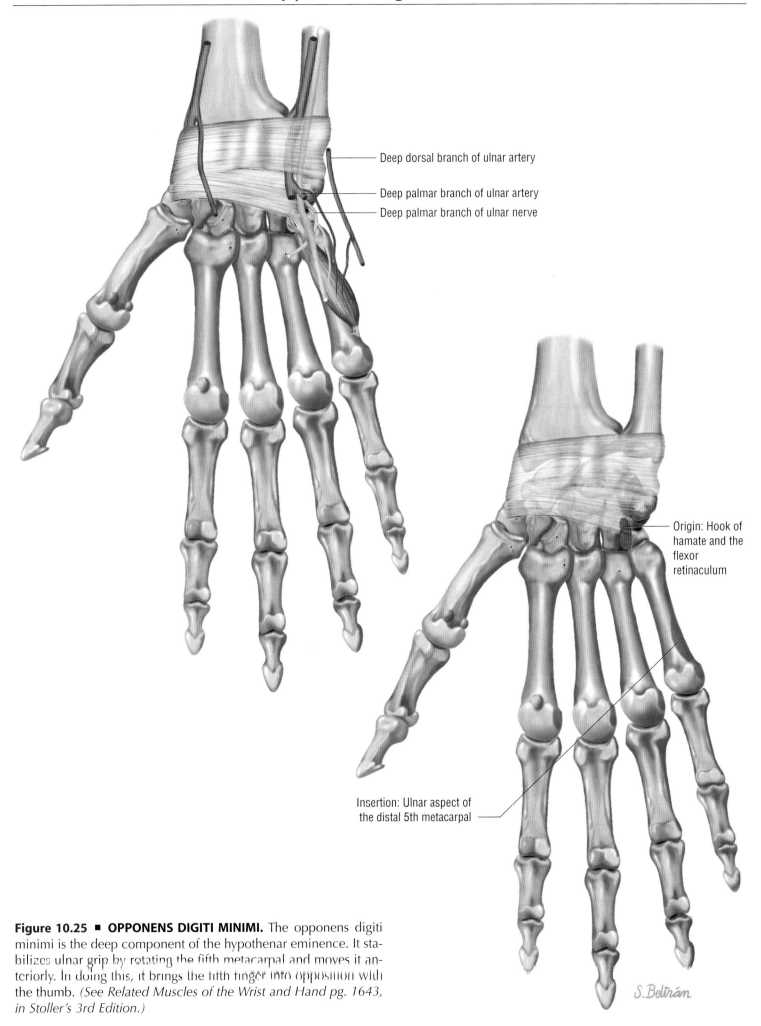

Deep dorsal branch of ulnar artery

Deep palmar branch of ulnar artery

Deep palmar branch of ulnar nerve

Origin: Hook of hamate and the flexor retinaculum

Insertion: Ulnar aspect of the distal 5th metacarpal

Figure 10.25 ■ OPPONENS DIGITI MINIMI. The opponens digiti minimi is the deep component of the hypothenar eminence. It stabilizes ulnar grip by rotating the fifth metacarpal and moves it anteriorly. In doing this, it brings the fifth finger into opposition with the thumb. *(See Related Muscles of the Wrist and Hand pg. 1643, in Stoller's 3rd Edition.)*

S.Beltrán

Lumbricals

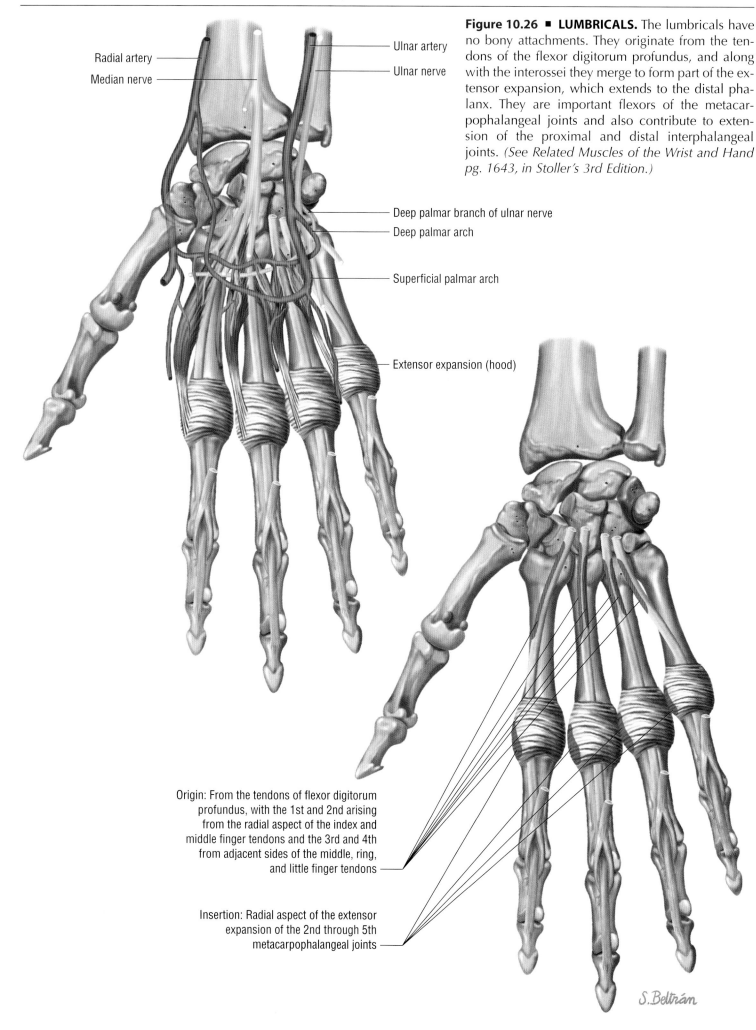

Radial artery

Median nerve

Ulnar artery

Ulnar nerve

Deep palmar branch of ulnar nerve

Deep palmar arch

Superficial palmar arch

Extensor expansion (hood)

Figure 10.26 ■ LUMBRICALS. The lumbricals have no bony attachments. They originate from the tendons of the flexor digitorum profundus, and along with the interossei they merge to form part of the extensor expansion, which extends to the distal phalanx. They are important flexors of the metacarpophalangeal joints and also contribute to extension of the proximal and distal interphalangeal joints. *(See Related Muscles of the Wrist and Hand pg. 1643, in Stoller's 3rd Edition.)*

Origin: From the tendons of flexor digitorum profundus, with the 1st and 2nd arising from the radial aspect of the index and middle finger tendons and the 3rd and 4th from adjacent sides of the middle, ring, and little finger tendons

Insertion: Radial aspect of the extensor expansion of the 2nd through 5th metacarpophalangeal joints

S.Beltrán

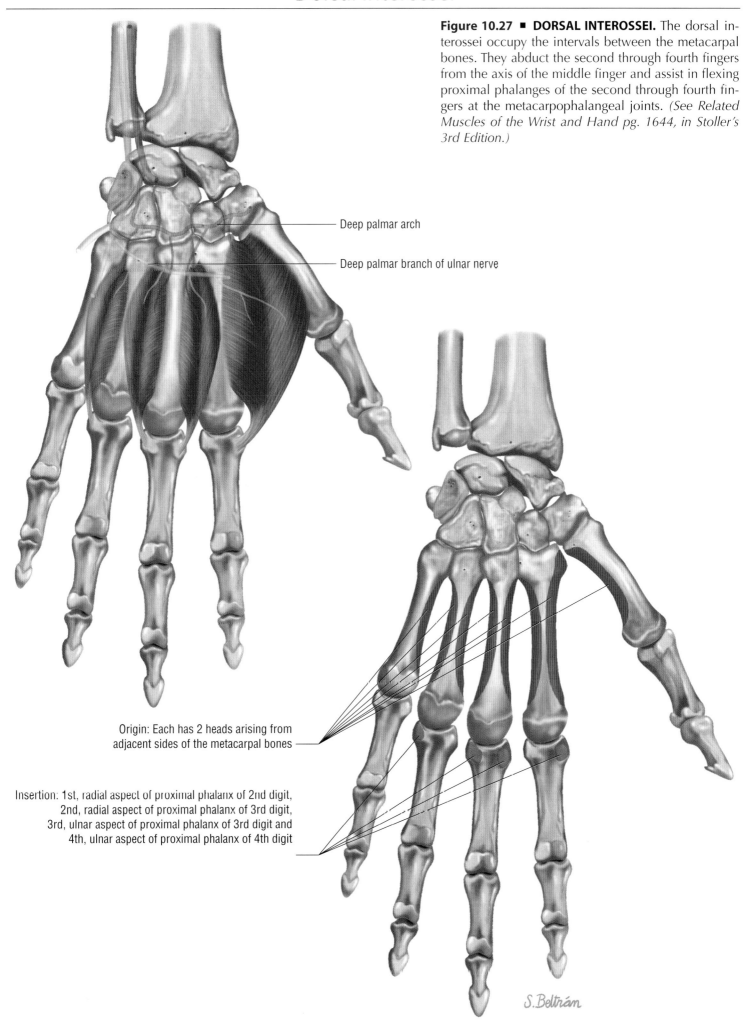

Figure 10.27 ▪ **DORSAL INTEROSSEI.** The dorsal interossei occupy the intervals between the metacarpal bones. They abduct the second through fourth fingers from the axis of the middle finger and assist in flexing proximal phalanges of the second through fourth fingers at the metacarpophalangeal joints. *(See Related Muscles of the Wrist and Hand pg. 1644, in Stoller's 3rd Edition.)*

Deep palmar arch

Deep palmar branch of ulnar nerve

Origin: Each has 2 heads arising from adjacent sides of the metacarpal bones

Insertion: 1st, radial aspect of proximal phalanx of 2nd digit, 2nd, radial aspect of proximal phalanx of 3rd digit, 3rd, ulnar aspect of proximal phalanx of 3rd digit and 4th, ulnar aspect of proximal phalanx of 4th digit

S. Beltrán

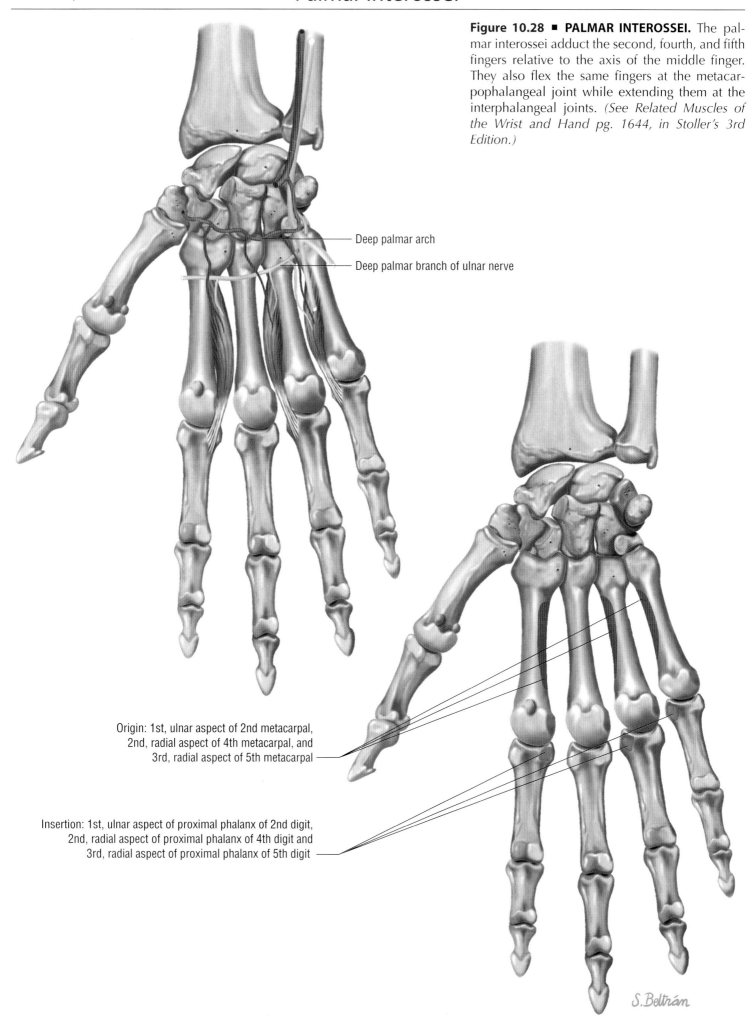

Figure 10.28 ▪ PALMAR INTEROSSEI. The palmar interossei adduct the second, fourth, and fifth fingers relative to the axis of the middle finger. They also flex the same fingers at the metacarpophalangeal joint while extending them at the interphalangeal joints. *(See Related Muscles of the Wrist and Hand pg. 1644, in Stoller's 3rd Edition.)*

Deep palmar arch

Deep palmar branch of ulnar nerve

Origin: 1st, ulnar aspect of 2nd metacarpal, 2nd, radial aspect of 4th metacarpal, and 3rd, radial aspect of 5th metacarpal

Insertion: 1st, ulnar aspect of proximal phalanx of 2nd digit, 2nd, radial aspect of proximal phalanx of 4th digit and 3rd, radial aspect of proximal phalanx of 5th digit

S. Beltrán

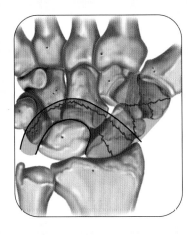

The Wrist and Hand

Anatomy and Pathology

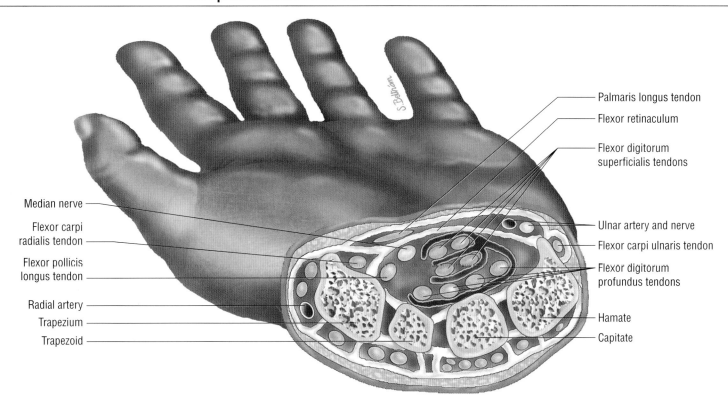

Palmaris longus tendon

Flexor retinaculum

Flexor digitorum superficialis tendons

Ulnar artery and nerve

Flexor carpi ulnaris tendon

Flexor digitorum profundus tendons

Hamate

Capitate

Median nerve

Flexor carpi radialis tendon

Flexor pollicis longus tendon

Radial artery

Trapezium

Trapezoid

Figure 10.29 ▪ The carpal tunnel in cross section. *(See Tendons of the Wrist and Hand pgs. 1691 and 1700, in Stoller's 3rd Edition.)*

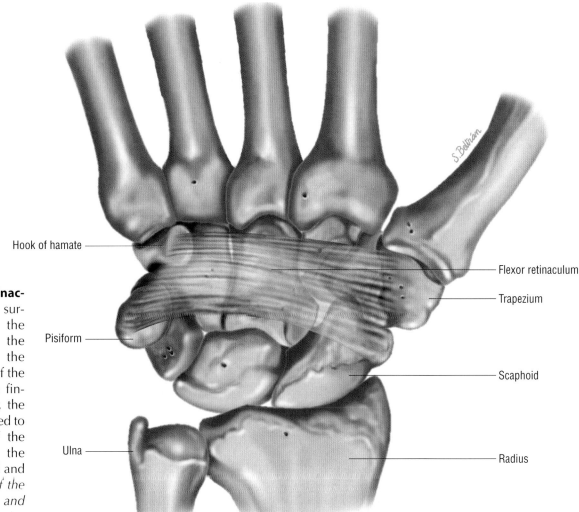

Hook of hamate

Flexor retinaculum

Trapezium

Pisiform

Scaphoid

Ulna

Radius

Figure 10.30 ▪ **Flexor retinaculum.** The concave volar surface of the carpus and the flexor retinaculum form the anatomic boundaries of the carpal tunnel (for passage of the long flexor tendons of the fingers and thumb). Medially, the flexor retinaculum is attached to the pisiform and hook of the hamate and laterally to the tuberosities of the scaphoid and trapezium. *(See Tendons of the Wrist and Hand pgs. 1691 and 1699, in Stoller's 3rd Edition.)*

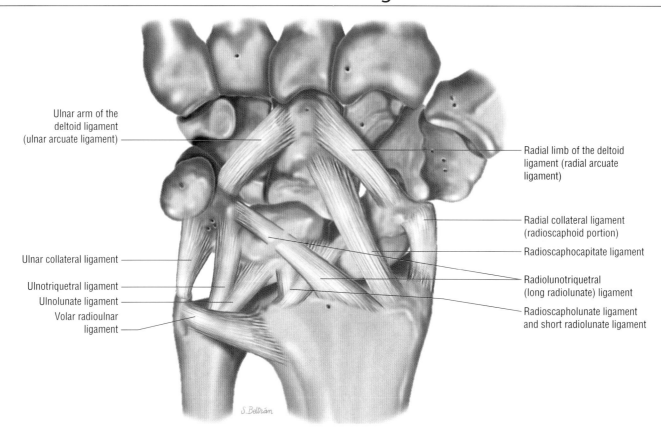

Ulnar arm of the
deltoid ligament
(ulnar arcuate ligament)

Radial limb of the deltoid
ligament (radial arcuate
ligament)

Radial collateral ligament
(radioscaphoid portion)

Radioscaphocapitate ligament

Ulnar collateral ligament

Ulnotriquetral ligament

Ulnolunate ligament

Volar radioulnar
ligament

Radiolunotriquetral
(long radiolunate) ligament

Radioscapholunate ligament
and short radiolunate ligament

Figure 10.31 ▪ The volar extrinsic ligaments. The radioscapholunate ligament courses between the short and long radiolunate (radiolunotriquetral) ligaments. The fibers of the short radiolunate ligament contribute to the floor of the radiolunate space. *Based on Lichtman DM, Alexander AH. The wrist and its disorders, ed 2. Philadelphia: WB Saunders, 1997. (See Extrinsic Ligaments pgs. 1684 and 1685, in Stoller's 3rd Edition.)*

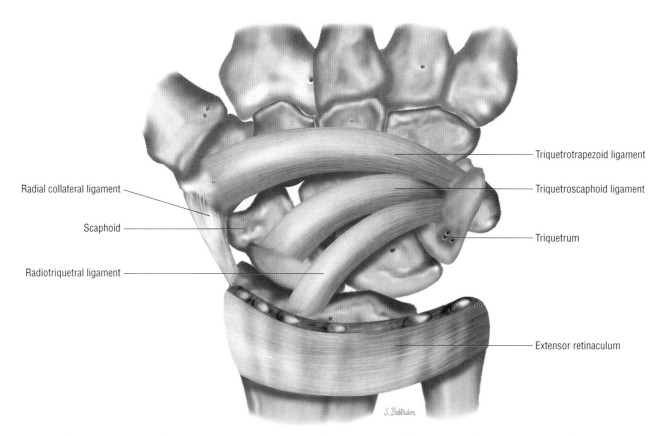

Radial collateral ligament

Scaphoid

Radiotriquetral ligament

Triquetrotrapezoid ligament

Triquetroscaphoid ligament

Triquetrum

Extensor retinaculum

Figure 10.32 ▪ The extensor retinaculum and dorsal carpal ligaments. The radiotriquetral ligament (an extrinsic dorsal capsular ligament) and the dorsal intercarpal ligament (an intrinsic dorsal capsular ligament) are illustrated. The dorsal intercarpal ligament is composed of separate triquetroscaphoid and triquetrotrapezoid fascicles. The radial collateral ligament and the bilaminar extensor retinaculum are also shown. *(See Dorsal Ligaments pgs. 1687 and 1694, in Stoller's 3rd Edition.)*

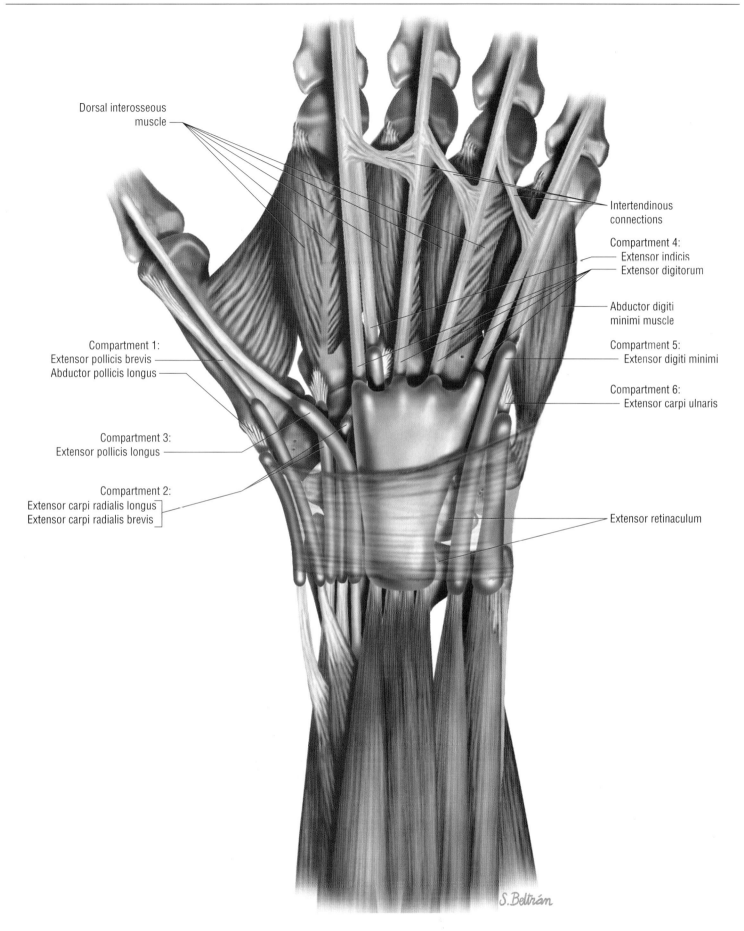

Dorsal interosseous muscle

Intertendinous connections

Compartment 4:
Extensor indicis
Extensor digitorum

Abductor digiti minimi muscle

Compartment 1:
Extensor pollicis brevis
Abductor pollicis longus

Compartment 5:
Extensor digiti minimi

Compartment 6:
Extensor carpi ulnaris

Compartment 3:
Extensor pollicis longus

Compartment 2:
Extensor carpi radialis longus
Extensor carpi radialis brevis

Extensor retinaculum

S. Beltrán

Figure 10.33 ■ The extensor tendons are arranged into six compartments on the dorsum of the wrist. *(See Dorsum of the Hand pgs. 1691 and 1706, in Stoller's 3rd Edition.)*

TFC Complex

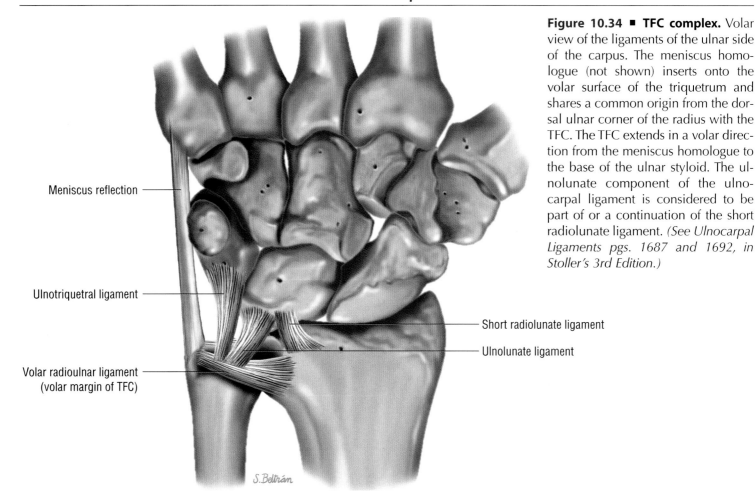

Meniscus reflection

Ulnotriquetral ligament

Volar radioulnar ligament
(volar margin of TFC)

S. Beltrán

Short radiolunate ligament

Ulnolunate ligament

Figure 10.34 ▪ TFC complex. Volar view of the ligaments of the ulnar side of the carpus. The meniscus homologue (not shown) inserts onto the volar surface of the triquetrum and shares a common origin from the dorsal ulnar corner of the radius with the TFC. The TFC extends in a volar direction from the meniscus homologue to the base of the ulnar styloid. The ulnolunate component of the ulnocarpal ligament is considered to be part of or a continuation of the short radiolunate ligament. *(See Ulnocarpal Ligaments pgs. 1687 and 1692, in Stoller's 3rd Edition.)*

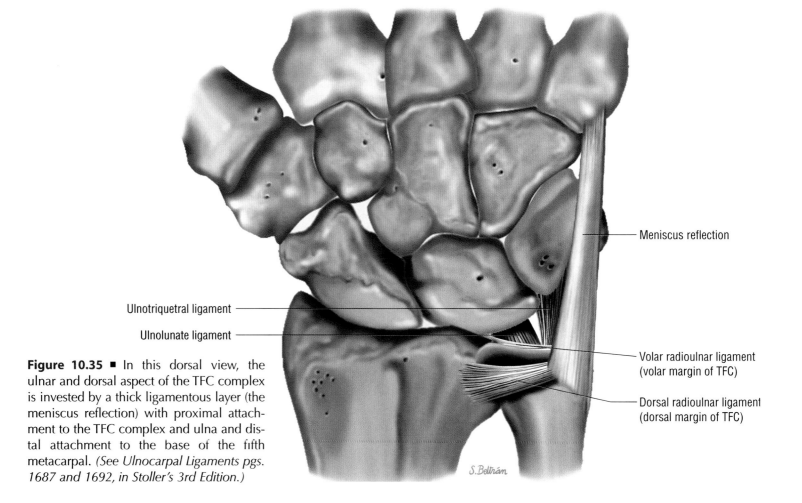

Ulnotriquetral ligament

Ulnolunate ligament

Meniscus reflection

Volar radioulnar ligament
(volar margin of TFC)

Dorsal radioulnar ligament
(dorsal margin of TFC)

S. Beltrán

Figure 10.35 ▪ In this dorsal view, the ulnar and dorsal aspect of the TFC complex is invested by a thick ligamentous layer (the meniscus reflection) with proximal attachment to the TFC complex and ulna and distal attachment to the base of the fifth metacarpal. *(See Ulnocarpal Ligaments pgs. 1687 and 1692, in Stoller's 3rd Edition.)*

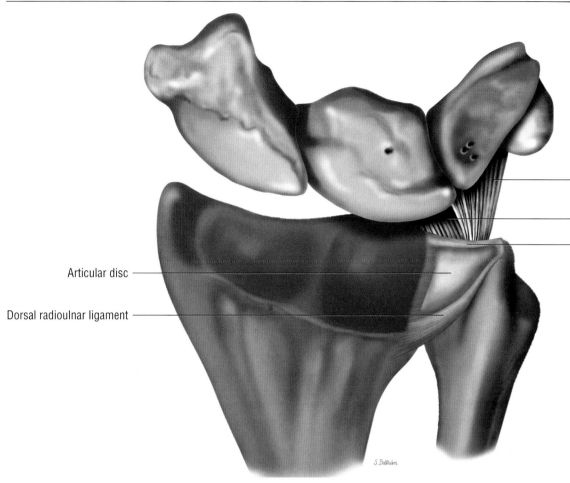

Figure 10.36 ■ Dorsal superior view of the TFC complex demonstrates the dorsal and volar radioulnar ligaments as separate from the articular disc of the TFC. *(See Ulnocarpal Ligaments pgs. 1687, 1692, and 1693, in Stoller's 3rd Edition.)*

Ulnotriquetral ligament

Ulnolunate ligament

Volar radioulnar ligament

Articular disc

Dorsal radioulnar ligament

Figure 10.37 ■ Dorsal view of the TFC complex. TFC refers to the central horizontal articular disc and adjoining volar and dorsal radioulnar ligaments. TFC complex refers to the TFC and any additional ulnar ligamentous structures, such as the meniscus homologue, ulnar collateral ligament, subsheath of the extensor carpi ulnaris tendon, and ulnolunate and ulnotriquetral ligaments. *(See Ulnocarpal Ligament pgs. 1687, 1692, and 1693, in Stoller's 3rd Edition.)*

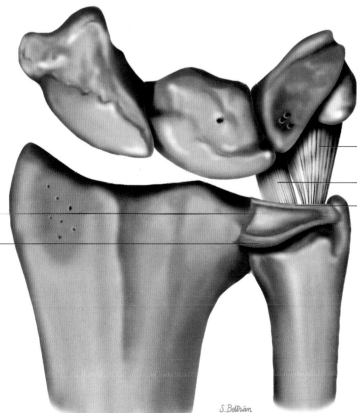

Articular disc

Dorsal radioulnar ligament (dorsal margin of TFC)

Ulnotriquetral ligament

Ulnolunate ligament

Volar radioulnar ligament (volar margin of TFC)

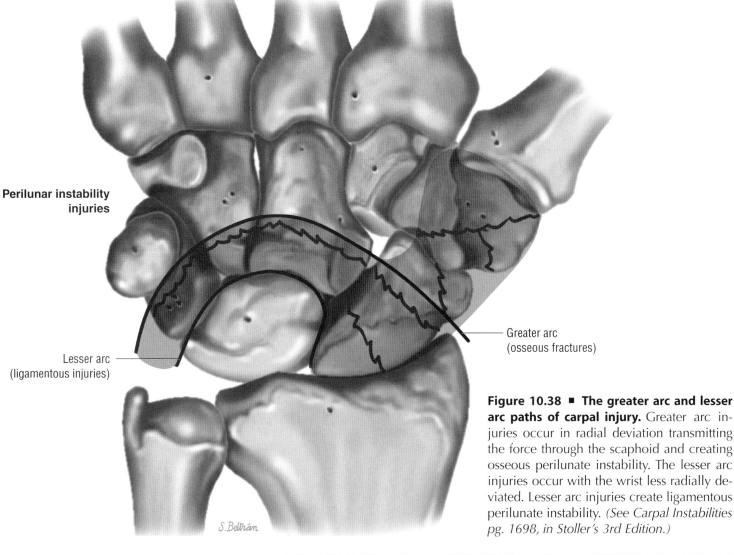

Perilunar instability injuries

Lesser arc (ligamentous injuries)

Greater arc (osseous fractures)

S.Beltrán

Figure 10.38 ■ **The greater arc and lesser arc paths of carpal injury.** Greater arc injuries occur in radial deviation transmitting the force through the scaphoid and creating osseous perilunate instability. The lesser arc injuries occur with the wrist less radially deviated. Lesser arc injuries create ligamentous perilunate instability. *(See Carpal Instabilities pg. 1698, in Stoller's 3rd Edition.)*

Figure 10.39 ■ **Membranous wedge-shaped component of the scapholunate ligament with direct proximal attachment to the articular surfaces of the scaphoid and lunate.** The distal apex is free without direct attachment and presents as a prominent distal protrusion into the scapholunate articulation. *(See Intrinsic Interosseous Ligaments pgs. 1688, 1689, and 1696, in Stoller's 3rd Edition.)*

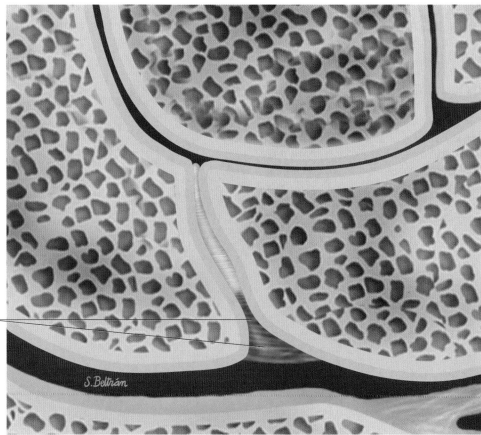

Membranous scapholunate ligament

S.Beltrán

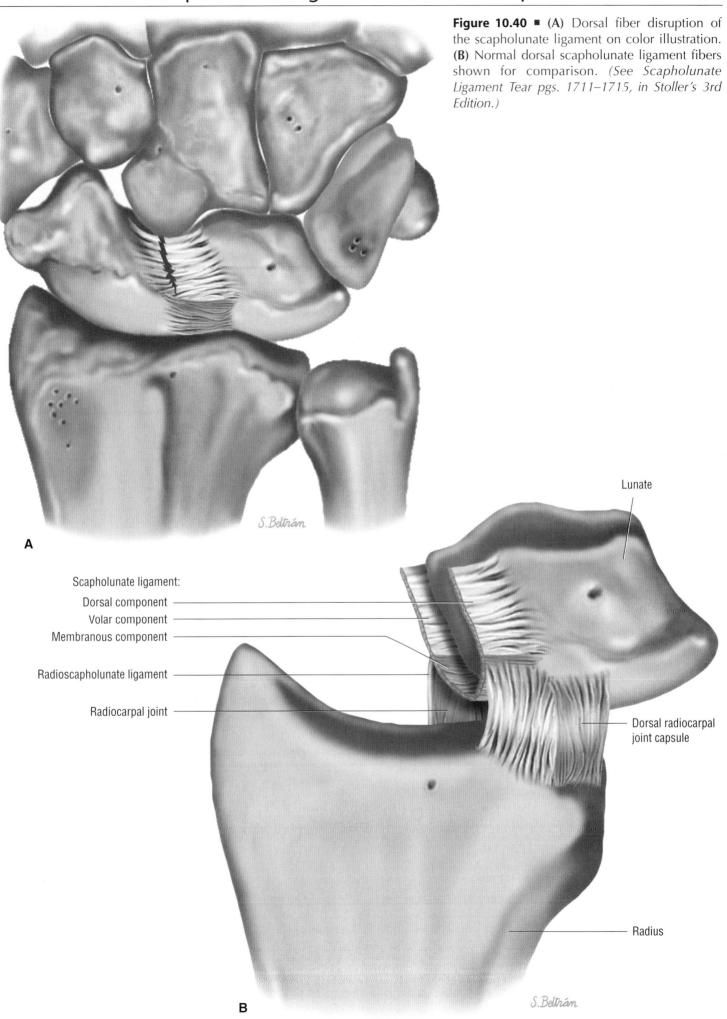

Figure 10.40 ■ **(A)** Dorsal fiber disruption of the scapholunate ligament on color illustration. **(B)** Normal dorsal scapholunate ligament fibers shown for comparison. *(See Scapholunate Ligament Tear pgs. 1711–1715, in Stoller's 3rd Edition.)*

A

Lunate

Scapholunate ligament:

Dorsal component

Volar component

Membranous component

Radioscapholunate ligament

Radiocarpal joint

Dorsal radiocarpal joint capsule

Radius

B

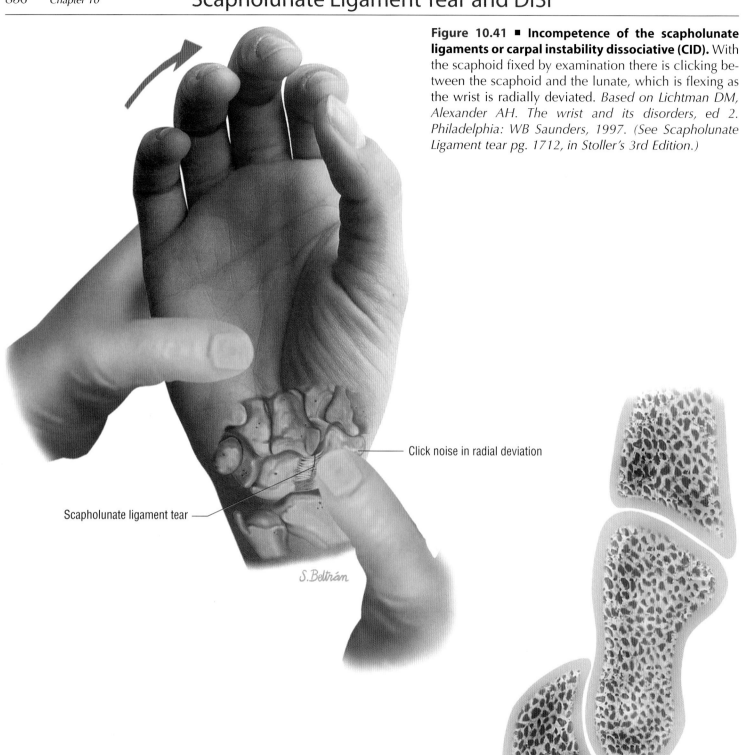

S. Beltrán

Click noise in radial deviation

Scapholunate ligament tear

Figure 10.41 ■ **Incompetence of the scapholunate ligaments or carpal instability dissociative (CID).** With the scaphoid fixed by examination there is clicking between the scaphoid and the lunate, which is flexing as the wrist is radially deviated. *Based on Lichtman DM, Alexander AH. The wrist and its disorders, ed 2. Philadelphia: WB Saunders, 1997. (See Scapholunate Ligament tear pg. 1712, in Stoller's 3rd Edition.)*

Figure 10.42 ■ **DISI deformity with lunate extension or dorsal tilting of the lunate and proximal movement of the capitate.** DISI deformity is characterized by a scapholunate angle greater than 70°, a capitolunate angle greater than 20°, and a dorsiflexed and volarly displaced lunate. DISI deformity is not pathognomonic for scapholunate instability and can be associated with unstable scaphoid fractures (bony DISI), and capsular/ligamentous pathology, including scapholunate instability (ligamentous DISI). Lateral graphic of DISI with dorsal tilting of the lunate. *(See Scapholunate Ligament Tear pg. 1718, in Stoller's 3rd Edition.)*

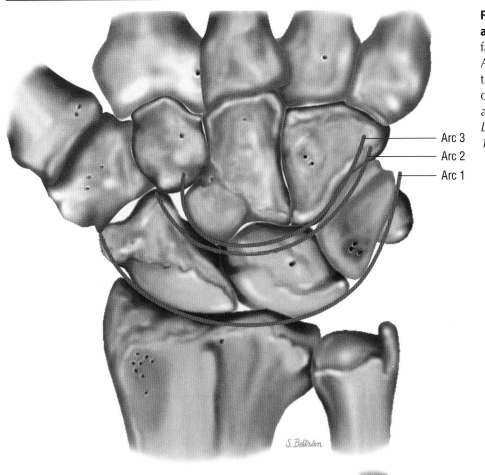

Figure 10.43 ■ Normal congruity of carpal arcs. Arc 1 connects the proximal articular surfaces of the scaphoid, lunate, and triquetrum. Arc 2 connects the distal concave surfaces of the scaphoid, lunate, and triquetrum. Arc 3 outlines the proximal convexity of the capitate and hamate. Coronal color illustration. *(See Lunotriquetral Ligament Tear pgs. 1721 and 1724, in Stoller's 3rd Edition.)*

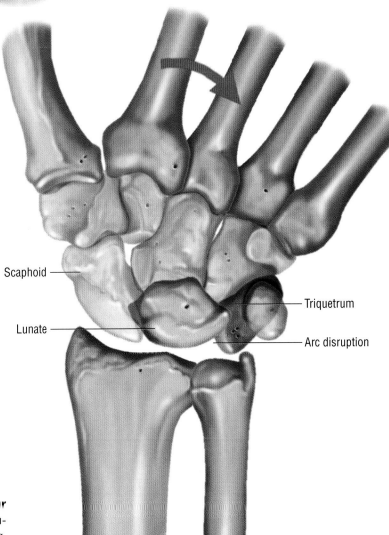

Figure 10.44 ■ Disruption of the smooth convex contour at the proximal carpal row. There is overlapping of the lunate and triquetrum. *(See Lunotriquetral Ligament Tear pg. 1724, in Stoller's 3rd Edition.)*

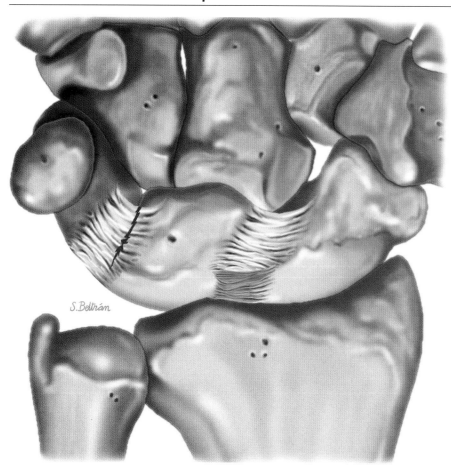

Figure 10.45 ■ Volar component tear of the lunotriquetral (LT) ligament. *(See Lunotriquetral Ligament pgs. 1720, 1721, and 1726, in Stoller's 3rd Edition.)*

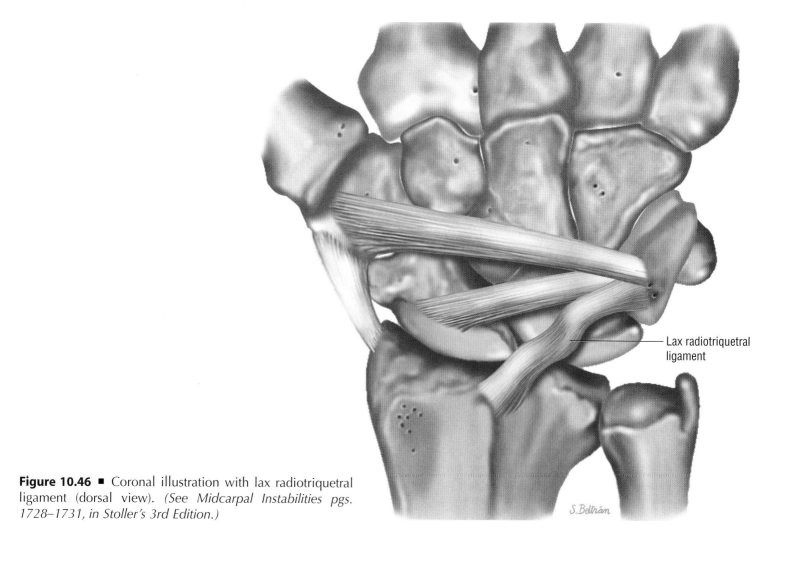

Lax radiotriquetral ligament

Figure 10.46 ■ Coronal illustration with lax radiotriquetral ligament (dorsal view). *(See Midcarpal Instabilities pgs. 1728–1731, in Stoller's 3rd Edition.)*

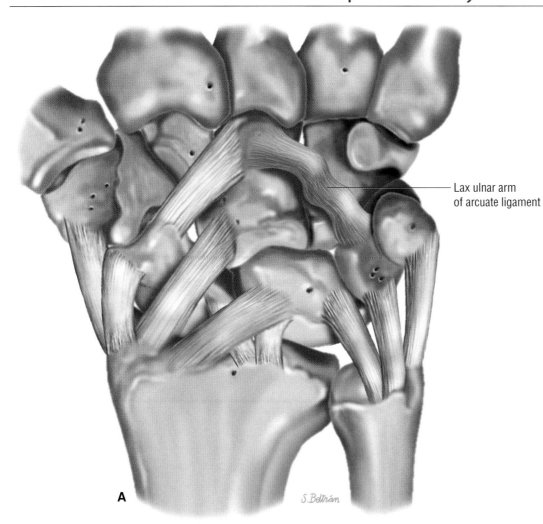

Lax ulnar arm
of arcuate ligament

A

S.Beltrán

Figure 10.47 ▪ Palmar midcarpal instability (MCI) is the most common pattern of midcarpal instability. Palmar MCI is associated with laxity of the ulnar arm of the arcuate ligament and the dorsal radiotriquetral ligament with palmar (volar) translation of the distal carpal row. **(A)** Coronal illustration of the lax ulnar arm of the arcuate ligament. **(B)** Coronal illustration of the lax radioscaphocapitate ligament as seen in dorsal midcarpal instability in contrast to palmar midcarpal instability. Dorsal midcarpal instability is a much less common variant of midcarpal instability. *(See Midcarpal Instabilities pgs. 1728–1730, in Stoller's 3rd Edition.)*

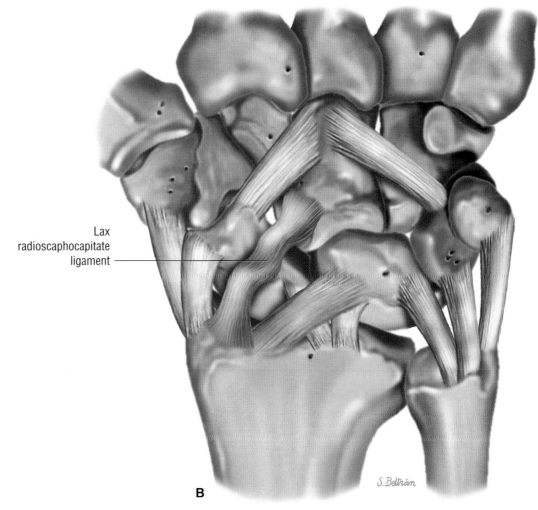

Lax
radioscaphocapitate
ligament

B

S.Beltrán

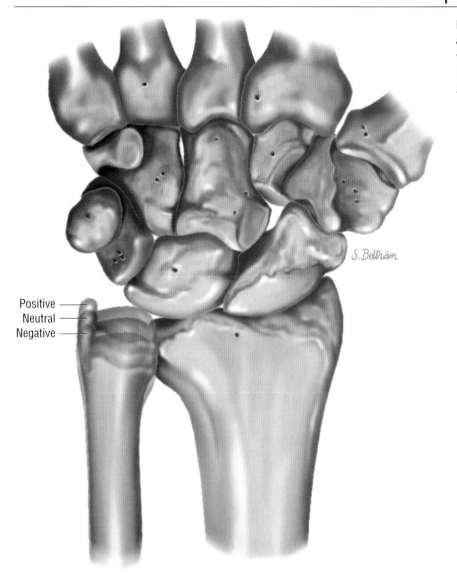

Positive —
Neutral —
Negative —

Figure 10.48 ■ Negative ulnar variance is associated with avascular necrosis of the lunate. Positive variance is associated with ulnocarpal impaction. *(See Ulnar Variance pg. 1733, in Stoller's 3rd Edition.)*

Figure 10.49 ■ Coronal color illustration of ulnocarpal (ulnolunate) abutment with associated lunotriquetral ligament tear. TFC perforation and reactive subchondral edema are shown in the lunate and triquetrum. *(See Ulnocarpal (Ulnolunate) Abutment (Impaction) Syndrome pgs. 1733–1735, in Stoller's 3rd Edition.)*

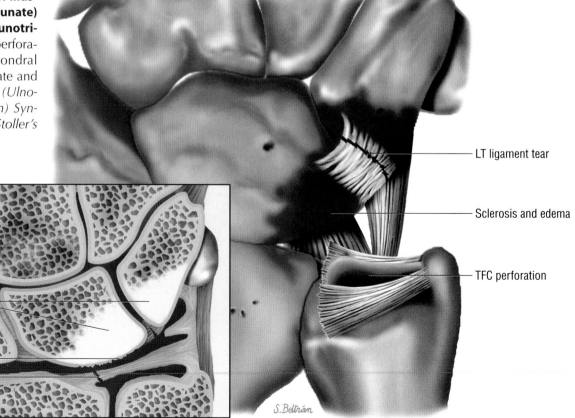

LT ligament tear

Sclerosis and edema

TFC perforation

Lunate and triquetral edema

Lunate chondromalacia

TFC perforation

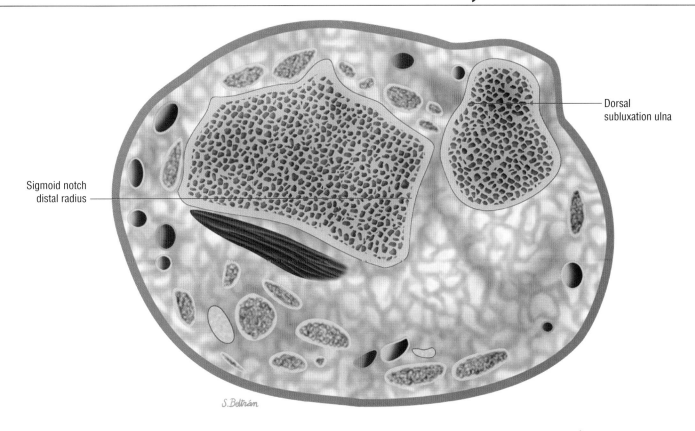

Figure 10.50 ▪ Dorsal subluxation of the ulna relative to the sigmoid notch. Axial color graphic. *(See Instability of the Distal Radioulnar Joint pgs. 1736 and 1739, in Stoller's 3rd Edition.)*

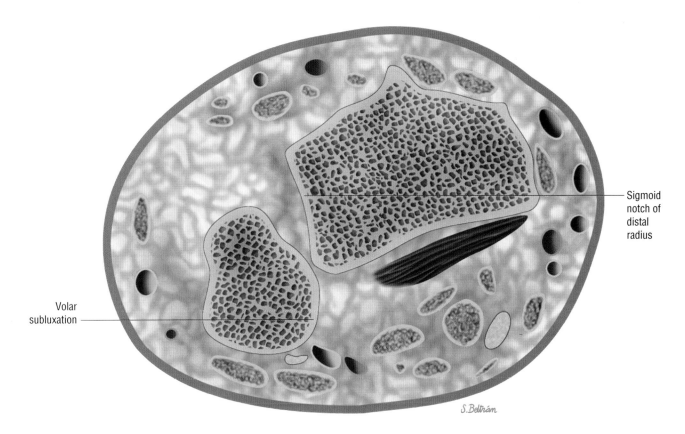

Figure 10.51 ▪ Volar subluxation of the distal ulna (dorsal subluxation of the distal radius) with disruption of the dorsal margin of the TFC (dorsal radioulnar ligament). Axial color graphic. *(See Instability of the Distal Radioulnar Joint pgs. 1736 and 1740, in Stoller's 3rd Edition.)*

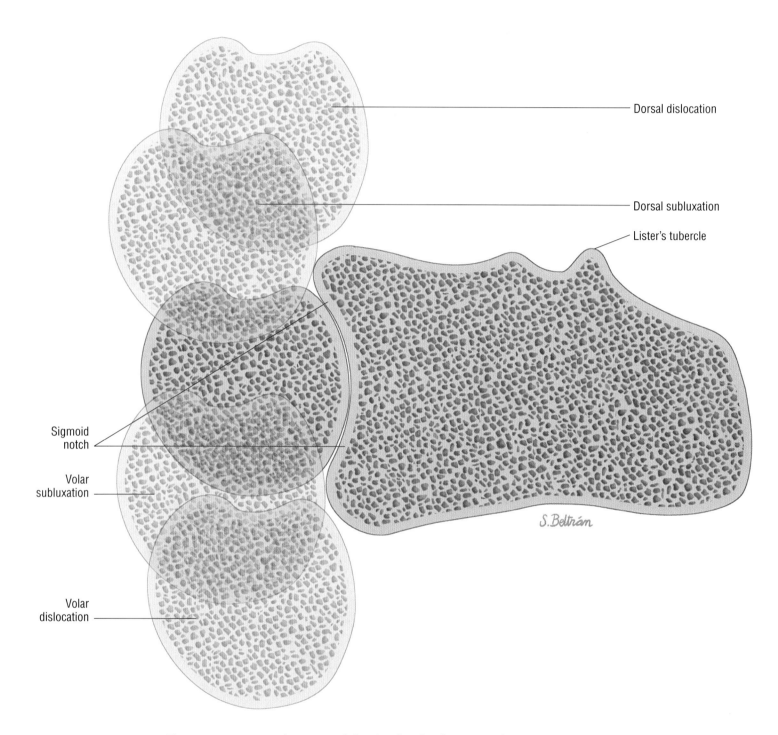

Dorsal dislocation

Dorsal subluxation

Lister's tubercle

Sigmoid notch

Volar subluxation

Volar dislocation

S. Beltrán

Figure 10.52 ■ Axial section of the distal radioulnar joint demonstrating the positions of subluxation and dislocation of the distal ulna relative to the sigmoid notch of the distal radius. *(See Instability of the Distal Radioulnar Joint pg. 1741, in Stoller's 3rd Edition.)*

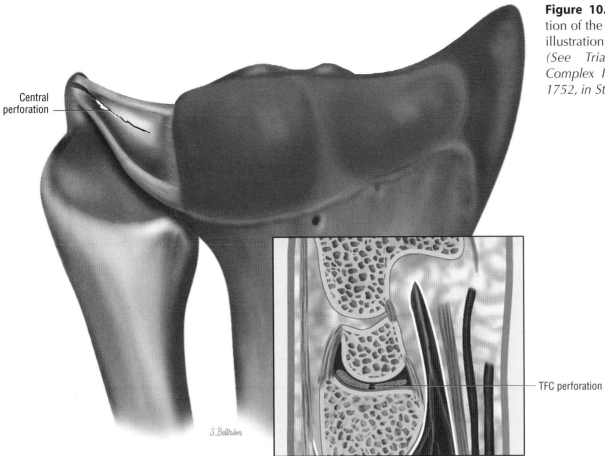

Figure 10.53 ▪ Central perforation of the TFC on a coronal color illustration with a sagittal inset. *(See Triangular Fibrocartilage Complex Injuries pgs. 1742 and 1752, in Stoller's 3rd Edition.)*

Central perforation

TFC perforation

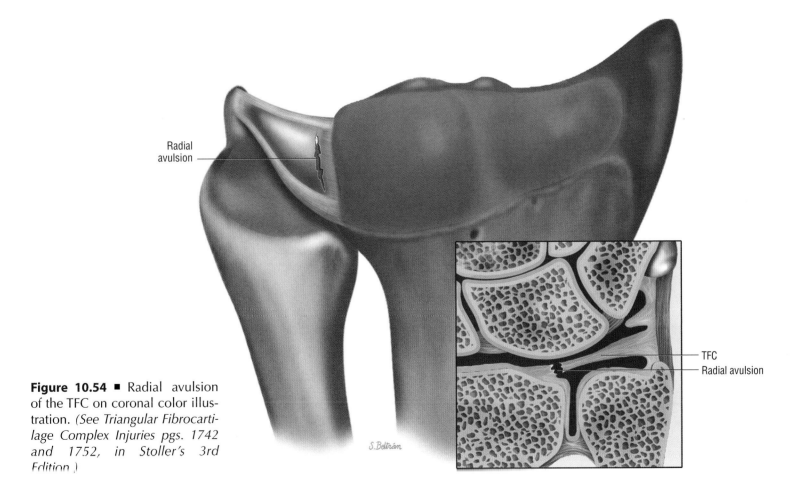

Radial avulsion

TFC

Radial avulsion

Figure 10.54 ▪ Radial avulsion of the TFC on coronal color illustration. *(See Triangular Fibrocartilage Complex Injuries pgs. 1742 and 1752, in Stoller's 3rd Edition.)*

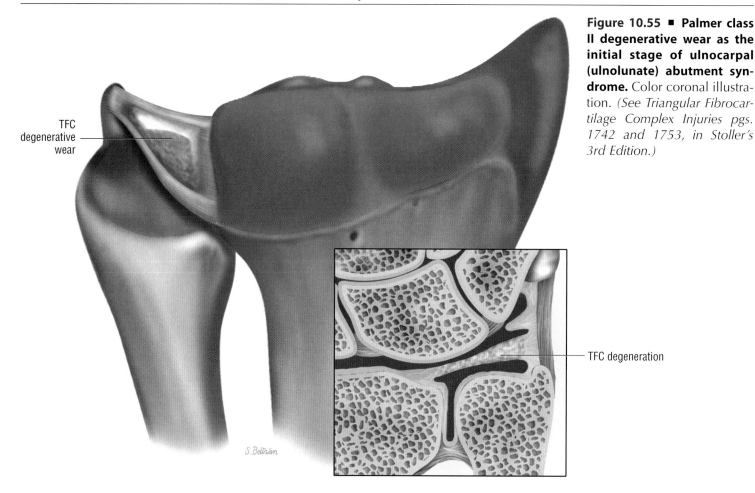

TFC
degenerative
wear

TFC degeneration

S.Beltrán

Figure 10.55 ■ **Palmer class II degenerative wear as the initial stage of ulnocarpal (ulnolunate) abutment syndrome.** Color coronal illustration. *(See Triangular Fibrocartilage Complex Injuries pgs. 1742 and 1753, in Stoller's 3rd Edition.)*

Figure 10.56 ■ **Advanced changes of ulnocarpal (ulnolunate) abutment (Palmer class II) with TFC tear, lunate, triquetral and ulnar chondromalacia, and lunotriquetral ligament tear**. Coronal color illustration. *(See Triangular Fibrocartilage Complex Injuries pgs. 1742 and 1754, in Stoller's 3rd Edition.)*

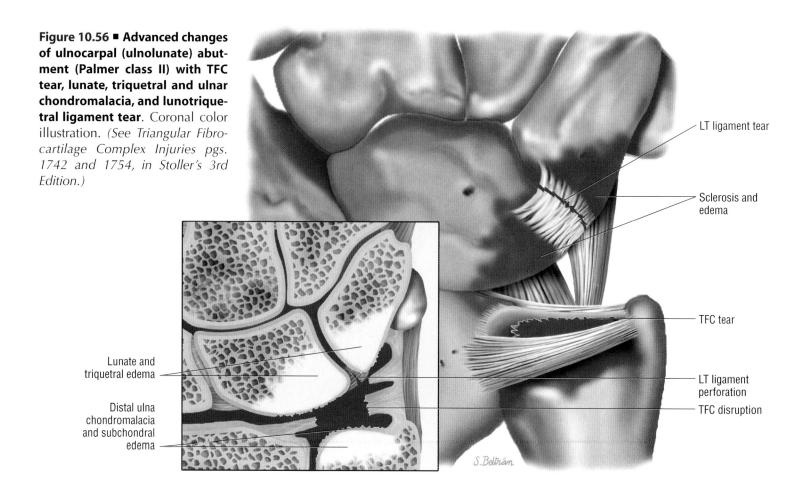

LT ligament tear

Sclerosis and
edema

TFC tear

LT ligament
perforation

TFC disruption

Lunate and
triquetral edema

Distal ulna
chondromalacia
and subchondral
edema

S.Beltrán

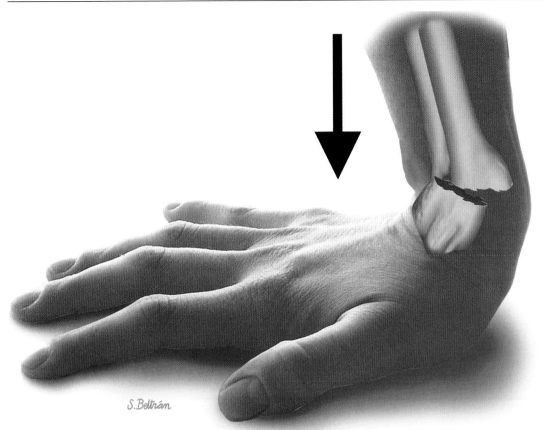

Figure 10.57 ■ Dorsal displacement of the distal radius in Colles' fracture resulting from a fall on an outstretched hand. *(See Colles' Fracture pg. 1756, in Stoller's 3rd Edition.)*

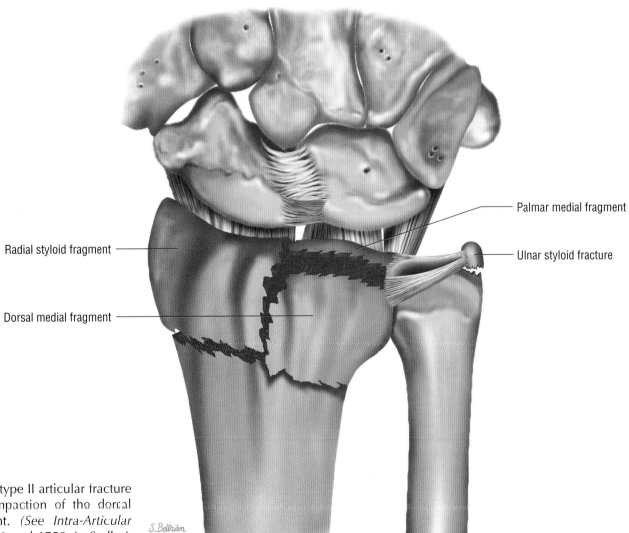

Radial styloid fragment

Dorsal medial fragment

Palmar medial fragment

Ulnar styloid fracture

Figure 10.58 ■ A type II articular fracture with die punch impaction of the dorsal medial component. *(See Intra-Articular Fractures pgs. 1756 and 1758, in Stoller's 3rd Edition.)*

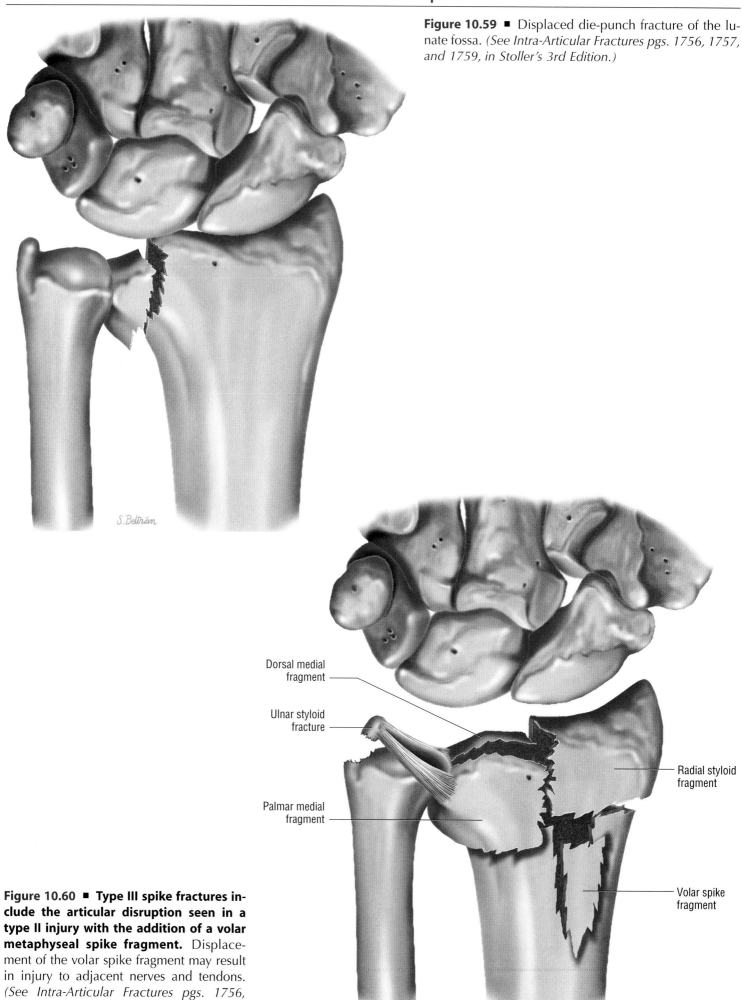

Figure 10.59 ■ Displaced die-punch fracture of the lunate fossa. *(See Intra-Articular Fractures pgs. 1756, 1757, and 1759, in Stoller's 3rd Edition.)*

Dorsal medial fragment

Ulnar styloid fracture

Palmar medial fragment

Radial styloid fragment

Volar spike fragment

Figure 10.60 ■ **Type III spike fractures include the articular disruption seen in a type II injury with the addition of a volar metaphyseal spike fragment.** Displacement of the volar spike fragment may result in injury to adjacent nerves and tendons. *(See Intra-Articular Fractures pgs. 1756, 1757, and 1759, in Stoller's 3rd Edition.)*

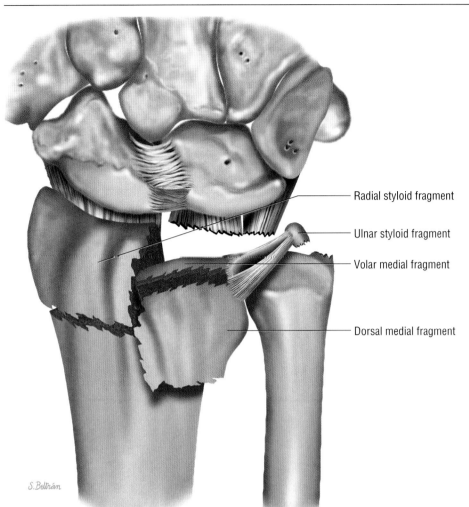

Radial styloid fragment

Ulnar styloid fragment

Volar medial fragment

Dorsal medial fragment

Figure 10.61 ■ Type IV fracture pattern with wide separation on rotation of the dorsal and palmar medial fragments. *(See Intra-Articular Fractures pgs. 1756, 1757, and 1760, in Stoller's 3rd Edition.)*

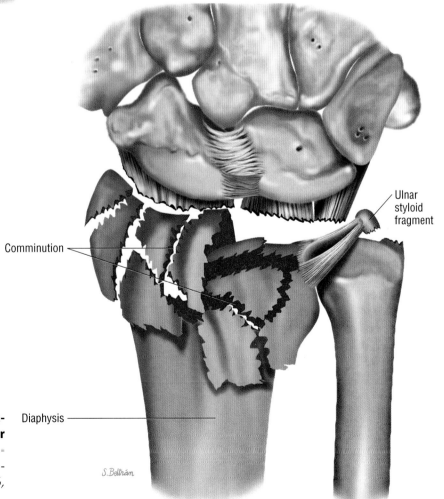

Ulnar styloid fragment

Comminution

Diaphysis

Figure 10.62 ■ **Type V explosion fracture with comminution extending from the distal radius articular surfaces to the diaphysis.** This injury pattern is associated with massive soft-tissue trauma. Coronal color illustration. *(See Intra-Articular Fractures pgs. 1756, 1756, and 1760, in Stoller's 3rd Edition.)*

Ulnar Styloid Fracture

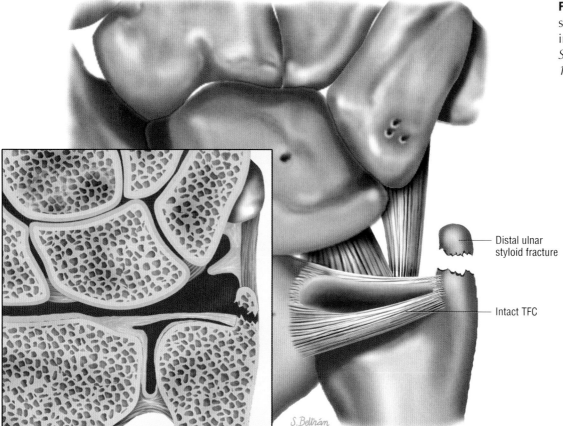

Figure 10.63 ■ Type 1 ulnar styloid fracture nonunion with intact TFC complex. *(See Ulnar Styloid Fractures pgs. 1760 and 1761, in Stoller's 3rd Edition.)*

Distal ulnar styloid fracture

Intact TFC

S. Beltrán

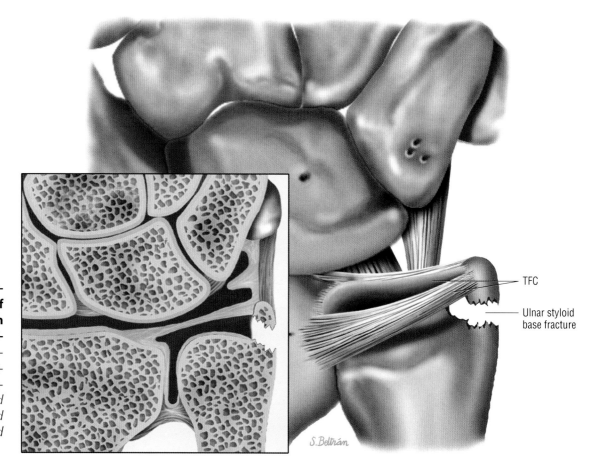

Figure 10.64 ■ **Ulnar styloid fracture at the base of the styloid associated with an unstable distal radioulnar joint.** The TFC and ulnocarpal ligaments are attached to the styloid fragment. *(See Ulnar Styloid Fractures pgs. 1760 and 1762, in Stoller's 3rd Edition.)*

TFC

Ulnar styloid base fracture

S. Beltrán

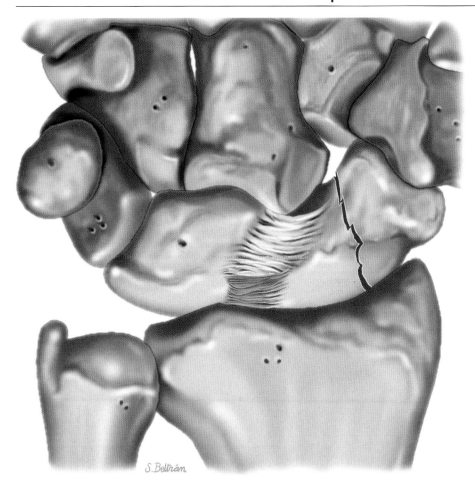

Figure 10.65 ■ **Middle-third scaphoid waist fracture.** The scaphoid is unique in its relationship to the distal radius, distal carpal row, and volar carpal ligaments and is more susceptible to injury than the other carpal bones. Coronal color illustration. *(See Scaphoid Fractures pgs. 1762–1765, in Stoller's 3rd Edition.)*

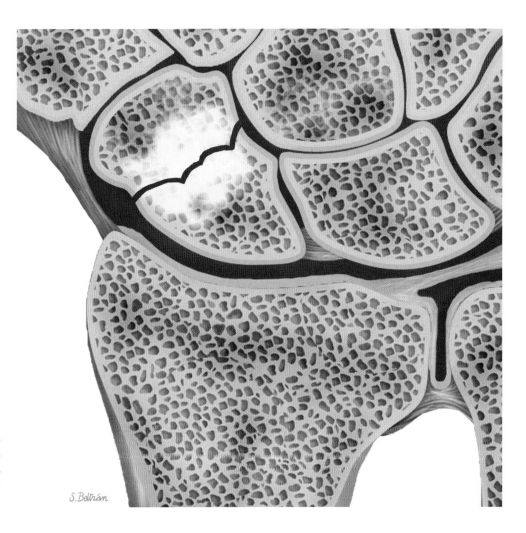

Figure 10.66 ■ **Marrow edema on proximal and distal sides of a scaphoid fracture.** Coronal color illustration. *(See Scaphoid Fractures pg. 1766, in Stoller's 3rd Edition.)*

Scaphoid Fracture and Flexion

Fracture patterns in the scaphoid

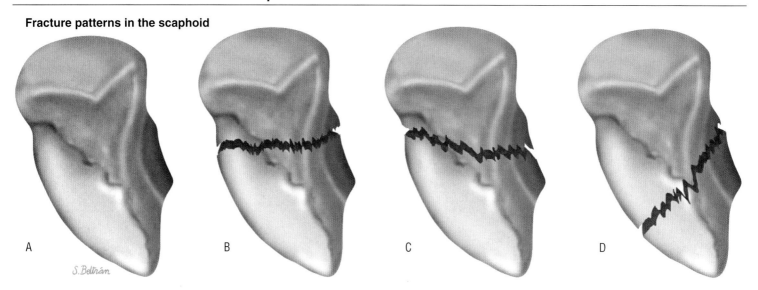

S.Beltrán

A   B   C   D

Figure 10.67 ▪ **Fracture patterns in the scaphoid. (A)** Scaphoid non-union may occur in the proximal, middle or distal third of the scaphoid. **(B)** Transverse fracture. **(C)** Horizontal oblique fracture pattern. **(D)** Vertical oblique fracture. *(See Scaphoid Fractures pgs. 1762–1767, in Stoller's 3rd Edition.)*

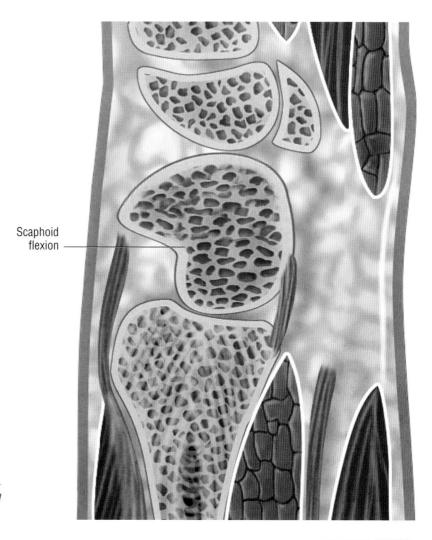

Scaphoid flexion

Figure 10.68 ▪ Scaphoid flexion on color sagittal illustration. *(See Scaphoid Fractures pg. 1767, in Stoller's 3rd Edition.)*

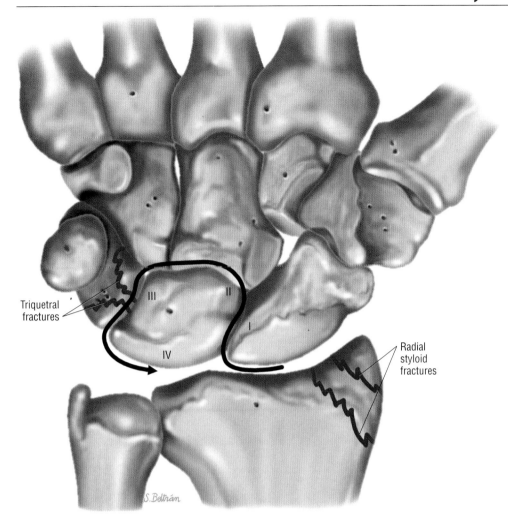

Figure 10.69 ■ Perilunate pattern of injury. There is a progression from Stage I to Stage IV. In Stage I there is partial disruption of the scapholunate interval. Stage II demonstrates a complete disruption of the scapholunate joint. In Stage III there is disruption of the scapholunate, capitolunate, and lunotriquetral joints. In Stage IV there is the addition of the dorsal radiocarpal ligaments, which allows volar lunate dislocation or dorsal perilunate dislocation. Radial styloid or triquetrum fractures may be associated with perilunate ligament injuries. *Based on Lichtman DM, Alexander AH. The wrist and its disorders, ed 2. Philadelphia: WB Saunders, 1997. (See Unstable Scaphoid Fracture Dislocations pgs. 1767 and 1769, in Stoller's 3rd Edition.)*

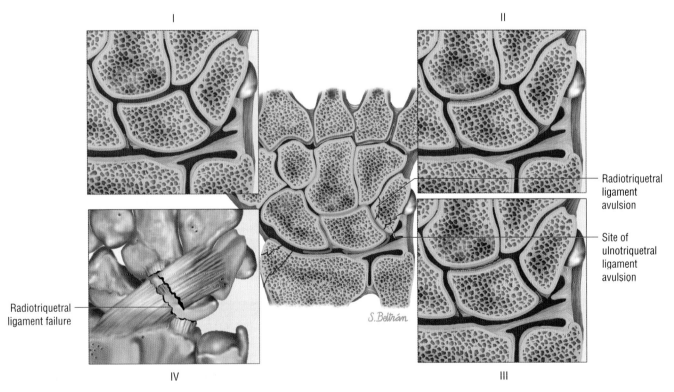

Figure 10.70 ■ Perilunate patterns of instability. Stage I is scapholunate failure, stage II is capitolunate failure, stage III is triquetrolunate failure (with triquetral dislocation and radiotriquetral ligament failure), and stage IV is dorsal radiocarpal ligament failure resulting in volar rotation of the lunate. Color coronal illustrations. *(See Unstable Scaphoid Fracture Dislocations pgs. 1767 and 1769, in Stoller's 3rd Edition.)*

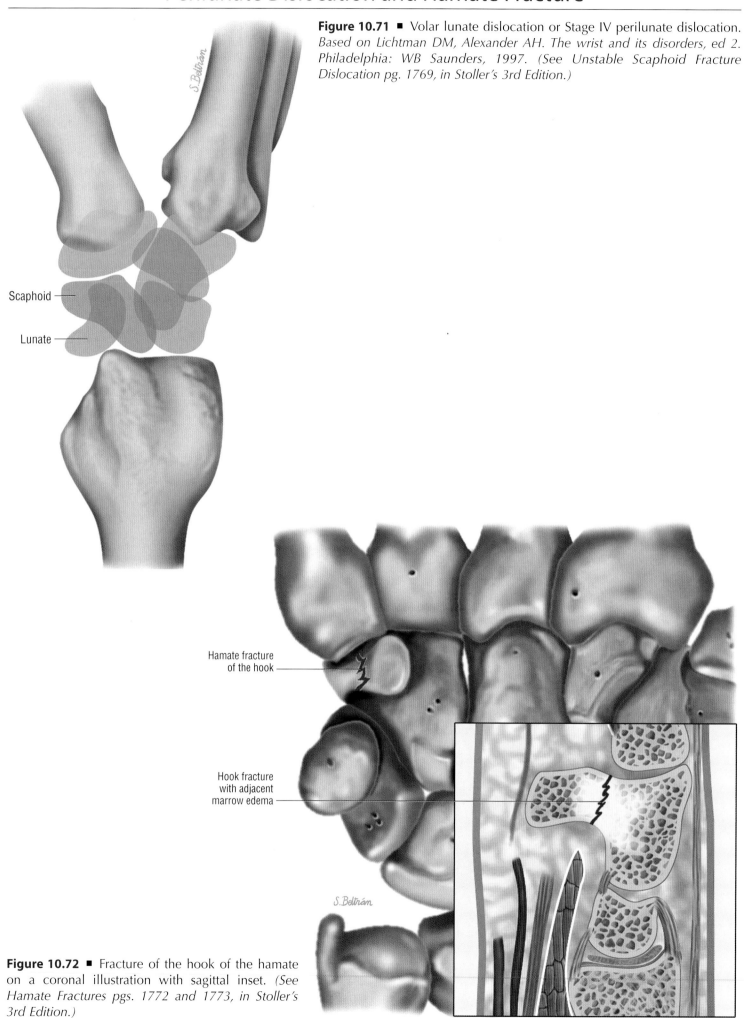

Scaphoid

Lunate

Figure 10.71 ■ Volar lunate dislocation or Stage IV perilunate dislocation. *Based on Lichtman DM, Alexander AH. The wrist and its disorders, ed 2. Philadelphia: WB Saunders, 1997. (See Unstable Scaphoid Fracture Dislocation pg. 1769, in Stoller's 3rd Edition.)*

Hamate fracture of the hook

Hook fracture with adjacent marrow edema

Figure 10.72 ■ Fracture of the hook of the hamate on a coronal illustration with sagittal inset. *(See Hamate Fractures pgs. 1772 and 1773, in Stoller's 3rd Edition.)*

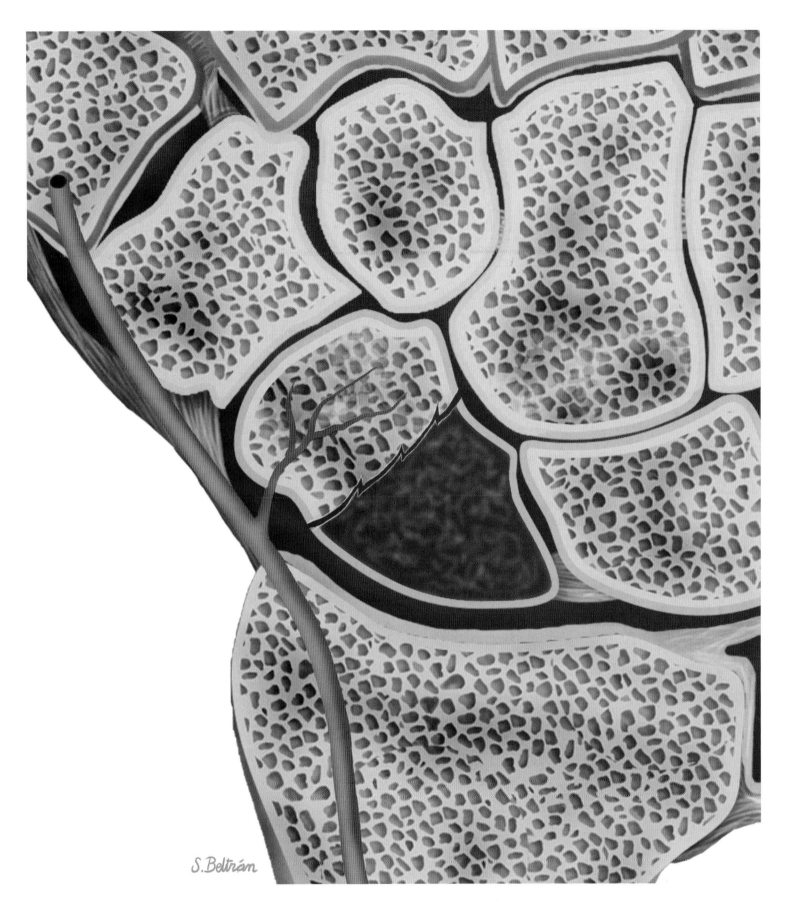

Figure 10.73 ▪ **Coronal illustration shows a fracture of the waist of the scaphoid with AVN of the proximal pole.** The vascular supply to the proximal pole occurs through the radial artery from the distal pole. *(See Avascular Necrosis and Nonunion of the Scaphoid pgs. 1774–1777, in Stoller's 3rd Edition.)*

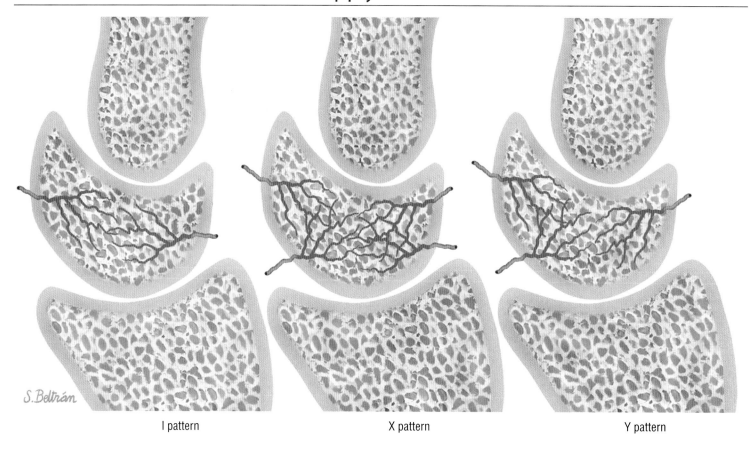

I pattern   X pattern   Y pattern

Figure 10.74 ■ Three patterns of the interosseous vascular supply of the lunate. Acute trauma or repeated microtrauma with excessive shear force results in interruption of the blood supply to a lunate susceptible to or at risk for Kienböck's disease. A single nutrient vessel or compromised intraosseous blood supply places the lunate at risk. Sagittal color illustrations. *(See Kienböck's Disease pgs. 1779 and 1782, in Stoller's 3rd Edition.)*

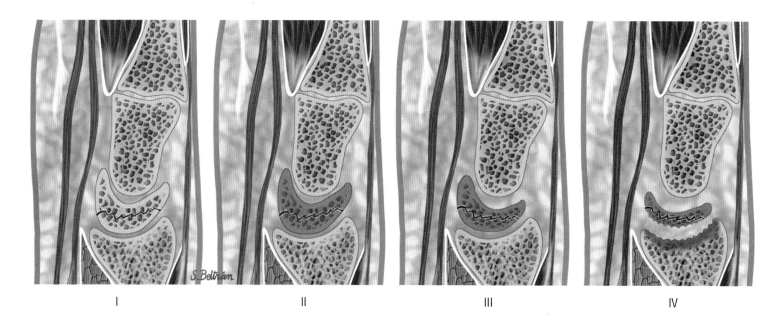

I   II   III   IV

Figure 10.75 ■ The four stages of Kienböck's disease. In contrast to stages I and II, stages III and IV are characterized by lunate collapse in the coronal plane and elongation of the lunate in the sagittal plane. Associated findings (in Stage III and IV) include proximal migration of the capitate, scapholunate dissociation, scaphoid flexion, and ulnar migration of the triquetrum. Stage IV has generalized degenerative changes of the carpus. Extensive lunate marrow edema is associated with Stage I Kienböck's disease. Sagittal color illustration. *(See Kienböck's Disease pgs. 1782 and 1783, in Stoller's 3rd Edition.)*

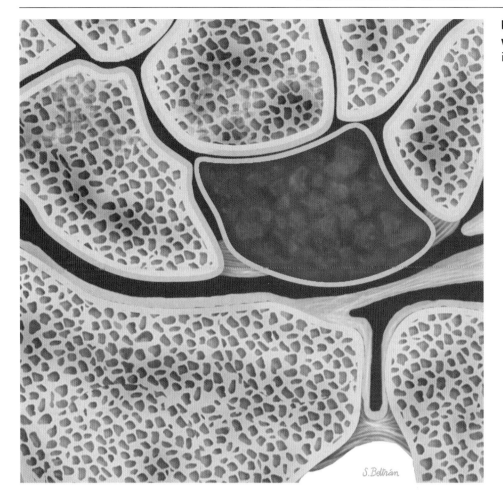

Figure 10.76 ■ **Stage I Kienböck's disease without visible fracture line.** Color coronal illustration. *(See Kienböck's Disease pgs. 1782 and 1784, in Stoller's 3rd Edition.)*

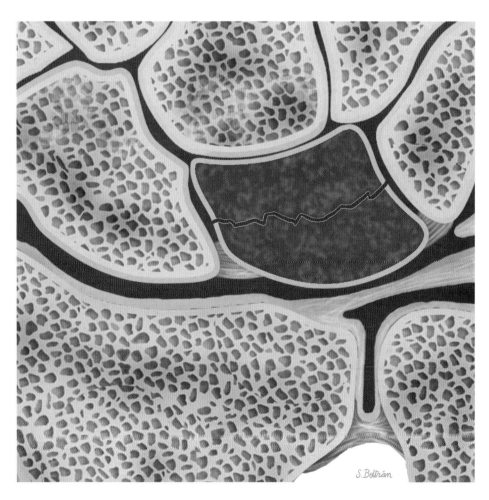

Figure 10.77 ■ **Discrete transverse fracture line associated with Stage I Kienböck's disease.** Coronal color illustration. *(See Kienböck's Disease pgs. 1779 and 1788, in Stoller's 3rd Edition.)*

Flexor Retinaculum and Carpal Tunnel

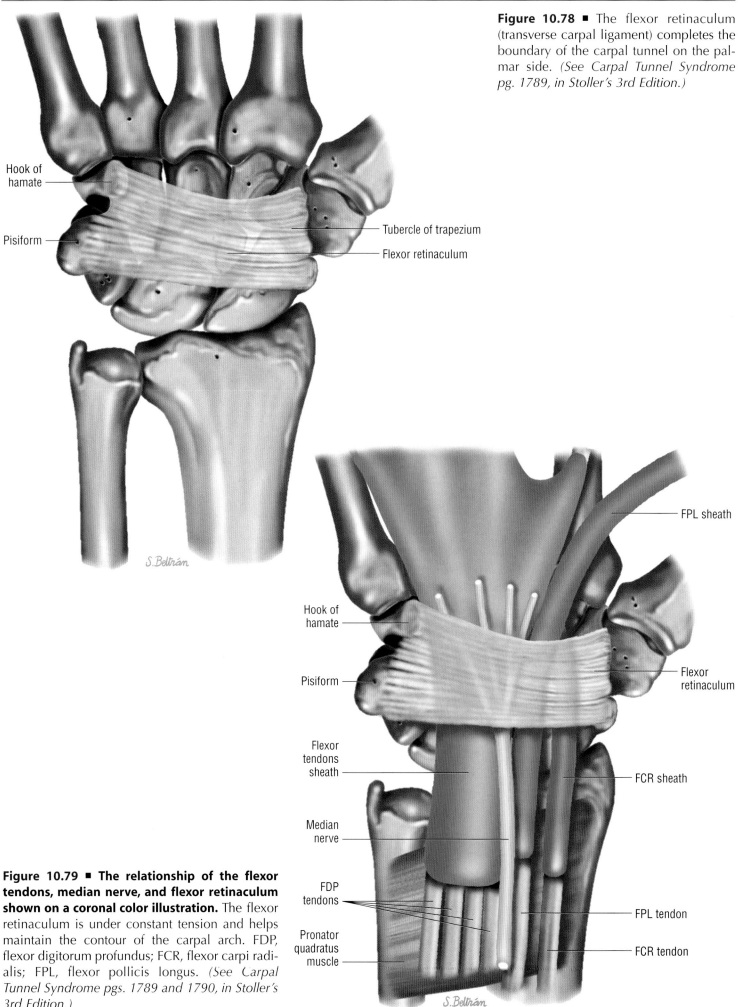

Figure 10.78 ▪ The flexor retinaculum (transverse carpal ligament) completes the boundary of the carpal tunnel on the palmar side. *(See Carpal Tunnel Syndrome pg. 1789, in Stoller's 3rd Edition.)*

Hook of hamate

Pisiform

Tubercle of trapezium

Flexor retinaculum

FPL sheath

Hook of hamate

Pisiform

Flexor retinaculum

Flexor tendons sheath

FCR sheath

Median nerve

FDP tendons

Pronator quadratus muscle

FPL tendon

FCR tendon

Figure 10.79 ▪ **The relationship of the flexor tendons, median nerve, and flexor retinaculum shown on a coronal color illustration.** The flexor retinaculum is under constant tension and helps maintain the contour of the carpal arch. FDP, flexor digitorum profundus; FCR, flexor carpi radialis; FPL, flexor pollicis longus. *(See Carpal Tunnel Syndrome pgs. 1789 and 1790, in Stoller's 3rd Edition.)*

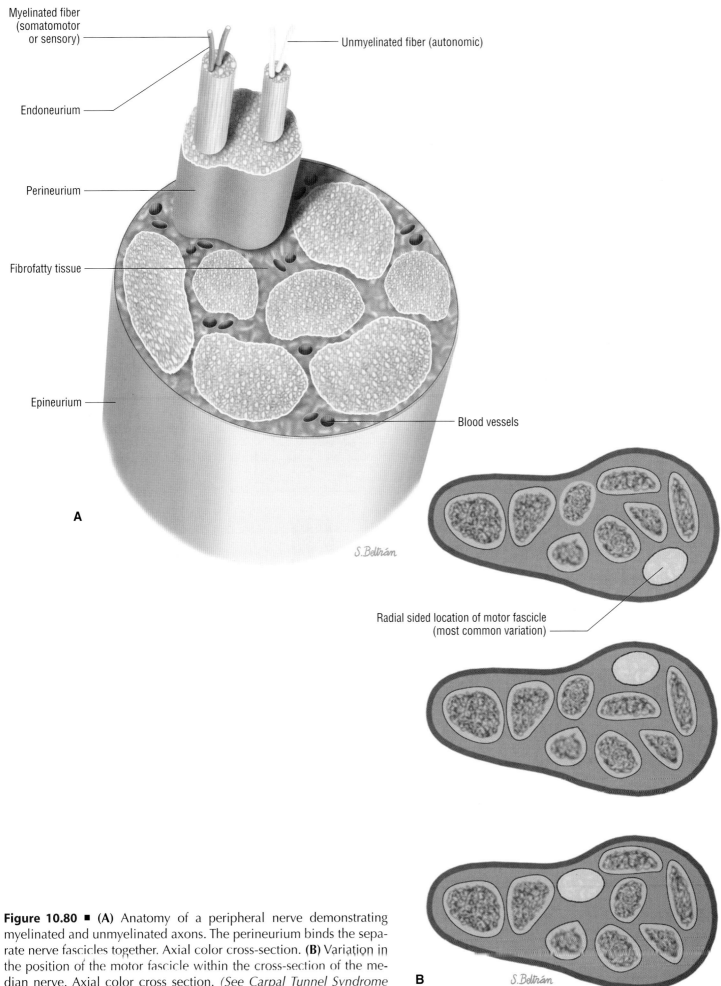

Figure 10.80 ■ **(A)** Anatomy of a peripheral nerve demonstrating myelinated and unmyelinated axons. The perineurium binds the separate nerve fascicles together. Axial color cross-section. **(B)** Variation in the position of the motor fascicle within the cross-section of the median nerve. Axial color cross section. *(See Carpal Tunnel Syndrome pg. 1791, in Stoller's 3rd Edition.)*

Carpal Tunnel Syndrome

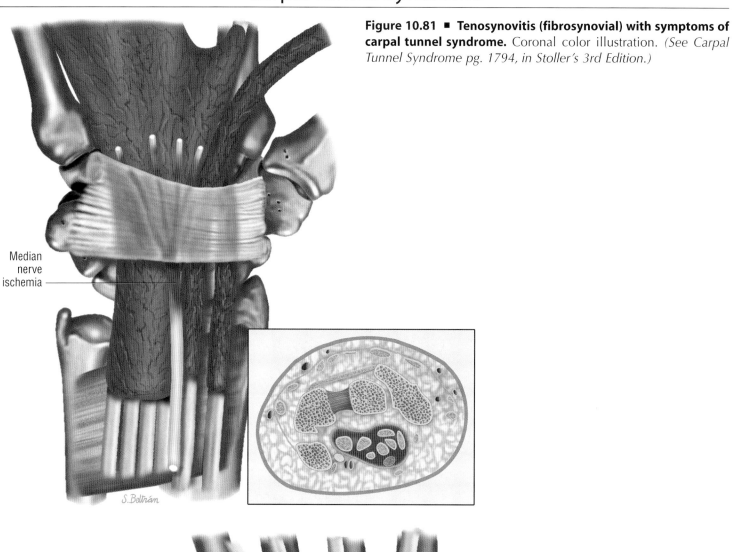

Figure 10.81 ▪ **Tenosynovitis (fibrosynovial) with symptoms of carpal tunnel syndrome.** Coronal color illustration. *(See Carpal Tunnel Syndrome pg. 1794, in Stoller's 3rd Edition.)*

Median nerve ischemia

S.Beltrán

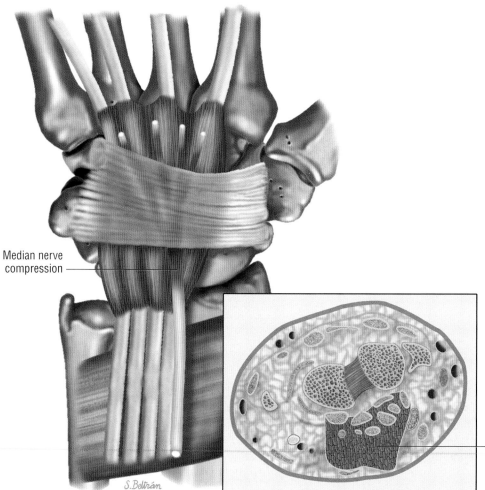

Median nerve compression

Accessory superficialis

Figure 10.82 ▪ Accessory flexor digitorum superficialis muscle resulting in median nerve compression on coronal color illustration. *(See Carpal Tunnel Syndrome pg. 1797, in Stoller's 3rd Edition.)*

S.Beltrán

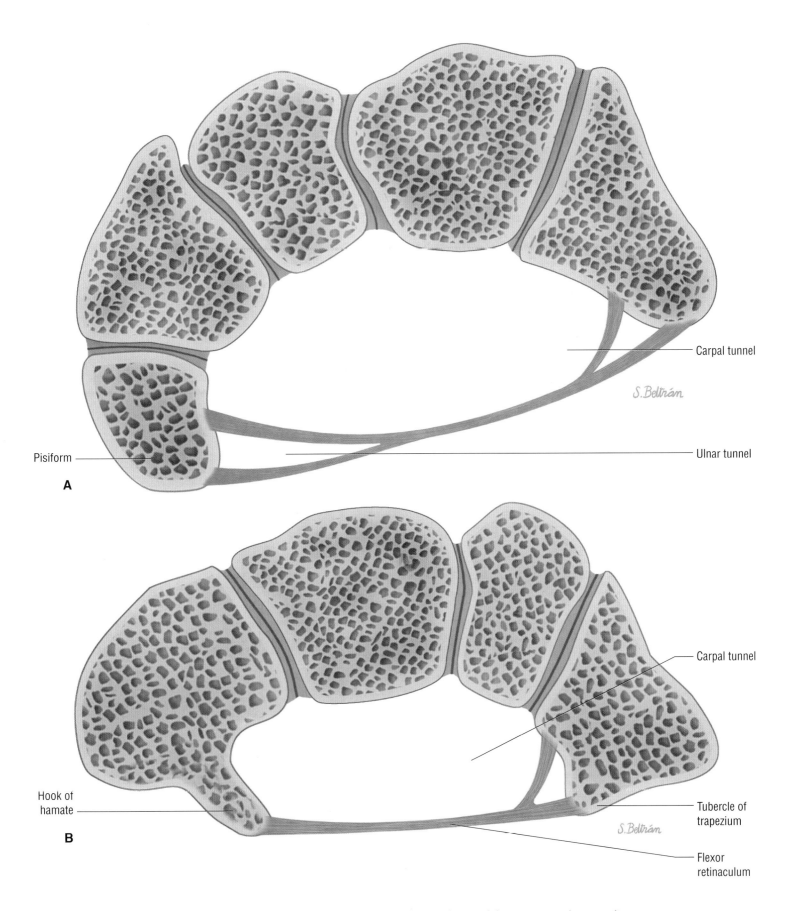

Carpal tunnel

S.Beltrán

Pisiform

Ulnar tunnel

A

Hook of
hamate

Carpal tunnel

S.Beltrán

Tubercle of
trapezium

B

Flexor
retinaculum

Figure 10.83 ▪ Progressive narrowing of the carpal tunnel from proximal **(A)** to distal **(B)**. Axial color cross sections. *(See Carpal Tunnel Syndrome pgs. 1797 and 1798, in Stoller's 3rd Edition.)*

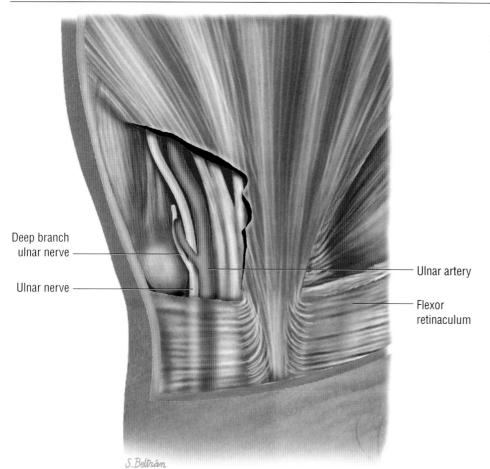

Deep branch
ulnar nerve

Ulnar nerve

Ulnar artery

Flexor
retinaculum

S.Beltrán

Figure 10.84 ■ Coronal color illustration showing ulnar tunnel or Guyon's canal and the relationship of the ulnar nerve. *(See Guyon's Canal/Ulnar Tunnel Syndrome pgs. 1798 and 1801, in Stoller's 3rd Edition.)*

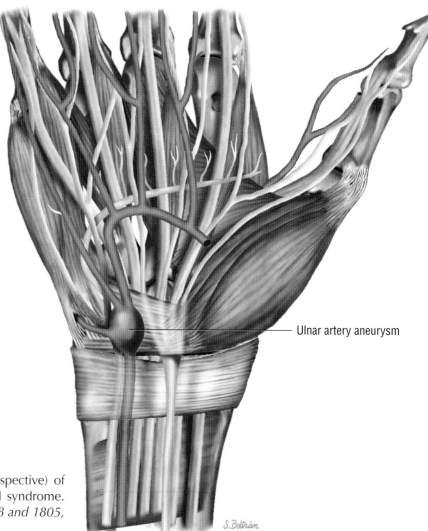

Ulnar artery aneurysm

S.Beltrán

Figure 10.85 ■ Coronal color illustration (volar perspective) of ulnar artery aneurysm as an etiology of ulnar tunnel syndrome. *(See Guyon's Canal Ulnar Tunnel Syndrome pgs. 1798 and 1805, in Stoller's 3rd Edition.)*

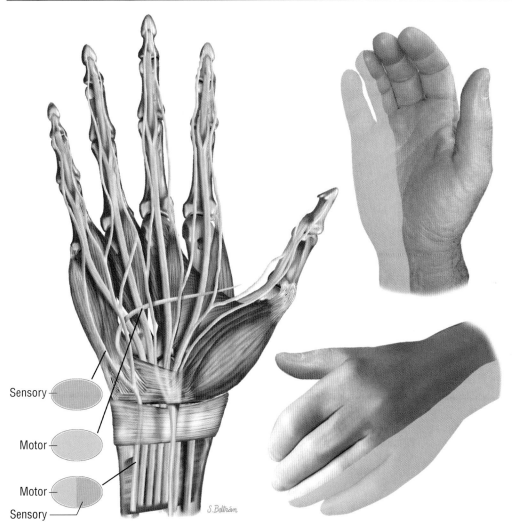

Sensory

Motor

Motor

Sensory

S.Beltrán

Figure 10.86 ▪ **Potential sites of ulnar nerve injury.** Orange represents sensory fibers, green represents motor fibers, and mixed orange-green represents both. Corresponding ulnar-side palmar and dorsal cutaneous innervation is shown. Coronal and oblique color illustrations. *(See Guyon's Canal/Ulnar Tunnel Syndrome pgs. 1799 and 1802, in Stoller's 3rd Edition.)*

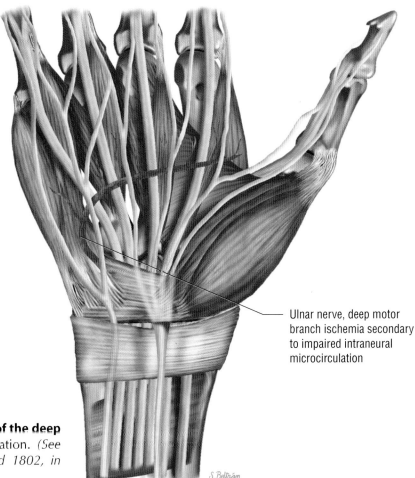

Ulnar nerve, deep motor branch ischemia secondary to impaired intraneural microcirculation

S.Beltrán

Figure 10.87 ▪ **Ulnar tunnel syndrome with ischemia of the deep motor branch of the ulnar nerve.** Coronal color illustration. *(See Guyon's Canal/Ulnar Tunnel Syndrome pgs. 1799 and 1802, in Stoller's 3rd Edition.)*

Ulnar Tunnel Syndrome

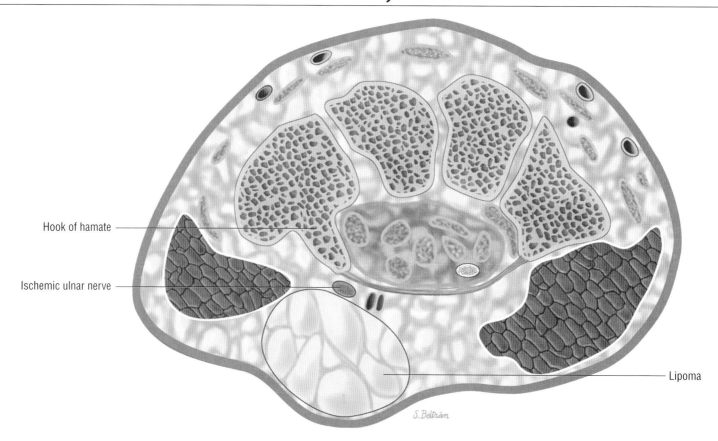

Hook of hamate

Ischemic ulnar nerve

Lipoma

S.Beltrán

Figure 10.88 ■ **Ulnar tunnel syndrome caused by extrinsic compression by a lipoma.** Color axial section. *(See Guyon's Canal Ulnar Tunnel Syndrome pgs. 1799 and 1803, in Stoller's 3rd Edition.)*

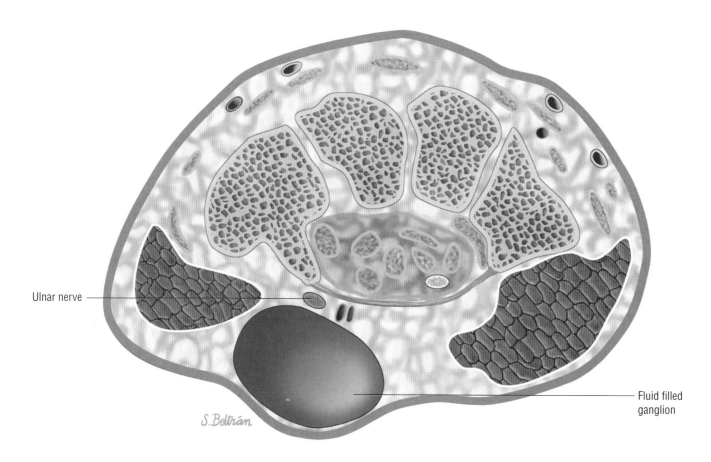

Ulnar nerve

Fluid filled ganglion

S.Beltrán

Figure 10.89 ■ Axial color illustration showing a ganglion compressing the ulnar nerve. *(See Guyon's Canal Ulnar Tunnel Syndrome pgs. 1799 and 1804, in Stoller's 3rd Edition.)*

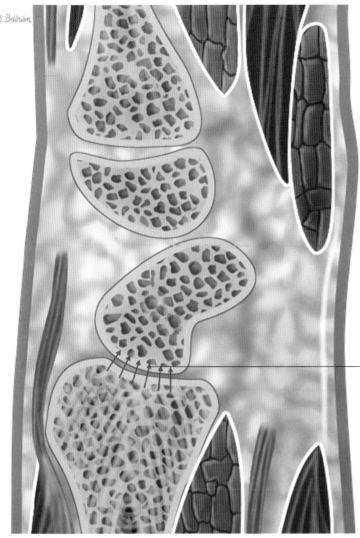

A

Congruous load distribution between the parallel curved surfaces of the scaphoid and scaphoid fossa of the distal radius

Figure 10.90 ■ **(A)** Normal radioscaphoid congruous joint surfaces. **(B)** The congruous joint surface contact between the scaphoid and radius is lost with rotational instability secondary to rotary subluxation of the scaphoid. There is an abnormal load transferred to the volar and dorsal margins of the radius and the center of the scaphoid. The rotation of the scaphoid thus accelerates the process of radioscaphoid joint degeneration. *(See Arthritis pgs. 1802 and 1806, in Stoller's 3rd Edition.)*

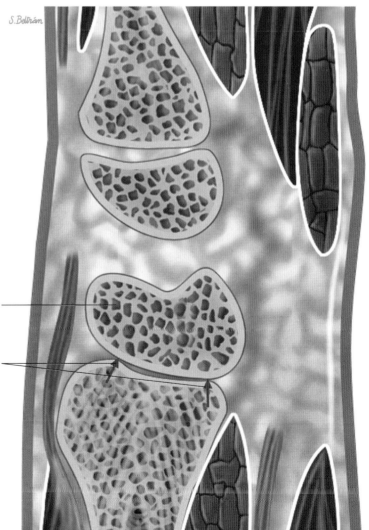

Scaphoid rotary subluxation

Abnormal load transference to the margins of the radius

B

SLAC Arthritis

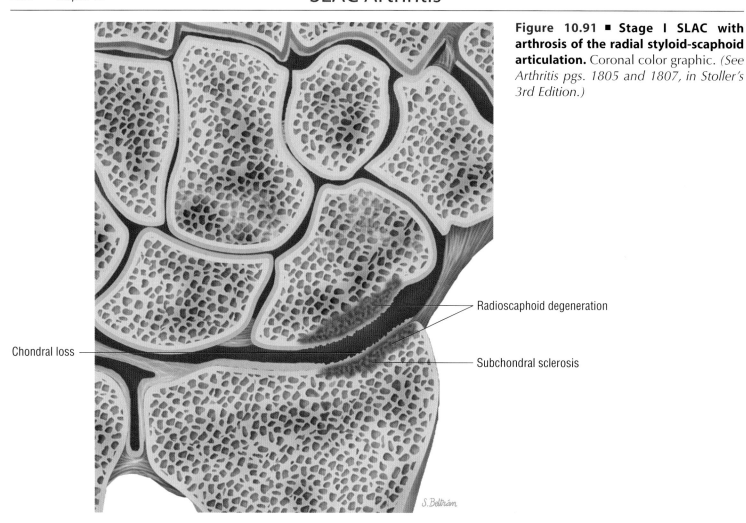

Chondral loss

Radioscaphoid degeneration

Subchondral sclerosis

Figure 10.91 ■ Stage I SLAC with arthrosis of the radial styloid-scaphoid articulation. Coronal color graphic. *(See Arthritis pgs. 1805 and 1807, in Stoller's 3rd Edition.)*

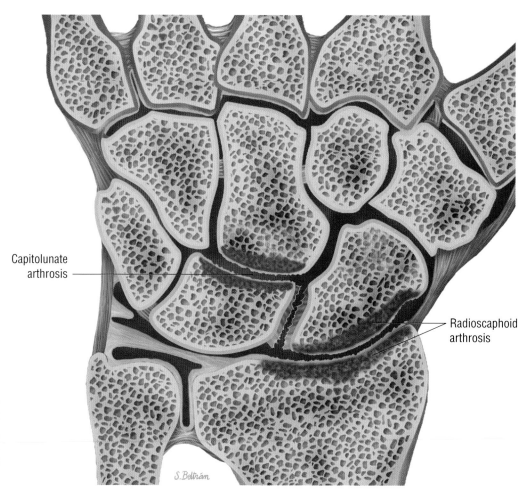

Capitolunate arthrosis

Radioscaphoid arthrosis

Figure 10.92 ■ Stage III SLAC with arthrosis of the entire radioscaphoid articulation and capitolunate joint. Color coronal graphic. *(See Arthritis pgs. 1805 and 1807, in Stoller's 3rd Edition.)*

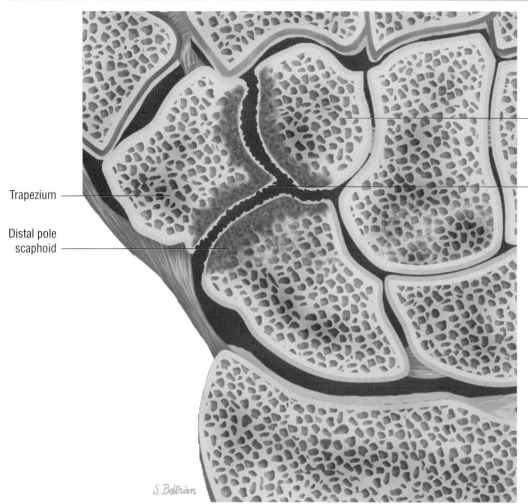

Trapezoid

Arthrosis secondary
to abnormal shear
stresses

Trapezium

Distal pole
scaphoid

S.Beltrán

Figure 10.93 ■ **Triscaphe arthritis
with arthrosis and destruction of the
trapezioscaphoid and trapezoido-
scaphoid joints.** There is disruption in
the ligamentous support of the
scaphoid distally. Coronal color
graphic. *(See Arthritis pgs. 1805 and
1809, in Stoller's 3rd Edition.)*

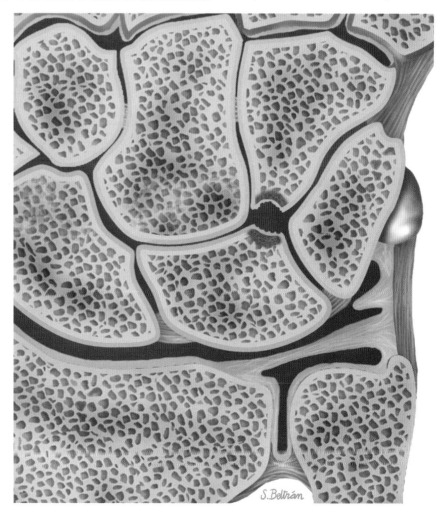

Figure 10.94 ■ **Type II lunate (medial lunate facet)
with subchondral erosion of the proximal pole of
the hamate and accessory lunate facet.** Coronal
color illustration. *(See Hamate-Lunate Impingement
pg. 1810, in Stoller's 3rd Edition.)*

S.Beltrán

Rheumatoid Arthritis

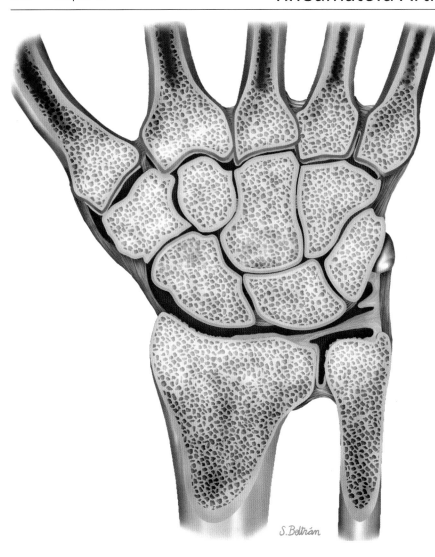

Figure 10.95 ■ Juxta-articular osteopenia with patchy marrow edema as shown on a coronal color graphic. *(See Rheumatoid Arthritis pgs. 181 and 1812, in Stoller's 3rd Edition.)*

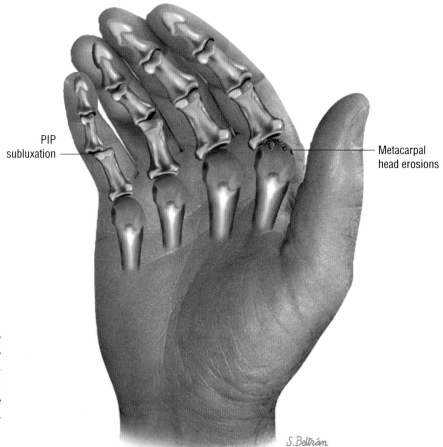

PIP subluxation

Metacarpal head erosions

Figure 10.96 ■ **Ulnar deviation at the metacarpophalangeal joints is associated with radial deviation at the radiocarpal joint.** Metacarpal head erosions are demonstrated. Soft-tissue swelling, marginal erosions (bare areas including the radial aspect of the second and third metacarpal heads), and joint deformities are common. *(See Rheumatoid Arthritis pgs. 1811 and 1812, in Stoller's 3rd Edition.)*

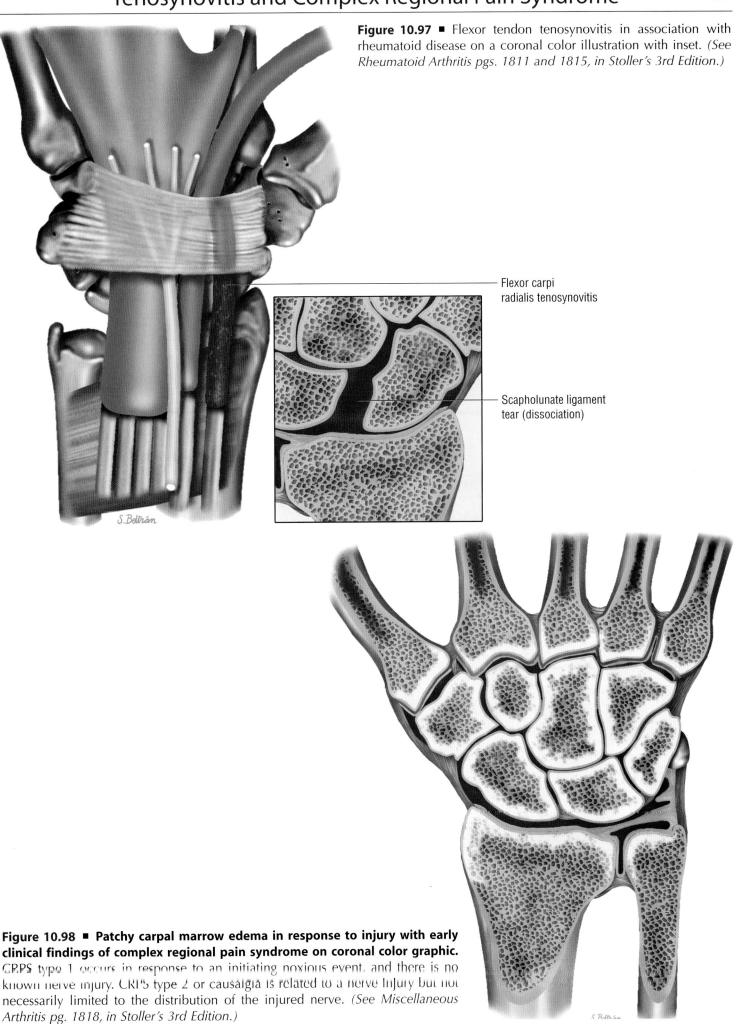

Figure 10.97 ■ Flexor tendon tenosynovitis in association with rheumatoid disease on a coronal color illustration with inset. *(See Rheumatoid Arthritis pgs. 1811 and 1815, in Stoller's 3rd Edition.)*

Flexor carpi radialis tenosynovitis

Scapholunate ligament tear (dissociation)

Figure 10.98 ■ **Patchy carpal marrow edema in response to injury with early clinical findings of complex regional pain syndrome on coronal color graphic.** CRPS type 1 occurs in response to an initiating noxious event, and there is no known nerve injury. CRPS type 2 or causalgia is related to a nerve injury but not necessarily limited to the distribution of the injured nerve. *(See Miscellaneous Arthritis pg. 1818, in Stoller's 3rd Edition.)*

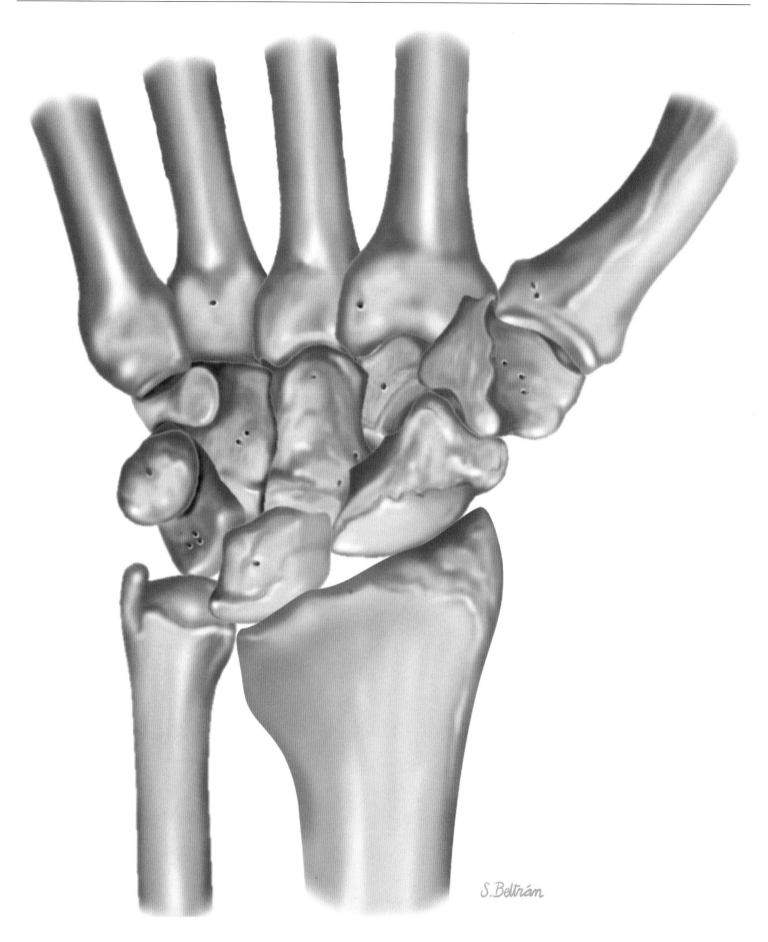

Figure 10.99 ■ **Madelung's deformity with medial angulation of the distal radial articular surface and triangulation of the carpus.** Coronal color illustration. *(See Madelung's Deformity pgs. 1817 and 1819, in Stoller's 3rd Edition.)*

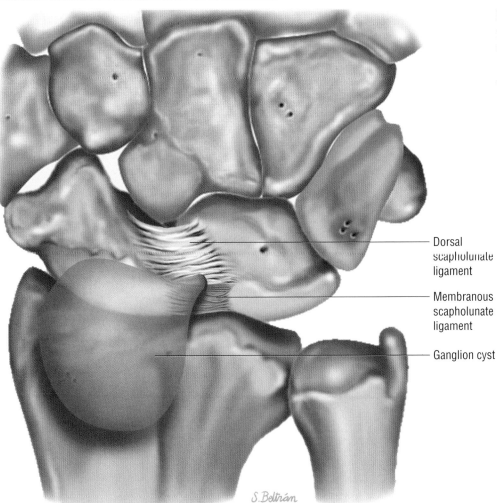

Figure 10.100 ■ Common location of a ganglion cyst relative to the dorsal scapholunate interval. Coronal color illustration. *(See Ganglion Cysts pgs. 1819 and 1820, in Stoller's 3rd Edition.)*

Dorsal scapholunate ligament

Membranous scapholunate ligament

Ganglion cyst

S.Beltrán

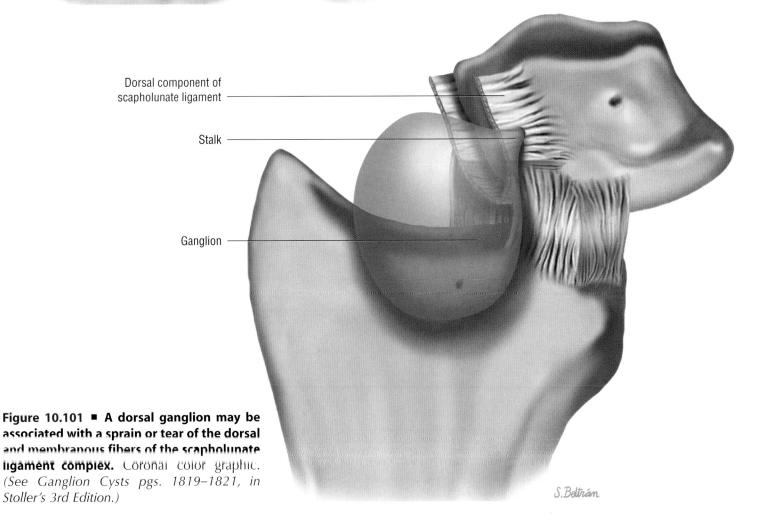

Dorsal component of scapholunate ligament

Stalk

Ganglion

Figure 10.101 ■ A dorsal ganglion may be associated with a sprain or tear of the dorsal and membranous fibers of the scapholunate ligament complex. Coronal color graphic. *(See Ganglion Cysts pgs. 1819–1821, in Stoller's 3rd Edition.)*

S.Beltrán

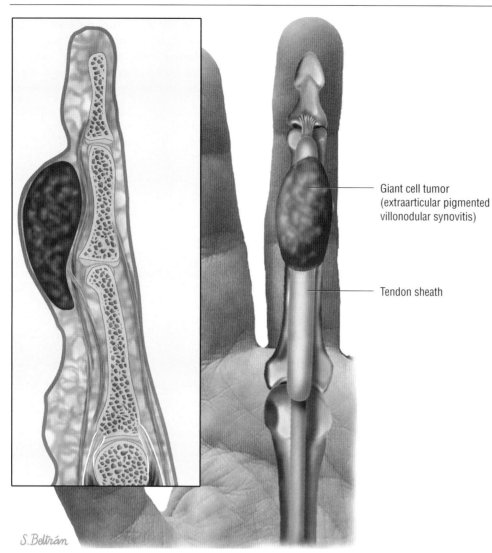

Figure 10.102 ■ **Coronal graphic and sagittal inset of a giant cell tumor of the flexor tendon sheath.** Characteristic lobulations and well-circumscribed fibrous morphology are shown. *(See Giant Cell Tumors of the Tendon Sheath pgs. 1822 and 1824, in Stoller's 3rd Edition.)*

Giant cell tumor (extraarticular pigmented villonodular synovitis)

Tendon sheath

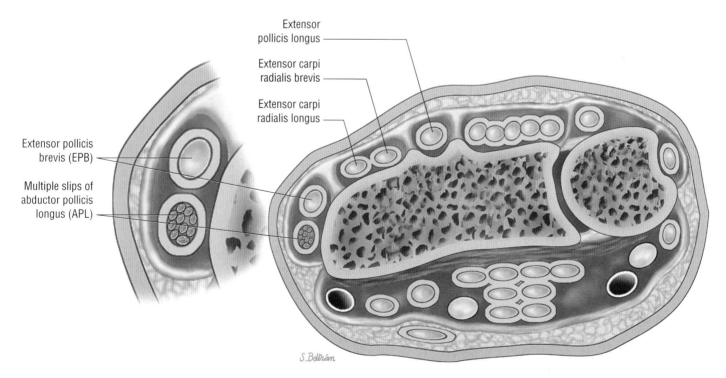

Extensor pollicis longus

Extensor carpi radialis brevis

Extensor carpi radialis longus

Extensor pollicis brevis (EPB)

Multiple slips of abductor pollicis longus (APL)

Figure 10.103 ■ **Multiple slips of the abductor pollicis longus (APL) tendon of the first dorsal compartment.** There may be between five to seven slips of the APL. The overlying extensor retinaculum forms a fibro-osseous tunnel for the EPB and APL tendons. As the first compartment tendons pass through the tunnel, their angle increases with ulnar deviation of the wrist. *(See De Quervain's Tenosynovitis pgs. 1826–1827, in Stoller's 3rd Edition.)*

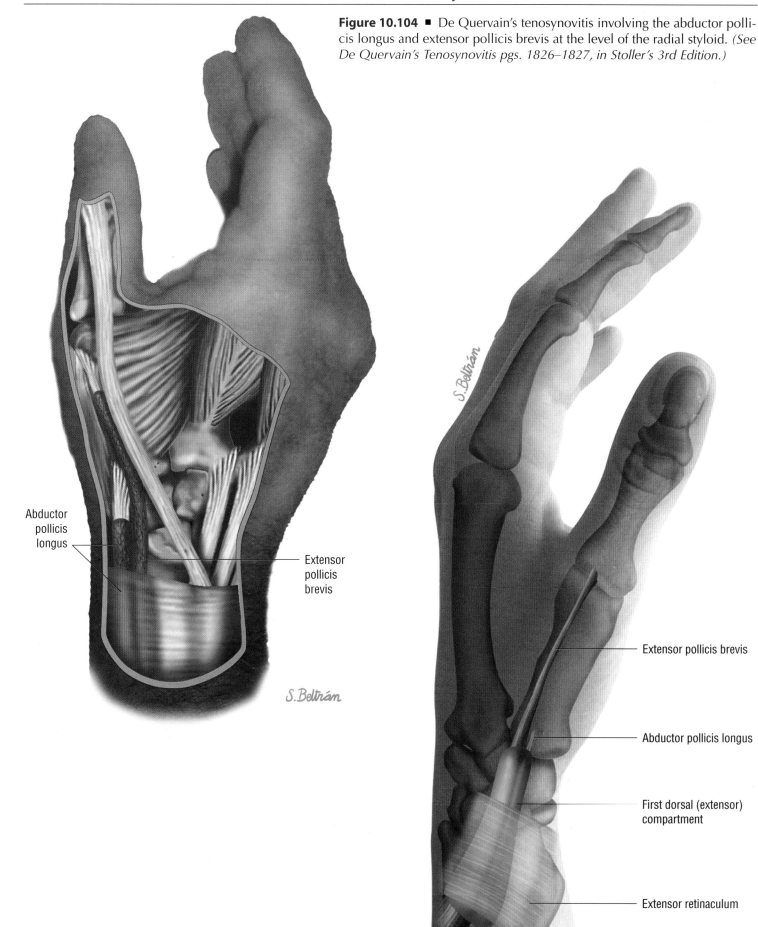

Figure 10.104 ■ De Quervain's tenosynovitis involving the abductor pollicis longus and extensor pollicis brevis at the level of the radial styloid. *(See De Quervain's Tenosynovitis pgs. 1826–1827, in Stoller's 3rd Edition.)*

Abductor pollicis longus

Extensor pollicis brevis

Extensor pollicis brevis

Abductor pollicis longus

First dorsal (extensor) compartment

Extensor retinaculum

Figure 10.105 ■ The fibro-osseous tunnel at the level of the radial styloid demonstrating the passage of the extensor pollicis of the extensor pollicis brevis and abductor pollicis longus tendons. *(See De Quervain's Tenosynovitis pgs. 1825–1827, in Stoller's 3rd Edition.)*

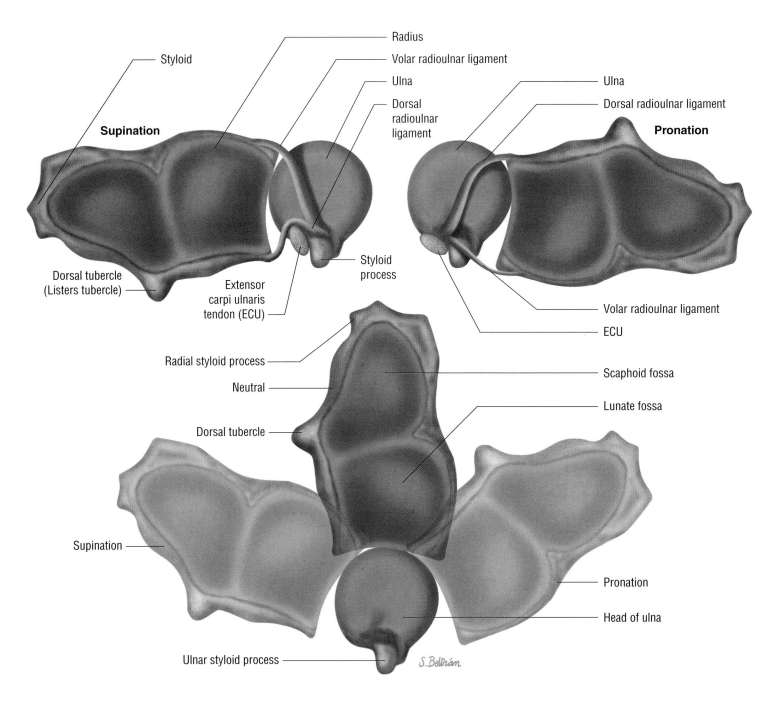

Styloid

Radius

Volar radioulnar ligament

Ulna

Supination

Dorsal radioulnar ligament

Ulna

Dorsal radioulnar ligament

Pronation

Dorsal tubercle (Listers tubercle)

Extensor carpi ulnaris tendon (ECU)

Styloid process

Volar radioulnar ligament

ECU

Radial styloid process

Neutral

Dorsal tubercle

Scaphoid fossa

Lunate fossa

Supination

Pronation

Head of ulna

Ulnar styloid process

S.Beltrán

Figure 10.106 ■ **Relationship of the dorsal and volar radioulnar ligaments in supination and pronation.** This ulnocarpal ligament complex stabilizes the distal radioulnar joint. *(See Distal Radioulnar Joint pg. 1732, in Stoller's 3rd Edition.)*

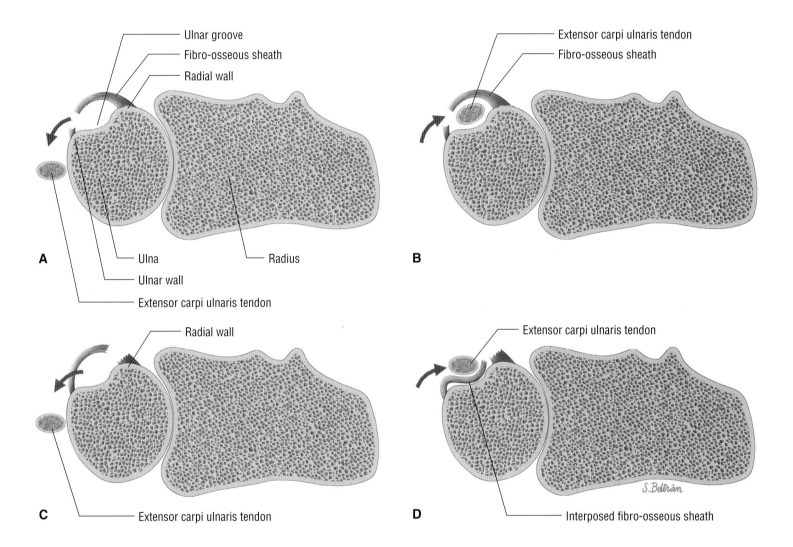

Figure 10.107 ■ **(A and B)** Disruption of the fibro-osseous sheath from the ulnar wall **(A)**. The extensor carpi ulnaris tendon may return to the ulnar groove deep to fibro-osseous sheath **(B)**. **(C and D)** Disruption of the fibro-osseous sheath from the radial wall **(C)**. The extensor carpi ulnaris (ECU) tendon is dorsal to the interposed fibro-osseous sheath preventing healing within the ulnar groove **(D)**. *Based on Inoue G, Tamura Y. Recurrent dislocation of the extensor carpi ulnaris tendon. Br J of Sports Med 1998 Jun;32(2):172-4. (See Extensor Carpi Ulnaris Tendinitis and Dysfunction pgs. 1828–1830, in Stoller's 3rd Edition.)*

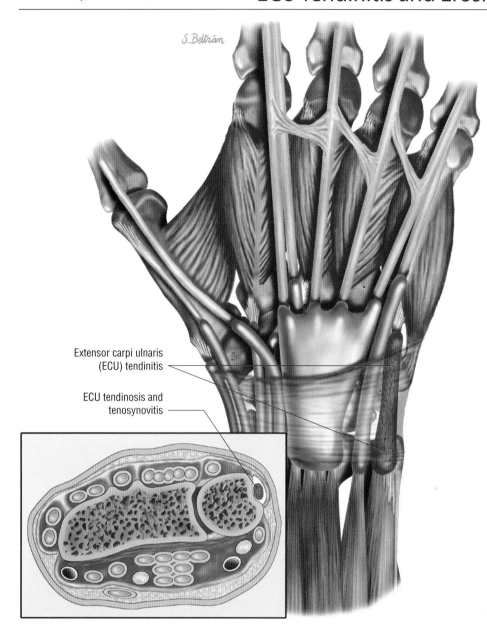

S.Beltrán

Extensor carpi ulnaris
(ECU) tendinitis

ECU tendinosis and
tenosynovitis

Figure 10.108 ■ **Extensor carpi ulnaris tendinitis represents an inflammation of the synovial lining of the extensor carpi ulnaris and frequently is associated with intrinsic tendon degeneration.** Color coronal illustration and axial inset. *(See Extensor Carpi Ulnaris Tendinitis and Dysfunction pgs. 1828 and 1829, in Stoller's 3rd Edition.)*

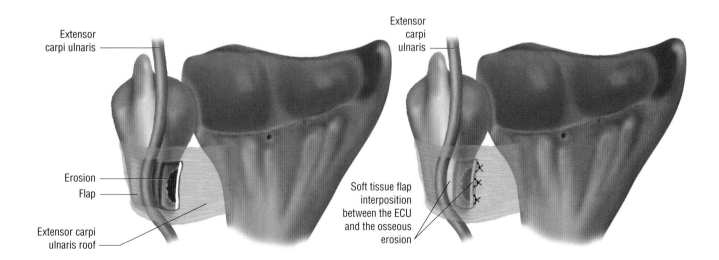

Extensor
carpi ulnaris

Extensor
carpi
ulnaris

Erosion
Flap

Extensor carpi
ulnaris roof

Soft tissue flap
interposition
between the ECU
and the osseous
erosion

Figure 10.109 ■ **A volar based flap from the ECU roof is interposed between the ECU tendon and distal ulnar erosion.** This interposition surgery is used to treat chronic ECU tendinosis associated with erosion of the sixth compartment floor. *Based on Carneiro RS, Fontana R, Mazzer N. Ulnar wrist pain in athletes caused by erosion of the floor of the sixth dorsal compartment: a case series. Am J of Sports Med 2005; 33: 1910-1913. (See Extensor Carpi Ulnaris Tendinitis and Dysfunction pgs. 1828–1830, in Stoller's 3rd Edition.)*

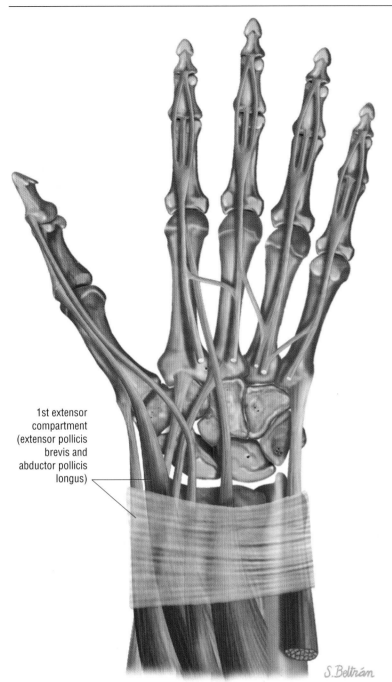

Figure 10.110 ■ **Area where tenosynovitis of the second dorsal compartment occurs in intersection syndrome.** Pain and swelling usually occur proximal to the wrist as inflammation occurs where the muscle belly of the abductor pollicis longus and extensor pollicis brevis cross the common wrist extensors of the second dorsal compartment. Coronal color graphic. *(See Intersection Syndrome pgs. 1831 and 1833, in Stoller's 3rd Edition.)*

1st extensor compartment (extensor pollicis brevis and abductor pollicis longus)

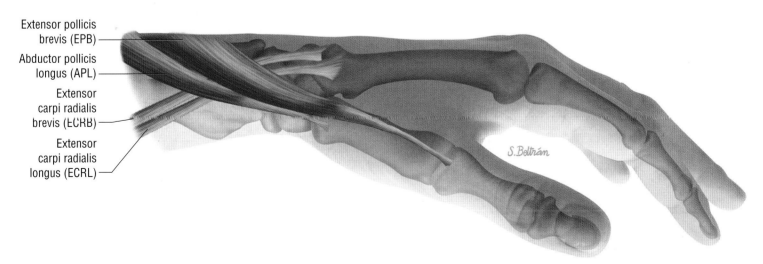

Extensor pollicis brevis (EPB)

Abductor pollicis longus (APL)

Extensor carpi radialis brevis (ECRB)

Extensor carpi radialis longus (ECRL)

Figure 10.111 ■ Intersection syndrome demonstrating the anatomy of the crossing of the APL and the EPB over the ECRL and the ECRB. *(See Intersection Syndrome pgs. 1831 and 1833, in Stoller's 3rd Edition.)*

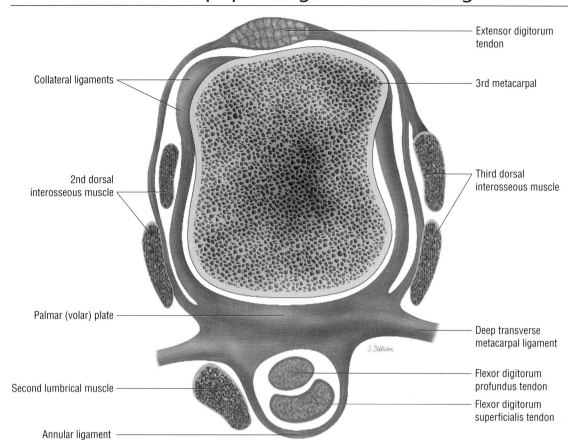

Extensor digitorum tendon

Collateral ligaments

3rd metacarpal

2nd dorsal interosseous muscle

Third dorsal interosseous muscle

Palmar (volar) plate

Deep transverse metacarpal ligament

Flexor digitorum profundus tendon

Second lumbrical muscle

Flexor digitorum superficialis tendon

Annular ligament

Figure 10.112 ■ Normal anatomy of the third metacarpal at the level of the metacarpophalangeal joint. Axial color graphic. *(See Pathology of the Finger and Thumb pgs. 1831 and 1834, in Stoller's 3rd Edition.)*

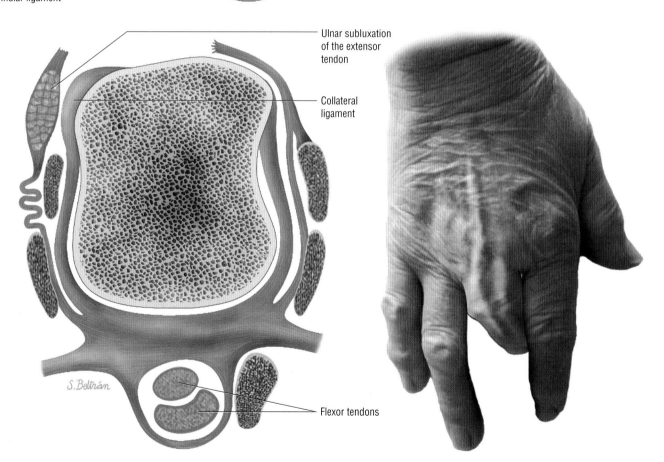

Ulnar subluxation of the extensor tendon

Collateral ligament

Flexor tendons

Figure 10.113 ■ Post-traumatic rupture of the sagittal band at the level of the metacarpophalangeal joint is associated with extensor tendon instability. When the extensor tendon is no longer centered over the dorsal MCP joint there is loss of finger extension. A common mechanism of sagittal band injury is a blow to the hand with the MCP joints flexed (e.g. boxing). *Based on Morrey BF, Strickland JW, Graham TJ. Master techniques in orthopaedic surgery, ed 2. The hand. Philadelphia: Lippincott, Williams & Wilkins, 2005. (See Pathology of the Finger and Thumb pg. 1834, in Stoller's 3rd Edition.)*

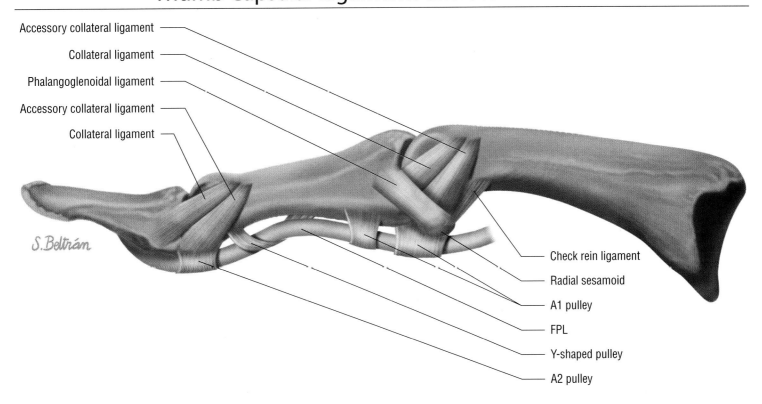

Accessory collateral ligament
Collateral ligament
Phalangoglenoidal ligament
Accessory collateral ligament
Collateral ligament

S.Beltrán

Check rein ligament
Radial sesamoid
A1 pulley
FPL
Y-shaped pulley
A2 pulley

Figure 10.114 ▪ Thumb capsular ligaments of the metacarpophalangeal and interphalangeal joints. Lateral color graphic. *(See Pathology of the Finger and Thumb pgs. 1831 and 1835, in Stoller's 3rd Edition.)*

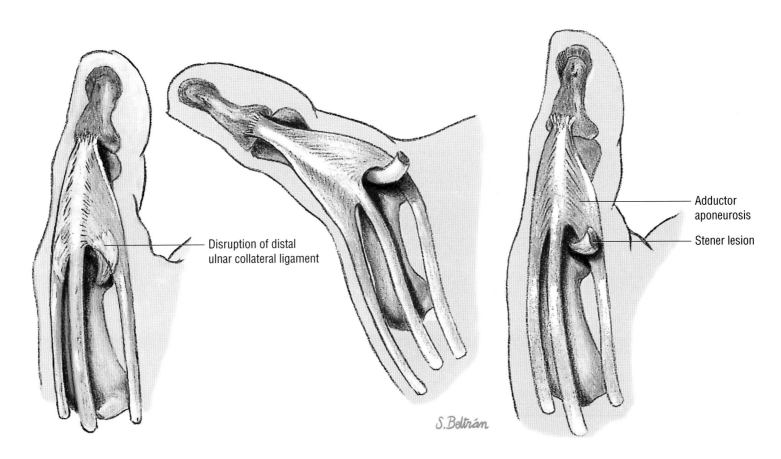

Disruption of distal
ulnar collateral ligament

S.Beltrán

Adductor
aponeurosis

Stener lesion

Figure 10.115 ▪ Progression of a displaced ulnar collateral ligament (UCL) forming Stener's lesion with the proximal margin of the adductor aponeurosis intersecting and entrapping the folded UCL. *(See Ulnar Collateral Ligament Tears of the Thumb pgs. 1836 and 1837, in Stoller's 3rd Edition.)*

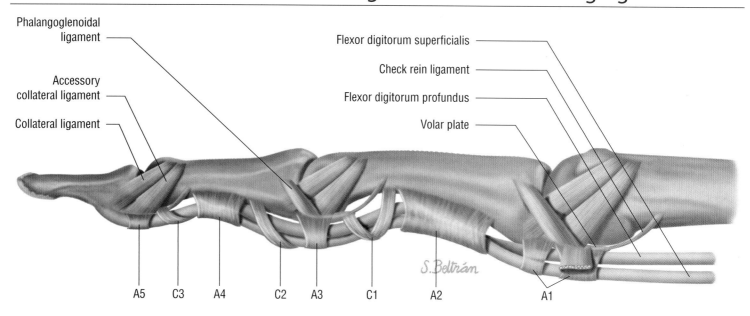

Phalangoglenoidal ligament

Accessory collateral ligament

Collateral ligament

Flexor digitorum superficialis

Check rein ligament

Flexor digitorum profundus

Volar plate

S. Beltrán

A5   C3   A4   C2   A3   C1   A2   A1

Figure 10.116 ▪ Normal anatomy of the ligaments reinforcing the digital tendon sheath. A1 through A5 represent the annular ligaments and C1 through C3 represent the cruciform ligaments. The longest annular ligament, the A2 pulley, is located on the proximal diaphysis of the proximal phalanx. Sagittal color graphic. *(See Flexor Annular Pulley Tears pgs. 1838 and 1839, in Stoller's 3rd Edition.)*

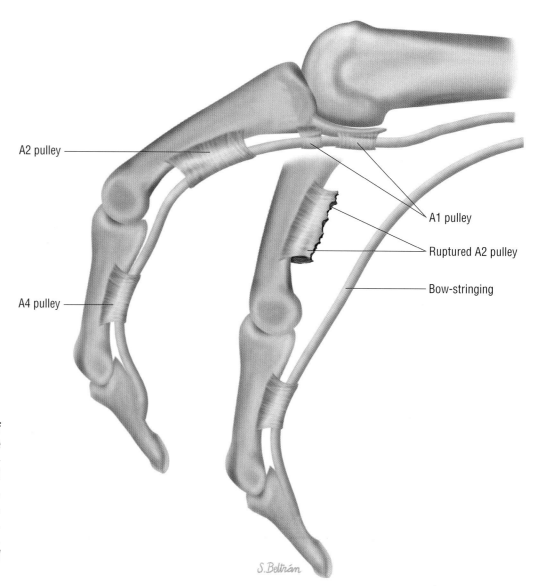

A2 pulley

A1 pulley

Ruptured A2 pulley

Bow-stringing

A4 pulley

S. Beltrán

Figure 10.117 ▪ Bowstringing of flexor tendons secondary to rupture of the A1 and A2 pulleys. Bowstringing of the flexor tendons is associated with rock-climbing pulley injuries. Ruptures may occur at the A3, A2, A4, or A1 pulleys. Sagittal color graphic. *(See Flexor Annular Pulley Tears pgs. 1839 and 1840, in Stoller's 3rd Edition.)*

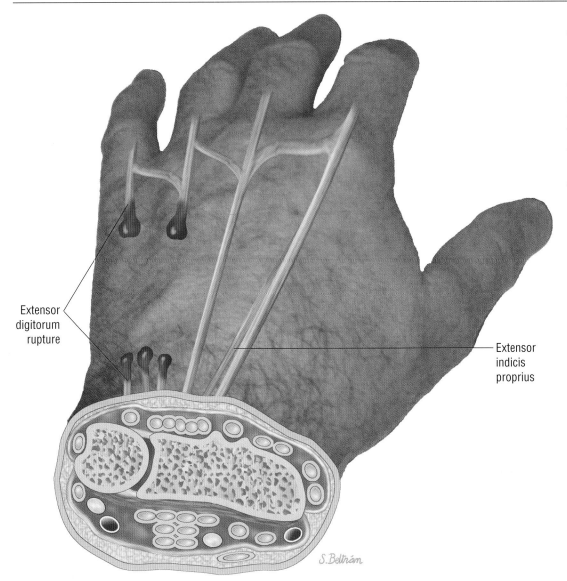

Figure 10.118 ■ Ruptured extensor tendons. The extensor indicis proprius (EIP) may be mobilized for transfer and the extensor hood is closed. The distal stump of the EIP is sutured onto the torn common extensor tendon. *Based on Morrey BF, Strickland JW, Graham TJ. Master techniques in orthopaedic surgery, ed 2. The Hand. Philadelphia: Lippincott, Williams & Wilkins, 2005. (See Rheumatoid Arthritis pgs. 1811–1815, in Stoller's 3rd Edition.)*

Extensor digitorum rupture

Extensor indicis proprius

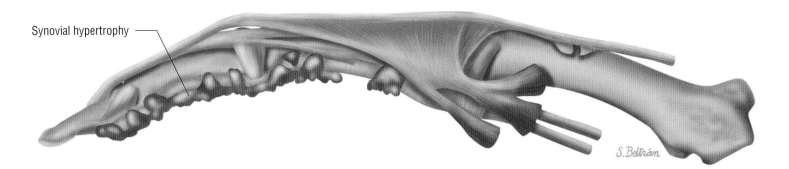

Figure 10.119 ■ Flexor tenosynovitis in a rheumatoid digit. The synovial thickening may be associated with attenuation of the annular pulleys and bulging of the cruciate ligaments compromising the tendons' efficiency at the proximal PIP joint. *(See Rheumatoid Arthritis pgs. 1811–1815, in Stoller's 3rd Edition.)*

Synovial hypertrophy

Swan-Neck Deformity

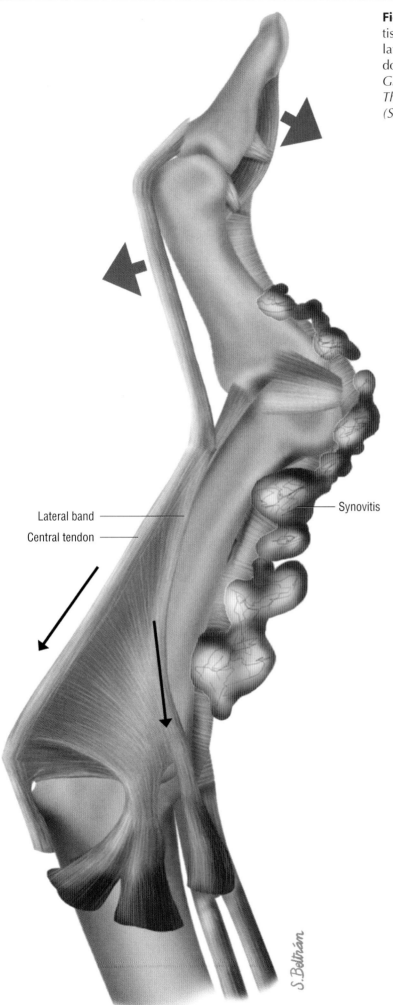

Lateral band ————

Central tendon ————

———— Synovitis

Figure 10.120 ▪ Swan-neck deformity associated with synovitis of the volar aspect of the PIP joint, dorsal subluxation of the lateral bands, and an increased extension pull of the central dorsal extensor tendon. *Based on Morrey BF, Strickland JW, Graham TJ., Master techniques in orthopaedic surgery, ed 2. The hand. Philadelphia: Lippincott, Williams & Wilkins, 2005. (See Tendon Injuries pg. 1839, in Stoller's 3rd Edition.)*

S. Beltrán

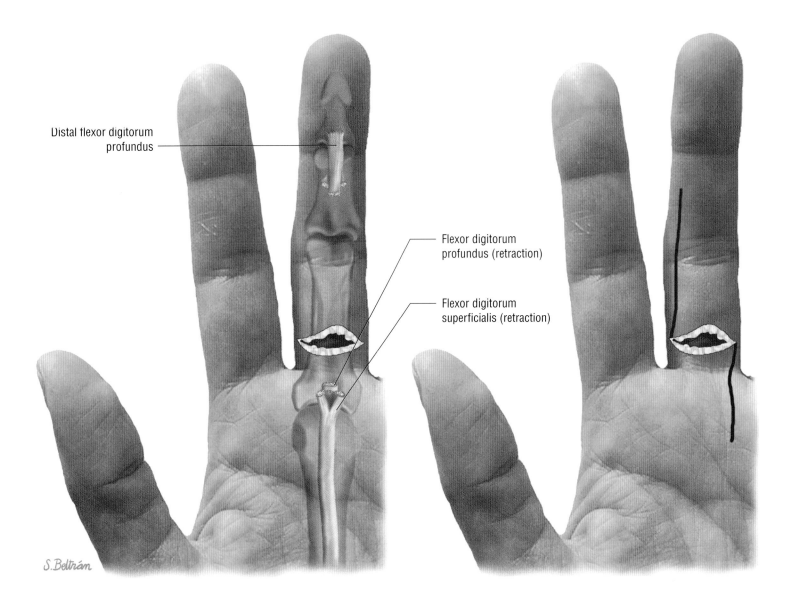

Figure 10.121 ■ Flexor tendon laceration involving the flexor digitorum superficialis and profundus tendons (a zone II injury) with surgical skin flap exposure.*Based on Morrey BF, Strickland JW, Graham TJ. Master techniques in orthopaedic surgery, ed 2. The hand. Philadelphia: Lippincott, Williams & Wilkins, 2005. (See Flexor Digitorum Profundus Avulsions pg. 1841, in Stoller's 3rd Edition.)*

Chapter

11

MR Imaging of the Fingers

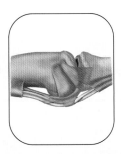

Pearls and Pitfalls & Color Illustrations

Pearls and Pitfalls

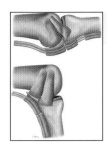

MR TECHNIQUES

- Routine examinations include T1 spin echo and STIR or fat-suppressed fast-spin-echo T2 sequences. The confidence level of diagnosis may be improved in post-traumatic cases by gadolinium-enhanced fat-suppressed T1 images.

- Axial images allow assessment of all the anatomic elements of the finger. Sagittal images are used to evaluate the flexor and extensor tendons, the volar plate, the pulleys, and the cartilage surfaces. The coronal plane images are useful in assessing the collateral ligaments and osteochondral lesions.

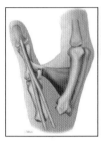

TRAUMATIC FINGER INJURIES – LIGAMENTS
(See Figs. 11.1–11.5)

- Injury of the UCL of the first MP joint is called gamekeeper's thumb or skier's thumb. Surgical repair is necessary if bony avulsion occurs, or the torn UCL retracts proximally and superficially above the adductor aponeurosis, creating a Stener's lesion.

- Injuries of the collateral ligaments of the II-V MP joints are rare and mainly involve the RCL.

- Forced valgus or varus stress of an extended PIP joint injures the collateral ligament, ranging from sprain to partial or complete tear. Treatment is usually conservative.

- Hyperextension injury of the PIP joint produces sagittal instability and usually dorsal subluxation.

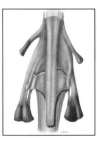

TRAUMATIC FINGER INJURIES – TENDONS
(See Figs. 11.6–11.16)

- MR imaging is useful to evaluate bony avulsion, locate retracted tendon ends, and measure the length of gap in tendon tears.

- Zone classifications are used to categorize extensor apparatus and flexor tendon injuries.

- Short TE sequences may produce magic angle phenomenon. Typical areas include the terminal band of the extensor tendon, the periarticular part of the flexor digitorum tendons, and the thenar eminence segment of the flexor pollicis longus tendon.

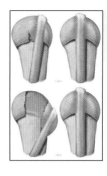

TRAUMATIC FINGER INJURIES – EXTENSOR TENDONS
(See Figs. 11.7–11.11)

- The most common closed extensor tendon injury in sports is mallet finger. With acute flexion of the DIP joint, the insertion of the terminal band of the extensor tendon on the distal phalanx is injured, with possible fracture of the base of the phalanx.

- Injury of the central slip of the extensor tendon at or close to its insertion on the base of the middle phalanx and volar displacement of the lateral bands, may cause flexion of the PIP joint. This can result in increased tension on the terminal band of the extensor tendon and subsequent extension of the DIP joint, forming a boutonniere deformity.

- A tear of the sagittal band of the extensor hood at the MP joint may result in subluxation or dislocation of the extensor tendon, assessed by axial stress imaging with the MP joint in flexion. The middle and little fingers are most frequently involved, and the radial sagittal band is usually injured with ulnar subluxation of the tendon.

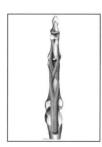

TRAUMATIC FINGER INJURIES – FLEXOR TENDONS AND PULLEY INJURIES
(See Figs. 11.12–11.16)

- Sudden hyperextension during active flexion can result in distal avulsion of the FDP, a "rugby" or "jersey finger." The ring finger is involved in 80% of cases.

- Annular pulley ruptures usually progress from A2 distal partial tears to complete tears, and then to A3, A4, and rarely A1 tears. The most commonly injured is the A2 pulley of the fourth finger of the non-dominant hand.

- Bowstringing on sagittal images is the most sensitive indirect sign of pulley injury.

- Trigger finger is a common stenosing tenosynovitis of the flexor tendons, which can be primary idiopathic, or secondary to rheumatoid arthritis, diabetes mellitus, gout, or connective tissue disorders.

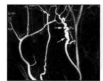

TRAUMATIC FINGER INJURIES - VASCULAR TRAUMA AND NERVE TRAUMA

- Dynamic 3D gradient-echo sequences after intravenous injection of gadolinium is more sensitive than T1 or T2 images in diagnosing post-traumatic AVFs.

- Hypothenar hammer syndrome involves the superficial branch of the ulnar artery where it is more exposed to injury as it emerges from Guyon's canal and runs superficially across the hypothenar musculature.

- Neuroma is a pseudotumor of the digital nerve that develops after injury or repetitive microtrauma.

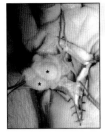

SOFT TISSUE PSEUDOTUMORS

- The majority of ganglion cysts are in the middle finger, at the weak point between the A1 and A2 pulleys.
- The differential of granulomatous inflammation of the synovium includes TB, other infections such as fungal or Brucella, inflammatory disease such as sarcoidosis or gout, or foreign body reactions.
- Tenosynovial chondromatosis is caused by cartilaginous metaplasia of the synovium of a tendon sheath.
- Dupuytren's contracture is a superficial palmar fibromatosis occurring in 1% to 2% of the population.

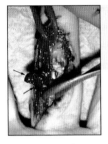

SOFT TISSUE TUMORS – VASCULAR MALFORMATIONS AND INTRAMUSCULAR HEMANGIOMAS

- Vascular malformations differ from hemangiomas. They are present at birth, and their growth follows that of the child and never regresses.
- In 1996 the ISSVA classified vascular malformations into low flow, including venous, lymphatic, and capillary malformations, and high flow represented by AVMs and AVFs.
- Venous malformations are the most common type of vascular malformation, frequently multifocal with intramuscular and subcutaneous components.
- Lymphatic malformations are more commonly seen in the cephalic, axillary, and thoracic regions.
- Intramuscular hemangioma is a rare entity found in teens and young adults. This lesion is distinguished from vascular malformation by the absence of soft tissue component.

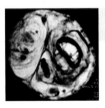

SOFT TISSUE TUMORS - NONVASCULAR

- Tenosynovial giant cell tumor is the second most common soft tissue tumor in the hand and is most commonly found in the palmar aspect of the first three fingers.
- Fibrolipohamartomas are rare tumors of children and young adults in which fatty and fibrous tissues infiltrate the epineurium and perineurium and surround the median nerve and its terminal branches.
- Neurogenic tumors, such as schwannomas and neurofibromas, may involve digital nerves. The main differential diagnosis is neuroma.
- Extraskeletal chondromas are well-defined cartilaginous masses located in the soft tissues with a predilection for the hand, appearing low on T1 and very high on T2, occasionally with low-signal areas reflecting calcifications.
- Malignant tumors are extremely rare in the hand. The most common malignant tumors of the hand are epithelioid sarcoma, synovial cell sarcoma, and malignant fibrous histiocytoma.

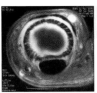

BONE TUMORS

- Majority of bone tumors in the hand are benign and are of cartilaginous origin, including enchondromas, juxtacortical chondromas, and osteochondromas.
- Enchondroma is the most common bone tumor of the hand. Multiple enchondromas in a predominantly unilateral distribution are seen in Ollier's disease, and in association with multiple hemangiomas of the skin in Maffuci's syndrome.
- Juxtacortical chondromas are located adjacent to and partially embedded in the shaft of the phalanx or metacarpal. MR confirms intralesional cartilage lobules and frequently displays marrow invasion.
- Osteochondromas are much less prevalent than enchondromas. Subungual exostoses, florid reactive periostitis, and bizarre paraosteal osteochondromatous proliferation (BPOP) have different clinical and imaging manifestations, but share similar histologic features.
- Subungual exostoses have a predilection for the thumb and the index finger, usually diagnosed with the triad of pain, ungual dystrophy, and distinctive radiographic pattern.
- Distinguishing between florid reactive periostitis and malignant bone tumor or infection is suggested by the presence of a large inflammatory soft tissue component with aggressive periosteal reaction but intact bony cortex.
- BPOP is usually a painless mass. Phalangeal bone edema reflects inflammatory reaction and should not be mistaken for bone tumor or infection.
- 8% of osteoid osteomas occur in the phalanges and often present with atypical clinical and radiographic features.
- Giant cell tumor in the hands usually presents as a metaepiphyseal osteolytic metacarpal lesion with a geographic pattern of bone destruction, and has higher recurrence than in other locations.
- Aneurysmal bone cyst most commonly occurs in the metacarpals but can occur in any bone, including the sesamoids.
- Malignant bone tumors of the hand are extremely rare and are almost always chondrosarcomas. In the hand, there is a high risk, up to 50%, of malignant transformation in patients with Ollier's disease.

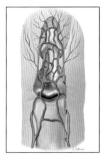

UNGUAL AND PERIUNGUAL PSEUDOTUMORS AND TUMORS
(See Figs. 11.17—-11.19)

- Mucoid pseudocysts or ganglia of the fingertip usually originate from the posterior nail fold, common in elderly patients. These are thin walled cysts usually associated with severe osteoarthritis and synovitis of the DIP joint.

- Epidermoid cysts may be located anywhere along the finger, but are most common in the distal phalanx. They are usually secondary to trauma and old penetrating injury.

- Giant cell reaction of bone is a rare reactive process usually in the distal phalanx. This osteolytic lesion can be expansile with partial destruction of the cortex and may mimic an epidermoid cyst or a glomus tumor.

- Glomus tumors can be considered hamartomas from hyperplasia of glomus bodies most commonly located in the subungual area.

- Keratoacanthoma is a rare benign tumor located in the most distal nail bed and may mimic subungual squamous carcinoma. Onychomatricomas have distinct MR features with low signal tumor core in the metrical area and invagination into a funnel-shaped nail plate.

- Fibrous tumors such as Koenen's tumor, acquired fibrokeratoma, and dermatofibroma, can present with a wide range of clinical patterns despite histologic uniformity.

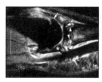

ARTHRITIS – OSTEOARTHRITIS

- Bone edema is the earliest manifestation and seems to correlate with pain and activity of OA.

- Subchondral bone cysts in OA develop in sclerotic bone and show absent or faint peripheral enhancement.

- Dorsal osteophytes of the DIP joint may be large, affect extensor tendons, and generate mucoid pseudocyst.

- The degree of synovitis in OA may help identify those patients who can benefit from synovium-targeted therapy.

- Heberden's nodes described at the DIP joint and Bouchard's nodes at the PIP joint are caused by overgrowth of the phalangeal condyles and capsular-ligamentous thickening.

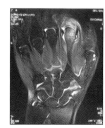

ARTHRITIS – RHEUMATOID ARTHRITIS

- MR diagnosis is based on the triad of synovitis, bone erosion, and bone edema.

- Early postcontrast images are useful for assessing true thickness of active synovitis.

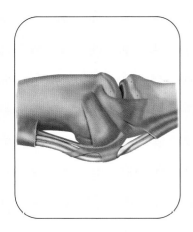

MR Imaging of the Fingers

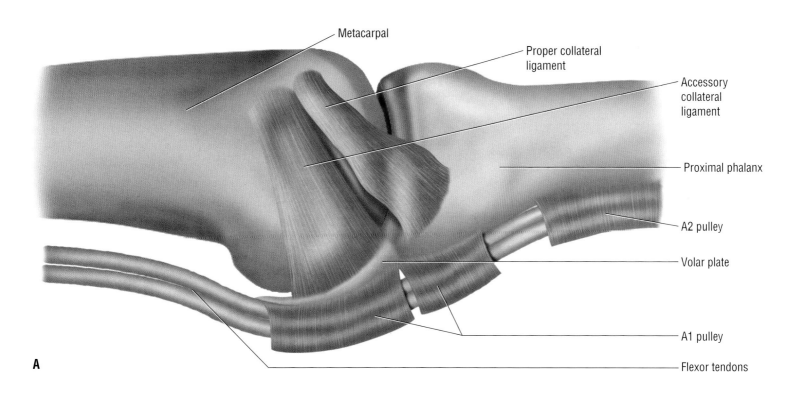

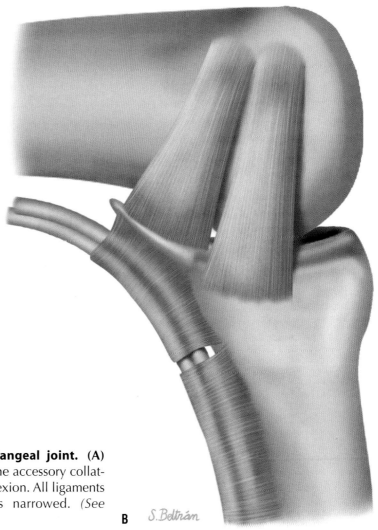

Figure 11.1 ▪ **Capsular ligaments of the metacarpophalangeal joint.** **(A)** Extension. The proper collateral ligament (PCL) is relaxed and the accessory collateral ligament (ACL) is under tension and limits extension. **(B)** Flexion. All ligaments are taut. The space between the A1 and A2 pulleys is narrowed. *(See Metacarpophalangeal Joint pg. 1848, in Stoller's 3rd Edition.)*

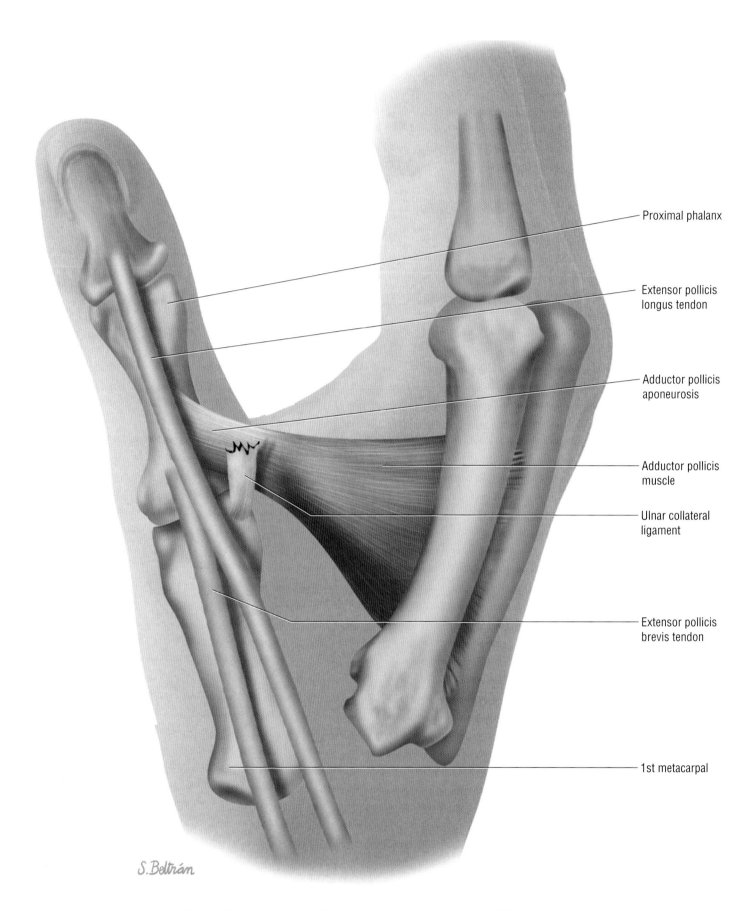

Proximal phalanx

Extensor pollicis longus tendon

Adductor pollicis aponeurosis

Adductor pollicis muscle

Ulnar collateral ligament

Extensor pollicis brevis tendon

1st metacarpal

S.Beltrán

Figure 11.2 ■ Stener's lesion. The ulnar collateral ligament (UCL) is torn from its distal insertion. The proximal UCL passes over the expansion of the adductor pollicis aponeurosis and cannot heal. *(See Gamekeeper's Thumb pg. 1850, in Stoller's 3rd Edition.)*

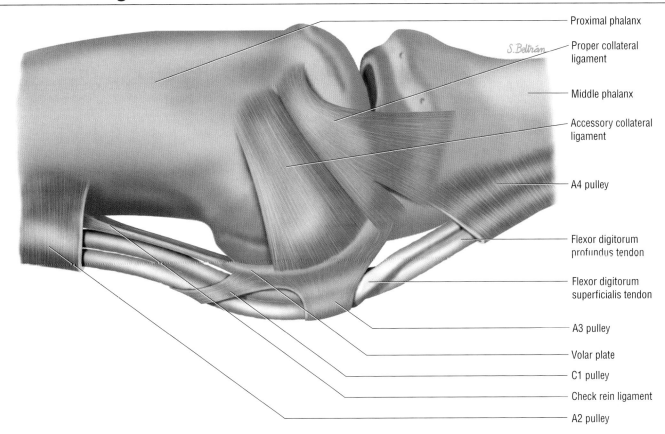

Proximal phalanx

Proper collateral ligament

Middle phalanx

Accessory collateral ligament

A4 pulley

Flexor digitorum profundus tendon

Flexor digitorum superficialis tendon

A3 pulley

Volar plate

C1 pulley

Check rein ligament

A2 pulley

Figure 11.3 ▪ **Capsular ligaments of the proximal interphalangeal joint.** The proper collateral ligament inserts on the base of the middle phalanx and partially on the volar plate. The accessory collateral ligament inserts on the lateral aspect of the volar plate and flexor tendon sheath. *(See Proximal Interphalangeal Joint pg. 1855, in Stoller's 3rd Edition.)*

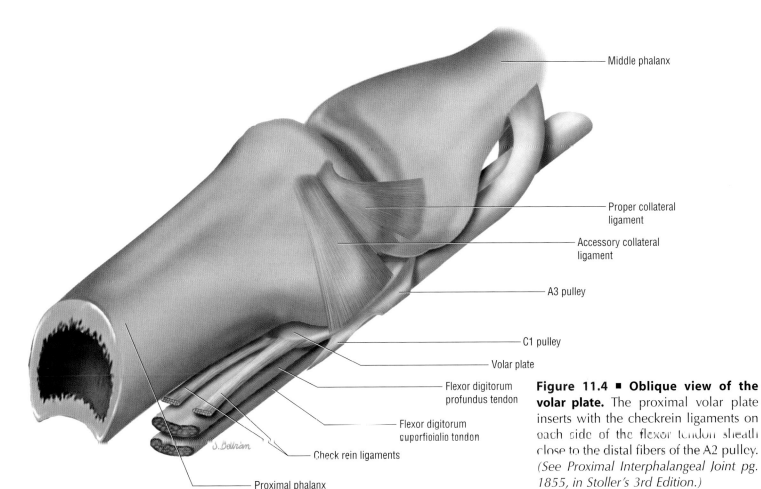

Middle phalanx

Proper collateral ligament

Accessory collateral ligament

A3 pulley

C1 pulley

Volar plate

Flexor digitorum profundus tendon

Flexor digitorum superficialis tendon

Check rein ligaments

Proximal phalanx

Figure 11.4 ▪ **Oblique view of the volar plate.** The proximal volar plate inserts with the checkrein ligaments on each side of the flexor tendon sheath close to the distal fibers of the A2 pulley. *(See Proximal Interphalangeal Joint pg. 1855, in Stoller's 3rd Edition.)*

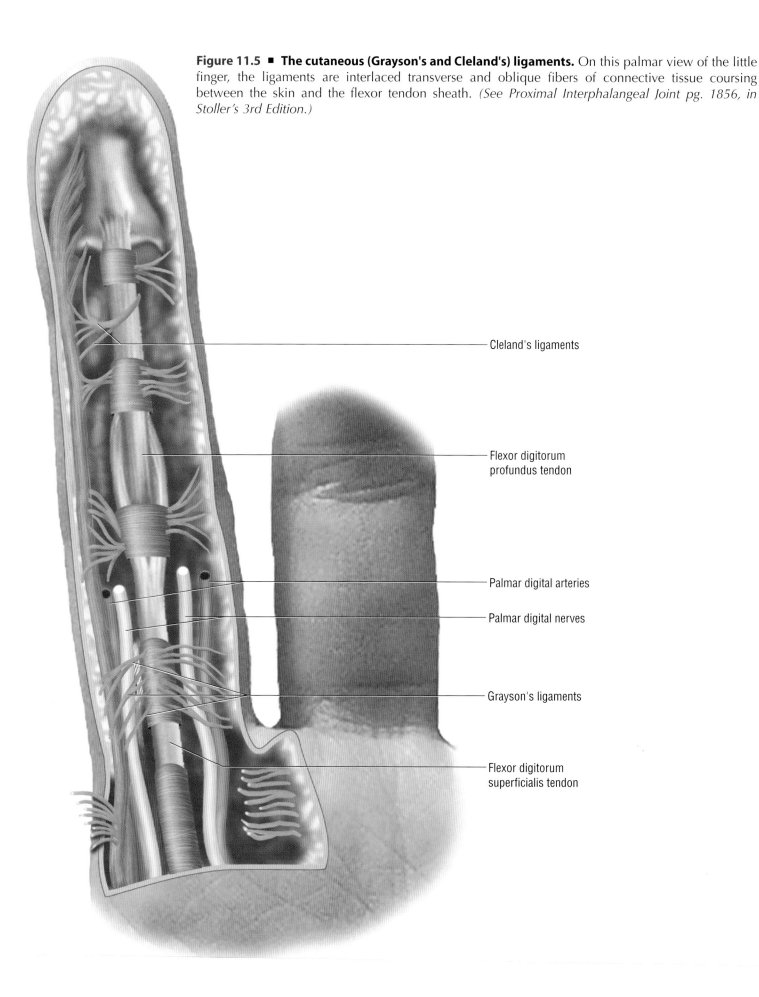

Figure 11.5 ■ The cutaneous (Grayson's and Cleland's) ligaments. On this palmar view of the little finger, the ligaments are interlaced transverse and oblique fibers of connective tissue coursing between the skin and the flexor tendon sheath. *(See Proximal Interphalangeal Joint pg. 1856, in Stoller's 3rd Edition.)*

Cleland's ligaments

Flexor digitorum profundus tendon

Palmar digital arteries

Palmar digital nerves

Grayson's ligaments

Flexor digitorum superficialis tendon

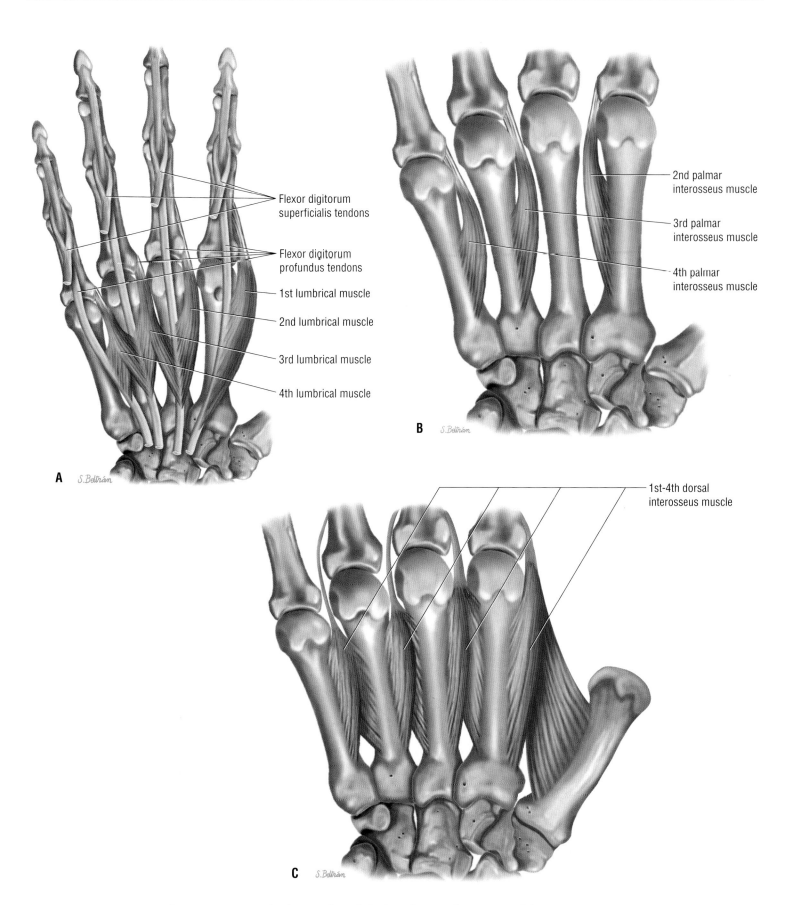

Figure 11.6 ■ **Intrinsic muscles of the hand.** (**A**) Palmar view of the most common configuration of the lumbrical muscles. (**B**) Palmar view of the palmar interossei muscles. (**C**) Palmar view of the dorsal interossei muscles. *(See Extensor Tendons pg. 1860, in Stoller's 3rd Edition.)*

Labels in figure A: Flexor digitorum superficialis tendons; Flexor digitorum profundus tendons; 1st lumbrical muscle; 2nd lumbrical muscle; 3rd lumbrical muscle; 4th lumbrical muscle

Labels in figure B: 2nd palmar interosseus muscle; 3rd palmar interosseus muscle; 4th palmar interosseus muscle

Labels in figure C: 1st-4th dorsal interosseus muscle

Extensor Tendons

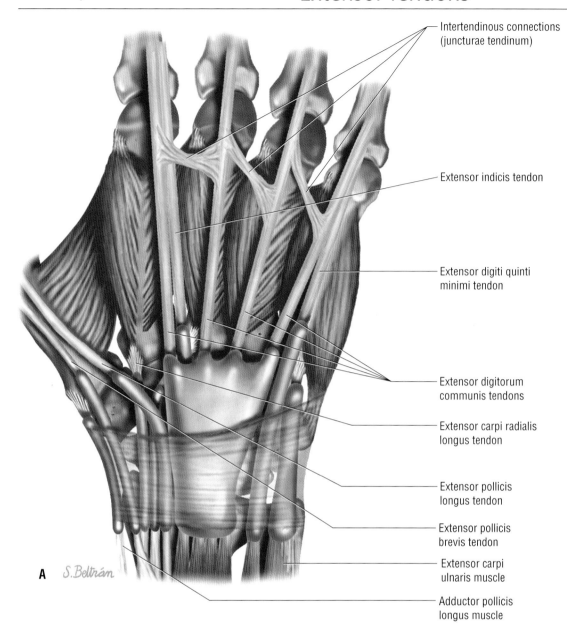

Intertendinous connections
(juncturae tendinum)

Extensor indicis tendon

Extensor digiti quinti
minimi tendon

Extensor digitorum
communis tendons

Extensor carpi radialis
longus tendon

Extensor pollicis
longus tendon

Extensor pollicis
brevis tendon

Extensor carpi
ulnaris muscle

Adductor pollicis
longus muscle

A   *S. Beltrán*

Figure 11.7 ▪ Extensor tendons and their interconnections (juncturae tendinum). (A) Dorsal aspect and (B) axial image at the metacarpal heads. The most common configuration is presented. The extensor indicis tendon (EIT) lacks a junctura tendinum. (*See Extensor Tendons pg. 1861, in Stoller's 3rd Edition.*)

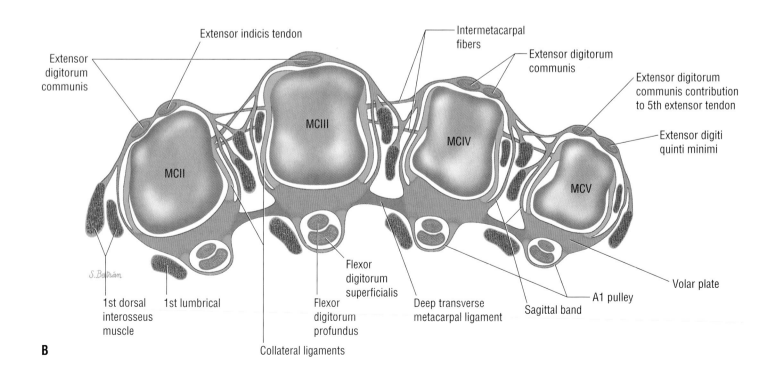

Extensor indicis tendon

Intermetacarpal
fibers

Extensor
digitorum
communis

Extensor digitorum
communis

Extensor digitorum
communis contribution
to 5th extensor tendon

Extensor digiti
quinti minimi

MCII

MCIII

MCIV

MCV

1st dorsal
interosseus
muscle

1st lumbrical

Flexor
digitorum
profundus

Flexor
digitorum
superficialis

Collateral ligaments

Deep transverse
metacarpal ligament

Sagittal band

A1 pulley

Volar plate

S. Beltrán

B

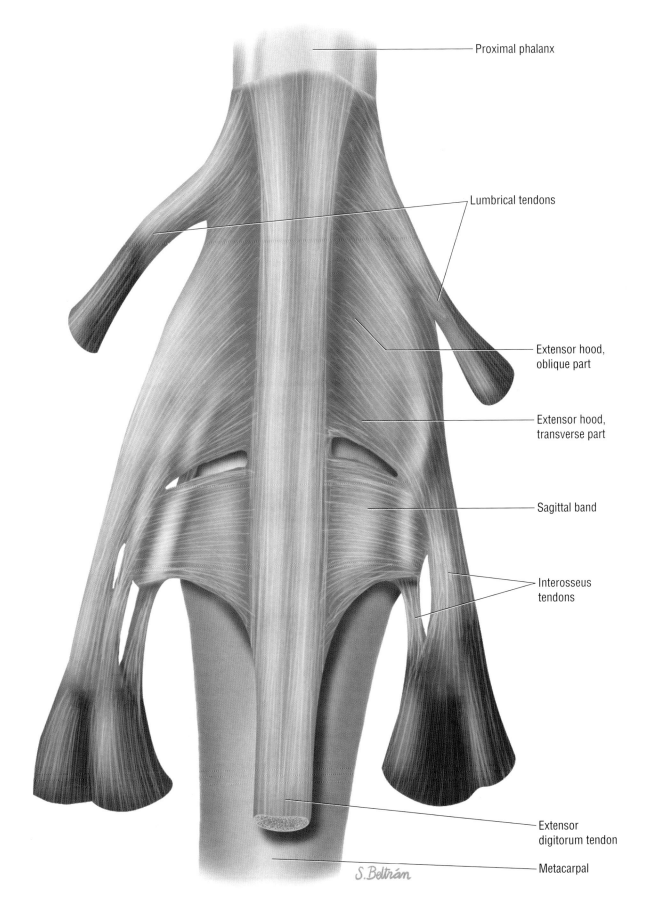

Proximal phalanx

Lumbrical tendons

Extensor hood, oblique part

Extensor hood, transverse part

Sagittal band

Interosseus tendons

Extensor digitorum tendon

Metacarpal

S.Beltrán

Figure 11.8 ■ Extensor hood and sagittal bands. Dorsal aspect. *(See Extensor tendons pg 1862, in Stoller's 3rd Edition.)*

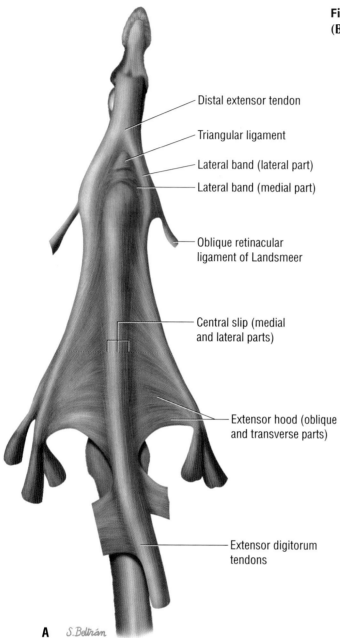

Figure 11.9 ▪ Extensor apparatus of the finger. (A) Dorsal aspect and **(B)** radial aspect. *(See Extensor Tendons pg. 1862, in Stoller's 3rd Edition.)*

Distal extensor tendon

Triangular ligament

Lateral band (lateral part)

Lateral band (medial part)

Oblique retinacular ligament of Landsmeer

Central slip (medial and lateral parts)

Extensor hood (oblique and transverse parts)

Extensor digitorum tendons

A   *S.Beltrán*

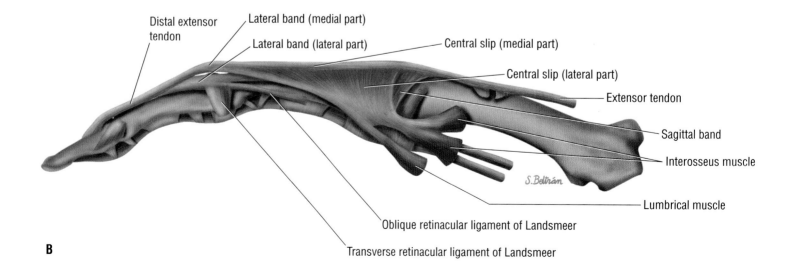

Distal extensor tendon

Lateral band (medial part)

Lateral band (lateral part)

Central slip (medial part)

Central slip (lateral part)

Extensor tendon

Sagittal band

Interosseus muscle

Lumbrical muscle

S.Beltrán

Oblique retinacular ligament of Landsmeer

Transverse retinacular ligament of Landsmeer

B

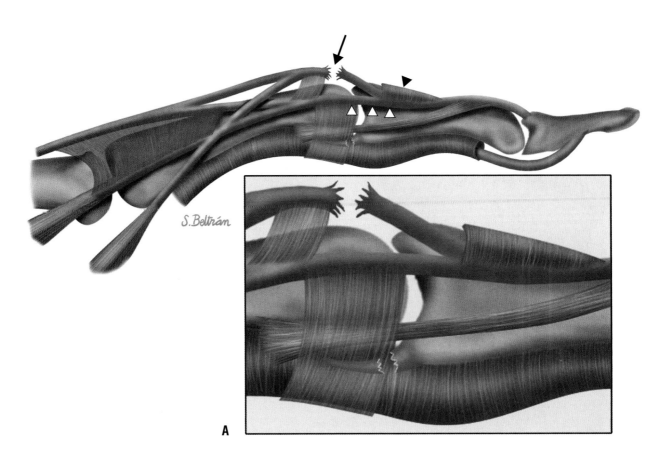

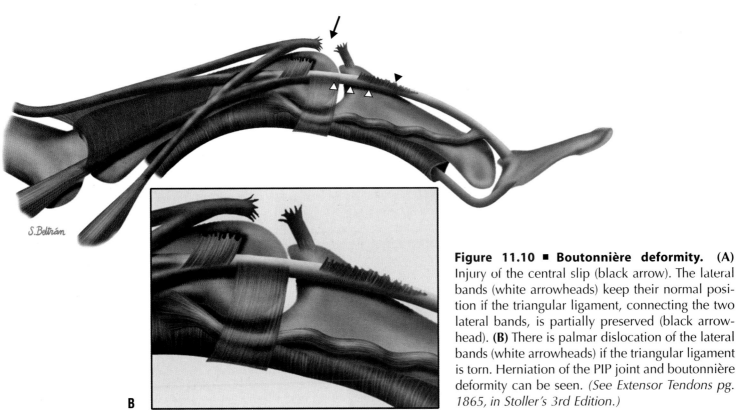

Figure 11.10 ■ Boutonnière deformity. (A) Injury of the central slip (black arrow). The lateral bands (white arrowheads) keep their normal position if the triangular ligament, connecting the two lateral bands, is partially preserved (black arrowhead). **(B)** There is palmar dislocation of the lateral bands (white arrowheads) if the triangular ligament is torn. Herniation of the PIP joint and boutonnière deformity can be seen. *(See Extensor Tendons pg. 1865, in Stoller's 3rd Edition.)*

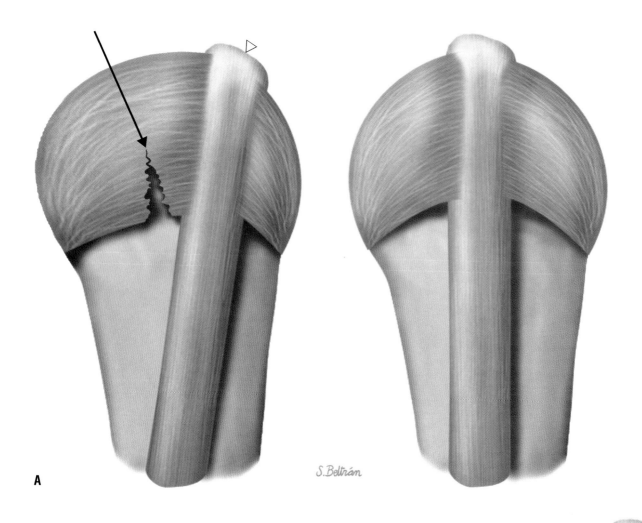

A

Figure 11.11 ■ Injury of the radial sagittal band (arrow) with ulnar subluxation of the extensor tendon (arrowhead). The degree of tendon instability is determined by the extent of sagittal band disruption. **(A)** In a partial tear, a proximal tear rather than a distal tear of the sagittal band contributes to instability. **(B)** In a complete tear, there is dislocation of the extensor tendon into the intermetacarpal space. *(See Extensor Tendon Injuries pg. 1867, in Stoller's 3rd Edition.)*

B

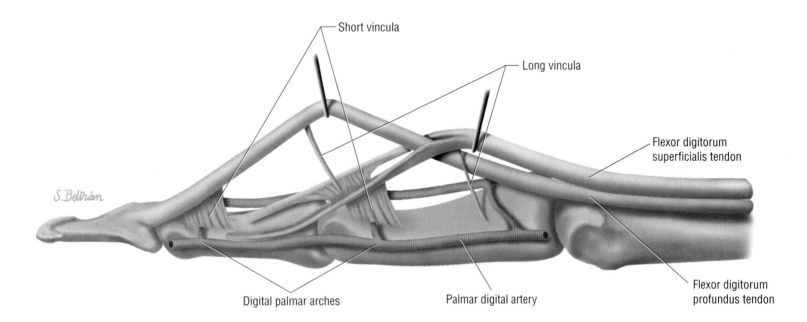

Figure 11.12 ■ Lateral aspect of the flexor digitorum tendons and their vascular supply. *(See Flexor Tendons pg. 1868 , in Stoller's 3rd Edition.)*

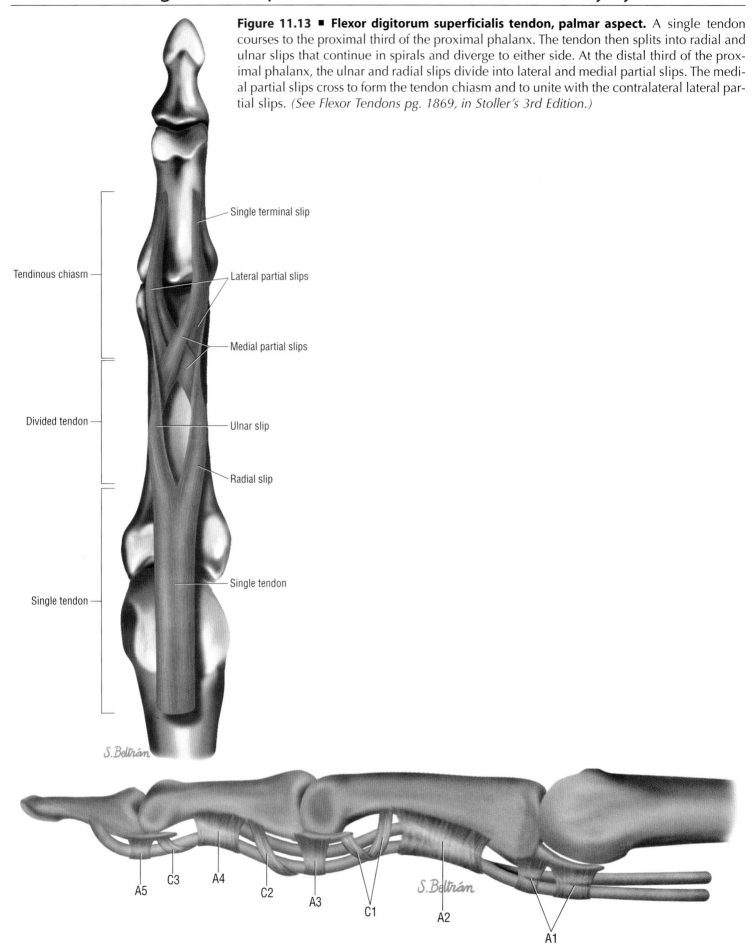

Figure 11.13 ■ **Flexor digitorum superficialis tendon, palmar aspect.** A single tendon courses to the proximal third of the proximal phalanx. The tendon then splits into radial and ulnar slips that continue in spirals and diverge to either side. At the distal third of the proximal phalanx, the ulnar and radial slips divide into lateral and medial partial slips. The medial partial slips cross to form the tendon chiasm and to unite with the contralateral lateral partial slips. *(See Flexor Tendons pg. 1869, in Stoller's 3rd Edition.)*

Tendinous chiasm

Divided tendon

Single tendon

Single terminal slip

Lateral partial slips

Medial partial slips

Ulnar slip

Radial slip

Single tendon

S. Beltrán

A5   C3   A4   C2   A3   C1   A2   A1   S. Beltrán

Figure 11.14 ■ Lateral view in extension of the pulley system of the digital flexor tendon sheaths. The flexor tendons undulate along the palmar aspect of the bones of the finger. *(See Flexor Tendons pg. 1869, in Stoller's 3rd Edition.)*

Figure 11.15 ■ **Classification of Jersey finger: (A)** type I, **(B)** type II, **(C)** type III, and **(D)** type IV. *(See Flexor Tendon Injuries pg. 1872, in Stoller's 3rd Edition.)*

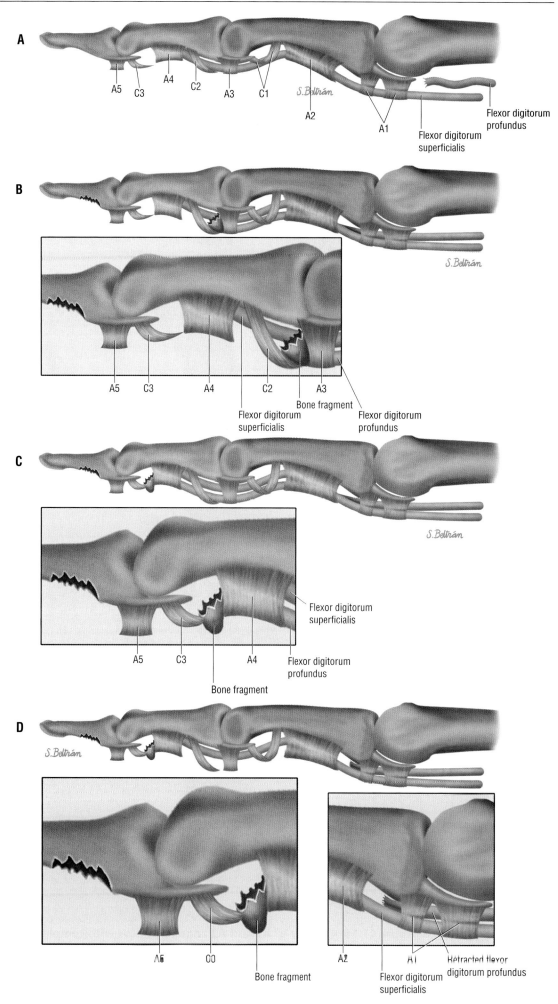

A1 and A2 Annular Pulley Injury

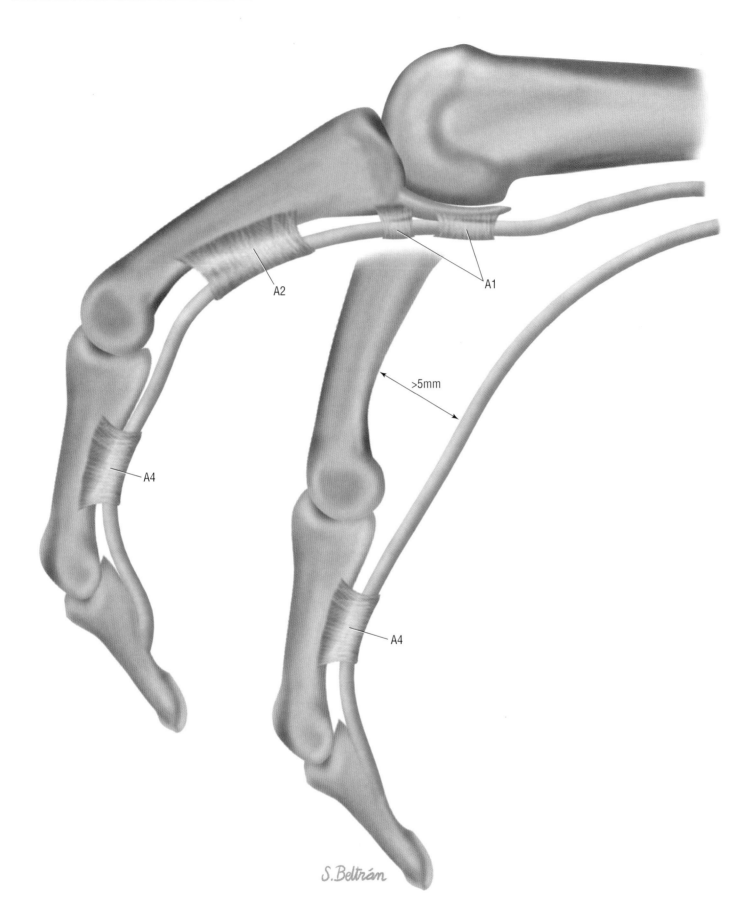

Figure 11.16 ■ **Injury of A1 and A2 annular pulleys with complete tear.** There is bowstringing of the flexor tendons during flexion. *(See Pulley Injuries pg. 1876, in Stoller's 3rd Edition.)*

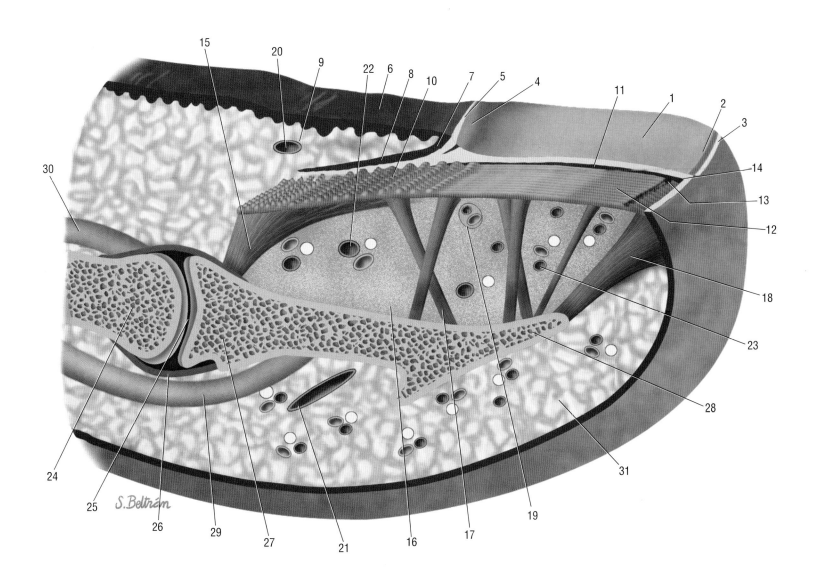

Figure 11.17 ▪ Sagittal anatomy of the nail unit. Dorsal oblique view of the nail unit: 1, nail plate; 2, onychodermal band; 3, free edge of plate; 4, lunula; 5, cuticle; 6, proximal nail fold; 7, inferior aspect of proximal nail fold or eponychium; 8, proximal or dorsal nail matrix; 9, cul-de-sac; 10, intermediate or ventral nail matrix; 11, nail bed epithelium ridges; 12, nail bed corium; 13, hyponychium; 14, distal groove; 15, matrix phalangeal ligament; 16, submatrical hypersignal area; 17, network of collagenous fibers; 18, hyponychio-phalangeal ligament; 19, glomus body; 20, proximal dorsal arterial arch; 21, distal dorsal arterial arch; 22, distal matrix arterial arch; 23, nail bed arterial arch; 24, middle phalanx; 25, distal interphalangeal joint; 26, volar plate; 27, distal phalanx; 28, tuberosity of distal phalanx; 29, flexor digitorum profundus tendon; 30, terminal band of extensor tendon; and 31, pulp. *(See Ungual and Periungual Pseudotumors and Tumors pg. 1907, in Stoller's 3rd Edition.)*

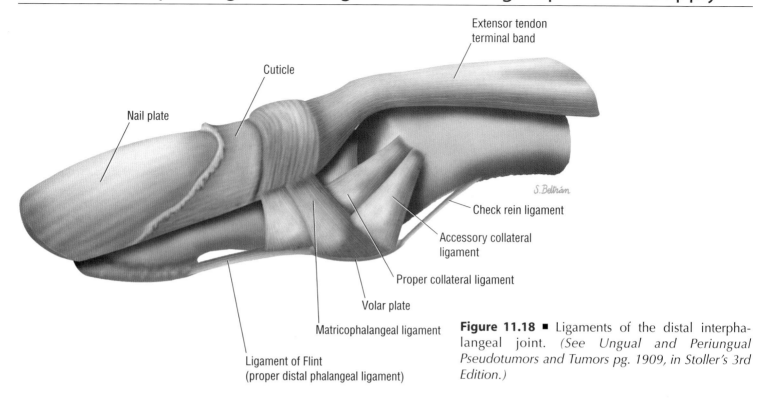

Extensor tendon
terminal band

Cuticle

Nail plate

Check rein ligament

Accessory collateral
ligament

Proper collateral ligament

Volar plate

Matricophalangeal ligament

Ligament of Flint
(proper distal phalangeal ligament)

Figure 11.18 ■ Ligaments of the distal interphalangeal joint. *(See Ungual and Periungual Pseudotumors and Tumors pg. 1909, in Stoller's 3rd Edition.)*

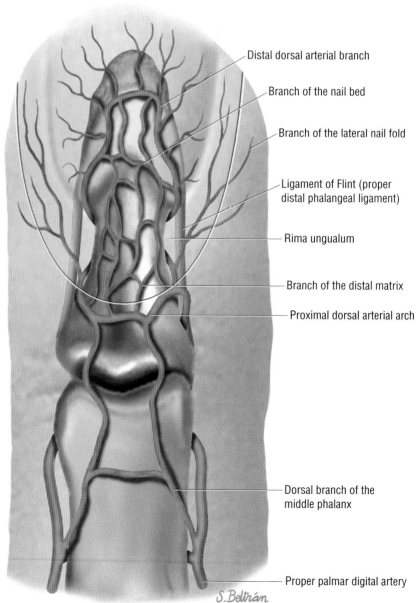

Distal dorsal arterial branch

Branch of the nail bed

Branch of the lateral nail fold

Ligament of Flint (proper
distal phalangeal ligament)

Rima ungualum

Branch of the distal matrix

Proximal dorsal arterial arch

Dorsal branch of the
middle phalanx

Proper palmar digital artery

Figure 11.19 ■ Dorsal aspect of the arterial supply of the fingertip. *(See Ungual and Periungual Pseudotumors and Tumors pg. 1910, in Stoller's 3rd Edition.)*

Chapter

12

Entrapment Neuropathies of the Upper Extremity

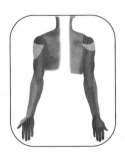

Pearls and Pitfalls & Color Illustrations

Pearls and Pitfalls

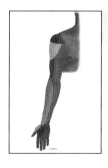

TERMINOLOGY

- Neuropraxia is a first-degree nerve injury with temporary loss of nerve conduction.
- Axonotmesis is a second-degree nerve injury characterized by interruption of the axon with intact connective tissue structures surrounding the axon and Schwann cells.

■ Neurotmesis is complete disruption of the nerve and supporting connective tissue structures.

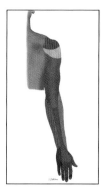

IMAGING TECHNIQUES

- STIR or FS PD FSE images are more sensitive than T2 FSE images in the detection of denervated muscle.

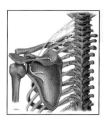

SHOULDER NEUROPATHIES
(See Figures 12.2–12.3)

- Suprascapular nerve syndrome
- Proximal entrapment associated with supraspinatus and infraspinatus muscle denervation.
- Distal entrapment associated with infraspinatus muscle denervation.

■ T1 or PD-weighted images are required to assess fatty atrophy.

■ FS PD FSE images are sensitive to muscle denervation.

■ Axillary neuropathy includes quadrilateral space syndrome and posttraumatic injury to the axillary nerve.

■ The Parsonage-Turner syndrome is primarily associated with suprascapular nerve disease, although the axillary, radial, or phrenic nerves or the entire brachial plexus may be affected.

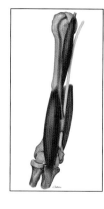

ARM AND ELBOW NEUROPATHIES
(See Figures 12.4–12.7)

- The cubital tunnel is the most common site of ulnar neuropathy.
- Ulnar neuropathy also occurs at the arcade of Struthers, the edge of the medial intermuscular septum, the ligament of Struthers, the arcuate ligament, and the deep flexor pronator aponeurosis.
- The pronator syndrome is the most common cause of median nerve entrapment. It is characterized by numbness in the median nerve distribution, occurring with repetitive forearm pronation/supination.

■ Potential sites of compression in the pronator syndrome include the supracondylar process/ligament of Struthers, the lacertus fibrosus, the pronator teres muscle, and the proximal arch of the flexor digitorum superficialis muscle.

■ The anterior interosseous syndrome affects only the motor branch of the median nerve and is less common than the pronator syndrome.

■ The radial tunnel syndrome involves compression of the posterior interosseous nerve without motor deficit.

■ The posterior interosseous nerve syndrome is a motor neuropathy with the same potential sites of compression as in the radial tunnel syndrome.

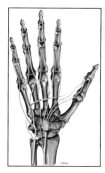

WRIST NEUROPATHIES
(See Figure 12.8)

- The carpal tunnel syndrome with compression of the median nerve occurs at the proximal aspect of the transverse carpal ligament or at the level of the hook of the hamate.
- In the ulnar tunnel syndrome, sensation to the dorsal ulnar hand is spared. In contrast, ulnar compressive neuropathy proximal to the wrist is associated with loss of sensation in this area.

■ The superficial radial nerve syndrome involves entrapment of the sensory branch of the radial nerve in the distal forearm.

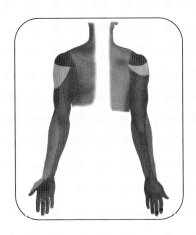

Entrapment Neuropathies of the Upper Extremity

Muscle

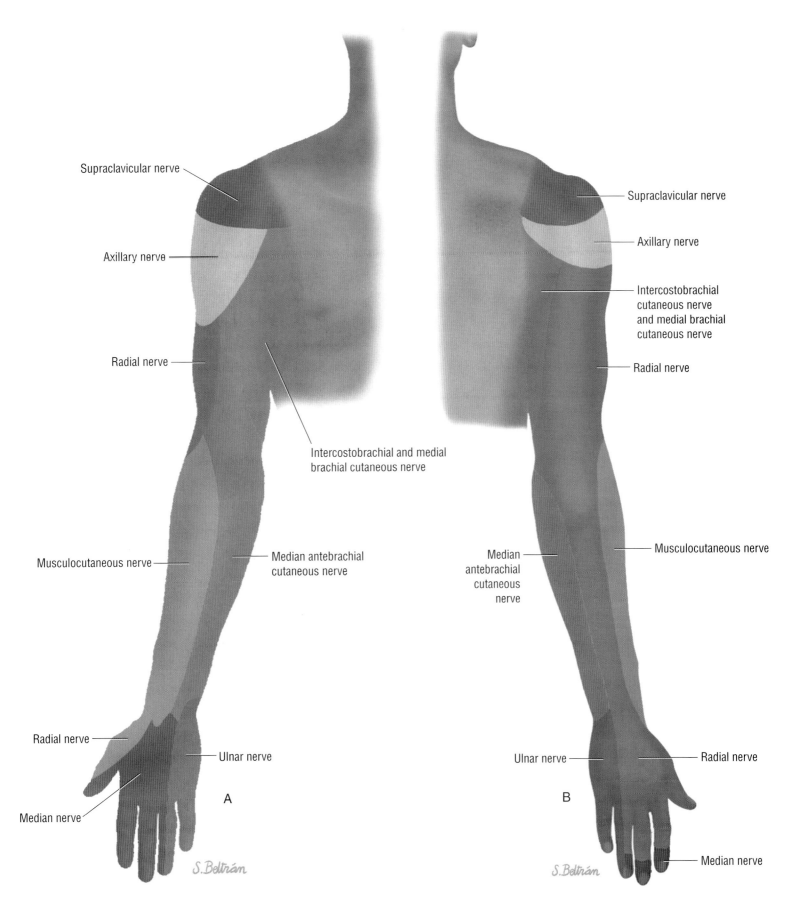

Figure 12.1 ■ **(A)** Upper extremity volar sensory innervation. **(B)** Upper extremity dorsal sensory innervation. *(See Entrapment Neuropathies of the Upper Extremity pg 1934, in Stoller's 3rd Edition.)*

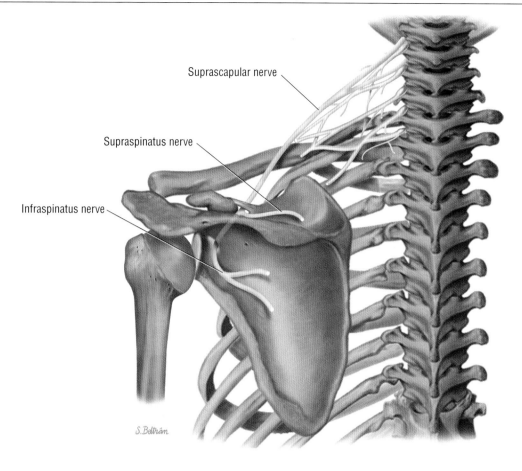

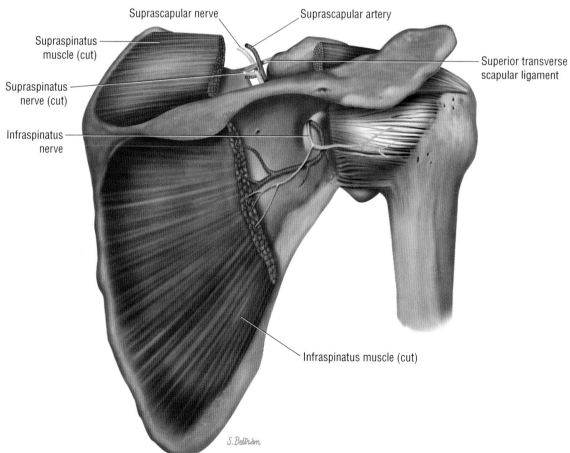

Figure 12.2 ■ The suprascapular nerve in the shoulder. *(See Suprascapular Nerve pg. 1937, in Stoller's 3rd Edition.)*

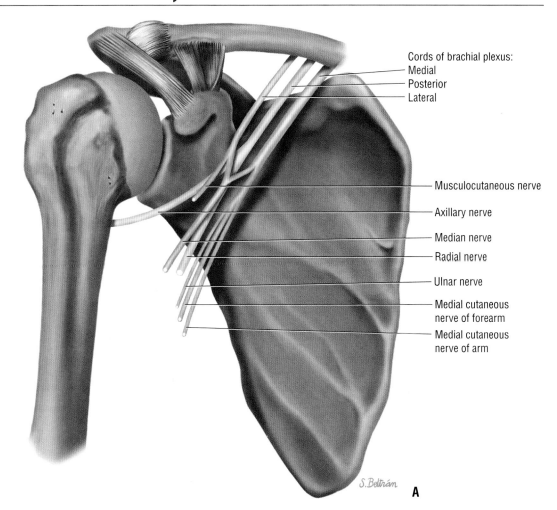

Cords of brachial plexus:
Medial
Posterior
Lateral

Musculocutaneous nerve

Axillary nerve

Median nerve

Radial nerve

Ulnar nerve

Medial cutaneous
nerve of forearm

Medial cutaneous
nerve of arm

A

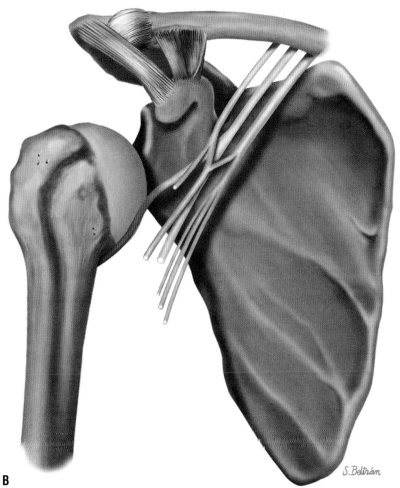

B

Figure 12.3 ▪ The axillary nerve. (A) The axillary nerve is seen coursing within the quadrilateral space in close relationship to the inferior glenoid rim. **(B)** Traction on the axillary nerve by a dislocated humeral head. *(See Axillary Neuropathy pgs. 1942–1943, in Stoller's 3rd Edition.)*

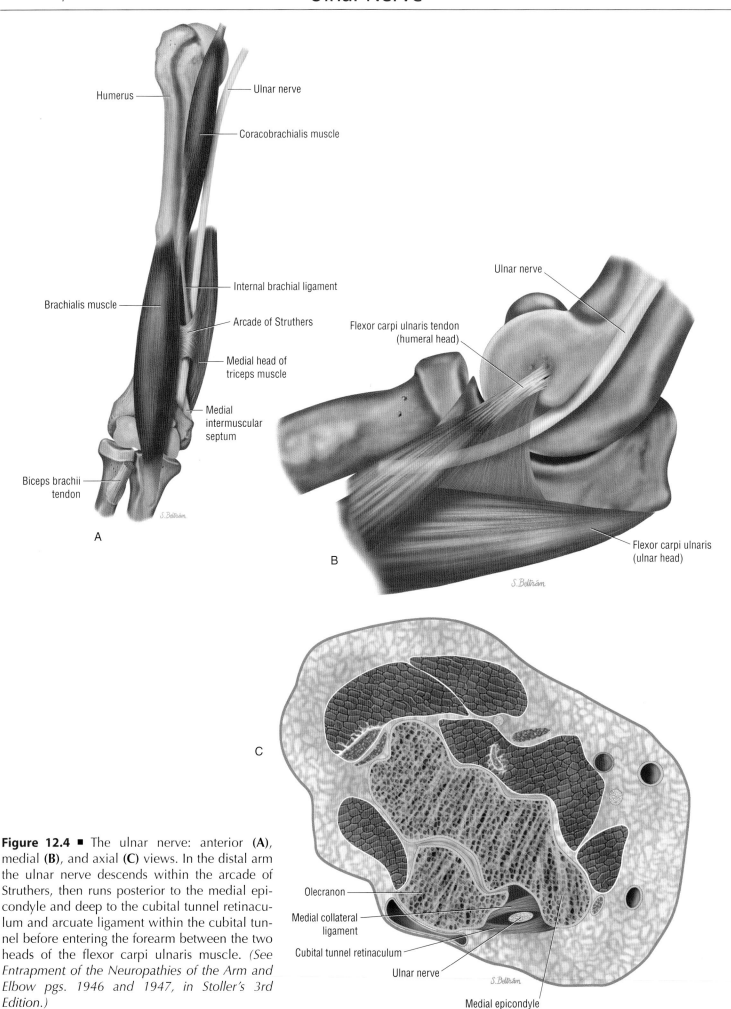

Figure 12.4 ■ The ulnar nerve: anterior **(A)**, medial **(B)**, and axial **(C)** views. In the distal arm the ulnar nerve descends within the arcade of Struthers, then runs posterior to the medial epicondyle and deep to the cubital tunnel retinaculum and arcuate ligament within the cubital tunnel before entering the forearm between the two heads of the flexor carpi ulnaris muscle. *(See Entrapment of the Neuropathies of the Arm and Elbow pgs. 1946 and 1947, in Stoller's 3rd Edition.)*

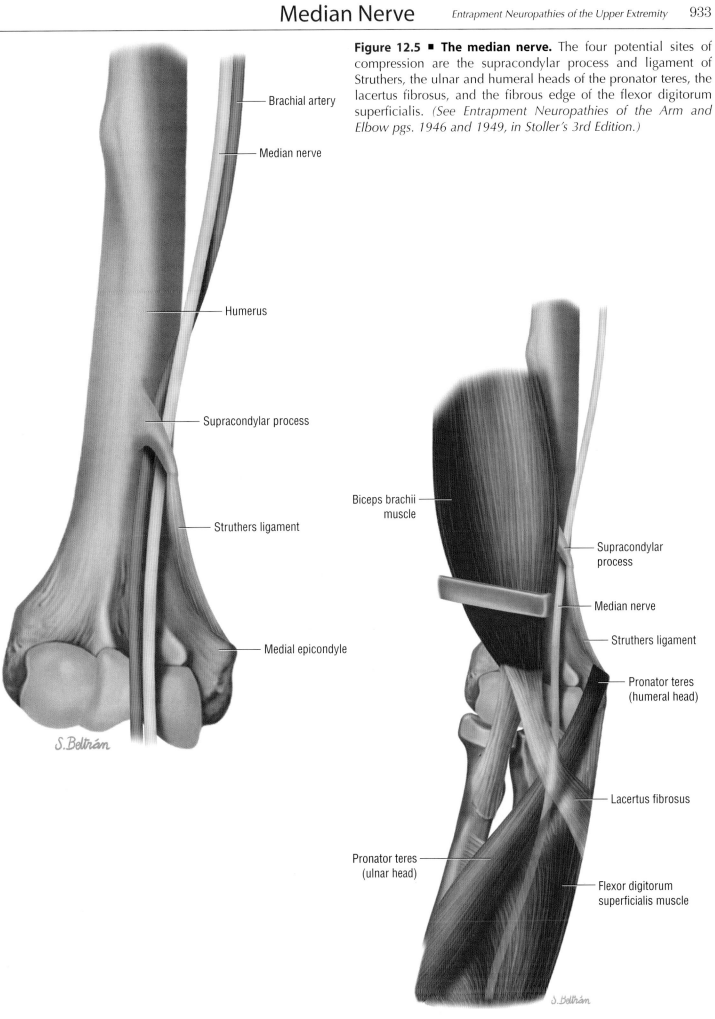

Figure 12.5 ■ **The median nerve.** The four potential sites of compression are the supracondylar process and ligament of Struthers, the ulnar and humeral heads of the pronator teres, the lacertus fibrosus, and the fibrous edge of the flexor digitorum superficialis. *(See Entrapment Neuropathies of the Arm and Elbow pgs. 1946 and 1949, in Stoller's 3rd Edition.)*

Brachial artery

Median nerve

Humerus

Supracondylar process

Struthers ligament

Medial epicondyle

Biceps brachii muscle

Supracondylar process

Median nerve

Struthers ligament

Pronator teres (humeral head)

Lacertus fibrosus

Pronator teres (ulnar head)

Flexor digitorum superficialis muscle

S.Beltrán

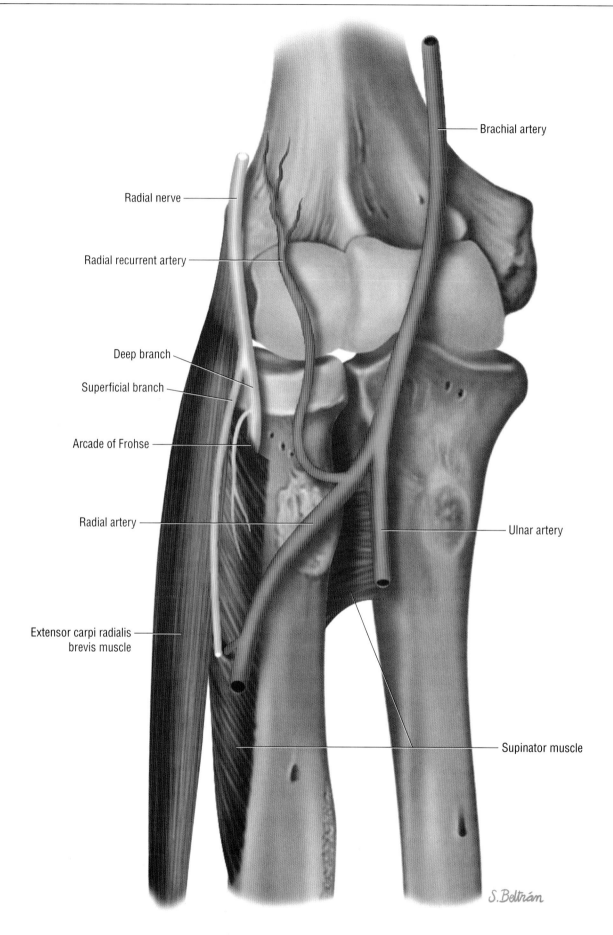

Brachial artery

Radial nerve

Radial recurrent artery

Deep branch

Superficial branch

Arcade of Frohse

Radial artery

Ulnar artery

Extensor carpi radialis
brevis muscle

Supinator muscle

S.Beltrán

Figure 12.6 ■ The radial nerve. The radial nerve splits into the superficial radial nerve and the posterior interosseous nerve at the radiocapitellar joint. The posterior interosseous branch courses between the deep and superficial heads of the supinator muscle. *(See Radial Nerve pgs. 1950 and 1951, in Stoller's 3rd Edition.)*

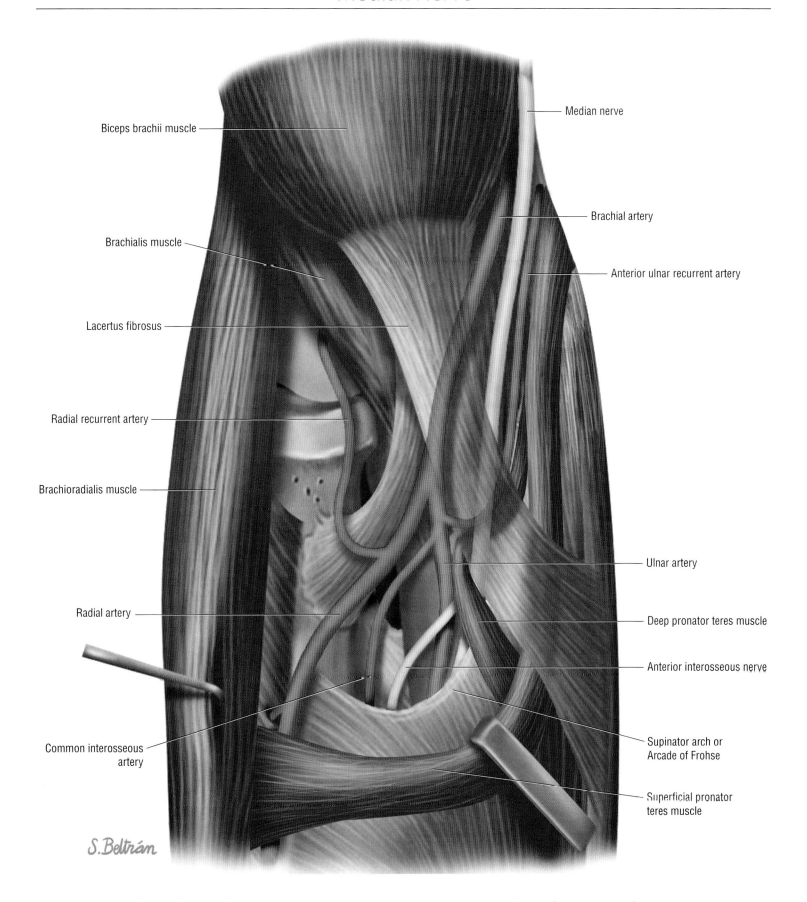

Biceps brachii muscle

Brachialis muscle

Lacertus fibrosus

Radial recurrent artery

Brachioradialis muscle

Radial artery

Common interosseous
artery

Median nerve

Brachial artery

Anterior ulnar recurrent artery

Ulnar artery

Deep pronator teres muscle

Anterior interosseous nerve

Supinator arch or
Arcade of Frohse

Superficial pronator
teres muscle

S. Beltrán

Figure 12.7 ▪ Median nerve in supination and pronation of the elbow. The nerve may become trapped between the two heads of the pronator teres in forearm pronation. This is the most common compression site in pronator syndrome. (Adapted from Pecina MM, Drmpotic-Nemanic J, Markiewitz AD. Tunnel syndromes in the upper extremities. In: Pecina MM, Krompotic-Nemanic J, Markiewitz AD, ed. Tunnel syndromes. New York: CRC Press, 1991:29-53). *(See Median Nerve Entrapment pgs. 1957-1960, in Stoller's 3rd Edition.)*

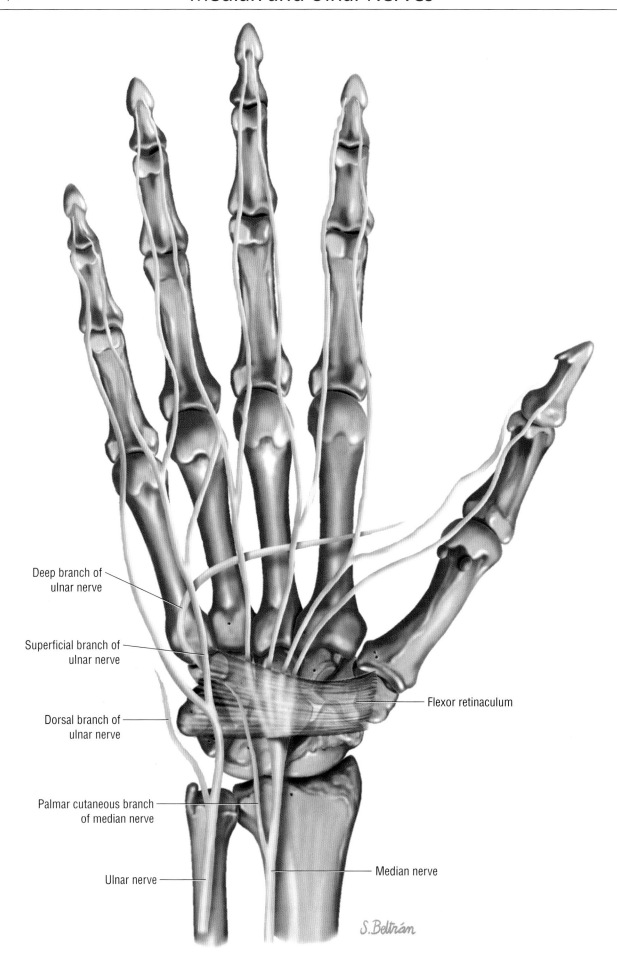

Deep branch of
ulnar nerve

Superficial branch of
ulnar nerve

Dorsal branch of
ulnar nerve

Palmar cutaneous branch
of median nerve

Ulnar nerve

Flexor retinaculum

Median nerve

S. Beltrán

Figure 12.8 ■ The median and ulnar nerves in the wrist and hand. *(See Entrapment Neuropathies of the Wrist pg. 1964, in Stoller's 3rd Edition.)*

13 Marrow Imaging

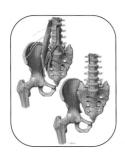

Pearls and Pitfalls & Color Illustrations

Pearls and Pitfalls

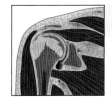

NORMAL BONE MARROW
(see Figures 13.1-13.3)

- Be aware of normal variations of red marrow patterns and recognize them as normal.
- Distribution of red marrow can vary from person to person but is usually symmetric in the same person.

- Subchondral red marrow can be seen in the proximal epiphyses of the humerus and femur.
- T1-weighted and STIR sequences are most useful in detecting marrow infiltrative processes.
- Normal red marrow signal is equal to or higher than muscle or disk on T1-weighted images.
- Abnormal marrow signal is equal to or lower than muscle or disk on T1-weighted images.
- Consider whole-body MR imaging for metastatic or myeloma survey and for staging of malignant neoplasms and lymphoma.

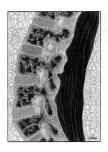

LEUKEMIA
(see Figures 13.4-13.6)

- Marrow involvement is usually diffuse in acute leukemia.
- Relapse can present with patchy areas of marrow infiltration.
- Abnormal marrow is darker than adjacent disk or muscle on T1-weighted images.

- Be aware of post-therapy marrow changes (edema, fibrosis, fatty infiltration) that can simulate residual or metastatic disease.
- Patients treated with G-CSF often develop reconversion from fatty to hematopoietic marrow.

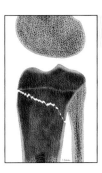

MALIGNANT LYMPHOMA
(see Figures 13.7-13.8)

- Lymphoma presents focally rather than diffusely.
- STIR imaging is useful in detecting marrow and mediastinal involvement.
- Whole-body MR imaging and whole-body FDG-PET imaging are sensitive and accurate in the detection and staging of lymphoma.

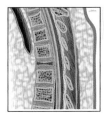

LANGERHANS CELL HISTIOCYTOSIS
(see Figure 13.9)

- Langerhans cell histiocytosis is the "great imitator" of various benign and malignant bone lesions.
- This disorder frequently presents with vertebral body collapse (vertebra plana).

- It is important to differentiate localized from disseminated disease (different prognosis).
- Consider CT-guided percutaneous steroid injection for treatment.

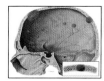

MULTIPLE MYELOMA
(see Figures 13.10-13.11)

- Multiple myeloma is the most common primary neoplasm of bone.
- Imaging is important for staging. More than one lesion changes the prognosis from stage I to stage III.

- MR imaging of the spine and pelvis and whole-body MR imaging are most sensitive for evaluating the extent of myelomatous involvement.
- STIR and T1-weighted sequences are most useful for lesion detection.

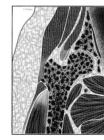

METASTATIC DISEASE
(see Figures 13.12-13.16)

- STIR and T1-weighted sequences with and without gadolinium are most useful in detecting metastatic disease.
- Consider whole-body MR imaging for staging.
- A halo sign on T2-weighted images indicates active disease, whereas a halo sign on T1-weighted images indicates response to therapy.

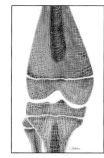

GAUCHER DISEASE
(see Figures 13.17-13.18)

- Gaucher disease lesions demonstrate decreased signal on T1- and T2-weighted images.
- Osteonecrosis is common.
- Erlenmeyer flask deformity of the femurs is characteristic.

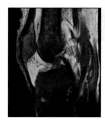

IRON STORAGE

- Increased iron stores cause decreased signal on T1- and T2-weighted images.

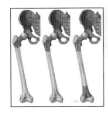

BONE MARROW IN SPECIAL POPULATIONS
(see Figure 13.19)

- Be aware of normal variations of red marrow patterns and recognize them as normal.

- Normal red marrow demonstrates T1 signal that is equal to or higher than muscle or disk.

- Marrow reconversion from yellow to red marrow occurs in the reverse order, as does conversion from red to yellow marrow.

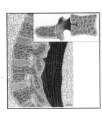

APLASTIC ANEMIA
(see Figure 13.20)

- Increased signal on T1-weighted images is caused by hypoplastic marrow.

- Marrow heterogeneity caused by hematopoiesis can be seen during recovery.

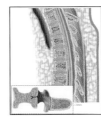

HEMOGLOBINOPATHIES
(see Figures 13.21-13.24)

- Expansion of marrow cavities is caused by an increased demand for hematopoiesis.

- Vascular occlusion leads to bone infarcts.

- H vertebrae in patients with sickle cell anemia are caused by infarcts.

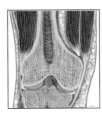

MISCELLANEOUS LESIONS
(see Figures 13.25-13.27)

- Enlarged bone with cortical and trabecular thickening is characteristic of Paget's disease.

- STIR images are most sensitive in evaluating the extent of hyperemic marrow in transient osteoporosis and reflex sympathetic dystrophy.

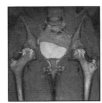

AIDS

- Patients with AIDS are at increased risk for infections and neoplasms, especially lymphoma.

- Complications of antiviral therapy include lipodystrophy.

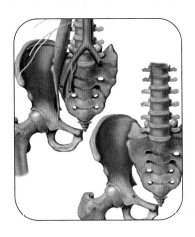

Marrow Imaging

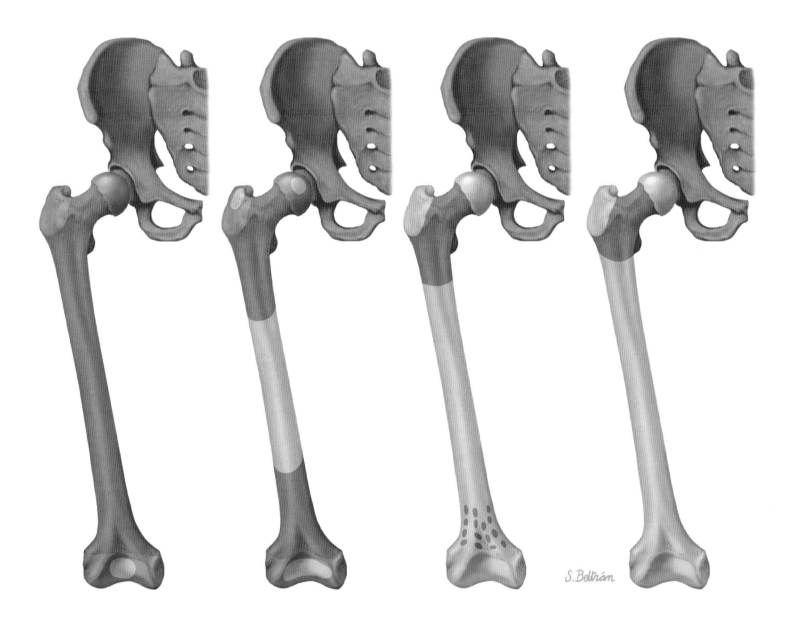

Figure 13.1 ■ **Bone marrow conversion from birth to adulthood.** Graphic illustration demonstrating marrow distribution as a function of age with conversion of red marrow to yellow marrow. *(See Red to Yellow Marrow Conversion pg. 1979, in Stoller's 3rd Edition.)*

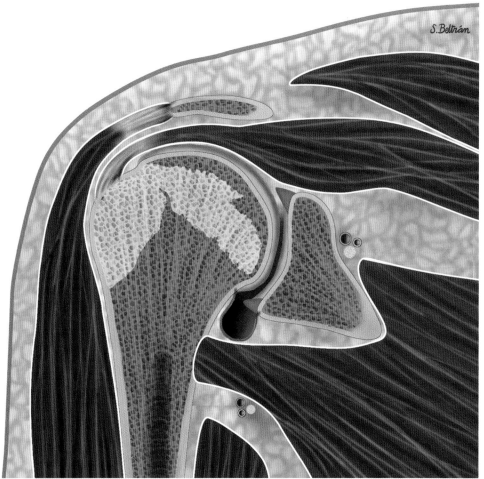

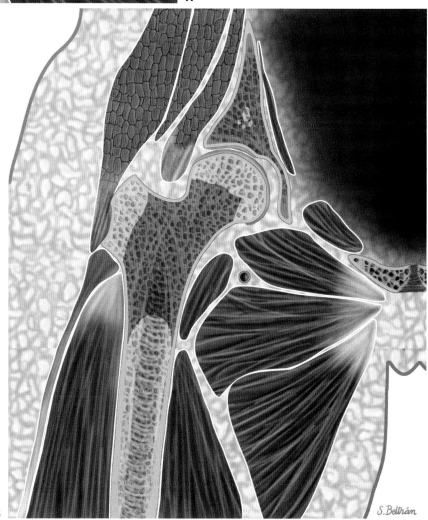

Figure 13.2 ▪ Normal red marrow. Coronal graphic illustrations of the shoulder **(A)** and hip **(B)** demonstrate the normal appearance of residual red marrow in the humeral (red color) and femoral (red color) metaphyses. Note the curvilinear distribution of red marrow involving the medial humeral head, a normal finding. *(See Normal Bone Marrow pg 1981, in Stoller's 3rd Edition.)*

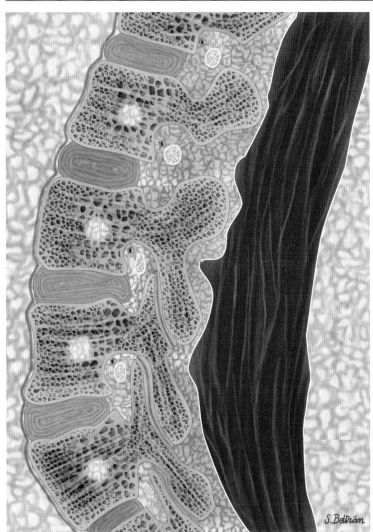

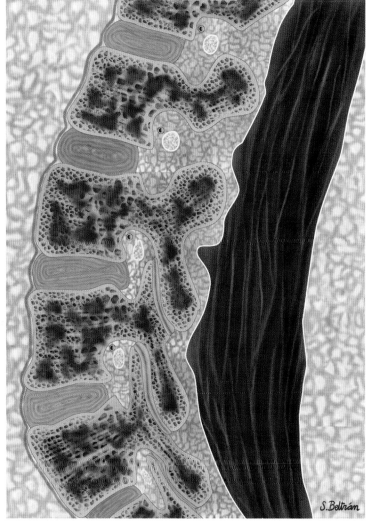

Figure 13.3 ▪ Sagittal graphic illustration of the lumbar spine shows normal marrow heterogeneity with foci of fatty marrow in the vertebral bodies. *(See Normal Bone Marrow pg. 1982, in Stoller's 3rd Edition.)*

Figure 13.4 ▪ Sagittal graphic illustration shows diffuse leukemic bone marrow infiltration of the lumbar spine (shown in brown). *(See Leukemia pg. 1985, in Stoller's 3rd Edition.)*

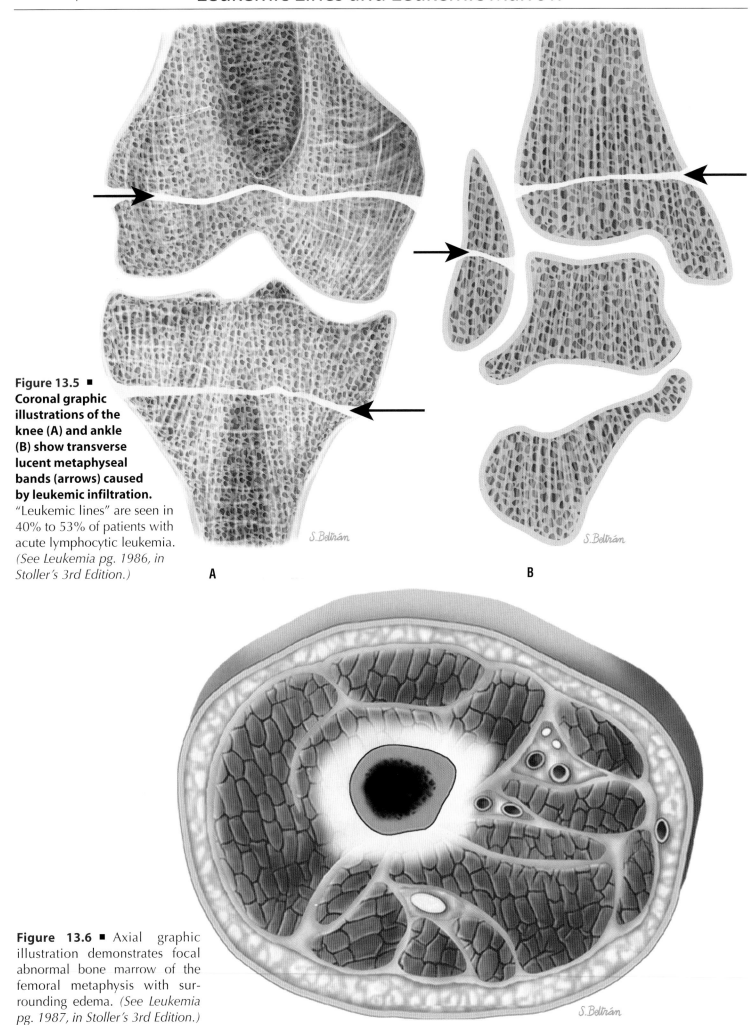

Figure 13.5 ▪ Coronal graphic illustrations of the knee (A) and ankle (B) show transverse lucent metaphyseal bands (arrows) caused by leukemic infiltration. "Leukemic lines" are seen in 40% to 53% of patients with acute lymphocytic leukemia. *(See Leukemia pg. 1986, in Stoller's 3rd Edition.)*

A

B

Figure 13.6 ▪ Axial graphic illustration demonstrates focal abnormal bone marrow of the femoral metaphysis with surrounding edema. *(See Leukemia pg. 1987, in Stoller's 3rd Edition.)*

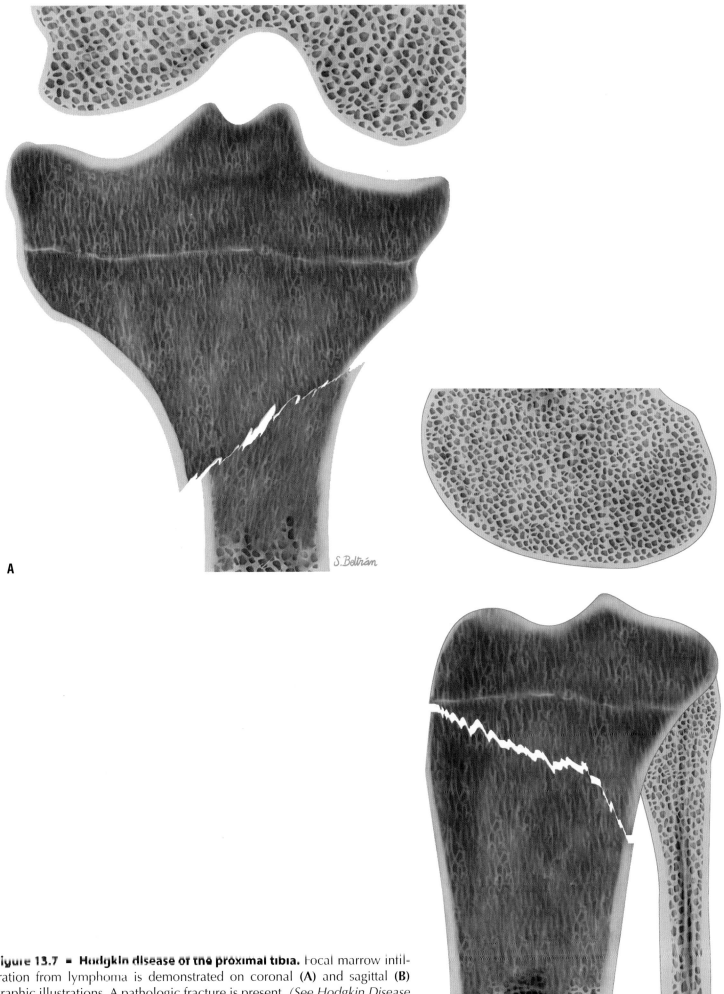

Figure 13.7 ▪ **Hodgkin disease of the proximal tibia.** Focal marrow infiltration from lymphoma is demonstrated on coronal (**A**) and sagittal (**B**) graphic illustrations. A pathologic fracture is present. *(See Hodgkin Disease pg. 1997, in Stoller's 3rd Edition.)*

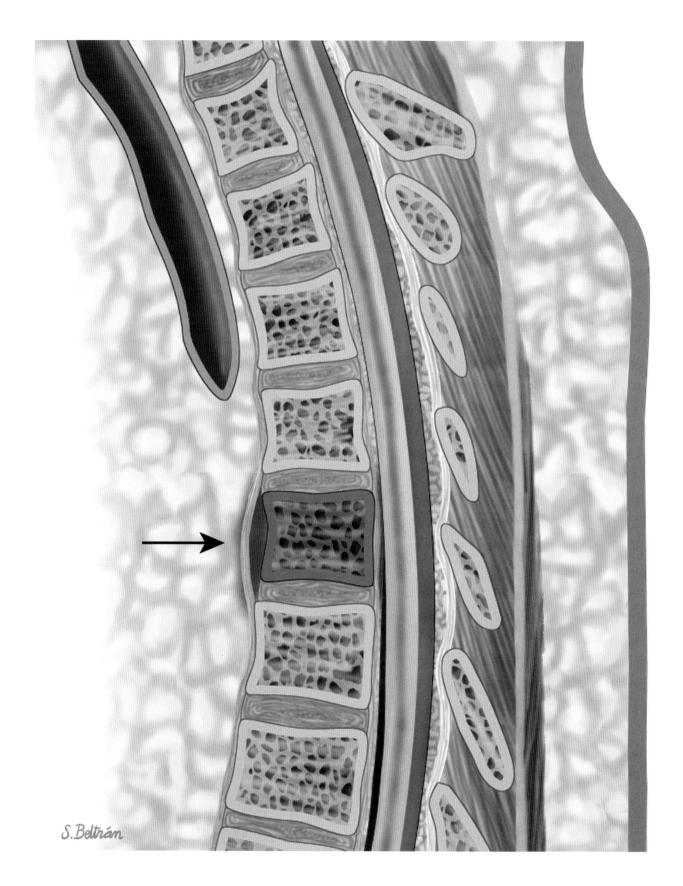

Figure 13.8 ▪ Spinal involvement in Hodgkin disease. Sagittal graphic illustration demonstrates sclerosis of a thoracic vertebral body ("ivory vertebral body") with associated soft-tissue component. *(See Hodgkin Disease pg. 1998, in Stoller's 3rd Edition.)*

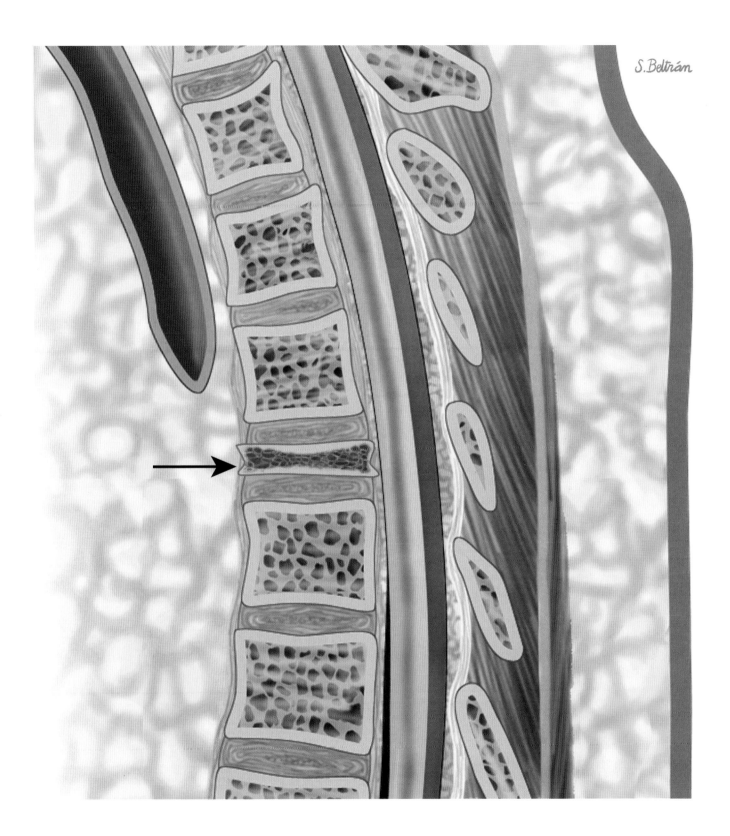

Figure 13.9 ■ Sagittal graphic illustration shows vertebra plana of the thoracic spine (arrow). *(See Langerhans Histiocytosis pg. 2005, in Stoller's 3rd Edition.)*

Multiple Myeloma

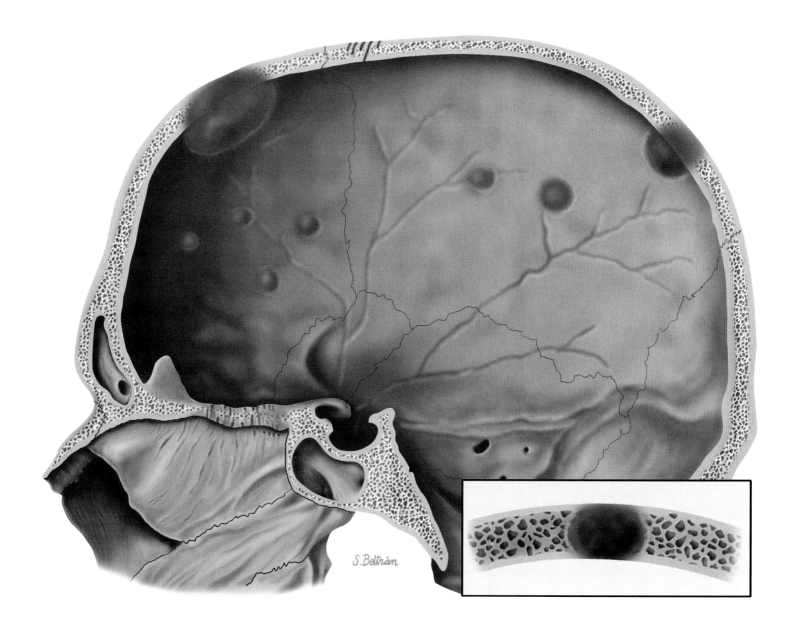

Figure 13.10 ■ Multiple punched-out lesions are seen as gray areas of the skull on this sagittal graphic illustration. *(See Multiple Myeloma pg. 2008, in Stoller's 3rd Edition.)*

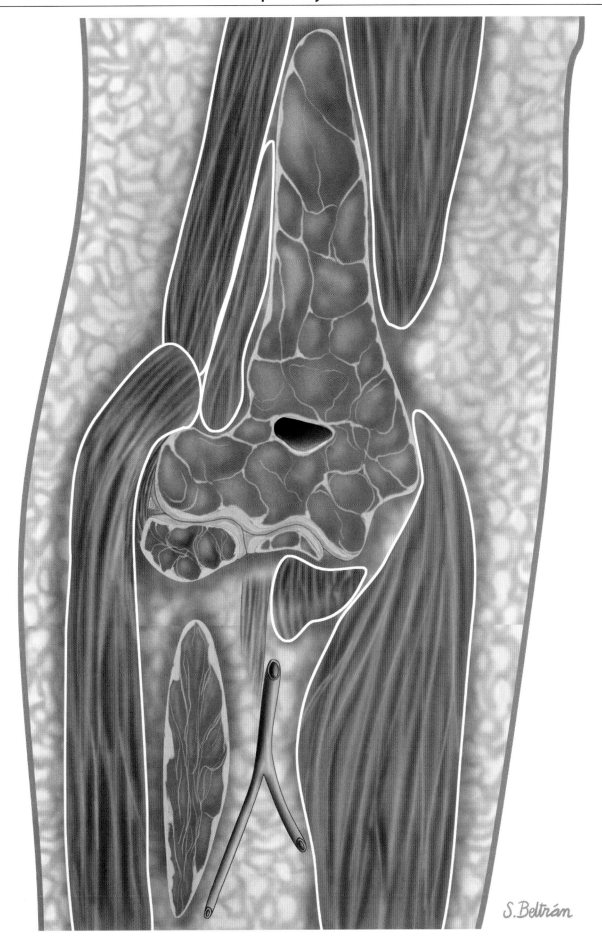

Figure 13.11 ■ A diffuse pattern of marrow replacement of the elbow is indicated in gray on this coronal graphic illustration. *(See Multiple Myeloma pg. 2010, in Stoller's 3rd Edition.)*

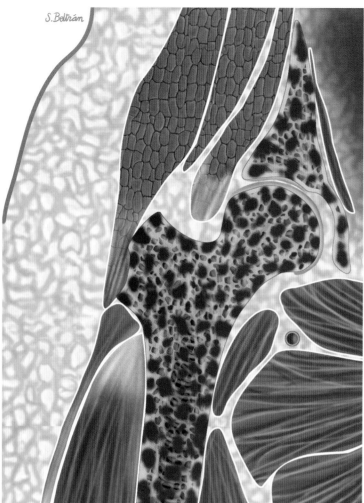

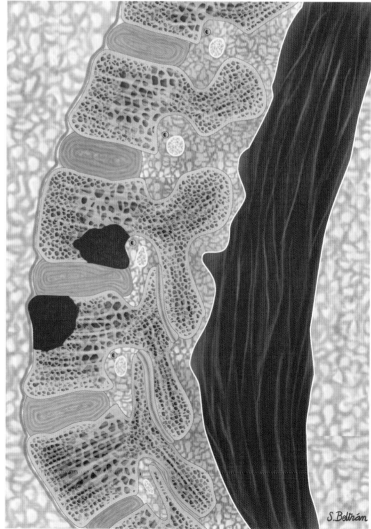

Figure 13.12 ▪ Coronal graphic illustration of the hip shows diffuse metastatic marrow replacement. The pelvic bones are a common site for metastatic disease because of their rich vascular supply. *(See Metastatic Disease of the Marrow pg. 2019, in Stoller's 3rd Edition.)*

Figure 13.13 ▪ Metastatic disease to the lumbar spine is shown in brown on a sagittal graphic illustration. The spine has a rich blood supply through the vertebral venous plexus and is therefore a common site for metastases. *(See Metastatic Disease of the Marrow pg. 2019, in Stoller's 3rd Edition.)*

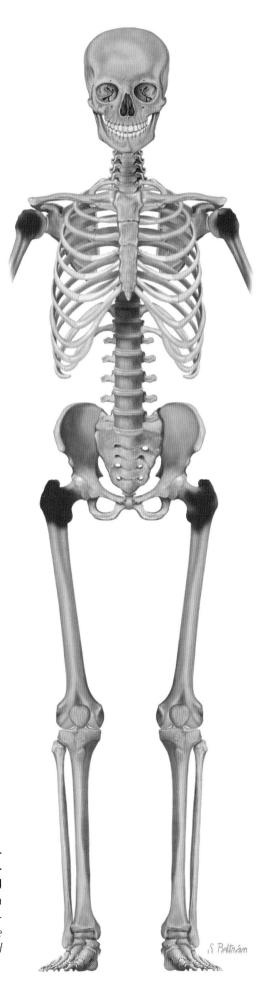

Figure 13.14 ■ **A coronal graphic illustration shows metastatic deposits involving the proximal femoral and humeral metaphyses in red.** These are common sites for metastatic disease in the appendicular skeleton. *(See Metastatic Disease of the Marrow pg. 2019, in Stoller's 3rd Edition.)*

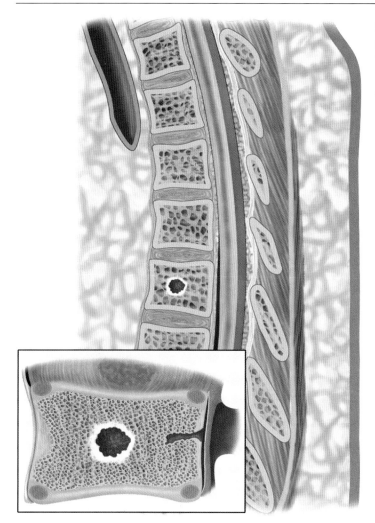

Figure 13.15 ■ **The halo sign is demonstrated on a sagittal graphic illustration.** A peripheral rim of T2 hyperintensity surrounding a lesion indicates active metastatic disease on MR images. *(See Metastatic Disease of the Marrow pg. 2024, in Stoller's 3rd Edition.)*

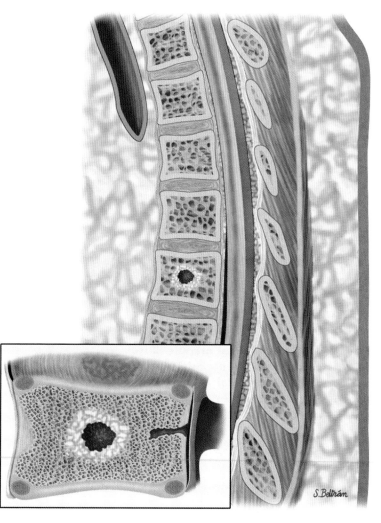

Figure 13.16 ■ **Sagittal graphic illustration showing a peripheral rim of yellow marrow surrounding a metastatic lesion.** High signal surrounding a metastatic lesion on T1-weighted images indicates response to therapy. *(See Metastatic Disease of the Marrow pg. 2024, in Stoller's 3rd Edition.)*

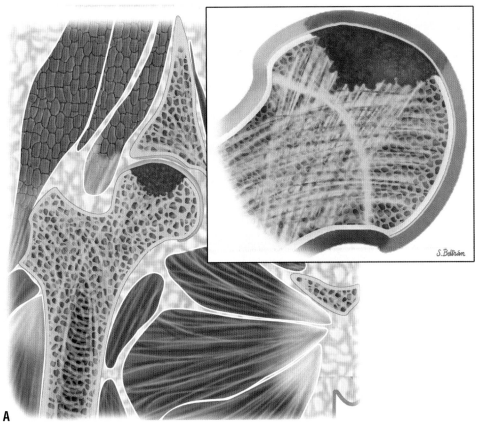

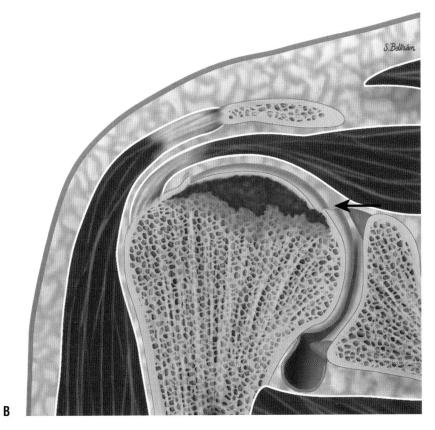

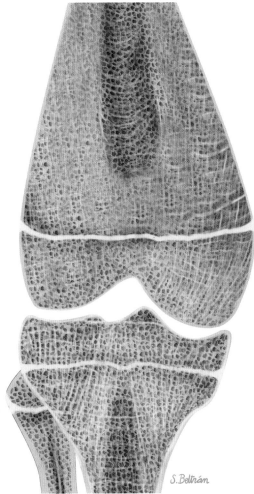

Figure 13.17 ■ **Avascular necrosis in Gaucher disease.** (A) Coronal graphic illustration of the hip shows a subchondral marrow abnormality (in brown) from osteonecrosis of the femoral head. (B) Coronal graphic illustration of the shoulder demonstrates osteonecrosis with a pathologic fracture (arrow) of the humeral head. *(See Gaucher Disease pg. 2025, in Stoller's 3rd Edition.)*

Figure 13.18 ■ Coronal graphic illustration shows characteristic Erlenmeyer flask deformity of the distal femur. *(See Gaucher Disease pg. 2027, in Stoller's 3rd Edition.)*

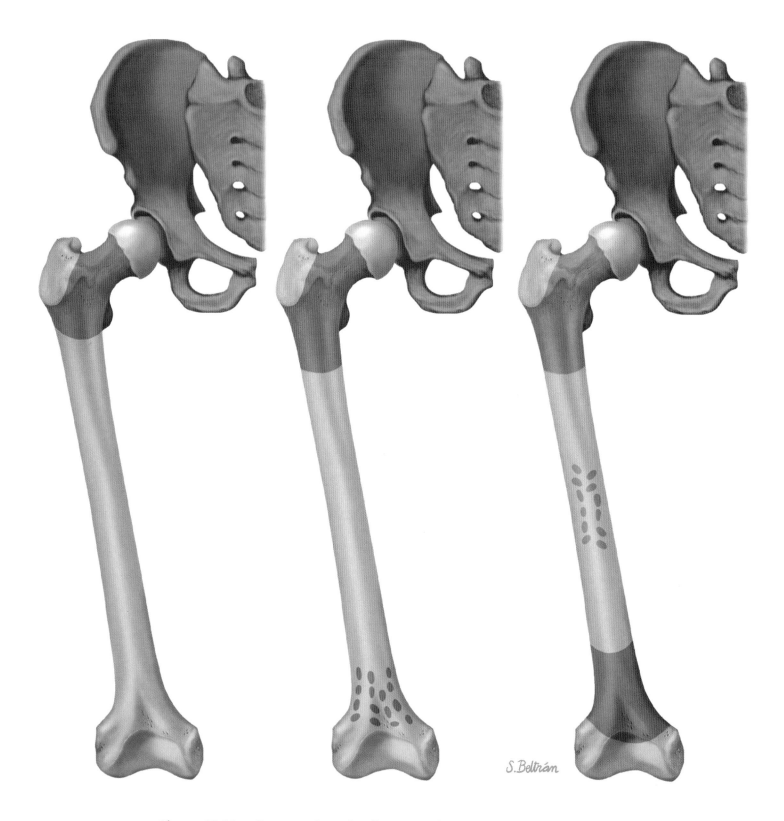

Figure 13.19 ■ Reconversion of yellow to red marrow caused by increased demand for hematopoiesis. Yellow to red reconversion occurs in the reverse order as does conversion from red to yellow marrow. *(See Bone Marrow Changes in Female Athletes and Smokers pg. 2030, in Stoller's 3rd Edition.)*

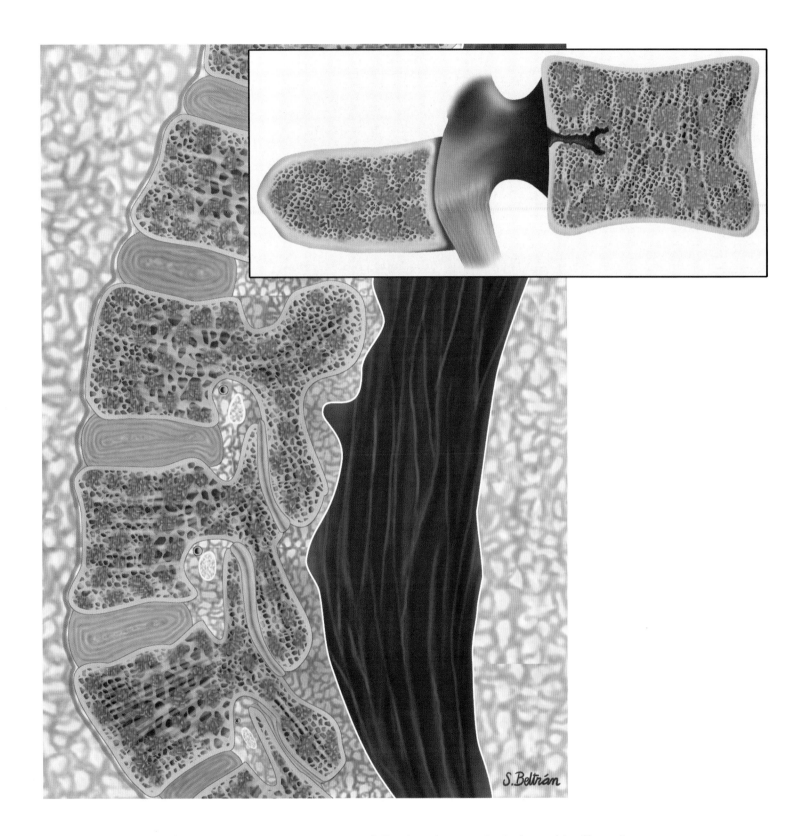

Figure 13.20 ■ **Aplastic anemia following therapy.** Sagittal graphic illustration shows heterogeneous marrow with islands of hematopoiesis (in red). *(See Aplastic Anemia pg. 2031, in Stoller's 3rd Edition.)*

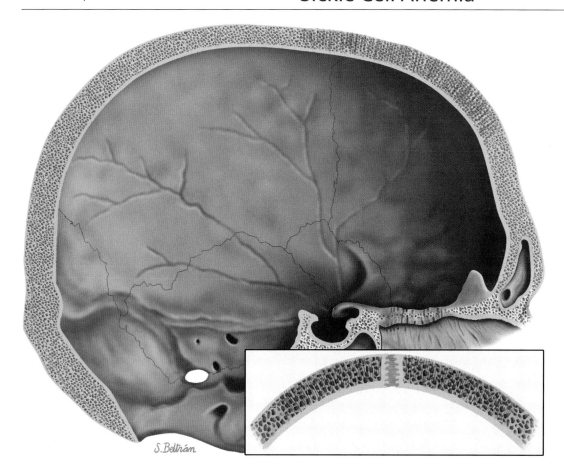

Figure 13.21 ■ Sagittal graphic illustration shows expansion of the marrow spaces of the skull in sickle cell anemia. *(See Sickle Cell Anemia pg. 2032, in Stoller's 3rd Edition.)*

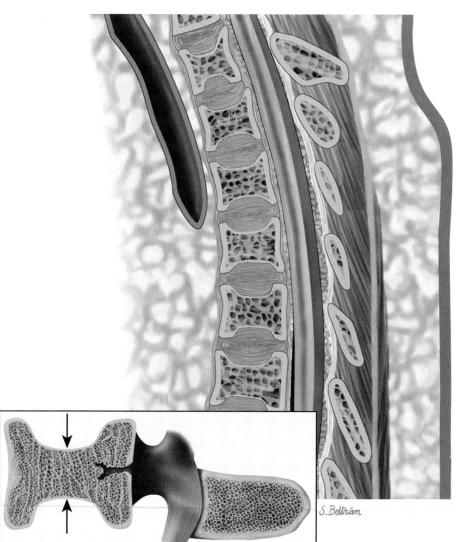

Figure 13.22 ■ **H vertebrae in sickle cell anemia.** Bone marrow ischemia of the central vertebral body leads to central squared-off endplate depressions (arrows). *(See Sickle Cell Anemia pg. 2033, in Stoller's 3rd Edition.)*

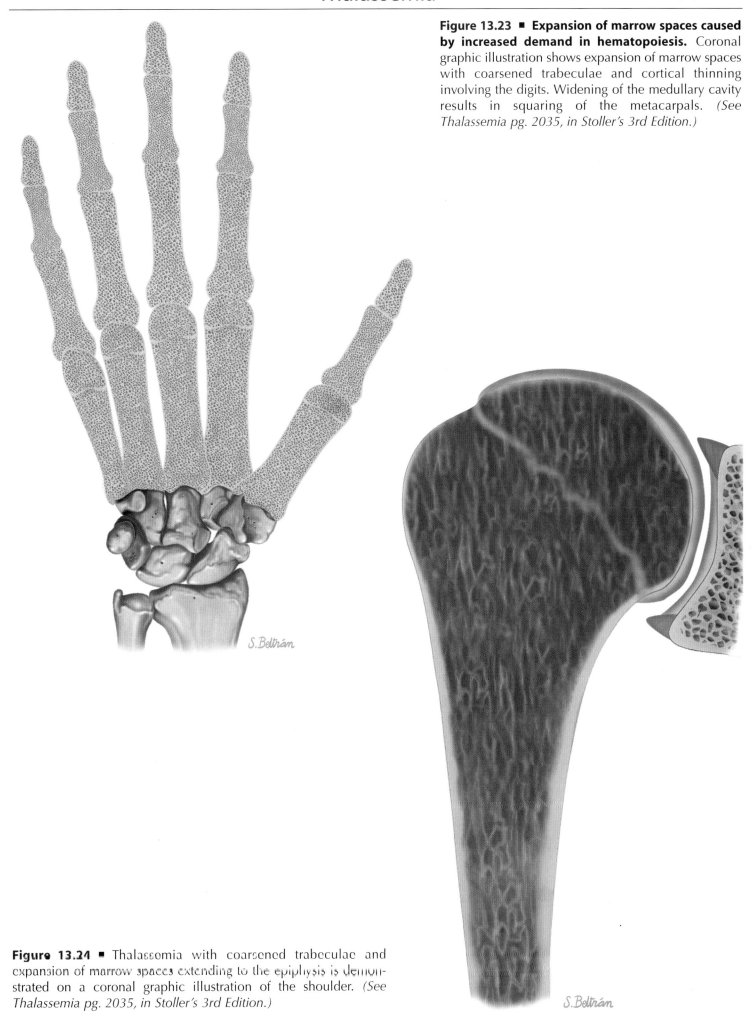

Figure 13.24 ■ Thalassemia with coarsened trabeculae and expansion of marrow spaces extending to the epiphysis is demonstrated on a coronal graphic illustration of the shoulder. *(See Thalassemia pg. 2035, in Stoller's 3rd Edition.)*

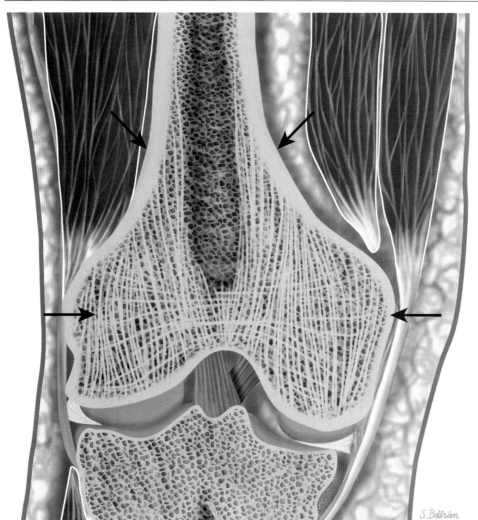

Figure 13.25 ■ Paget's disease of the femur. Coronal graphic illustration shows enlargement of the distal femur with cortical thickening and coarsened trabeculae (arrows). *(See Paget's Disease pg. 2036, in Stoller's 3rd Edition.)*

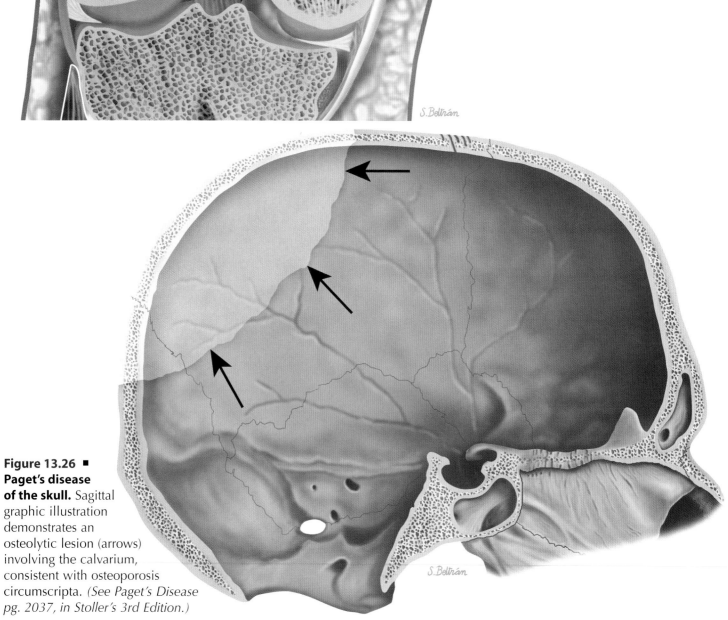

Figure 13.26 ■ Paget's disease of the skull. Sagittal graphic illustration demonstrates an osteolytic lesion (arrows) involving the calvarium, consistent with osteoporosis circumscripta. *(See Paget's Disease pg. 2037, in Stoller's 3rd Edition.)*

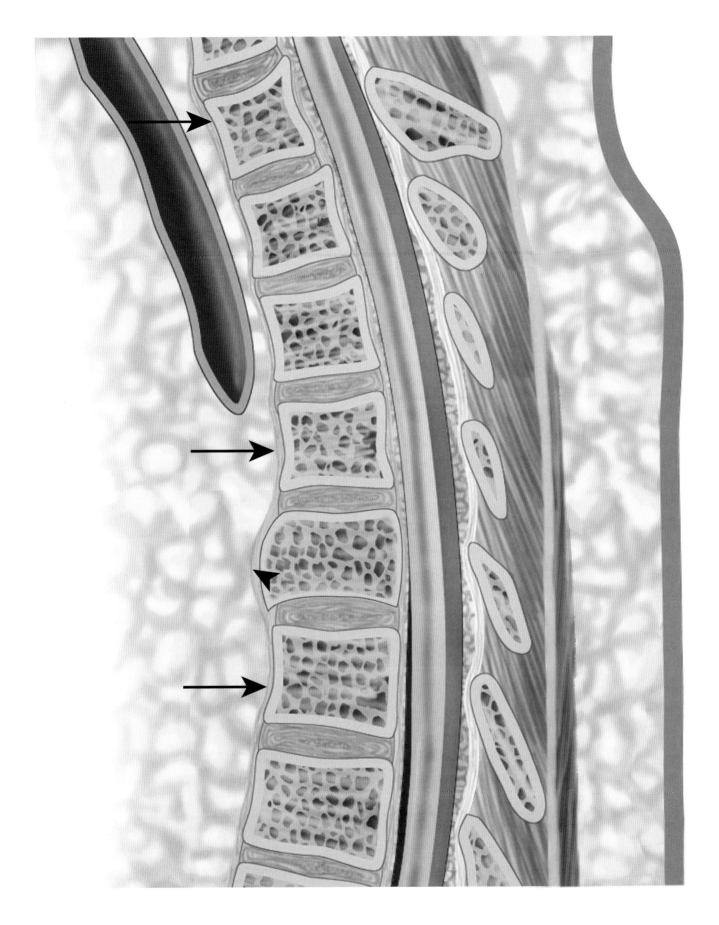

Figure 13.27 ▪ Paget's disease of the spine. Sagittal graphic illustration shows coarse trabecular pattern (arrows) and expansion of a thoracic vertebral body (arrowhead). (See *Paget's Disease* pg. 2037, in *Stoller's 3rd Edition*.)

14

Bone and Soft-Tissue Tumors

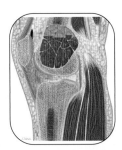

Pearls and Pitfalls & Color Illustrations

Pearls and Pitfalls

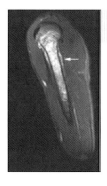

IMAGING TECHNIQUES

- Radiographs are essential for evaluating bone tumors and some soft-tissue tumors.
- MR imaging features are usually nonspecific in differentiating benign from malignant processes.
- MR imaging is important in the evaluation of tumor extent, staging, and response to therapy.

- Gadolinium administration is useful in the evaluation of nonenhancing necrotic or hemorrhagic tumor components.

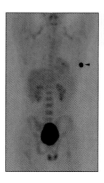

STAGING

- MR imaging is the method of choice in staging musculoskeletal neoplasms.
- MR images should be read in conjunction with radiographs.
- MR imaging is accurate in determining the local extent of tumor and involvement of muscle compartments, joints, and neurovascular bundles.

- Evaluation of intra- and extraosseous extent, joint invasion, neurovascular bundle involvement, skip metastases, and local adenopathy, as well as distant metastases, is important for accurate staging and subsequent therapy.
- Consider FDG-PET for staging and evaluation of therapy response in equivocal cases.

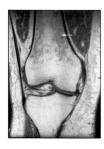

GENERAL MR APPEARANCE

- MR imaging features are usually nonspecific in differentiating benign from malignant processes.
- Benign and malignant tumors usually demonstrate low signal on T1- and high signal on T2-weighted images.

- Infiltration of neurovascular bundles is seen more commonly in malignant tumors.
- Both benign and malignant tumors can present with fluid–fluid levels.

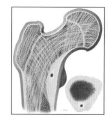

BENIGN OSTEOBLASTIC LESIONS
(see Figures 14.1–14.4)

- Osteoid osteomas may present with extensive marrow edema on MR imaging, obscuring the nidus, and may therefore be mistaken for osteomyelitis or malignant tumor.

- CT is most sensitive in detecting the nidus in osteoid osteomas.
- Consider image-guided therapy for the treatment of osteoid osteomas.
- Osteoblastomas frequently involve the posterior elements of the spine.
- Osteoblastomas can present with fluid–fluid levels.

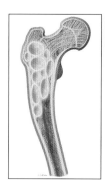

BENIGN CHONDROBLASTIC LESIONS
(see Figures 14.5–14.10)

- On T2-weighted and STIR images, chondroid matrix is markedly hyperintense.
- Enchondromas can be confused with bone infarcts. Infarcts show central fat signal and serpiginous borders.
- Syndromes associated with multiple enchondromas have an increased risk of malignant transformation.

- Osteochondromas show continuity with the marrow cavity of host bone.
- Osteochondromas have their own growth plate and stop growing with skeletal maturity.
- MR imaging is useful in determining the thickness of the cartilage cap.
- Chondroblastomas involve the epiphyses/epiphysis equivalents.

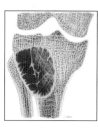

BENIGN FIBROUS AND RELATED LESIONS
(see Figures 14.11–14.15)

- Fibrous lesions demonstrate low signal intensity on T1-, and intermediate to high signal intensity on T2-weighted images.
- Central fat signal can be seen during involution of lesions.

- Periosteal desmoids likely occur from traction on inserting muscle groups and should not be biopsied.

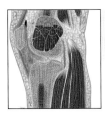

BENIGN TUMORS AND NON-NEOPLASTIC LESIONS
(see Figures 14.16–14.20)

- Unicameral bone cysts demonstrate fluid signal on MR imaging without evidence of enhancement.

- Unicameral and aneurysmal bone cysts can be treated with CT-guided percutaneous injections.

- Fluid–fluid levels are characteristic of aneurysmal bone cysts.

- Secondary aneurysmal bone cysts can be seen in a variety of benign and malignant tumors.

- Intraosseous hemangiomas are characterized by fat signal intensity.

- Intraosseous lipomas follow the signal intensity of fat on all pulse sequences.

- Langerhans cell histiocytosis is a "great imitator" of various benign and malignant lesions.

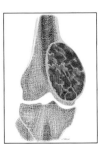

GIANT CELL TUMOR
(see Figures 14.21–14.22)

- Giant cell tumors originate in the metaphysis and extend into the epiphysis to subchondral bone.

- Typically, giant cell tumors occur in skeletally mature patients.

- Giant cell tumors can be aggressive and recur locally.

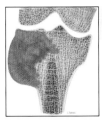

MALIGNANT LESIONS
(see Figures 14.23–14.30)

- MR imaging is nonspecific in differentiating benign from malignant processes.

- Most benign and malignant tumors show increased T1 and T2 signal.

- Cortical destruction, soft-tissue masses, and involvement of neurovascular bundles are more common in malignant tumors.

- MR imaging findings suggestive of tumor recurrence include new edema, convex margins of the treatment site, and nodular enhancement.

- With MR imaging, intramedullary marrow involvement, soft-tissue extension, areas of necrosis, skip-lesions, metastases, and postoperative recurrence can be accurately assessed.

- Osteosarcoma can arise de novo (primary osteosarcoma), or in association with preexisting lesions of bone such as Paget's disease, prior radiation, or bone infarcts.

- Telangiectatic osteosarcoma can simulate an aneurysmal bone cyst.

- Frank cortical disruption, soft-tissue extension, and periosteal reaction in a preexisting enchondroma or osteochondroma are suspicious for malignant transformation to chondrosarcoma.

- Ewing sarcoma predominately involves the flat bones and diaphyses of long bones.

- The tibia is involved in 90% of cases of adamantinoma.

- MR imaging should be performed if there is suspicion of metastatic disease and radiographs are normal.

- Distinguishing primary lymphoma of bone from secondary involvement is important because the latter has a worse prognosis and is treated differently.

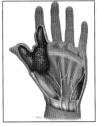

BENIGN SOFT-TISSUE NEOPLASMS
(see Figures 14.31–14.37)

- Benign soft-tissue tumors are usually homogeneous and well marginated.

- Lipomas follow the signal intensity of fat on all pulse sequences. Low-signal-intensity septations may be present.

- Hemangiomas are ill defined, with areas of high T1 signal caused by fat or slow-flowing blood.

- If MR imaging is nondiagnostic for hemangioma, it is important to obtain radiographs because phleboliths can be missed on MR examinations.

- Fibromatosis represents a group of benign disorders characterized by fibrous growth and a tendency to infiltrate adjacent tissues and recur. They may appear very aggressive and may be mistaken for sarcoma.

- Juvenile fibromatosis demonstrates low signal on T1- and T2-weighted images.

- Benign peripheral nerve sheath tumors are best seen on long axis (coronal or sagittal) imaging planes and appear as fusiform masses entering and exiting a nerve.

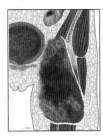

MALIGNANT SOFT-TISSUE NEOPLASMS
(see Figures 14.38–14.45)

- Liposarcomas often do not contain visible fat on MR images.

- Myxoid liposarcomas may appear as cystic lesions on T2-weighted images, so gadolinium contrast is necessary to diagnose solid lesions.

- Consider malignant transformation when a preexisting neurofibroma enlarges.

- FDG-PET is useful in detecting malignant change in plexiform neurofibromas.

- Synovial sarcomas do not arise from synovium or joints.

- Synovial sarcomas can be misdiagnosed as benign lesions, such as ganglions, if no intravenous contrast is administered.

- Malignant fibrous histiocytoma often presents as a hemorrhagic mass, and extensive areas of hemorrhage can obscure the underlying neoplasm. Therefore, intravenous contrast is required for evaluation of suspected hematomas.

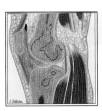

TUMOR-LIKE LESIONS
(see Figures 14.46–14.48)

- Myositis ossificans may be mistaken for soft-tissue tumor on MR imaging.

- CT scans or radiographs are often more helpful in showing peripheral calcifications and diagnosing myositis ossificans.

- Central fatty marrow signal is characteristic for bone infarcts.

- Subacute hemorrhage is hyperintense on T1-weighted images.

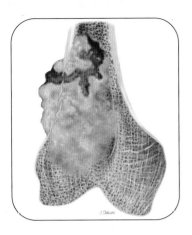

Bone and Soft-Tissue Tumors

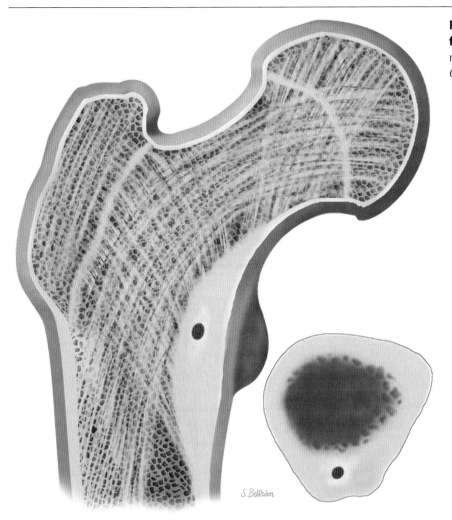

Figure 14.1 ▪ Osteoid osteoma of the proximal femur. Coronal graphic illustration shows tumor nidus in red with surrounding sclerosis. *(See Osteoid Osteoma pg. 2051, in Stoller's 3rd Edition.)*

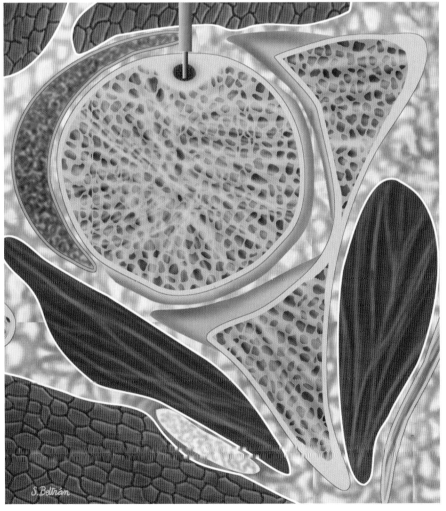

Figure 14.2 ▪ Axial graphic illustration shows radiofrequency ablation of an osteoid osteoma. Nidus is shown in red with surrounding cortical thickening. The radiofrequency probe is positioned within the nidus. *(See Osteoid Osteoma pg. 2054, in Stoller's 3rd Edition.)*

Osteoblastoma

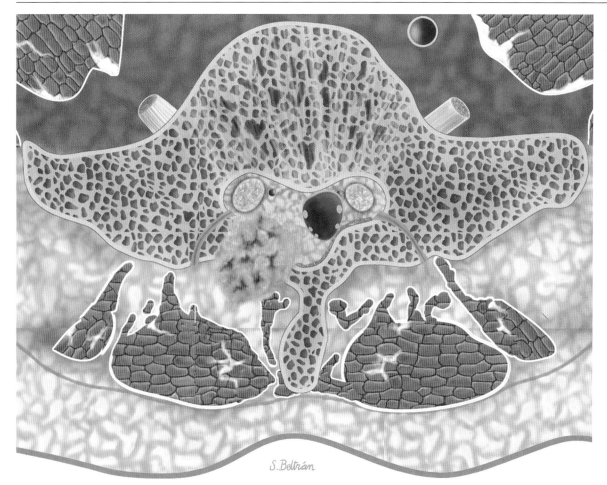

S.Beltrán

Figure 14.3 ▪ Osteoblastoma of the spine. Axial graphic illustration shows expansile tumor in red arising from the posterior elements. *(See Osteoblastoma pg. 2055, in Stoller's 3rd Edition.)*

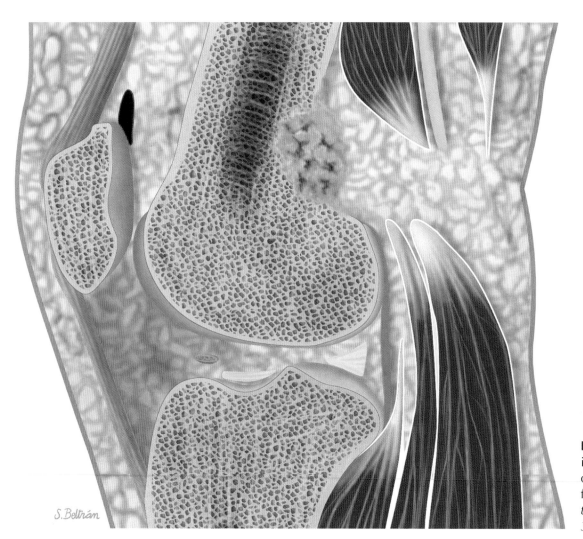

S.Beltrán

Figure 14.4 ▪ Sagittal graphic illustration shows cortical osteoblastoma of the distal femur in red. *(See Osteoblastoma pg. 2055, in Stoller's 3rd Edition.)*

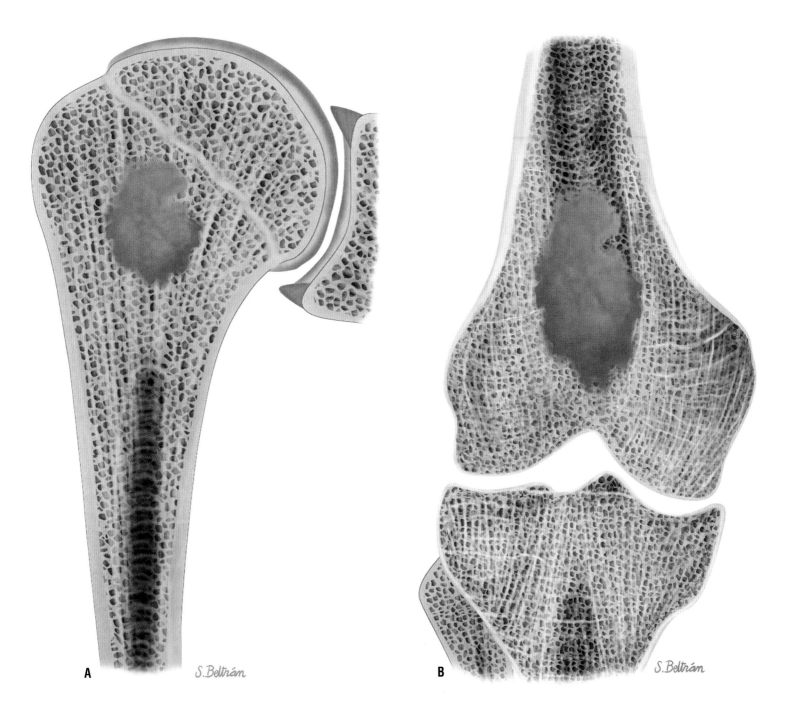

Figure 14.5 ■ Coronal graphic illustration of the humerus **(A)** and femur **(B)** shows a well-defined lobulated metaphyseal enchondroma in purple. *(See Enchondroma pg. 2058, in Stoller's 3rd Edition.)*

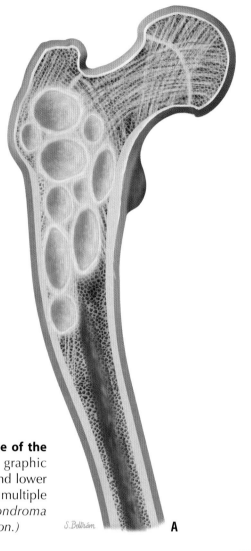

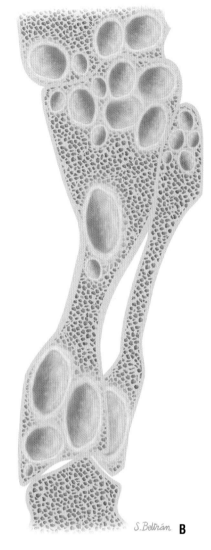

Figure 14.6 ■ Ollier's disease of the lower extremity. Coronal graphic illustration of the femur **(A)** and lower leg **(B)** shows deformity with multiple enchondromas. *(See Enchondroma pg. 2059, in Stoller's 3rd Edition.)*

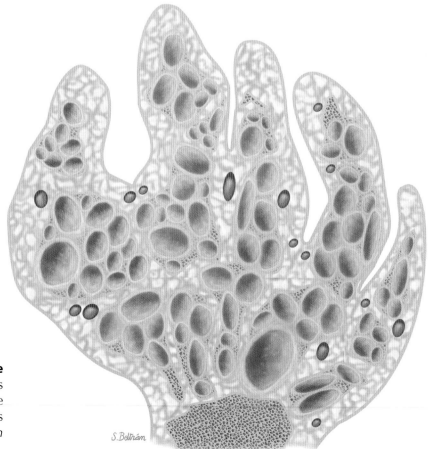

Figure 14.7 ■ Maffucci's syndrome of the hand. Coronal graphic illustration shows marked deformity of the hand with multiple enchondromas in purple and hemangiomas in red. *(See Enchondroma pg. 2059, in Stoller's 3rd Edition.)*

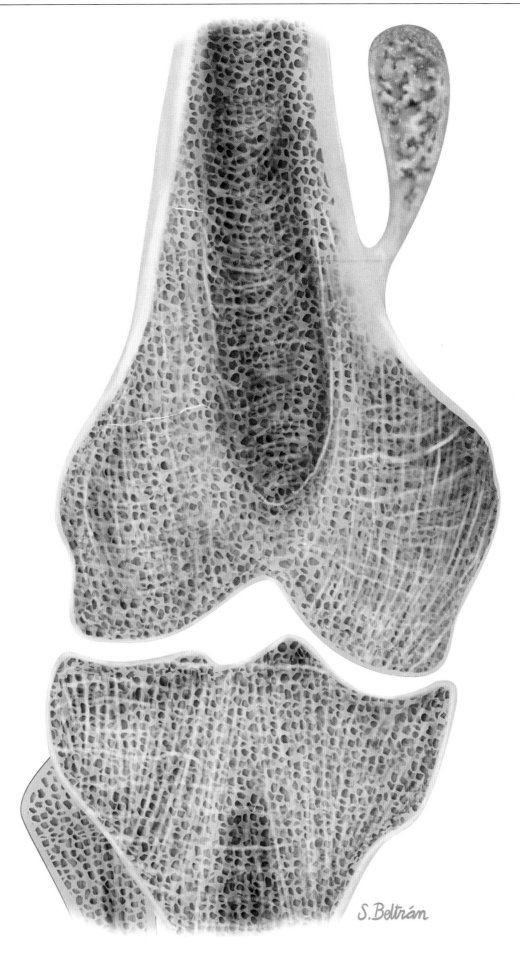

Figure 14.0 ■ **Coronal graphic illustration demonstrates an osteochondroma arising from the distal femur.** Note the continuity of the lesion with the marrow cavity of the host bone. Calcifications within the osteochondroma are shown in red, and the cartilage cap is shown in blue. *(See Osteochondroma pg. 2065, in Stoller's 3rd Edition.)*

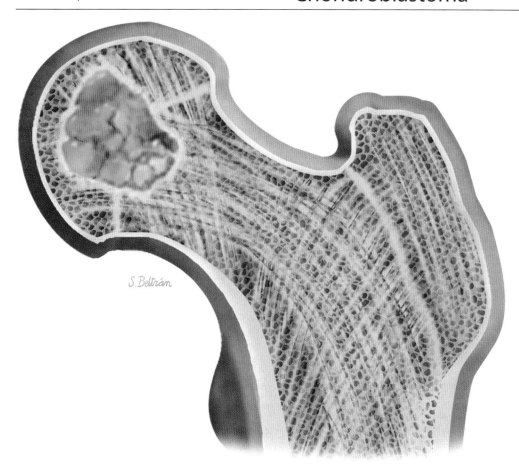

Figure 14.9 ▪ Chondroblastoma of the proximal femur. A well-defined lobulated lesion involving the femoral epiphysis is shown in red. *(See Chondroblastoma pg. 2070, in Stoller's 3rd Edition.)*

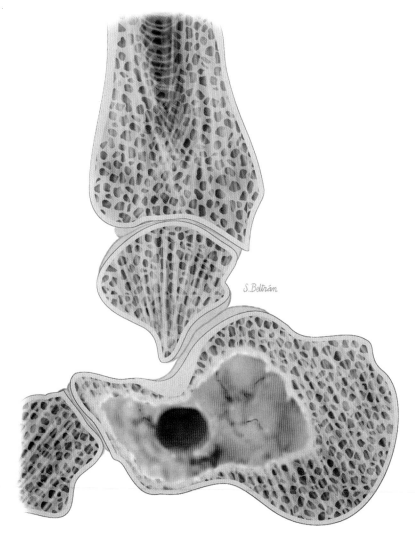

Figure 14.10 ▪ A chondroblastoma of the calcaneus is shown in red on a sagittal graphic illustration. Areas of calcification are shown in white, and a hemorrhagic cyst is shown in red. *(See Chondroblastoma pg. 2070, in Stoller's 3rd Edition.)*

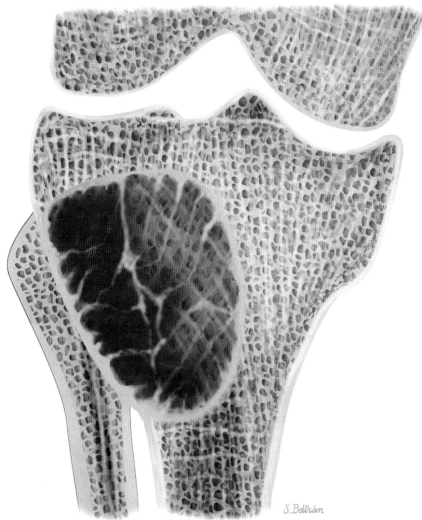

Figure 14.11 ■ **Coronal graphic illustration demonstrates a well-defined nonossifying fibroma of the proximal tibia in reddish-brown.** Note the sclerotic scalloped borders. *(See Nonossifying Fibroma pg. 2074, in Stoller's 3rd Edition.)*

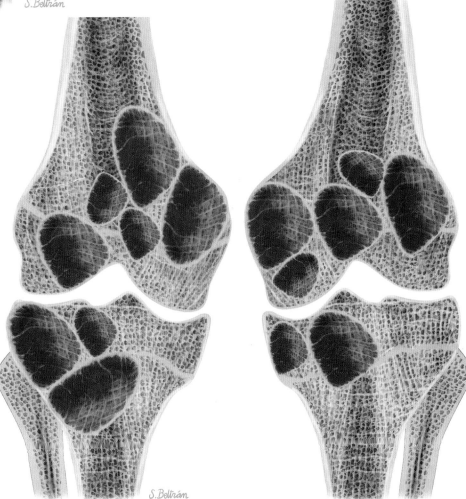

Figure 14.12 ■ **Coronal graphic illustration of the knees shows multiple bilateral nonossifying fibromas in a patient with Jaffe-Campanacci syndrome.** Patients with this syndrome also have extraskeletal abnormalities, such as café-au-lait spots, mental retardation, and hypogonadism. *(See Nonossifying Fibroma pg. 2076, in Stoller's 3rd Edition.)*

Figure 14.13 ▪ Fibrous dysplasia of the facial bones. Coronal graphic illustration shows an expansile, well-defined lesion involving the angle of the mandible. *(See Fibrous and Osteofibrous Dysplasia pg. 2079, in Stoller's 3rd Edition.)*

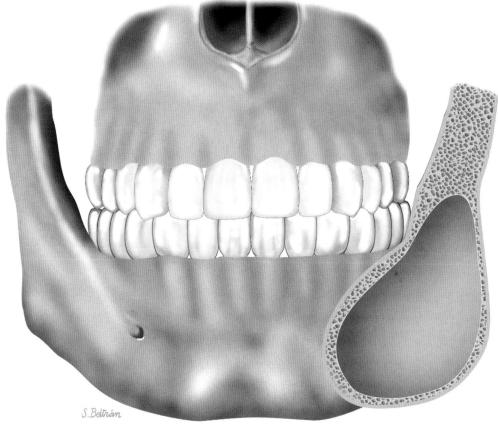

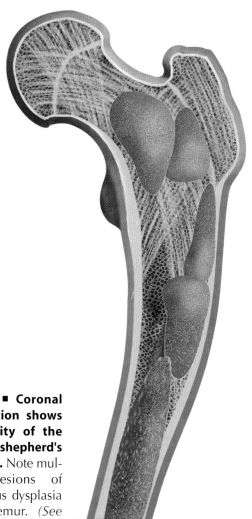

Figure 14.14 ▪ Coronal graphic illustration shows bowing deformity of the proximal femur (shepherd's crook deformity). Note multiple lucent lesions of polyostotic fibrous dysplasia involving the femur. *(See Fibrous and Osteofibrous Dysplasia pg. 2079, in Stoller's 3rd Edition.)*

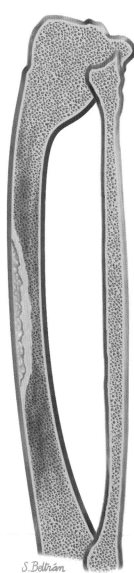

Figure 14.15 ▪ Osteofibrous dysplasia of the tibia is shown in blue on a sagittal graphic illustration. Surrounding sclerosis is shown in light brown. Note the anterior bowing of the tibia, often seen in osteofibrous dysplasia. *(See Fibrous and Osteofibrous Dysplasia pg. 2079, in Stoller's 3rd Edition.)*

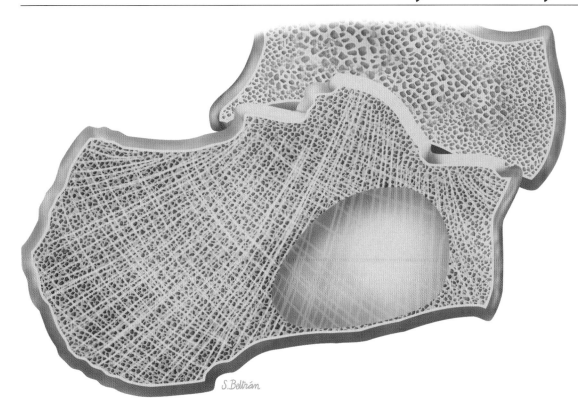

Figure 14.16 ▪ Unicameral bone cyst of the calcaneus. Sagittal graphic illustration demonstrates a well-defined lytic lesion with intact adjacent cortex. *(See Unicameral Bone Cyst pg. 2081, in Stoller's 3rd Edition.)*

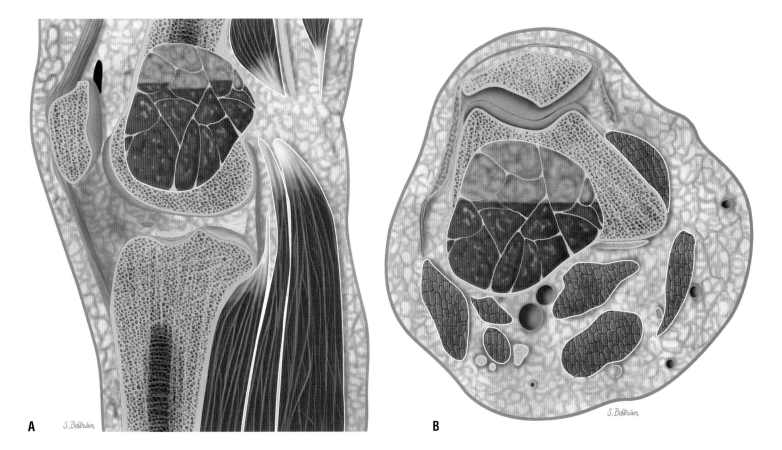

A

B

Figure 14.17 ▪ Aneurysmal bone cyst of the distal femur. (A) Sagittal and (B) axial graphic illustrations show an expansile blood-filled lesion with fluid-fluid levels in red. *(See Aneurysmal Bone Cyst pg. 2083, in Stoller's 3rd Edition.)*

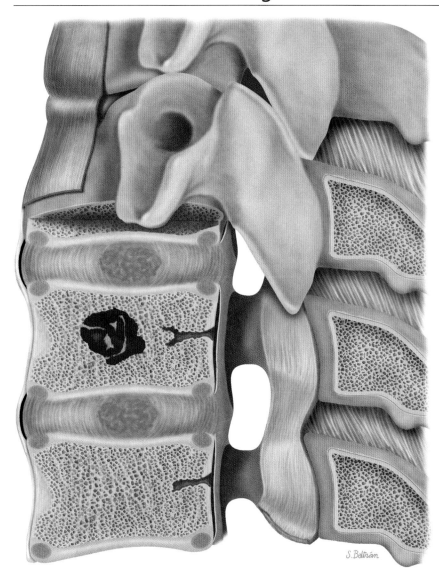

Figure 14.18 ▪ Hemangioma of the spine is shown in red on a sagittal graphic illustration. *(See Hemangioma pg. 2085, in Stoller's 3rd Edition.)*

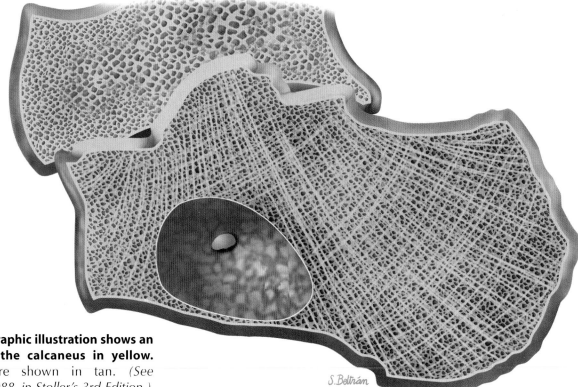

Figure 14.19 ▪ **Sagittal graphic illustration shows an intraosseous lipoma of the calcaneus in yellow.** Central calcifications are shown in tan. *(See Intraosseous Lipoma pg. 2088, in Stoller's 3rd Edition.)*

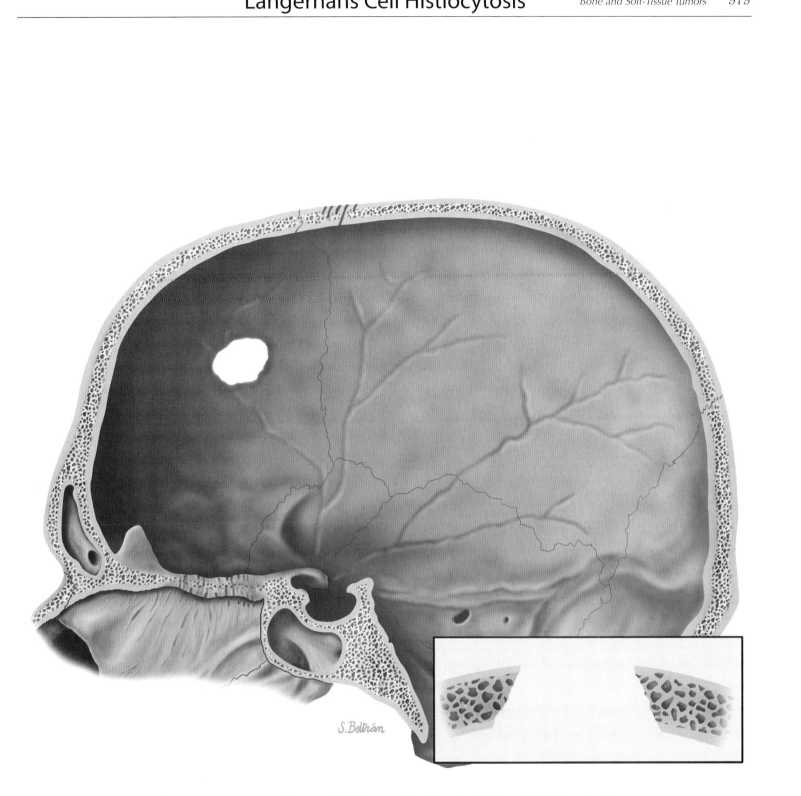

Figure 14.20 ■ **Langerhans cell histiocytosis of the skull.** Osteolytic lesion in the frontal bone with sharp margins, giving it a punched-out appearance. Uneven involvement of the inner and outer tables results in beveled appearance. *(See Langerhans Cell Histiocytosis pg. 2089, in Stoller's 3rd Edition.)*

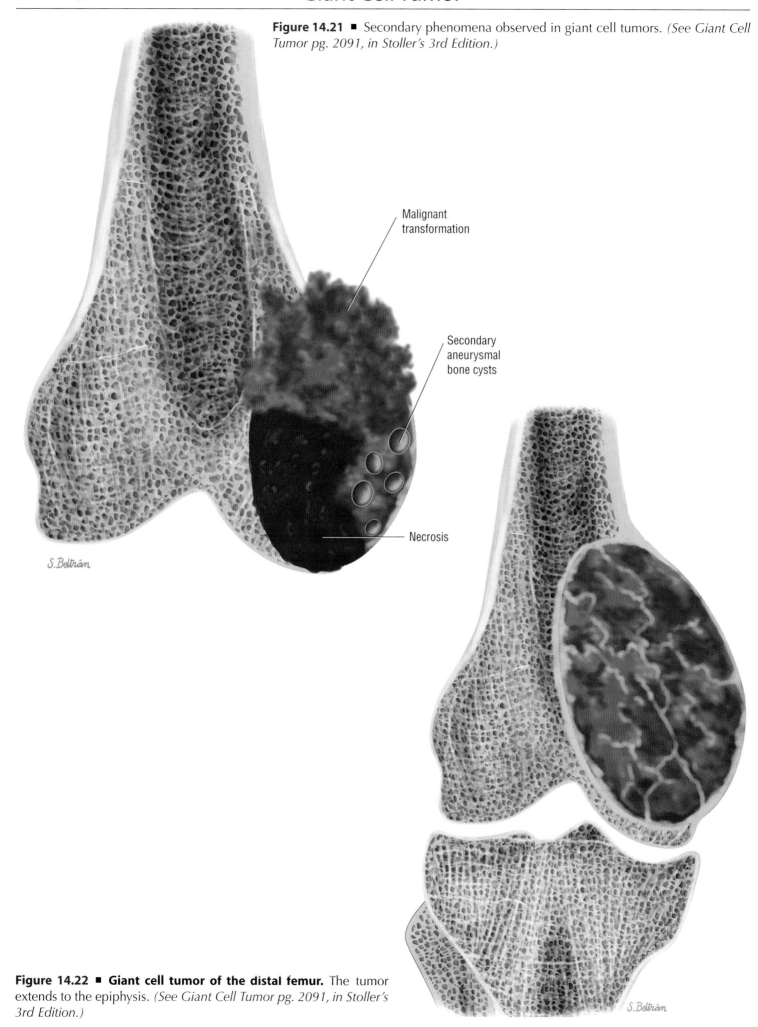

Figure 14.21 ■ Secondary phenomena observed in giant cell tumors. *(See Giant Cell Tumor pg. 2091, in Stoller's 3rd Edition.)*

Malignant transformation

Secondary aneurysmal bone cysts

Necrosis

S.Beltrán

Figure 14.22 ■ **Giant cell tumor of the distal femur.** The tumor extends to the epiphysis. *(See Giant Cell Tumor pg. 2091, in Stoller's 3rd Edition.)*

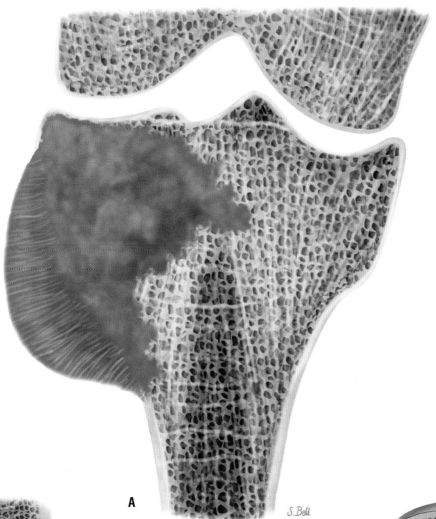

Figure 14.23 ■ Primary osteosarcoma of bone. Coronal graphic illustrations of the knee and shoulder show osteosarcoma with sclerotic and lytic areas and aggressive periosteal reaction involving the proximal tibia **(A)**, distal femur **(B)**, and proximal humerus **(C)**. (*See Primary Osteosarcoma pg. 2096, in Stoller's 3rd Edition.*)

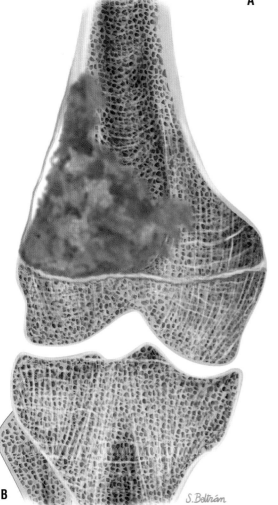

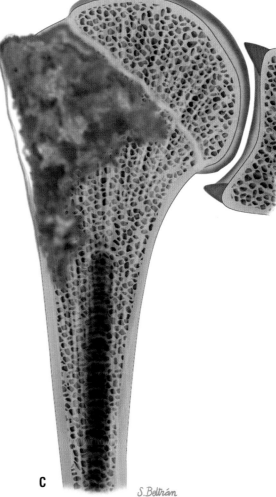

Telangiectatic Osteosarcoma

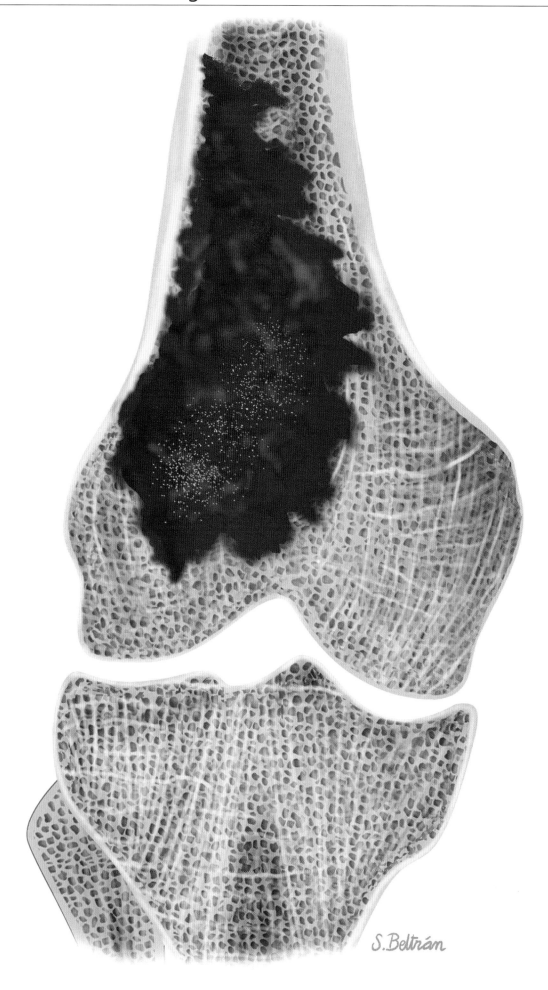

Figure 14.24 ■ **Coronal graphic illustration shows telangiectatic osteosarcoma of the distal femur.** Hemorrhagic areas are shown in red. *(See Osteosarcoma pg. 2096, in Stoller's 3rd Edition.)*

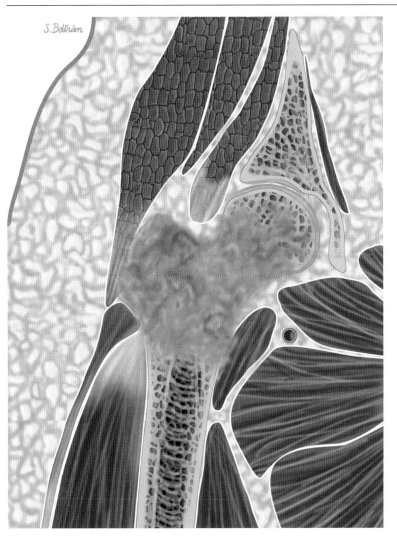

A

B

Figure 14.25 ■ Chondrosarcoma of the proximal femur (A) and calcaneus (B). Chondroid tissue is shown in blue. Note cortical destruction and soft-tissue extension. *(See Chondrosarcoma pg. 2105, in Stoller's 3rd Edition.)*

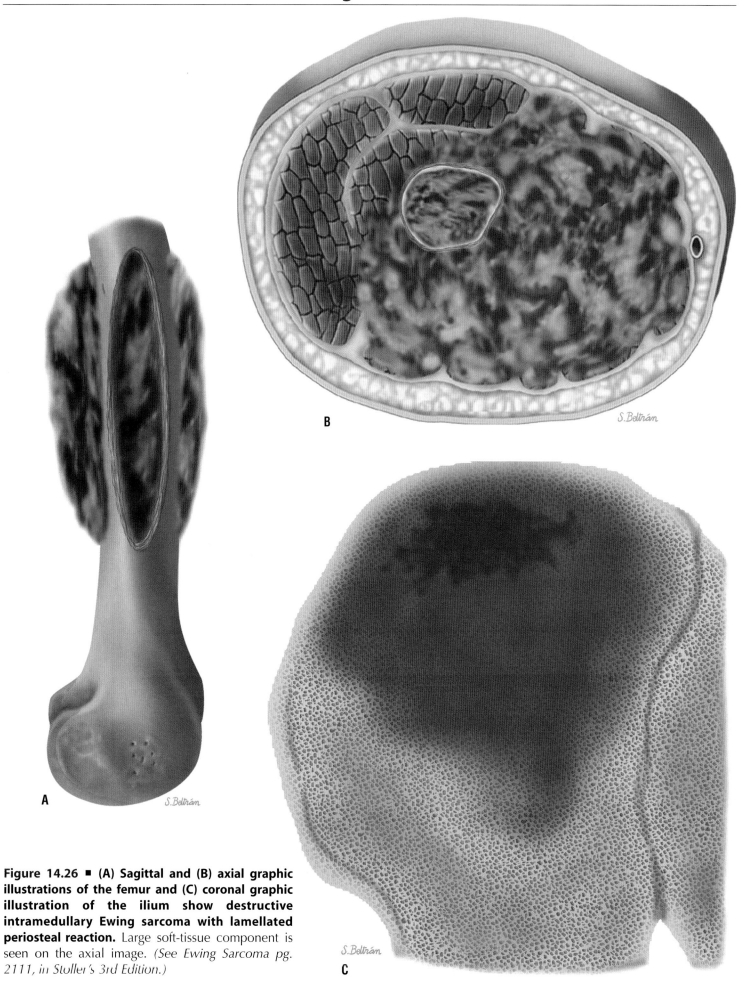

Figure 14.26 ▪ (A) Sagittal and (B) axial graphic illustrations of the femur and (C) coronal graphic illustration of the ilium show destructive intramedullary Ewing sarcoma with lamellated periosteal reaction. Large soft-tissue component is seen on the axial image. *(See Ewing Sarcoma pg. 2111, in Stoller's 3rd Edition.)*

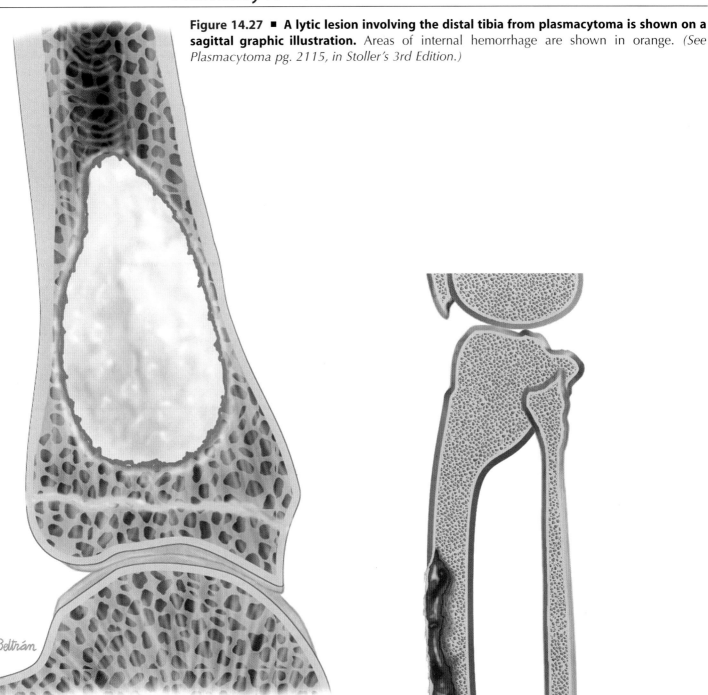

Figure 14.27 ■ **A lytic lesion involving the distal tibia from plasmacytoma is shown on a sagittal graphic illustration.** Areas of internal hemorrhage are shown in orange. *(See Plasmacytoma pg. 2115, in Stoller's 3rd Edition.)*

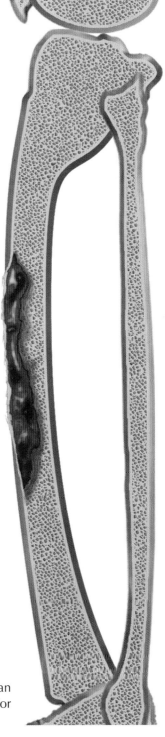

Figure 14.28 ■ **Adamantinoma of the tibia.** Sagittal graphic illustration shows an adamantinoma involving the anterolateral cortex of tibia with associated anterior bowing. *(See Adamantinoma pg. 2116, in Stoller's 3rd Edition.)*

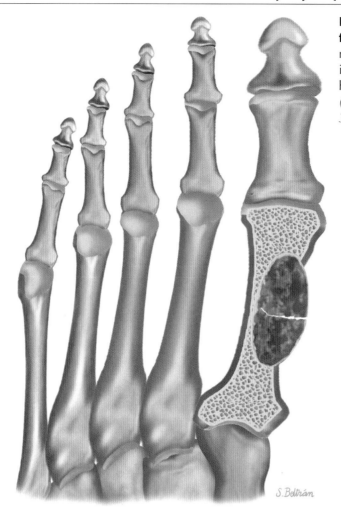

Figure 14.29 ▪ Metastatic lung cancer to the foot. Coronal graphic illustration shows a metastatic lesion with a pathologic fracture involving the metatarsal. Metastases to the hands and feet are usually from lung cancer. *(See Metastatic Disease pg. 2118, in Stoller's 3rd Edition.)*

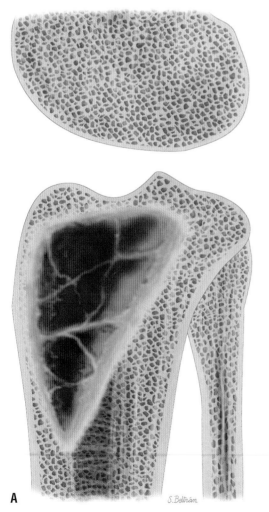

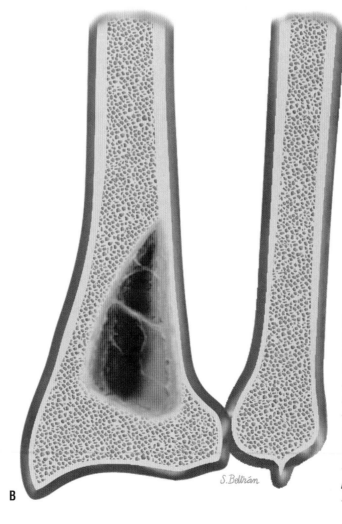

Figure 14.30 ▪ Primary lymphoma of bone is shown as a hemorrhagic intramedullary mass in red on coronal graphic illustrations of the knee **(A)** and distal forearm **(B)**. *(See Primary Lymphoma of Bone pg. 2121, in Stoller's 3rd Edition.)*

A

B

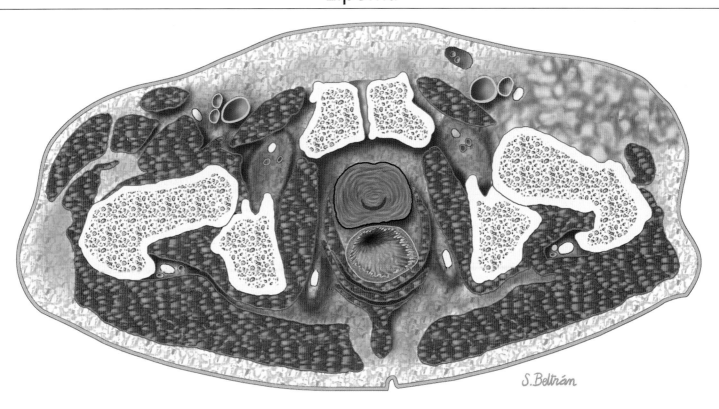

Figure 14.31 ▪ Subcutaneous lipoma, shown in yellow, of the anterior thigh. *(See Lipoma pg. 2123, in Stoller's 3rd Edition.)*

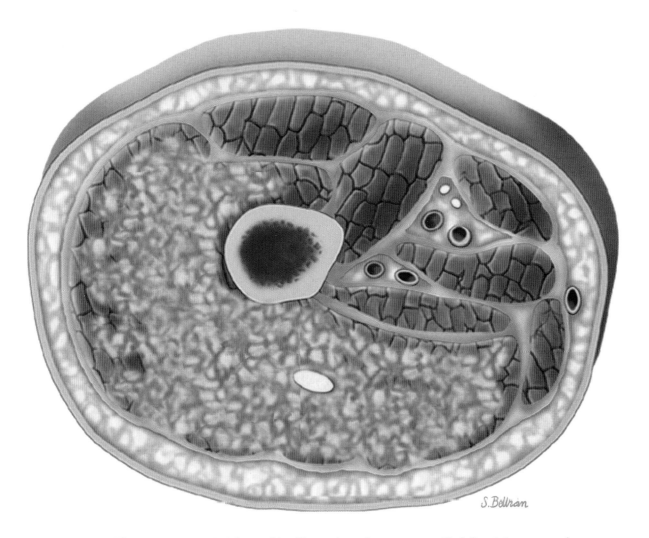

Figure 14.32 ▪ Axial graphic illustration demonstrates ill-defined intramuscular lipoma (in yellow) of the thigh. *(See Lipoma pg. 2126, in Stoller's 3rd Edition.)*

Lipomatosis

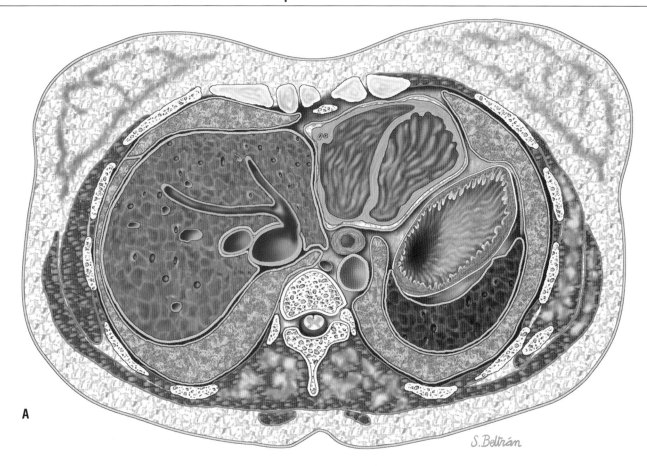

A

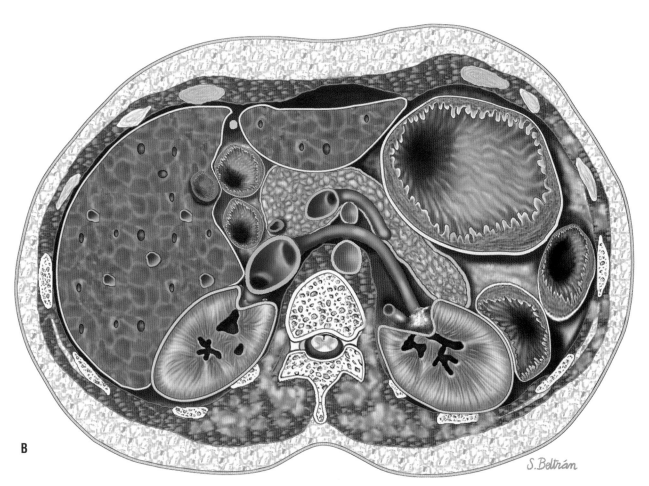

B

Figure 14.33 ▪ Axial graphic illustrations showing lipomatosis of the chest and abdominal wall in yellow. (A) Diffuse infiltration of the paraspinal muscles and left chest wall and **(B)** infiltration of the paraspinal muscles and left abdominal wall. *(See Lipoma pg. 2127, in Stoller's 3rd Edition.)*

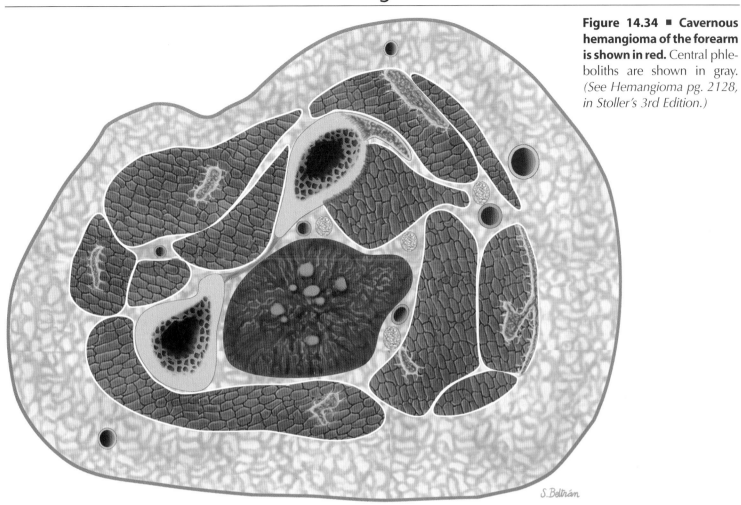

Figure 14.34 ■ **Cavernous hemangioma of the forearm is shown in red.** Central phleboliths are shown in gray. *(See Hemangioma pg. 2128, in Stoller's 3rd Edition.)*

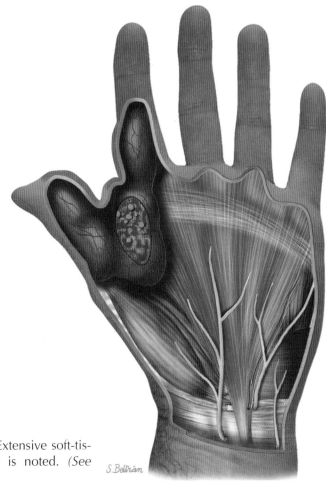

Figure 14.35 ■ **Hemangioma of the hand with calcified phleboliths.** Extensive soft-tissue swelling involving the thumb, index finger, and thenar region is noted. *(See Hemangioma pg. 2128, in Stoller's 3rd Edition.)*

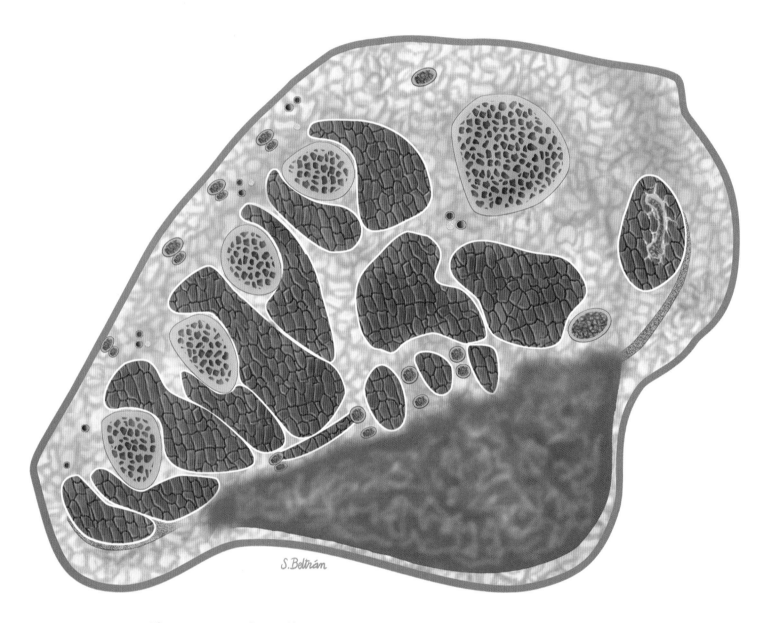

Figure 14.36 ■ Plantar fibromatosis is seen as a heterogeneous mass in gray infiltrating the adjacent muscles. *(See Fibromatosis pg. 2132, in Stoller's 3rd Edition.)*

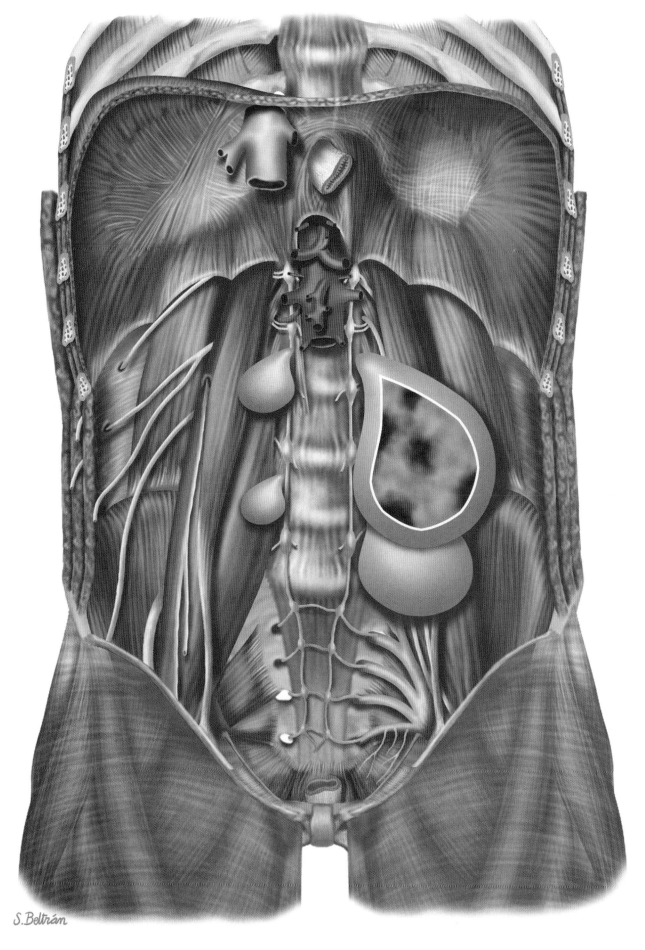

Figure 14.37 ■ Multiple spinal plexiform neurofibromas in a patient with neurofibromatosis type 1. Hemorrhage within a lesion is shown in red. *(See Benign Peripheral Nerve Sheath Tumor pg. 2137, in Stoller's 3rd Edition.)*

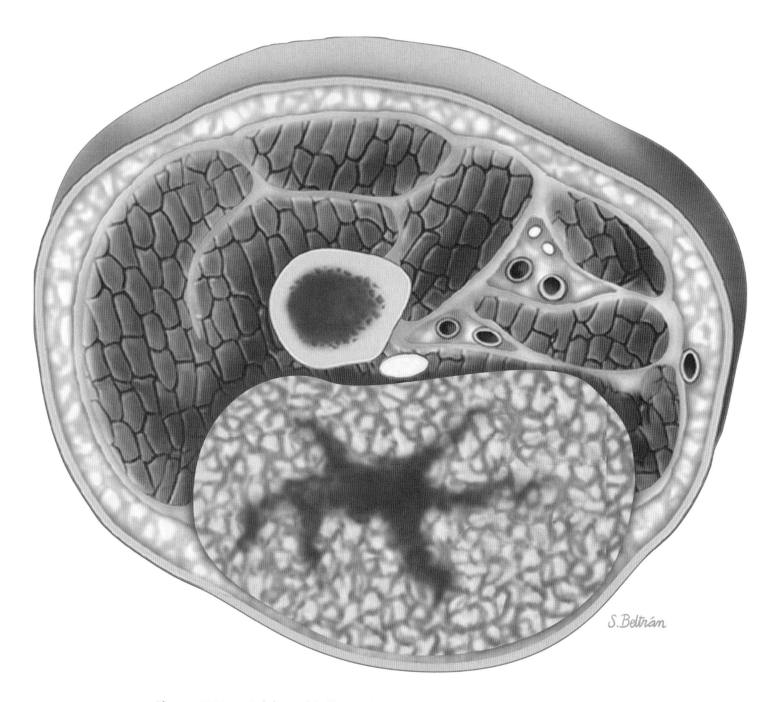

Figure 14.38 ■ Axial graphic illustration showing liposarcoma in yellow. Central areas of necrosis are shown in brown. *(See Liposarcoma pg. 2140, in Stoller's 3rd Edition.)*

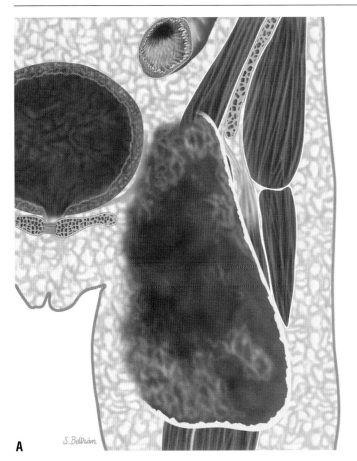

A

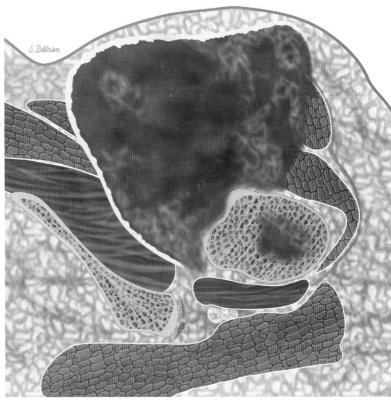

B

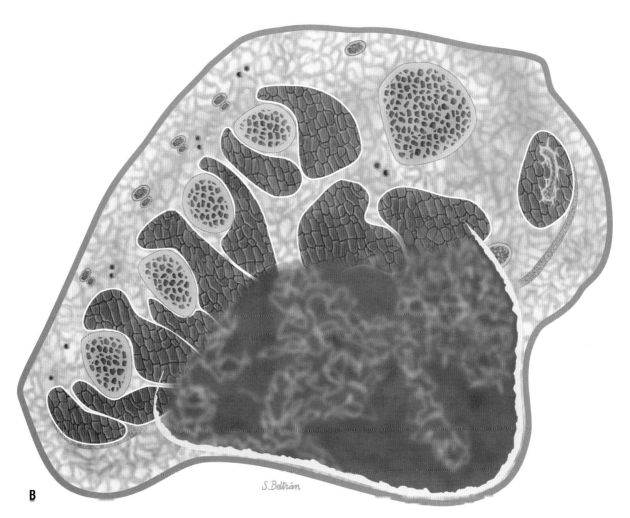

B

Figure 14.39 ▪ **Leiomyosarcoma of the thigh on coronal (A) and axial (B) graphic illustrations.** Bone metastasis is shown in brown. Axial graphic illustration **(C)** shows leiomyosarcoma of the foot. *(See Leiomyosarcoma pg. 2143, in Stoller's 3rd Edition.)*

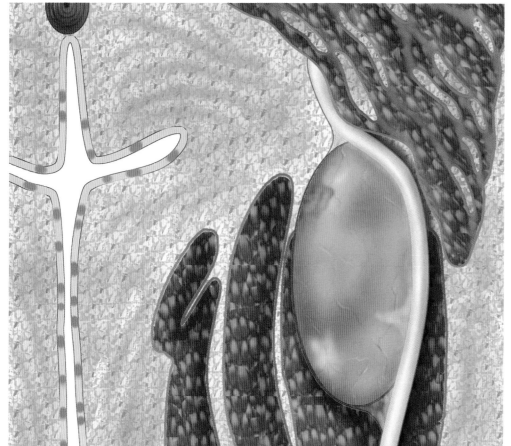

Figure 14.40 ▪ **Malignant peripheral nerve sheath tumor associated with neurofibromatosis.** Coronal graphic illustration shows a large fusiform mass in the thigh. The sciatic nerve is seen entering and exiting the mass. Numerous superficial neurofibromas are present. *(See Malignant Peripheral Nerve Sheath Tumor pg. 2144, in Stoller's 3rd Edition.)*

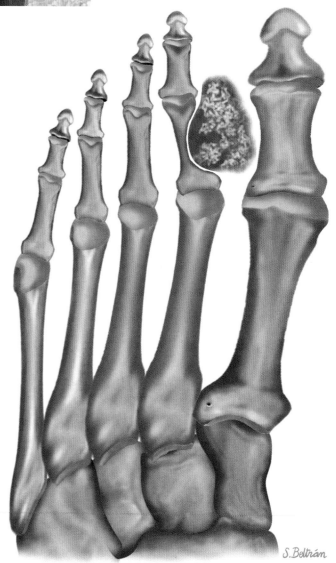

Figure 14.41 ▪ **Coronal graphic illustration shows a synovial sarcoma of the foot in gray.** Internal calcifications are present. The mass erodes the proximal phalanx of the second toe. *(See Synovial Sarcoma pg. 2146, in Stoller's 3rd Edition.)*

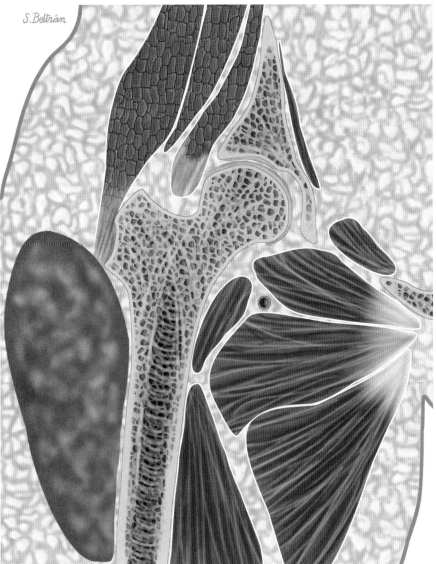

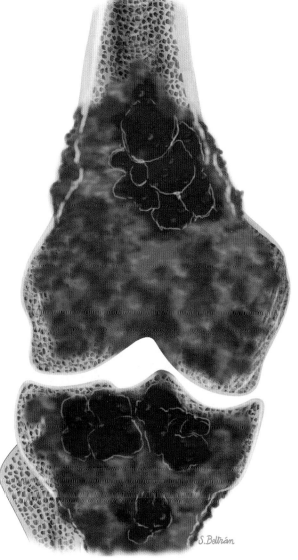

Figure 14.42 ▪ Pleomorphic malignant fibrous histiocytoma. Coronal graphic illustration shows a large soft-tissue mass in the lateral thigh. *(See Malignant Fibrous Histiocytoma pg. 2149, in Stoller's 3rd Edition.)*

Figure 14.43 ▪ Malignant fibrous histiocytoma of bone. Coronal graphic illustration shows an intramedullary tumor of the distal femur and proximal tibia with hemorrhagic and necrotic changes and cortical disruption. *(See Malignant Fibrous Histiocytoma pg. 2149, in Stoller's 3rd Edition.)*

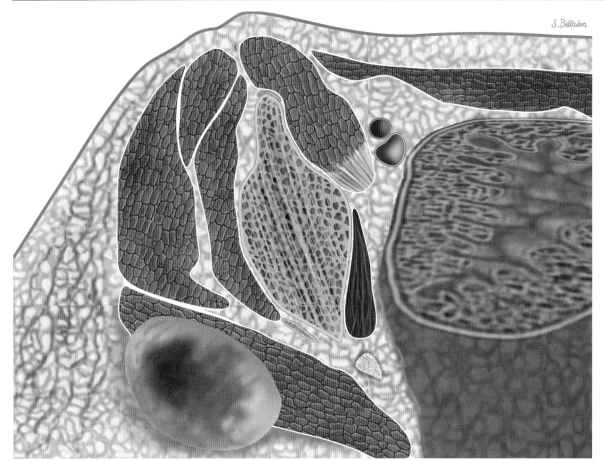

S.Beltrán

Figure 14.44 ▪ Fibrosarcoma of soft tissues. Axial graphic illustration shows a heterogeneous mass in the gluteus maximus with central necrosis. *(See Fibrosarcoma pg. 2152, in Stoller's 3rd Edition.)*

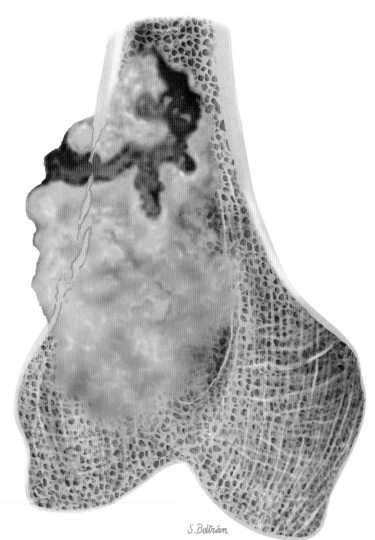

S.Beltrán

Figure 14.45 ▪ Fibrosarcoma of bone. Coronal graphic illustration shows a gray-white to tan mass in the distal femur with cortical destruction and soft-tissue extension. Internal hemorrhage is shown in red. *(See Fibrosarcoma pg. 2152, in Stoller's 3rd Edition.)*

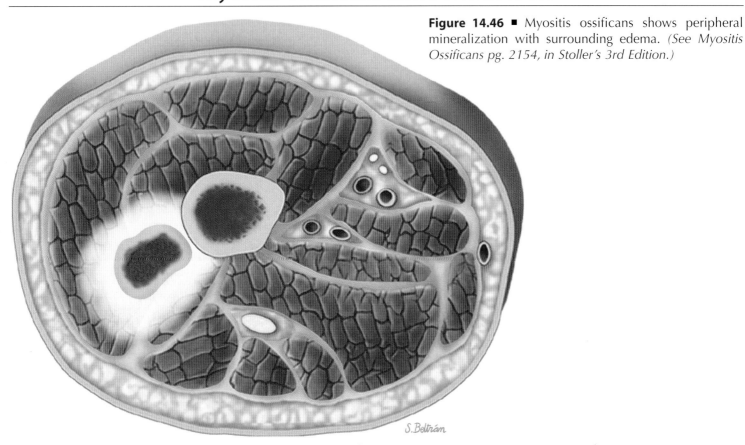

Figure 14.46 ■ Myositis ossificans shows peripheral mineralization with surrounding edema. *(See Myositis Ossificans pg. 2154, in Stoller's 3rd Edition.)*

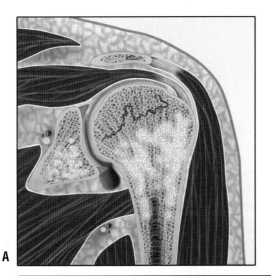

Figure 14.47 ■ Bone infarcts of the shoulder (**A**) and knee (**B** and **C**) with characteristic serpentine lines. *(See Bone Infarct pg. 2156, in Stoller's 3rd Edition.)*

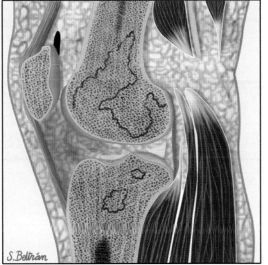

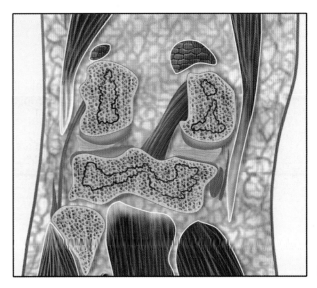

Hematoma

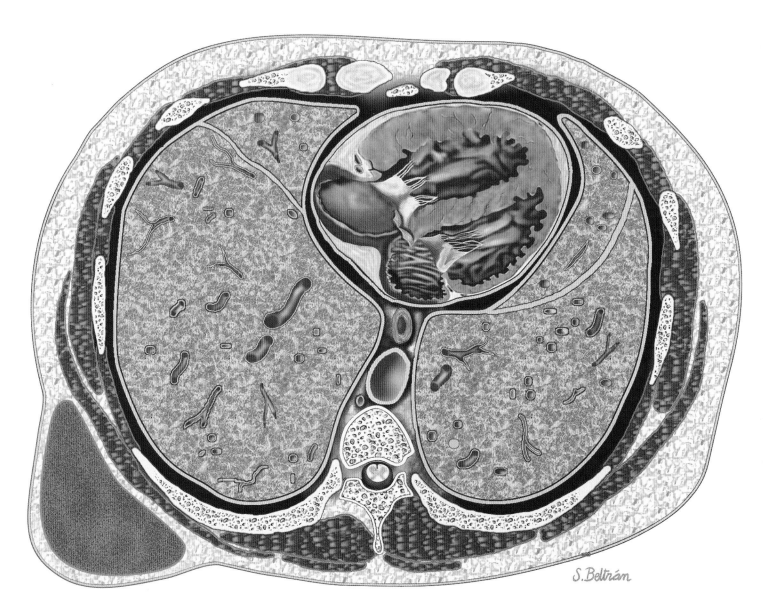

Figure 14.48 ▪ Axial graphic illustration shows organized hematoma of the chest wall in red. *(See Hematoma pg. 2157, in Stoller's 3rd Edition.)*

Index